GOTH'S MEDICAL PHARMACOLOGY

GOTH'S MEDICAL
PHARMACOLOGY

WESLEY G. CLARK, Ph.D.
Associate Professor
Department of Pharmacology
Southwestern Medical School
The University of Texas Southwestern Medical Center at Dallas
Dallas, Texas

D. CRAIG BRATER, M.D.
Professor, Director of Clinical Pharmacology
Department of Medicine
Indiana University School of Medicine
Indianapolis, Indiana

ALICE R. JOHNSON, Ph.D.
Professor, Department of Biochemistry
The University of Texas Health Center at Tyler
Tyler, Texas

TWELFTH EDITION

With 377 illustrations

The C. V. Mosby Company
ST. LOUIS • WASHINGTON, D.C. • TORONTO   1988

MOSBY

A TRADITION OF PUBLISHING EXCELLENCE

Editor: Stephanie Bircher
Assistant editor: Anne Gunter
Project manager: Kathleen L. Teal
Manuscript editor: Carl Masthay
Cover design: Susan E. Lane
Production: Teresa Breckwoldt, Ginny Douglas

TWELFTH EDITION

Previous editions copyrighted 1961, 1964, 1966, 1968, 1970, 1972, 1974,
1976, 1978, 1981, 1984

Printed in the United States of America

The C.V. Mosby Company
11830 Westline Industrial Drive, St. Louis, Missouri 63146

Library of Congress Cataloging in Publication Data
Goth, Andres, 1914-
    Goth's medical pharmacology.
    Rev. ed. of: Medical pharmacology/Andres Goth.
11th ed. 1984.
    Includes bibliographies and index.
    1. Pharmacology.   I. Clark, Wesley G.   II. Brater,
D. Craig.   III. Johnson, Alice R.   IV. Title.   V. Title:
Medical pharmacology.   [DNLM: 1. Pharmacology.
QV 4 G684m]
RM300.G65   1988   615'.1   87-24714
ISBN 0-8016-1167-9

GW/VH/VH   9 8 7 6 5 4 3 2 1

Contributors

Burnell R. Brown, Jr., M.D., Ph.D.
Professor and Head
Department of Anesthesiology
University of Arizona Health Science Center
Tucson, Arizona

William B. Campbell, Ph.D.
Associate Professor
Department of Pharmacology
Southwestern Medical School
The University of Texas Southwestern Medical Center at Dallas
Dallas, Texas

Gregory G. Dimijian, M.D.
Clinical Assistant Professor
Department of Psychiatry
Southwestern Medical School
The University of Texas Southwestern Medical Center at Dallas
Dallas, Texas

Barton A. Kamen, M.D., Ph.D.
Associate Professor
Departments of Pediatrics and Pharmacology
Southwestern Medical School
The University of Texas Southwestern Medical Center at Dallas
Dallas, Texas

Bill H. McAnalley, Ph.D.
Research Director
Carrington Laboratories, Inc.
Dallas, Texas

James W. Smith, M.D.
Professor
Department of Internal Medicine
Southwestern Medical School
The University of Texas Southwestern Medical Center at Dallas;
Chief, Infectious Diseases
Dallas Veteran's Administration Medical Center
Dallas, Texas

Alvin Taurog, Ph.D.
Professor
Department of Pharmacology
Southwestern Medical School
The University of Texas Southwestern Medical Center at Dallas
Dallas, Texas

Preface

Since publication of the eleventh edition of *Medical Pharmacology* in 1984, Dr. Andres Goth, Chairman of the Department of Pharmacology of Southwestern Medical School for over 30 years, has retired. The orientation of this widely used textbook, which he defined with the original publication in 1961, is being continued, with Dr. Goth's blessing and encouragement, by former colleagues, most of whom were either students or faculty members in his department.

We continue in this twelfth edition the original intent of this textbook, expressed in the preface to the first edition, "to present current pharmacologic knowledge with particular reference to principles and concepts . . . written primarily for students and practitioners." The general format of previous editions also has been preserved, but all chapters have been extensively revised. The bibliographies have been updated and expanded to provide additional sources of information. To improve the flow of the discussion in many chapters, information regarding dosage, dosage forms, trade names, and so forth has been removed from the text and incorporated into tables, where such details can be located more readily. Information on the pharmacokinetic characteristics of many drugs is now included in an appendix.

We especially thank Mrs. Yvonne Clark, who provided the starting point for our revisions by transcribing the eleventh edition.

Wesley G. Clark
D. Craig Brater
Alice R. Johnson

Contents

1   Introduction, 1

section one   *General aspects of pharmacology*

2   Drug-receptor interactions, 6

3   Pharmacokinetic principles in the use of drugs, 12

4   Drug metabolism and enzyme induction, 28

5   Drug safety and effectiveness, 39

6   Pharmacogenetics: the individual response to drugs, 48

7   Effects of age on drug disposition, 57

8   Effects of diet on drug disposition, 63

9   Effects of occupation and disease on drug disposition, 69

section two   *Drug effects on the nervous system and neuroeffectors*

10   General aspects of neuropharmacology, 82

11   Cholinergic drugs, 102

12   Cholinergic (muscarinic) blocking agents, 114

13   Ganglionic blocking agents, 127

14   Neuromuscular blocking agents and muscle relaxants, 132

15   Adrenergic (sympathomimetic) drugs, 142

16   Adrenergic blocking agents, 163

17   Drugs acting on the adrenergic neuron, 172

18   Antihypertensive drugs, 177

19   Histamine, 197

20   Antihistaminic drugs, 206

21 Serotonin, kinins, and miscellaneous autacoids, 214

22 Prostaglandins and leukotrienes, 227

---

section three   Psychopharmacology

23 General concepts of psychopharmacology, 242

24 Antipsychotic and antianxiety drugs, 250

25 Antidepressant and psychotomimetic drugs, 268

---

section four   Depressants and stimulants of the central nervous system

26 Hypnotic drugs and alcohol, 280

27 Central nervous system stimulants of the convulsant type, 302

28 Antiepileptic drugs, 308

29 Narcotic (opioid) analgesic drugs, 319

30 Contemporary drug abuse, 337
GREGORY G. DIMIJIAN

31 Nonsteroidal anti-inflammatory antipyretic analgesics, 364

---

section five   Anesthetics

32 Pharmacology of general anesthesia, 384
BURNELL R. BROWN, Jr.

33 Pharmacology of local anesthesia, 407
BURNELL R. BROWN, Jr.

---

section six   Drugs used in cardiovascular disease

34 Digitalis, 418

35 Antiarrhythmic drugs, 433

36 Antianginal drugs, 450

37 Drugs that affect hemostasis, 459

38 Diuretic drugs, 477

39 Pharmacologic approaches to atherosclerosis, 493

section seven   *Drug effects on the respiratory and gastrointestinal tracts*

40   Drug effects on the respiratory tract, 506

41   Drug effects on the gastrointestinal tract, 518

section eight   *Drugs that influence metabolic and endocrine functions*

42   Insulin, glucagon, and oral hypoglycemic agents, 530

43   Adrenal steroids, 543
WILLIAM B. CAMPBELL

44   Thyroid hormones and antithyroid drugs, 557
ALVIN TAUROG

45   Parathyroid extract and vitamin D, 567

46   Posterior pituitary hormones—vasopressin and oxytocin, 573

47   Anterior pituitary gonadotropins and sex hormones, 580

48   Pharmacologic approaches to gout, 599

49   Antianemic drugs, 605

50   Vitamins, 614

section nine   *Chemotherapy*

51   Introduction to chemotherapy; mechanisms of antibiotic action, 626
JAMES W. SMITH

52   Sulfonamides, 632
JAMES W. SMITH

53   Antibiotic drugs, 642
JAMES W. SMITH

54   Antiviral agents, 667
JAMES W. SMITH

55   Drugs used to treat mycobacterial and fungal infections, 672
JAMES W. SMITH

56   Antiseptics and disinfectants, 683
JAMES W. SMITH

57   Drugs used to treat amebiasis and other intestinal protozoal infections, 687
JAMES W. SMITH

58 Drugs used to treat malaria and other extraintestinal protozoal
infections, 690
JAMES W. SMITH

59 Anthelmintic drugs, 697
JAMES W. SMITH

60 Drugs used in chemotherapy of neoplastic disease, 702
BARTON A. KAMEN

section ten   *Principles of immunopharmacology*

61 Principles of immunopharmacology, 716

section eleven   *Poisons and antidotes*

62 Poisons and antidotes, 730
BILL H. McANALLEY

section twelve   *Drug interactions*

63 Drug interactions, 748

section thirteen   *Prescription writing and drug compendia*

64 Prescription writing and drug compendia, 758

appendixes

A Drug concentrations in blood, 766
1. Therapeutic drug concentrations, 768
2. Toxic and lethal blood concentrations, 769
BILL H. McANALLEY

B Comparison of selected effects of commonly abused drugs, 773
GREGORY G. DIMIJIAN

C Pharmacokinetic characteristics of drugs, 776

Chapter 1

Introduction

Chemical agents not only provide the structural basis and energy supply of living organisms but also regulate their functional activities. Interactions between potent chemicals and living systems contribute to our knowledge of biologic processes and provide effective methods for treatment, prevention, and diagnosis of many diseases. Compounds used for these purposes are called *drugs*, and their actions on living systems lead to *drug effects*.

Pharmacology deals with the properties and effects of drugs and, in a more general sense, with interactions between chemical compounds and living systems. It is a discipline of biology that is closely related to physiology and biochemistry. Nevertheless, pharmacology is unique in that it deals especially with the mechanism of action of biologically active substances.

Although the specific aim of many pharmacologists is to define the biologic activity of chemical compounds, the use of such agents can also contribute greatly to knowledge of living systems. This contribution to the understanding of life processes is valuable to biologic sciences in general and to medicine in particular. However, some aspects of pharmacology are of less relevance to the study of medicine. To emphasize this distinction, the title *Medical Pharmacology* was chosen for this book.

SUBDIVISIONS OF PHARMACOLOGY AND RELATED DISCIPLINES

There are several fields of study that may be considered subdivisions of pharmacology or disciplines related to it.

Pharmacodynamics is the study of drug actions and effects, whereas *pharmacokinetics* deals with the handling of drugs by the body. These aspects of pharmacology are perhaps nearest to the basic science of medicine.

Emphasis on mode of action of chemical compounds distinguishes pharmacology from other basic medical sciences. As used in medicine, the term *pharmacology* is essentially synonymous with pharmacodynamics.

Chemotherapy is the subdivision of pharmacology that, according to the definition first proposed by Paul Ehrlich, deals with drugs that are capable of destroying invading organisms without destroying the host.

Pharmacy is concerned with the preparation and dispensing of drugs. Today the physician seldom needs to prepare or dispense drugs. Even the pharmacist has very little to do with preparation of drugs, most of which are manufactured by large companies. The pharmacist may provide useful services, however, as a member of the health team with special knowledge about drug preparations.

Therapeutics refers to the treatment of disease. *Pharmacotherapeutics* is the application of drugs for treatment of disease.

Toxicology is the science of poisons and poisonings. Although toxicology may be viewed as a special extension of pharmacology, it has developed into a separate discipline for a variety of reasons. Forensic and environmental medicine requires the services and knowledge of toxicologists with special training in drug identification and poison control.

HISTORICAL DEVELOPMENT OF PHARMACOLOGY	Although no detailed discussion will be attempted, the history of pharmacology can be divided into two periods. The early period extends to antiquity and was characterized by empiric observations in the use of crude medicinal preparations. It is interesting that even primitive people discovered relationships between drugs and disease. The use of drugs has been so prevalent throughout history that Sir William Osler stated (1894) with some justification that "man has an inborn craving for medicine."

In contrast to this ancient period, modern pharmacology is based on experimental investigations concerning the site and mode of action of drugs. The application of the scientific method to study drugs was initiated in France by François Magendie and was expanded by Claude Bernard (1813-1878). The name of Oswald Schmiedeberg (1838-1921) is commonly associated with the development of experimental pharmacology in Germany, and John Jacob Abel (1857-1938) played a similar role in the United States.

The growth of pharmacology was greatly stimulated by the rise of synthetic organic chemistry, which provided new tools and new therapeutic agents. More recently, pharmacology has benefited from developments in other basic sciences and in turn has contributed to their growth.

One of the most dynamic areas of pharmacologic research deals with drug receptors and related areas; for example, the discovery of the endorphins occurred shortly after the existence of related drug receptors was recognized. One of the basic functions of pharmacology is to map out and characterize such receptors in the body.

Some of the greatest changes in medicine during the last few decades are directly attributable to the discovery of new drugs. Progress in this field has not been without its problems, however. Sometimes new therapeutic agents are found to be unsafe. Studies during development of new drugs do not include large enough numbers of patients to identify rare but serious adverse effects. As a consequence, it is inevitable that some new drugs will be found lacking when used in sufficient numbers of patients to identify all their effects. Furthermore, it has proved difficult for the practicing physician to stay abreast of rapid developments in the field of pharmacology. Hence all physicians must have a solid understanding of basic principles. These shortcomings notwithstanding, in the recent history of pharmacology the successes have more than made up for problems that occur with drugs.

There are several reasons for considering pharmacology an increasingly important basic science in medicine. Some of these are obvious; others are not yet generally recognized.

Large numbers of drugs are used in the practice of medicine. They cannot be administered intelligently or safely without an understanding of their mode of action, side effects, toxicity, and metabolism. As powerful new drugs are introduced, adequate pharmacologic knowledge on the part of the physician is mandatory. Pharmacologic terms and concepts are used so commonly in clinical journals that a physician without a good grounding in the subject will find it difficult to read and evaluate the current medical literature.

Pharmacology is taught in medical schools for other reasons. As a basic science it contributes important concepts to the understanding of health and disease. In research, drugs are used increasingly as chemical tools for elucidating basic mechanisms. Also drugs are being used more frequently for diagnostic purposes.

Pharmacology is also important in medicine because of commercial influences that are exerted on the physician in the selection of drugs. A knowledge of the principles of pharmacology will provide the physician with the ability to evaluate critically and rationally the claims made for new drug preparations.

Finally, it is increasingly recognized that numerous functions in the body are regulated by endogenous compounds that interact with specific receptors. Many commonly used drugs mimic or oppose the action of these endogenous compounds or alter their metabolism. When viewed in this light, pharmacology is not only the scientific basis of drug therapy but also contributes to our understanding of bodily functions.

PLACE OF PHARMACOLOGY IN MEDICINE

Although pharmacology is concerned with drug effects in all species of animals, in medicine there is increasing interest in clinical pharmacology, which directly concerns itself with drug actions in human beings.

There are many reasons for this interest. For instance, results of studies on animals cannot always be applied to human beings because of species differences in the response to a drug or in its metabolism. Clinical pharmacology also provides scientific methods for the determination of usefulness, potency, and toxicity of new drugs in humans.

CLINICAL PHARMACOLOGY

section one

General aspects of pharmacology

2   Drug-receptor interactions, 6

3   Pharmacokinetic principles in the use of drugs, 12

4   Drug metabolism and enzyme induction, 28

5   Drug safety and effectiveness, 39

6   Pharmacogenetics: the individual response to drugs, 48

7   Effects of age on drug disposition, 57

8   Effects of diet on drug disposition, 63

9   Effects of occupation and disease on drug disposition, 69

Chapter 2

Drug-receptor interactions

Most drugs exert potent and specific actions in the body by forming a bond, generally reversible, with a cellular constituent termed a *receptor*. Drugs that interact with a receptor to elicit a response are termed *agonists;* compounds that interact with a receptor to prevent the action of agonists are referred to as *specific pharmacologic antagonists*. Those that can act either as an agonist or an antagonist, depending on circumstances, are called partial agonists or antagonists.

The existence of cellular receptors for a drug can be deduced from (1) relationships between structure and activity in a homologous or congeneric series, (2) quantitative studies on agonist-antagonist pairs, and (3) selective binding of radioactive drugs to isolated cells or membranes.

The function of a receptor is to recognize a specific chemical signal and to discriminate between this appropriate structural signal and other molecules. The drug-receptor interaction is then coupled, usually through a second messenger such as cyclic AMP or the phosphoinositide system, to an effector mechanism to cause a cellular response.[1,2,5,8] The presence of receptors at an anatomic site is one determinant of the selective nature of many drug actions. For example, acetylcholine applied directly to a motor end plate produces an action potential. When the same drug is applied a short distance from the end plate, where there are no receptors, it has no effect.

Not all drug actions are mediated by receptors. For example, volatile anesthetics, metal-chelating agents, and osmotic diuretics exert effects that are not mediated by specific receptors. On the other hand, drugs of the autonomic nervous system, the opiate narcotics, and most antipsychotic drugs act on specific receptors.

RECEPTOR THEORY

The *receptor concept* was first proposed by Langley in 1878 and was used extensively by Paul Ehrlich in his studies on chemotherapy. While investigating the opposing actions of pilocarpine and atropine on salivary secretion, Langley hypothesized the presence of some substance in the nerve endings or glands with which the drugs combine. As conceived by Ehrlich, receptors are groups of protoplasmic macromolecules with which drugs combine *reversibly* or *irreversibly*.

According to current concepts, there are several types of drug receptors.[1,7,8,10] Some are on the external surface of the plasma membrane of target cells. Examples are those that interact with peptide hormones and releasing factors or with drugs that mimic or block the actions of autonomic mediators, such as the catecholamines.[7,10]

Other receptors are located in the cytoplasm of target cells, for example, those that combine with drugs that mimic or block the actions of steroid hormones;[1] the drug-receptor combination is translocated to the nucleus where it may regulate the concentration of a specific messenger ribonucleic acid (RNA) and, ultimately, the synthesis of proteins. Still other receptors are initially in the nucleus. Thyroid hormone is an important example of an agent that interacts with nuclear receptors.

The binding forces in the drug-receptor interaction consist of covalent, ionic, and hydrogen bonds as well as van der Waals forces. Covalent binding, because of its high energy, causes essentially irreversible effects. If the drug is an antagonist such as phenoxybenzamine, formation of a covalent bond results in noncompetitive antagonism. Ionic bonds are important because most drugs contain cationic and anionic groups. Consequently, pH may influence their interaction with receptors. The van der Waals bond is a weak interaction between dipoles. Although the bond energy is only about 0.5 kcal per mole—compared with 100 kcal per mole for the covalent bond—van der Waals bonds are very important in drug-receptor interactions for several reasons. First, the binding forces are summed over a large number of interacting atoms. Second, since drugs and receptors "fit" in three-dimensional space, interatomic distances allow the receptor to discriminate between a specific drug and a related compound with a different conformation. Finally, the relatively weak van der Waals bond allows for reversible interactions and thereby drug effects of short duration.

The basic requirement for a receptor is the ability to discriminate signal from noise.[1] To receive the signal, the receptor must have an affinity for the drug. At the same time, receptors must have specificity, in other words, an appropriately low affinity for less active drugs.

DRUG-RECEPTOR INTERACTIONS

Log dose-response curves illustrating the difference between potency and efficacy. **A,** *Drug A is much more potent than drug B, but both have the same maximum effect.* **B,** *Drug A is not only more potent but also has greater efficacy; it produces a greater peak effect than drug B.*

FIG. 2-1

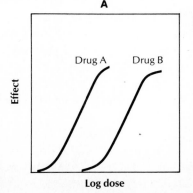
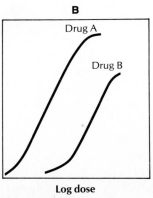

Affinity is quantified when one studies the dose-response relationship between a drug and a receptor, using one of several methods. In systems in which only dose and response can be determined, the log of the dose is plotted against the response (Fig. 2-1). In such studies, the dose of a drug that produces a response that is 50% of the maximum is referred to as the "ED_{50}" (effective dose$_{50}$).

With newer methods, usually requiring radioactive drugs, the relationships between free and specifically bound drugs can be quantified, and much additional information can be obtained.

The binding of a drug (D) and a receptor (R) can be represented as follows:

$$[D] + [R] \xrightarrow{k_1} [DR]$$

The rate at which they combine is described by the rate constant k_1. Since most drug-receptor interactions are reversible, it is also true that

$$[DR] \xrightarrow{k_2} [D] + [R]$$

At equilibrium the rates of the forward and backward reactions are equal, and

$$k_1[D][R] = k_2[DR]$$

The concept of K_d emerges if the above equation is rewritten:

$$\frac{[D][R]}{[DR]} = \frac{k_2}{k_1} = K_d$$

K_d is the equilibrium dissociation constant, and it is related to affinity. In the above equation, if half of the receptors are bound to a drug, the concentrations of R and DR are equal and cancel. Under such conditions $K_d = [D]$. This means that the concentration of drug necessary to bind 50% of the receptors equals the K_d. If this concentration is low, affinity is high.

Affinity and intrinsic activity

Affinity then is the tendency of a drug to combine with the receptor, and the magnitude of response is a function of the number of receptors occupied. One drug may not only have a higher affinity than another compound but may also produce a greater maximum effect (Fig. 2-1, *B*); that is, there are *partial agonists* that act on the same receptor as a full agonist but that cannot produce the same maximum effect, regardless of concentration. Therefore the response not only is a function of the concentration of the drug-receptor complex but also depends on what is termed *intrinsic activity*, or efficacy. This concept may be defined as the capacity to stimulate relative to a given receptor occupancy.

In summary, an agonist is a drug that has both affinity for a receptor and intrinsic activity. A competitive antagonist has affinity for the receptor but lacks intrinsic activity.

Drugs that do not act on specific receptors

The biologic activity of anesthetics and alcohol is believed to depend not on drug-receptor interactions but on the *relative saturation* at some cellular phase (Ferguson's principle).[3] Whenever chemically unrelated drugs give the same effect at the same relative saturation, they are unlikely to act on specific receptors. It is probable that by reaching a certain level of saturation at some cellular site (the so-called biophase) they hinder some metabolic function.

Receptor regulation

The response to a drug depends partially on the number of available receptors, and this number may be affected by the continued presence of the drug. Generally, receptors that activate adenylate cyclase and insulin receptors tend to decrease in number or undergo *downregulation* with continued drug administration. This phenomenon is sometimes referred to as *desensitization,* or *tachyphylaxis*.[7,9] Although there is great interest in downregulation, it should be pointed out that most drugs can be administered repeatedly or continuously without development of much desensitization. Furthermore, only agonists produce homologous downregulation. Lastly, tachyphylaxis to some drugs (for example, nitrates) occurs through mechanisms unrelated to receptors.

There are a few examples of increased receptor numbers. Thyroid hormone increases the number of β-adrenergic receptors in the myocardium, consistent with the clinical impression that hyperthyroid persons are more sensitive to catecholamines.

Receptor-related diseases

There is great interest in the role of receptor changes in certain diseases.[6] Practically all patients with myasthenia gravis have antibodies to acetylcholine receptors. In some forms of insulin-resistant diabetes, there are antibodies to insulin receptors.[4] Other interesting examples of receptor-related diseases are testicular feminization (androgen insensitivity), familial hypercholesterolemia (decrease in receptors for low-density lipoproteins), and several endocrine diseases that may represent receptor insensitivity rather than hormonal deficiencies.

QUANTITATIVE ASPECTS OF DRUG POTENCY AND EFFICACY

A drug is said to be "potent" when it has great biologic activity per unit weight. When the dose of a drug is plotted on a logarithmic scale against a measured effect, a sigmoid curve is obtained, usually referred to as a *log dose-response curve*. Any point on such a curve could indicate the potency of a drug, but for comparative purposes the ED_{50} is most often selected. In Fig. 2-1, *A*, drugs A and B produced parallel dose-response curves. The ED_{50} of drug B may be 10 times greater than that of drug A. As a consequence, it may be said that drug A is 10 times more potent than drug B. *It is essential to remember that potencies are compared on the basis of doses that produce the same effect and not by comparison of the magnitudes of effects elicited by the same dose*.

A clinically relevant example of a potency relationship, typical of that illustrated in Fig. 2-1, *A*, is that of the diuretic drugs chlorothiazide and hydrochlorothiazide. It takes about 1 g of chlorothiazide to achieve the same effect as 100 mg of hydrochlorothiazide. As a consequence, hydrochlorothiazide is 10 times more potent than chlorothiazide.

Fig. 2-1, *B*, illustrates another property of a drug that should not be confused with potency. Drug A is not only 10 times more potent than drug B, but it also has a higher maximum or "ceiling" of activity. The maximum effect is commonly referred to as *efficacy*, or *power*. It is an expression of intrinsic activity and can be illustrated by another example. Both chlorothiazide and hydrochlorothiazide have equal ceilings of activity. Furosemide, however, has not only greater potency than these two drugs but also a higher ceiling. It can cause the excretion of a larger amount of sodium chloride. Consequently, furosemide not only is more potent than chlorothiazide but also has greater efficacy.

Potency and efficacy are often confused in medical terminology. Potency alone is an overrated advantage in therapeutics. If drug A is 10 times more potent than drug B but has no other virtues, this means only that the patient will take smaller tablets. Pharmaceutical companies often emphasize that a drug is more potent than some other drug. This in itself has little importance to the physician. On the other hand, if the drug has greater efficacy, it may accomplish results that are unattainable with a less efficacious compound.

AGONIST, ANTAGONIST, AND PARTIAL AGONIST

An agonist is a drug that has affinity and efficacy. It interacts with receptors and elicits a response. Acetylcholine is a good example of an agonist. However, if a log dose-response curve to acetylcholine is obtained in the presence of atropine (an antagonist), it will be found that atropine alone causes no effects but shifts the log dose-response curve of acetylcholine to the right.

Atropine is viewed as competing with acetylcholine for the same receptors; in other words, the antagonist has affinity but lacks efficacy. This is an example of *competitive* or *surmountable* antagonism. The key feature of this kind of antagonism is *parallel displacement of the log dose-response curve to the right without a shift in the maximum* (Fig. 2-2, A).

FIG. 2-2 *Log dose-response curves illustrating differences between a competitive antagonist and a noncompetitive antagonist. A, A competitive antagonist decreases potency but not efficacy; there is a parallel shift of the log dose-response curve to the right. B, A noncompetitive antagonist decreases both efficacy and potency; the log dose-response curve is not only shifted to the right but the maximal effect is also reduced.*

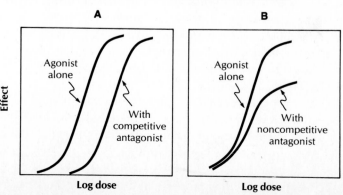

Somewhere between pure agonists and pure antagonists are the drugs termed *partial agonists*. They have affinity and some efficacy but may antagonize the action of other agonists that have a greater efficacy.

In the case of atropine and acetylcholine the antagonist and agonist were competing for the same receptor, as evidenced by the parallel shift in the log dose-response curve without a shift in the maximum. In some instances the antagonist may combine irreversibly with the receptor, in which case increasing the concentration of the agonist can never fully overcome the inhibition. The net effect will be a decrease in the maximum height of the log dose-response curve, which is believed to reflect a decrease in the number of drug-receptor complexes (Fig. 2-2, *B*).

NONCOMPETITIVE ANTAGONISM

PROBLEM 2-1. *The graph below depicts the linear segment of a typical log dose-response curve. What is the dose (X) that induces Y units of response? How many units is Y ?*

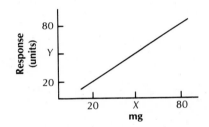

Since dosage is plotted on a *log* scale, equal increments on the abscissa represent equal *multiples* so that X = 40 mg. In contrast, the magnitude of the response is plotted on a *linear* scale, so that equal increments on the ordinate represent *equal* changes in response; Y therefore equals 50 units.

REFERENCES

1. Baxter, J.D., and Funder, J.W.: Hormone receptors, N. Engl. J. Med. **301**:1149, 1979.
2. Berridge, M.J., and Irvine, R.F.: Inositol trisphosphate, a novel second messenger in cellular signal transduction, Nature **312**:315, 1984.
3. Ferguson, J.: Use of chemical potentials as indices of toxicity, Proc. R. Soc. Lond. [Biol.] **127**:387, 1939.
4. Flier, J.S., Kahn, C.R., and Roth, J.: Receptors, antireceptor antibodies and mechanisms of insulin resistance, N. Engl. J. Med. **300**:413, 1979.
5. Hurwitz, L., and Suria, A.: The link between agonist action and response in smooth muscle, Annu. Rev. Pharmacol. **11**:303, 1971.
6. Jacobs, S., and Cuatrecasas, P.: Cell receptors in disease, N. Engl. J. Med. **297**:1383, 1977.
7. Lefkowitz, R.J.: Direct binding studies of adrenergic receptors: biochemical, physiologic, and clinical implications, Ann. Intern. Med. **91**:450, 1979.
8. Motulsky, H.J., and Insel, P.A.: Adrenergic receptors in man: direct identification, physiologic regulation, and clinical alterations, N. Engl. J. Med. **307**:18, 1982.
9. Overstreet, D.H., and Yamamura, H.I.: Receptor alterations and drug tolerance, Life Sci. **25**:1865, 1979.
10. Snyder, S.H.: Drug and neurotransmitter receptors in the brain, Science **224**:22, 1984.

Chapter 3

Pharmacokinetic principles in the use of drugs

Pharmacokinetics is the study of the time course of absorption, distribution, metabolism, and excretion of drugs and their metabolites in the intact organism. A schema of pharmacokinetics is shown below:

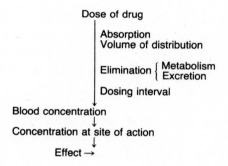

It should be apparent that understanding and quantification of the different pharmacokinetic parameters will allow better selection of a dose and dosing interval to achieve the desired effect (while avoiding toxicity) in an individual patient.

PASSAGE OF DRUGS ACROSS BODY MEMBRANES

For a drug to reach its site of action it must pass through various body membranes. Fig. 3-1 depicts the general course of a drug in the body. Absorption, capillary transfer, penetration into cells, and excretion are basic examples of the movement of drugs across body membranes.

Because of its lipoid nature, the cell membrane is highly permeable to lipid-soluble substances. Since water and other small lipid-insoluble substances such as urea also readily enter cells, it is believed that the lipid membrane has pores or channels that allow passage of lipid-insoluble molecules of small dimensions.

In addition to passive movement of many substances across body membranes, it is necessary to postulate more complex processes for the passage of glucose, amino acids, and some inorganic ions and drug substances. A simplified summary of the various mechanisms follows:

1. Passive transfer
   a. Simple diffusion
   b. Filtration
2. Specialized transport
   a. Active transport
   b. Facilitated diffusion
   c. Pinocytosis

The essential features of these transfer mechanisms will be described briefly.

Simple *diffusion* of a substance across a membrane is characterized by a rate of transfer that is directly proportional to the concentration gradient across the membrane. Both lipid-soluble substances and lipid-insoluble molecules of small size may cross membranes by this process. *Filtration* through a porous membrane refers to bulk flow of a solvent along with substances dissolved in it, except for molecules that are larger than the pores. The glomerular membrane of the kidney is a good example of a filtering membrane.

A special situation exists in the case of weak electrolytes, including most drugs. Cell membranes are more permeable to the nonionized and therefore more lipid-soluble (lipophilic) form of a given drug than to its ionized and more water-soluble (hydrophilic) form. As a consequence, the passage of many drugs across membranes and into cells is a function of the pH of the environment and the pK_a of the drug.

Passive transfer

Movement of drug in the body. After absorption, drug in the plasma can be bound to protein; only unbound drug is accessible to the site of action and to routes of metabolism and excretion. Metabolized products or excreted drug in renal tubular fluid or intestinal tract may reenter the plasma space before final elimination.

FIG. 3-1

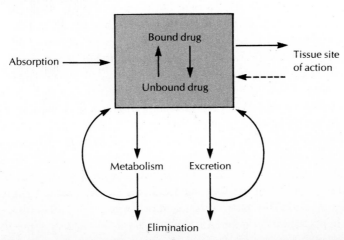

TABLE 3-1	pK$_a$ values for some weak acids and bases (at 25° C)			
Weak acids	pK$_a$		Weak bases	pK$_a$
Salicylic acid	3.00		Reserpine	6.6
Aspirin	3.49		Codeine	7.9
Sulfadiazine	6.48		Quinine	8.4
Barbital	7.91		Procaine	8.8
Boric acid	9.24		Ephedrine	9.36
			Atropine	9.65

The concept of pK$_a$ is derived from the Henderson-Hasselbalch equation. For an acid:

$$pK_a = pH + Log \frac{\text{Molecular concentration of nonionized acid}}{\text{Molecular concentration of ionized acid}}$$

For a base:

$$pK_a = pH + Log \frac{\text{Molecular concentration of ionized base}}{\text{Molecular concentration of nonionized base}}$$

It follows from these equations that the pH resulting in equal portions of the ionized and nonionized forms of a drug is the same as its pK$_a$. In other words, a substance is half-ionized in an environment in which the pH is equal to its pK$_a$.

Although these concepts may seem academic, they explain several clinically important observations. For example, weak acids are well absorbed from the stomach, whereas weak bases are not appreciably absorbed until they reach the less acidic intestine. The influence of urinary pH on excretion of salicylic acid or phenobarbital is another example of the dependence of diffusion on the pK$_a$ of drugs. Once these drugs enter the urine, an alkaline pH increases the ionized form of the drug. This decreases the tendency for the drug to be passively reabsorbed across the tubular epithelium and enhances its excretion, hence the rationale for alkalinizing the urine in treating salicylate or phenobarbital intoxication.

The pK$_a$ values for a number of drugs are listed in Table 3-1. It should be remembered that for acidic drugs the lower the pK$_a$, the stronger the acid, whereas for basic drugs the higher the pK$_a$, the stronger the base.

Relationships between pH, pK$_a$, and ionization of an acidic drug are exemplified with salicylic acid in Table 3-2.

Specialized transport   The passage of many substances into cells and across body membranes cannot be explained simply on the basis of diffusion or filtration. As examples, compounds may be taken up against a concentration gradient, selectivity can be shown for

TABLE 3-2	Effect of pH on the ionization of salicylic acid (pK$_a$ 3)
pH	Percent nonionized
1	99.0
2	90.9
3	50.0
4	9.1
5	1.0
6	0.1

compounds of the same size, competitive inhibition can occur among substances transported by the same mechanism, and in some instances metabolic inhibitors can block transport processes.

To explain these phenomena, the existence of specific *carriers* in membranes has been postulated. *Active transport* refers to transport of substances against a concentration or electrochemical gradient. For example, many drugs are actively secreted into the urine. *Facilitated diffusion* is a special form of carrier transport that has many of the characteristics of active transport, except that the substrate does not move against a concentration gradient. The uptake of glucose by cells is an example of facilitated diffusion. *Pinocytosis* refers to the ability of cells to engulf small droplets. Aminoglycoside antibiotics enter the proximal tubule of the kidney by this mechanism.

PRINCIPLES OF PHARMACO-KINETICS

Pharmacokinetic parameters

For use of drugs in patients, the important pharmacokinetic parameters are bioavailability, half-life, volume of distribution, and clearance.[2,4,6,8] *Bioavailability* determines how much of a dose gets into the body.[7] This parameter is designated *F*, the fraction of drug absorbed. If administered intravenously, bioavailability is 100% (*F* = 1.0). Drugs administered by other routes may have incomplete bioavailability (*F* = <1.0). The clinician must have a quantitative estimate of bioavailability to correctly decide the dose a patient should receive.

The most commonly used pharmacokinetic term has been *half-life*. This is unfortunate because, as will be shown subsequently, half-life is a hybrid function of both clearance and volume of distribution. An alteration in half-life attributable to clearance has therapeutic implications different from those of a change secondary to volume of distribution. Unfortunately, historically we have used half-life uncritically without realizing its limitations.

Half-life is important primarily as an indication of the time it takes for a dosing regimen to achieve steady-state concentrations of drug in blood. If a loading dose is not administered, 4 to 5 half-lives must elapse before the drug reaches steady-state concentrations in the patient. To be more precise, after 4 half-lives the drug will have reached 94% of its steady-state concentration. For a drug such as digoxin then, which has a half-life of about 36 hours in patients with normal renal function, approximately 1 week must elapse before steady state is achieved. Likewise, if the dose of drug is changed, whether increased or decreased, 4 to 5 times the half-life must elapse to reattain steady state. Similarly, if drug half-life changes, as is common with a change in the patient's disease state, a new steady state will be reached after 4 to 5 times the *new* half-life.

One must always try to be aware whether a patient is at steady state. Interpreting drug concentrations and clinical end points of response is very difficult, if not impossible, without considering this factor. Changing dosage of a drug before the patient has reached steady state with one regimen can be a confusing and potentially hazardous exercise.

The *volume of distribution* (V_d) of a drug describes the relationship between the blood concentration attained and the dose of drug given; that is,

$$\text{Concentration achieved} = \text{Dose}/V_d$$

This volume should *not* be ascribed physiologic meaning or interpretation; it is a derived parameter. Clinically, the volume of distribution is used to calculate the loading dose of a drug required to reach an initial target blood concentration. For example, if a concentration of 10 µg/ml is needed and the volume of distribution is 100 liters, the loading dose would be 1000 mg:

$$\text{Concentration achieved} = \frac{\text{Dose}}{V_d}$$

$$10 \ \mu g/ml = \frac{\text{Dose}}{100,000 \ ml}$$

This calculation is independent of clearance and half-life. Importantly, diseases can affect the volume of distribution and thereby alter the loading dose needed. In this example, if a disease had decreased the volume of distribution of the drug from 100 to 50 L, and the patient was given the same 1000 mg loading dose, the serum concentration would predictably be 1000/50, or 20 µg/ml, and could result in toxicity.

To reemphasize, a loading dose is administered to achieve therapeutic concentrations of a drug quickly. Otherwise, one must wait 4 to 5 times the half-life for steady state to occur.

Clearance is usually referred to as blood, plasma, or serum clearance, depending on the particular fluid assayed. Clearance is equivalent to an amount of body fluid sufficient to account for all drug removed per unit of time. Therefore a serum clearance of 100 ml/min means that in 1 minute all of the drug could have been eliminated from 100 ml of serum. This removal can occur through distribution to tissues, metabolism, or excretion.

Clinically, clearance is important for determination of the amount of drug needed to *maintain* a steady-state concentration. By definition, at steady state:

$$\text{Rate in} = \text{Rate out}$$

The rate of drug entering is a function of the dose administered, the fraction, F, of that dose absorbed if administered orally or intramuscularly and the time interval over which it is administered:

$$\text{Rate in} = F \times \text{Dose/Dosing interval}$$

The rate of drug leaving the body is a function of its steady-state concentration (Cp_{ave}) and its clearance (Cl):

$$\text{Rate out} = Cp_{ave} \times Cl$$

Therefore at steady state:

$$F \times \text{Dose/Dosing interval} = Cp_{ave} \times Cl$$

or with the equation rearranged:

$$Cp_{ave} = \frac{F \times \text{Dose}}{\text{Dosing interval} \times Cl}$$

It is obvious from this relationship that changes or individual differences in bioavailability, in dosing regimen (dose and dosing interval), and in clearance can influence the steady-state concentration of a drug. Disease effects on drug clearance must be compensated for by the maintenance regimen; by a change in the dose or the frequency with which it is administered, or both. The method selected for adjusting the dosage regimen influences the magnitude of difference between peak and trough concentrations of drug, that is, the fluctuation above and below the average drug concentration. The more frequently a drug is administered, the less fluctuation and vice versa.

No best method can be promulgated for adjustment of the maintenance regimen of a drug.[2,4,6,8] Knowing the general relationship between dosing frequency and fluctuation of drug concentrations must be coupled with knowledge of the influence of specific disease states on the pharmacokinetics and dynamics of specific drugs. This allows approximation of a starting point for adjustment of dosage regimens that must then be tailored to the individual patient by assessment of clinical end points of response and by measurement of serum concentrations of drugs.

Table 3-3 summarizes the clinically most important pharmacokinetic principles.

To reiterate, volume of distribution is important for loading dose, clearance for maintenance dose, and half-life for determining the time required to reach steady state. It is important to note that half-life can be affected by changes in volume of distribution or clearance. Therefore, knowing only that the half-life of a drug is altered in a particular disease state does not allow one to decide upon the appropriate adjustment of therapy. One must dissect this parameter into its component terms of volume of distribution and clearance and alter therapy accordingly.

Table 3-4 illustrates these points with the drugs digoxin and lidocaine and shows how changes in volume of distribution or clearance affect therapeutic decisions. As can be appreciated from the table, the actual quantitative effect on half-life will be

TABLE 3-3   Pharmacokinetic principles

$$\text{Initial concentration achieved} = \frac{\text{Loading dose}}{\text{Volume of distribution}}$$

$$\text{Steady-state concentration maintained} = \frac{\text{Fraction absorbed} \times \text{Maintenance dose}}{\text{Dosing interval} \times \text{Clearance}}$$

$$\text{Half-life} = \frac{0.693 \times \text{Volume of distribution}}{\text{Clearance}}$$

a function of the relative magnitude of change of each of its determinants. For example, assessing the effect of congestive heart failure only on the half-life of lidocaine would result in no dose adjustment whereas, clearly, both loading and maintenance doses of this drug should be reduced in this therapeutic setting.

Studies on drug distribution, absorption, and excretion have led to the concept that the body may be considered as if it consists of different compartments. In the simplest form, a drug passes from one compartment to another in direct proportion to its concentration gradient. In other words, a constant fraction (rather than a constant amount) of drug moves between compartments. Drugs with this characteristic are said to obey *first-order* kinetics as opposed to zero-order, saturable, or Michaelis-Menten kinetics. In a *one-compartment model*, it is assumed that drugs are homogeneously distributed throughout the tissues and fluids of the body (Fig. 3-1).

In most instances a graphic representation of the time course of both absorption and elimination of drugs describes an exponential decay curve (Fig. 3-2, *A*). If the same data are graphed on semilogarithmic paper, the result is a straight line (Fig. 3-2, *B*). The intercept of the extrapolated line on the ordinate indicates the initial concentration that would have been achieved if the drug had been administered and distributed instantaneously throughout the body. This hypothetical concentration is used experimentally to calculate volume of distribution (see equation on p. 16). Clearance is calculated from the dose administered divided by the *area under the curve* (AUC) of the graph shown. Lastly, half-life, the time required for a 50% decrease in concentration of the drug, can also be derived from the graph. It is apparent from Fig. 3-2, *B*, that, in this model, half-life is independent of the concentration of the drug.

For some drugs elimination is a *zero-order* process; that is, a fixed quantity of drug is eliminated per unit of time. The best example is alcohol. It is assumed that saturation of the metabolizing enzymes is responsible for the deviation from first-order kinetics. For a few drugs, such as aspirin and phenytoin, the type of elimination is dose related. At low concentrations first-order kinetics prevail; saturation of elimination processes by higher concentrations results in zero-order elimination. For such

TABLE 3-4   Clinical illustration of pharmacokinetic principles

Clinical setting	Kinetic parameter			Dosing	
	V_d	Cl	$T_{1/2}$	Load	Maintenance
Digoxin in mild to moderate renal failure	—*	↓	↑	—	↓
Digoxin in end-stage renal failure	↓	↓ ↓	↑	↓	↓ ↓
Lidocaine in liver disease	—	↓	↑	—	↓
Lidocaine in congestive heart failure	↓	↓	—	↓	↓

*No change.

Schematic representation of drug disappearance curves and biologic half-life. The y *axis is on the linear scale in* **A** *and on the logarithmic scale in* **B**. *Drug A has a biologic half-life of 1 hour. The biologic half-life of drug B is 2 hours.*   FIG. 3-2

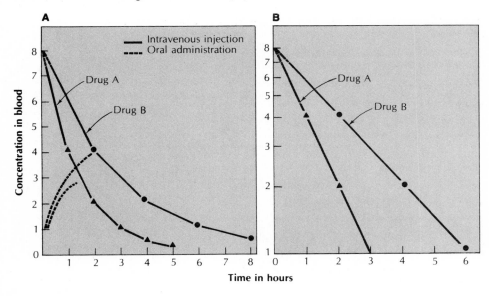

drugs, the half-life at higher concentrations is longer than at low concentrations because clearance is lower at high concentrations and, as shown previously, half-life is inversely related to clearance.

The single-compartment model assumes an instantaneous and homogeneous distribution of drugs throughout the body. This is obviously an oversimplification. A *two-compartment open model* more adequately describes the distribution of many drugs (Fig. 3-3). The plasma concentration profile that occurs with this type of model is shown in Fig. 3-4 where the curve has two distinct components; usually the first

Two-compartment open model

FIG. 3-3 *Diagram of two-compartment open model.*

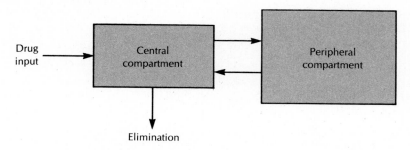

FIG. 3-4 *Logarithm of drug concentration in blood plotted against time (solid line) after intravenous administration of a drug whose disposition can be described by a two-compartment model. Broken line (----) represents extrapolation of terminal (B) phase. The ·····- line was obtained by method of residuals.*

From Dvorchik, B.H., and Vesell, E.S.: Clin. Chem. **22**:868, 1976.

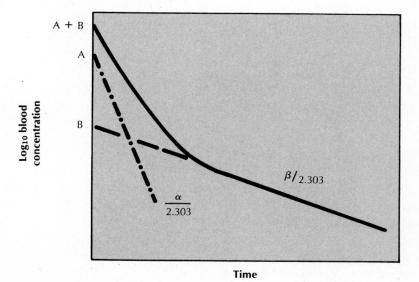

is related to distribution and the second to elimination. Transforming the curve as shown in the figure allows derivations of values for A, B, α, and β, from which relevant pharmacokinetic parameters can be calculated.

The two-compartment model incorporates a small central compartment and a larger peripheral compartment. Although no specific anatomic spaces are implied, the central compartment usually corresponds to the blood and extracellular fluid of highly perfused organs. The peripheral compartment consists of less well perfused tissues such as skin, fat, and muscle. It is further assumed that drugs initially enter and are eventually eliminated from the central compartment though some reversible transfer occurs to the peripheral compartment, which thus can act as a reservoir.[2,4,6,8]

Importantly, these different models allow calculation of volume of distribution, clearance, and half-life, which can then be used to derive dosage regimens to achieve the desired concentration of drug in individual patients.

ABSORPTION

The process whereby a drug initially enters body fluids is referred to as *absorption*. The rate of this process depends on the route of administration, drug solubility and other physical properties of the drug, disease states affecting absorptive processes, and so on.

Absorption from the gastrointestinal tract

Drugs are administered by the oral route in many different forms—solutions, suspensions, capsules, and tablets with various coatings.[3] For absorption a drug must be in solution in molecular form. When a drug is not given in solution, its rate of absorption will be slowed by the time necessary for the tablet or capsule to release the drug (dissolution) and for the drug to dissolve in the gastrointestinal fluid. The rate of dissolution is determined by the pharmaceutic formulation, which thus influences absorption. Once a drug is in solution, absorption is a basic characteristic of the membranes of the gastrointestinal tract and can be accounted for by simple diffusion across a membrane having the characteristics of a lipoid structure with water-filled pores.

As discussed previously, the gastrointestinal membrane is permeable to nonionized lipid-soluble forms of drugs and is virtually impermeable to the ionized form. Weak acids, such as salicylates and barbiturates, are largely nonionized in the acidic gastric fluid and are therefore well absorbed from the stomach. Despite this, factors such as gastric emptying time and surface area may result in absorption of a greater fraction of weak acids from the intestine than from the stomach. In contrast, weak bases, such as quinine or ephedrine, and ionized quaternary amines, such as tetraethylammonium, are poorly absorbed from the stomach. Alkalinization of gastric contents will decrease absorption of weak acids from the stomach and increase that of weak bases.

Absorption from the small intestine is similar in principle to that from the stomach, except that the surface area is so much greater in the gut and the pH of intestinal contents is more alkaline. Weakly acidic and weakly basic drugs are well absorbed from the small intestine, but highly ionized acids and bases are not.

The mucosal membrane of the small intestine appears to be more permissive or porous than that of the stomach in addition to having a greater surface area. Hence many drugs, whether they are acids or bases, are absorbed primarily in the proximal small intestine. How soon the stomach empties its contents into the intestine therefore can greatly influence how quickly drugs are absorbed. For example, if quinine is retained in the stomach, its absorption may be considerably delayed. Several drugs and diseases can affect gastric emptying and thereby greatly influence absorption. For example, opioid analgesics slow emptying, whereas metoclopramide hastens it.

Passive intestinal absorption does not account for uptake of all substances. Special mechanisms exist for the absorption of sugars, amino acids, and compounds related to normal nutrients. Similarly, some inorganic ions, such as sodium and chloride, are well absorbed despite the fact that they are charged.

In the oral cavity the mucosa also behaves as a lipid-pore membrane, and drugs may be absorbed after sublingual administration. Nitroglycerin is administered in this manner.

Absorption with parenteral administration	When injected intravenously, a drug is rapidly distributed to various compartments of the body.

When injected intravenously, a drug is rapidly distributed to various compartments of the body.

The rate of absorption after subcutaneous or intramuscular injection depends largely on two factors: the solubility of the preparation and the blood flow through the region. Suspensions or colloidal preparations are absorbed more slowly than aqueous solutions. Advantage can be taken of this fact when prolonged absorption is desirable. For example, protamine is added to insulin to form a suspension and thereby slow absorption from the subcutaneous depot. Various penicillin suspensions also illustrate prolongation of a therapeutic action by slowing the absorption.

Local blood flow also has much to do with the speed of drug absorption from a tissue. Absorption from a subcutaneous site may be very slow in the presence of peripheral circulatory failure. This has been observed after administration of morphine to patients in shock. Similarly, greater blood flow per unit weight of muscle is responsible for more rapid absorption of drugs from this tissue than from subcutaneous fat. In addition, muscle groups receive various rates of blood flow, and absorption can depend on the particular muscle chosen for injection.

Certain consequences of these facts may be of clinical importance. Cooling an area of subcutaneous injection will slow absorption, a desirable effect if an excessive dose has been inadvertently injected or if untoward reactions begin to develop. On the other hand, massage of the site will increase blood flow and hasten absorption.

Rate-controlled drug delivery

There is increasing interest in methods of administration that maintain a fairly uniform drug concentration at its site of action. Examples are constant-infusion pumps, sustained-release gastrointestinal delivery systems, and transdermal devices.[3] Pumps can be worn externally or implanted under the skin. Insulin-infusion pumps are being used in diabetics. When pilocarpine is used in eyedrops, frequent administration is necessary because of rapid clearance. A device that releases the drug uniformly can now be placed under the lower eyelid. Skin patches are used increasingly for transdermal administration of scopolamine, nitroglycerin, and clonidine. Whether such an approach is feasible depends greatly on the physicochemical characteristics of the drug itself and the structure (for example, the skin) through which the drug is absorbed.

Some drugs are completely absorbed, some little or not at all, and still others are partially absorbed. The importance of bioavailability is readily appreciated if one considers its impact on the steady-state concentration achieved with chronic dosing (Table 3-3). Examples of well-absorbed drugs are most sulfonamides, digitoxin, aspirin, and barbiturates. Drugs not absorbed include streptomycin, neomycin, and kanamycin. Examples of partially or variably absorbed drugs are penicillin G, certain digitalis glycosides, and dicumarol.

Clinical pharmacology of absorption

The dosage form of a drug has a major influence on absorption.[3] Solutions are absorbed most rapidly and coated tablets most slowly. Enteric-coated tablets are commonly used to provide a sustained level of drug in the body, but this dosage form cannot generally be considered a predictable method of administering drugs despite its popularity. There are great individual variations in gastric emptying and rate of dissolution of such preparations. They may even be eliminated unchanged in the feces.

When administered orally, drugs must pass through the intestinal wall, and they ordinarily traverse the liver before reaching systemic sites. Even with complete gastrointestinal absorption a fraction of the dose may not reach the sampling site because of metabolism within the gut or liver. This concept is referred to as the "first-pass effect" and is important for many drugs, one of the best studied being propranolol. Occasionally, it is important clinically to circumvent this first-pass effect. For example, swallowed nitroglycerin does not reach the systemic circulation because the first-pass effect is so great. Consequently, this drug is administered under the tongue where it is absorbed into vessels that do not drain into the liver.

FIRST-PASS EFFECT

Once a drug reaches the plasma, it must cross various barriers to reach its site of action.[5] The first of these barriers is the capillary wall. Through diffusion and filtration most drugs rapidly cross the capillary wall, which has the usual characteristics of biologic membranes. Lipid-soluble substances diffuse through the endothelium, whereas lipid-insoluble drugs pass through pores that represent a relatively larger fraction of the total surface area. The capillary transfer of lipid-insoluble substances is inversely related to molecular size. Large molecules such as dextran are transferred so slowly that they can be used as plasma substitutes to retain fluid within the vascular compartment.

DISTRIBUTION OF DRUGS IN THE BODY

Factors that affect distribution of drugs in the body include (1) binding to plasma proteins, (2) cellular binding, (3) concentration in fatty tissues, and (4) the blood-brain barrier.

Factors contributing to unequal distribution of drugs

Binding of drugs to plasma proteins increases the concentration of drug in blood relative to that in extracellular fluid. It also provides a depot, since the bound portion of the drug is in equilibrium with the free form. As the unbound fraction is excreted or metabolized, additional amounts dissociate from the protein. Protein binding can prolong the half-life of a drug in the body, since the bound fraction is not filtered through renal glomeruli and is protected from biotransformation. The protein-bound fraction of a drug also is restricted from reaching its site of action and is inactive. The protein responsible for binding of acidic drugs is usually albumin; basic drugs are bound to α_1-acid glycoprotein; and many hormonal agents are bound to other types of proteins, for example, transcortin for glucocorticoids.

The binding capacity of proteins is not unlimited. Once binding becomes saturated, a small increase in dose can result in a large increase in unbound drug with a concomitant increase in effect, including the precipitation of toxicity. In hypoalbuminemia, toxic manifestations of drugs may develop because of the deficiency of binding protein.

Drugs may influence protein binding of other substances or drugs. Thus salicylates decrease the binding of thyroxin to proteins. The binding of bilirubin to albumin may be inhibited by a variety of drugs, such as sulfisoxazole or salicylates. This can be particularly hazardous in neonates by increasing the accessibility of bilirubin to the brain. Fatal kernicterus has occurred in premature infants who were given sulfisoxazole. Other examples of drug interactions based on displacement from protein binding are discussed in Chapter 63.

The *cellular binding* of drugs is usually a result of affinity for some cellular constituent. The high concentration of the antimalarial drug quinacrine in liver or muscle is probably caused by its affinity for nucleoproteins.

The *concentration of drug in fatty tissues* also affects distribution. Highly lipid-soluble drugs like glutethimide distribute into fat, which then serves as a depot. Removal of such drugs from plasma results in egress from fat into blood with restoration of the circulating concentration. In contrast, the rapid but short action of drugs such as the thiobarbiturate intravenous anesthetics has been explained on the basis of rapid uptake by fatty tissues of the brain. As the concentration of drug in the blood falls, the anesthetic rapidly distributes out of the brain and the patient awakens.

The *blood-brain barrier* provides a unique example of unequal distribution of drugs. Even if injected intravenously, many drugs fail to reach the central nervous system, the cerebrospinal fluid, or the aqueous humor, or they enter much less rapidly than they enter other tissues. There are, however, some brain regions with a weak blood-brain barrier; these include the neurohypophysis and the area postrema.

The capillaries in the central nervous system are enveloped by glial cells, which present a barrier to many water-soluble compounds, though they are permeable to lipid-soluble substances. Thus quaternary amines penetrate the central nervous system poorly, whereas general anesthetics do so with ease.

Of great importance in clinical medicine is the increase produced by inflammation in permeability of barriers. For example, administration of large doses of penicillin to normal persons fails to produce detectable levels of the antibiotic in cerebrospinal fluid. By such data alone, one might conclude a lack of potential efficacy of the drug in meningitis. However, penicillin can penetrate readily into the spinal fluid of patients with inflamed meninges and is commonly used in some forms of meningitis.

Although many drugs do not penetrate the cerebrospinal fluid well, they can move efficiently in the reverse direction when administered by intracisternal injection, by filtration across the arachnoid villi. In addition, the choroid plexus is capable of pumping certain substances from the cerebrospinal fluid, for example, penicillin. The peritoneal membrane exhibits similar parallels in which transport from the peritoneum into blood is much greater than the reverse.

The passage of drugs into *milk* may be explained by diffusion of the nonionized, non–protein bound fraction. Sufficient amounts may reach the milk to exert adverse effects on the breast-fed infant. On the other hand, many drugs appear in milk only in small quantities and are generally of no clinical significance for the infant. In general, large doses of drugs should not be administered to a mother who is breast-feeding her child without considering the potential danger to the infant.

EXCRETION (CLEARANCE) OF DRUGS

The most important route of excretion for most drugs is the kidney.[1] Many drugs are also excreted into bile, but they can then be reabsorbed from the intestine (so-called enterohepatic circulation), making this route quantitatively unimportant. Elimination of drugs in the feces or through the lungs and the salivary and sweat glands is important only in special cases to be discussed under individual drugs. The elimination of a drug will also be influenced by such extrarenal factors as plasma protein binding, the existence of tissue depots, and, most important, the rate of drug metabolism (see Chapter 4).

Three major mechanisms are involved in the renal handling of drugs: glomerular filtration, variable tubular reabsorption, and tubular secretion. The usual course of a drug is filtration through the glomeruli and partial reabsorption in the tubules. Since water is reabsorbed to a much greater extent than most drugs are, the concentration of drugs in the urine is usually greater than that in plasma.

Just as in the gastrointestinal tract, the fraction of drug in tubular fluid that is uncharged will be a function of the urinary pH and the pK_a of the drug. Drugs that are bases are excreted to a greater extent if the urine is acidic, whereas acidic compounds are excreted more favorably if the urine is alkaline. A practical application of this principle is used in treatment of phenobarbital poisoning. Since phenobarbital is a weak acid, an alkaline urine will increase the relative amount of ionized drug, thereby decreasing its capacity for reabsorption and increasing excretion. Administration of sodium bicarbonate can cause a clinically significant increase in excretion of phenobarbital.

Since urine is normally acidic, the elimination of weakly acidic drugs by excretion alone would require a very long time. Fortunately, metabolism tends to transform these drugs into stronger electrolytes, thereby increasing the percentage in the ionic form and limiting tubular reabsorption.

In addition to glomerular filtration with passive tubular reabsorption, the renal tubule can actively secrete organic anions and cations. The classic examples of organic anions are penicillin and probenecid; examples of organic cations are cimetidine and procainamide. These active-transport pathways also secrete other agents, and competition for active tubular secretion occurs among the various anions and cations.

Drugs, such as penicillins, that are secreted by the tubules, in general, have very short half-lives. To slow elimination, tubular secretion can be inhibited by a drug like probenecid, a compound specifically developed for this purpose. Usually, however, it is simpler to maintain a drug in the body for longer periods of time by prolonging its absorption rather than by impairing elimination. This is the reason for the development of penicillin preparations that are absorbed slowly after intramuscular injection.

DOSAGE SCHEDULES AND PHARMACO- KINETICS

Drugs may be administered in a single dose or in a repetitive fashion. Fig. 3-2, A, shows two drug-concentration curves, to which a two-compartment model applies, after administration of a single intravenous dose. If the drug is administered orally in a single dose, the curve will have an ascending limb, a peak, and a descending limb. Variations in absorption and elimination may greatly influence the concentration

FIG. 3-5 *Plot of concentration of a drug in blood after repetitive oral administration of equal doses at equal time intervals.*

From Dvorchik, B.H., and Vesell, E.S.: Clin. Chem. **22:**868, 1976.

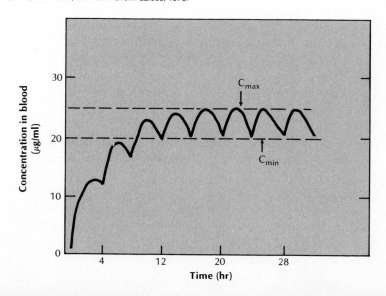

curve, reflecting changes in the peak effect, the time required to achieve peak effect, and the duration of action of the drug.

If a drug is given repeatedly at intervals shorter than the time necessary for its complete elimination, it will accumulate in the body. A typical plot is depicted in Fig. 3-5. It can be seen that the drug concentration rises until it reaches a *plateau*. The curve also shows *fluctuations*.

The fluctuations in drug concentration depend on the maintenance dose, the dosage interval, and the elimination half-life. Frequent administration of a drug tends to minimize these fluctuations, since the ratio of dosage interval to half-life is decreased. The importance of fluctuations depends on the drug and on the clinical setting. With some drugs, such as penicillin, large fluctuations are acceptable, whereas with drugs used to treat abnormal cardiac rhythms relatively constant blood concentrations are necessary to achieve a therapeutic objective while avoiding toxicity.

In general, if a drug has a short duration of action, the following methods are available for prolonging its action:

1. *Frequent administration*. Most sulfonamides are administered every 4 hours.
2. *Slowing absorption*. Enteric coating and other pharmaceutic maneuvers may accomplish this.
3. *Interfering with renal secretion*. Probenecid blocks the excretion of penicillin.
4. *Inhibiting drug metabolism*. Allopurinol was originally developed for blocking the metabolic degradation of mercaptopurine.

PROBLEM 3-1 *A sleeping medication has a half-life of 1 hour. It is administered in a dose of 100 mg, and the patient wakes up when only 12.5 mg remain in the body. How many hours will the patient sleep? If 200 mg of the same drug is administered, how much longer will the patient sleep? The answer can be found by comparison with Fig. 3-2. Doubling the dose simply adds one half-life to the duration of sleep.*

---

1. Bennett, W.M., Singer, I., and Coggins, C.H.: A practical guide to drug usage in adult patients with impaired renal function, J.A.M.A. **214**:1468, 1970.
2. Gibaldi, M., and Levy, G.: Pharmacokinetics in clinical practice. I. Concepts, J.A.M.A. **235**:1864, 1976.
3. Goldman, P.: Rate-controlled drug delivery, N. Engl. J. Med. **307**:286, 1982.
4. Greenblatt, D.J., and Koch-Weser, J.: Clinical pharmacokinetics, N. Engl. J. Med. **293**:702 and 964, 1975.
5. La Du, B.N., Mandel, H.G., and Way, E.L.: Fundamentals of drug metabolism and drug disposition, Baltimore, 1971, The Williams & Wilkins Co.
6. Rowland, M., and Tozer, T.N.: Clinical pharmacokinetics: concepts and applications, Philadelphia, 1980, Lea & Febiger.
7. Ther, L., and Winne, D.: Drug absorption, Annu. Rev. Pharmacol. **11**:57, 1971.
8. Winter, M.E.: Basic clinical pharmacokinetics, San Francisco, 1980, Applied Therapeutics, Inc.

Chapter 4

Drug metabolism and enzyme induction

If the body depended solely on excretory mechanisms for ridding itself of drugs, lipid-soluble compounds would be retained almost indefinitely. Drug metabolism generally results in the formation of more polar water-soluble metabolites that are either filtered or secreted by the kidney and are not well reabsorbed passively by the renal tubules; hence they are more efficiently excreted (Fig. 4-1). Drug metabolism varies greatly among different species and among individuals of the same species.

DRUG METABOLISM
Chemical reactions in drug metabolism

The chemical reactions involved in drug metabolism or *biotransformation* are classified as microsomal oxidations, nonmicrosomal oxidations, reductions, hydrolyses, and conjugations.[4] These pathways of metabolism will each be discussed, with specific examples. Since microsomal enzymes play a predominant role in biotransformation (Table 4-1), their functions are summarized first.

MICROSOMAL ENZYMES

The microsomal enzymes of the liver, which are part of the smooth endoplasmic reticulum, convert many lipid-soluble drugs and foreign compounds into more water-soluble metabolites.[4]

The microsomal drug-metabolizing enzymes constitute a mixed-function oxidase system. In the presence of nicotinamide adenine dinucleotide phosphate (NADPH) and oxygen, the enzyme system transfers one atom of oxygen to the drug while another atom of oxygen is reduced to form water. The general scheme is as follows:

$$NADPH + A + H_2 \rightarrow AH_2 + NADP^+$$

$$AH_2 + O_2 \rightarrow \text{``Active oxygen''}$$

$$\text{``Active oxygen''} + \text{Drug} \rightarrow \text{Oxidized drug} + A + H_2O$$

Result: $$NADPH + O_2 + \text{Drug} = NADP^+ + H_2O + \text{Oxidized drug}$$

In this scheme, A is cytochrome P-450, which is the terminal oxidase for a variety of drug-oxidative reactions. Cytochrome P-450 is so named because this hemoprotein in its reduced state can combine with carbon monoxide to form a product with an absorption peak at 450 nm. Other essential enzymes in the reaction include NADPH cytochrome P-450 reductase, which reduces the oxidized P-450.

Reactions catalyzed by microsomal drug-metabolizing enzymes include hydroxylation of aromatic rings, aliphatic hydroxylations, N-dealkylations, O-dealkylations, deaminations, sulfoxidations, and N-oxidations.

Elimination of drugs.   *FIG. 4-1*

From Remmer, H.: Am. J. Med. **49**:617, 1970.

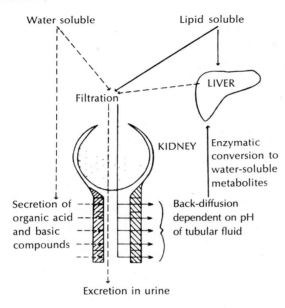

TABLE 4-1   Drug metabolism and enzymes of the endoplasmic reticulum*

Drug metabolism	Enzyme
Oxidations of aliphatic and aromatic groups Barbiturates Benzodiazepines Phenothiazines Meprobamate Phenytoin Antihistamines Acetophenetidin Aminopyrine Some synthetic steroids	Cytochrome P-450
Reductions of azo and nitro groups	Flavin enzymes
Hydrolyses of esters and amides	Esterases
Conjugations with glucuronic acid Alcohols Phenols	Transferases

*Modified from Remmer, H.: Am. J. Med. **49**:617, 1970.

Induction and inhibition of microsomal hydroxylase. Phenobarbital, rifampin, and many other lipid-soluble drugs may cause hypertrophy of the smooth endoplasmic reticulum and increase the amount of microsomal hydroxylase.[1,2,6] Clinically this results in increased clearance of the drug, which may be sufficient to require an increase in dose.

Premature infants and persons with liver disease may have a deficiency of microsomal enzymes. Some drugs, such as cimetidine, inhibit drug-metabolizing enzymes.[5,6] In such settings, drug clearance is decreased, often necessitating a decrease in dose to avoid toxic concentrations.

MICROSOMAL OXIDATIONS   *Hydroxylation of aromatic rings.* Acetanilide is changed to active *p*-hydroxyacetanilide, more commonly known as acetaminophen. Phenobarbital is converted to inactive *p*-hydroxyphenobarbital.

Phenobarbital   *p*-Hydroxyphenobarbital

Side-chain oxidation (aliphatic hydroxylation). Pentobarbital is metabolized to pentobarbital alcohol. Meprobamate is oxidized to hydroxymeprobamate.

Pentobarbital   Pentobarbital alcohol

N-dealkylation. Mephobarbital is demethylated to phenobarbital. A clinically important caveat with this pathway is that it appears to be less if at all subject to induction and inhibition by other drugs as compared to hydroxylation reactions.

Mephobarbital   Phenobarbital

N-oxidation. Trimethylamine is oxidized to trimethylamine oxide.

$$(CH_3)_3N \xrightarrow{[O]} (CH_3)_3N=O$$

Trimethylamine   **Trimethylamine oxide**

Sulfoxidation. Chlorpromazine is converted to chlorpromazine sulfoxide.

Chlorpromazine   **Chlorpromazine sulfoxide**

O-dealkylation. Acetophenetidin (phenacetin) is changed to acetaminophen.

Phenacetin   **Acetaminophen**

S-dealkylation. 6-Methylthiopurine is demethylated to 6-mercaptopurine.

6-Methylthiopurine   **6-Mercaptopurine**

Deamination. Amphetamine is oxidized to phenylacetone.

Amphetamine   **Phenylacetone**

Desulfuration. Parathion is oxidized to paraoxon.

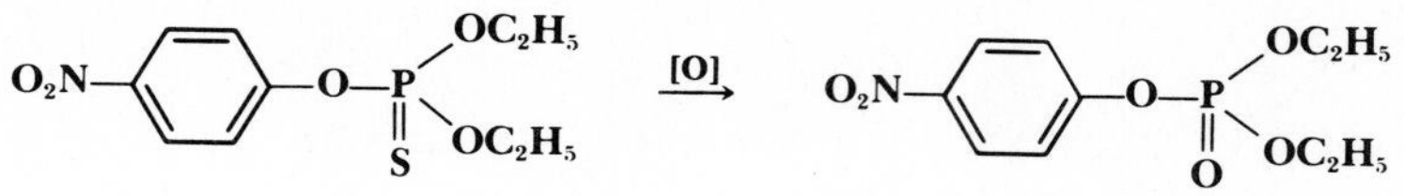

Parathion $\xrightarrow{[O]}$ Paraoxon

NONMICROSOMAL (ALCOHOL) OXIDATION

p-Nitrobenzyl alcohol is changed to *p*-nitrobenzaldehyde.

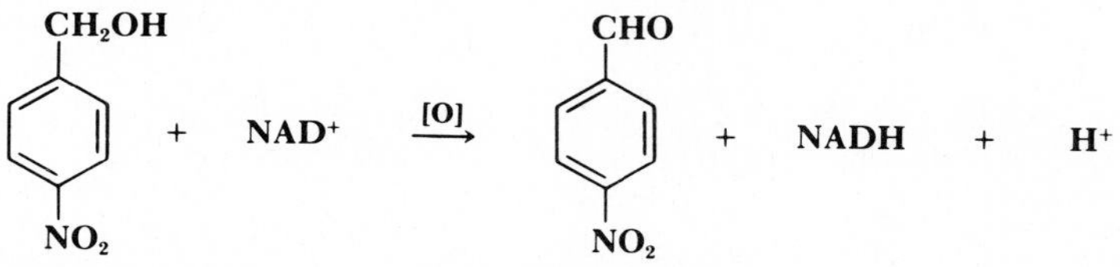

p-Nitrobenzyl alcohol + NAD$^+$ $\xrightarrow{[O]}$ *p*-Nitrobenzaldehyde + NADH + H$^+$

REDUCTIONS

Nitroreduction. Chloramphenicol is reduced to the arylamine.

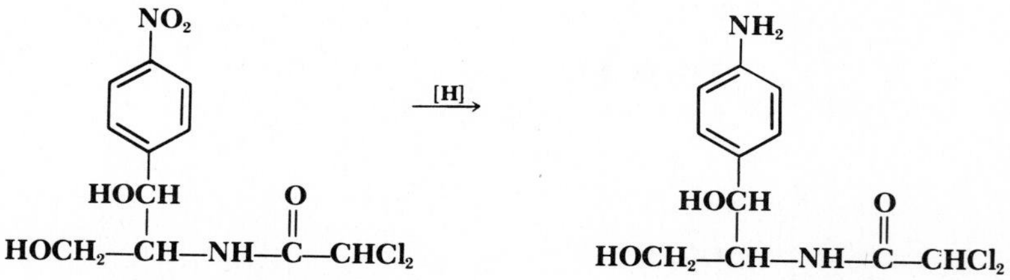

Chloramphenicol $\xrightarrow{[H]}$ "Arylamine"

Azoreduction. Prontosil is reduced to sulfanilamide.

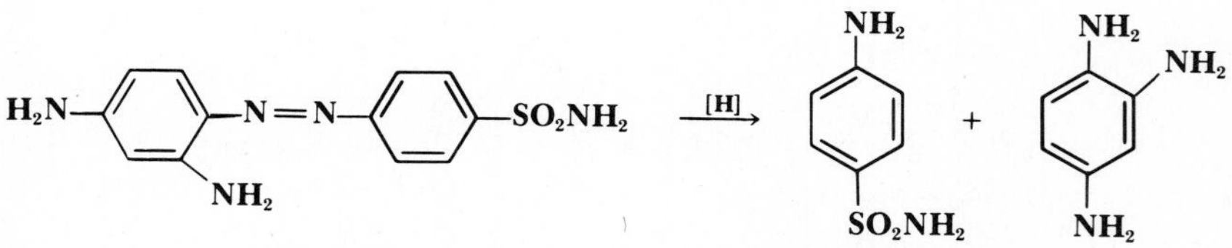

Prontosil $\xrightarrow{[H]}$ Sulfanilamide +

Alcohol dehydrogenation. Chloral hydrate is changed to trichloroethanol, the active moiety.

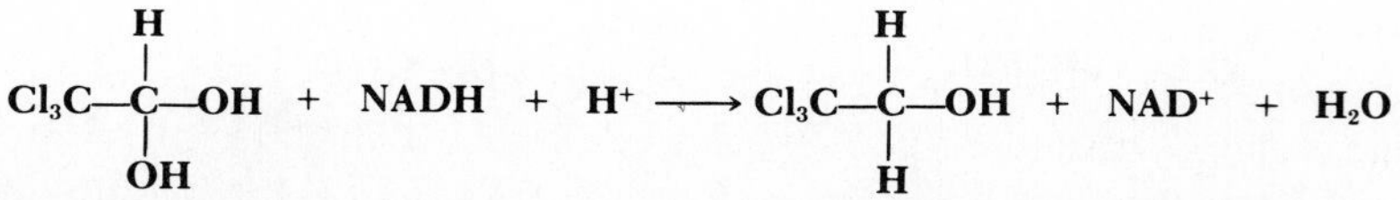

Chloral hydrate + NADH + H$^+$ $\longrightarrow$ Trichloroethanol + NAD$^+$ + H$_2$O

Procaine is hydrolyzed to *p*-aminobenzoic acid and diethylaminoethanol.

| Procaine | *p*-Aminobenzoic acid | Diethylaminoethanol |

The most important conjugation reactions are glucuronide synthesis, glycine conjugation, sulfate conjugation, acetylation, mercapturic acid synthesis, and methylation.

Glucuronide synthesis. Phenols, alcohols, carboxylic acids, and compounds containing amino or sulfhydryl groups may undergo glucuronide conjugation. Glucuronide formation is one of the most common routes of drug metabolism. Not only does
this process occur with parent compounds, but many metabolites formed by the
pathways discussed on pp. 30 to 32 are in turn conjugated to a glucuronide before
excretion. The mechanism of the reaction is as follows:

$$\text{Uridine diphosphoglucuronate} + \text{ROH} \xrightarrow[\text{transferase}]{\text{Glucuronyl}} \text{RO glucuronide} + \text{Uridine diphosphate}$$

An example of a drug excreted almost entirely as the glucuronide is salicylamide.

Salicylamide   Salicylamide glucuronide

Glycine conjugation. Glycine conjugation is characteristic for certain aromatic acids.
It depends on the availability of coenzyme A, glycine, and glycine-*N*-acylase. A typical
reaction is as follows:

$$\text{Benzoic acid} \xrightarrow{\text{ATP} + \text{CoA}} \text{Benzoyl CoA} \xrightarrow{\text{Glycine}} \text{Hippuric acid}$$

Drugs conjugated with glycine in humans include salicylic acid, isonicotinic acid,
and *p*-aminosalicylic acid. These drugs are also metabolized by other pathways that
may be more important quantitatively than glycine conjugation.

Sulfate conjugation. Phenols, alcohols, or aromatic amines may undergo sulfate
conjugation. The sulfate donor is 3′-phosphoadenosine-5-phosphosulfate (PAPS).

Acetylation. Derivatives of aniline are acetylated in the body. In addition to sulfanilamide and related compounds, widely used drugs such as *p*-aminosalicylic acid,

isoniazid, and procainamide are transformed by this mechanism. The general reaction involving an amine, acetyl coenzyme A, and a specific acetylating enzyme may be depicted as follows:

$$RNH_2 + CoASCOCH_3 \xrightarrow{\text{Acetylase}} RNHCOCH_3 + CoASH$$

The acetylating ability of individuals may differ considerably and shows a bimodal distribution; patients can be grouped as slow acetylators as opposed to rapid acetylators.[3] In the case of isoniazid, a low degree of acetylation shows some correlation with the incidence of toxic reactions such as peripheral neuritis.

Isoniazid → **Acetylated isoniazid**

Mercapturic acid synthesis. Mercapturic acid synthesis is not a common pathway in humans, though it may occur. Some drugs containing an active halogen or a nitro group may be changed to mercapturates. In fact, the thiol derivative of nitrates is the active intermediate that causes vasodilatation.

Methylation. Norepinephrine and epinephrine are metabolized in part to normetanephrine and metanephrine by O-methylation, whereas nicotinic acid is metabolized to *N*-methylnicotinic acid, an example of N-methylation. The source of methyl groups for drug methylations is *S*-adenosylmethionine.

Norepinephrine → **Normetanephrine**

Drug metabolism and detoxification

Drug metabolism, for the most part, changes a drug to more water-soluble metabolites that are usually, but not necessarily, inactive. The term *detoxification* is not accurate, since the body can also form a toxic metabolite from a less toxic drug. For example, a normally minor intermediate step in acetaminophen metabolism is formation of a reactive compound that can damage hepatocytes. With usual doses the liver is protected from this metabolite because it is neutralized by a sulfhydryl group. Overdoses, however, can exhaust the sulfhydryl groups and thereby allow exposure of hepatocytes to the toxic metabolite that causes cell necrosis. Hence the morbidity and mortality of acetaminophen intoxication are attributable to hepatic failure. Thus treatment is logically aimed at replenishing thiol donors by administering *N*-acetylcysteine.

Another example of possible deleterious effects of the so-called detoxification process is the liver damage caused by carbon tetrachloride. The finding that newborn rats are relatively resistant to the toxic action of this drug,[1] together with observations that phenobarbital increases not only the metabolism of this halogenated hydrocarbon but also its toxicity, indicates that metabolism may be involved in its hepatotoxicity. It is believed that free radicals are formed from the interaction of some drugs and drug-metabolizing enzymes. The free radicals may be directly toxic, perhaps through an interaction with membrane phospholipids. They may also make endogenous proteins antigenic, thus accounting for some forms of drug allergy.

Drugs are usually metabolized at rates proportional to their plasma concentrations because at therapeutic levels their concentrations are not high enough to saturate drug-metabolizing enzymes. Conditions that lower the concentration of a drug at the site of metabolizing enzymes or that decrease the amount or activity of the enzymes would be expected to decrease clearance of the drug. Several of these factors are of great importance, whereas others may become significant only in particular diseases or in the presence of certain drug combinations. The following are some examples:

Factors that delay the metabolism of drugs

1. Reversible protein binding limits drug metabolism. Phenylbutazone, for example, is highly protein bound—up to 98% at therapeutic doses. If the dose is increased so that only 88% of the drug is protein bound, the free portion is metabolized much more rapidly. As a consequence, one gains little by increasing the dose.
2. Localization of the drug in the adipose tissue (thiopental) or in the liver (quinacrine) protects it against metabolic degradation.
3. Diseases of the liver and immaturity of drug-metabolizing enzymes during the neonatal period can interfere with the biotransformation of some drugs.
4. A drug may inhibit the metabolism of another drug and thus may prolong and intensify the effect of the latter.[5,6] This is why monoamine oxidase inhibitors can cause alarming reactions when tyramine-containing foods or beverages are ingested. Cimetidine, an antihistamine used to treat a variety of acid-peptic disorders, inhibits microsomal enzymes that metabolize a large number of drugs. Isoniazid is another potent inhibitor of drug-metabolizing enzymes. Co-administration of these and other drugs metabolized by the microsomal system can cause dramatic increases in serum drug concentrations and mandate dose adjustment.
5. With age, the capacity for drug metabolism in general decreases.[7] Hence the elderly usually require lower doses of medications.

When several drugs are used simultaneously in a patient, it is difficult to keep in mind their various pharmacodynamic interactions. An additional difficulty is that some drugs can induce the formation of microsomal drug-metabolizing enzymes, that is, a pharmacokinetic interaction. Some cases of tolerance to a drug may be caused by microsomal enzyme induction. There are well-authenticated cases in both experimental and clinical literature of such drug interactions.

ENZYME INDUCTION

Stimulation of drug
metabolism in
humans

The following examples of enhanced drug metabolism have been demonstrated in humans.

Phenobarbital stimulates the metabolism of phenytoin, griseofulvin, and dicumarol (Fig. 4-2). Barbiturates stimulate glucuronide conjugation of bilirubin in mice; this finding led to the use of phenobarbital in treatment of congenital nonhemolytic jaundice in infants. Administration of phenobarbital two or three times daily lowered the free serum bilirubin concentration in the infants. In addition, it improved the conjugation of salicylamide in the same infants, another example of glucuronide formation.

Phenytoin, meprobamate, and **carbamazepine** may induce tolerance to their own action by enzyme induction; that is, they stimulate their own metabolism (autoinduction). Smoking increases the metabolism of theophylline and most likely a variety of other drugs.[7]

One should also remember that inducers may promote the metabolism of certain hormones as well as that of drugs and foreign compounds. Oxidative drug-metabolizing enzymes hydroxylate such endogenous compounds as testosterone, estradiol, progesterone, and hydrocortisone.

**PHARMACO-
GENETICS**

The systematic study of pharmacogenetics is recent,[3] but several abnormal drug reactions in inherited diseases are well known. The drugs include barbiturates, which may precipitate attacks in congenital porphyria; salicylates, which are dangerous in persons whose glucuronyl transferase is congenitally absent (Crigler-Najjar syndrome); atropine, to which hypersensitivity occurs in patients suffering from Down's

FIG. 4-2 *Effect of phenobarbital on plasma levels of dicumarol and on prothrombin time in a human subject treated chronically with 75 mg/day of dicumarol.*

From Cucinell, S.A., Conney, A.H., Sansur, M., and Burns, J.J.: Clin. Pharmacol. Ther. 6:420, 1965.

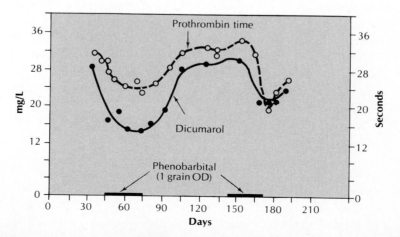

syndrome; epinephrine and glucagon, which fail to produce hyperglycemia in those who are deficient in glucose-6-phosphatase (von Gierke's disease).

A broad classification of pharmacogenetic abnormalities[3] would attribute most genetically conditioned anomalous drug responses to (1) receptor-site abnormalities, (2) drug-metabolism disorders, (3) tissue-metabolism disorders, and (4) anatomic abnormalities.

Although there are not many well-established examples of *receptor-site abnormalities*, they undoubtedly contribute to variation in drug responses. The resistance of some individuals to coumarin anticoagulants is probably an example. The best known examples of pharmacogenetics are provided by *drug-metabolism disorders*, in which abnormal blood concentrations of a drug can be measured after administration of a normal dose. In *tissue-metabolism disorders* an individual may show an adverse reaction at a normal blood concentration of a drug because of a special vulnerability caused by an abnormality in tissue metabolism. For example, in glucose-6-phosphate dehydrogenase (G-6-PD) deficiency a usual dose of primaquine may cause hemolytic anemia. Hemolytic anemia after ingestion of the bean *Vicia fava* and reactions to several other drugs have similarly been traced to a deficiency of G-6-PD. As discussed on p. 55, G-6-PD in the red blood cell is responsible for formation of NADPH, which is a cofactor for glutathione reductase. When there is a genetically determined deficiency of glucose-6-phosphate in the red cell, severe hemolytic episodes may be caused by administration of oxidant drugs. Finally, an *anatomic abnormality* may cause adverse drug reactions. For example, in a patient with hypertrophic subaortic stenosis, digitalis may cause fatal reactions.[3]

Schematic illustration of continuous *and* discontinuous *variation. When a standard dose of a drug is given to a large number of persons and a drug effect or metabolism is measured, the usual finding is a normal frequency distribution as in* **A**. *On the other hand, a discontinuous variation, as exemplified by the bimodal distribution shown in* **B**, *may indicate a genetically determined abnormality in drug action or metabolism.*   *FIG. 4-3*

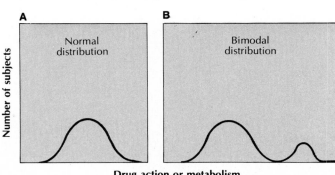

Drug action or metabolism

Continuous and discontinuous variation

It is generally recognized that the response to a drug in a population shows *continuous variation*. The LD_{50} or ED_{50} (pp. 39 and 40) and the rate of destruction of a drug in the body generally show a normal distribution in a population, as shown in Fig. 4-3, *A*. Some of the important discoveries in pharmacogenetics have occurred when the response to some drug or the metabolism of a drug indicated a *discontinuous variation*, as shown in Fig. 4-3, *B*. Follow-up study of such a bimodal distribution often reveals a genetic basis and provides an explanation for unusual responses to drugs.

REFERENCES

1. Anders, M.W.: Enhancement and inhibition of drug metabolism, Annu. Rev. Pharmacol. **11**:37, 1971.
2. Gelehrter, T.D.: Enzyme induction, N. Engl. J. Med. **294**:589, 1976.
3. La Du, B.N., Jr.: The genetics of drug reactions, Hosp. Pract. **6**:97, June 1971.
4. La Du, B.N., Mandel, H.G., and Way, E.L.: Fundamentals of drug metabolism and drug disposition, Baltimore, 1971, The Williams & Wilkins Co.
5. Sedman, A.J.: Cimetidine-drug interactions, Am. J. Med. **76**:109, 1984.
6. Vasko, M.R., and Brater, D.C.: Drug-drug interactions. In Chernow, B., and Lake, C.R., editors: The pharmacologic approach to the critically ill patient, Baltimore, 1983, The Williams & Wilkins Co., p. 22.
7. Vestal, R.E., and Wood, A.J.J.: Influence of age and smoking on drug kinetics in man: studies using model compounds, Clin. Pharmacokinet. **5**:309, 1980.

Chapter 5

Drug safety and effectiveness

With the large number of effective and potent drugs and with recognition of their complex effects and interactions with each other, it is necessary for the physician to have a high level of awareness and considerable knowledge of drug actions, toxicity, and interactions.

Since the most extensive studies on drug action are usually carried out with the development of *new* drugs, this subject is discussed in some detail along with factors that modify drug safety and effectiveness.

New drugs originate from many different sources. Accidental observations with natural products, unexpected clinical observations with the use of known compounds, physiologic or biochemical investigations, and basic pharmacologic experiments have provided leads for therapeutic discoveries. However, today most new drugs are discovered by screening. Large numbers of natural products or synthetic compounds are tested for a variety of possible biologic activities. A highly effective drug that seems safe enough in preliminary testing is then carried through the following series of steps:

DEVELOPMENT OF A NEW DRUG

1. Animal studies
   a. Acute, subacute, and chronic toxicity
   b. Therapeutic index
   c. Pharmacokinetics and metabolic pathways
2. Human studies
   a. Phase 1: preliminary pharmacologic evaluation
   b. Phase 2: controlled clinical evaluation
   c. Phase 3: extended clinical evaluation
   d. Phase 4: postmarketing surveillance for some drugs

The most common measure of acute toxicity is the median lethal dose (LD_{50}), that is, the dose that is lethal to 50% of the animals tested. The LD_{50} is determined when various doses of a drug are given to groups of animals. Ordinarily only a single dose is given to each animal. The percentage of animals dying in each group is plotted against the dose. From this curve the dose that kills 50% of the animals is estimated. This particular dose-mortality figure is chosen because it can be determined more precisely; the curve approximates a straight line at the LD_{50}. It should be obvious

Animal studies
ACUTE, SUBACUTE, AND
CHRONIC TOXICITY

that the LD_{50} of any drug is of interest only to experimental pharmacologists, not to clinicians.

Customarily, at least three different species are used for acute toxicity determinations, and observations are made not only on the LD_{50} but also on the types of toxic symptoms that the animals develop.

In subacute toxicity studies the mode of administration and the dosage depend on the proposed clinical trial. Usually the drug is administered orally. Several doses are used, some within the range of the estimated human dose and others that produce toxic manifestations. Careful observations include a variety of laboratory studies such as hematologic examinations, renal and hepatic function tests, and many others.

The chronic toxicity studies are of long duration. They may last many months and may be extended through several generations to detect the possible teratogenic effects of a drug. Again several species are used because some species are more suitable than others for the demonstration of adverse effects. At various intervals selected animals are killed, and thorough pathologic examinations are performed.

THERAPEUTIC INDEX The LD_{50} of a drug is not nearly so important as its therapeutic index, or therapeutic ratio. This concept in *animal experiments* refers to the ratio of the LD_{50} to the median effective dose (ED_{50}), as illustrated in Fig. 5-1.

$$\text{Therapeutic index} = \frac{LD_{50}}{ED_{50}}$$

In clinical medicine the therapeutic index based on median lethal doses has no use. Sometimes the ratio of a toxic dose to the effective dose is used. Even in animal

FIG. 5-1 *Illustrating concept of therapeutic index (TI).*

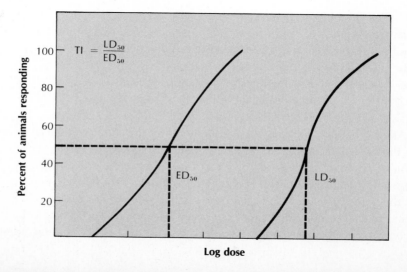

experiments, the ratio of LD_1/ED_{100} (the dose lethal to 1% over the dose effective in all) would give a better idea of safety, but it has no particular application. The concept of effectiveness in relation to toxicity (margin of safety) is more important than any specific ratio. A physician may not be interested in the number of milligrams of a drug that will produce toxic effects but, indeed, is greatly interested in knowing how far the usual therapeutic dose can be exceeded before adverse effects are likely to be encountered.

Animal studies provide a general profile of the toxicity, pharmacologic activity, and pharmacokinetics of a new drug. Even with this information, the initiation of clinical studies is risky. There are numerous examples of drugs that passed all the preclinical criteria for safety but caused serious adverse effects in humans. The lack of correlation often seen between toxicity data in animals and adverse effects in humans is well known. Not only is there great species variation in toxicity, an example of comparative pharmacology, but also many adverse effects simply cannot be ascertained in animals. Zbinden[8] has claimed that of the 45 most frequent drug-related symptoms observed in 11,000 patients treated with 77 different drugs or drug combinations, at least half would probably not be recognized in animal experiments. Such symptoms include drowsiness, nausea, dizziness, nervousness, epigastric distress, headache, weakness, insomnia, fatigue, tinnitus, heartburn, skin rash, depression, dermatitis, increased energy, vertigo, lethargy, nocturia, abdominal distention, flatulence, stiffness, and even urticaria.

Because of these discrepancies between animal data and human responses, initial clinical studies on any drug must be undertaken with great care, with the methodology meticulously planned and with special attention to *relevance* (pertinence of data), *representativeness* (selection of material to eliminate bias) and *reliability* (repeatability of results). A *new drug application* (NDA) must be filed before any clinical evaluation is initiated.

HUMAN STUDIES: CLINICAL PHARMACOLOGY

Very small doses of the drug are administered to human volunteers to obtain a preliminary estimate of its safety. With increasing doses, an attempt is made to extend to humans the results previously demonstrated in animals. In most instances it is essential to determine blood concentrations of the new drug. Otherwise the investigator cannot tell whether lack of effectiveness is a consequence of lack of absorption or of rapid metabolism or excretion.

Ethical aspects of human experimentation have been the subject of much discussion in recent years and will not be considered in detail here. The important points, however, are that the volunteer must be truly a volunteer (that is, not subjected to coercion and able to give informed consent) and that the investigator must be competent.

Phase 1: preliminary pharmacologic evaluation

Whereas the phase 1 studies are usually performed by one or two clinical investigators, in phase 2 a larger number of investigators obtain as much information

Phase 2: controlled clinical evaluation

as possible about the safety and efficacy of the new drug in blind or double-blind studies. Adverse effects must be reported promptly to the sponsoring company and to the Food and Drug Administration (FDA), and specific studies are sometimes initiated to ascertain the significance of any unexpected findings.

Phase 3: extended clinical evaluation	As many as 50 to 100 physicians may participate in large-scale clinical trials of a new drug, many of them performing the same study. The investigators must not only be competent clinicians but must also have experience and training in the field of drug evaluation. Assuming that the phase 3 studies demonstrate to the satisfaction of the FDA that the drug is safe and effective, the investigational drug may be approved for distribution and use.
Phase 4: postmarketing surveillance	It would seem that with all these safeguards approval of a drug by the FDA would be free of hazard. Unfortunately, there are many unusual side effects, idiosyncrasies, and allergies that are observed only after extensive use by large numbers of patients. As a result, some drugs now undergo postmarketing surveillance in which data concerning efficacy and toxicity are systematically gathered after the drug has been marketed. In this manner effects can be assessed from a much larger data base in terms of patient exposure. It is hoped that this approach will allow early detection of adverse effects that were not detected in studies of fewer patients over shorter periods of time.
FACTORS INFLU-ENCING THE SAFETY AND EFFECTIVENESS OF DRUGS *Biologic variation*	Experimental studies in animals show that the dose of a drug that will give an all-or-nothing response (such as death of the animal) varies considerably. Fig. 5-2 illustrates the gaussian distribution of susceptibility, which can be demonstrated easily in animals. The biologic variation in drug effect is an important reason dosage must be individualized and treatment adjusted to the requirements of a given patient.
Hypersusceptibility	Because of biologic variation, disease, or the presence of another medication, some persons may show a much greater than normal response to an ordinary dose of a drug. For example, a thyrotoxic patient may have an exaggerated cardiovascular response to injected epinephrine. Such patients are at the sensitive end of a gaussian frequency-distribution curve, and their responses are quantitatively greater than in normal persons. A patient with subclinical asthma may evidence symptoms of bronchial constriction from doses of histamine or β-adrenergic antagonists that are innocuous in normal persons. Hypersusceptibility is sometimes referred to as *drug intolerance*.
Drug idiosyncrasy and drug allergy	The term *idiosyncrasy* has been used rather vaguely in medicine to apply to drug reactions that are *qualitatively* different from the effects obtained in the majority of patients and that cannot be attributed to drug allergy. Occasionally extreme susceptibility of an individual to an expected pharmacologic action of a drug has also been

Biologic variation in susceptibility to drugs. FIG. 5-2

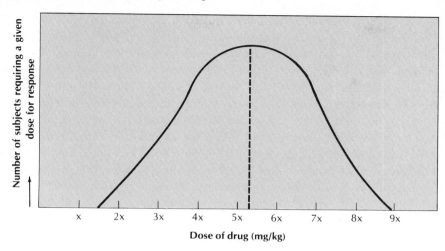

With increasing knowledge of pharmacogenetics, many drug idiosyncrasies have been found to be genetically determined enzymatic deficiencies. Such deficiencies can interfere with the metabolic degradation of a drug, as in prolonged apnea caused by succinylcholine, or they may make certain cells more vulnerable to an adverse action of a drug, as is the case in drug-induced hemolytic anemia in patients whose red cells are deficient in glucose-6-phosphate dehydrogenase.

Drug allergy is a response to a drug that results from a previous sensitizing exposure and is mediated by an immunologic mechanism. It differs from drug toxicity in a number of respects: (1) The reaction occurs in only a fraction of the population. (2) Its dose response is unusual in that a minute amount of an otherwise safe drug can elicit a severe reaction. (3) The manifestations of the reaction are different from the usual pharmacologic effects of the drug. (4) There is a primary sensitizing period before the individual responds with the unusual reaction. (5) When the sensitizing drug is a protein or a compound that forms covalent bonds with proteins, circulating antibodies may be demonstrated in sensitized individuals, and skin tests, though hazardous, may show a positive reaction to the offending drug.

In most drug allergies, the complete antigen is not known nor is the form in which the drug acts as a hapten. For example, a patient may react to ingestion of a sulfonamide by developing a skin rash and still show no reaction to the same drug injected intracutaneously. This is generally true for drugs of small molecular weight and the *immediate* type of allergies elicited by them. In *contact dermatitis*, on the other hand, positive skin tests are regularly obtained.

The terms *immediate* and *delayed reactions* originated from observations of the rapidity with which the positive skin test to allergens becomes manifest. Thus in anaphylactic hypersensitivity, skin-test results are immediate; in delayed reactions,

IMMEDIATE AND DELAYED

DRUG ALLERGIES

in the skin where the antigen was injected. In addition, there are profound differences in the immunologic bases of the two types of hypersensitivities. Circulating antibodies are believed to be important in immediate but not in delayed hypersensitivities. The latter can be transferred to normal individuals only by means of sensitized cells.

Among the many types of drug allergies, some are considered immediate, others are delayed, and still others are not classifiable at present. *Anaphylaxis, urticaria, angioneurotic edema, drug fever,* and *asthma* clearly belong in the category of immediate reactions. *Serum sickness* reactions are characterized by a delay in their appearance. This same delay is observed after the first administration of a foreign serum. Once sensitized, however, an individual often reacts rapidly to the same drug. For example, methyldopa may be taken daily by an individual for 1 to 2 weeks before fever and joint pain develop. The subsequent administration of a small dose of the drug will produce the same reaction in a matter of hours. *Contact dermatitis* is undoubtedly a delayed allergy. Many other cutaneous reactions and *some* severe hematologic disturbances elicited by drugs probably also belong in the delayed category.

Age and weight of patient

In experimental investigations, drugs are administered on the basis of a certain number of milligrams per kilogram of body weight, since the volume of distribution of a drug often is roughly a function of body mass. For the same reason the weight of the patient should be taken into consideration when a dose is calculated. Certain formulas allow adjustment of dosage according to weight. For example, Clark's rule is as follows:

$$\text{Dose for child} = \text{Adult dose} \times \frac{\text{Weight of child in pounds}}{150}$$

It is assumed in this formula that a child needs a smaller dose because the weight is less, but this is only an approximation. It has been pointed out that the child is not simply a "small adult" and that reactions to drugs in children may result from problems in growth and development rather than size.[5] Catastrophes have resulted from routine adaptation of adult dosages for children. The gray-baby syndrome caused by chloramphenicol, kernicterus by vitamin K, and blindness by the use of oxygen in premature infants are examples of special problems of drug use in pediatrics.

DOSE FOR CHILDREN BASED ON SURFACE AREA

The dose of a drug for children is proportional to weight to the 0.7 power.[2] Since body surface is similarly related to body weight, it has been suggested that pediatric dosages should be calculated on the basis of surface area of the body in square meters (m^2). Tables relating the weight of a child in pounds to surface area in square meters and approximate percentage of adult dose are available. These are based on a surface area in adults of 1.73 m^2. Thus a 22-pound child having a surface area of 0.46 m^2 should receive 27% of the adult dose. Another child weighing 121 pounds with a surface area of 1.58 m^2 would receive 91% of the adult dose.

Pathologic processes can influence susceptibility to drugs. In some instances this can be explained by disease-induced changes in drug elimination, but in other cases the explanation may be obscure.

Disease processes influencing susceptibility

It is obvious that in severe renal disease one must use with caution those drugs that depend on the kidney for excretion.[3] For example, if the dose of digoxin is not adjusted in patients with renal insufficiency, fatal toxicity can occur. In severe liver disease, similar care must be exercised in the use of drugs that are normally inactivated by hepatic processes.[6,7]

When more than one drug is given to the same patient, their actions may be completely independent of one another. Often, however, the combined effect may be greater than that which could have been obtained with a single drug; on the other hand, a drug may have less effect than if it were given alone (see Chapter 63).

Presence of other drugs

When the combined effect of two drugs is the algebraic sum of the individual actions, it is sometimes referred to as *summation* or an *additive effect*. However, a better way to consider additivity is in terms of doses rather than effects. If a certain dose of drug A and a certain dose of drug B produce the same effect quantitatively (that is, are *equieffective*), the drugs are considered additive if half of each of these doses used simultaneously elicits the same effect as the full dose of either drug alone. *Synergism* is defined in various ways. Although more precisely it means a greater than additive effect, to some it implies additivity. Some reserve the term for cases in which one drug increases the potency of another by interfering with its destruction or disposition, thus increasing the effect of a given dose. *Potentiation* is a better term for the latter case in which a drug that appears to have no action when given alone increases the potency of the second drug. Since each of these terms is interpreted differently by different people, one should ask for clarification if the meaning is not specified.

ADDITIVE EFFECT, SYNERGISM, AND POTENTIATION

Drug antagonism may be of several types: chemical, physiologic, pharmacologic, and pharmacokinetic.

ANTAGONISM

Chemical antagonism. A drug may actually combine with another in the body. This is the basis of action of chemical antidotes. For example, dimercaprol (British antilewisite, BAL) can combine with mercury, lead, or arsenic in the body.

Physiologic antagonism. Two drugs may influence a physiologic system in opposite directions, one drug canceling the effect of another. The simultaneous injection of properly adjusted doses of vasodilator and vasoconstrictor drugs may cause no change in blood pressure. Similarly, stimulants and depressants of the central nervous system can antagonize each other.

Pharmacologic antagonism. Two drugs may bind reversibly or irreversibly to the same receptor site; the inactive or weaker member of the pair inhibits access of the potent drug (see Chapter 2). Examples of pharmacologic antagonism are the histamine–antihistaminic drug relationships and also atropine-acetylcholine antagonism.

Pharmacokinetic antagonism. One drug may reduce the potency of another drug by mechanisms enumerated below.

COMPLEX DRUG INTERACTIONS IN CLINICAL PHARMACOLOGY

In addition to the large variety of pharmacodynamic interactions that can occur as noted above, one drug may also interact with another by several pharmacokinetic mechanisms. These include (1) altered absorption from the gastrointestinal tract,[1,4] (2) reduced binding to plasma proteins, (3) altered renal excretion,[3] (4) inhibition of metabolic degradation, and (5) promotion of metabolic degradation by enzyme induction. Potentiation or antagonism can result from such interactions, and they have acquired such importance in clinical pharmacology that the problem is discussed in detail in Chapter 63. Examples of pharmacokinetic antagonism include the binding of tetracycline to milk products or antacids precluding absorption,[1,4] enhanced metabolism of a number of drugs by phenobarbital or rifampin and increased renal excretion of weakly acidic compounds in an alkaline urine.

Cumulation, tolerance, and tachyphylaxis

Response to dosage can be greatly influenced by certain special features of drug metabolism such as cumulation, tolerance, and tachyphylaxis.

CUMULATION

Most drugs are eliminated from the body by a first-order reaction. This means that a constant fraction of the drug in the body is eliminated per unit of time. It also means that it takes 4 half-lives to eliminate 94% of the drug. If the drug is administered repeatedly and frequently in relation to its half-life, it will accumulate in the body. Eventually, however, a *plateau* is reached when elimination equals the amount of drug being administered. Digitoxin is a good example of a drug having a long half-life (7 days), leading to cumulation when administered daily.

When one is dealing with drugs that accumulate, the dosage will vary greatly, depending on whether loading or maintenance doses are administered. The former must be large enough to reach a therapeutically effective level in the body, whereas maintenance doses are adjusted to match daily metabolic and excretory rates.

TOLERANCE

Tolerance is an interesting phenomenon characterized by the need for increasing amounts of a drug to obtain the same therapeutic effect. Drugs vary greatly in their tendency to induce tolerance; perhaps the best-known examples are the opium alkaloids. The adult therapeutic dose of morphine is ordinarily about 10 mg, but if the drug is administered repeatedly to a patient, increasing doses are necessary to obtain the same analgesic effect. Finally, enormous doses are used by an addict who has developed pronounced tolerance. Although it is a well-studied phenomenon, the actual mechanisms of tolerance remain mysterious.

Tachyphylaxis is a term reserved for rapidly developing tolerance. This is noted in laboratory experiments with certain drugs, for example, vasopressin, nitrates, or certain adrenergic compounds such as amphetamine. In these experiments the first injection of vasopressin or amphetamine produces a much greater elevation of blood pressure than subsequent injections given after only a brief interval. *TACHYPHYLAXIS*

The mechanism of tachyphylaxis is understood only in some cases. Indirectly acting sympathomimetic amines such as amphetamine release norepinephrine from adrenergic nerve endings. Tachyphylaxis probably is a consequence of depletion of available norepinephrine. The same mechanism plays a role in tachyphylaxis to histamine releasers. In other instances the action of a drug may persist at the receptor site, but its overt manifestations are concealed by compensatory reflexes or by desensitization of the receptor.

Drug effects are greatly influenced by genetically determined variations in susceptibility. Idiosyncrasies in some cases are related to pharmacogenetic abnormalities. This subject is discussed in detail in Chapter 6. *Pharmacogenetics*

REFERENCES

1. Azarnoff, D.L., and Huffman, D.H.: Therapeutic implications of bioavailability, Annu. Rev. Pharmacol. Toxicol. **16**:53, 1976.
2. Done, A.K.: Drugs for children, In Modell, W., editor: Drugs of choice 1972-1973, St. Louis, 1972, The C.V. Mosby Co.
3. Fabre, J., Fox, H.M., Dayer, P., and Balant, L.: Differences in kinetic properties of drugs: implications as to the selection of a particular drug for use in patients with renal failure with special emphasis on antibiotics and β-adrenoceptor blocking agents, Clin. Pharmacokinet. **5**:441, 1980.
4. Koch-Weser, J.: Bioavailability of drugs, N. Engl. J. Med. **291**:233 and 503, 1974.
5. Shirkey, H.C., and Ericson, A.J.: Adverse reactions to drugs—their relation to growth and development, In Shirkey, H.C., editor: Pediatric therapy, ed. 6, St. Louis, 1980, The C.V. Mosby Co.
6. Williams, R.L.: Drug administration in hepatic disease, N. Engl. J. Med. **309**:1616, 1983.
7. Williams, R.L., and Mamelok, R.D.: Hepatic disease and drug pharmacokinetics, Clin. Pharmacokinet. **5**:528, 1980.
8. Zbinden, G.: Animal toxicity studies: a critical evaluation, Appl. Ther. **8**:128, 1966.

Chapter 6

Pharmacogenetics: the individual response to drugs

VARIABILITY IN DRUG RESPONSE

A perplexing problem for both pharmacologists and physicians is the variation that occurs among normal subjects as well as among patients in response to a particular drug. This interindividual variability necessitates a correspondingly wide range of doses among patients. Differences in clearance of a drug among individuals can range from fourfold to fortyfold. The clinical consequences of concomitant differences in dose requirement cannot be overemphasized.

Drug elimination rates and drug toxicity

Every physician learns to take into account variations among patients in rates of drug elimination by individualizing the dose of certain drugs, particularly drugs with narrow margins of safety. If the dose of such a drug is not individualized, a given dose administered by the same route may produce toxicity in some patients, the desired pharmacologic effect in other patients, and no effect in still others. In contrast, with some drugs a beneficial effect occurs at doses much lower than those that cause toxicity; hence the physician has less concern about administering relatively large doses to ensure efficacy. A similar strategy with a drug having a narrow margin of safety is impossible because the cost would be a high incidence of adverse effects.

Determining causes of variations in drug elimination rates

The frequency at which adverse drug reactions occur demonstrates the need to understand the causes of differences among patients in drug response. Understanding the mechanisms should lead to safer use of drugs. Many adverse reactions probably arise from failure to tailor the dosage of drugs to widely different individual needs.

PHARMACOGENETICS

Pharmacogenetics deals with genetically caused variations in drug response. Some pharmacogenetic conditions in humans that affect either drug metabolism or the interaction of drugs at different sites (including receptor sites) are listed in Table 6-1. Pharmacogenetic conditions transmitted by genes at a single locus are divided for convenience into those that affect drug pharmacokinetics and those that affect pharmacodynamics.

In pharmacogenetics the ultimate goal is the ability to screen populations by a simple, rapid, safe test to ascertain how a particular trait is inherited, its incidence in a given group, and differences in frequency among various patient populations.

In pharmacogenetic studies the plasma half-life or clearance of a drug has been conveniently employed as the principal test of gene structure and function. However, such measurements may not be a sensitive enough index of variations in genes that control proteins that are directly involved in the disposition of certain drugs.

Several types of curve can be generated when a dose of drug is given to a large population of normal subjects and a specific quantitative response to the drug is measured and plotted. The three most common shapes of this distribution curve are *unimodal, bimodal,* and *trimodal.* For most drugs, when a population is tested, a unimodal, gaussian distribution curve of drug response is obtained. This curve can arise from purely environmental differences, such as a dose-related effect of smoking on the metabolism of a certain drug. In addition, genetic differences in which genes at multiple loci contribute to the variation may be responsible. This

DISTRIBUTION CURVES OF DRUG RESPONSE

TABLE 6-1   Genetic conditions, probably transmitted as single factors, that alter drug response

Condition	Aberrant enzyme and location	Mode of inheritance*	Agent provoking response
Altering the way the body acts on drugs			
Acatalasia	Catalase in erythrocytes	AR	Hydrogen peroxide
Succinylcholine sensitivity or atypical cholinesterase	Cholinesterase in plasma	AR	Succinylcholine
Slow inactivation of isoniazid	Isoniazid acetylase in liver	AR	Isoniazid, dapsone, hydralazine, phenelzine, procainamide, sulfamethazine
Phenacetin-induced methemoglobinemia	?Mixed-function oxidase in liver microsomes that de-ethylates phenacetin	AR	Phenacetin
Deficient N-glucosidation of amobarbital	?Mixed-function oxidase in liver microsomes that N-glucosidates amobarbital	AR	Amobarbital
Polymorphic hydroxylation of debrisoquin	Mixed-function oxidase in liver microsomes that 4-hydroxylates debrisoquin	AR	Debrisoquin, amitriptyline, encainide, mephenytoin, mephobarbital, metoprolol, nortriptyline, perhexiline, propranolol, timolol
Altering the way drugs act on the body			
Warfarin resistance	?Altered receptor or enzyme in liver with increased affinity for vitamin K	AD	Warfarin
Inability to taste phenylthiourea or phenylthiocarbamide	Unknown	AR	Drugs containing N—C—S group such as phenyl-, methyl-, and propylthiourea
Glucose-6-phosphate dehydrogenase deficiency, favism, or drug-induced hemolytic anemia	Glucose-6-phosphate dehydrogenase	XL incomplete codominant	Various analgesics (aspirin, aminopyrine, antipyrine, phenacetin); sulfones and sulfonamides (sulfisoxazole); antimalarials (primaquine, quinacrine); nonsulfonamide antibacterial agents (furazolidone, nitrofurantoin, chloramphenicol, *p*-aminosalicylic acid); miscellaneous agents (dimercaprol, probenecid, quinidine, quinine, vitamin K)

*AR, Autosomal recessive; AD, autosomal dominant; XL, X linked.

latter type of control is called *polygenic*. Polygenic control, for example, is at least partially involved in regulation of such traits as blood pressure, intelligence, and intensity of skin color. Bimodal or trimodal curves of drug response are usually produced by monogenically controlled conditions, such as those listed in Table 6-1, but can also arise from environmental differences; for example, one mode representing metabolism of theophylline by normal persons and another mode representing subjects receiving an inhibitor of theophylline metabolism like cimetidine.

FIG. 6-1   *Plasma half-lives of bishydroxycoumarin and antipyrine were measured separately at an interval of more than 6 months in healthy monozygotic (identical) and dizygotic (fraternal) twins. Values for each set of twins for each drug are joined by a solid line. Notice that intratwin differences in plasma half-life of both bishydroxycoumarin and antipyrine are smaller (as indicated by a shorter line joining the circles) in monozygotic than in dizygotic twins.*

Based on data from Vesell, E.S., and Page, J.G.: J. Clin. Invest. **47**:2657, 1968; and Vesell, E.S., and Page, J.G.: Science **161**:72, 1968.

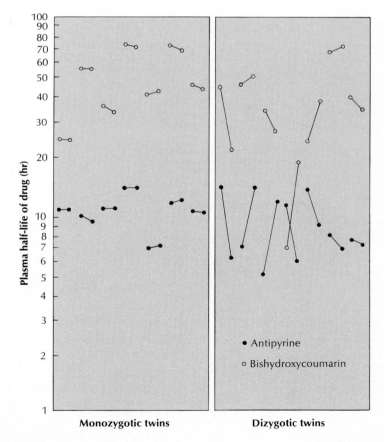

The second critical step in exploring pharmacogenetics is to perform family studies on individuals located at the extremes of the distribution curve. Individuals at the extremes are most likely to exhibit a sufficiently distinctive response to drugs to permit clear-cut identification and tracing through several generations. By determining whether this particular type of drug response is in fact transmitted through several generations in conformity to mendelian laws for inheritance of dominant and recessive traits, investigators can tell whether a genetic mechanism controls the variation in drug response observed in the population. Furthermore, the specific kind of genetic control (autosomal dominant or recessive; X-linked dominant or recessive) can be discovered.

Studies with twins have demonstrated that fivefold to tenfold interindividual variations in disposition of antipyrine, phenylbutazone, and bishydroxycoumarin are genetically controlled (Fig. 6-1). For these purposes, twins may be considered representative of partial family units, since monozygotic twins are identical with respect to all their genes, whereas dizygotic twins have approximately 50% of their genes in common, just as do any siblings. Genetic factors controlling interindividual variations in rates of drug elimination proved, unlike most conditions listed in Table 6-1, to occur commonly and to involve several drugs.

Although precise genetic mechanisms responsible for variations in hepatic metabolism of drugs have not yet been firmly established, techniques to measure the major metabolites of many drugs are now being used in family studies that should provide definitive answers to this important question.[4]

PHARMACOGE-NETIC DIFFER-ENCES IN ELIMI-NATION RATES OF COMMONLY USED DRUGS

Disease states, other drugs, diet, smoking, and other environmental factors (see Chapters 7 to 9 and 63) also can alter rates of drug elimination in patients. Their relative roles in influencing rates of metabolism can change even in the same subject with time. Hence it is difficult to identify the specific contribution of each factor to total drug-metabolizing capacity in a person. For these reasons, the role of single factors is generally investigated separately in normal, nonmedicated volunteer subjects in a near basal state with respect to most of the variables known to alter hepatic drug-metabolizing capacity.[10] Measurements with a test drug (such as antipyrine) are performed to quantify this basal capacity in each volunteer subject; a single environmental alteration is then introduced, during which the subject's drug-metabolizing activity is remeasured; and the change from basal values is taken to quantitate the effect exerted by the single environmental perturbation. This approach clearly has limitations, since results cannot always be extrapolated with accuracy to other drugs. On the other hand, environmental factors that alter the disposition of other drugs may not always alter pharmacokinetics of the test compound.

GENETIC AND ENVIRONMENTAL CAUSES OF VARIATIONS IN DRUG RESPONSE

PHARMACOGENET-IC CONDITIONS (SINGLE-LOCUS TRANSMISSION) THAT ALTER DRUG METABOLISM

In several pharmacogenetic conditions an enzyme controlling the metabolism of a drug has been identified. Mutations decrease the ability to metabolize the drug so that it accumulates, causing toxicity. Thus one can identify the condition by measuring decreased clearance of the parent compound or decreased appearance of a metabolite or by documenting a greatly increased concentration of parent drug relative to metabolite. If persons possessing such genetic abnormalities can be identified *before* they receive the drug, one can avoid toxicity by not giving the drug or by giving a much reduced dose. For these reasons, familiarity with pharmacogenetic conditions can help physicians administer drugs more safely and can reduce the incidence of drug toxicity.

Acatalasia

The condition acatalasia was discovered in a patient during application of hydrogen peroxide to the gums to sterilize a wound after surgery.[9] Instead of bubbles of oxygen forming by the action of the enzyme catalase as occurs in normal persons, the peroxide remained unchanged and caused toxicity by denaturing tissue proteins. The patient lacked catalase in her oral mucosa and erythrocytes, as did three of her five siblings. The parents were second cousins—consanguinity is a risk factor for autosomal recessive inheritance, the mode of transmission of acatalasia. The incidence of this condition reaches 1% in certain regions of Japan, and the deficiency also occurs in Switzerland. Only sporadic cases have been reported in the United States. An impressive lesson from the discovery of acatalasia is that an observant clinician (in this case, the Japanese oral surgeon Takahara[10]) made an important contribution by being alert to the possibility that genetic differences can cause unusual reactions to drugs. Takahara postulated that his patient responded inappropriately to the peroxide because she lacked the normal form of the enzyme required to eliminate the drug. He proved his theory to be correct by gathering similar cases from 27 Japanese families.

Atypical plasma cholinesterase

Another example of a pharmacogenetic lesion that can produce drug toxicity is that of atypical plasma cholinesterase. Individuals homozygous for the mutant gene cannot adequately hydrolyze succinylcholine, a compound administered during anesthesia to produce muscle relaxation. Normally, succinylcholine is rapidly metabolized by plasma cholinesterase. However, in homozygous patients the drug remains active in the body for much longer periods than usual. Succinylcholine can then produce prolonged respiratory failure and, if mechanical respiration is not available, death. When succinylcholine was introduced in 1952 and administered widely in England as a preanesthetic agent, several deaths occurred in persons who had inherited from each parent a mutant gene at the cholinesterase locus. Although 1 in 25 persons is a heterozygote, homozygotes occur only once among 2500 persons.

Studies on the plasma cholinesterase activity of affected persons, their families, and normal persons showed considerable overlap until a refinement in technique utilizing the "dibucaine number" was introduced. This number represents the percent inhibition of plasma cholinesterase by the local anesthetic dibucaine. The dibucaine numbers of 135 individuals of seven unrelated families gave a trimodal curve with no overlap. It has been postulated that plasma cholinesterase activity is determined by two genes (alleles) at a single locus, one responsible for the *usual* and the other for the *atypical* form of the enzyme. Most persons, with a dibucaine number of about 80, have two of the usual alleles. Persons of the atypical phenotype, with dibucaine numbers of about 22, have two atypical genes. Finally, an intermediate group, with dibucaine numbers of about 62, may have one of each allele.

Isoniazid is used to treat tuberculosis. Persons with the genetically transmitted trait of fast acetylation of isoniazid may not be adequately treated on a fixed low dose because of rapid biotransformation. By contrast, slow acetylators receiving a normal dose may develop toxic effects. Isoniazid-induced polyneuritis—pain and tingling and possibly muscular weakness in the upper and lower extremities—occurs more frequently in slow than in rapid acetylators of isoniazid.[1] Fortunately, the neuritis can be effectively treated with vitamin B_6 (pyridoxine).

Genetic differences in rates of acetylation of isoniazid, hydralazine, procainamide, and other drugs

Isoniazid is metabolized by a liver acetylase. Approximately 50% of the population in the United States are slow acetylators, being homozygous for a recessive form of the gene at this locus. Fast acetylators are either heterozygous or homozygous for the dominant allele. Like several other genetically controlled variations in humans, this hereditary variation in acetylation exhibits pronounced geographic differences in gene frequency. For example, slow inactivation is uncommon in Eskimos, 95% of whom are rapid acetylators, and only slightly more common in Japanese, 90% of whom are rapid acetylators. In Latin America, approximately 67% of the population are rapid acetylators.

Isoniazid is also an example of how toxicity can develop not only from drug accumulation but also from the metabolites themselves. For example, rapid acetylators of isoniazid are more liable than slow acetylators to develop hepatitis after chronic isoniazid administration; presumably a metabolite is the offending agent. Thus all metabolites cannot be considered innocuous.

Fast and slow acetylation also occurs for several other drugs, including certain sulfonamides, the antihypertensive drug hydralazine, the antiarrhythmic procainamide and the antidepressant phenelzine. Continued administration of high doses of hydralazine in slow, but not fast, acetylators can lead to severe toxicity in the form of a lupus erythematosus–like syndrome. However, several other drugs metabolized by acetylation, such as the antitubercular drug *p*-aminosalicylic acid, do not show this difference in metabolic rate; a different enzyme must acetylate these drugs.

Severe methemoglobinemia and hemolysis occurred in a 17-year-old girl after ingesting the analgesic phenacetin. As much as one half of the patient's hemoglobin was occasionally in the form of methemoglobin. After administration of phenacetin, large amounts of the 2-hydroxyphenetidin metabolite and its conjugates appeared in her urine. In normal persons more than 70% of a single 2 g dose of phenacetin can be accounted for in the urine as acetaminophen, with only minute amounts of the hydroxylated product that predominated in this patient's urine. One sister, a brother,

Phenacetin-induced methemoglobinemia

and both parents of the patient had a normal response to phenacetin, but another sister responded abnormally. These facts indicated a probable autosomal recessive mode of inheritance of a defect in which the patient's hepatic drug-metabolizing enzymes were deficient in de-ethylating capacity. In this patient and her sister, toxicity after phenacetin administration was probably caused by the abnormal hydroxylated products, since induction of hepatic phenacetin-hydroxylating enzymes by phenobarbital exacerbated the condition. In contrast, in a normal volunteer, phenacetin administration after the same pretreatment with phenobarbital failed to elicit the syndrome.

Deficient N-glucosidation of amobarbital

A twin study suggested that large interindividual variations in elimination rates of amobarbital were under genetic control.[2] Pursuing their initial observations, Kalow and associates investigated the family of one set of twins with a deficiency in N-hydroxylation, but not C-hydroxylation, of amobarbital.[4] The family study of these twins disclosed that this deficiency probably arose from autosomal recessive transmission of a mutant gene.

Polymorphic hydroxylation of debrisoquin

The antihypertensive drug debrisoquin is used in England but not in the United States. It was observed that patients receiving debrisoquin vary widely in their hypotensive responses to the adrenergic-blocking action of the drug and that there is a close correlation between debrisoquin plasma concentration and the resultant decline in blood pressure.[8] In 94 unrelated volunteers the urinary ratio of the parent drug to the primary metabolite, 4-hydroxydebrisoquin, was measured after a single oral dose of 10 mg of debrisoquin.[6] In three of these 94 subjects the ratio was very high, suggestive of a deficiency of the hepatic cytochrome P-450–dependent monooxygenase that 4-hydroxylates debrisoquin. Furthermore, family studies of these three volunteers suggested transmission of the metabolic deficiency as an autosomal recessive trait.[6] Most side effects as well as the most pronounced antihypertensive activity of debrisoquin occurred in these slow metabolizers.

Another fundamental pharmacogenetic principle is underscored by the work of the British group on the control of debrisoquin metabolism and by the previously described example of genetic differences in isoniazid metabolism. When a genetically controlled variation is discovered in the disposition of a particular drug, a search should be undertaken to determine if disposition of structurally related drugs is similarly affected by the same genes. The British group and others have reported that metabolism of a number of agents in addition to debrisoquin is regulated by this same genetic locus; these other metabolic reactions include O-de-ethylation of phenacetin and hydroxylation of nortriptyline, amitriptyline, metoprolol, timolol, propranolol, perhexiline, mephenytoin, mephobarbital, and encainide.[3,5,7,11]

Resistance to warfarin is one of several mutations in humans that modify the pharmacologic response to a drug by altering the drug receptor (Table 6-1). In subjects with the mutant gene, anticoagulation occurs only after many times the normal dose of warfarin.

Warfarin inhibits production of several blood components necessary for clotting, probably by competing with vitamin K for a receptor. In cases of warfarin resistance the mutant receptor may be envisioned as a structurally altered molecule that fails to bind warfarin as strongly as the normal one and therefore does not produce anticoagulation; this alteration also results in a stronger than normal binding of vitamin K.

PHARMACOGENET-IC CONDITIONS (SINGLE-LOCUS TRANSMISSION) THAT ALTER DRUG INTERACTIONS
Warfarin resistance

Most persons are able to taste dilute solutions of phenylthiocarbamide (PTC, phenylthiourea) and chemically related compounds containing the thiocyanate group, whereas others cannot. This difference in ability to taste PTC, in addition to the fact that metabolism of some thiocyanate compounds appears to be no different in tasters and nontasters, indicates that a receptor mutation may exist in nontasters. Interestingly, this difference in taste threshold may influence food preferences and thus consumption of potential goitrogenic compounds. Enlargement of the thyroid gland, called *goiter*, can be produced in rats by PTC. Several common vegetables including turnips, brussels sprouts, and kale contain a goiter-producing chemical, and nodular goiters are more common among nontasters than among tasters of PTC.

Genetic differences in capacity to taste phenylthiocarbamide

A more complicated condition is glucose-6-phosphate dehydrogenase (G-6-PD) deficiency, which affects about 100 million people in the world, primarily in areas where malaria is endemic. In the United States one in 10 black males is affected. Individuals with any one of 80 different mutations that occur at a specific site on the X chromosome develop hemolytic anemia after exposure to a large number of drugs, some of which are listed in Table 6-1. Some dietary constituents, such as fava beans (of the plant *Vicia fava*), can also cause hemolysis in susceptible subjects. The mechanism believed responsible for hemolysis is complex but probably initially involves a shortage of NADPH. NADPH is produced by the enzyme G-6-PD. NADPH itself then serves as a cofactor for glutathione reductase. Thus G-6-PD deficiency ultimately leads to a deficiency of reduced glutathione.

In normal persons, the red cell membrane is maintained in a functional state by having a supply of reduced glutathione adequate to keep membrane proteins in a reduced and operative condition. Highly reactive drug metabolites oxidize membrane proteins; if these oxidized proteins are not rapidly reduced by glutathione, hemolysis ensues. Thus a genetically induced enzyme deficiency results in decreased usable glutathione, thereby allowing reactive drug metabolites to produce hemolysis.

Genetic control of glucose-6-phosphate dehydrogenase deficiency

REFERENCES

1. Drayer, D.E., and Reidenberg, M.M.: Clinical consequences of polymorphic acetylation of basic drugs, Clin. Pharmacol. Ther. **22**:251, 1977.
2. Endrenyi, L., Inaba, T., and Kalow, W.: Genetic study of amobarbital elimination based on its kinetics in twins, Clin. Pharmacol. Ther. **20**:701, 1976.
3. Jacqz, E., Hall, S.D., Branch, R.A., and Wilkinson, G.R.: Polymorphic metabolism of mephenytoin in man: pharmacokinetic interaction with a co-regulated substrate, mephobarbital, Clin. Pharmacol. Ther. **39**:646, 1986.
4. Kalow, W., Kadar, D., Inaba, T., and Tang, B.K.: A case of deficiency of N-hydroxylation of amobarbital, Clin. Pharmacol. Ther. **21**:530, 1977.
5. Lennard, M.S., Tucker, G.T., and Woods, H.F.: The polymorphic oxidation of β-adrenoceptor antagonists: clinical pharmacokinetic considerations, Clin. Pharmacokinet. **11**:1, 1986.
6. Mahgoub, A., Idle, J.R., Dring, L.G., et al.: Polymorphic hydroxylation of debrisoquine in man, Lancet **2**:584, 1977.
7. Mellström, B., Säwe, J., Bertilsson, L., and Sjöqvist, F.: Amitriptyline metabolism: association with debrisoquin hydroxylation in nonsmokers, Clin. Pharmacol. Ther. **39**:369, 1986.
8. Silas, J.H., Lennard, M.S., Tucker, G.T., et al.: Why hypertensive patients vary in their response to oral debrisoquine, Br. Med. J. **1**:422, 1977.
9. Takahara, S., Sato, H., Doi, M., and Mihara, S.: Acatalasemia. III. On the heredity of acatalasemia, Proc. Jpn. Acad. **28**:585, 1952.
10. Vesell, E.S., and Page, J.G.: Genetic control of the phenobarbital-induced shortening of plasma antipyrine half-lives in man, J. Clin. Invest. **48**:2202, 1969.
11. Woosley, R.L., Roden, D.M., Dai, G., et al.: Co-inheritance of the polymorphic metabolism of encainide and debrisoquin, Clin. Pharmacol. Ther. **39**:282, 1986.

Chapter 7

Effects of age on drug disposition

For many years physicians have recognized that elderly patients receiving drugs with low therapeutic indices frequently need lower doses to avoid toxicity. Only recently have some mechanisms responsible for changed dosage requirements of such patients been firmly established. For almost every drug investigated, rates of drug absorption, distribution, metabolism, or excretion have differed in geriatric subjects compared to young adults.[4,9] Unfortunately, many earlier studies assessed kinetics only by measuring half-life. Hence the changes noted could not be ascribed clearly to changes either in volume of distribution or in clearance. For example, early studies of some benzodiazepines showed an increase in half-life with aging, assumed to represent a decrease in metabolic capacity, that is, clearance. Subsequent studies have shown this effect to represent primarily an increase in volume of distribution with some benzodiazepines (for example, diazepam and chlordiazepoxide) and a decrease in clearance with others. Hence the physician should be aware of limitations of much of the data in this area.

In addition, geriatric subjects, compared to middle-aged subjects, present other problems of definition to the pharmacologist and the clinician. To identify how drugs are handled in "normal" geriatric subjects, such subjects must be carefully examined to exclude concomitant pathologic conditions. However, the very changes that occur in drug disposition in geriatric subjects occur largely because of degenerative alterations in the structure and function of the heart, liver, and kidney. Cardiac output declines approximately 1% per year from 19 to 86 years of age, and with age a decreased proportion of the cardiac output is distributed to the liver and kidneys. The liver's metabolic capacity and the kidney's excretory capacity both decrease with age. Moreover, circulating albumin concentrations (to which many drugs bind) decline with age,[1,5,7,11] the proportion of body fat relative to muscle increases and total body water decreases, all of which can influence distribution patterns of drugs. Age-induced changes in the structure and function of critical organs probably occur at different rates in different subjects. Accordingly, subjects of the same chronologic age exhibit varied degrees of cardiovascular, hepatic, or renal impairment in physiologic function.

PROBLEMS OF INVESTIGATING

Although complete data concerning effects of age on gastrointestinal absorption of drugs are presently unavailable, certain changes that occur with age should, from a purely theoretical point of view, alter drug absorption from the gastrointestinal

DRUG ABSORPTION

tract. For example, with age gastric emptying time decreases, probably as a result of increased stomach pH. Shortened retention of drugs in the stomach would be anticipated to accelerate their delivery to absorption sites in the small intestine and hasten overall absorption.

Another critical factor that affects gastrointestinal drug absorption is intestinal blood perfusion, which has been demonstrated to decrease by 40% to 50% from rates measured in young adults. This reduction should slow absorption from the gut by decreasing transfer of drugs across the serosal membrane. Passive absorption of xylose in the gut declines by 40% from ages 18 to 40 years to ages 70 to 80 years.[4]

Despite these theoretical considerations suggestive of reduced rates of gastrointestinal drug absorption with age, no effect has been observed on either the rate or amount of gastrointestinal absorption of aspirin, an acidic drug, or the β-adrenergic blocker practolol, a basic drug absorbed from the small intestine.

DRUG DISTRIBUTION

As noted above, with aging there is a change in the composition of fluid compartments of the body such as total body water, extracellular water, and intracellular water. This change and decreases in drug binding are undoubtedly responsible for alterations in volume of distribution with age.

Albumin concentrations decline with age (Fig. 7-1).[5] Whether this decrease occurs as a consequence of reduced albumin synthesis, increased albumin catabolism, or a combination of these is uncertain. From a theoretical viewpoint reduced albumin concentration per se would exert no pharmacokinetic or pharmacodynamic effect for drugs not highly bound to albumin. In contrast, one would predict that for highly bound drugs the unbound (free) fraction would increase, thereby increasing distribution into tissues and the volume of distribution; similarly, more drug would be available to metabolizing and excreting sites, thus increasing elimination. This scenario would seem to make the elderly eliminate highly bound drugs more quickly. However, if these effects are coupled with decreased functional ability of eliminating organs, an increase in unbound, pharmacologically active drug can occur and cause an increased effect.[10] Lower doses would then be needed to avoid toxicity.

When the percent binding of specific drugs to albumin has been compared in geriatric subjects and normal, middle-aged adults, a variety of results (often conflicting) has been obtained. For example, no changes were observed for binding of phenobarbital, penicillin G, or phenytoin, though albumin concentrations declined, from 4.0 to 3.4 g/dl in those over 50 years of age.[1] Likewise, in other studies the percent binding of warfarin or diazepam did not change with age. In contrast, another report showed reduced plasma binding of phenylbutazone and naproxen with age but no change in plasma binding of sulfadiazine or salicylate. In still another study, phenytoin binding declined with age when subjects less than 45 years of age who had a mean serum albumin concentration of 4.1 g/dl were compared with subjects over 65 years of age whose mean albumin concentration was 2.9 g/dl.[11] In this and confirmatory papers on phenytoin from different laboratories,[7,8] the decrease in drug

Change in mean (±SE) serum albumin concentrations according to age in 11,090 hos- **FIG. 7-1**
pitalized medical patients.

From Greenblatt, D.J.: Am. Geriatr. Soc. 27:20, 1979.

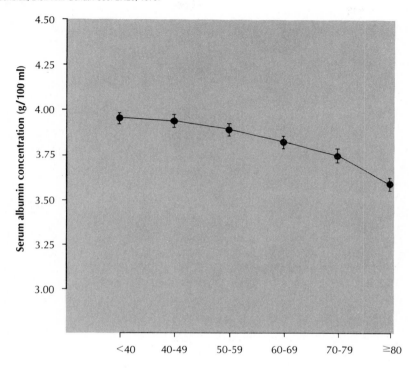

binding with age paralleled the decline in plasma albumin concentration. The net result of these data is that it is difficult to predict whether an individual elderly patient will manifest a change in drug binding. The physician should be alert to this possibility and monitor all elderly patients accordingly.

Other practical consequences of decreased albumin concentrations in geriatric subjects are noteworthy. Wallace, Whiting, and Runcie showed that the magnitude of interactions involving displacement from albumin of one drug by another was greater in older than in younger subjects.[11] Binding of plasma proteins of three drugs—phenylbutazone, salicylate, and sulfadiazine—was measured in young and geriatric subjects. In subjects receiving one or more other drugs, geriatric subjects exhibited much higher concentrations of the free form of these drugs than the concentrations in geriatric subjects not taking other drugs or in younger subjects taking other drugs. The increase in free drug concentration in plasma of geriatric subjects correlated with the number of drugs taken. These authors suggested that geriatric subjects are more susceptible than younger subjects to displacement of one drug from albumin by another.

TABLE 7-1 Effects of age on drug disposition

Drug	Elimination rate — Young adult	Elimination rate — Geriatric	Volume of distribution	Apparent mechanism for age-related change
Acetanilide	$t_{1/2}$ = 1.45 hr	$t_{1/2}$ = 2.07 hr	—	↓ metabolism
Aminopyrine	$t_{1/2}$ = 3.0 hr	$t_{1/2}$ = 10.0 hr	—	—
Amitriptyline	$t_{1/2}$ = 16 hr	$t_{1/2}$ = 22 hr	↑ in geriatric subjects	—
Ampicillin	$t_{1/2}$ = 1.0 hr	$t_{1/2}$ = 1.2 hr	—	↓ renal function
Amobarbital	Urinary metabolite excretion = 14.2% Plasma drug level = 1.3 µg/ml	Urinary metabolite excretion = 4.3% Plasma drug level = 1.0 µg/ml	—	↓ metabolism
Antipyrine	First study: $t_{1/2}$ = 12 hr Second study: MCR* unchanged in nonsmokers; MCR* decreased with age in smokers	First study: $t_{1/2}$ = 17.4 hr	—	—
Chlordiazepoxide	Clearance† = 26.6 ml/min	Clearance† = 46.3 ml/min	↑ in geriatric subjects	—
Diazepam	$t_{1/2}$ = 20 hr	$t_{1/2}$ = 80 hr	×3 in geriatric subjects	—
Digoxin	$t_{1/2}$ = 51 hr	$t_{1/2}$ = 73 hr	—	↓ renal function
Doxycycline	$t_{1/2}$ = 12 hr	$t_{1/2}$ = 18 hr	—	↓ renal function
Flurazepam	Incidence of flurazepam toxicity increased with age			—
Indocyanine green	MCR* decreased with age			↓ liver blood flow
Isoniazid	$t_{1/2}$ = 2.5 hr	$t_{1/2}$ = 2.9 hr	—	—
Kanamycin	$t_{1/2}$ = 107 min	$t_{1/2}$ = 282 min	—	↓ renal function
Lithium	Clearance = 41.5 ml/min	Clearance = 7.7 ml/min	—	↓ renal function
Lorazepam	Clearance = 0.99 ml/min/kg	Clearance = 0.77 ml/min/kg	×2.5 in geriatric subjects	—
Meperidine	Plasma levels twice as high in geriatric subjects			—
Nitrazepam	Men: Clearance = 0.95 ml/min/kg Women: Clearance = 1.09 ml/min/kg	Clearance = 0.84 ml/min/kg Clearance = 1.19 ml/min/kg	↑ 20% in geriatric subjects No change	—
Penicillin	$t_{1/2}$ = 33 min (penicillin G) $t_{1/2}$ = 10 hr (procaine penicillin)	$t_{1/2}$ = 60 min (penicillin G) $t_{1/2}$ = 18 hr (procaine penicillin)	—	↓ renal function
Phenobarbital	$t_{1/2}$ = 71 hr	$t_{1/2}$ = 107 hr	—	—
Phenylbutazone	First study: $t_{1/2}$ = 81 hr Second study: $t_{1/2}$ = 87 hr	$t_{1/2}$ = 105 hr $t_{1/2}$ = 110 hr	—	↓ metabolism
Phenytoin	Clearance = 26 ml/hr/kg	Clearance = 42 ml/hr/kg	—	—
Practolol	$t_{1/2}$ = 7.1 hr	$t_{1/2}$ = 8.6 hr	—	↓ renal function
Propranolol	Clearance decreases with age only in smokers			—
Quinidine	Clearance = 4.04 ml/min/kg	Clearance = 2.64 ml/min/kg	No change	↓ metabolism and renal function
Tetracycline	$t_{1/2}$ = 3.5 hr	$t_{1/2}$ = 4.5 hr	—	↓ metabolism
Theophylline	$t_{1/2}$ = 7 hr	$t_{1/2}$ = 10 hr	—	↓ metabolism
Valproic acid	67% Increase in plasma concentration of free drug in the elderly			↓ metabolism of free drug

*MCR, Metabolic clearance rate.

†Clearance of total drug; clearance of unbound drug is not altered.

Table 7-1 summarizes studies that show the influence of age on drug metabolism in human subjects. Effects of age on drug metabolism had previously been demonstrated in rodents.[4] With increasing age rats exhibited reduced activity of several hepatic cytochrome P-450–dependent monooxygenases, the system most responsible for biotransformation of drugs in mammals. Heterogeneity of cytochrome P-450 may be responsible in part for the complex, age-associated changes observed in both rodents and humans; in general, the hepatic drug-metabolizing capacity is very low during the fetal and neonatal periods, reaches a peak in the pediatric age range, and declines thereafter. Different forms of cytochrome P-450 may display different developmental patterns. Hence drugs metabolized by one set of isozymes would behave differently with age compared to another isozyme system. To this end, it appears that benzodiazepines eliminated by hepatic microsomal oxidative isozymes show decreased clearance with age, whereas those involving nitro reduction show no change.[6]

DRUG METABOLISM

Many drugs and their metabolites are eliminated from the body by renal excretion. If the extent to which renal mechanisms contribute to drug elimination from the body is 40% or greater, it is likely that dosing of the drug needs to be modified in the elderly.[3] Examples include digoxin, aminoglycoside antibiotics, and penicillins. Estimates of the degree of renal impairment are made from creatinine clearance. Importantly, in the elderly serum creatinine concentrations become a poor estimate of renal function unless adjusted for age as in the following, commonly used, algorithm[2]:

DRUG EXCRETION

$$\text{Creatinine clearance corrected to a 72 kg body weight} = \frac{140 - \text{Age}}{\text{Serum creatinine (in mg/dl)}} \quad \text{(Women} = 85\% \text{ of this value)}$$

From an estimate of creatinine clearance, various nomograms permit selection of appropriately lowered doses of drugs in patients with renal insufficiency, including the elderly.[3]

Effects of age on drug absorption, distribution, metabolism, elimination, and various combinations of these have been the subject of recent reviews.[9] The magnitude of such age-related changes depends on both the pharmacologic profile of the particular drug and environmental and genetic characteristics of each geriatric subject. Because so many diverse factors that can influence drug disposition change concomitantly in elderly subjects, it is often difficult to determine specific mechanisms responsible for the pharmacokinetic characteristics of a given drug in a particular geriatric patient. For these reasons and because of the incompleteness of our present knowledge, physicians need to exercise special care to avoid toxicity when drugs are administered singly or in combination to geriatric patients. In general the best approach is to start with lower doses than in the young and to increase dosage slowly and in small increments.

CONCLUSIONS

REFERENCES

1. Bender, A.D., Post, A., Meier, J.P., et al.: Plasma protein binding of drugs as a function of age in adult human subjects, J. Pharm. Sci. 64:1711, 1975.
2. Cockcroft, D.W., and Gault, M.H.: Prediction of creatinine clearance from serum creatinine, Nephron 16:31, 1976.
3. Dettli, L.: Drug dosage in renal disease, Clin. Pharmacokinet. 1:126, 1976.
4. Gorrod, J.W.: Absorption, metabolism, and excretion of drugs in geriatric subjects, Gerontol. Clin. 16:30, 1974.
5. Greenblatt, D.J.: Reduced serum albumin concentration in the elderly: a report from the Boston Collaborative Drug Surveillance Program, J. Am. Geriatr. Soc. 27:20, 1979.
6. Greenblatt, D.J., Abernethy, D.R., Locniskar, A., et al.: Age, sex, and nitrazepam kinetics: relation to antipyrine disposition, Clin. Pharmacol. Ther. 38:697, 1985.

7. Hayes, M.J., Langman, M.J.S., and Short, A.H.: Changes in drug metabolism with increasing age. I. Warfarin binding and plasma protein, Br. J. Clin. Pharmacol. 2:69, 1975.
8. Hooper, W.D., Bochner, F., Eadie, M.J., and Tyrer, J.H.: Plasma protein binding of diphenylhydantoin: effects of sex hormones, renal and hepatic disease, Clin. Pharmacol. Ther. 15:276, 1974.
9. Richey, D.P., and Bender, A.D.: Pharmacokinetic consequences of aging, Annu. Rev. Pharmacol. Toxicol. 17:49, 1977.
10. Upton, R.A., Williams, R.L., Kelly, J., and Jones, R.M.: Naproxen pharmacokinetics in the elderly, Br. J. Clin. Pharmacol. 18:207, 1984.
11. Wallace, S., Whiting, B., and Runcie, J.: Factors affecting drug binding in plasma of elderly patients, Br. J. Clin. Pharmacol. 3:327, 1976.

Chapter 8

Effects of diet on drug disposition

Relationships between diet and drug response in human subjects were not even suspected until carefully designed studies clearly established such interactions and indicated the need for future investigations.[4,6,7,12] A few examples illustrate the influence of dietary factors on rates of metabolism of drugs such as antipyrine and theophylline.

Of all dietary manipulations, the extreme form—starvation—would be expected to produce the most pronounced pharmacokinetic alterations. When drugs were administered to fasting rodents, the rate of hepatic metabolism of some drugs was greatly reduced.[3,8] In contrast, there were no major changes in rates of drug metabolism in obese, otherwise healthy, human subjects after 7 to 10 consecutive days on a diet in which the total daily carbohydrate intake was less than 15 g.[14] This diet was sufficient to cause ketosis as well as weight loss that ranged from 3.6 to 15 kg. When uncorrected for body weight, the volume of distribution (V_d) of both antipyrine and tolbutamide was significantly lower after fasting than before, presumably because the early loss of body weight during fasting is mainly body water rather than reduced fat or muscle mass. The extent of decrease in V_d was proportional in each subject to the weight lost so that, when correction was made for body weight, fasting had no effect on the V_d of either drug. Other drugs metabolized by hepatic microsomal oxidations, including sulfisoxazole, isoniazid, and procaine, were also studied.[13] When allowance was made for body weight, neither half-life nor clearance of the five above drugs was changed in obese subjects. Although fasting decreased sulfisoxazole excretion, this was probably secondary to a decline in urine flow and in urinary pH, both of which favor nonionic diffusion of the drug back into the circulation.

General conclusions regarding the failure of acute fasting to alter hepatic metabolism were further extended by a study of seven female patients with anorexia nervosa. In these patients prolonged refusal to eat had produced differing degrees of dehydration, hyponatremia, hypochloremia, hypokalemia and anemia.[2] Compared with age- and sex-matched normal controls, the patients exhibited normal antipyrine pharmacokinetics when values were corrected for body weight.

A study in India revealed that in 15 men suffering from nutritional edema—a severe manifestation of protein deficiency and resultant hypoalbuminemia—the mean plasma antipyrine half-life of 12.8 hours was not significantly different from that of age- and sex-matched nonsmoking controls (11.2 hours) but was higher than that of age- and sex-matched smoking controls (8.9 hours).[9] This same study examined another group of 13 undernourished, hypoalbuminemic men without edema. Their short mean antipyrine half-life of 8.6 hours, similar to that of smoking controls (8.9 hours), could be because some of them smoked cigarettes, some drank ethanol, and some were agricultural laborers exposed to pesticides known to induce hepatic drug-metabolizing enzymes (see Chapter 9). Thus in this study severe malnutrition did not by itself greatly alter antipyrine disposition. However, it is important to note that antipyrine is a probe of hepatic metabolism by microsomal oxidation. It is conceivable that other metabolic pathways might be affected.

| EFFECTS OF DIET ON DRUG ABSORPTION | Food can have considerable effects on drug absorption. In general, ingestion of food delays gastric emptying. This in turn delays delivery of ingested drugs to absorption sites in the small intestine and can delay the appearance of drug in the serum. Usually, ingestion of drugs with food also prolongs their absorption so that a lower peak concentration is reached. Lastly, some foodstuffs decrease the bioavailability of specific drugs if they are coingested. The classic example of this phenomenon is the chelation of tetracycline by milk products, which prevents absorption of the antibiotic. It should be clear that food can affect drug absorption in many ways. If there is concern about this possibility, patients should be instructed to take their medications 1 hour before or 2 or more hours after a meal. |

An interesting additional effect of food on absorption has been the recent description of "dose-dumping" of a sustained-release theophylline product caused by a high fat meal.[5] Ingestion of this formulation with a high-fat meal resulted in loss of the sustained-release characteristics by unknown mechanisms.

EFFECTS OF DIET ON DRUG BINDING

Decreased albumin concentrations per se would undoubtedly affect the volume of distribution and clearance of many drugs with a high degree of binding to albumin. In fact, this scenario has been demonstrated with phenylbutazone, a highly bound nonsteroidal anti-inflammatory drug. The pharmacokinetics of this drug were examined in four normal male controls and five undernourished, hypoalbuminemic male subjects, none of whom smoked cigarettes or consumed ethanol chronically. Compared to controls, the malnourished group exhibited increased V_d and clearance.[1] These changes in phenylbutazone disposition in undernutrition presumably arose from reduced binding of phenylbutazone to albumin, with a corresponding increase in availability of drug for metabolism and elimination. As discussed in Chapter 7, if decreased binding cannot be compensated for by increased excretion or metabolism, then the free, pharmacologically active concentration will increase, necessitating a decrease in dosage. Clearly, with the scant data available, it is difficult to predict an appropriate dosage adjustment. Therefore, as with the elderly, the physician must monitor the patient appropriately.

Renal elimination of certain drugs can be altered by fasting or starvation as in the case of sulfisoxazole, for which renal excretion decreases during fasting. Renal excretion of drugs eliminated by glomerular filtration might also be affected by nutrition. Protein loads increase glomerular filtration rate. In settings of parenteral or enteral nutrition, this increase may be sufficient to enhance the renal elimination of drugs such as aminoglycosides to a clinically important degree, thereby requiring larger than usual doses.

EFFECTS OF DIET ON DRUG EXCRETION

The most dramatic change in drug metabolism caused by dietary manipulation was described by Kappas and associates,[7] who showed that on an isocaloric diet the rate of antipyrine and theophylline metabolism was prolonged twofold as the percentage of total calories as carbohydrate doubled from 35% to 70% and the percentage of protein decreased from 44% to 10%, the remainder being fat. The switch from high to low protein with a reverse change in carbohydrate content affected antipyrine and theophylline half-life (Fig. 8-1) by decreasing clearance, with no effect on the volume of distribution.

It is not understood why starvation produces a negligible change in antipyrine metabolism, whereas with an isocaloric diet simply switching the proportion of carbohydrate to protein greatly alters antipyrine metabolism.

Many patients who receive drugs are debilitated and chronically ill; they may have inadequate nutrition and the proportion of their diet that is carbohydrate, protein, or fat may change. For such patients drug elimination may be affected. Furthermore, some of the normal population use various weight-reduction diets; these persons could also be susceptible to changes in drug-metabolizing capacity.

ALTERATIONS IN DRUG METABOLISM CAUSED BY DIETARY MANIPULATION

The way in which food is prepared can also affect drug disposition. Isolated intestinal preparations from rats fed charcoal-broiled beef (rather than beef cooked while covered with foil, which prevents formation of polycyclic hydrocarbons) exhibited an elevenfold increase in intestinal metabolism of phenacetin.[10] Plasma antipyrine and theophylline half-lives in eight healthy human volunteers were measured before and after 7 days on a charcoal-broiled beef diet.[6] The pharmacokinetics of these drugs were likewise assessed before and after another 7-day course on a diet containing the same amount of beef cooked while covered with foil. After eating charcoal-broiled beef, the plasma antipyrine and theophylline half-lives were shortened by 22%. This observation was attributable to an increase in metabolism, since no change occurred in the volume of distribution of either drug while clearance of both increased.

EFFECTS OF CHARCOAL BROILING ON DRUG DISPOSITION

FIG. 8-1 *Theophylline half-lives in six normal subjects maintained on their usual home diets and on two test-diet periods. Each bar represents mean ± SE for the six subjects. P, Protein; C, carbohydrate; F, fat. Values for diets 1, 3, and 4, are not significantly different from each other. Value for diet 2 is significantly different from that of diet 1 (p = 0.05) and diet 3 (p = 0.01).*

From Kappas, A., Anderson, K.E., Conney, A.H., and Alvares, A.P.: Clin. Pharmacol. Ther. 20:643, 1976.

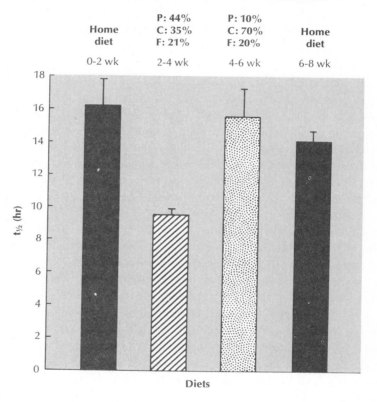

STIMULATORY EFFECT OF BRUSSELS SPROUTS AND CABBAGE

In rats a diet containing certain cruciferous vegetables, such as brussels sprouts, cabbage, turnips, broccoli, cauliflower, or spinach, induced intestinal benzo[*a*]pyrene hydroxylase activity and the intestinal enzymes that metabolize 7-ethoxycoumarin, hexobarbital, and phenacetin.[11,15] Certain indoles present in these vegetables are potent inducers of these enzymes. A similar study in 10 healthy volunteers showed that on a 7-day diet rich in brussels sprouts and cabbage antipyrine clearance increased by 11% and mean plasma phenacetin concentrations decreased by 34% to 67%.[12] This effect with antipyrine is unlikely to be clinically important. However, as reflected by the change with phenacetin, with some drugs such an effect may require dosage modification.

Decay of a single oral dose of theobromine (6 mg/kg) before and after 2-week dietary   **FIG. 8-2**
abstention from methylxanthines.

From Drouillard, D.D., Vesell, E.S., and Dvorchik, B.H.: Clin. Pharmacol. Ther. **23:**296, 1978.

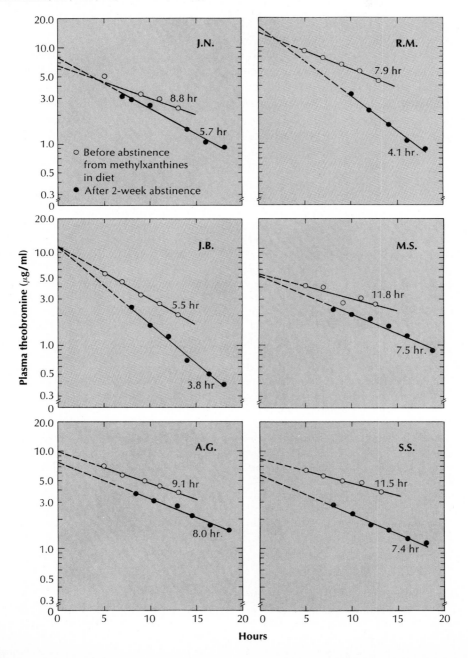

Hours

THEOBROMINE AS A METABOLIC INHIBITOR

Studies with the methylxanthine theobromine, a nutritional constituent of such dietary staples as chocolate and cocoa, revealed that daily dietary theobromine intake decreases the capacity to eliminate theobromine itself.[4] After 2 weeks on a methylxanthine-free diet, each of six healthy male subjects increased his capacity to eliminate a test dose of theobromine (Fig. 8-2).

Although theobromine is not used as a drug, closely related methylxanthines such as theophylline are. In a given patient, it is commonly observed that theophylline doses may need to be changed frequently. Chronic dosing with theophylline may affect its own metabolism, but it is also possible that dietary theobromine intake might influence theophylline dosage requirements and account for these clinical observations. Support for this possibility is the demonstration that in human subjects theobromine inhibits theophylline elimination.

REFERENCES

1. Adithan, C., Gandhi, I.S., and Chandrasekar, S.: Pharmacokinetics of phenylbutazone in undernutrition, Indian J. Pharmacol. **10**:301, 1978.
2. Bakke, O.M., Aanderud, S., Syversen, G., et al.: Antipyrine metabolism in anorexia nervosa, Br. J. Clin. Pharmacol. **5**:341, 1978.
3. Dixon, R.L., Shultice, R.W., and Fouts, J.R.: Factors affecting drug metabolism by liver microsomes. IV. Starvation, Proc. Soc. Exp. Biol. Med. **103**:333, 1960.
4. Drouillard, D.D., Vesell, E.S., and Dvorchik, B.H.: Studies on theobromine disposition in normal subjects: alterations induced by dietary abstention from or exposure to methylxanthines, Clin. Pharmacol. Ther. **23**:296, 1978.
5. Hendeles, L., Thakker, K., and Weinberger, M.: Food-induced dose dumping of Theo-24, Am. Pharm. NS25:592, 1985.
6. Kappas, A., Alvares, A.P., Anderson, K.E., et al.: Effect of charcoal-broiled beef on antipyrine and theophylline metabolism, Clin. Pharmacol. Ther. **23**:445, 1978.
7. Kappas, A., Anderson, K.E., Conney, A.H., and Alvares, A.P.: Influence of dietary protein and carbohydrate on antipyrine and theophylline metabolism in man, Clin. Pharmacol. Ther. **20**:643, 1976.
8. Kato, R., and Gillette, J.R.: Sex differences in the effects of abnormal physiological states on the metabolism of drugs by rat liver microsomes, J. Pharmacol. Exp. Ther. **150**:285, 1965.
9. Krishnaswamy, K., and Naidu, A.N.: Microsomal enzymes in malnutrition as determined by plasma half life of antipyrine, Br. Med. J. **1**:538, 1977.
10. Pantuck, E.J., Hsiao, K.-C., Kuntzman, R., and Conney, A.H.: Intestinal metabolism of phenacetin in the rat: effect of charcoal-broiled beef and rat chow, Science **187**:744, 1975.
11. Pantuck, E.J., Hsiao, K.-C., Loub, W.D., et al.: Stimulatory effect of vegetables on intestinal drug metabolism in the rat, J. Pharmacol. Exp. Ther. **198**:278, 1976.
12. Pantuck, E.J., Pantuck, C.B., Garland, W.A., et al.: Stimulatory effect of brussels sprouts and cabbage on human drug metabolism, Clin. Pharmacol. Ther. **25**:88, 1979.
13. Reidenberg, M.M.: Obesity and fasting: effects on drug metabolism and drug action in man, Clin. Pharmacol. Ther. **22**:729, 1977.
14. Reidenberg, M.M., and Vesell, E.S.: Unaltered metabolism of antipyrine and tolbutamide in fasting man, Clin. Pharmacol. Ther. **17**:650, 1975.
15. Wattenberg, L.W.: Studies of polycyclic hydrocarbon hydroxylases of the intestine possibly related to cancer: effect of diet on benzpyrene hydroxylase activity, Cancer **28**:99, 1971.

Chapter 9

Effects of occupation and disease on drug disposition

OCCUPATIONAL FACTORS THAT ALTER RESPONSE OF DRUG-METABOLIZING ENZYMES

As discussed in Chapter 6, genetic factors contribute appreciably to large interindividual variations in drug pharmacokinetics. In addition, we are chronically exposed to numerous environmental compounds and conditions that can induce or inhibit the activity of hepatic mixed-function oxidases. Hence a dynamic interaction exists between the genes that control these oxidases and environmental factors. Chemicals such as DDT, polychlorinated biphenyls, and polycyclic hydrocarbons can induce a subject's hepatic drug-metabolizing enzyme activity. As shown later in this chapter, disease states can also greatly change a subject's ability to eliminate drugs. Overall, then, a host of factors can influence drug handling in an individual patient.

OCCUPATIONAL CHEMICALS THAT ALTER DRUG-METABOLIZING CAPACITY

In recent years, the field of occupational medicine has expanded greatly as it was recognized that various human diseases develop from chronic exposure to certain chemicals. This association was first documented in the eighteenth century by Percival Potts. He reported that English chimney sweeps were at high risk of developing cancer of the scrotum. In the twentieth century it has been learned that exposure at work to asbestos, benzene, phenol, vinyl chloride, radium, and x rays also increases the risk of developing certain forms of cancer. Prolonged, chronic intake of combination analgesics to relieve headaches, produced by long hours of eyestrain, greatly increased the risk of watchmakers in Switzerland of developing renal disease. Likewise, coal miners had a much higher incidence of pulmonary disease than age-matched controls who did not work in the mines. An additional new aspect of occupational medicine is the influence of chemicals encountered at work on a subject's capacity to metabolize drugs. Many chemicals to which subjects are chronically exposed can probably change their rates of drug elimination.

Because ours is a pill-oriented society, exposure to potent chemicals that can alter a subject's clearance of drugs is rarely limited solely to occupational exposure. Such chemicals are more commonly ingested for medicinal, recreational, or nutritional purposes than as a result of occupational exposure only. Overall, the physician must be aware of myriad possible influences on drug handling and response in an individual patient.

69

EFFECTS OF DISEASE ON DRUG DISPOSITION

A single disease may cause multiple changes in the separate processes of drug absorption, distribution, metabolism, excretion, and receptor action. When each of the individual effects is measured and all effects are summated, the net change in "drug response" may be negligible as a result of the balancing of one action by another in an opposite direction. Changes in the patient's condition or treatment may upset this balance to expose a major effect of the disease on a single pharmacokinetic or pharmacodynamic process.

A critical point to remember is that a disease process may affect the disposition of different drugs in different ways. Each drug has a distinct pharmacologic profile, and the way a disease process alters the disposition of a particular drug depends on its specific pharmacologic characteristics. For example, in hypoalbuminemia the disposition of drugs that are extensively bound to albumin, such as warfarin and phenylbutazone, will be changed, whereas the disposition of isoniazid and kanamycin, which bind negligibly to albumin, will not be altered. As another example, hepatocellular disease affects the disposition of drugs such as barbital but does not affect the majority of antibiotics.

Table 9-1 presents a partial list of drugs for which elimination is altered by diseases of the liver or kidney. To illustrate how diseases can influence handling of and response to drugs, it is useful to consider the effects of several prototypical disease states on each of the pharmacokinetic processes. It is important to reemphasize that changes are often reported as an alteration in drug half-life. Such data do not provide sufficient information for adjustment of dosage in the patient because a change in volume of distribution of a drug (important for loading dose) can alter its half-life without affecting clearance (important for maintenance dose). Furthermore, large changes can occur in both clearance and volume of distribution of a drug without an effect on half-life.

Many disorders and pathologic states can alter the normal rates and pathways for drug absorption, distribution, biotransformation, excretion, interaction with receptor sites, or various combinations of these. The extent to which a disease affects these processes will depend on the particular drug. It is hazardous to extrapolate from observations with one drug to the effect of pathosis on others.

The clinical consequences of an alteration in drug disposition produced by disease will also be determined by the drug's margin of safety as well as by certain genetic and environmental characteristics of the patient. For example, a change of 200% in the clearance of antipyrine, low-dose salicylates, or penicillin will probably have little or no clinical consequence, whereas a shift of 20% in the clearance of digoxin, procainamide, or lidocaine may prove critical. By the same token, a decrease in albumin binding of warfarin from 99% to 98% may, at first, seem trivial. However, it may have profound toxicologic results since the pharmacologically active free concentration has doubled (from 1% to 2%). In contrast, a decrease of 1% in albumin binding of probenecid, from the normal of 75% to 74%, has negligible clinical consequences. Here the crucial factor is the percent change in the unbound portion of the drug.

TABLE 9-1   A partial list of drugs whose clearances have been reported to be altered by hepatic or renal dysfunction

Drug	Change in clearance		Drug	Change in clearance	
	Hepatic dysfunction	Renal dysfunction		Hepatic dysfunction	Renal dysfunction
Acetaminophen	↓		Indocyanine green	↓	
Amiloride		↓	Isoniazid	↓	
Aminopyrine	↓	No change	Lidocaine	↓	
Ampicillin		↓	Meperidine	↓	No change
Antipyrine	↓	No change	Methicillin		↓
Carbenicillin	↓	↓	Nafcillin	↓	↓
Cefazolin		↓	Niridazole	↓	
Cephacetrile		↓	Oxacillin		↓
Cephalexin		↓	Penicillin G		↓
Cephaloridine		↓	Pentobarbital	↓	No change
Cephalothin		↓	Phenacetin	No change	↓
Chloramphenicol	↓	No change	Phenylbutazone	↓ or no change	
Chlorpropamide		↓	Phenytoin	↓	
Clindamycin	↓	↓	Prednisone		↓
Cloxacillin		↓	Procainamide		↓
Colchicine	↑	↓	Propranolol	↓	↑ or no change
Colistimethate		↓	Rifampin	↓	
Diazepam	↓		Streptomycin		↓
Diazoxide		↓	Sulfadimethoxine		↓
Dicloxacillin		↓	Sulfamethazine		↓
Digitoxin		↑ or no change	Sulfamethoxazole		↓ or no change
Digoxin		↓	Sulfamethoxy-pyridazine		↓
Doxorubicin	↓	↓	Tetracycline		↓
Erythromycin		↓	Tobramycin		↓
Ethambutol		↓	Trimethoprim		↓
Flucytosine		↓	Vancomycin		↓
Furosemide		↓			
Gentamicin		↓			
Hydrocortisone	↓				

Data derived from reviews by Creasey,[5] Pagliaro and Benet,[14] Reidenberg,[19] and Vesell.[24]

Drug absorption   Effects of disease states on absorption depend on many factors, including the site of drug administration. If the drug is administered orally, the influence of disease will depend on the nature of the disease process, whether it affects the areas in the gut where the drug is normally absorbed, and how the disease alters the normal physiologic volume, pH, temperature, viscosity, surface tension, and composition of gastrointestinal secretions and contents.[9] Rates of drug absorption may also be influenced by the presence of food, the nature and quantity of bile salts and bacterial flora, the rate of splanchnic blood flow, prior diet and food intake, and gastrointestinal motility. Until recently little was known about how disease alters these factors in man. Large differences in rates of absorption of many orally administered drugs occur in patients and in normal volunteers. For example, a sevenfold range in the amount of tetracycline absorbed was reported in six fasting, healthy subjects.[17] Acetaminophen plasma concentrations were significantly higher after oral administration of the drug to 12 convalescent hospital patients in bed than to seven healthy ambulatory volunteers matched for age and sex.[16] Variations in gastric emptying may contribute significantly to interindividual differences in drug absorption rate because numerous physiologic and pathologic conditions plus pharmacologic effects of other drugs can change gastric emptying time. Grossly impaired absorption of acetaminophen occurs in patients with delayed gastric emptying and pyloric stenosis. In patients with slow gastric emptying, levodopa may be ineffective.[3] Therapeutic failure of orally administered drugs can accompany gastric stasis.[13,15] On the other hand, in patients with achlorhydria, aspirin was absorbed significantly faster and plasma salicylate concentrations were higher than those in control subjects.[15]

It is interesting that absorption of *p*-aminosalicylic acid and isoniazid was unchanged by gastrectomy for peptic ulcer though complete failure of ethionamide absorption occurred in some patients.[12] Furthermore, partial gastrectomy failed to alter the absorption of sulfisoxazole, quinidine, or ethambutol unless vagotomy had been performed, thereby slowing gastric emptying.

Rates of absorption from orally administered pills and capsules depend on rates of dissolution and dispersion, and some of the factors enumerated above can alter the latter, thereby contributing to variations in drug absorption.

In jejunal disease folic acid absorption is diminished.[7] In ileal disease the transport of bile acids may be impaired. This can reduce enterohepatic transport of many lipid-soluble drugs because bile acids promote absorption of fat and certain fat-soluble compounds, including many drugs and vitamins A, D, K, and E. Ileal disease may also impair vitamin B_{12} absorption, since this vitamin is absorbed from the ileum after it forms a complex with intrinsic factor produced by the gastric parietal cell. Surgical removal or defective function of the ileum attributable to a process such as inflammatory bowel disease can cause vitamin B_{12} malabsorption and pernicious anemia. Vitamin B_{12} absorption can also be impaired in gastric diseases in which parietal cell function is abnormal, so that intrinsic factor is deficient. In some patients with pernicious anemia, precipitating or blocking antibodies to intrinsic factor have been identified. In addition, regional enteritis as well as tropical sprue, celiac disease, and Whipple's disease can produce vitamin B_{12} malabsorption. In steatorrhea, fat-soluble drugs and vitamins may be lost in the feces.

Some inactive drugs are converted to an active form by gut bacteria, the best example being cleavage of sulfasalazine, a drug used to treat chronic ulcerative colitis. Diseases or drugs that change the nature of the gastrointestinal flora can affect the disposition of drugs metabolized by gut bacteria. In some patients, absorption of digoxin is reduced by neomycin administration, perhaps because of an effect on gut flora.[10] On the other hand, approximately 10% of patients have a gastrointestinal flora that inactivates digoxin, thereby decreasing its bioavailability. Eradication of these bacteria with broad-spectrum antibiotics can decrease digoxin inactivation, increase absorption (bioavailability), and result in a higher serum concentration.[11]

Drug distribution

Binding of many drugs to albumin can be altered, particularly in diseases of the liver and kidney associated with decreased concentrations of serum albumin. In cirrhosis and nephrosis there is an elevation in the unbound fraction of many drugs compared with conditions of normal protein and albumin concentrations.

In addition, in uremia endogenous competitors for albumin binding sites accumulate and can decrease binding. For example, phenytoin binding to protein was decreased in 15 uremic patients.[18] The percent unbound correlated well with blood urea nitrogen and serum creatinine. Other organic acids, including clofibrate, sulfonamides, thyroxin, and tryptophan, have also exhibited decreased protein binding in uremia. In addition to disease-associated *quantitative* changes in drug binding to albumin, *qualitative* changes can occur in the nature of the binding. In uremia the avidity of phenytoin binding to albumin is reduced.[20]

In contrast, organic bases bind to plasma proteins other than albumin; hence they bind normally in plasma from uremic patients. Many basic drugs bind to α_1-acid glycoprotein, an acute-phase reactant. The concentration of this protein can increase substantially in acute clinical syndromes such as myocardial infarction. Lidocaine, for example, is bound to this protein; binding can increase and the free fraction can decrease in patients with acute myocardial infarction.[21]

These situations illustrate the danger of selecting drug dose solely on the basis of total drug concentration in plasma rather than on the free concentration, since only the free form is pharmacologically active.

Hepatic drug metabolism

It is not unusual for drugs metabolized in the liver to have numerous metabolites. Several enzymes responsible for the multiple reactions are cytoplasmic; others are associated with specific subcellular organelles. Under normal conditions the cytochrome P-450–dependent monooxygenases, located in the smooth endoplasmic reticulum and responsible for many drug oxidations, exist in at least three and possibly six or more molecular forms. Diseases of the liver can differentially affect these enzymes and isozymes. Hence one can anticipate that it is not possible to generalize concerning effects of liver disease on drug metabolism.

Aside from these physiologic considerations, pathophysiologic changes in liver diseases are relevant. The most common form of liver disease in this country, alcoholic cirrhosis, is characterized by remissions and exacerbations and by variable progression over time. During the early stage of the disease, the metabolism of many drugs in alcoholic subjects may actually be faster than in normal subjects because multiple doses of ethanol induce the cytochrome P-450–dependent monooxygenases.[24] However, with time the disease converts functional hepatocytes into fibrous bands incapable of metabolizing drugs.

Since it is difficult to predict precisely how a particular patient with cirrhosis will eliminate a drug whose disposition depends largely on hepatic metabolism, the best course is to give these patients lower than normal doses of such drugs initially and to observe them closely to make certain that toxicity does not occur.

Fig. 9-1 illustrates how patients with different forms of liver disease metabolize aminopyrine, a relatively safe test drug, compared to patients with normal cardiovascular, hepatic, and renal function. In humans, aminopyrine is eliminated mainly by N-demethylation accomplished by cytochrome P-450–dependent monooxygenases.[8] Subsequently, the methyl group removed by these enzymatic reactions is converted to CO_2, is excreted in the breath, and can be measured as $^{14}CO_2$ if a single tracer dose of [dimethylamine-^{14}C]-aminopyrine is initially administered. Fig. 9-1 shows that patients with fatty liver and cholestasis do not exhibit sharp reductions in their hepatic N-demethylating capacity. On the other hand, patients with hepatocellular diseases, such as cirrhosis, infectious hepatitis, and certain metastatic cancers or hepatomas, show reduced N-demethylating capacity.

These observations are in agreement with others that liver disease is accompanied by reduced rates of antipyrine metabolism.[4] In contrast, warfarin disposition during acute viral hepatitis is unchanged,[25] and oxazepam disposition is normal during acute viral hepatitis and cirrhosis.[22] Between these extremes, a group of drugs of which clindamycin is an example exhibit intermediate or moderate changes in disposition in liver disease.[1] It should be apparent then that a wide range of alterations has been reported in liver disease, depending on the drug studied and its particular dispositional characteristics.

There are drugs that are avidly removed by the liver (high hepatic extraction ratio) and those with slower rates of removal (low extraction ratio), even though both types are eliminated by hepatic metabolism. For drugs with a high hepatic extraction ratio (greater than 0.8), such as propranolol and lidocaine, in the simplest terms the liver can remove nearly all of the drug presented to it. Therefore alterations in blood flow accompanying liver disease can produce large changes in hepatic clearance of the compound. In contrast, for drugs with a very low hepatic extraction ratio (less than 0.2), such as antipyrine and aminopyrine, the metabolic capacity of the liver is the determinant of drug removal, and blood flow has little influence on metabolism. Variability among drugs within this class may be attributed in part to multiple mo-

Excretion of $^{14}CO_2$ in breath of patients with various forms of liver disease compared to control patients 2 hours after oral administration of a single tracer dose of [^{14}C]aminopyrine.

FIG. 9-1

From Hepner, G.W., and Vesell, E.S.: Ann. Intern. Med. **83**:632, 1975.

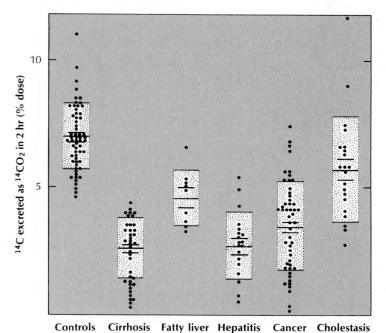

lecular forms of hepatic cytochrome P-450 that are differentially affected by a particular hepatic disorder.

In addition to the primary diseases of the liver shown in Fig. 9-1, which are associated with reduced aminopyrine N-demethylation, certain disorders of other organs may secondarily involve the liver. For example, in congestive heart failure, liver function may become impaired as a result of pooling of blood in the liver and reduced hepatic perfusion. Reduced blood flow to the liver should decrease hepatic uptake of drugs with a high hepatic extraction. Hence congestive heart failure reduces elimination of lidocaine.[23] However, for drugs with low hepatic extraction, it would not be anticipated that congestive heart failure would affect elimination unless hepatic congestion was sufficient to impair metabolic functions. Fig. 9-2 shows that patients admitted to the hospital with acute congestive heart failure were unable to eliminate aminopyrine as rapidly as they could after 7 to 10 days of treatment. Thus the hemodynamic changes associated with congestive heart failure can be sufficient to impair hepatic drug metabolism.

FIG. 9-2 *Excretion of* $^{14}CO_2$ *2 hours after an oral tracer dose of [^{14}C]aminopyrine in breath of 8 patients who received [^{14}C]aminopyrine before and 7 or 10 days after treatment of congestive heart failure. Notice improvement in hepatic capacity to N-demethylate aminopyrine with treatment of congestive heart failure as indicated by greatly increased* $^{14}CO_2$ *output in breath after 7 or 10 days of treatment.*

From Hepner, G.W., Vesell, E.S., and Tatum, K.R.: Am. J. Med. 65:271, 1978.

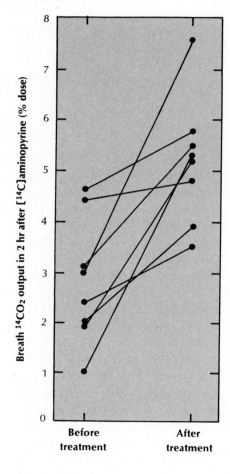

Several drugs are eliminated primarily by renal excretion, and renal disease slows removal of these drugs. Therefore the dose of these drugs must be reduced, the extent of reduction depending on the severity of the renal disease. Methods for dose adjustment in such patients have been promulgated by several investigators.[2,6] In a simple version, a linear relationship exists between the overall elimination rate constant (k_e) and the endogenous creatinine clearance (Cl_{cr}):

Renal excretion of drugs

$$k_e = k_{nr} + \delta \cdot Cl_{cr}$$

In this equation, k_{nr} is the mean extrarenal elimination rate constant in anuric patients (which is assumed to remain constant) and δ is a constant relating Cl_{cr} to the renal elimination rate constant (k_r) of the drug. This equation can be used for numerous drugs; simple nomograms have been devised to allow estimation of the rate of drug elimination in a patient with kidney disease from the value of Cl_{cr}.[6]

The information provided in Chapters 6 to 9 was selected to illustrate the extreme plasticity and sensitivity of human pharmacokinetic processes to perturbation by numerous factors. A physician who is aware of the principles illustrated will be more successful in selecting a dosage regimen that is therapeutic rather than toxic or ineffective. Several steps are available to help the physician make the right choice: (1) close clinical observation of the patient for qualitative therapeutic, as well as toxic, signs of drug action; (2) assessment of quantitative clinical end points for certain drugs (such as anticoagulants or antihypertensive agents) against which the dose can be titrated; (3) measurement of drug concentrations in biologic fluids (see Appendix A). Thus, despite the fact that dynamic interactions occur among the many factors influencing rates of drug elimination in individual patients and render dosage selection difficult, the physician can proceed in a rational, deliberate manner to choose the correct dose and to derive the maximal therapeutic benefit from available drugs, while minimizing risks of toxicity.

PERSPECTIVE

REFERENCES

1. Avant, G.R., Schenker, S., and Alford, R.H.: The effect of cirrhosis on the disposition and elimination of clindamycin, Am. J. Dig. Dis. **20**:223, 1975.

2. Bennett, W.M., Singer, I., and Coggins, C.H.: Guide to drug usage in adult patients with impaired renal function: a supplement, J.A.M.A. **223**:991, 1973.

3. Bianchine, J.R., Calimlim, L.R., Morgan, J.P., et al.: Metabolism and absorption of L-3,4-dihydroxyphenylalanine in patients with Parkinson's disease, Ann. N.Y. Acad. Sci. **179**:126, 1971.

4. Branch, R.A., Herbert, C.M., and Read, A.E.: Determinants of serum antipyrine half-lives in patients with liver disease, Gut **14**:569, 1973.

5. Creasey, W.A.: Drug disposition in humans: the basis of clinical pharmacology, New York, 1979, Oxford University Press.

6. Dettli, L.: Individualization of drug dosage in patients with renal disease, Med. Clin. North Am. **58**:977, 1974.

7. Hepner, G.W., Booth, C.C., Cowan, J., et al.: Absorption of crystalline folic acid in man, Lancet **2**:302, 1968.

8. Hepner, G.W., and Vesell, E.S.: Assessment of aminopyrine metabolism in man by breath analysis after oral administration of ^{14}C-aminopyrine: effects of phenobarbital, disulfiram and portal cirrhosis, N. Engl. J. Med. **291**:1384, 1974.

9. Levine, R.R.: Factors affecting gastrointestinal absorption of drugs, Am. J. Dig. Dis. **15**:171, 1970.

10. Lindenbaum, J., Maulitz, R.M., and Butler, V.P., Jr.: Inhibition of digoxin absorption by neomycin, Gastroenterology **71**:399, 1976.

11. Lindenbaum, J., Rund, D.G., Butler, V.P., Jr., et al.: Inactivation of digoxin by the gut flora: reversal by antibiotic therapy, N. Engl. J. Med. **305**:789, 1981.

12. Mattila, M.J., Friman, A., Larmi, T.K., and Koskinen, R.: Absorption of ethionamid, isoniazid and aminosalicylic acid from the post-resection gastrointestinal tract, Ann. Med. Exp. Biol. Fenn. **47**:209, 1969.

13. Nimmo, J., Heading, R.C., Tothill, P., and Prescott, L.F.: Pharmacological modification of gastric emptying: effects of propantheline and metoclopramide on paracetamol absorption, Br. Med. J. **1**:587, 1973.

14. Pagliaro, L.A., and Benet, L.Z.: Critical compilation of terminal half-lives, percent excreted unchanged, and changes of half-life in renal and hepatic dysfunction for studies in humans with references, J. Pharmacokinet. Biopharm. **3**:333, 1975.

15. Prescott, L.F.: Gastrointestinal absorption of drugs, Med. Clin. North Am. **58**:907, 1974.

16. Prescott, L.F.: Pathological and physiological factors affecting drug absorption, distribution, elimination, and response in man, Handb. Exp. Pharmacol. **28**(part 3):234, 1975.

17. Prescott, L.F. and Nimmo, J.: Generic inequivalence—clinical observations, Acta Pharmacol. Toxicol. (Copenh.) **29**(suppl. 3):288, 1971.

18. Reidenberg, M.M.: Kidney disease and drug metabolism, Med. Clin. North Am. **58**:1059, 1974.

19. Reidenberg, M.M., and Drayer, D.E.: Effects of renal disease upon drug disposition, Drug. Metab. Rev. **8**:293, 1978.

20. Reidenberg, M.M., Odar-Cederlöf, I., von Bahr, C., et al.: Protein binding of diphenylhydantoin and desmethylimipramine in plasma from patients with poor renal function, N. Engl. J. Med. **285**:264, 1971.

21. Routledge, P.A., Stargel, W.W., Wagner, G.S., and Shand, D.G.: Increased alpha-1-acid glycoprotein and lidocaine disposition in myocardial infarction, Ann. Intern. Med. **93**:701, 1980.

22. Shull, H.J., Wilkinson, G.R., Johnson, R., and Schenker, S.: Normal disposition of oxazepam in acute viral hepatitis and cirrhosis, Ann. Intern. Med. **84**:420, 1976.

23. Thomson, P.D., Melmon, K.L., Richardson, J.A., et al.: Lidocaine pharmacokinetics in advanced heart failure, liver disease, and renal failure in humans, Ann. Intern. Med. **78**:499, 1973.

24. Vesell, E.S., Page, J.G., and Passananti, G.T.: Genetic and environmental factors affecting ethanol metabolism in man, Clin. Pharmacol. Ther. **12**:192, 1971.

25. Williams, R.L., Schary, W.L., Blaschke, T.F., et al.: Influence of acute viral hepatitis on disposition and pharmacologic effect of warfarin, Clin. Pharmacol. Ther. **20**:90, 1976.

section two

Drug effects on the nervous system and neuroeffectors

10   General aspects of neuropharmacology, 82

11   Cholinergic drugs, 102

12   Cholinergic (muscarinic) blocking agents, 114

13   Ganglionic blocking agents, 127

14   Neuromuscular blocking agents and muscle relaxants, 132

15   Adrenergic (sympathomimetic) drugs, 142

16   Adrenergic blocking agents, 163

17   Drugs acting on the adrenergic neuron, 172

18   Antihypertensive drugs, 177

19   Histamine, 197

20   Antihistaminic drugs, 206

21   Serotonin, kinins, and miscellaneous autacoids, 214

22   Prostaglandins and leukotrienes, 227

Chapter 10

General aspects of neuropharmacology

The more than 10 billion neurons that constitute the human nervous system communicate with each other by means of chemical mediators. They also exert their effects on peripheral structures by release of these mediators and not by electrical impulses.

In the periphery acetylcholine and norepinephrine play the predominant roles in the autonomic nervous system. They act on postjunctional membranes, producing excitation or inhibition as a consequence of depolarization or hyperpolarization of these membranes. The role of presynaptic *autoreceptors* that influence release of neurotransmitters, exemplified by α_2-adrenergic receptors, in short- and long-term effects of drugs is of relatively recent interest and is likely to become of increasing importance in development of new drugs.

Amines, acetylcholine, certain amino acids, adenosine, and numerous peptides serve as neurotransmitters and modulators within the central nervous system. Among the amines, norepinephrine, dopamine, serotonin (5-hydroxytryptamine), and probably histamine and epinephrine play a role. Amino acids such as glutamic and aspartic acids excite postsynaptic membranes of many neurons, whereas γ-aminobutyric acid (GABA) and glycine are inhibitory transmitters. Substance P, the endorphins, and the enkephalins are among at least 30 peptides under consideration as neurotransmitters.[11] As improved techniques for assessing ligand binding to membrane recognition sites (putative receptors) have been developed, the number of known and postulated receptor types and subtypes has proliferated considerably.[18] The recent discovery that neurons may release more than one neurotransmitter, for example, an amine and a peptide, adds another level of complexity to be unraveled when one is trying to understand drug actions.[15]

Numerous drugs mimic or influence the action of chemical mediators and are classified as neuropharmacologic agents. Others that act by less well understood mechanisms may be classified according to their clinical usage as hypnotics, analgesics, anticonvulsants, and general or local anesthetics.

THE CHEMICAL NEUROTRANSMISSION CONCEPT

Similarities between responses to certain drugs and those to nerve stimulation were noted before this century. Muscarine, obtained from mushrooms, was known to slow heart rate, just like vagal stimulation. Adrenal extracts produced effects similar to those occurring after stimulation of sympathetic nerves (Oliver and Shafer, 1895).

Definitive proof of chemical neurotransmission was provided in 1921 by experiments of Loewi and of Cannon and Uridil. In his classic experiment Otto Loewi demonstrated that when the vagus nerve of a perfused frog heart was stimulated, a substance was released that could slow a second frog heart that had no neural connections to the first.[13] Cannon and Uridil found that sympathetic nerve stimulation of the liver released a substance that was similar to epinephrine in many respects.[3] This mediator, at first named "sympathin," is now known to be norepinephrine. Identification of the neurotransmitter in adrenergic axons as norepinephrine was provided by von Euler.[23]

Acetylcholine was first studied systematically by Dale.[4] The "quantum hypothesis" of acetylcholine release and of the role of synaptic vesicles in neuromuscular and synaptic transmission is a contribution of Katz and co-workers.[6,9] The discovery by Brodie and Shore[2] of monoamine release by reserpine led to a great expansion of knowledge regarding the metabolism and functions of catecholamines in the nervous system. The concept of uptake of catecholamines by sympathetic nerves was mainly developed by Axelrod.[1] The importance of these discoveries is attested to by the Nobel prizes that have been awarded to most of the investigators just cited.

After these developments, it was apparent that drugs need not act through nerves to influence an effector organ. In fact, it was then clear that nerves release chemical compounds that in turn influence the effectors. Instead of classifying drugs as sympathomimetic and parasympathomimetic, it was often more useful to classify nerves on the basis of the mediator released from them. This led to the concept of *cholinergic* and *adrenergic* nerve fibers.

The role of neurotransmitters at various anatomic sites is well established in some cases and is surmised in others. The generally accepted information on the site of action of these compounds may be summarized as follows:

SITES OF ACTION OF CHEMICAL MEDIATORS

1. Postganglionic parasympathetic nerve endings on smooth muscle, cardiac muscle, and exocrine glands: acetylcholine
2. Postganglionic sympathetic nerve endings on smooth muscle, cardiac muscle, and exocrine glands: norepinephrine (except for sweat glands)
3. All autonomic ganglionic synapses: acetylcholine
4. Motor fiber terminals at skeletal neuromuscular junctions: acetylcholine
5. Central nervous system synapses: acetylcholine, norepinephrine, dopamine, serotonin, histamine, glutamic and aspartic acids, GABA, glycine, adenosine, and numerous peptides

Although in the following discussion the postjunctional sites of drug action are emphasized, there is growing evidence for presynaptic actions of many drugs, particularly in relation to catecholamine release (see p. 144).

The sites of action of mediators in the autonomic nervous system are the most firmly established. The situation is much more complex in the central nervous system where neurophysiologic techniques are not sufficient for establishing the role of transmitters at a given site. Selective localization of active compounds in the brain with the use of immunofluorescence and biochemical identification of their binding sites are among newer approaches to establishing transmitter roles.

Mediators to sweat glands, adrenal medulla, and vascular smooth muscle

An important exception exists to the generalization that norepinephrine is the chemical mediator to sympathetically innervated structures. Sweat glands, which receive sympathetic innervation, are activated by cholinergic drugs and inhibited by anticholinergic drugs, such as atropine. This anomaly has been explained by the demonstration that postganglionic fibers innervating sweat glands are cholinergic rather than adrenergic.

The adrenal medulla primarily secretes epinephrine when cholinergic drugs are injected, a response inhibited by ganglionic blocking agents. Embryologically the adrenal medulla can be considered a modified sympathetic ganglion. It is therefore not surprising that it responds to acetylcholine, the normal ganglionic mediator to both sympathetic and parasympathetic postganglionic neurons.

Most vascular regions do not receive parasympathetic innervation so that direct control of vascular tone is mediated by variations in sympathetic input to the vessels. Nevertheless, stimulation of muscarinic receptors, possibly located in the vascular endothelium rather than on the smooth muscle, by circulating agonists can dilate blood vessels and cause pronounced hypotension.

RECEPTOR CONCEPT IN NEUROPHARMA-COLOGY

Neurotransmitters affect membranes by interacting with specific receptors. The existence of these receptors may be deduced from structure-activity studies on congeneric series of chemicals or from shifts of dose-response curves in the presence of specific antagonists. The following receptors may be postulated for some of the neurotransmitters:

1. Acetylcholine acts on muscarinic and nicotinic receptors. Cholinergic receptors in smooth muscles, cardiac muscle, and exocrine glands are termed *muscarinic* because muscarine, a quaternary amine alkaloid, has an action similar to that of acetylcholine at these sites. The muscarinic receptor is competitively blocked by atropine.

Nicotine acts on so-called *nicotinic* receptors for acetylcholine located in autonomic ganglia and at skeletal neuromuscular junctions. However, the receptors at these two sites are not identical. The action of acetylcholine in ganglia is antagonized by hexamethonium, whereas receptors in the end-plate regions of skeletal muscle are blocked by tubocurarine. At nicotinic sites, unlike muscarinic sites, an excess of agonist can cause persisting depolarization and blockade of transmission.

There are muscarinic and nicotinic receptors in the central nervous system also. For instance, the synapse between the collaterals of motor axons and the Renshaw cell is nicotinic. Muscarinic receptors are indicated by the ability of atropine to prevent many effects of central cholinergic stimulation.

2. Norepinephrine acts on adrenergic receptors that are classified as *alpha* (α)

and *beta* (β). Drugs that block these receptors are known as α- and β-*adrenergic blocking agents*. In addition, α-receptors are divided into α_1- and α_2-receptors, and β-receptors are divided into β_1- and β_2-receptors (see p. 144).

3. Dopamine acts on dopaminergic receptors in the central nervous system, in ganglia, and in the kidney. Dopaminergic receptors are blocked specifically by antipsychotic drugs such as the phenothiazines and butyrophenones. Dopamine also acts on β_1-receptors in the heart and in higher doses on α-receptors.

4. Serotonin acts on serotonergic receptors in the central nervous system and in some peripheral organs. Its action is blocked by antagonists such as methysergide.

5. Histamine acts on histaminergic receptors classified as H_1 and H_2. The antihistamines commonly used for hay fever are H_1-receptor antagonists, for example, diphenhydramine. H_2-receptor antagonists are relatively newer. A typical example is cimetidine.

Little is known about receptors for the amino acid transmitters, but glycine is antagonized by strychnine. GABA acts in a multireceptor complex that controls chloride ion permeability and is antagonized by bicuculline. Many other receptors are being investigated by radioligand binding techniques.[18]

The presence of receptors does not always denote neurotransmission, since hormones can also act on receptors. Furthermore, muscarinic receptors in most vascular smooth muscle and peripheral histamine receptors do not receive neuronal input.

Current understanding of the structure and function of this receptor derives to a large extent from studies of nicotinic receptors from eels and rays that have electric organs with an extremely high density of receptors. The binding sites for acetylcholine reside on components of a funnel-shaped ion channel (Fig. 10-1) that extends beyond both sides of the cell membrane and is composed of five subunits designated α, α, β, γ, and δ.[14] Binding of acetylcholine to both α subunits maximally opens the channel. The exact arrangement of the subunits is controversial, but the α subunits are not adjacent.

Newer concepts of the end-plate receptor

PROBLEM 10-1. *What accounts for the muscarinic or nicotinic nature of a cholinergic agent? Crystallographic analysis of acetylcholine and related agonists provides a tentative answer to this question. Acetylcholine is a flexible molecule, and rotation is possible at two different bonds. Muscarinic and nicotinic drugs differ from acetylcholine in the degree of rotation at the sites of torsion. Thus acetylcholine has both muscarinic and nicotinic activities, whereas purely muscarinic or nicotinic congeners have constraints imposed on them by conformational factors.*

The following steps may be distinguished in junctional transmission: (1) synthesis of the mediator, (2) binding (storage) of the mediator in a potentially active form, (3) release of the mediator, (4) binding of the mediator to a postjunctional receptor, (5) depolarization of the postjunctional membrane with a subsequent change in effector activity, (6) removal or inactivation of the mediator, and (7) repolarization of the postjunctional membrane. Theoretically, at least, drugs could influence transmission

SEQUENCE OF CHEMICAL EVENTS AT SYNAPSES AND NEUROEFFECTOR JUNCTIONS

FIG. 10-1 *Three-dimensional model of the funnel-shaped acetylcholine receptor from* Torpedo californica. Left, *Side view;* right, *view of extracellular surface with tentative assignment of subunit types.*

From McCarthy, M.P., Earnest, J.P., Young, E.F., Choe, S., and Stroud, R.M. Reproduced, with permission, from Annu. Rev. Neurosci. 9:387, copyright 1986 by Annual Reviews Inc.

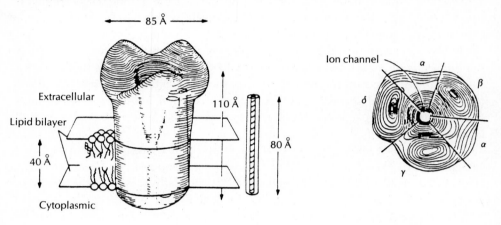

TABLE 10-1 Sites of drug action in relation to junctional transmission

Site of drug action	Mediator involved	
	Acetylcholine	Norepinephrine
Synthesis of mediator inhibited by	Hemicholinium	Metyrosine
Binding of mediator in granules inhibited by		Reserpine, guanethidine
Release of mediator enhanced by	Carbachol	Tyramine, amphetamine
Release of mediator inhibited by	Botulinus toxin	Bretylium, quanethidine

Depolarization of postsynaptic membrane promoted by	A. Muscarine
	  Choline esters
	  Pilocarpine
	B. Nicotine
	  Choline esters
	C. Nicotine
	  Choline esters
		Catecholamine and related amines

Depolarization of postsynaptic membrane inhibited by	A. Atropine
	B. Hexamethonium
	C. *d*-Tubocurarine
		α-Receptor blocking agents: e.g.,
		  phenoxybenzamine
		β-Receptor blocking agents: e.g.,
		  propranolol

Removal or inactivation of mediator inhibited by	Anticholinesterases	Cocaine, tricyclic antidepressants

A, Cholinergic neuroeffector site.
B, Ganglionic site.
C, Skeletal neuromuscular site.

Cholinergic nerve terminal depicting the synthesis, storage, and release of acetylcholine   **FIG. 10-2**
(ACh), its hydrolysis by acetylcholinesterase, and its action on cholinergic receptors on
the effector cell and presynaptic membrane.

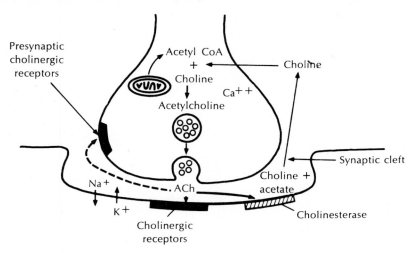

by acting at any of these steps, and, indeed, we have examples of many such inter-actions, as shown in Table 10-1.

A synapse is the site of transmission of the nerve impulse between two neurons. The axonal terminal is separated from the postsynaptic membrane by a synaptic cleft of about 20 nm in width. Electron micrographs show that the presynaptic element contains numerous vesicles in which the transmitter is stored.

Transmission of the nerve impulse across a synapse is quite different from axonal conduction. First, transmission is unidirectional. Second, when the axon is stimulated electrically, there is a delay of about 0.2 second before the postsynaptic element is depolarized.

At a skeletal neuromuscular junction an axon terminal of the somatic motoneuron lies within the gutters of the end-plate region (Fig. 10-2). An action potential causes Ca^{++} influx, which releases acetylcholine from vesicles in the axon terminal.[17] The acetylcholine diffuses across the gap and changes the permeability of the postjunctional membrane to Na^+ and K^+. The release process is inhibited by Mg^{++}.

At the termination of autonomic nerve fibers at neuroeffector junctions in smooth muscles, cardiac muscle, and exocrine glands, there are no specialized structures analogous to the motor end plate. The transmitters apparently are discharged from varicosities along the terminal plexuses into the extracellular space to reach receptors by diffusion.

FIG. 10-3   *Autonomic innervation of various organs.*

Redrawn from a Sandoz Pharmaceuticals publication.

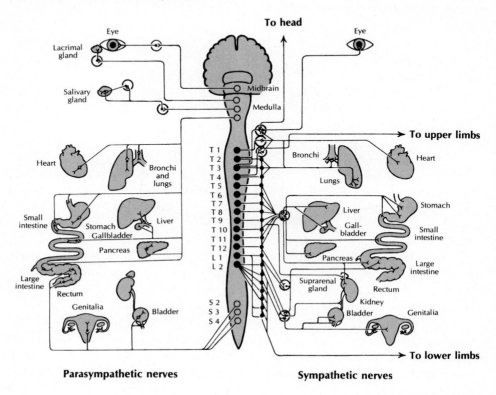

FIG. 10-4   *Schematic representation of autonomic innervation of neuroeffector cells. Ach, Acetylcholine; NE, norepinephrine.*

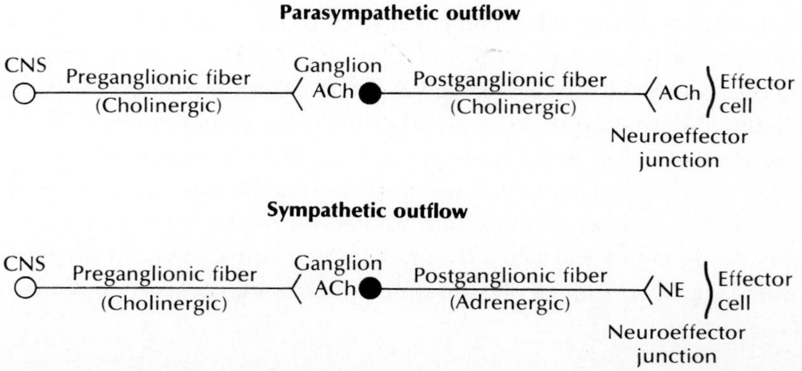

See Figs. 10-3 and 10-4 for a display of organs innervated by the autonomic nervous system and a schema of parasympathetic and sympathetic outflows to the neuroeffector cells.

The role of a mediator in neurotransmission is suggested or established by some or all of the following:

1. Presence of the transmitter in the axon along with enzymes responsible for its production and destruction
2. Similarity of the mediator's effect to that of nerve stimulation
3. Release of the transmitter by nerve stimulation
4. Blockade of the effect of nerve stimulation by drugs that block the transmitter's action

Most of these criteria can be met in studies of neuromuscular and ganglionic transmission. There are formidable difficulties in proving the transmitter role of a substance in the central nervous system by these same criteria. A chemical is often, at least tentatively, accepted as a transmitter in the central nervous system if it is present naturally in relatively high concentrations in brain regions that exhibit the capacity for high affinity, preferably stereospecific, binding of the substance, especially if local electrical stimulation and microinjection of the compound elicit similar responses. Prime examples are the opioid peptides, the enkephalins. Agents that selectively deplete the brain of a particular compound can be very useful for assessment of the physiologic roles of probable neurotransmitters.

EVIDENCE FOR CHOLINERGIC AND ADRENERGIC NEUROTRANSMISSION

The response of effector cells may be altered remarkably under certain circumstances. The conditions that have received the most attention are sensitization after denervation and sensitization in the presence of other drugs.

FACTORS INFLUENCING RESPONSE OF EFFECTORS TO CHEMICAL MEDIATORS

The supersensitivity of surgically or chemically denervated structures develops by various mechanisms. Supersensitivity to catecholamines has been studied mostly on the nictitating membrane where two types of supersensitivity may develop.[22] Supersensitivity after postganglionic surgical denervation is correlated with degeneration of adrenergic nerve terminals. It is specific for catecholamines and related amines, develops within 48 hours after denervation, and is undoubtedly related to disappearance of the catecholamine uptake mechanism (see p. 94). Preganglionic denervation, or *decentralization*, is much less effective in increasing the susceptibility of effectors to neurotransmitters. This type of supersensitivity appears to be postjunctional on the effector and requires weeks for its development. It is a consequence of chronically reduced levels of transmitter. Such denervation need not be surgical.

Denervation supersensitivity

Chronic administration of a ganglionic blocking agent to a guinea pig can increase the sensitivity of its isolated ileum to histamine, potassium, and serotonin as well as to the normal postganglionic mediator acetylcholine.[7] Similarly, chronic administration of reserpine can cause supersensitivity to catecholamines by sustained depletion of transmitter.

A specialized supersensitivity develops in denervated skeletal muscle. A week or two after denervation, the surface of the entire muscle fiber becomes responsive to externally applied acetylcholine, whereas only the end-plate region was sensitive before denervation. New acetylcholine receptors have spread as a consequence of denervation.[19]

Sensitization by drugs

In contrast to supersensitivity induced by denervation or prolonged inactivity, more rapid sensitization to neurotransmitters and related drugs can be produced by certain other agents.

Enzyme inhibitors may be quite effective. Inhibitors of acetylcholinesterase immediately potentiate the actions of acetylcholine.

Drugs may interfere with reflex mechanisms and thereby allow greater fluctuation in a physiologic parameter such as blood pressure when a neuropharmacologic agent is administered. Ganglionic blocking agents increase the effectiveness of injected vasopressor drugs by interfering with buffering reflexes.

Cocaine and tricyclic antidepressants enhance sensitivity by interfering with prejunctional catecholamine reuptake by adrenergic terminals (see p. 94). These same compounds can block the actions of guanethidine and indirectly acting sympathomimetic drugs such as tyramine that must be actively pumped into sympathetic nerve endings to reach their site of action.

Direct radioligand studies indicate that the *number* of receptors may change under various circumstances. An increase in receptor number is referred to as *upregulation* and a decrease in receptor number as *downregulation*.[12] High concentrations of adrenergic agents can lead to decreased numbers of receptors, whereas a reduction in the tissue or serum levels of catecholamines has the opposite effect. These concepts may explain changes in sensitivity to mediators in various disease states. They may also explain changes in sensitivity to various mediators induced by hormones and drugs. For example, it is tempting to attribute the propranolol withdrawal syndrome (see p. 169) to an increase in receptor number and increased responsiveness to endogenous catecholamines.[12]

NEUROTRANSMITTER KINETICS AND THE NERVOUS SYSTEM

Aside from acetylcholine, the best studied neurotransmitters are nitrogenous bases synthesized by neurons from precursors and stored in vesicles for release by exocytosis. The active amines do not cross the blood-brain barrier efficiently, whereas their precursor amino acids do.

Acetylcholine is present in certain autonomic nerves and in nerve endings in the brain, where its vesicular localization has been demonstrated. Acetylcholine is synthesized by the cytoplasmic enzyme choline acetyltransferase (CAT).

$$\text{Choline} + \text{Acetyl coenzyme A} \xrightarrow{\text{CAT}} \text{Acetylcholine} + \text{Coenzyme A}$$

Acetylcholine

The compound *hemicholinium* blocks synthesis of the mediator by interfering with transport of choline across the neuronal membrane. Botulinus toxin blocks release of acetylcholine.

During nerve stimulation, recently synthesized acetylcholine appears to be preferentially released.[5] Acetylcholine released by a nerve impulse must be destroyed rapidly so that the acetylcholine released by the next impulse can act within a few milliseconds on a repolarized postsynaptic membrane. Hydrolysis of acetylcholine reduces the potency of the compound a hundred-thousandfold.

Destruction of acetylcholine is accomplished by *cholinesterases*, which are of two types. *Acetylcholinesterase*, or specific cholinesterase, hydrolyzes acetyl esters of choline more rapidly than butyryl esters. On the other hand, *pseudocholinesterase*, or nonspecific cholinesterase, is also called butyrylcholinesterase because it hydrolyzes butyrylcholine more rapidly than it hydrolyzes the acetyl ester. Acetylcholinesterase is localized within neuronal membranes and, surprisingly, also in membranes of red blood cells where its function is unknown. Nonspecific cholinesterase is widely distributed in the body. Plasma cholinesterase is of the nonspecific type. Its presence in plasma is not related to neural activity. Its low titer after exposure to anticholinesterase pesticides is a useful indication of such poisonings. The titer of plasma cholinesterase is depressed also in advanced liver disease, since the enzyme is manufactured in the liver.

The collective term for norepinephrine, epinephrine, and dopamine is *catecholamine*, since these neurotransmitters are catechols (*ortho*-dihydroxybenzenes) and contain an amine group in their aliphatic side chain.

Catecholamines

The distribution of catecholamines in the body is well understood, thanks to suitable methods for their determination, such as fluorometric assay. In addition, histochemical fluorescence microscopy techniques developed by Swedish investigators allow an actual visualization of catecholamine-containing structures (see Fig. 15-1), their precise localization, and their susceptibility to drug actions.

Localization

Norepinephrine is present in adrenergic fibers and in certain pathways within the central nervous system. *Epinephrine* constitutes most of the catecholamine in the human adrenal medulla, though adrenal medullary tumors (pheochromocytomas) may contain primarily norepinephrine. Small amounts of epinephrine may exist also in various organs and in the central nervous system, but its main recognized source is the adrenal medulla. *Dopamine* is present in relatively high concentrations in the brain, particularly in the caudate nucleus and the putamen (Table 10-2).

TABLE 10-2   Distribution of norepinephrine and dopamine in the human brain (micrograms/gram)

	Norepinephrine	Dopamine
Frontal lobe	0.00-0.02	0.00
Caudate nucleus	0.04	3.12
Putamen	0.02	5.27
Hypothalamus (anterior part)	0.96	0.18
Substantia nigra	0.04	0.40
Pons	0.04	0.00
Medulla oblongata (dorsal part)	0.13	0.00
Cerebellar cortex	0.02	0.02

Based on data from Bertler, Å.: Acta Physiol. Scand. 51:97, 1961.

The distribution of norepinephrine in various organs corresponds well with their adrenergic innervation. Although there is considerable species variation, the heart, arteries, and veins of most mammals contain norepinephrine of the order of 1 μg/g of tissue.[23] The liver, lungs, and skeletal muscle contain considerably less, whereas the vas deferens has about five to 10 times as much.

BIOSYNTHESIS   The biosynthesis of catecholamines represents a small but very important portion of the metabolism of tyrosine. Other pathways lead to the formation of thyroxin, melanin, protein, and peptides. Tyrosine is taken up directly by neurons for catecholamine synthesis.

The steps in biosynthesis of catecholamines are shown in Fig. 10-5.

Tyrosine hydroxylase, a cytoplasmic enzyme, catalyzes the rate-limiting step in catecholamine biosynthesis. Inhibition of this enzyme by the amino acid analog metyrosine (α-methyl-*p*-tyrosine) leads to depletion of catecholamines from brain and sympathetic nerves.

Aromatic L-amino acid decarboxylase is a cytoplasmic enzyme that decarboxylates several substrates besides dopa (3,4-dihydroxyphenylalanine), for example, 5-hydroxytryptophan to serotonin.

Dopamine-β-hydroxylase, a copper-containing enzyme bound to membranes of the axoplasmic granules, catalyzes the conversion of dopamine to norepinephrine. This enzyme is inhibited by copper reagents such as disulfiram and diethyldithiocarbamate. The enzyme is associated primarily with larger catecholamine vesicles, and sufficient sympathetic stimulation leads to the appearance of dopamine-β-hydroxylase activity in the circulation.[8]

Phenylethanolamine-N-*methyltransferase* is a cytoplasmic enzyme present largely in the adrenal medulla where it catalyzes the transfer of a methyl group from *S*-adenosylmethionine to norepinephrine for the formation of epinephrine.

Pathway of synthesis of catecholamines. Enzymes catalyzing various reactions are as **FIG. 10-5**
follows: 1, tyrosine hydroxylase; 2, aromatic L-amino acid decarboxylase; 3, dopamine-β-
hydroxylase; 4, phenylethanolamine-N-methyltransferase. Dopa, 3,4-Dihydroxyphenyl-
alanine.

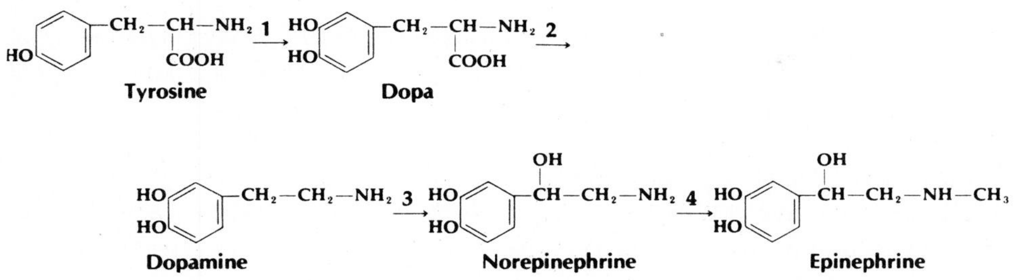

Negative feedback of catecholamine biosynthesis. Sympathetic nerve stimulation does not cause catecholamine depletion in the axon; this means synthesis can keep up with loss. With the discovery of tyrosine hydroxylase as the rate-limiting enzyme in catecholamine biosynthesis, the relative constancy of catecholamine stores can be explained. Norepinephrine inhibits tyrosine hydroxylase. It becomes understandable, then, that increased catecholamine release through sympathetic activity, by decreasing intraneuronal norepinephrine, will accelerate synthesis of catecholamines in nerve terminals. On the other hand, monoamine oxidase (MAO) inhibitors, which elevate catecholamine levels in adrenergic neurons, reduce catecholamine biosynthesis. Thus regulation of norepinephrine synthesis in adrenergic neurons is achieved by end-product inhibition. In addition to these intraneuronal influences, stimulation of receptors on the axon terminals (presynaptic α_2-autoreceptors, see p. 144) by endogenous or exogenous norepinephrine or related agents also inhibits subsequent release of the neurotransmitter. Stimulation of presynaptic receptors for neurotransmitters other than the one released by a particular neuron may also affect transmitter release.

Catecholamines are stored in both large and small vesicles in association with **STORAGE AND RELEASE** adenosine triphosphate.[8] The large vesicles, formed originally in the cell body and then transported to the endings by axoplasmic flow, also contain dopamine-β-hydroxylase, the soluble protein *chromogranin*, and opioid peptides. These vesicles appear primarily responsible for the conversion of dopamine to norepinephrine, some of which escapes into the cytoplasm to be taken up by the smaller vesicles or metabolized.

Release of catecholamines is generally believed to take place by exocytosis. Adenosine triphosphate, chromogranin, and dopamine-β-hydroxylase, in addition to the catecholamine, are released by sympathetic nerve stimulation. Although these findings indicate that the larger vesicles empty their contents, other evidence indicates that recently synthesized catecholamine is released preferentially, probably from the small vesicles.[21] Catecholamine release requires calcium and in this respect is similar to acetylcholine release from cholinergic nerves and to histamine release from mast cells.

In contrast to release by exocytosis, reserpine "releases" catecholamines from granules into the axoplasm, where they are deaminated by MAO (see below) present in the axonal mitochondria.

DISPOSITION OF THE
RELEASED
CATECHOLAMINE

Reuptake. The relative constancy of catecholamine stores in adrenergic or dopaminergic neurons not only is a consequence of feedback regulation of its biosynthesis, but it is also an expression of a remarkable ability to transport the amine back into these neurons. This "reuptake," which may conserve more than half the released catecholamine, is achieved by an amine pump that is located in the nerve membrane and requires sodium.

Several observations indicate that uptake of catecholamines by nerves is the most important mechanism for termination of their action. First, injection of small, physiologic doses of tritiated norepinephrine results in its rapid clearance from the blood by the heart and other organs innervated by adrenergic fibers. That this uptake is into adrenergic fibers has been demonstrated by histochemical techniques in vitro. Furthermore, subsequent sympathetic nerve stimulation or reserpine treatment causes release of tritiated catecholamine in vivo.

Denervated organs take up only very small quantities of tritiated norepinephrine. Such organs, however, are supersensitive to catecholamines. Cocaine, tricyclic antidepressants such as desipramine, ouabain, and even certain antihistamines can block uptake of norepinephrine and enhance the potency of catecholamines.

The relatively nonspecific amine pump transports not only catecholamines but also other amines, including tyramine, amphetamine, and even serotonin. Some of these, such as metaraminol, are retained by the axon terminal and released on nerve stimulation, thereby acting as *false transmitters*. Such false transmitters may be relatively weak agonists, and so transmission is impaired (octopamine, metaraminol), or they may be potent agonists and effectively mimic norepinephrine. The antihypertensive amino acid α-methyldopa is actively taken up by the neuron and transformed to α-methylnorepinephrine, which acts as a potent false transmitter.

Despite the low specificity of the amine pump, the adrenergic neuron is protected against the accumulation of numerous amines by the much greater specificity of the granular storage mechanism. Thus, when tyramine is taken up, it is not only deaminated by MAO but is also rejected by the granules, since only β-hydroxylated amines are stored. After the use of MAO inhibitors, however, tyramine, which is then protected against deamination, is transformed by the fairly nonspecific dopamine-β-hydroxylase into the β-hydroxy derivative *octopamine*, which is stored in the granules and acts as a false transmitter.

Adrenergic nerve terminals also take up compounds that may be injurious to them. The experimental agent 6-*hydroxydopamine* causes degenerative changes in

Fate of norepinephrine released from adrenergic nerve. 1, Release and interaction with   **FIG. 10-6**
receptor on effector cell; 2, reuptake into the nerve of a portion of released norepinephrine; 3, metabolism by COMT and MAO; 4, metabolic degradation within the nerve by MAO of norepinephrine released within the axoplasm (as after ingestion of reserpine).

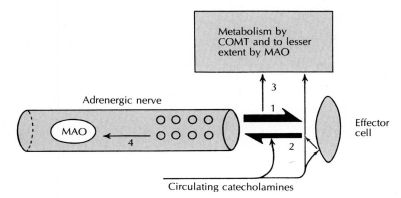

adrenergic nerve terminals, leading to *chemical sympathectomy*. Desipramine, a blocker of the amine pump, prevents these effects.

Extraneuronal metabolism. The portion of the released catecholamine that diffuses away to escape reuptake by the amine pump is metabolized extraneuronally by two enzymes: *catechol-O-methyltransferase* (COMT) and monoamine oxidase (MAO).[10] The latter is widely distributed in the body, not only in adrenergic axonal mitochondria, where it metabolizes cytoplasmic norepinephrine, but also in nonneural structures, in particular the liver and kidneys. MAO-A, the form primarily involved in metabolism of norepinephrine, is found in adrenergic neurons and adrenergic nuclei in the brain. MAO-B is localized to serotonergic neurons and astrocytes. COMT is also widely distributed and is concentrated in the liver and kidneys. Although the precise relationship of these enzymes to sympathetic function is not understood, it is clearly not so crucial as the acetylcholine-cholinesterase interdependence. For example, inhibition of COMT by catechol or pyrogallol does not significantly increase sympathetic activity or potentiate the action of injected catecholamines. Similarly, drugs that inhibit MAO fail to potentiate the action of catecholamines and do not increase sympathetic functions in the periphery. These relationships may become clearer by an examination of Fig. 10-6.

The detailed metabolic pathways of norepinephrine and epinephrine are shown in Fig. 10-7. MOPEG, metanephrine, and normetanephrine are excreted primarily as conjugates. The role of many of these pathways may be appreciated from data on urinary elimination of the metabolites; the proportions of norepinephrine metabolites have been estimated as follows[10]:

Normetanephrine	3%-5%
4-Hydroxy-3-methoxyphenyl(ethylene) glycol (MOPEG)	30%-40%
4-Hydroxy-3-methoxymandelic acid (VMA)	55%-65%

Pathways of metabolism of norepinephrine and epinephrine. Enzymes catalyzing various reactions are as follows: **FIG. 10-7**
1, Monoamine oxidase (MAO) and aldehyde dehydrogenase; 2, MAO and aldehyde reductase; 3, catechol-O-methyltransferase; DOPEG, 3,4-dihydroxyphenyl(ethylene) glycol; DOMA, 3,4-dihydroxymandelic acid; MOPEG, MHPG, 4-hydroxy-3-methoxyphenyl(ethylene) glycol; VMA, vanillylmandelic acid, 4-hydroxy-3-methoxymandelic acid.

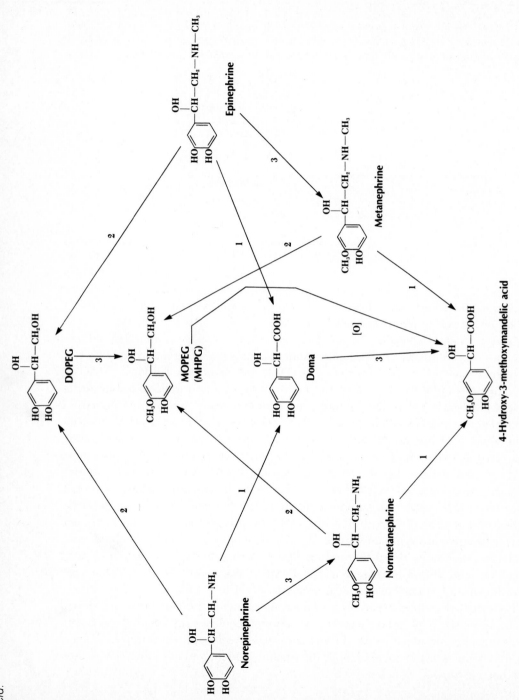

The 24-hour excretion of VMA in normal persons is about 3 mg. Much larger amounts may be eliminated by patients with adrenal medullary tumors (p. 152). Small amounts of unmetabolized catecholamines are also excreted. The particular pattern of metabolites in the urine depends on the source of amines, that is, neuronal, adrenal medullary, or exogenous.

The administration of 6-hydroxydopamine, an interesting experimental tool, causes an extremely long-lasting depletion of catecholamines from sympathetically innervated organs. Electron microscopic studies indicate that the drug causes a selective destruction of adrenergic nerve terminals. In newborn animals the entire neuron is destroyed irreversibly, whereas in adults only the terminals are affected so that regeneration of the fibers is possible.[20] Because 6-hydroxydopamine does not cross the blood-brain barrier, it must be injected into the cerebral ventricles to destroy adrenergic terminals in the central nervous system.

CHEMICAL SYMPATHECTOMY: 6-HYDROXYDOPAMINE

Serotonin, or 5-hydroxytryptamine, is present in high concentrations in the enterochromaffin cells of the intestinal tract and in the pineal gland. It is also present in the brain, in platelets, and in mast cells of rats and mice. Serotonin occurs also in some fruits, such as bananas.

Serotonin

The steps in the biosynthesis of serotonin are as follows:

$$\text{Tryptophan} \xrightarrow{\text{Tryptophan hydroxylase}} \text{5-Hydroxytryptophan} \xrightarrow[\text{decarboxylase}]{\text{Aromatic L-amino acid}} \text{5-Hydroxytryptamine}$$

Serotonin is degraded to 5-hydroxyindolacetic acid (5-HIAA) by the enzyme MAO. The daily excretion of 5-HIAA in humans is about 3 mg. This may increase greatly in patients with malignancy of enterochromaffin cells or after administration of reserpine. Ingestion of bananas also increases the concentration of 5-HIAA in urine to a minor extent.

In the pineal gland, in addition to a high concentration of serotonin, there is also melatonin (5-methoxy-*N*-acetyltryptamine), a biosynthetic product of the amine. Melatonin lightens skin color by affecting melanocytes, and its synthesis is greatly influenced by light.

In addition to the neurotransmitters discussed above, several other compounds may play a role in neural function, though the evidence for characterizing them as mediators of neurotransmission is less than complete.

Histamine is present in the hypothalamus along with serotonin and catecholamines. The brain can form histamine from histidine and is rich in the methylating enzyme that inactivates this amine.

Glutamic and **aspartic acids** are remarkably potent in depolarizing nerve cells when applied by iontophoresis. Furthermore, analogs of these acids, such as kainic acid, ibotenic acid, and *N*-methyl-D-aspartic acid, are also powerful agonists on central neurons.

MISCELLANEOUS POTENTIAL NEUROTRANS- MITTERS

Autonomic and related drugs

Classification by site of action *and* mode of action

I. Drugs acting on autonomic receptors in end organs
  A. Agonists mimicking postganglionic transmitters
    1. Cholinergic drugs (parasympathomimetics)
      a. Direct action on effector cell (effective after denervation)—acetylcholine, pilocarpine
      b. Indirect action (potentiate endogenous ACh; ineffective after denervation)
        (1) Competitive cholinesterase inhibitors—physostigmine
        (2) Noncompetitive cholinesterase inhibitors—isoflurophate (DFP) (enzyme reactivated by pralidoxime)
    2. Adrenergic drugs (sympathomimetics)
      a. Direct action on effector cell (effective after denervation)—norepinephrine, epinephrine, isoproterenol
      b. Indirect action (release norepinephrine from adrenergic nerve endings; ineffective peripherally after denervation)—tyramine, amphetamine
      c. Mixed action (direct and indirect)—ephedrine, metaraminol
  B. Antagonists acting on end-organ receptors
    1. Cholinergic receptor antagonists (cholinergic blocking drugs)
      a. Competitive antagonists at muscarinic receptors—atropine
    2. Adrenergic receptor antagonists (adrenergic blocking drugs)
      a. Antagonize at α-adrenergic receptors
        (1) Competitive—phentolamine
        (2) Noncompetitive—phenoxybenzamine
      b. Antagonize at β-adrenergic receptors
        (1) Competitive—propranolol
II. Drugs acting on autonomic nerve endings
  A. Agonists that cause the release of transmitters
    1. Cholinergic neurons—carbachol
    2. Adrenergic neurons—indirect and mixed acting sympathomimetics
  B. Drugs that inhibit the release of transmitters
    1. Cholinergic neurons—botulin toxin
    2. Adrenergic neurons—bretylium, guanethidine
  C. Drugs that inhibit the synthesis of transmitters
    1. Cholinergic neurons (inhibits synthesis of ACh)—hemicholinium
    2. Adrenergic neurons (inhibits synthesis of norepinephrine)—metyrosine
  D. Drugs that inhibit the storage of transmitters in neurons
    1. Cholinergic neurons—none
    2. Adrenergic neurons (deplete norepinephrine)—reserpine, guanethidine
  E. Drugs that cause the formation of false transmitters in neurons
    1. Cholinergic neurons—none
    2. Adrenergic neurons—methyldopa, metaraminol
  F. Drugs that inhibit the uptake of transmitters into neurons
    1. Cholinergic neurons—none
    2. Adrenergic neurons—cocaine, tricyclic antidepressants
III. Drugs acting on autonomic ganglia
  A. Agonists that stimulate postganglionic neurons ("nicotinic" stimulants)
    1. Both cholinergic and adrenergic neurons—nicotine
  B. Antagonists that inhibit nicotinic receptors or postganglionic neurons
    1. Both cholinergic and adrenergic neurons (competitive antagonists)—hexamethonium, mecamylamine

---

Nonautonomic drugs

  I. Drugs acting on the skeletal muscle neuromuscular junction
    A. Agonists mimicking the motor nerve transmitter acetylcholine
      1. Direct action on muscle cell—neostigmine
      2. Indirect action (cholinesterase inhibitors)
        a. Competitive—neostigmine, physostigmine
        b. Noncompetitive—isoflurophate
    B. Antagonists that block skeletal muscle receptors
      1. Depolarizing—succinylcholine
      2. Nondepolarizing (competitive)—tubocurarine
  II. Drugs acting on sensory nerve endings
    A. "Sensitize" stretch receptors monitoring blood pressure—*Veratrum* alkaloids
  III. Drugs acting on all nerves to block conduction of action potentials
    A. Local anesthetics
  IV. Drugs acting on vascular smooth muscle
    A. Vasoconstrictors—angiotensin, vasopressin
    B. Vasodilators—nitrites, papaverine
    C. Antihypertensive drugs—hydralazine, diazoxide
  V. Other endogenous biologically active compounds
    A. Serotonin, histamine, bradykinin, prostaglandins, peptides, etc.

Glycine is recognized increasingly as a major inhibitory transmitter in the spinal cord. This simple amino acid is present in high concentration in the spinal cord and causes hyperpolarization of motoneurons. Since strychnine is known to antagonize the naturally occurring inhibitory transmitter released from Renshaw cells onto motoneurons, it was of great interest to examine the possible relationship between the alkaloid and glycine. Antagonism of the hyperpolarizing effect of glycine by strychnine, applied by microelectrophoresis, has been clearly demonstrated. Interestingly, tetanus toxin in the same system does not antagonize glycine, implying a presynaptic site of action for the toxin.

γ-Aminobutyric acid (GABA) is now believed to be the primary inhibitory neurotransmitter in the brain and has been postulated to be released at up to 50% of all brain synapses. This compound is formed by decarboxylation of glutamic acid and is destroyed by transamination. Brain tissue contains significant quantities of GABA.

$$\underset{\textbf{Glutamic acid}}{\text{HOOC—}\overset{\overset{\textstyle\textbf{NH}_2}{|}}{\text{CH}}\text{—CH}_2\text{—CH}_2\text{—COOH}} \qquad \underset{\textbf{γ-Aminobutyric acid}}{\text{H}_2\text{N—CH}_2\text{—CH}_2\text{—CH}_2\text{—COOH}}$$

Several **peptides** are implicated as important neurotransmitters in the central nervous system.[11] Much of the impetus in this area was provided by discoveries with the opioid peptides (see Chapter 29). Substance P, somatostatin, cholecystokinin, and other peptides are present in spinal ganglia and the spinal cord,[16] as shown by immunocytochemical studies. Substance P contains 11 amino acids and appears to be a sensory neurotransmitter with an important role in nociception. Capsaicin, obtained from red pepper, depletes substance P from the spinal cord and elevates the threshold to painful stimuli.

CLASSIFICATION OF NEUROPHARMACOLOGIC AGENTS

The rational classification of neuropharmacologic agents should be based on their site and mode of action, reflecting drug-receptor interactions. This can be done satisfactorily for drugs acting on autonomic end organs, nerve endings, and ganglia and at skeletal neuromuscular junctions. At each site we have agonists and antagonists or drugs that promote or inhibit the release of neurotransmitters.

For the sake of simplicity, autonomic drugs are classified in the succeeding chapters as cholinergic drugs, anticholinergic drugs (various types), adrenergic drugs, and adrenergic blocking drugs (alpha [α] and beta [β]).

REFERENCES

1. Axelrod, J.: The metabolism of catecholamines *in vivo* and *in vitro*, Pharmacol. Rev. **11**:402, 1959.
2. Brodie, B.B., Spector, S., and Shore, P.A.: Interaction of drugs with norepinephrine in the brain, Pharmacol. Rev. **11**:548, 1959.
3. Cannon, W.B., and Uridil, J.E.: Studies on the conditions of activity in endocrine glands. VIII. Some effects on the denervated heart of stimulating the nerves of the liver, Am. J. Physiol. **58**:353, 1921.
4. Dale, H.H.: The action of certain esters and ethers of choline, and their relation to muscarine, J. Pharmacol. Exp. Ther. **6**:147, 1914.
5. Dunant, Y.: On the mechanism of acetylcholine release, Prog. Neurobiol. **26**:55, 1986.
6. Fatt, P., and Katz, B.: Spontaneous subthreshold activity at motor nerve endings, J. Physiol. (London) **117**:109, 1952.
7. Fleming, W.W.: Nonspecific supersensitivity of the guinea-pig ileum produced by chronic ganglion blockade, J. Pharmacol. Exp. Ther. **162**:277, 1968.
8. Fried, G., Lagercrantz, H., Klein, R., and Thureson-Klein, Å.: Large and small noradrenergic vesicles—origin, contents, and functional significance. In Usdin, E., Carlsson, A., Dahlström, A., and Engel, J., editors: Catecholamines. Part A: Basic and peripheral mechanisms, New York, 1984, Alan R. Liss, Inc., p. 45.
9. Katz, B., and Miledi, R.: Propagation of electric activity in motor nerve terminals, Proc. R. Soc. Lond. [Biol.] **161**:453, 1965.
10. Kopin, I.J.: Catecholamine metabolism: basic aspects and clinical significance, Pharmacol. Rev. **37**:333, 1985.
11. Krieger, D.T.: Brain peptides, Vitam. Horm. **41**:1, 1984.
12. Lefkowitz, R.J.: Direct binding studies of adrenergic receptors: biochemical, physiologic, and clinical implications, Ann. Intern. Med. **91**:450, 1979.
13. Loewi, O.: Über humorale Übertragbarkeit der Herznervenwirkung, Pflugers Arch. Ges. Physiol. **189**:239, 1921.
14. McCarthy, M.P., Earnest, J.P., Young, E.F., et al.: The molecular neurobiology of the acetylcholine receptor, Annu. Rev. Neurosci. **9**:383, 1986.

15. O'Donohue, T.L., Millington, W.R., Handelmann, G.E., et al.: On the 50th anniversary of Dale's law: multiple neurotransmitter neurons, Trends Pharmacol. Sci. **6:**305, 1985.

16. Schoenen, J., Lotstra, F., Vierendeels, G., et al.: Substance P, enkephalins, somatostatin, cholecystokinin, oxytocin, and vasopressin in human spinal cord, Neurology (N.Y.) **35:**881, 1985.

17. Silinsky, E.M.: The biophysical pharmacology of calcium-dependent acetylcholine secretion, Pharmacol. Rev. **37:**81, 1985.

18. Snyder, S.H.: Drug and neurotransmitter receptors in the brain, Science **224:**22, 1984.

19. Thesleff, S.: Effects of motor innervation on the chemical sensitivity of skeletal muscle, Physiol. Rev. **40:**734, 1960.

20. Thoenen, H., and Tranzer, J.P.: The pharmacology of 6-hydroxydopamine, Annu. Rev. Pharmacol. **13:**169, 1973.

21. Thureson-Klein, Å.: The roles of large and small noradrenergic vesicles in exocytosis. In Usdin, E., Carlsson, A., Dahlström, A., and Engel, J., editors: Catecholamines, Part A: Basic and peripheral mechanisms, New York, 1984, Alan R. Liss, Inc., p. 79.

22. Trendelenburg, U.: I. Mechanisms of supersensitivity and subsensitivity to sympathomimetic amines, Pharmacol. Rev. **18:**629, 1966.

23. von Euler, U.S.: Noradrenaline: chemistry, physiology, pharmacology and clinical aspects, Springfield, Ill., 1956, Charles C Thomas, Publisher.

Chapter 11

Cholinergic drugs

Cholinergic agents can be divided into two major groups: directly acting cholinergic agonists and indirectly acting cholinesterase inhibitors (anticholinesterases).

DIRECTLY ACTING
CHOLINERGIC
AGONISTS
Choline esters

Although acetylcholine is essential for normal neural control of function of many organs in the body, two characteristics render it unsuitable as a drug. First, its action is very brief, even when it is injected intravenously, because of rapid destruction by ubiquitous cholinesterases. Second, it causes such diverse effects that no selective therapeutic end point is possible. Derivatives of acetylcholine, however, are more resistant to the action of cholinesterases and exhibit greater selectivity in their sites of action.

As the acetylcholine-cholinesterase interaction is depicted in Fig. 11-1, it is apparent that changes in the structure of the ester should alter its union with the enzyme. Relatively slight modifications can reduce or prevent hydrolysis of the molecule but still allow the ester to stimulate cholinergic receptors. Important agents in this category are as follows:

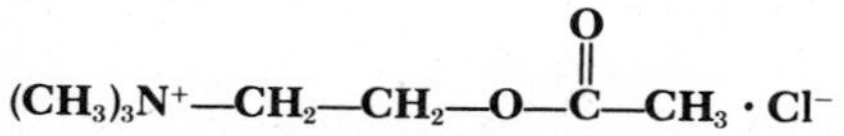

$$(CH_3)_3N^+—CH_2—CH_2—O—\overset{\overset{\textstyle O}{\|}}{C}—CH_3 \cdot Cl^-$$
Acetylcholine chloride

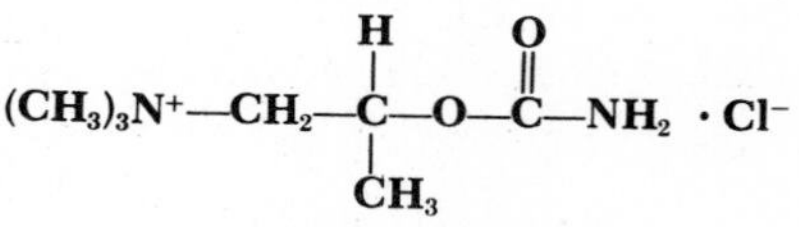

$$(CH_3)_3N^+—CH_2—\overset{\overset{\textstyle H}{|}}{\underset{\underset{\textstyle CH_3}{|}}{C}}—O—\overset{\overset{\textstyle O}{\|}}{C}—NH_2 \cdot Cl^-$$
Bethanechol chloride

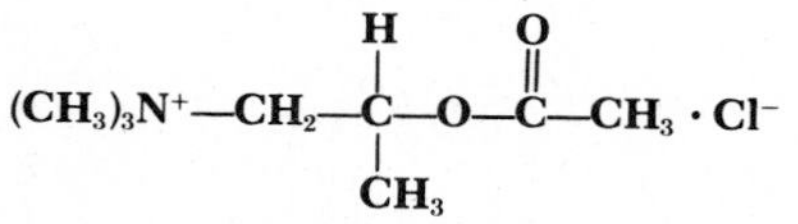

$$(CH_3)_3N^+—CH_2—\overset{\overset{\textstyle H}{|}}{\underset{\underset{\textstyle CH_3}{|}}{C}}—O—\overset{\overset{\textstyle O}{\|}}{C}—CH_3 \cdot Cl^-$$
Methacholine chloride

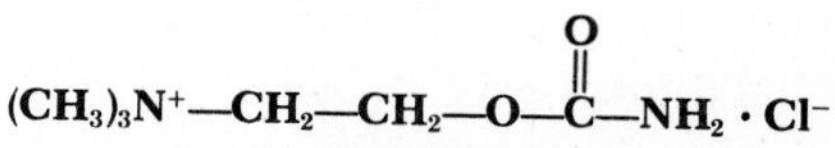

$$(CH_3)_3N^+—CH_2—CH_2—O—\overset{\overset{\textstyle O}{\|}}{C}—NH_2 \cdot Cl^-$$
Carbachol chloride

All drugs in this group are quaternary amines. Substitution on the β carbon, as in acetyl-β-methylcholine (methacholine), protects preferentially against the action of nonspecific cholinesterase. Because methacholine is an acetyl ester, it is still hydrolyzed by acetylcholinesterase, though more slowly than acetylcholine. Replacement of the acetyl group by carbamate protects the drug (bethanechol or carbachol) from both types of cholinesterase.

Bethanechol and methacholine exhibit the action of acetylcholine on smooth muscles and exocrine glands without significantly affecting ganglionic and skeletal neuromuscular transmission. Methacholine was previously used for management of paroxysmal atrial tachycardia and as a diagnostic test for the presence of adrenal

Interaction of acetylcholine and acetylcholinesterase. The quaternary nitrogen of acetyl-   **FIG. 11-1**
choline forms an ionic bond with the negatively charged anionic site, and the other portion
of the molecule covalently acetylates a serine residue, G, at the esteratic site. After initial
hydrolysis of choline from the molecule, the acetate in turn is rapidly hydrolyzed from the
enzyme.

From Wilson, I.B.: Neurology 8(suppl. 1):41, 1958.

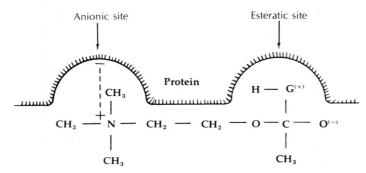

medullary tumors (pheochromocytoma). Other agents have supplanted this usage.

Bethanechol chloride (Urecholine, others) relatively selectively affects the gastrointestinal and urinary tracts and is the cholinergic drug of choice for treatment of postoperative, postpartum, or neurogenic urinary retention.[3] It has also been used to relieve reflux esophagitis and postoperative abdominal distention. The usual cholinergic side effects include sweating, cutaneous vasodilatation with flushing, salivation, nausea, vomiting, and diarrhea. There are variable changes in heart rate and blood pressure. There may be a precipitous fall in the pressure of some persons, whereas in others alterations in blood pressure and heart rate are slight because of more effective compensatory reflexes. It must be remembered that asthmatic patients are particularly susceptible to the bronchoconstrictor action of these compounds.

Contraindications to the use of bethanechol include asthma, peptic ulcer, parkinsonism, pregnancy, severe cardiac disease, hyperthyroidism (wherein atrial fibrillation may occur), and mechanical obstruction or impairment of the structural integrity of the gastrointestinal or urinary tracts. These contraindications generally apply to all the cholinergic agents discussed in this chapter. Preparations include tablets of 5 to 50 mg and a solution for subcutaneous injection, 5 mg/ml. The recommended dosage for adults is 10 to 50 mg by mouth or 2.5 to 5 mg by subcutaneous injection, three or four times daily, but more frequent or larger doses may be necessary.[3]

Carbachol (Carbacel, Isopto Carbachol) is a very potent choline ester with both muscarinic and nicotinic activity. Its only use at present is in treatment of glaucoma. Solutions of 0.75% to 3%, 1 or 2 drops at 4- to 8-hour intervals, applied to the conjunctiva cause miosis and reduce intraocular pressure. A very dilute solution (Miostat Intraocular, 0.01%) may also be instilled into the anterior chamber of the

FIG. 11-2   *Effect of acetylcholine on blood pressure before and after atropine. The following drugs were administered intravenously to a dog anesthetized with pentobarbital: A, acetylcholine, 10 µg/kg; between A and B, atropine, 1 mg/kg; B, acetylcholine, 10 µg/kg; C, acetylcholine, 100 µg/kg; between C and D, phentolamine, 5 mg/kg; D, acetylcholine, 100 µg/kg. Notice that atropine prevented the decrease in blood pressure in response to the low dose of acetylcholine. The larger dose of acetylcholine then increased blood pressure because of its nicotinic action in ganglia. This hypertensive response was blocked by phentolamine, an α-adrenergic blocking agent.*

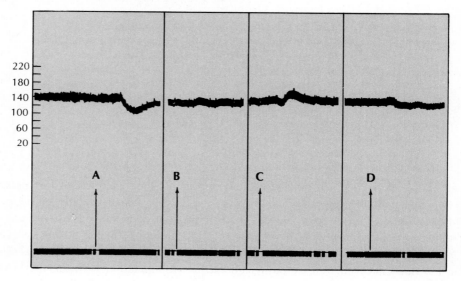

eye to induce miosis after cataract removal. Acetylcholine chloride (Miochol Intra-ocular, 20 mg, to be reconstituted in 2 ml amounts when needed) is also used for this purpose.

The muscarinic and nicotinic actions of choline esters can be illustrated by a simple experiment. Fig. 11-2 shows the effect of acetylcholine injection on the blood pressure of a dog before and after atropine administration.

Pilocarpine and muscarine   The alkaloids pilocarpine and muscarine have the curious property of acting like acetylcholine on receptors of smooth muscles, exocrine glands, and heart. Muscarine is present in the mushrooms *Amanita muscaria* and *Inocybe patouillard*,[16] whereas pilocarpine is found in the leaves of the plant *Pilocarpus jaborandi*.

Muscarine

Pilocarpine

Both alkaloids elicit the so-called muscarinic effects of acetylcholine without having significant nicotinic action. As one would expect, atropine blocks these muscarinic

TABLE 11-1	Pharmacologic approaches to management of glaucoma
Drug or class	Postulated mechanism
Muscarinic agonists, anticholinesterases	Improved drainage of aqueous humor
Epinephrine	Improved drainage of aqueous humor
β-Adrenergic antagonists	Decreased formation of aqueous humor
Carbonic anhydrase inhibitors	Decreased formation of aqueous humor

effects. It is not surprising that muscarine, a quaternary ammonium compound, shows some similarity to acetylcholine, but it is puzzling why pilocarpine, a tertiary amine, should also be similar. It is well established, however, that this is not the result of cholinesterase inhibition.

Of these two agents, muscarine has only historic and toxicologic interest. However, **pilocarpine hydrochloride** (Isopto Carpine; others) or nitrate (P.V. Carpine Liquifilm), in concentrations ranging from 0.25% to 10%, is employed in ophthalmology to reverse the effects of mydriatic and cycloplegic agents and is the cholinergic agent most often used to lower intraocular pressure in glaucoma.[6] In open-angle glaucoma pilocarpine is taken every 6 to 8 hours as drops, initially in a 1% solution. Concentrations above 4% are not usually more effective but increase the likelihood of toxicity.[5] Contraction of the ciliary muscle by cholinergic drugs is believed to enhance outflow of aqueous humor from the anterior chamber of the eye (Table 11-1) by an improvement in flow through the trabecular network.[5,6] The precise mechanism is not entirely clear.[7] Two controlled-release preparations are also available. One (Ocusert Pilo-20 or -40) is placed into the conjunctival sac for release of pilocarpine over a 7-day period. The other (Pilopine H.S. Gel) is used once daily at bedtime.

Acute angle-closure glaucoma is a much more serious disorder in which the trabecular network is obstructed by the iris. The miotic effect of cholinergic drugs is useful as a temporary, emergency measure to lower intraocular pressure until iridectomy can be performed. There appears to be little advantage to the practice of concurrent administration of two miotics, such as physostigmine with pilocarpine or echothiophate. Application of 2% pilocarpine four times at 5-minute intervals and then once every 3 hours should be maximally effective, if the pupil can respond at all, with minimal toxicity.[5]

Pilocarpine was once used to promote salivation in patients who complained of dryness of the mouth during therapy with ganglionic blocking agents.

PROBLEM 11-1. The fixed dilated pupil may be an ominous sign caused by involvement of the third nerve in an intracranial disease. How can this be distinguished from accidental application to the eye of an anticholinergic drug? Topical application of pilocarpine has been used to establish the diagnosis.[14] The pupil responds well to pilocarpine in the case of nerve damage, whereas it is unresponsive if dilatation is caused by application of a muscarinic antagonist. Could an anticholinesterase such as physostigmine be substituted for pilocarpine in this diagnostic test?

TABLE 11-2   Anticholinesterase preparations

Drug	Preparations*	Usual route of administration
For glaucoma:		
Demecarium bromide (Humorsol)	S: 0.125%, 0.25%	Topical
Echothiophate (Phospholine) iodide	P: 1.5-12.5 mg	Topical
Isoflurophate (Floropryl)	O: 0.025%	Topical
Physostigmine salicylate (Isopto Eserine)	S: 0.25%, 0.5%	Topical
Physostigmine (Eserine) sulfate	O: 0.25%	Topical
For myasthenia gravis:		
Ambenonium chloride (Mytelase)	T: 10 mg	Oral
Edrophonium chloride (Tensilon)	I: 10 mg/ml	Intravenous
Neostigmine bromide (Prostigmin)	T: 15 mg	Oral
Neostigmine methylsulfate (Prostigmin)	I: 0.25-1.0 mg/ml	Intravenous, intramuscular
Pyridostigmine bromide (Mestinon)	T: 60, 180 mg	Oral
	Sy: 60 mg/5 ml	Oral
(Mestinon, Regonol)	I: 5 mg/ml	Intravenous, intramuscular

*I, Injectable; O, ointment; P, powder for reconstitution to 0.06% or 0.125%; S, ophthalmic solution; Sy, syrup; T, tablet.

ANTICHOLIN-ESTERASES

Some drugs indirectly enhance cholinergic transmission by inhibiting destruction of acetylcholine, thereby increasing its potency and prolonging its effects. They can also potentiate the action of some synthetic choline esters. Cholinesterase inhibitors are useful in management of glaucoma and myasthenia gravis (Table 11-2), especially the latter. This group also includes some of our most potent insecticides and several potential chemical warfare agents.

From studies on anticholinesterases, much has been learned about cholinesterases. Since plasma cholinesterase can be reduced to very low levels by an anticholinesterase without important consequences, the physiologic role of this esterase is unknown. Nevertheless, it is important in metabolism of exogenous acetylcholine, the neuromuscular blocker succinylcholine (see p. 52), and local anesthetics of the ester type (see Chapter 33). Plasma cholinesterase activity may be reduced by liver disease or by previous administration of anticholinesterases. Measurements of this activity are useful in industrial medicine to evaluate the extent of exposure to anticholinesterases, thus minimizing risk of poisoning.

Whereas moderate decreases of the specific acetylcholinesterase may have little physiologic consequence, a severe reduction of brain acetylcholinesterase can be lethal. Although the acetylcholinesterase in red blood cells has no obvious physiologic role, its measurement can be used to assess the severity of anticholinesterase intoxication.[9] Regeneration of activity in red blood cells after administration of an irreversible anticholinesterase is directly proportional to production of new cells.

Physostigmine and neostigmine, like acetylcholine, are esters that bind to cho- *Reversible*
linesterases. However, they are more slowly hydrolyzed from the enzyme, which is *anticholinesterases*
unavailable to inactivate acetylcholine so long as the inhibitor remains attached.
Physostigmine is a tertiary amine used to treat glaucoma, to improve postoperative
intestinal tone and peristalsis, and to act as an antidote to poisoning caused by
atropine-like drugs. Neostigmine is a quaternary ammonium compound used to treat
myasthenia gravis, to reverse skeletal muscle paralysis caused by curare-like drugs,
and to act as a urinary tract stimulant.

Physostigmine, an alkaloid obtained from seeds of the calabar or ordeal bean
Physostigma venenosum, has been familiar to pharmacologists since the latter part
of the nineteenth century. In 1934 the British physician Mary Walker[15] successfully
used physostigmine to treat myasthenia gravis because of the clinical similarity of
this disease to a curarized state. Synthesis of compounds related to physostigmine
led to development of neostigmine in 1931.

Physostigmine   Neostigmine bromide

The effects of physostigmine are attributable virtually entirely to cholinesterase *PHYSOSTIGMINE*
inhibition on the basis of the following considerations. The drug inhibits cholinesterase in vitro. Its affinity for the enzyme is about 10,000 times greater than that of
acetylcholine. It has a potent action on structures with normal innervation because
of its ability to protect released acetylcholine, but it lacks an action on the denervated
pupil or on denervated skeletal muscle, even when given by close intra-arterial
injection. After combination with the enzyme, physostigmine is first hydrolyzed to
leave a carbamyl group covalently attached to the enzyme. As this group, in turn,
is gradually hydrolyzed from the enzyme, enzymatic activity is restored. Consequently, the drug is a reversible inhibitor of the cholinesterases.

Physostigmine salicylate (Antilirium, 1 mg/ml) injection or infusion, the specific
antidote for anticholinergic intoxication, can be of benefit when added to supportive
management of poisoning by atropine and other agents, such as tricyclic antidepressants, that have appreciable anticholinergic activity. However, this antidote
should be reserved for severe intoxications and must be given carefully to avoid
seizures, excessive cardiac slowing, or other manifestations of too much cholinergic
stimulation.[8] Physostigmine is also used topically to treat primary open-angle glaucoma, though pilocarpine is preferred.

Some of the effects of neostigmine are caused solely by cholinesterase inhibition, whereas others result from a combination of enzyme inhibition plus a direct acetylcholine-like action. On the denervated eye, for example, neostigmine acts like physostigmine, producing no pupillary constriction. On the other hand, intra-arterially injected neostigmine will stimulate the neuromuscular junction even after the nerves have degenerated and all cholinesterase has been destroyed by isoflurophate. This evidence indicates that muscarinic effects of neostigmine are caused by cholinesterase inhibition, whereas the nicotinic effect at the neuromuscular site is in part caused by direct stimulation.

The intramuscular or subcutaneous injection of 0.5 to 1 mg of **neostigmine methylsulfate** into a normal human will elicit common cholinergic effects. Intestinal contractions and contraction of smooth muscle of the urinary bladder can alleviate postoperative abdominal distention or urinary retention. Other responses may include elevation of skin temperature, sweating, salivation, slowing of the heart rate with possible hypotension, and skeletal muscle fasciculations. Atropine will inhibit the muscarinic, but not the nicotinic, effects of neostigmine. *As a general rule, atropine pretreatment or simultaneous parenteral administration is recommended whenever cholinergic drugs are injected for their* nicotinic *effects* (for example, to reverse paralysis induced by a nondepolarizing neuromuscular blocking agent), to avoid unnecessary and potentially dangerous muscarinic effects. *When cholinergic agents are injected for their* muscarinic *effects* (for instance, to relieve urinary retention), *a syringe containing atropine should be available* as a precaution against overdose.

For chronic therapy, **neostigmine bromide** is given. An oral dose of 15 to 30 mg is necessary because much of the drug is inactivated in the gastrointestinal tract. Absorption may be quite variable, and untoward reactions will occur if too much is suddenly absorbed.

Neostigmine substitutes. **Pyridostigmine bromide** is used in chronic management of myasthenia gravis and may be preferred by patients.[12] Its duration of action is 3 to 6 hours. Sustained-release tablets (Mestinon Timespan) containing 180 mg are also available for administration at bedtime. Preparations for injection can be used to treat acute myasthenia gravis or to reverse paralysis caused by nondepolarizing neuromuscular antagonists.

Ambenonium is also used to treat myasthenia gravis. Its duration of action is 4 to 6 hours.

Pyridostigmine bromide

Ambenonium chloride

Edrophonium differs structurally from neostigmine primarily in not being an *Edrophonium*
ester. It does not bind covalently to the enzyme, and the action of a typical intravenous
dose lasts only 5 to 10 minutes in a normal subject. Although edrophonium was
introduced as an antagonist of neuromuscular blockade by nondepolarizing agents
such as tubocurarine, it is especially useful as a diagnostic and investigative tool in
myasthenia. In an untreated myasthenic patient intravenous injection of 2 mg of
edrophonium may cause a rapid but transient increase in muscular strength. If there
is no immediate improvement, after a brief pause an 8 mg dose is given. This test
may be used for diagnostic purposes and also for assessment of the status of therapy.
Because myasthenia is a disorder of nicotinic receptors, either too little or too much
neurotransmitter can cause weakness. Extreme cases have been termed *myasthenic
crisis* and *cholinergic crisis* respectively. In the latter there are likely to be muscarinic
indications of intoxication as well. The physician may be uncertain whether to increase
or to decrease the dosage of neostigmine for a myasthenic patient. If edrophonium
improves strength, it is likely that previous therapy was inadequate. On the other
hand, if the reaction to this "edrophonium test" is unfavorable, indicative of overtreatment, a reduction in neostigmine dosage should be beneficial. The action of
edrophonium in this test usually lasts only a few minutes. If the patient is in crisis
with respiratory difficulty, measures to normalize respiration, such as assisted ventilation, must be instituted first and the dose of edrophonium is reduced to 1 mg,
given twice if necessary with a 1-minute interval. An alternative diagnostic approach
that has been recommended for respiratory difficulties is simply stopping anticholinesterase medication while beginning mechanical ventilation.[12] If respiration improves spontaneously, the patient was receiving too much drug; if respiration does
not improve, therapy can be reinstituted at a higher dosage.

$$HO-C_6H_4-N^+(CH_3)_2(C_2H_5) \cdot Cl^-$$

Edrophonium chloride

Edrophonium is an effective antidote to curare. It acts more rapidly than neostigmine, but because its action is brief, multiple injections are often needed. Although the mechanism is not understood, an intravenous bolus of edrophonium has
been proposed as a diagnostic test to elicit chest pain arising from the esophagus.[11]

Isoflurophate (diisopropyl fluorophosphate, DFP) and a variety of other organ- *Irreversible*
ophosphates are highly toxic compounds that produce irreversible inactivation of the *organophosphorus*
cholinesterases. They were developed as potential chemical warfare agents and have *anticholinesterases*
had some therapeutic application, but their principal interest is toxicologic because
of their widespread use as insecticides. Except for echothiophate, most of these

compounds are highly lipid soluble, can be absorbed through the skin as well as after inhalation or ingestion, and readily enter the central nervous system.

The structural formulas of some of the organophosphorus compounds are as follows:

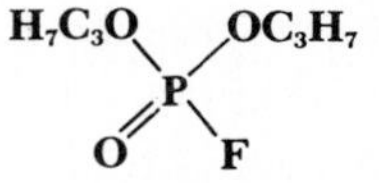

Isoflurophate

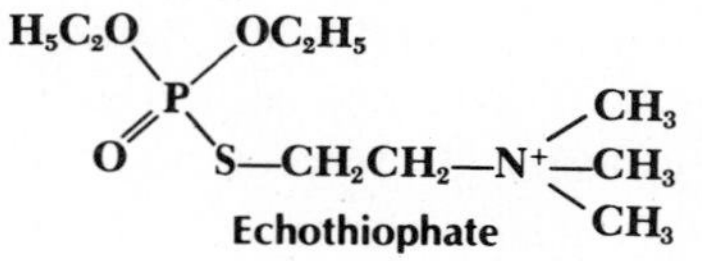

Echothiophate

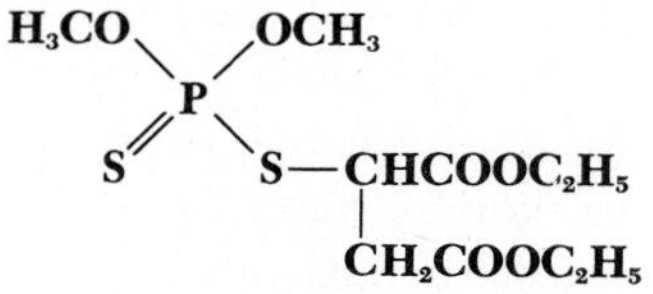

Malathion

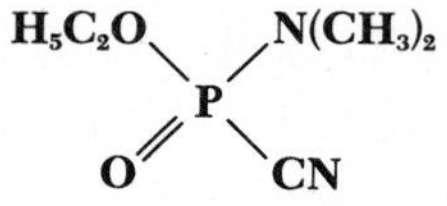

Tabun

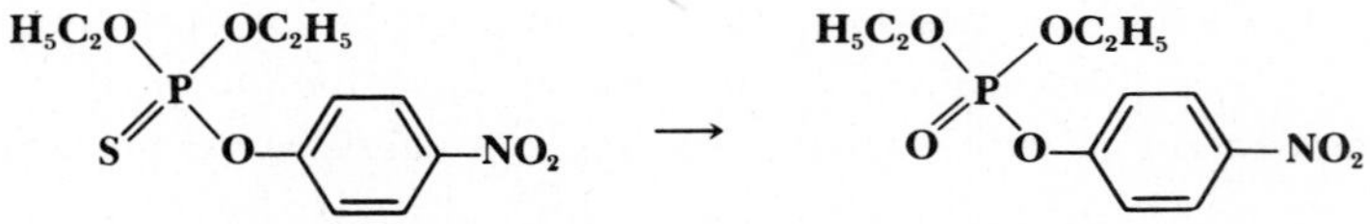

Parathion → Paraoxon

Whereas reversible anticholinesterases depress enzymatic activity up to a few hours after a single administration, the effect of organophosphorus compounds may persist for weeks or months. When the organophosphorus compounds combine with cholinesterase, the enzyme becomes permanently phosphorylated and is inactive against acetylcholine. As a consequence, enzymatic activity is reduced until new enzyme can be synthesized, unless a reactivator of cholinesterase is employed as an antidote.

MEDICAL USES OF
ORGANOPHOSPHATES

Isoflurophate, echothiophate, and **demecarium** are used for treatment of open-angle glaucoma mainly because their prolonged action improves compliance. Echothiophate, the preferred agent in this group, is usually applied twice a day. Their action should remain localized if administered correctly to minimize drainage through the lacrimal ducts into the nasal passages, where systemic absorption can occur. Discomfort associated with ciliary spasm is more of a problem with these drugs than with pilocarpine and in younger than in older patients. The risk of cataract development appears increased with these agents, but they can be very useful after a lens has been removed. The ocular effects of isoflurophate and echothiophate may be

TABLE 11-3	Signs and symptoms of organophosphate poisoning	
Muscarinic manifestations	Nicotinic manifestations	CNS manifestations
Bronchoconstriction	Muscular fasciculation	Restlessness
Increased bronchial secretions	Tachycardia	Insomnia
Sweating	Hypertension	Tremors
Salivation		Confusion
Lacrimation		Ataxia
Bradycardia		Convulsions
Miosis		Respiratory depression
Blurring of vision		Circulatory collapse
Urinary incontinence		Hypotension

Modified from Namba, T., Nolte, C.T., Jackrel, J., and Grob, D.: Am. J. Med. **50:**475, 1971.

partially inhibited by prior application of physostigmine. Although most often used as an insecticide, **malathion** can be applied to the scalp as a lotion (Prioderm) to eliminate head lice.

Organophosphates are used most widely as insecticides (**malathion, parathion, and diazinon**) so that acute and chronic poisoning by these agents is not uncommon. Many extremely potent, potential chemical warfare agents (**soman** and **tabun**) also are organophosphates. When an organophosphate anticholinesterase is injected or inhaled, the nonspecific cholinesterase of plasma is affected preferentially. With a sufficient dose, however, there is also inactivation of acetylcholinesterase in red blood cells and in neural tissue. Whereas plasma cholinesterase may be regenerated by the liver in 2 weeks to 2 months,[9] it may take 3 months to completely restore acetylcholinesterase activity at synapses and neuromuscular junctions. The clinical picture in intoxication is a combination of peripheral cholinergic effects and involvement of the central nervous system (Table 11-3). Death is usually secondary to respiratory complications.[10] In a group of 16 intoxicated field workers, nausea, dizziness, vomiting, abdominal pain, weakness, blurred vision, and headache were the most common symptoms initially; the last two tended to persist for more than a month.[9] A delayed, often permanent, neurotoxicity may also follow exposure to many organophosphates.[1]

GENERAL PHARMACOLOGIC EFFECTS AND TOXICITY

Pralidoxime (*N*-methylpyridinium-2-aldoxime, 2-PAM) is a tailor-made molecule developed on the basis of a mechanism postulated by Wilson[17] to explain the action of organophosphate anticholinesterases. Experimental studies had shown that hydroxylamine and oximes are capable of regenerating the enzyme after it has been phosphorylated. With this in mind, a molecule was designed that would act more efficiently as a regenerator than would an ordinary oxime.

ANTIDOTAL ACTION OF PRALIDOXIME

$$\left[\begin{array}{c} \underset{\underset{N^+}{|}}{\overset{CH_3}{|}} \quad CH=NOH \\ \end{array}\right] Cl^-$$

Pralidoxime chloride

Pralidoxime (Protopam) chloride must be administered parenterally in severe intoxications. It is supplied in 20 ml vials containing 1 g, and 1 to 2 g is usually dissolved in sterile water for intravenous infusion. Administration may be repeated if necessary after an hour and again later if symptoms persist. Tablets containing 500 mg may be useful in mild cases in which gastrointestinal symptoms such as vomiting are absent. Pralidoxime has some anticholinesterase activity of its own and is not used in intoxication by reversible anticholinesterases.

TREATMENT OF
ORGANOPHOSPHORUS
INTOXICATION

If the patient is cyanotic, mechanical ventilation should be started even before atropine is given. In an adult an intravenous test dose of 2 mg of atropine can be repeated or increased at 15- to 60-minute intervals as needed, with careful observation to avoid excessive administration.[4] Atropine protects against the peripheral muscarinic actions and involvement of the central nervous system. It exerts no protective effect against muscle fasciculations and skeletal muscle weakness. Pralidoxime is administered primarily to reverse the neuromuscular involvement. Pralidoxime, a quaternary amine, is of no benefit against the central nervous system symptoms. The skin, stomach, and eyes should be decontaminated. Other measures are symptomatic and supportive.

PHARMACOLOGIC
ASPECTS OF
MYASTHENIA
GRAVIS

Myasthenia gravis is an autoimmune neuromuscular disease characterized by muscle fatigability. The density of acetylcholine receptors at the neuromuscular junction is reduced, and the neuromuscular junction undergoes extensive morphologic modifications.[2,13]

Repetitive stimulation of a motor nerve in a myasthenic patient leads to a rapid decrease in the force of contraction of muscles innervated by that particular nerve. Intra-arterial injection of acetylcholine, neostigmine, or edrophonium increases the strength of such fatigued muscles. In normal persons the intra-arterial injection of these drugs produces fasciculation and weakness, probably as a result of persistent depolarization of the neuromuscular end plates. Myasthenic patients are susceptible to the relaxant activity of doses of tubocurarine or quinine that scarcely affect normal persons.

Reversible anticholinesterases are useful for diagnosis and management of myasthenia. For diagnostic purposes, edrophonium may be used as discussed above. Alternatively, neostigmine may be injected by the intramuscular route or intravenously.

For chronic management of weakness, oral administration of neostigmine and related drugs is most useful (Table 11-2). Neostigmine bromide is administered orally in doses of 15 to 30 mg, sometimes as often as every 3 hours. Much smaller doses of neostigmine as the methylsulfate suffice when given by the intramuscular route. Atropine may be necessary initially to minimize unwanted muscarinic effects.

The following drugs require special caution and are probably best avoided when possible in myasthenic patients, since they may aggravate the symptoms of the disease:

Drug interactions

1. Aminoglycoside antibiotics and perhaps bacitracin and tetracyclines
2. Quinidine, quinine, and procainamide
3. Local anesthetics, such as procaine and lidocaine
4. Inhalational anesthetics, particularly ether
5. Skeletal muscle relaxants, such as curare and succinylcholine
6. Respiratory depressants, such as opioid analgesics and hypnotics

REFERENCES

1. Abou-Donia, M.B.: Organophosphorus ester-induced delayed neurotoxicity, Annu. Rev. Pharmacol. Toxicol. **21**:511, 1981.
2. Drachman, D.B.: Myasthenia gravis: immunobiology of a receptor disorder, Trends Neurosci. **6**:446, 1983.
3. Finkbeiner, A.E., and Bissada, N.K.: Drug therapy for lower urinary tract dysfunction, Urol. Clin. North Am. **7**:3, 1980.
4. Haddad, L.M.: The organophosphate insecticides. In Haddad, L.M., and Winchester, J.F., editor: Clinical management of poisoning and drug overdose, Philadelphia, 1983, W.B. Saunders Co., p. 704.
5. Havener, W.H.: Ocular pharmacology, ed. 5, St. Louis, 1983, The C.V. Mosby Co.
6. Johnson, D.H., and Brubaker, R.F.: Glaucoma: an overview, Mayo Clin. Proc. **61**:59, 1986.
7. Kaufman, P.L., Wiedman, T., and Robinson, J.R.: Cholinergics, Handb. Exp. Pharmacol. **69**:149, 1984.
8. Kulig, K., and Rumack, B.H.: Anticholinergic poisoning. In Haddad, L.M., and Winchester, J.F., editors: Clinical management of poisoning and drug overdose, Philadelphia, 1983, W.B. Saunders Co., p. 482.
9. Midtling, J.E., Barnett, P.G., Coye, M.J., et al.: Clinical management of field worker organophosphate poisoning, West. J. Med. **142**:514, 1985.
10. Namba, T., Nolte, C.T., Jackrel, J., and Grob, D.: Poisoning due to organophosphate insecticides: acute and chronic manifestations, Am. J. Med. **50**:475, 1971.
11. Richter, J.E., Hackshaw, B.T., Wu, W.C., and Castell, D.O.: Edrophonium: a useful provocative test for esophageal chest pain, Ann. Intern. Med. **103**:14, 1985.
12. Rowland, L.P.: Controversies about treatment of myasthenia gravis, J. Neurol. Neurosurg. Psychiatry **43**:644, 1980.
13. Seybold, M.E.: Myasthenia gravis: a clinical and basic science review, J.A.M.A. **250**:2516, 1983.
14. Thompson, H.S., Newsome, D.A., and Loewenfeld, I.E.: The fixed dilated pupil. Sudden iridoplegia or mydriatic drops? A simple diagnostic test, Arch. Ophthalmol. **86**:21, 1971.
15. Walker, M.B.: Case showing effect of prostigmin on myasthenia gravis, Proc. R. Soc. Med. **28**:759, 1935.
16. Wieland, T.: Poisonous principles of mushrooms of the genus Amanita, Science **159**:946, 1968.
17. Wilson, I.B.: A specific antidote for nerve gas and insecticide (alkylphosphate) intoxication, Neurology **8**(suppl. 1):41, 1958.

Chapter 12

Cholinergic (muscarinic) blocking agents

GENERAL
CONCEPTS

Atropine and scopolamine are competitive antagonists of acetylcholine at muscarinic receptors in organs innervated by postganglionic nerves. They have been extremely useful as pharmacologic tools. These alkaloids and related drugs find application in ophthalmology and anesthesia and in cardiac and gastrointestinal diseases. In addition to their peripheral anticholinergic activity, many of these agents act on the central nervous system. They are used for treatment of Parkinson's disease and for prevention of motion sickness and were once found in many over-the-counter sleep aids. As antidotes for anticholinesterase intoxication, both peripheral and central actions of atropine are of great benefit.

ATROPINE AND
SCOPOLAMINE
*Origin and
chemistry*

Atropine and scopolamine are among the oldest drugs in medicine. Many solanaceous plants have been used for centuries because of their active principles *l*-hyoscyamine and *l*-hyoscine (scopolamine). Atropine is *dl*-hyoscyamine; racemization occurs during the extraction process. The name *hyoscyamine* is derived from *Hyoscyamus niger* (henbane; literally 'black hog-bean'). It is of toxicologic interest that the common jimson weed, *Datura stramonium*, contains these alkaloids. They are also found in the deadly nightshade, *Atropa belladonna*. Hence these compounds are often referred to collectively as *belladonna alkaloids*. Just as acetylcholine is an ester of an amino alcohol, blocking drugs of the belladonna group are esters of complex organic bases with tropic acid. Atropine and scopolamine differ only slightly in the structure of the organic base part of the molecule.

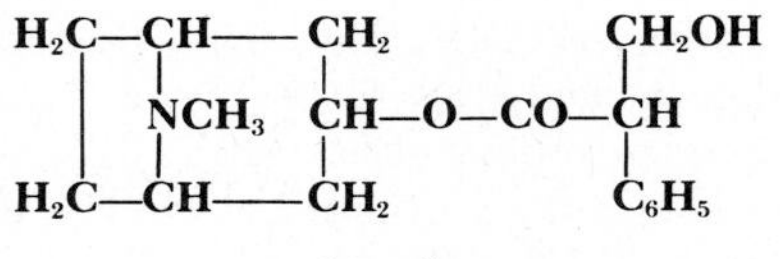

$$H_2C-CH-CH_2 \quad CH_2OH$$
$$NCH_3 \quad CH-O-CO-CH$$
$$H_2C-CH-CH_2 \quad C_6H_5$$

Atropine

$$O< \begin{matrix} HC-CH-CH_2 \\ HC-CH-CH_2 \end{matrix} \quad NCH_3 \quad \begin{matrix} CH_2OH \\ CH-O-CO-CH \end{matrix} \quad C_6H_5$$

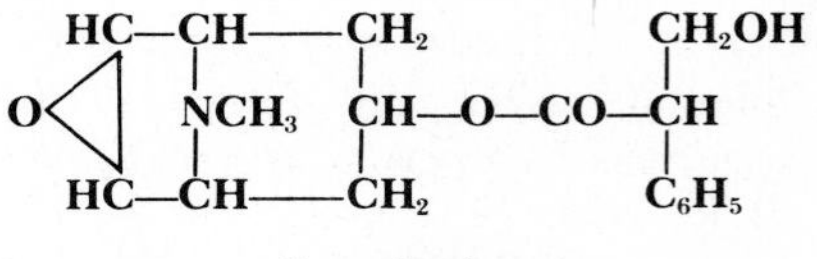

Scopolamine

*Pharmacologic
effects*

Atropine and scopolamine compete with acetylcholine for binding to receptor sites in smooth and cardiac muscles and in exocrine glands (Fig. 12-1). They tend to inhibit muscarinic responses to injected cholinergic drugs more easily than vagally mediated responses. There is a definite gradation in the sensitivity to inhibition by these alkaloids of the various peripheral functions mediated by acetylcholine. An oral dose of 0.6 mg of atropine may dry the mouth and inhibit sweating, whereas

Effect of acetylcholine on tension development of guinea pig ileum. Atropine, a competitive   **FIG. 12-1**
antagonist, causes a parallel shift of the log dose-response curve.

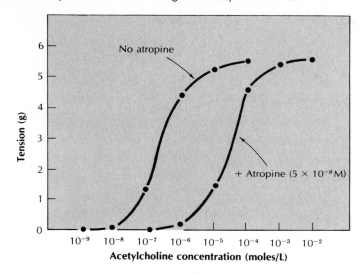

blockade of parasympathetic input to the eye and heart requires somewhat larger doses. Gastrointestinal and urinary tract smooth muscles are even more resistant. Because of such differences in sensitivity, use of atropine for inhibition of gastric secretion, the most resistant, is generally impractical; the dose required will cause side effects from more sensitive organs. Atropine and scopolamine differ mainly in that, relative to other organs, the eye is more sensitive to scopolamine and that at therapeutic doses scopolamine, unlike atropine, may produce considerable sleepiness and even amnesia. In large enough doses both cause central nervous system stimulation, which may progress to delirium. Finally, after very high doses of either drug, coma may supervene.

Cardiovascular system. The effect of atropine on heart rate in humans is complex. With high therapeutic or slightly larger doses tachycardia develops, as expected, from blockade of the vagal influence on the sinoatrial node. With smaller doses, paradoxical as it may seem, the heart rate may decrease slightly. Ablation experiments have shown that atropine stimulates vagal nuclei in the medulla. This stimulation results in bradycardia unless enough drug is given to block the peripheral action of acetylcholine at cardiac muscarinic receptors. Similarly bradycardia has been observed in subjects given a small intravenous bolus of scopolamine or during recovery from larger doses after the tachycardia has dissipated.[8]

The effects of atropine and scopolamine on blood pressure are not impressive because most vascular regions in the body do not receive parasympathetic innervation. It is a common experience in the laboratory to inject atropine into a dog without observing a significant change in pressure. Flushing of the skin may be very

FIG. 12-2   *Autonomic innervation of iris.*

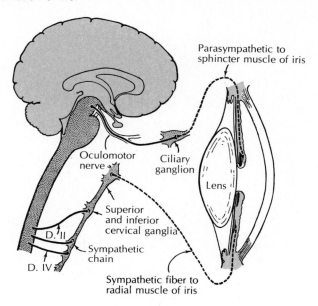

noticeable after large doses of atropine and occurs by two mechanisms: (1) In a hot environment cutaneous vasodilatation may be a heat-loss response to hyperthermia that is secondary to inhibition of sweating; (2) in addition, atropine has an unexplained vasodilator action.

Gastrointestinal and urinary tracts. In large enough doses the belladonna alkaloids reduce motility and tone of the gastrointestinal tract and may even reduce the volume of its secretions. Gastric motility is more easily reduced by therapeutic doses than secretion is, particularly if a peptic ulcer is present. Atropine has little effect on the ureters. It relaxes the fundus of the bladder but promotes contraction of the sphincter, thus favoring urinary retention.

Eye. Atropine and scopolamine produce prolonged (up to 2 weeks) mydriasis and paralysis of accommodation (cycloplegia). The sphincter muscle of the iris receives cholinergic innervation from the third cranial nerve (Fig. 12-2). Atropine blocks the action of acetylcholine on this muscle, and the resulting dominance of the radial muscle causes mydriasis. The atropinized pupil does not react to light. Cycloplegia is caused by paralysis of the ciliary muscle, which is also innervated by cholinergic fibers. It should be noted that adrenergic agonists can also produce mydriasis. They act, however, by contracting the radial muscle of the iris and do not impair accommodation.

Muscarinic blocking drugs are contraindicated for topical use in patients subject to glaucoma. However, systemic anticholinergic medication for other purposes will seldom be harmful to patients already receiving therapy for glaucoma.[10] The subject most at risk from such medication is one with an undiagnosed narrow angle. In narrow-angle glaucoma the increased intraocular pressure is attributed to impeded drainage of aqueous humor from the anterior chamber caused by the retracted iris. Hence administration of an anticholinergic drug may precipitate an acute attack with catastrophic increases in intraocular pressure.

Central nervous system. In anticholinergic poisoning central nervous system effects are very striking; patients most often become excited and may hallucinate or be delirious. As discussed in the previous chapter, the central anticholinergic action of large doses of atropine may be life saving in intoxication by organophosphate cholinesterase inhibitors. Anticholinergic drugs were once the primary therapy in management of Parkinson's disease. Scopolamine in particular is valuable in the prevention of motion sickness,[4] and, when given by injection for preanesthetic medication, it promotes a state of sedation and may cause amnesia.[6]

Atropine and scopolamine are well absorbed from the gastrointestinal tract and after injection. Scopolamine is even applied topically to the skin. Systemic toxicity may occur in ophthalmologic use, particularly in children, if the drug reaches the nasal mucosa through the nasolacrimal duct after application to the conjunctival sac.

Absorption, excretion, and metabolism

Atropine is rapidly excreted and about half of an injected dose appears in the urine as metabolites and unchanged drug within 4 hours. The remainder is excreted within 24 hours. The duration of pharmacologic action reflects the rapidity of excretion except for dilatation of the pupils and paralysis of accommodation, which may persist for a long time, particularly when the alkaloids are applied to the conjunctiva.

Belladonna alkaloids are used either in pure form or in galenic preparations. (Galenic preparations contain one or more active botanical ingredients as contrasted with pure chemical substances.) Belladonna tincture is given orally in a dose of 0.6 to 1.0 ml, equivalent to 0.18 to 0.3 mg of the alkaloids. Tablets of atropine sulfate contain 0.3 to 0.6 mg for administration to adults at 4- to 6-hour intervals. Atropine can be inhaled with a nebulizer (Dey-Dose, Dey-Lute). It is instilled into the conjunctival sac as an ointment or in solution (Atropisal, Isopto Atropine). The usual strength is 0.5% or 1%, though higher concentrations are available in solution. Hyoscyamine sulfate is available in several forms. Scopolamine hydrobromide is available as tablets (0.3 to 0.6 mg) and capsules (Triptone, 0.25 mg). The usual dose is 0.4 to 0.8 mg. For a more rapid action and preanesthetic medication, injectable solutions of atropine sulfate (0.05 to 1.2 mg/ml) and scopolamine hydrobromide (0.3 to 1 mg/ml) are used.

Preparations and clinical uses

Ophthalmologic use. Anticholinergic drugs are applied topically to produce mydriasis and cycloplegia. Atropine has such a long action that its use in ophthalmology is often impractical. However, it is used to produce maximal cycloplegia for refraction in young children with accommodative esotropia and to break adhesions (synechiae) between the iris and the lens in iridocyclitis.

Perioperative uses. When ether was a commonly used anesthetic, it was necessary to premedicate surgical patients with atropine or scopolamine to protect them from salivary and bronchial secretions and from reflex vagal bradycardia. Ether has been replaced by anesthetics that do not cause excessive secretions, and the need for routine preanesthetic anticholinergics has greatly lessened.[9] However, they are still given intravenously during surgery to prevent bradycardia. Scopolamine is used in obstetrics for its sedative and amnesic effects. When an anticholinesterase is administered near the end of anesthesia to reverse muscle paralysis induced by a neuromuscular blocking agent, atropine or a related agent is also given to prevent muscarinic effects.

Cardiac uses. Atropine is used after myocardial infarction if the heart rate falls below 60[9] and the bradycardia is associated with hypotension or arrhythmias. Atropine can cause dangerous tachycardia and ventricular arrhythmias in cardiac patients and should be used cautiously. The drug may also be useful in digitalis-induced heart block.

Uses in gastrointestinal disease. Anticholinergic drugs were once commonly used to treat peptic ulcer. They can diminish vagally mediated secretion, relieve spasm, and, by slowing gastric emptying, prolong the time during which antacids remain in the stomach. However, to be effective, the anticholinergics must be administered in doses that usually cause unpleasant side effects.

Motion sickness. Scopolamine was the first drug to be administered by means of a patch placed behind one ear. To prevent motion sickness, the disk (Transderm Scōp) is designed to release a priming dose and then about 5 μg/hour for 72 hours. The disk should be applied a minimum of 4 hours and preferably longer before exposure to an emetic stimulus, and the hands should be thoroughly washed to avoid transfer of the drug to the eyes. Clinical trials indicated that this preparation is as effective as oral dimenhydrinate and less sedative. Dry mouth is a common side effect.

Other uses. The antidotal benefit of atropine in anticholinesterase intoxication is discussed in Chapter 11. Treatment of Parkinson's disease is discussed below. Atropine-like drugs also counteract parkinsonian side effects of neuroleptic agents. Atropine is included in an antidiarrheal preparation (Lomotil) to prevent abuse of the opioid diphenoxylate. Asthmatics may benefit from judicious use of antimuscarinic drugs, though several other modalities of treatment are preferred (see Chapter 40).

Toxicity and antidotes   The belladonna alkaloids and other atropine-like drugs are generally safe medications. Large therapeutic doses in a normal person may cause unpleasant effects but are not life threatening. Normal persons have survived doses as high as 1 g taken by mouth. Blurred vision, tachycardia, dry mouth, constipation, and urinary retention are among the effects. However, patients with glaucoma and prostatic hypertrophy may have disastrous reactions, even to therapeutic doses.

Severe anticholinergic poisoning[16] is characterized by hot dry skin and hyperthermia,[3] hyperactivity, confusion, delirium, and hallucinations and eventually by coma, respiratory depression, and cardiovascular collapse. Infants have died after application of eye drops. Intoxication with antihistamines and tricyclic antidepressants, which also have antimuscarinic activity, may mimic atropine poisoning.

Patients with atropine intoxication should be managed with supportive care, including gastric lavage or induction of emesis if the agent was ingested. Sedatives such as chlordiazepoxide or diazepam may help control violent excitement. The use of physostigmine as an antidote to atropine poisoning is discussed on p. 107.

PROBLEM 12-1. Why is physostigmine preferable to neostigmine in reversing the CNS effects of atropine? The answer undoubtedly has some connection with the relative rates of penetration of the two drugs across the blood-brain barrier. Physostigmine is not a quaternary compound, but neostigmine is.

Atropine substitutes fall into three groups based to a certain extent on indications for their use: the mydriatics, the antispasmodics, which are of minimal usefulness today, and the antiparkinsonian drugs. *ATROPINE SUBSTITUTES*

For examination of the fundus and measurement of refractive errors, relatively short-acting agents are usually preferred. Alternatively, topical application of α-adrenergic agonists, such as phenylephrine, produces mydriasis without cycloplegia. Combinations of phenylephrine with scopolamine or cyclopentolate are also available. *Atropine-like mydriatics*

Homatropine hydrobromide (Isopto Homatropine), the oldest of the atropine-like mydriatic drugs, differs from atropine only in that it is an ester of mandelic rather than of tropic acid. It is applied to the eye in 2% or 5% solutions. Mydriasis develops fairly rapidly and may persist up to 4 days.

Homatropine

Cyclopentolate hydrochloride (Cyclogyl, Ak-Pentolate, Pentolair) produces mydriasis and cycloplegia in 15 to 45 minutes, with return of normal vision in less than 24 hours. It is used in 0.5% and 1% solutions, though for deeply pigmented eyes a 2% solution may be necessary. However, adverse effects are not uncommon with the latter concentration, which has evoked generalized seizures in children.

Tropicamide (Mydriacyl, Mydriafair), a more short-acting mydriatic and cycloplegic, is effective in less than 30 minutes and lasts less than 4 to 6 hours. It is used in 0.5% and 1% solutions.

A large group of atropine substitutes has been synthesized in an attempt to obtain some selective action on the gastrointestinal tract. The rationale for development of such agents includes the prevalence of peptic ulcer, the idea that reduction of smooth muscle tone and hypersecretion are beneficial in its management, and the need to *Anticholinergic smooth muscle relaxants*

FIG. 12-3   *Effect of atropine sulfate and atropine methylbromide on maternal and fetal heart rates. The lesser effect of the quaternary anticholinergic drug on fetal heart rate illustrates a basic difference between the two types of drugs as regards their passage across biologic membranes.*

From dePadua, C.B., and Gravenstein, J.S.: J.A.M.A. **208**:1022, 1969.

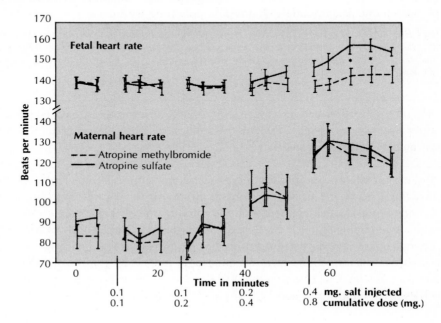

minimize side effects. These agents have been replaced by more effective and better tolerated agents, including histamine H_2-receptor antagonists (see Chapter 20) and sucralfate (see Chapter 41).

Conversion of tertiary atropine-like drugs to quaternary amines converts them to less lipid-soluble agents that do not readily cross the blood-brain barrier. Thus atropine methylbromide does not enter the central nervous system as efficiently as atropine sulfate. The difference between the two in regard to passage across biologic membranes is illustrated in Fig. 12-3. The quaternary agents also cause some ganglionic blockade that may reinforce their action on muscarinic receptors in the gastrointestinal tract but also contributes to unwanted side effects. Methscopolamine bromide, propantheline bromide, and the tertiary compound dicyclomine are examples of these agents. The quaternary drug glycopyrrolate (Robinul, 0.2 mg/ml) is a popular anticholinergic for perioperative use.

PIRENZEPINE   Pirenzepine, first marketed in Germany in 1971, is similar in structure to the tricyclic antidepressants but without appreciable central nervous system action. Unlike other muscarinic antagonists, which often induce unacceptable side effects when used to treat peptic ulcer, pirenzepine can reduce the volume of gastric acid and pepsin secretions at doses that cause minimal change in gastrointestinal motility or other antimuscarinic side effects, dry mouth being the most common.[2] Pirenzepine is a more potent antagonist of vagally mediated secretion than of bethanechol-induced secretion. This has been attributed to its blockade of *ganglionic* muscarinic receptors (subtype M_1) in the stomach rather than to a direct action on the muscarinic receptors (subtype M_2) on parietal cells. Although histamine H_2-antagonists and antacids now constitute the primary therapy for peptic ulcer, pirenzepine may prove useful for management of this problem in some patients. Not yet approved for use in the United States, pirenzepine is taken in doses of 100 to 150 mg per day, divided at bedtime and before breakfast.

Pirenzepine

Antiparkinsonian drugs

The pharmacology of Parkinson's disease was revolutionized by the discovery in the 1960s of the therapeutic effectiveness of levodopa (L-dopa)[15] and by elucidation of the role of dopamine in extrapyramidal function. Before the introduction of levodopa, the treatment of this common and disabling condition was based on the empiric use of (1) belladonna alkaloids and their synthetic congeners, (2) drugs with both anticholinergic and antihistaminic properties, and (3) dextroamphetamine.

Parkinsonism, characterized by tremor, rigidity, and bradykinesia, includes idiopathic paralysis agitans, postencephalitic parkinsonism, and other disturbances of the extrapyramidal system. It may also be caused by drugs. It was suggested more than 100 years ago that belladonna alkaloids might be useful in management of the syndrome, and drugs have also been extremely useful in the development of current concepts of its pathophysiology (Table 12-1).

CHOLINERGIC AND DOPAMINERGIC MECHANISMS IN PARKINSONISM

Parkinson's disease is believed to result from an imbalance between cholinergic and dopaminergic contributions to extrapyramidal control of motor function.[18] The effectiveness of belladonna alkaloids in treatment of parkinsonism suggested a contribution of cholinergic mechanisms to the pathologic process, a role supported by experiments in which *tremorine*, a muscarinic agonist, produced a syndrome in animals resembling parkinsonism. The injection of acetylcholine into the globus pallidus of patients undergoing stereotaxic surgery increased tremor contralaterally. Furthermore, physostigmine was found to exacerbate the symptoms of parkinsonian patients, and the suggestion was made that the cholinergic system may interact with a dopaminergic mechanism.[5]

TABLE 12-1 Drug effects in parkinsonism	
Drugs that aggravate or cause parkinsonism	Drugs that relieve parkinsonism
Reserpine	Belladonna alkaloids
Chlorpromazine (phenothiazines)	Synthetic anticholinergic drugs
Haloperidol	Antihistamines
Methyldopa	Drugs having both anticholinergic and antihistaminic properties
MPTP	Levodopa
	Amantadine
	Bromocriptine
	Deprenyl

The nigrostriatal dopaminergic system plays an important pathogenetic role in parkinsonism. Histochemical fluorescence techniques have shown[1] that the characteristic green fluorescence of catecholamines is present in nerve cell bodies in the *substantia nigra* and in nerve terminals in the *striatum,* two regions rich in dopamine. Lesions in the substantia nigra of rats decrease the dopamine concentration in the ipsilateral striatum.[1] In idiopathic parkinsonism conspicuous lesions are found in the substantia nigra, and the level of dopamine is greatly reduced in the striatum where the nigral axons terminate.[11] The effectiveness of levodopa in the treatment of Parkinson's disease indicates that this precursor can overcome the deficiency of dopamine that exists in the nigrostriatal dopaminergic pathway. Recently, MPTP (1-methyl-4-phenyl-1,2,3,6-tetrahydropyridine) has been added to the tools available for study of parkinsonism.[17] This compound, a contaminant in certain "designer drug" preparations, has caused a syndrome nearly identical to Parkinson's disease in a few drug abusers. The syndrome is irreversible, responds to dopaminergic therapy, and is characterized by damage to the substantia nigra. MPTP apparently acts through a metabolite, the 1-methyl-4-phenylpyridinium ion.

Drugs that aggravate parkinsonism. Both reserpine and neuroleptics aggravate the symptoms of parkinsonism. Reserpine depletes dopamine from the striatum and disturbs the dopaminergic-cholinergic balance. Neuroleptic drugs, such as chlorpromazine and haloperidol, are dopamine antagonists.

MAJOR ANTIPARKINSONIAN AGENTS

Antiparkinsonian drugs fall into the following groups on the basis of their pharmacologic properties:
1. Levodopa
2. Belladonna alkaloids and synthetic anticholinergics
3. Drugs with both anticholinergic and antihistaminic properties
4. Miscellaneous drugs that act on dopaminergic mechanisms, such as amantadine and bromocriptine

Levodopa. Levodopa is considered the most effective medication for parkinsonism.[15] Since it is an amino acid, levodopa is actively transported from the gut into the circulation and from the blood into the brain where it serves as a substrate for conversion to dopamine. When administered orally in increasing doses, it is likely to benefit well over half of the patients, though it may take several weeks for the improvement to become manifest. It is not necessary to discontinue the usual anticholinergic medications, though the dosage may be gradually decreased as the dosage of levodopa is increased. Anticholinergics can delay levodopa absorption by their effect on gastric emptying. The initial daily dose of levodopa is 500 mg to 1 g. To allow tolerance to minimize side effects, dosage is increased gradually, usually to no more than 8 g, until noticeable improvement occurs or adverse reactions make further increases impractical. Levodopa (Dopar, Larodopa) is available in tablets and capsules containing 100 to 500 mg.

Levodopa is most often given in a combination (Sinemet) with carbidopa, an inhibitor of aromatic L-amino acid decarboxylase. Carbidopa does not enter the central nervous system so that it inhibits decarboxylation of levodopa only in the periphery. As a consequence more levodopa is available for transport to the brain, and the dosage of levodopa can be reduced by about 75%. An additional benefit is that side effects caused by peripheral conversion to dopamine, in particular nausea and vomiting, are minimized. The decrease in required dose is also partially attributable to increased absorption of levodopa because in the absence of carbidopa the vitamin pyridoxine, a cofactor of intestinal decarboxylase, greatly reduces levodopa absorption. Patients receiving levodopa alone must discontinue their medication at least 8 hours before beginning the levodopa-carbidopa combination. The preparation is available in tablets of three strengths: Sinemet 10/100, 25/100, and 25/250. The first number indicates the dose of carbidopa and the second of levodopa, both in milligrams. Dosage must be determined by careful titration for each patient.

After 2 to 5 years of therapy the beneficial effect may begin to wane (undergo "wearing off") before the next dose is scheduled. Eventually akinesis may develop rather abruptly. Such fluctuations between symptom control and lack of control have been termed the "on-off phenomenon."[14] Administration of smaller but more frequent doses of levodopa may alleviate this problem for a time, and addition of bromocriptine to the regimen may also help. The mechanism of this phenomenon is poorly understood, but diminished conversion of levodopa to dopamine or reduced storage of the latter has been suggested. Periods in which levodopa is withheld for 2 to 10 days have been advocated to allow sensitivity to be restored, though such "drug holidays" require hospitalization and may be very stressful to the patient.[12] Bromocriptine or anticholinergic medication may alleviate symptoms during the levodopa vacation. Overall, though, management of this phenomenon is often only marginally effective and can be very frustrating to the patient and physician alike.

In addition to nausea and vomiting, orthostatic hypotension and cardiac arrhythmias may occur initially with levodopa therapy, but tolerance gradually develops as therapy continues. More serious adverse effects of levodopa are choreiform and other involuntary movements and psychiatric disturbances that tend to present an increasing problem as therapy is prolonged.[14,15] At this stage the on-off phenomenon may take the form of swings between dyskinesias and the parkinsonian state. Particularly because of the dyskinesias, the use of levodopa should be reserved, with reliance on administration of other agents, such as the anticholinergics or amantadine, until the parkinsonian disability becomes relatively severe.

Inhibitors of monoamine oxidase A, typically used as antidepressants (see Chapter 25), may cause a hypertensive crisis when used concomitantly with levodopa and should be discontinued 2 to 4 weeks before giving the latter. In contrast, **deprenyl,** an inhibitor of the monoamine oxidase (type B) that metabolizes dopamine, does not interact adversely with levodopa and is used in other countries to treat Parkinson's disease. The effects of sympathomimetic amines may be enhanced in patients treated with levodopa. Antihypertensive drugs should also be used with caution because orthostatic hypotension can be a reaction to levodopa. Neuroleptic-induced parkinsonian-like symptoms may be resistant to levodopa.

Belladonna alkaloids and synthetic anticholinergics. The naturally occurring alkaloids atropine and scopolamine were used for years to treat parkinsonism. They were replaced by synthetics that produce less peripheral anticholinergic symptoms for equal relief of parkinsonian disability, especially rigidity and to a lesser extent tremor. These latter agents are still useful early in therapy, so that the use of levodopa can be postponed.

Trihexyphenidyl hydrochloride (Artane, others) is available in tablets of 2 and 5 mg, timed-release capsules of 5 mg, and an elixir at 2 mg/5 ml. Dosage ranges from 1 mg initially to a maximum of 15 mg daily.

Biperiden (Akineton) **hydrochloride** is available in 2 mg tablets; **biperiden lactate** is available in solution, 5 mg/ml, for injection.

Procyclidine hydrochloride (Kemadrin) is available in 5 mg tablets.

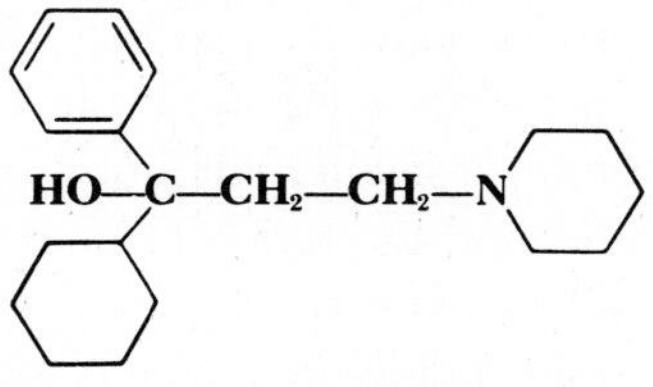

Trihexyphenidyl

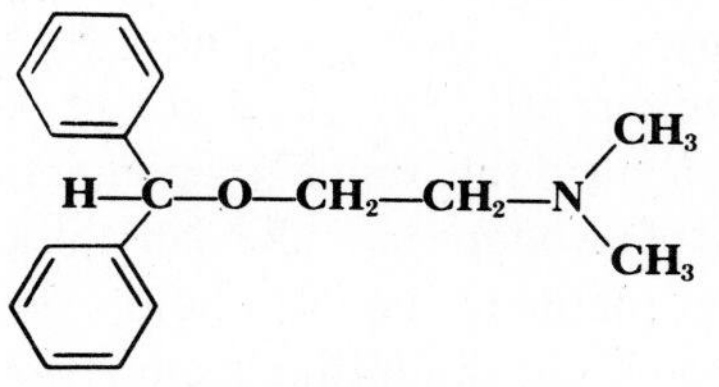

Diphenhydramine

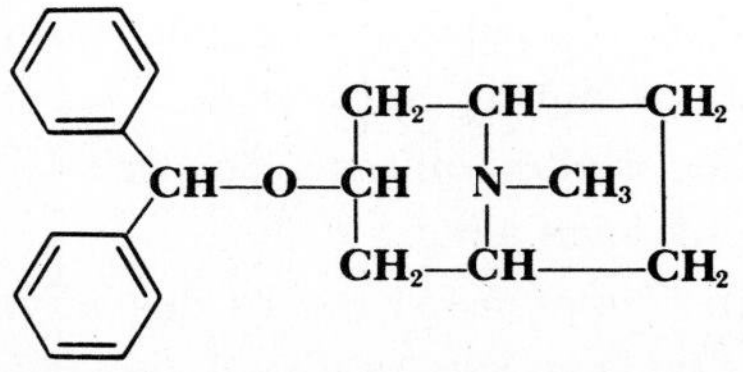

Benztropine

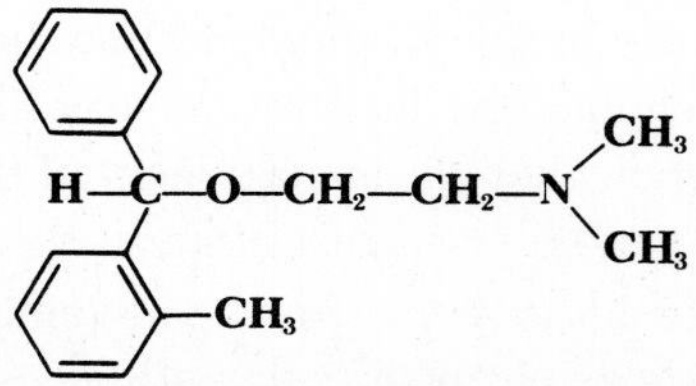

Orphenadrine

Drugs with both anticholinergic and antihistaminic properties. Many H_1-antihistamines (see Chapter 20) also have appreciable antimuscarinic activity, which probably accounts for their usefulness in Parkinson's disease. The major representative of this class is benztropine. An examination of its structure reveals similarities to atropine and to a typical antihistamine. Its pharmacologic properties resemble those of atropine, not only with regard to adverse effects but also from the standpoint of its prolonged duration of action.

Benztropine mesylate (Cogentin) is available in tablets of 0.5 to 2 mg and in solution for intramuscular or, occasionally, intravenous injection, 1 mg/ml.

Ethopropazine hydrochloride (Parsidol), a phenothiazine, may be a useful adjunct. Drowsiness is common, and it can cause muscle cramps, paresthesias, hypotension, or, rarely, agranulocytosis. It is supplied as tablets of 10 and 50 mg.

Diphenhydramine and the closely related **orphenadrine** have some usefulness in treatment of parkinsonism including that induced by drugs such as the phenothiazines. They are not so effective as the above agents but produce fewer atropine-like untoward effects. On the other hand, they produce considerable drowsiness.

Miscellaneous agents. The antiviral agent **amantadine** produces clinical improvement in some patients with parkinsonian symptoms and does so much more rapidly than levodopa. However, tolerance to the beneficial effect develops in 6 to 8 weeks in about 20% of patients. Although its mode of action is uncertain, enhancement of dopamine release, inhibition of dopamine reuptake, and an increase in the number of postsynaptic dopamine receptors have all been proposed.[7]

Adverse effects of amantadine include mottling of the skin (livedo reticularis) and ankle edema. Other effects are anxiety, irritability, insomnia, and gastrointestinal disturbances. A few cases of congestive heart failure have been associated with amantadine, and convulsions have occurred after excessive doses.

Amantadine hydrochloride (Symmetrel) is available in capsules of 100 mg and in a syrup containing 50 mg/5 ml. The initial dose for use alone is 100 mg twice daily.

The dopamine agonist **bromocriptine mesylate** (Parlodel) appears most useful as an adjunct to minimize the on-off fluctuations associated with levodopa therapy.[13]

Dopamine   **Bromocriptine**   **Amantadine**

Adverse reactions to bromocriptine include nausea, vomiting, orthostatic hypotension, and psychiatric complications. Bromocriptine also inhibits prolactin secretion (see p. 582) and is contraindicated in pregnancy. It is available either as 2.5 mg tablets or in 5 mg capsules. Therapy is started with half a tablet twice a day and has been increased to as much as 300 mg daily. The best dosage regimen has not yet been established. Other potentially useful agonists, which act directly on the dopamine receptor and are currently under investigation, include piribedil, lisuride, and pergolide.[15]

REFERENCES

1. Andén, N.-E., Carlsson, A., Dahlström, A., et al.: Demonstration and mapping out of nigro-neostriatal dopamine neurons, Life Sci. **3**:523, 1964.
2. Carmine, A.A., and Brogden, R.N.: Pirenzepine: a review of its pharmacodynamic and pharmacokinetic properties and therapeutic efficacy in peptic ulcer disease and other allied diseases, Drugs **30**:85, 1985.
3. Clark, W.G., and Lipton, J.M.: Drug-related heatstroke, Pharmacol. Ther. **26**:345, 1984.
4. Clissold, S.P., and Heel, R.C.: Transdermal hyoscine (scopolamine): a preliminary review of its pharmacodynamic properties and therapeutic efficacy, Drugs **29**:189, 1985.
5. Duvoisin, R.C.: Cholinergic-anticholinergic antagonism in parkinsonism, Arch. Neurol. **17**:124, 1967.
6. Frumin, M.J., Herekar, V.R., and Jarvik, M.E.: Amnesic actions of diazepam and scopolamine in man, Anesthesiology **45**:406, 1976.
7. Gianutsos, G., Chute, S., and Dunn, J.P.: Pharmacological changes in dopaminergic systems induced by long-term administration of amantadine, Eur. J. Pharmacol. **110**:357, 1985.
8. Gravenstein, J.S., and Thornby, J.I.: Scopolamine on heart rates in man, Clin. Pharmacol. Ther. **10**:395, 1969.
9. Greenblatt, D.J., and Shader, R.I.: Anticholinergics, N.Engl. J. Med. **288**:1215, 1973.
10. Havener, W.H.: Ocular pharmacology, ed. 5, St. Louis, 1983, The C.V. Mosby Co.
11. Hornykiewicz, O.: Brain neurotransmitter changes in Parkinson's disease. In Marsden, C.D., and Fahn, S., editors: Movement disorders, Neurology 2, London, 1981, Butterworth Scientific, p. 41.
12. Kaye, J.A., and Feldman, R.G.: The role of L-DOPA holiday in the long-term management of Parkinson's disease, Clin. Neuropharmacol. **9**:1, 1986.
13. Lieberman, A.N., and Goldstein, M.: Bromocriptine in Parkinson disease, Pharmacol. Rev. **37**:217, 1985.
14. Marsden, C.D., Parkes, J.D., and Quinn, N.: Fluctuations of disability in Parkinson's disease: clinical aspects. In Marsden, C.D., and Fahn, S., editors: Movement disorders, Neurology 2, London, 1981, Butterworth Scientific, p. 96.
15. Quinn, N.P.: Anti-parkinsonian drugs today, Drugs **28**:236, 1984.
16. Shader, R.I., and Greenblatt, D.J.: Uses and toxicity of belladonna alkaloids and synthetic anticholinergics, Semin. Psychiatry **3**:449, 1971.
17. Snyder, S.H., and D'Amato, R.J.: MPTP: a neurotoxin relevant to the pathophysiology of Parkinson's disease, Neurology (N.Y.) **36**:250, 1986.
18. Stahl, S.M.: Neuropharmacology of movement disorders: comparison of spontaneous and drug-induced movement disorders. In Shah, N.S., and Donald, A.G., editors: Movement disorders, New York, 1986, Plenum Medical Book Co.

Chapter 13

Ganglionic blocking agents

GENERAL CONCEPT

Neurotransmission at nicotinic receptors can be blocked either by compounds that prevent depolarization by acetylcholine (mecamylamine in ganglia, tubocurarine at the skeletal neuromuscular junction) or by agents that produce initial stimulation and depolarization followed by persistent receptor desensitization (nicotine).[10] Evidence has recently been presented that the classical ganglionic blocking agent hexamethonium is not an antagonist at these receptors but, rather, has a channel-blocking action; that is, it becomes trapped within ionic channels, thereby preventing sodium ion influx.[4]

In concentrations that have little action at other sites, the currently used ganglionic blocking agents competitively inhibit the action of acetylcholine at nicotinic receptors on postganglionic neurons. It is these receptors that are mainly responsible for transmission through intact ganglia. In certain experimental circumstances, muscarinic, adrenergic, and peptide receptors have also been demonstrated in ganglia[5,8] (Fig. 13-1). Although pharmacologic blockade of muscarinic and catecholamine receptors alters ganglionic action potentials, fast excitation of autonomic neuroeffectors is unimpeded. Sympathetic ganglia are relatively accessible and simple structures that have been remarkably useful for research on neurotransmission.

Impulse transmission in sympathetic autonomic ganglia. Acetylcholine (ACh) interacts with nicotinic receptors (N) on postganglionic neurons (Principal cells) to cause rapid depolarization, the fast excitatory postsynaptic potential (f-EPSP). ACh also binds to muscarinic receptors (M) on these cells to cause a late (l-) EPSP and on small intensely fluorescent (SIF) interneurons,[2] which release dopamine (DA). Dopamine interaction with catecholamine receptors (C) initiates an inhibitory postsynaptic potential (IPSP). Sites of action of the antagonists are also shown. GF, Ganglionic fiber.

FIG. 13-1

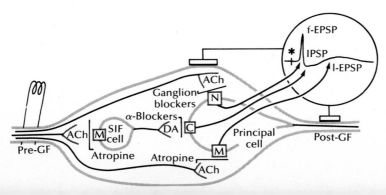

GANGLIONIC STIMULANTS   Certain ganglionic stimulants, such as tetra*methyl*ammonium, and small doses of nicotine cause vasoconstriction and raise blood pressure as a consequence of their action on sympathetic ganglia. This type of drug effect has not found therapeutic application. However, some drugs that were used in the past to diagnose pheochromocytoma (for example, methacholine) cause catecholamine release from the adrenal. This is analogous to ganglionic stimulation.

Nicotine   Nicotine is a highly toxic liquid that is absorbed readily through the skin. It is found in some insecticides. Symptoms of intoxication, which include nausea, vomiting, sweating, diarrhea, skeletal muscular fasciculations and weakness, fluctuations in blood pressure and heart rate, seizures, and eventually respiratory depression, result from sequential stimulation and then inhibition of transmission at nicotinic receptors in ganglia, at the neuromuscular junction, and in the central nervous system.

Chewing gum (Nicorette) containing 2 mg of nicotine per piece is available by prescription as an aid for persons stopping cigarette smoking. In nonsmokers this dose is sufficient to increase heart rate and blood pressure. Contraindications include recent myocardial infarction, life-threatening arrhythmias, severe angina, and pregnancy.

GANGLIONIC BLOCKING AGENTS
Development   The curious ability of nicotine to block ganglionic transmission after initial stimulation has been known for many years. During the latter part of the nineteenth century, Langley and Dickinson[6] charted the distribution of fibers emanating from sympathetic ganglia by selectively blocking the ganglia with local applications of nicotine.

The ability of tetra*ethyl*ammonium to prevent the effect of ganglionic stimulants was also known for many years. This received little attention, however, until 1946, when the mode of action of tetraethylammonium on mammalian circulation was thoroughly investigated.[1] This study indicated the possibility of blocking ganglionic transmission in a fairly selective manner. Several ganglionic blocking agents were then developed and used to treat hypertension or to produce controlled hypotension. Among these were hexamethonium, pentolinium, chlorisondamine, trimethaphan, pempidine, and mecamylamine.

Chemistry   The chemical formulas of some of these agents are as follows:

$$(C_2H_5)_3 N^+ - CH_2 - CH_3 \cdot Cl^-$$

Tetraethylammonium chloride

$$(CH_3)_3 N^+ - CH_2 - (CH_2)_4 - CH_2 - N^+(CH_3)_3 \cdot 2Cl^-$$

Hexamethonium chloride

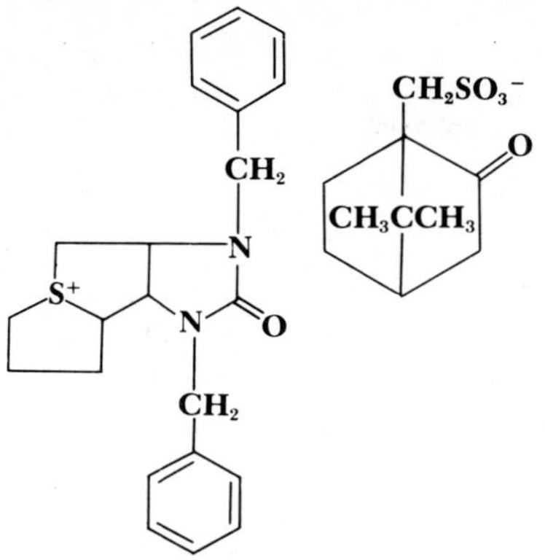

Trimethaphan camsylate

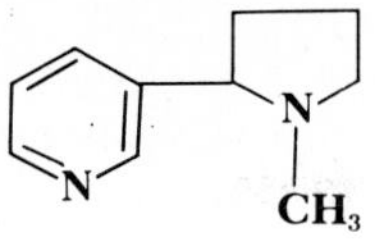

Nicotine

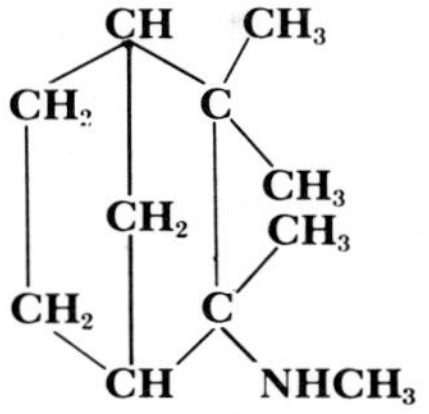

Mecamylamine

Like acetylcholine, most ganglionic blocking drugs have been quaternary ammonium compounds. However, of the two agents in current though infrequent use, trimethaphan contains a tertiary sulfur, and so it too is a strong electrolyte, and mecamylamine is a secondary amine.

Ganglionic blocking agents have been used principally to decrease sympathetic control of vascular smooth muscle tone. They were first-line drugs for management of hypertension until more specific and less toxic compounds became available. Although ganglionic blockers are selective in that they have little if any action elsewhere, they are nonspecific by comparison with other antihypertensive drugs because they block transmission in both sympathetic and parasympathetic ganglia. For this reason their effects depend on the autonomic tone prevailing in each organ at the time of administration.

Clinical pharmacology

PROBLEM 13-1. *Before reading the rest of this chapter, predict the effects of a typical ganglionic blocking agent in a resting subject. Keep in mind that in the resting state the parasympathetic influence is usually dominant in organs innervated by both parasympathetic and sympathetic branches of the autonomic nervous system. How did your predictions compare with Paton's description below?*

A picturesque description of a person without a functioning autonomic nervous system was given by Paton in his account of the "hexamethonium man."

He is a pink-complexioned person, except when he has stood in a queue for some time, when he may get pale and faint. His handshake is warm and dry. He is a placid and relaxed companion; he may laugh, but he can't cry because the tears cannot come. Your rudest story will not make him blush and the most unpleasant circumstances will fail to make him turn pale. His . . . collars and socks stay very clean and sweet. He wears corsets and may, if you meet him out, be rather fidgety (the corsets compress his splanchnic vascular pool, the fidgets keep the venous return going from his legs). He dislikes speaking much unless helped with something to moisten his dry mouth and throat. He is rather long-sighted and easily blinded by bright light. The redness of his eye-balls may suggest irregular habits and in fact his head is rather weak. But he always behaves like a gentleman and never belches nor hiccups. He tends to get cold and keeps well wrapped up. But his health is good; he does not have chilblains and those diseases of modern civilization, hypertension and peptic ulcer, pass him by. He is thin because his appetite is modest; he never feels hunger pains and his stomach never rumbles. He gets rather constipated so that his intake of liquid paraffin is high. As old age comes on, frequency, precipitancy and strangury will not worry him, but he will suffer from retention of urine and impotence. One is uncertain how he will end, but perhaps, if he is not careful, by eating less and less and getting colder and colder, he will sink into a symptomless, hypoglycemic coma and (like the universe) die a sort of entropy death.*

Circulatory effects. Ganglionic blocking drugs lower blood pressure primarily by decreasing sympathetic tone to various vascular regions. The intensity of this hypotensive action depends on several factors, in particular the position of the patient. There may be only a slight lowering of pressure while the patient is in the recumbent position. Upon standing, however, the patient may experience a precipitous fall in blood pressure and may faint. This orthostatic (postural) hypotension results from pooling of blood in the extremities, in the absence of compensatory venoconstriction.

Other side effects and complications. Reduction of smooth muscle tone of the gastrointestinal and urinary tracts by ganglionic blocking agents can cause constipation or difficulty in voiding. The pupils may dilate, and accommodation for near vision is impaired. Salivary secretion is inhibited, and dry mouth may be sufficiently uncomfortable to require administration of pilocarpine. Sweating is also inhibited (not an atropine-like effect) because of decreased sympathetic activity. Impotence is another problem. The high incidence of such effects contributes to poor compliance by patients. Although many of the adverse effects can be alleviated by concurrent management with cholinergic drugs, such as pilocarpine, by laxatives, and by physical measures such as supportive stockings, newer antihypertensive drugs (see Chapter 18) have nearly eliminated the use of these unpleasant agents.

Absorption and elimination	The quaternary ammonium blocking agents are poorly and erratically absorbed from the gastrointestinal tract. Yet they must be given orally for chronic management of hypertension. The oral:intravenous LD_{50} ratio of several of these drugs in mice is about 20:1. On the other hand, the secondary amine mecamylamine is much better absorbed, with an oral:intravenous LD_{50} ratio of about 4:1.[9] Trimethaphan camphorsulfonate cannot be used by mouth because of poor absorption and rapid excretion.

As would be expected from their ionic character, the quaternary agents cause no central nervous system effects and are eliminated through the kidney. Their distribution in the body is largely extracellular.

---

* From Paton, W.D.M.: The principles of ganglionic block. In Lectures on the scientific basis of medicine, vol. 2, London, 1954, Athlone Press.

Because **mecamylamine hydrochloride** (Inversine) is a secondary amine, it is well absorbed from the gastrointestinal tract and may cause central nervous system effects, including insomnia, confusion, depression, and even seizures. It has a duration of action of 4 to 12 hours. The initial oral dose is 2.5 mg twice daily. This dose is gradually increased until a satisfactory response is obtained, usually at about 25 mg/day. It is available in 2.5 and 10 mg tablets.

Mecamylamine and trimethaphan

Trimethaphan camsylate (Arfonad) is a very short-acting ganglionic blocking agent that is actively secreted by the kidney. It is used to reduce blood pressure rapidly in hypertensive emergencies and in cases of acute dissecting aneurysm of the aorta and to minimize bleeding during certain types of surgery.[7] Although histamine release by an intravenous bolus of trimethaphan can cause feelings of warmth, dizziness, headache, and flushing of the face, this release does not contribute to the hypotensive response.[3] Intravenous infusion at rates from 0.3 to 6 mg/min can effectively lower blood pressure, but elevation of the head of the patient's bed is usually required so that pooling of blood in the extremities can occur. When the infusion is stopped, blood pressure returns to its normal level in about 10 minutes. Trimethaphan camsylate is available as a 50 mg/ml solution, which must be diluted fiftyfold before intravenous infusion.

Nowadays mecamylamine is rarely if ever used. Trimethaphan is used solely for the indications mentioned above and then only by some physicians. For the most part, ganglionic blocking agents are of historic interest.

REFERENCES

1. Acheson, G.H., and Moe, G.K.: The action of tetraethylammonium ion on the mammalian circulation, J. Pharmacol. Exp. Ther. **87:**220, 1946.
2. Eränkö, O.: Small intensely fluorescent (SIF) cells and nervous transmission in sympathetic ganglia, Annu. Rev. Pharmacol. Toxicol. **18:**417, 1978.
3. Fahmy, N.R., and Soter, N.A.: Effects of trimethaphan on arterial blood histamine and systemic hemodynamics in humans, Anesthesiology **62:**562, 1985.
4. Gurney, A.M., and Rang, H.P.: The channel-blocking action of methonium compounds on rat submandibular ganglion cells, Br. J. Pharmacol. **82:**623, 1984.
5. Kawatani, M., Rutigliano, M., and de Groat, W.C.: Depolarization and muscarinic excitation induced in a sympathetic ganglion by vasoactive intestinal polypeptide, Science **229:**879, 1985.
6. Langley, J.N., and Dickinson, W.L.: On the local paralysis of peripheral ganglia, and on the connexion of different classes of nerve fibres with them, Proc. R. Soc. Lond. [series A] **46:**423, 1889.
7. Miller, E.D., Jr.: Deliberate hypotension. In Miller, R.D., editor: Anesthesia, vol. 3, ed. 2, New York, 1986, Churchill Livingstone, p. 1949.
8. Skok, V.I.: Ganglionic transmission: morphology and physiology, Handb. Exp. Pharmacol. **53:**9, 1980.
9. Stone, C.A., Torchiana, M.L., Navarro, A., and Beyer, K.H.: Ganglionic blocking properties of 3-methylaminoisocamphane hydrochloride (mecamylamine): a secondary amine, J. Pharmacol. Exp. Ther. **117:**169, 1956.
10. Volle, R.L.: Nicotinic ganglion-stimulating agents, Handb. Exp. Pharmacol. **53:**281, 1980.

Chapter 14

Neuromuscular blocking agents and muscle relaxants

GENERAL CONCEPT Neuromuscular blocking agents act on nicotinic receptors located in the specialized end-plate region of skeletal muscle. Most clinically useful neuromuscular blockers (the *nondepolarizing* agents) compete with acetylcholine for these receptors, whereas succinylcholine depolarizes the end-plate region and initially stimulates the muscle.

Skeletal muscle relaxation may be achieved by other mechanisms as well. Centrally acting agents, including mephenesin and antianxiety drugs such as diazepam, produce relaxation primarily by actions within the central nervous system. Dantrolene, in contrast, acts within the muscle fiber to interfere with excitation-contraction coupling.

Many other drugs impair neuromuscular transmission as an unwanted side effect.[1] For example, local anesthetics and certain antibiotics may cause postoperative respiratory depression or may aggravate myasthenia gravis.

NEUROMUSCULAR BLOCKING AGENTS
Development Experimentation with the South American arrow poison *curare* was one of the earliest examples of scientific pharmacology. In the nineteenth century Magendie and his pupil Claude Bernard studied its effects on nerve-muscle preparations. Bernard demonstrated that the drug prevented the response of skeletal muscle to nerve stimulation. Its inability to prevent the muscle from responding to electrical stimulation and its failure to block conduction in the nerve indicated an action at the junction of nerve and muscle.

The active principle of *Chondodendron tomentosum* roots is *d*-tubocurarine, a bulky molecule in which two nitrogen atoms are separated by a distance of about 1.1 nm.[11] Most nondepolarizing blockers in current use exhibit a similar separation between paired quaternary structures. Much of the current knowledge regarding the structure of muscular nicotinic receptors (see Fig. 10-1) has been derived from study of electric organs from rays and eels. It appears that two molecules of acetylcholine are required for the ion channel to open, one acting on each of the α subunits. Binding of a nondepolarizing antagonist to either of these subunits therefore prevents influx of sodium ions.

Unlike curare, succinylcholine mimics the neurotransmitter in stimulating the receptor and paralyzes much like an excess of acetylcholine, as in a myasthenic patient during anticholinesterase overtreatment.

Clinical pharmacology

The first consideration in choosing a neuromuscular blocker is the duration of paralysis needed. For brief paralysis to allow endotracheal intubation succinylcholine is most often used. For longer paralysis a nondepolarizing agent is generally preferred. The drugs are usually given intravenously, though tubocurarine and succinylcholine can be injected intramuscularly. Respiration must be assisted or controlled by the anesthetist. The most important antidotal measure is to maintain mechanical respiration until recovery. None of these agents appreciably affect the central nervous system because of the blood-brain barrier to quaternary ammonium compounds. Therefore they are not anesthetic or analgesic. Since the paralyzed patient cannot speak or otherwise indicate perception of pain, the anesthetist must pay careful attention to other indications of the depth of anesthesia. The beneficial effect on pain in conditions such as strychnine intoxication or tetanus is ascribed to relaxation of contracted muscles.

Intravenous injection of 5 to 10 mg of tubocurarine produces flaccid paralysis. Doubling the dose may produce apnea. There is a characteristic progression of effects, with the extrinsic muscles of the eye affected first, then those of the face, the extremities, and finally the diaphragm. This progression parallels the sequence of muscle involvement in myasthenia gravis.

NONDEPOLARIZING NEUROMUSCULAR BLOCKING AGENTS

Mode of action. Packets, or quanta, of acetylcholine are released from synaptic vesicles of motoneurons spontaneously or with the arrival of a nerve impulse.[5] These quanta stimulate receptors in the end-plate region of muscle fibers to produce an electrical change known as the *end-plate potential*. If depolarization is sufficient to reach threshold, a propagated *action potential* leads to muscle contraction. In a partially curarized preparation the small end-plate potential is clearly visible, since it is not followed by the larger action potential. The effect of curare on the end-plate potential and the anticurare action of physostigmine are illustrated in Fig. 14-1.

General characteristics. Certain characteristics of individual neuromuscular blocking agents are listed in Table 14-1. Maximum paralysis develops within 2 to 5 minutes after intravenous administration. The first four agents are relatively long acting (30 to 90 minutes), though the duration of paralysis can vary considerably with dosage, whereas atracurium and vecuronium, introduced in 1983 and 1984 respectively, provide paralysis for intermediate durations of 20 to 40 minutes. Increasing the dose beyond that necessary for paralysis prolongs relaxation but also increases the likelihood of side effects. To prolong paralysis, it is better to give a supplemental bolus as needed. Such supplements are limited to a fraction, ranging from one eighth to one half, of the initial dose because they are given before the previous dose is completely inactivated.

Interactions with other agents that enhance paralysis are of great importance. General anesthetics such as halothane, enflurane, and isoflurane have some relaxant

FIG. 14-1 *Effect of tubocurarine on the end-plate potential of the frog sartorius muscle and the antagonistic action of physostigmine. 1, After 6 μM of curarine; 2, after 9 μM of curarine; 3, after 9 μM of curarine plus physostigmine 10^{-5}.*

From Eccles, J.C., et al.: J Neurophysiol. **5:**211, 1942.

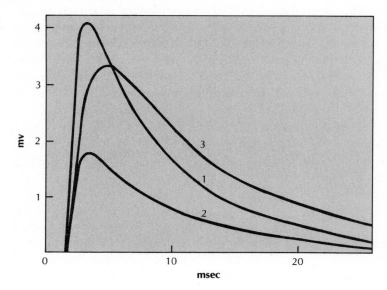

TABLE 14-1 Characteristics of neuromuscular blocking agents

Type	Initial dose (mg/kg)	Commercial preparation (mg/ml)	Typical duration (minutes)	Histamine release	Vagal block	Prolonged by renal impairment
Nondepolarizing (competitive)						
Tubocurarine	0.165	3	60	+ +		+
Metocurine	0.1-0.3	2	60	+		+
Pancuronium	0.04-0.1	1, 2	60		+	+
Gallamine	1.0	20, 100	60		+ +	+
Atracurium	0.4-0.5	10	30	±		
Vecuronium	0.08-0.1	2	30			
Depolarizing						
Succinyl-choline	0.3-1.1	20, 50, 100	5	+		

activity of their own, so that less neuromuscular blocker is necessary. The dose of relaxant is generally reduced about 20% to 30% with halothane and somewhat more with the other two anesthetics. Diethyl ether, though now seldom used in the United States, is such a good relaxant that the dose of tubocurarine was typically reduced by two thirds when they were used together. Aminoglycosides and some other antibiotics, such as polymyxin B, colistin, and lincomycin, also potentiate neuromuscular blockade, as do quinidine and magnesium salts. Finally, patients with myasthenia gravis or acidosis react excessively to usual doses of neuromuscular blockers. The older nondepolarizing blockers are excreted to a large extent unmetabolized in urine[10] and should be used cautiously in patients in shock or with impaired renal function. Pancuronium and tubocurarine are partially metabolized and excreted in bile so that caution is advised with patients who have liver damage.

Adverse reactions to nondepolarizing neuromuscular blocking drugs include prolonged apnea, bronchospasm, hypotension, and tachycardia. A major advantage of these agents over succinylcholine is that, in addition to mechanical respiration, reversible anticholinesterases are usually effective antagonists.[4] However, one must monitor the patient to be certain apnea does not recur. This can happen if anticholinesterase activity wears off before the blocker is inactivated. Atropine is given before or with the anticholinesterase to prevent muscarinic effects. Those agents that release histamine (Table 14-1) are generally contraindicated in patients with asthma or who have previously experienced an anaphylactoid reaction. Fentanyl, an opioid analgesic used in balanced anesthesia, does not release histamine[9] and is probably safer than morphine, which can release histamine, for combination with tubocurarine. Patients with severe cardiovascular disease may also suffer adverse responses to some of these agents. Histamine release and ganglionic blockade are both believed to contribute to hypotension. Gallamine in particular can block the cardiac vagus to elicit tachycardia. This action is not always a disadvantage, since it tends to minimize bradycardia induced by agents such as fentanyl or β-adrenergic antagonists.

Specific agents. **Tubocurarine** (*d*-tubocurarine) **chloride** is given initially as a divided dose with the first two thirds over a minute or so and the remainder 3 to 5 minutes later. This reduces histamine release and ganglionic blockade, which are favored by rapid administration and larger doses. About half of the drug is excreted unchanged in the urine, whereas the rest is metabolized. Although curare is still an important neuromuscular blocking agent, newer agents have reduced its use considerably. Occasionally, if an edrophonium test is not conclusive, low doses of tubocurarine (4 to 33 μg/kg) are given intravenously, very cautiously with facilities for mechanical respiration, for diagnosis of myasthenia gravis. Nondepolarizing blockers are also used to facilitate mechanical ventilation, as in patients with tetanus, and to prevent motor manifestations of electroconvulsive therapy. The derivative of tubocurarine **metocurine** (Metubine) **iodide** is also available.

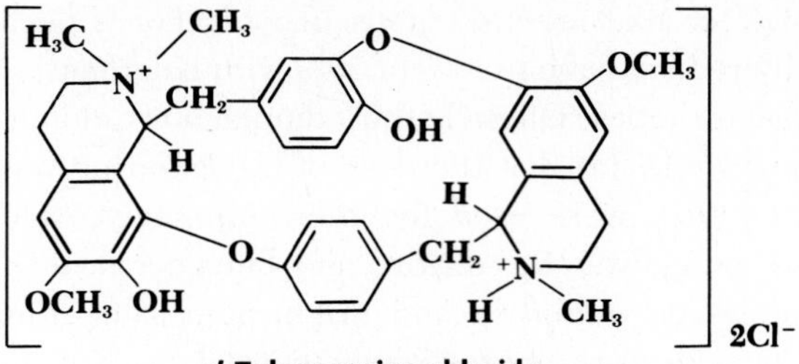

d-Tubocurarine chloride

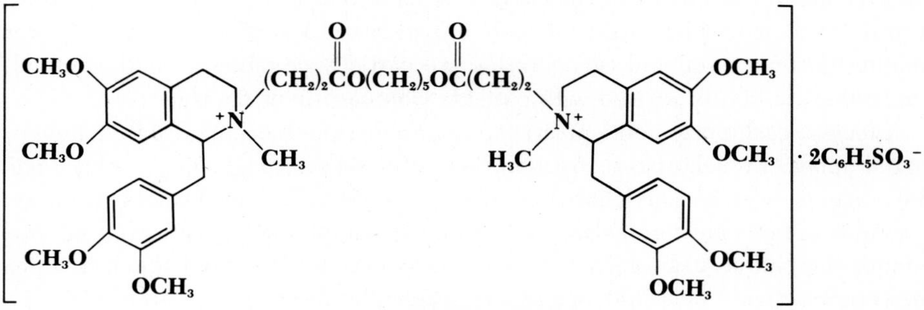

Atracurium besylate

Pancuronium bromide (Pavulon) differs from tubocurarine in its greater potency and lack of histamine-releasing or ganglionic blocking actions. It may cause a slight increase in heart rate because of vagal blockade. The drug has a steroid nucleus with two quaternary amines attached.

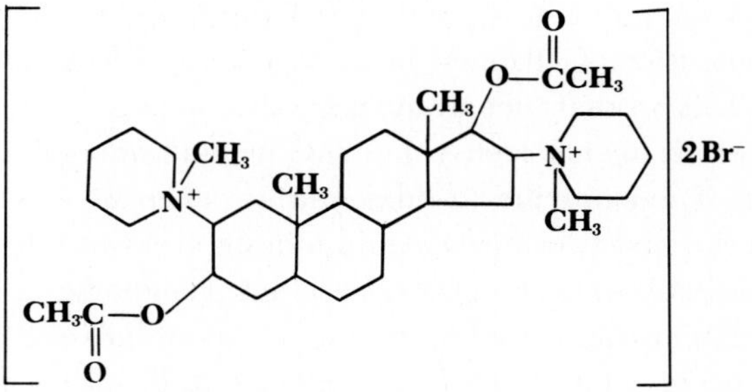

Pancuronium bromide

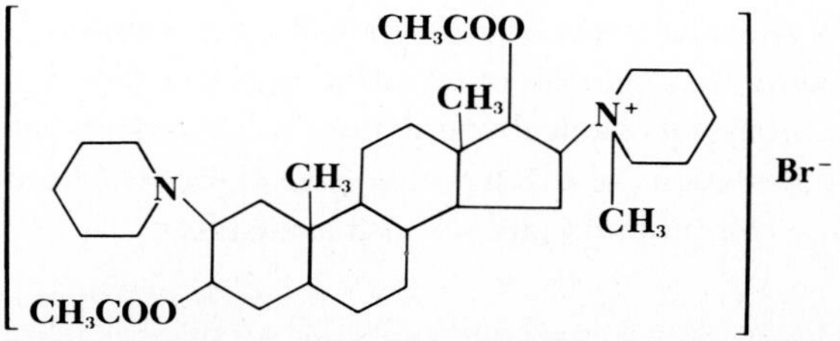

Vecuronium bromide

Gallamine triethiodide (Flaxedil) may have a slightly shorter duration of action then tubocurarine. It has an atropine-like effect at the cardiac branch of the vagus nerve and can induce considerable tachycardia, a disadvantage in some patients.

Atracurium besylate (Tracrium) is structurally related to tubocurarine. Advantages include an intermediate duration of action and minimal vagolytic activity or tendency to release histamine. Furthermore atracurium is inactivated in plasma so that it can be used safely in patients with impairment of either liver or renal function. Its inactivation is slowed in patients undergoing controlled hypothermia.

Vecuronium bromide (Norcuron), like pancuronium, has a steroid nucleus. It has an intermediate duration of action and lacks significant ganglionic blocking, vagolytic, or histamine-releasing activity. Its pharmacokinetics are unaffected by renal impairment, but its action may be prolonged in patients with cirrhosis.

The only available short-acting neuromuscular blocking agent is the depolarizing drug succinylcholine, which consists of two acetylcholine molecules joined together. When this drug is injected intravenously, there may be considerable muscular fasciculation for several seconds before paralysis. Many patients will later experience muscle soreness. The muscles remain paralyzed for about 5 minutes and resume their function in another 5 minutes.

Succinylcholine chloride

Succinylcholine is rapidly hydrolyzed by plasma cholinesterase to choline and succinylmonocholine. The latter is then hydrolyzed to succinic acid and choline. In patients with quantitative or qualitative differences in plasma cholinesterase, because of a genetic abnormality (p. 52), succinylcholine can produce apnea for hours.

The action of succinylcholine is inhibited by prior administration of a nondepolarizing blocker. When succinylcholine is used to facilitate endotracheal intubation, a sufficient interval should be allowed for it to wear off before a nondepolarizing blocker is given.

Neostigmine is not an antidote to succinylcholine during depolarization but rather tends to enhance early paralysis. *Mixed* or *dual block*, however, can result with prolonged exposure to succinylcholine. After initial stimulation, paralysis occurs during depolarization (phase I block) and is sustained for a period after repolarization (phase II block). In the latter phase, usually attributed to receptor desensitization, neostigmine can be an effective antidote, in contrast to phase I. The depth and phase of blockade can be assessed by peripheral nerve stimulation.[12]

Succinylcholine can also contribute to certain other problems.[7] In the absence of atropine, stimulation of ganglionic receptors may elicit bradycardia, whereas tachycardia may occur with large doses or after adequate treatment with atropine. Life-

SUCCINYLCHOLINE

FIG. 14-2   *Innervation of skeletal muscle.*

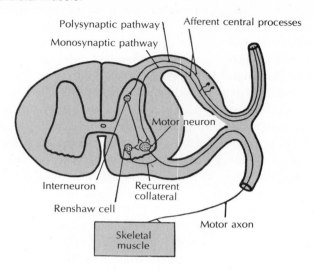

threatening hyperkalemia caused by tissue loss of potassium during depolarization can occur after extensive trauma (burns, spinal cord transection, crush injury).[2] The potential for development of *malignant hyperthermia*, a fulminant and often fatal disorder characterized by myoglobinuria and a rapid increase in temperature, is enhanced when succinylcholine is used with potent inhalational anesthetics.[8]

Succinylcholine chloride (Anectine) may be given in single intravenous doses or by infusion. Preparations for injection include powder, 0.1 to 1 g for reconstitution, and solutions of 20 to 100 mg/ml. Facilities for mechanical respiration are essential, since this is the only certain antidotal measure to apnea.

SKELETAL MUSCLE RELAXANTS THAT ACT ON THE SPINAL CORD

Some drugs may relax muscle by acting on internuncial spinal neurons to depress polysynaptic pathways (Fig. 14-2). Such relaxants also act on higher centers, and some, such as the benzodiazepines (see Chapters 24 and 26), are commonly used to relieve anxiety or to induce sleep. Although experimentally these drugs depress the spinal cord at doses that do not cause sleep or anesthesia, it is unclear to what extent the clinical benefit is attributable to their antianxiety or sedative effects. Only those agents that have been promoted primarily as relaxants are mentioned below. Indications for these drugs include treatment of muscle spasm resulting from sprains, arthritis, myositis, and fibrositis. They may also cause drowsiness, lethargy, ataxia, and allergic manifestations.

Mephenesin[6] and mephenesin carbamate were the first drugs introduced as centrally acting muscle relaxants. Their selective action on spinal neurons was shown by abolition of strychnine convulsions in animals by doses that did not cause sleep. **Methocarbamol** (Robaxin, others), closely related to mephenesin carbamate, is available in tablets of 500 and 750 mg and in a solution of 100 mg/ml in 50% polyethylene glycol for injection. **Chlorphenesin carbamate** (Maolate), also related to mephenesin, is available in tablets, 400 mg.

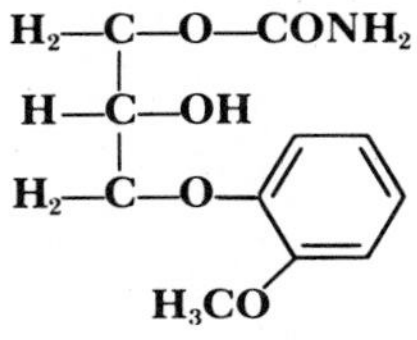

Methocarbamol

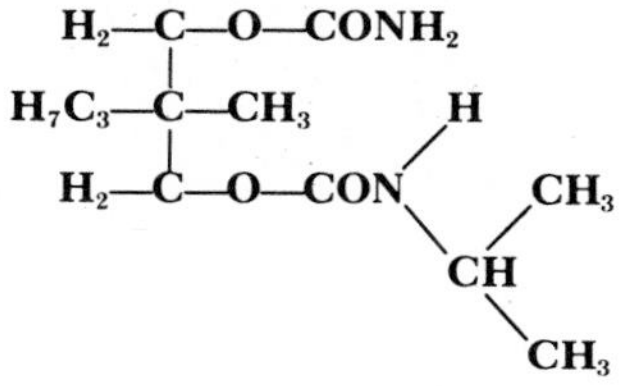

Carisoprodol

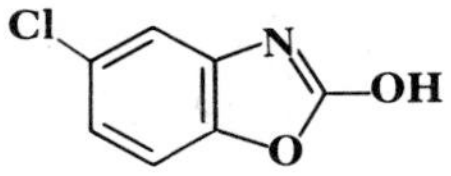

Chlorzoxazone

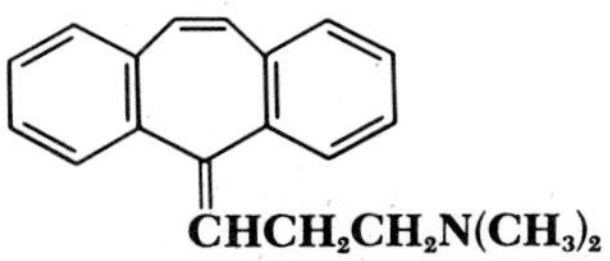

Cyclobenzaprine

Carisoprodol (Soma, others) is provided as tablets, 350 mg.

The relaxants zoxazolamine and chlorzoxazone were developed on the basis of the observation that benzimidazole depressed polysynaptic spinal pathways. Zoxazolamine is hepatotoxic and was removed from the market. **Chlorzoxazone** (Paraflex) may also cause jaundice in an occasional patient. It is available in tablets, 250 mg.

Metaxalone (Skelaxin) is available in tablets, 400 mg.

Cyclobenzaprine hydrochloride (Flexeril) is used for short-term treatment of acute, painful musculoskeletal conditions. It has numerous side effects just as tricyclic antidepressants have (see Chapter 25), to which it is related. It should be avoided by patients receiving monoamine oxidase inhibitors. Cyclobenzaprine is available in tablets, 10 mg.

Baclofen is a relatively new skeletal muscle relaxant that mimics GABA (γ-aminobutyric acid) at so-called GABA-B (bicuculline-insensitive) receptors. Unlike the agents above, it appears to inhibit transmission in monosynaptic as well as in polysynaptic spinal pathways. Baclofen is useful in treating spasticity associated with multiple sclerosis and in conditions related to spinal cord injury.[14] Side effects include drowsiness, weakness, and a variety of gastrointestinal effects. Baclofen (Lioresal) is supplied in tablets, 10 mg.

NEW APPROACHES TO MANAGEMENT OF SPASTICITY

Baclofen

$$H_2NCH_2—CH—CH_2—COOH$$

$$H_2NCH_2CH_2CH_2COOH$$

γ-Aminobutyric acid

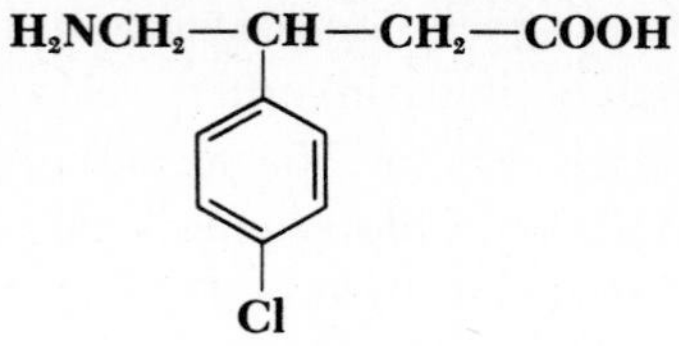

Cl

Baclofen

O_2N

CH=N

O

N

NH

O

Dantrolene

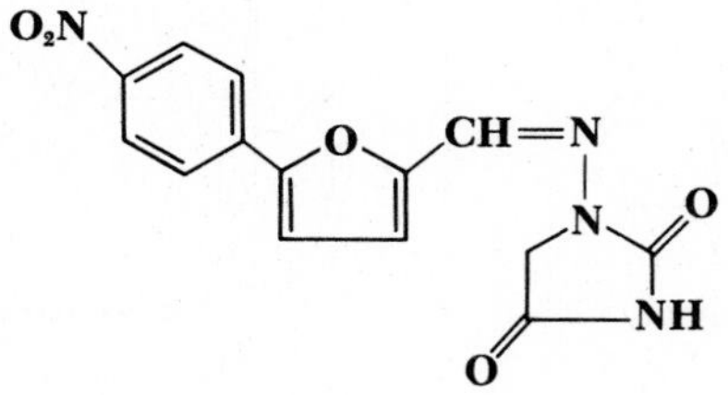

Dantrolene

Dantrolene is a hydantoin derivative that acts on skeletal muscle beyond the neuromuscular junction.[3,13] It reduces the availability of cytoplasmic calcium ions for muscle contraction. Dantrolene has produced improvement in patients with spinal cord injury, cerebral palsy, and, less consistently, multiple sclerosis. The drug has become the agent of choice for reducing heat production by muscle in anesthetic-induced malignant hyperthermia and has also been beneficial in the *neuroleptic malignant syndrome*.

Dantrolene can cause numerous serious reactions and side effects. When used chronically, hepatic damage, seizures, pleural effusion with pericarditis, and skin reactions suggestive of hypersensitivity have been noted. Drowsiness, dizziness, weakness, and gastrointestinal effects have been relatively common.

For oral administration of dantrolene sodium (Dantrium), capsules of 25 to 100 mg are available. The starting dose in adults of 25 mg a day can be increased gradually to 100 mg two to four times daily. Relief of spasticity may require treatment for a week. For more rapid action the drug is available in vials containing 20 mg. It has also been given before surgery to patients susceptible to malignant hyperthermia (4 to 8 mg/kg/day orally for 1 to 2 days or 2.5 mg/kg intravenously).

1. Argov, Z., and Mastaglia, F.L.: Disorders of neuromuscular transmission caused by drugs, N. Engl. J. Med. **301**:409, 1979.

2. Azar, I.: The response of patients with neuromuscular disorders to muscle relaxants: a review, Anesthesiology **61**:173, 1984.

3. Britt, B.A.: Dantrolene, Can. Anaesth. Soc. J. **31**:61, 1984.

4. Cronnelly, R., and Morris, R.B.: Antagonism of neuromuscular blockade, Br. J. Anaesth. **54**:183, 1982.

5. Drachman, D.B.: Myasthenia gravis, N. Engl. J. Med. **298**:136, 1978.

6. Henneman, E., Kaplan, A., and Unna, K.: A neuropharmacological study on the effect of myanesin (Tolserol) on motor systems, J. Pharmacol. Exp. Ther. **97**:331, 1949.

7. Katz, R.L., and Katz, L.E.: Complications associated with the use of muscle relaxants. In Orkin, F.K., and Cooperman, L.H., editors: Complications in anesthesiology, Philadelphia, 1983, J.B. Lippincott Co., p. 557.

8. Ørding, H.: Incidence of malignant hyperthermia in Denmark, Anesth. Analg. **64**:700, 1985.

9. Rosow, C.E., Moss, J., Philbin, D.M., and Savarese, J.J.: Histamine release during morphine and fentanyl anesthesia, Anesthesiology **56**:93, 1982.

10. Shanks, C.A.: Pharmacokinetics of the nondepolarizing neuromuscular relaxants applied to calculation of bolus and infusion dosage regimens, Anesthesiology **64**:72, 1986.

11. Sobell, H.M., Sakore, T.D., Tavale, S.S., et al.: Stereochemistry of a curare alkaloid: O,O',N-trimethyl-*d*-tubocurarine, Proc. Natl. Acad. Sci. U.S.A. **69**:2212, 1972.

12. Viby-Mogensen, J.: Clinical assessment of neuromuscular transmission, Br. J. Anaesth. **54**: 209, 1982.

13. Ward, A., Chaffman, M.O., and Sorkin, E.M.: Dantrolene: a review of its pharmacodynamic and pharmacokinetic properties and therapeutic use in malignant hyperthermia, the neuroleptic malignant syndrome and an update of its use in muscle spasticity, Drugs **32**:130, 1986.

14. Young, R.R., and Delwaide, P.J.: Spasticity, N. Engl. J. Med. **304**:96, 1981.

Chapter 15

Adrenergic (sympathomimetic) drugs

The adrenergic or sympathomimetic drugs comprise a large group of compounds that act *directly* on adrenergic receptors or that act presynaptically, and thus *indirectly*, to release catecholamines from nerve endings. Some of these drugs have a *mixed effect*, acting directly on receptors and also releasing catecholamines. The adrenergic group includes the endogenous catecholamines, ephedrine, and many synthetic amines. These agents are used for their cardiovascular effects and as bronchodilators, central nervous system stimulants, mydriatics, and appetite suppressants (anorexiants).

The effects of these drugs can be predicted from a knowledge of (1) the type of adrenergic receptor with which they interact, (2) the direct, indirect, or mixed nature of their action, and (3) their penetration or lack of penetration into the central nervous system.

CATECHOLAMINES

Norepinephrine, epinephrine, and dopamine occur naturally in the body, whereas isoproterenol is a synthetic analog. These substances are termed *catecholamines* because their structure includes catechol (*ortho*-dihydroxybenzene) and an amino group on the side chain.

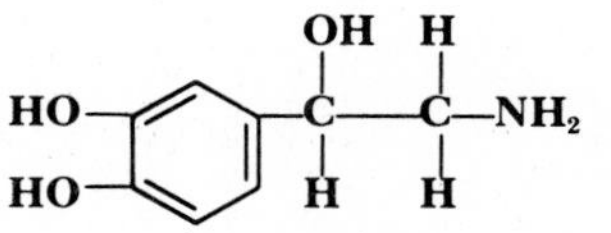

Norepinephrine

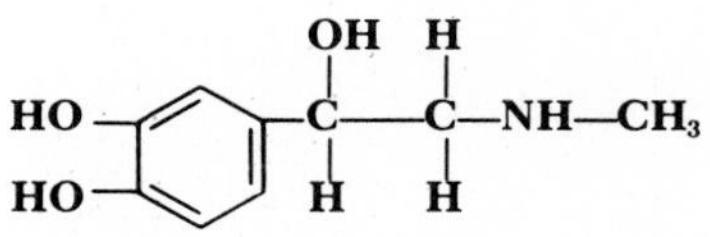

Epinephrine

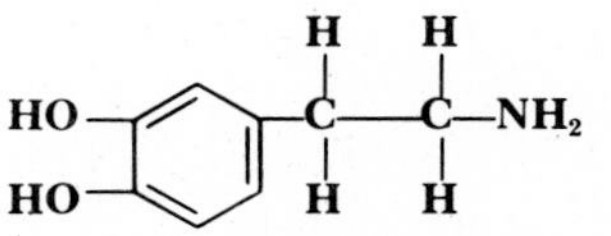

Dopamine

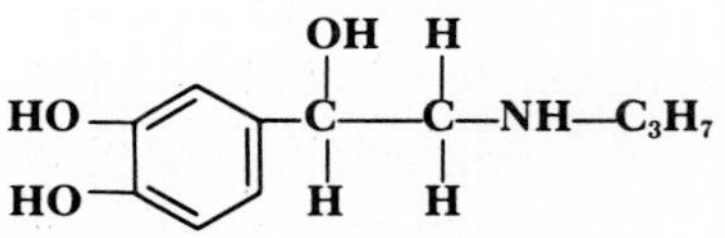

Isoproterenol

Epinephrine differs from norepinephrine in having a methyl group on the nitrogen, whereas isoproterenol has an isopropyl group on the nitrogen and dopamine lacks the β-hydroxyl on the side chain. The prefix *nor-* in norepinephrine is derived from German chemical terminology. It is the abbreviation of *Nitrogen ohne Radikal* ('nitrogen without radical'), which means that some attached group has been removed

Fluorescent adrenergic terminals around small arteries and a vein in the rat mesentery.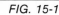

From Falck, B.: Acta Physiol. Scand. *56(suppl. 197):19, 1962.*

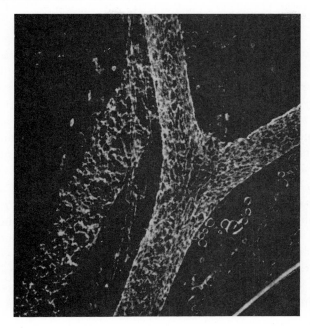

from the nitrogen. In the body, however, epinephrine is formed from norepinephrine (rather than the other way around as the nomenclature implies) by addition of a methyl group to the nitrogen.

The presence of norepinephrine in adrenergic nerve fibers was demonstrated by von Euler in 1946. It had been suspected that the "sympathin" released after adrenergic nerve stimulation was norepinephrine.

Occurrence and physiologic functions

The relationship between adrenergic nerves and blood vessels and the presence of catecholamine in the nerves is strikingly demonstrated by the fluorescence technique of the Swedish investigators Falck, Hillarp, and Carlsson, as shown in Fig. 15-1.

Epinephrine is highly concentrated in *chromaffin* granules of the adrenal medulla. It is also present in many other organs, probably also in chromaffin cells. Sympathetic denervation affects the norepinephrine content of an organ without a significant decrease in epinephrine concentration. From this observation it is believed that epinephrine is limited to chromaffin cells and is not located in adrenergic neurons.

Adrenal medullary granules and adrenergic axonal vesicles contain catecholamines along with adenosine triphosphate, in the proportion of 4:1 or perhaps higher in the nerve terminals.[3] They also contain a special soluble protein, *chromogranin*, and the enzyme dopamine β-hydroxylase.

In the human adrenal medulla, norepinephrine contributes as much as 20% to the total catecholamine content. It may constitute a much higher percentage in the medulla of the newborn infant and in pheochromocytoma, a tumor of the adrenal medulla.

The main functions of norepinephrine are maintenance of normal sympathetic tone and adjustment of circulatory dynamics. Epinephrine, in contrast, is the emergency hormone that stimulates metabolism and promotes blood flow to skeletal muscles, preparing the individual for "fight or flight."

Dopamine is localized in certain regions of the central nervous system where it is an important transmitter. It is also the precursor of norepinephrine and epinephrine at other sites and may contribute to peripheral control of renal and mesenteric blood flow. The role of dopamine in Parkinson's disease and in the actions of psychoactive drugs is discussed on pp. 121 and 242.

Adrenergic and dopaminergic receptors	The classification of adrenergic receptors as *alpha* (α) and *beta* (β), originally proposed by Ahlquist[1] in 1948, is now generally accepted. The concept was based on the order of activity of a series of sympathomimetic drugs at various effector sites and was greatly strengthened when specific blocking agents were developed for each receptor. Functions associated with α-adrenergic receptors include vasoconstriction, mydriasis, and intestinal relaxation (Table 15-1). β-Adrenergic receptors mediate bronchial and intestinal relaxation, vasodilatation, cardioacceleration, and a positive inotropic effect.

Norepinephrine acts on α- and some β-receptors. Epinephrine also acts on both receptor types, but in an organ with both types (such as vascular smooth muscle in skeletal muscle) the β-receptors are more sensitive at physiologic concentrations. Isoproterenol is a virtually pure β-receptor agonist, and its action is blocked by propranolol, a β-adrenergic receptor antagonist. Drugs such as methoxamine and phenylephrine act selectively on α-receptors and are antagonized by the α-adrenergic blocking agents phenoxybenzamine and phentolamine. Thus there is a gradation from essentially pure α-agonists to pure β-agonists.

SUBCLASSES OF α- AND β-ADRENERGIC RECEPTORS	In addition to postsynaptic α-receptors that mediate vasoconstriction and mydriasis, there are *presynaptic* α-receptors on adrenergic and other neurons that mediate inhibition of neurotransmitter release[6] (Fig. 15-2). This finding, based on the relative potencies of a series of agonists,[9] led to division of α-receptors into α_1 and α_2 subtypes. The decreasing order of selectivity of agonists for α_2- versus α_1-receptors is clonidine, epinephrine, norepinephrine, and phenylephrine.[10] For antagonists this order is yohimbine, phentolamine, phenoxybenzamine, and prazosin. These facts have practical importance in antihypertensive therapy and probably explain why tachycardia is a greater problem with phentolamine than with prazosin (see p. 165). It was later found that there are also *postsynaptic* α_2-receptors that mediate other effects: vasoconstriction and inhibition of lipolysis and insulin release.[10] Drugs, such as clonidine, methyldopa, and guanabenz, that stimulate central nervous

Autoinhibition of norepinephrine release from sympathetic nerves mediated by presynaptic α_2-receptors and facilitation of release through presynaptic β_2-receptors. Epinephrine (A) from the adrenal medulla is taken up by the neuron (dotted arrows) and acts as a false transmitter when released together with norepinephrine (NA). Notice that the facilitatory influence of β_2-receptor stimulation is indicated as weak relative to the effect of α_2-receptor stimulation. +, Facilitation of release; −, inhibition of release.

FIG. 15-2

From Göthert, M.: Arzneimittelforschung **35**:1909, 1985.

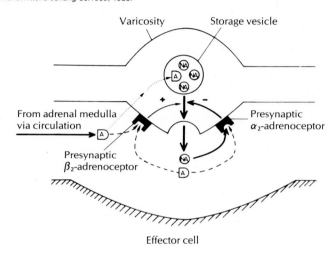

TABLE 15-1   Receptors mediating various adrenergic drug effects

Effector organ	Receptor	Response
Heart		
Sinoatrial node	β_1	Tachycardia
Atrioventricular node	β_1	Increase in conduction rate and shortening of functional refractory period
Atria and ventricles	β_1	Increased contractility
Blood vessels		
To skeletal muscle	α and β_2	Contraction or relaxation
To skin	α	Contraction
Bronchial muscle	β_2	Relaxation
Gastrointestinal smooth muscle		
To stomach	β	Decreased motility
To intestine	α and β	Decreased motility
Gastrointestinal sphincters		
To stomach	α	Contraction
To intestine	α	Contraction
Urinary bladder		
Detrusor	β	Relaxation
Trigone and sphincter	α	Contraction
Eye		
Radial muscle, iris	α	Contraction (mydriasis)
Ciliary muscle	β	Relaxation

system α_2-receptors have found use in management of hypertension (see Chapter 18).

β-Adrenergic receptors are also of two subtypes,[6] β_1 and β_2. β_1-Receptors mediate the cardiac effects of catecholamines and also lipolysis. β_2-Receptors mediate bronchodilatation and vasodilatation and on presynaptic membranes may have a facilitatory role in norepinephrine release (Fig. 15-2). β_2-Agonists are especially useful in treatment of asthma (see p. 158 and Chapter 40) and may prevent premature labor (see p. 578). The relative potencies of the three prototypic catecholamines on these receptors are as follows:

$$\alpha: \text{epinephrine} \geq \text{norepinephrine} >>> \text{isoproterenol}$$
$$\beta_1: \text{isoproterenol} > \text{epinephrine} = \text{norepinephrine}$$
$$\beta_2: \text{isoproterenol} \geq \text{epinephrine} >>> \text{norepinephrine}$$

Antagonists may be nonselective for β_1- and β_2-receptors (propranolol), or they may have a greater effect on β_1-receptors (metoprolol). Evidence has been presented that postsynaptic α_2- and β_2-receptors are located in proximity to the vascular lumen so that, rather than responding primarily to neuronal norepinephrine, they may be hormonal receptors for circulating epinephrine.[2,10] Events believed to occur after stimulation of α- and β-receptors are depicted in Fig. 15-3.[8] From a biochemical standpoint, the α_2- and β-receptors mediate changes in adenylate cyclase (Fig. 15-3 and p. 150), the α_2-receptor mediating inhibition and the β-receptor mediating activation.

Norepinephrine and epinephrine	Various aspects of the pharmacology of norepinephrine (levarterenol) and epinephrine (adrenaline) are discussed first, followed by those of dopamine, ephedrine, and other adrenergic drugs.

CARDIOVASCULAR EFFECTS	The effects of norepinephrine and epinephrine on the cardiovascular system are quite different physiologically or when the drugs are administered in small doses. The differences are a consequence of the minimal influence of norepinephrine on β_2-receptors at which epinephrine is a potent agonist.

Net effects of small doses in humans. When norepinephrine is infused intravenously into a normal person so that the subject receives about 10 to 20 $\mu g/min$, the hemodynamic changes listed in Table 15-2 are observed. If epinephrine is infused at the same rate, the changes listed in Table 15-3 are generally observed. These changes in heart rate and blood pressure are illustrated in Fig. 15-4.

Norepinephrine has widespread vasoconstrictor (α-receptor) properties, in skeletal muscle as well as elsewhere, and increases blood pressure. This effect elicits, by baroreceptors, a reflex bradycardia that is prevented by atropine. On the other hand, epinephrine constricts (α-receptor) some vascular beds and dilates (β_2-receptor) others. At the low concentration produced by such infusions, in blood vessels of skeletal muscle epinephrine primarily stimulates β_2-receptors. The vasodilatation and increased blood flow to the muscle is beneficial for "fight or flight" and tends to offset the effect on peripheral resistance of α-receptor–mediated constriction in other

Postulated α_1-, α_2-, and β-adrenergic receptor-coupled signal-transduction mechanisms   **FIG. 15-3**
leading to cellular responses. Agonist binding to the α_1-receptor activates hydrolysis
of phosphatidylinositol-4,5-bisphosphate (PIP$_2$) to myo-inositol-1,4,5-trisphosphate (IP$_3$)
and diacylglycerol (DG). IP$_3$ releases intracellular Ca^{++}, which activates responses
such as actin-myosin coupling or together with diacylglycerol promotes protein kinase
(C-kinase) activation. The latter may limit (broken arrow) further signal transduction through
the α_1-receptor. Activation of α_2- or β-receptors inhibits or stimulates, respectively, the
membrane-bound enzyme adenylate cyclase (not shown); responses are mediated by
independent inhibitory (G$_i$) and stimulatory (G$_s$) guanine nucleotide-binding regulatory
proteins. Increased adenylate cyclase activity promotes hydrolysis of ATP to cyclic aden-
osine 3',5'-monophosphate (cAMP), which activates cAMP-dependent protein kinase
(A-kinase).

From Homcy, C.J., and Graham, R.M.: Circu. Res. **56**:635, 1985, by permission of the American Heart Association, Inc.

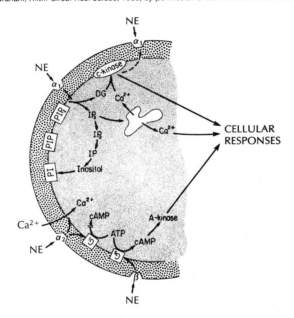

vascular beds, and so mean blood pressure may not be greatly affected. Blood is shunted to skeletal muscle from splanchnic and other regions of the body. If epinephrine does not elevate mean pressure, no reflex mechanism comes into play to slow the heart, and the direct stimulant action of the drug (β_1-receptor) increases the cardiac rate. These differences between epinephrine and norepinephrine tend to disappear when large, unphysiologic doses are administered. In this case, epinephrine will also stimulate α-receptors in skeletal muscle. Both drugs will then reduce blood flow through skeletal muscles and will increase total peripheral resistance and diastolic pressure.

Response of heart and various vascular areas. The actions of epinephrine on the heart increase rate, force of contraction, irritability, and coronary blood flow. Norepinephrine has a cardiac accelerator action also, but this is opposed, as noted above, by reflex slowing secondary to elevated blood pressure.

TABLE 15-2	Cardiovascular effects of small dose of norepinephrine in humans
Systolic pressure	Increased
Diastolic pressure	Increased
Mean pressure	Increased
Heart rate	Slightly decreased
Cardiac output	Slightly decreased
Peripheral resistance	Increased

TABLE 15-3	Cardiovascular effects of small dose of epinephrine in humans
Systolic pressure	Increased
Diastolic pressure	Decreased (increased by large dose)
Mean pressure	Unchanged
Heart rate	Increased
Cardiac output	Increased
Peripheral resistance	Decreased

attributable to increased cardiac work and metabolism. The drug has no usefulness in relieving anginal pain and may even precipitate attacks in patients with coronary atherosclerosis.

The effects of epinephrine on renal hemodynamics have received considerable attention. It is generally accepted that the drug decreases renal plasma flow but does not influence glomerular filtration. Large doses of epinephrine, however, may decrease glomerular filtration also.

Cerebral blood flow is affected in a complex manner by norepinephrine and epinephrine. They can directly constrict cerebral vessels. At low doses, however, the primary effect is secondary to elevation of systemic pressure, and so no significant change or even an increase in cerebral blood flow occurs.

BRONCHODILATOR EFFECT   Epinephrine dilates bronchial smooth muscle by stimulation of β_2-receptors.[12] As would be expected from its lack of appreciable action on β_2-receptors elsewhere, norepinephrine is not a useful bronchodilator. Isoproterenol is a somewhat more potent dilator than epinephrine. Bronchodilatation is not important when β_2-receptor agonists are administered to a normal person. It becomes prominent when the bronchi are constricted by agents such as histamine or methacholine or in bronchial asthma. In the latter condition epinephrine is a time-honored remedy.

Effect of norepinephrine and epinephrine infusion on blood pressure and heart rate in humans. Notice increased mean pressure and decreased heart rate after infusion of nor-epinephrine and essentially unchanged mean pressure, increase in pulse pressure, and elevated heart rate after infusion of epinephrine.   **FIG. 15-4**

From Barcroft, H., and Konzett, H.: Lancet 1:147, 1949.

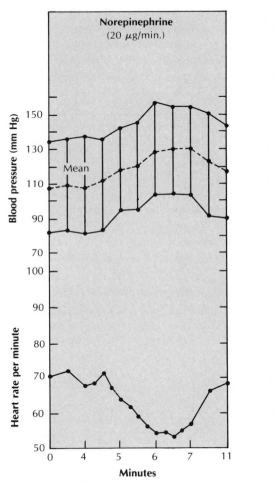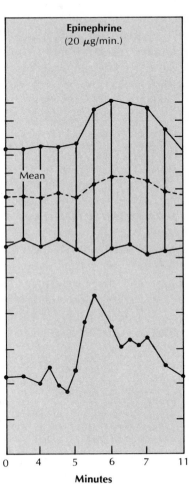

Epinephrine causes mydriasis by contracting the radial muscle of the iris. This effect is not usually prominent with direct application of the drug. Drops of epinephrine and related agents, including the prodrug dipivefrin, reduce intraocular pressure in open-angle glaucoma, apparently by improving drainage of aqueous humor.[7,15]   *OTHER SMOOTH MUSCLE EFFECTS*

The catecholamines can have a modest inhibitory action on gastrointestinal smooth muscle. This action has little physiologic and no therapeutic importance. The same may be said for the complex and variable effects of epinephrine on the uterus.

NEURAL EFFECTS

Injected catecholamines do not efficiently cross the blood-brain barrier. Alterations in norepinephrine content in the central nervous system can be associated with altered brain function and behavior, but injected catecholamines do not exert prominent effects. Nevertheless, injection of epinephrine into normal humans may produce anxiety and weakness. On the other hand, less polar adrenergic drugs such as the amphetamines have a pronounced stimulant action on the central nervous system.

METABOLIC EFFECTS

Oxygen consumption may be increased by 25% after injection of a therapeutic dose of epinephrine. Norepinephrine has considerably weaker effects on both oxygen consumption and lactic acid production in man.

Epinephrine and isoproterenol, and to a lesser degree norepinephrine, exert complex effects on carbohydrate metabolism. They elevate blood glucose by glycogenolysis and also inhibit glucose utilization. Glucose is released from the liver and lactic acid from muscle. The influence on phosphorylase has been studied extensively by Sutherland and Rall.[18] Epinephrine in many tissues, acting on β-receptors, promotes formation of the cyclic nucleotide adenosine 3',5'-monophosphate, or cyclic AMP, which has been termed a *second messenger* because of its involvement between receptor stimulation and the eventual cellular response. Characterization of the membrane components involved in control of adenylate cyclase, which catalyzes the conversion of ATP to cyclic AMP, has progressed considerably in recent years.[4]

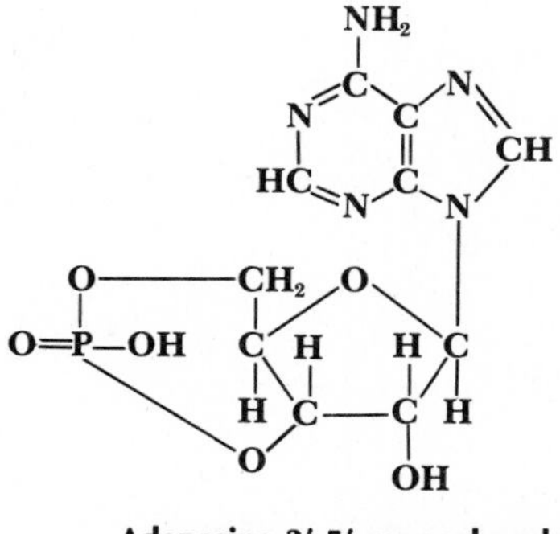

Adenosine 3',5'-monophosphate

Catecholamines promote release of fatty acids from adipose tissue and elevate the level of unesterified fatty acids in the blood. Thus the sympathetic nervous system, through catecholamine release, provides not only glucose but also free fatty acids as energy sources. The important effect on fatty acid release can be blocked by β-adrenergic blocking agents.

The distribution of potassium between extracellular and intracellular spaces is influenced by catecholamines. β_2-Receptor agonists cause distribution into cells, thereby decreasing serum potassium. In contrast, α-receptor agonists do the reverse. Transient elevations of serum potassium that may occur after injection of epinephrine imply predominance of α-receptor–mediated potassium efflux.

The therapeutic uses of epinephrine and norepinephrine are based primarily on their vasoconstrictor, cardiac stimulant, and bronchodilator properties.

THERAPEUTIC APPLICATIONS

Vasoconstriction. Epinephrine is commonly added to local anesthetic solutions to delay absorption of the anesthetic and to restrict its action to a limited region. Epinephrine is also widely used to treat urticaria and angioneurotic edema, and it can be applied topically to reduce superficial bleeding.

Norepinephrine infusions have been given for management of hypotension and shock. The initial enthusiasm decreased considerably once it was realized that sympathetic activity is already greatly increased in shock and that correction of underlying abnormalities such as decreased blood volume is more important. On the other hand, epinephrine is very useful for reversing hypotension associated with anaphylactic shock, and pressor amines are also used to maintain blood pressure during spinal anesthesia.

Cardiac. Either epinephrine or isoproterenol is indicated in management of heart block (Stokes-Adams syndrome). These drugs act partly to improve atrioventricular conduction but mostly by increasing ventricular automaticity, thus increasing ventricular rate. Caution should be exercised in so-called states of prefibrillation, since the drug may precipitate ventricular arrhythmias. Epinephrine can be injected directly into the heart in asystole in an attempt to achieve resuscitation. However, external cardiac massage and electrical defibrillation are now favored before epinephrine resuscitation is tried.

Bronchodilatation. For relief of asthmatic attacks epinephrine may be given subcutaneously in the amount of 0.2 to 1.0 ml of a 1:1000 solution. It is also given by inhalation, primarily for chronic or intermittent therapy. For this purpose a stronger solution is employed in a nebulizer. Currently, more specific agents are more frequently used.

Overdosage with norepinephrine or epinephrine may cause severe hypertension with possible cerebral hemorrhage, pulmonary edema, and arrhythmias, including ventricular fibrillation. Reactions that are less serious, such as palpitation, headache, tremor, and difficult breathing, may be very distressful to a patient who has not been forewarned. In addition, extravasation can cause ischemia at the site of intravenous infusions of norepinephrine. Such damage may be reduced by infiltration of phentolamine, an α-adrenergic blocking agent, or a local anesthetic.

ADVERSE REACTIONS

Patients receiving tricyclic antidepressants or guanethidine, which block the amine uptake mechanism in adrenergic nerves, may show exaggerated responses to norepinephrine and epinephrine.

PHEOCHROMOCYTOMA   A rare form of hypertension is caused by tumors of adrenomedullary tissue that secrete norepinephrine with variable amounts of epinephrine. Although pheochromocytoma is a rare tumor, its detection is very important because it represents one of the few forms of curable hypertension. Most of these tumors that have been examined by chemical methods have contained very high concentrations of norepinephrine and smaller amounts of epinephrine. There may be as much as 10 to 15 mg/g of tissue, and the total catecholamine content of a large tumor may be more than 1 g.

Several methods have been used to diagnose pheochromocytoma. Some of these are based on neuropharmacologic principles and others on determination of catecholamines in urine or plasma. Although it is rare to use pharmacologic tests today because they are less accurate and relatively hazardous as compared with chemical tests, they illustrate interesting principles.

Pharmacologic tests. Drug tests for pheochromocytoma have been of two types: those that inhibit the action of norepinephrine to lessen the increase in pressure and those that promote secretion of catecholamines from the tumor and further increase blood pressure. Among the latter agents have been histamine, methacholine, and tetraethylammonium, each of which causes hypotension in normal persons.

Drugs that lower blood pressure in patients with pheochromocytoma are the α-blockers phenoxybenzamine and phentolamine. The latter is now the most widely used drug for diagnosis of pheochromocytoma. A dose of 5 mg is injected intravenously. If systolic blood pressure falls more than 35 mm Hg and diastolic pressure more than 25 mm Hg, the test is considered positive. However, false positive and negative reactions may occur.

Chemical tests. The diagnosis of pheochromocytoma is now most often established by determination of (1) plasma amine concentrations or (2) the amount of the amines, their metabolites (normetanephrine, metanephrine, and vanillylmandelic acid), or a combination of these in a 24-hour urine specimen. Methyldopa, tetracycline, and quinidine may falsely increase norepinephrine and epinephrine values. MAO inhibitors will increase normetanephrine and metanephrine. Anxiety and excitement do not elevate the excretion of catecholamines sufficiently to cause diagnostic errors. On the other hand, acute myocardial infarction, surgical trauma, and shock may cause abnormally high urinary outputs of catecholamines and their metabolites.

Another diagnostic procedure is sort of a hybrid between the pharmacologic and chemical tests. Clonidine normally lowers circulating concentrations of catecholamines through its action on central α_2-receptors (see Chapter 18). However, this usually does not occur in patients with pheochromocytoma. Hence lack of suppression of amine concentrations by clonidine can indicate the presence of the tumor.

PREPARATIONS   **Norepinephrine** (Levophed) **bitartrate** is available for injection as 1 mg of base per milliliter in 4 ml ampules. For intravenous infusion in adults the contents of one ampule are added to 1 liter of 5% dextrose injection.

Epinephrine hydrochloride is provided in solutions containing 0.01 to 1 mg/ml epinephrine for injection, 1 mg/ml for nasal administration, and 10 mg/ml for nebulization.

Epinephrine bitartrate is available as aerosols (Medihaler-Epi, Primatene Mist Suspension, others) to deliver 160 μg per metered spray.

Epinephrine itself is available as an aqueous suspension for injection (Sus-Phrine) containing 5 mg/ml and as aerosols to deliver 200 (Primatene Mist) or 270 μg (Bronkaid Mist) per metered spray.

Epinephrine bitartrate (2%) and epinephrine hydrochloride (0.1% to 2%) are also available in solution for ophthalmic use.

Epinephryl borate (Epinal, Eppy/N) is used in ophthalmic solutions of 0.25% to 2%.

Dipivefrin hydrochloride (Propine), a prodrug that is hydrolyzed to epinephrine, is used as an 0.1% solution for management of glaucoma.[15] Because both phenolic hydroxyls of epinephrine are esterified in this agent, it penetrates more readily into ocular tissues.

This catecholamine is an important neurotransmitter in certain parts of the central nervous system (see Chapter 23). In the periphery dopamine acts on β_1-receptors in the heart to increase contractility and, to a lesser degree, heart rate. In large doses it acts on α-receptors to cause vasoconstriction. On the other hand, dopamine-induced dilatation of renal and mesenteric vessels is inhibited by haloperidol and phenothiazines rather than by propranolol. These results indicate the presence of dopaminergic receptors that have been designated DA_1 (D_1).[5] Other peripheral dopamine receptors in ganglia or receptors that function presynaptically to inhibit norepinephrine release have been designated DA_2 (D_2).

Dopamine

The hemodynamic effects of dopamine depend on the dose with some individual variation. Intravenous infusion of 1 to 5 μg/kg/min increases cardiac contractility, cardiac output, and renal blood flow. Heart rate and mean blood pressure do not change significantly. With higher rates of infusion arterial pressure rises and heart rate reflexly decreases.

Dopamine infusion is used in some cases of shock, in which its lack of constrictor action in the kidney and mesentery is an advantage. In this setting dopamine should be administered only if blood volume is adequate. Several orally effective dopaminergic agonists are potentially of benefit in therapy of congestive heart failure or hypertension.[5,11]

Ventricular arrhythmia is the most serious adverse effect. Nausea, vomiting, and hypertension may also occur. If blood pressure does become elevated, the action of the drug lasts only a few minutes.

Dopamine hydrochloride (Intropin, Dopastat) is available in 5 mg ampules, vials, or syringes that contain 200 to 800 mg. The drug should be diluted in 250 or 500 ml of a sterile intravenous solution. Usually an infusion of 2 to 5 μg/kg/min of the drug is given initially, with subsequent adjustment of the dose as needed.

Dobutamine hydrochloride (Dobutrex) is related to dopamine but has a selectivity for β_1-receptors as well as α_1-receptors. It is used in acute myocardial infarction with congestive failure and after coronary bypass operations. Since the half-life of the drug is very short, it is given by intravenous infusion, usually at rates of 2.5 to 10 μg/kg/min. Dobutamine is available in 20 ml vials containing 250 mg, for eventual dilution to 250 to 1000 μg/ml.

MISCELLANEOUS
ADRENERGIC
DRUGS
Classification based
on mechanism of
action

The various sympathomimetic drugs may act *directly* on α- and β-receptors, or they may act *indirectly* by releasing endogenous catecholamines. Some also have a *mixed* action, both direct and indirect. Some important examples are given below:

	α-RECEPTOR AGONISTS	β-RECEPTOR AGONISTS
Direct-acting drugs	Methoxamine	Isoproterenol
Mixed-acting drugs	Metaraminol	Ephedrine (indirect on α-receptors)
Indirect-acting drugs	Tyramine	
	Amphetamine	

This classification is based mainly on two types of experiments. In one type, drugs are administered to animals in which tissue norepinephrine content has been depleted by reserpine. In these animals responses to some adrenergic drugs are normal or augmented. Drugs of this type include norepinephrine, epinephrine, and phenylephrine. They act directly on receptors. Other adrenergic drugs, such as tyramine, amphetamine, and hydroxyamphetamine, act indirectly and are therefore inactivated by norepinephrine depletion (Fig. 15-5). The infusion of norepinephrine restores the capacity of animals to react to these drugs. Other adrenergic drugs are intermediate (mixed) in that some but not all of their effects are prevented by reserpine pretreatment. Ephedrine and phenylpropanolamine are examples.

The other line of support for norepinephrine release as the mode of action of indirectly acting amines is the observation that they are inactive on chronically denervated organs. Such organs become supersensitive to directly acting amines.

Classification based
on clinical usage

A discussion of sympathomimetic amines may be simplified if one places them into categories based on their clinical usage (Table 15-4). These are three major categories: **vasoconstrictors,** some of which are used primarily as nasal decongestants, **bronchodilators,** and **central nervous system stimulants,** which are commonly used as appetite suppressants. There is some overlap in these activities, especially in the case of ephedrine, which is used for its cardiovascular, bronchodilator, and stimulant properties. It is considered separately.

Ephedrine

Used in China for centuries and introduced into the United States in 1923, ephedrine is a naturally occurring sympathomimetic drug now used primarily in over-the-counter products. Ephedrine is similar to epinephrine and norepinephrine

Blood pressure response to tyramine. **A,** *Reserpinized cat.* **B,***Control cat. Dose of reserpine:*   **FIG. 15-5**
*7 mg/kg subcutaneously. Dose of tyramine: 0.5 mg/kg intravenously. Arrows indicate
times of tyramine injection.*

From Carlsson, A., Rosengren, E., Bertler, Å., and Nilsson, J.: In Garattini, S., and Ghetti, V., editors: Psychotropic drugs, Amsterdam, 1957, Elsevier Publishing Co.

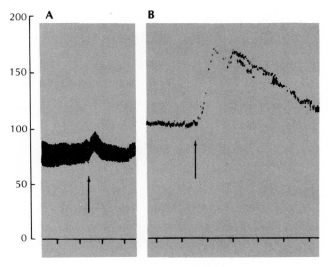

Tyramine (0.5 mg/kg)

except for a much longer duration of action, effectiveness by the oral route, penetration into the central nervous system leading to stimulation, and the occurrence of tachyphylaxis on frequent administration. On a weight basis it is about one hundredth as potent as the catecholamines. It is well absorbed from the gastrointestinal tract, and its action lasts for hours.

Ephedrine acts partially indirectly. Many of its peripheral actions are reduced by pretreatment with reserpine or by sympathetic denervation. Its bronchodilatory action must be direct, since norepinephrine is not a potent agonist at β_2-receptors.

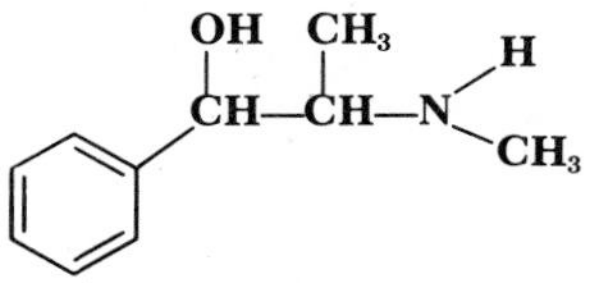

Ephedrine

In addition to its vasopressor effects, ephedrine can increase heart rate. It causes mydriasis when applied to the eye and stimulates the central nervous system.

TABLE 15-4   Indications and dosage forms for miscellaneous adrenergic drugs

Use	Drug	Tablets (mg)	Capsules (mg)	Nose drops (or spray) (%)	Eye drops (%)	Injection (mg/ml)	Miscellaneous* (mg)
Vasoconstriction							
	Ephedrine sulfate (Vatronal, others)		15-60	0.5, 1		5-50	J: 0.6%; S: 11, 20/5 ml
	Phenylephrine hydrochloride (Neo-Synephrine, others)			0.125-1	0.08-10	10	J: 0.5%
	Methoxamine hydrochloride (Vasoxyl)					20	
	Mephentermine (Wyamine) sulfate					15, 30	
	Metaraminol bitartrate (Aramine)					10	
	Hydroxyamphetamine hydrobromide (Paredrine)				1		
Nasal decongestion							
	Phenylpropanolamine hydrochloride	25-75	37.5-75				L: 25; S: 12.5/5 ml
	Propylhexedrine (Benzedrex, Dristan)						I: 250
	Oxymetazoline hydrochloride (Afrin, others)			0.025, 0.05			
	Naphazoline hydrochloride (Privine)			0.05	0.012-0.1		
	Tetrahydrozoline hydrochloride (Tyzine, Murine)			0.05, 0.1	0.05		
	Xylometazoline hydrochloride (Otrivin, others)			0.05, 0.1			
	Pseudoephedrine hydrochloride (Sudaphed, others)	30, 60	120				DO: 30/ml; S: 15, 30/5 ml
	Pseudoephedrine sulfate (Afrinol)	120					
Appetite suppression							
	Amphetamine sulfate	5, 10					
	Dextroamphetamine sulfate (Dexedrine, others)	5, 10	5-15				S: 5/5 ml
	Methamphetamine hydrochloride (Desoxyn, Methampex)	5-15					
	Diethylpropion hydrochloride (Tenuate, others)	25, 75					
	Phenmetrazine hydrochloride (Preludin)	25-75					
	Benzphetamine hydrochloride (Didrex)	25, 50					
	Phentermine (Ionamin)		15, 30				
	Phentermine hydrochloride (Fastin, others)	8-37.5	8-37.5				
	Phendimetrazine tartrate (Obalan, others)	35	35, 105				
	Fenfluramine hydrochloride (Pondimin)	20					
	Mazindol (Sanorex, Mazanor)	1, 2					

*DO, Drops (oral); I, inhaler; J, jelly; L, lozenge; S, solution or syrup (oral).

Phenylephrine is primarily a direct-acting α-receptor agonist. Subcutaneous or intramuscular injection of 2 to 5 mg is used to prevent hypotension during spinal anesthesia and for the management of orthostatic hypotension. It is also added to local anesthetic solutions to prolong anesthesia and is used topically as a nasal decongestant and as a mydriatic.

Adrenergic vasoconstrictors related to epinephrine or ephedrine

Methoxamine is a direct-acting α-receptor agonist that lacks cardiac stimulant properties. Both methoxamine and phenylephrine may be given intravenously to induce a reflex reduction in heart rate in patients with paroxysmal supraventricular tachycardia.

Mephentermine is both a direct and indirect vasoactive drug acting on both α- and β-receptors. The duration of its vasoconstrictor and myocardial stimulant actions is about 60 minutes after subcutaneous injection of 10 to 30 mg.

Metaraminol resembles phenylephrine in its properties, but it acts both directly and indirectly. It is taken up by sympathetic fibers and is released as a false transmitter. The drug is usually administered subcutaneously or intramuscularly in doses of 2 to 10 mg.

Hydroxyamphetamine resembles ephedrine in its action except for having little central nervous system effect. The drug is available as an ophthalmic preparation.

Phenylephrine

Methoxamine

Mephentermine

Metaraminol

Nasal vasoconstrictors or decongestants are symptomatic medications that have some usefulness but are not harmless. Their continued use may actually induce chronic rhinitis and congestion of the nasal mucosa, probably because ischemia leads to rebound swelling. In excessive doses these decongestants can evoke systemic effects, such as increased blood pressure, dizziness, palpitation, and in some cases central nervous system stimulation. Several of these agents are available over the counter. Oxymetazoline and xylometazoline are relatively longer acting and need to be taken no more than two or three times daily, respectively.

NASAL DECONGESTANTS

The decongestants are frequently combined with antihistamines. Thus preparations containing phenylephrine and an antihistamine have become very popular as nasal decongestants that are taken orally.

Commonly used nasal decongestants (Table 15-4) include phenylephrine, oxymetazoline, xylometazoline, pseudoephedrine, and the following.

Phenylpropanolamine is also used as an anorexiant. This over-the-counter drug has been very widely used, and moderate overdosage can cause severe hypertension.[14] **Propylhexedrine** is commonly administered by inhalation. It has many of the properties of amphetamine but less pressor activity and much less central nervous system stimulation. **Naphazoline,** an imidazoline derivative, may cause profound drowsiness and coma in children and also rebound swelling of the mucosa and cardiac irregularities when used excessively. **Tetrahydrozoline** is similar to naphazoline chemically and in its adverse effects.

Propylhexedrine

Oxymetazoline

Naphazoline

Tetrahydrozoline

Adrenergic bronchodilators

ISOPROTERENOL

Isoproterenol (isopropylnorepinephrine) is a potent β-receptor agonist. It dilates bronchial smooth muscle and increases heart rate and contractility. It also dilates blood vessels, particularly in skeletal muscle.

Isoproterenol is used primarily for treatment of bronchial asthma, atrioventricular block, and cardiac arrest. Palpitation, tachycardia, arrhythmias, hypotension, angina, and headache may occur after its administration. Some instances of sudden death in asthmatic persons have been attributed to excessive use of isoproterenol.[17] Cyclopropane, halogenated anesthetics, and propellants can sensitize the myocardium to isoproterenol. The effects of the drug are blocked by propranolol.

Isoproterenol (Isuprel) hydrochloride is available in solutions of 0.25% to 1% for oral inhalation, solutions containing 0.05 or 0.2 mg/ml for injection, and sublingual tablets of 10 and 15 mg. The effects of the tablets are somewhat unpredictable because of erratic absorption. The drug can also be taken as an aerosol that delivers 120 or 131 μg per metered spray. The sulfate is available as an aerosol (80 μg per spray) and a powder for oral insufflation (45 or 110 μg per inhalation).

Other

BRONCHODILATORS

Theophylline derivatives and several adrenergic drugs besides isoproterenol are also used as bronchodilators. Epinephrine and ephedrine have already been discussed. More selective β$_2$-receptor agonists, such as albuterol and metaproterenol, are increasingly employed in management of asthma because of fewer adverse cardiac effects. These agents are discussed in Chapter 40 in connection with drug effects on the respiratory tract.

Nylidrin and isoxsuprine are structurally related to isoproterenol and can dilate peripheral blood vessels experimentally. They appear to act primarily as direct vasodilators with perhaps some β-receptor agonist activity. These drugs have been used in dementia and in peripheral vascular disease to increase blood flow. There is no evidence that they have any salutary effect, and their use for these conditions should be abandoned.

The amphetamines are powerful stimulants of the central nervous system. *Dextro*amphetamine has considerably more central, and somewhat less cardiovascular, activity than the *levo* isomer has. Medically the drug is used and is also abused for its anorexiant effect, an indication questioned by many authorities. In addition, dextroamphetamine finds application in the management of children with attention-deficit disorder, as an adjunct in parkinsonism and other extrapyramidal disorders, and as a stimulant in the treatment of narcolepsy. Amphetamine, which lacks the phenolic hydroxyl groups of the catecholamines, is well absorbed from the gastrointestinal tract and readily reaches the brain. Its main metabolite is phenylacetone, a product of microsomal deamination. A minor metabolite, *p*-hydroxyamphetamine, is taken up by adrenergic nerves and transformed to *p*-hydroxynorephedrine, which is stored in vesicles, thus becoming a false transmitter.

Numerous anorexiants have been developed and are used by the medical profession, often without the realization that these drugs are essentially relatives of dextroamphetamine without significant advantages over the prototype. Evidence for a common receptor for these anorexiant drugs has recently been presented.[13] Except for phenylpropanolamine, which is a component of many over-the-counter "diet pills," these agents are controlled substances placed in Schedules II, III, or IV (see Table 64-1). In addition, numerous mixtures of adrenergic stimulants with barbiturates and other depressants have been prepared and are used widely. Despite their popularity, such mixtures are generally not recommended.

The disadvantages in use of anorexiants are related to development of psychic dependence, to untoward effects resulting from adrenergic actions, and to rapid development of tolerance, and so the anorexiant action is useful for only a week or two. Hence these agents at best are likely to serve only as a short-term adjunct to management of obesity. Large and repeated doses of amphetamines may produce a psychosis that has many of the characteristics of paranoid schizophrenia (see p. 348).

Amphetamine

The vascular effects of amphetamines may be attributed to endogenous catecholamine release, since they do not elevate blood pressure in a reserpinized animal.

In contrast, the central effects of amphetamine are not inhibited by catecholamine depletion, but blockade of catecholamine synthesis quickly inhibits its behavioral effects. These findings indicate that these effects may be mediated through a newly synthesized fraction of brain catecholamines.

Dextroamphetamine is available with amphetamine in a 50:50 resin complex that contains 12.5 or 20 mg of total amine. **Methamphetamine** is closely related from a structural standpoint to both ephedrine and amphetamine. It is a potent central nervous system stimulant and has considerable pressor action on blood vessels. It is used for the same purposes as amphetamine. **Diethylpropion** is basically an amphetamine-like drug, though it is claimed to cause less jitteriness and insomnia and also fewer cardiovascular effects than amphetamine does. The drug is considerably weaker than dextroamphetamine.

Other appetite suppressants include **phenmetrazine, benzphetamine, phentermine,** its hydrochloride, and **phendimetrazine.** See Table 15-4 for the available forms of these drugs.

MISCELLANEOUS
ANOREXIANTS

Fenfluramine and **mazindol** are comparable to other anorexiants in suppressing appetite. They may be used as short-term adjuncts to other measures that include caloric restriction, exercise, and psychotherapy. Fenfluramine is unusual in causing mild sedation along with appetite suppression. It is said to affect appetite control centers in the hypothalamus in common with other phenethylamines, but its mech-

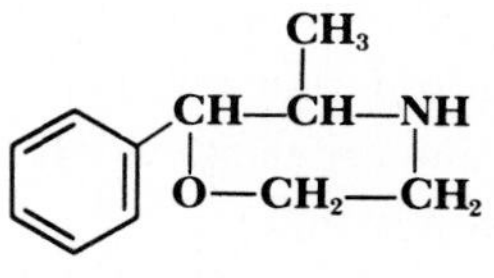

Phenmetrazine

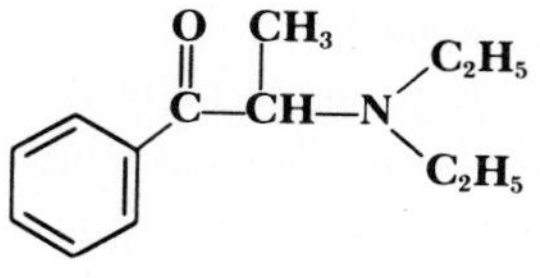

Diethylpropion

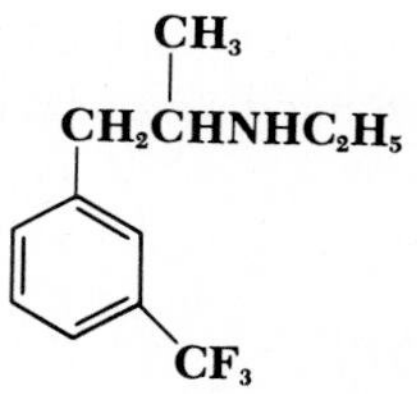

Fenfluramine

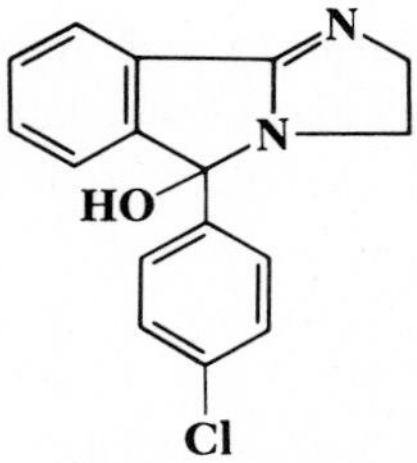

Mazindol

anism of action is not well understood.[16] Mazindol is not a phenethylamine and is claimed to have a different mode of action from the other anorexiants.

DRUG INTERACTIONS

All of these central nervous system stimulants and anorexiants may cause hypertensive crises in patients taking MAO inhibitors. All, except fenfluramine, antagonize the antihypertensive action of guanethidine. Fenfluramine may instead potentiate the antihypertensive action of guanethidine and methyldopa. Fenfluramine, being sedative, may enhance depression by alcohol and other central nervous system depressants. Mazindol potentiates the vasopressor effect of norepinephrine in dogs, and vasopressor medications must be used with great caution in patients taking mazindol.

Structure-activity relationships in adrenergic series

A great deal is known about the relationships between structure and activity of adrenergic drugs. Such knowledge in general is important to the pharmaceutical chemist as a guide to synthesis of new drugs. Structure-activity relationships are also of fundamental importance in that they should reflect basic characteristics of receptor-drug interactions. In the case of adrenergic drugs the problem is complicated by the fact that many sympathomimetic drugs act indirectly through release of endogenous catecholamines. The differences in action of these drugs may be related to the predominant site of catecholamine release. A few generalities may serve to illustrate the concept of structure-activity relationships.

The basic adrenergic structure is β-phenethylamine.

β-Phenethylamine

Hydroxyl groups on the benzene ring or on the side chain influence the metabolism and absorption of the drugs as well as their actions on receptors. Sympathomimetics that are not catechols are generally less polar and therefore absorbed better and are, of course, not O-methylated by COMT.

Substitutions on the nitrogen have a great influence on the type of receptor with which the drug will interact. Thus norepinephrine, lacking substitutions, acts on α- and β_1-receptors, epinephrine with one methyl group acts on α-receptors and both types of β-receptors, and isoproterenol acts almost entirely on β-receptors.

Substitutions on the α carbon tend to prolong the action of the drug by protecting against enzymatic destruction by MAO. The hydroxyl group on the β carbon is necessary for granular storage in adrenergic neurons.

REFERENCES

1. Ahlquist, R.P.: A study of the adrenotropic receptors, Am. J. Physiol. **153**:586, 1948.

2. Ariëns, E.J., and Simonis, A.M.: Physiological and pharmacological aspects of adrenergic receptor classification, Biochem. Pharmacol. **32**:1539, 1983.

3. Fried, G., Lagercrantz, H., Klein, R., and Thureson-Klein, Å.: Large and small noradrenergic vesicles: origin, contents, and functional significance. In Usdin, E., Carlsson, A., Dahlström, A., and Engel, J., editors: Catecholamines. Part A: Basic and peripheral mechanisms, New York, 1984, Alan R. Liss, Inc., p. 45.

4. Gilman, A.G.: G proteins and dual control of adenylate cyclase, Cell **36**:577, 1984.

5. Goldberg, L.I.: Dopamine: receptors and clinical applications, Clin. Physiol. Biochem. **3**:120, 1985.

6. Göthert, M.: Role of autoreceptors in the function of the peripheral and central nervous system, Arzneimittelforsch, **35**:1909, 1985.

7. Havener, W.H.: Ocular pharmacology, ed. 5, St. Louis, 1983, The C.V. Mosby Co.

8. Homcy, C.J., and Graham, R.M.: Molecular characterization of adrenergic receptors, Circ. Res. **56**:635, 1985.

9. Langer, S.Z.: Presynaptic regulation of catecholamine release, Biochem. Pharmacol. **23**:1793, 1974.

10. Langer, S.Z., Duval, N., and Massingham, R.: Pharmacologic and therapeutic significance of α-adrenoceptor subtypes, J. Cardiovasc. Pharmacol. **7**(suppl. 8):S1, 1985.

11. Lokhandwala, M.F., and Barrett, R.J.: Dopamine receptor agonists in cardiovascular therapy, Drug Dev. Res. **3**:299, 1983.

12. Nadel, J.A., and Barnes, P.J.: Autonomic regulation of the airways, Annu. Rev. Med. **35**:451, 1984.

13. Paul, S.M., Hulihan-Giblin, B., and Skolnick, P.: (+)-Amphetamine binding to rat hypothalamus: relation to anorexic potency of phenylethylamines, Science **218**:487, 1982.

14. Pentel, P.: Toxicity of over-the-counter stimulants, J.A.M.A. **252**:1898, 1984.

15. Remis, L.L., and Epstein, D.L.: Treatment of glaucoma, Annu. Rev. Med. **35**:195, 1984.

16. Rowland, N.E., and Carlton, J.: Neurobiology of an anorectic drug: fenfluramine, Prog. Neurobiol. **27**:13, 1986.

17. Stolley, P.D.: Asthma mortality. Why the United States was spared an epidemic of deaths due to asthma, Am. Rev. Respir. Dis. **105**:883, 1972.

18. Sutherland, E.W., and Rall, T.W.: The relation of adenosine-3′,5′-phosphate and phosphorylase to the actions of catecholamines and other hormones, Pharmacol. Rev. **12**:265, 1960.

Chapter 16

Adrenergic blocking agents

Adrenergic blocking agents are, with one exception, drugs that competitively antagonize the actions of catecholamines and other adrenergic agonists on their specific receptors. They are classified as *alpha* (α)- or *beta* (β)-receptor antagonists, reflecting their selective action on one or the other of the two major types of adrenergic receptors. In blood vessels that possess both receptor types, α-receptor stimulation causes contraction and β-receptor stimulation causes relaxation. In vivo the α-adrenergic blocking drugs cause vasodilatation by reducing sympathetic tone. In contrast, β-receptor blockers usually have little effect because β_2-receptors are not stimulated by epinephrine at rest, but they prevent the vasodilator action of epinephrine or isoproterenol. In organs, such as the heart, that are controlled primarily by β-receptor activation, the β-receptor blockers oppose the excitatory action of norepinephrine.

Drugs that deplete catecholamines or prevent their release from adrenergic nerves are considered in the next chapter and should not be confused with the antagonists, which act on α- and β-receptors.

The most characteristic feature of α-adrenergic blocking agents is their ability to convert the pressor effect of pharmacologic doses of epinephrine into a depressor response. This *epinephrine reversal* by phentolamine is shown in Fig. 16-1. Vascular smooth muscle, particularly in skeletal muscle, has both α- and β_2-receptors. Since epinephrine acts on both receptors, it causes vasodilatation if the α-receptors are blocked. On the other hand, norepinephrine has no action on β_2-receptors in vascular smooth muscle; thus its pressor effect is decreased by an α-blocker but is not converted to a depressor response.

The various drugs in this group differ from each other in potency, duration of action, and relative ability to block α_1- and α_2-receptors. They may also possess pharmacologic properties entirely unrelated to adrenergic blockade.

Phenoxybenzamine hydrochloride (Dibenzyline), administered in doses of 20 to 100 mg, lowers blood pressure and inhibits the reflex vasoconstriction that normally occurs in the capacitance vessels upon standing, and so orthostatic hypotension may occur. The effects of the drug last more than 24 hours. It is available in capsules, 10 mg.

The long duration of phenoxybenzamine action is a consequence of a stable combination between the drug and the α-receptor. Although there is competition

FIG. 16-1 *Epinephrine reversal by phentolamine. Effect of epinephrine on blood pressure before and after injection of phentolamine. A dog was anesthetized with pentobarbital. At A, epinephrine was injected intravenously, 1 μg/kg. At B, phentolamine was injected, 5 mg/kg. At C, epinephrine injection was repeated. Notice the lowering of pressure by epinephrine after the adrenergic blocking agent. The increased pulse pressure under these circumstances is an indication that the adrenergic blocking agent does not prevent the cardiac stimulant effect of epinephrine.*

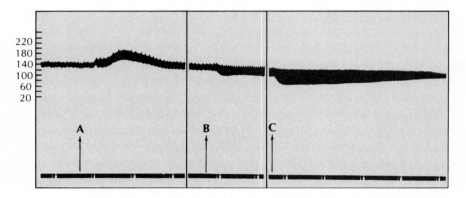

between the drug and catecholamines for the receptor during the early stage of blockade, competition becomes ineffective as blockade develops fully. The term *nonequilibrium blockade* has been applied to such an interaction between agonist and antagonist. Phenoxybenzamine is converted to a highly reactive aziridinium-ion intermediate that spontaneously forms a covalent bond with the α-receptor.[4]

Phenoxybenzamine

Phenoxybenzamine is used in management of pheochromocytoma both before and during surgical removal. Patients with this tumor are often treated for several days or weeks to allow stabilization before surgery. Phenoxybenzamine is particularly useful in this setting because of its availability in oral form and its long duration of action.

Among the many adverse effects that may be caused by phenoxybenzamine, orthostatic hypotension, tachycardia, nasal congestion, and miosis are common and predictable. Phenoxybenzamine can also block histamine, serotonin, and cholinergic receptors.

Tolazoline (Priscoline) hydrochloride, a weak α-receptor blocker, causes periph- *Tolazoline* eral vasodilatation largely by a direct relaxant effect on vascular smooth muscle. In addition, the drug is a direct cardiac stimulant, and its use is often accompanied by tachycardia. Other adverse effects of the drug include pilomotor stimulation (goose-flesh) and increased gastrointestinal motility and hydrochloric acid secretion. Tolazoline is related structurally to histamine.

Although used infrequently, tolazoline relieves vasospasm in peripheral vascular diseases. It is available as a solution for injection, 25 mg/ml.

Tolazoline

Phentolamine

Phentolamine is an α-receptor blocker used almost exclusively for diagnosis of *Phentolamine* pheochromocytoma (see p. 152) and for prevention of hypertension during operative removal of the tumor. Phentolamine mesylate (Regitine) is available for reconstitution and injection, 5 mg. In addition to its receptor-blocking action, the drug has other actions similar to those of tolazoline, to which it is chemically related. Adverse effects include orthostatic hypotension, tachycardia, nasal stuffiness, and gastrointestinal disturbances such as nausea, vomiting, and diarrhea. This drug cannot be used for chronic treatment of pheochromocytoma because it is poorly absorbed after oral administration.

Prazosin was initially believed to act by a direct relaxant effect on vascular smooth *Prazosin* muscle. It was later found, however, to be an effective but unusual α-receptor blocking agent.[16] It is a useful antihypertensive with fewer side effects than other α blockers, probably because of its selective action on postsynaptic α_1-receptors. The drug does not cause the pronounced tachycardia seen, for example, with phenoxy-benzamine. Blockade of presynaptic receptors by phenoxybenzamine prevents re-leased norepinephrine from reducing subsequent transmitter release. Consequently, norepinephrine release is enhanced and further stimulates unprotected cardiac β-receptors. The weak action of prazosin on presynaptic receptors does not greatly enhance norepinephrine release so that less cardiac stimulation results.

Prazosin hydrochloride (Minipress) is available in 1 to 5 mg capsules. Adverse effects include headache, drowsiness, and orthostatic hypotension after the first dose.

TABLE 16-1	Effects of β-adrenergic receptor blockade	
Heart rate		Decreased
Myocardial contractility		Decreased
Cardiac output		Decreased
Arterial blood pressure		Unaffected or decreased
Effect of exercise on heart rate and cardiac output		Decreased
β-Adrenergic drug effects (myocardial, arterial, bronchial, metabolic)		Blocked

Unlike other α blockers, however, this latter effect does not generally persist with continued drug use.

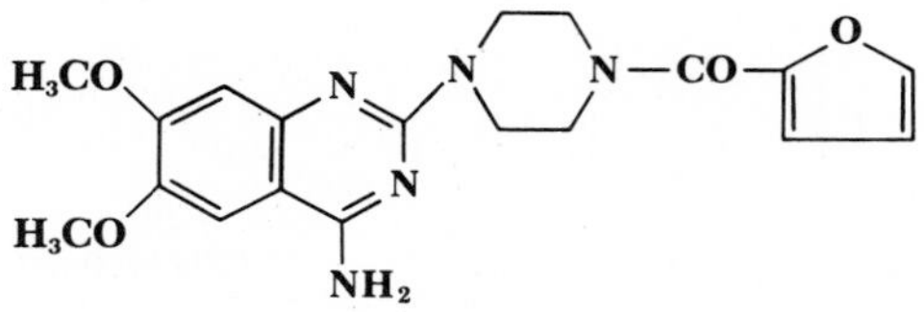

Prazosin

Ergot alkaloids

Certain alkaloids of ergot, such as ergotamine, have an α-adrenergic blocking action. However, they are used for their direct vasoconstrictor and oxytocic actions rather than as adrenergic blocking agents, and their pharmacology is discussed in Chapters 21 and 46.

β-ADRENERGIC BLOCKING AGENTS

These drugs are competitive inhibitors of catecholamines at β-adrenoceptors.[13] Their general effects are listed in Table 16-1. Some of them have a relatively greater potency at β_1-receptors in the heart, and they differ from each other in their duration of action. A summary of their properties is given in Table 16-2.

Although β-receptor blockers were first approved to treat angina pectoris, they have numerous other clinical indications. These include hypertension, arrhythmias, thyrotoxicosis, hypertrophic cardiomyopathy, migraine, and glaucoma. The first β-blocker, dichloroisoproterenol, was made by substitution of chlorine for both phenolic hydroxyls on the ring of the agonist isoproterenol. Propranolol, however, was the first agent sufficiently selective for β-receptor blockade to be useful clinically, and it has been one of the most often prescribed drugs ever since.

Propranolol

PHARMACOLOGIC EFFECTS

Propranolol competitively antagonizes the action of catecholamines on all β-receptors. As a consequence the drug exerts negative chronotropic and inotropic effects on the heart, slows atrioventricular conduction, promotes bronchoconstriction, lowers plasma renin activity, and may cause hypoglycemia. It also exerts some quinidine-like (membrane-stabilizing) actions on the heart at high doses. Propranolol is

TABLE 16-2 β-Receptor blockers: properties, uses, and dosage forms

	Relative cardio-selectivity (β₁)	β-Receptor agonist activity	Half-life (hours)	Therapeutic uses*	Dosage forms† (mg)
Propranolol hydrochloride‡ (Inderal)	0	0	3-4	HT, AN, MI, AR	T: 10-90; C: 80-160; I: 1/ml
Nadolol (Corgard)	0	0	20-24	HT, AN	T: 40-160
Pindolol (Visken)	0	+	3-4	HT	T: 5, 10
Timolol maleate (Blocadren, Timoptic)	0	0	4-5	HT, MI, GL	T: 5-20; D: 0.25%, 0.5%
Labetalol hydrochloride (Normodyne, Trandate)	0	0	6-8	HT	T: 200, 300; I: 5/ml
Metoprolol tartrate (Lopressor)	+	0	3-7	HT, AN, MI	T: 50, 100; I: 1/ml
Atenolol (Tenormin)	+	0	6-7	HT, AN	T: 50, 100
Acebutolol hydrochloride (Sectral)	+	+	3-4	HT, AR	C: 200, 400
Betaxolol (Betoptic)	+			GL	D: 0.5%
Levobunolol (Betagan)	0			GL	D: 0.5%

*AN, Angina pectoris; AR, cardiac arrhythmias; GL, glaucoma; HT, hypertension; MI, myocardial infarction.
†C, Capsules; D, eye drops; I, injection; T, tablets.
‡Also marketed for use in patients with hypertrophic subaortic stenosis, migraine, and pheochromocytoma.

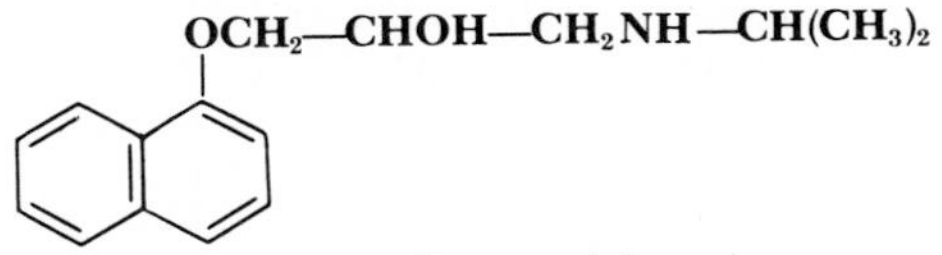

Propranolol

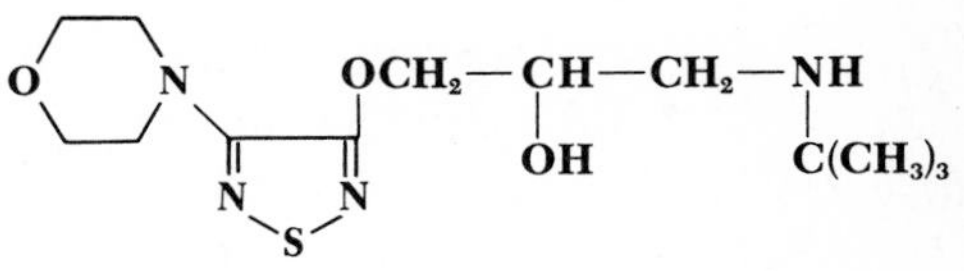

Timolol

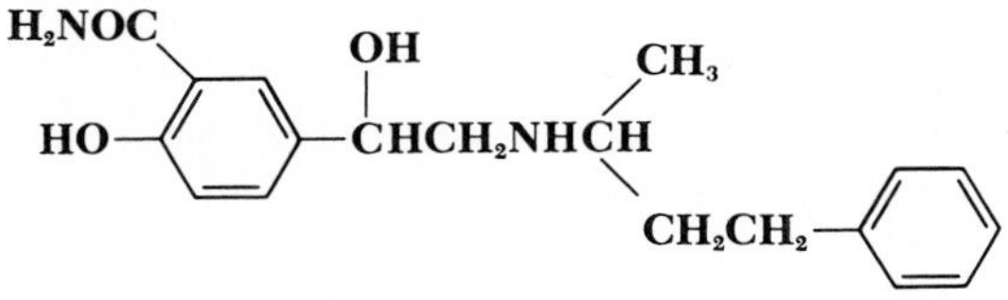

Labetalol

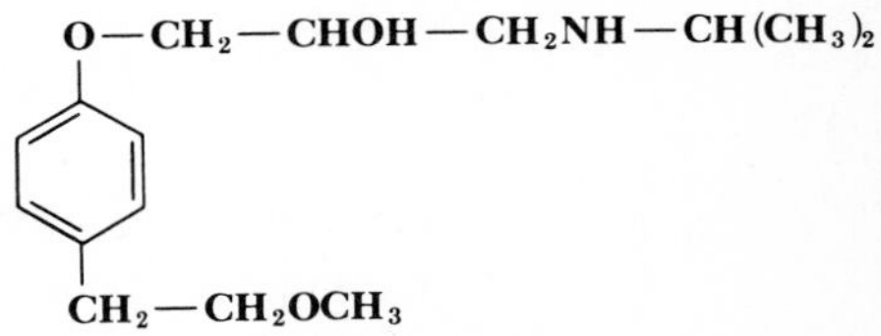

Metoprolol

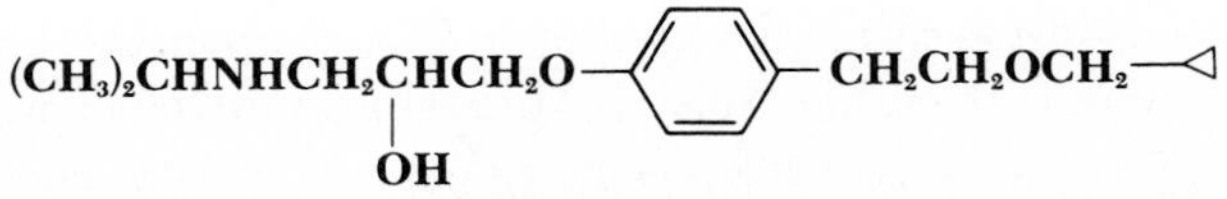

Betaxolol

a racemic mixture. The *levo* form is the β-blocker, but the *dextro* form has a greater membrane effect.

The effects of propranolol may be overcome by sufficiently large doses of β-agonists, such as isoproterenol, or by glucagon, which acts on a different receptor but also activates adenylate cyclase.

PHARMACOKINETICS

Propranolol is absorbed completely from the gastrointestinal tract, but about 50% is inactivated by the liver as the drug is absorbed, the first-pass effect. Plasma concentrations are low and variable. Its major metabolite, 4-hydroxypropranolol, is active as a β-receptor blocker but has an even shorter half-life.[9]

Despite its short half-life, propranolol may be administered at 6- to 12-hour intervals, depending partially on the indication. Altered renal function has little effect on the dosage regimen. On the other hand, phenobarbital (by induction of liver enzymes) further increases the clearance of the drug, whereas cirrhosis and drugs like cimetidine that diminish hepatic metabolism not only decrease clearance but also increase the bioavailability of propranolol (by decreasing the first-pass effect).

CLINICAL USES

The *antiarrhythmic effect* of propranolol results largely from β-receptor blockade. The drug is used in supraventricular tachyarrhythmias, as in thyrotoxicosis. Ventricular tachycardias caused by catecholamines or digitalis are also important indications, but propranolol is not the first choice in other types of ventricular tachycardias.

Angina pectoris is relieved by propranolol in selected patients who do not respond to conventional measures such as sublingual nitroglycerin. The benefit derives from the decrease in heart rate and reductions in left ventricular contractility and wall tension, all of which diminish myocardial oxygen demand.

The *antihypertensive effect* of propranolol has not been explained in a completely satisfactory manner. Reduction of cardiac output is most likely primary, but inhibition of renin release and some central nervous system effects have been suggested as other possible mechanisms of its antihypertensive action. Blockade of presynaptic β-receptors with a subsequent decrease in norepinephrine release over long-term therapy has also been proposed.[12] When propranolol is used with a peripheral vasodilator such as hydralazine, its beneficial effect is more easily understandable. Peripheral vasodilatation leads to reflex cardiac stimulation, which is blocked by propranolol.

Hypertrophic subaortic stenosis is accompanied by symptoms, such as angina, that are made worse by increased cardiac contractility. The usefulness of propranolol then becomes obvious.

Propranolol may be needed, as an adjunct to α-receptor blockade, to minimize cardiac stimulation during surgical removal or chronic management of *pheochromocytoma*. β-Receptor blockade alone, by preventing catecholamine-induced vasodilatation (mediated by β$_2$-receptors), may cause a dangerous rise in arterial pressure in these patients,[14] so that therapy with an α-receptor antagonist must be initiated beforehand.

In *myocardial infarction*, treatment with β-receptor blockers for a year or more after an infarction has been shown to have favorable effects on the likelihood of death or a recurrence of infarction.[20] Immediate intravenous administration of metoprolol or atenolol[8] upon admission followed by oral treatment for 7 days also appears beneficial, with a reduction in mortality primarily occurring within the first 2 days after infarction.

Propranolol is also used for prophylactic management of migraine and can reduce action tremors and autonomic symptoms of anxiety.

The major adverse effects of propranolol result from bronchial constriction, heart block, and depression of cardiac contractility. β-Adrenergic antagonists are generally contraindicated in patients with asthma.[17]
Propranolol may cause hypoglycemia or interfere with recovery from hypoglycemia after insulin administration, and it can prevent the tachycardia that is an indication to diabetics of hypoglycemia.[3] Central nervous system effects of β-blockers include drowsiness, fatigue, lethargy, and sleep disturbances, such as nightmares, hallucinations, and depression,[1,10] These effects appear to be less common with less lipid-soluble β-blockers.[7] Propranolol can increase the hypotensive action of phenothiazines, and it inhibits the β-adrenergic effects of dopamine, administered as such or formed from levodopa. Propranolol may aggravate the negative inotropic effects of quinidine and calcium antagonists. It is used in treatment of digitalis-induced arrhythmias but can exaggerate bradycardia caused by digitalis. Bradycardia induced by propranolol responds to atropine.

ADVERSE EFFECTS AND DRUG INTERACTIONS

Abrupt withdrawal of propranolol and other β-receptor blockers can lead to increased cardiac excitability, exacerbation of angina, or even myocardial infarction.[19] These changes begin within 2 days, and the patient's condition returns to normal in 10 to 14 days. This syndrome is generally attributed to upregulation of β-receptors as a consequence of prolonged suppression by the drugs. It is important to withdraw β-blockers very gradually and to warn patients not to interrupt therapy. β-Blockers may also mask thyrotoxicosis, which can then emerge in an exaggerated form (thyroid storm) when the drug is withdrawn.

PROPRANOLOL WITHDRAWAL

More recently developed β-blockers may differ from propranolol in several respects.[5,13] Those that are *cardioselective*, that is, exhibit preferential blockade of β_1- as opposed to β_2-receptors, potentially have advantages in asthmatic and diabetic patients. Those that are less lipid soluble (atenolol, nadolol, acebutolol) may cause less central nervous system side effects and are excreted to a greater extent unmetabolized. Overall the advantages of such differences are not well established clinically, and, despite differences in half-lives, once or twice daily

Newer β-adrenergic receptor blocking drugs

administration of any of these agents is usually effective for antihypertensive therapy.

Nadolol and **pindolol,** like propranolol, are not cardioselective and readily block both β_1- and β_2-receptors. Pindolol has some intrinsic β-receptor agonist and membrane-stabilizing activity.[10] The former action may cause tachycardia if sympathetic tone is minimal. **Labetalol** is an unusual antihypertensive agent in that, besides being a nonspecific β-receptor blocker, it also blocks α_1-receptors.

Timolol also is not cardioselective. In addition to their usefulness for cardiovascular indications, β-receptor blockers can reduce the formation of aqueous humor. It is uncertain if this effect is related to β-receptor blockade and whether it is attributable to an action on the ciliary processes or on the vasculature.[11] Propranolol is not used on the eye because of its local anesthetic action, but timolol has been considered the drug of choice by many opthalmologists for initial treatment of open-angle glaucoma.[6]

Metoprolol,[2] **atenolol,** and **acebutolol**[15] differ from the above agents in their relative cardioselectivity. Such agents are safer in asthmatics than those without β_1-receptor selectivity but still constitute considerable risk because they may block β_2-receptors in therapeutic doses. Even if they are used cautiously in patients with bronchospastic disease, concomitant administration of a β_2-receptor agonist may be necessary. Because cardioselective antagonists have less activity on the β_2-receptors that mediate vasodilatation, the use of these agents may be associated with a smaller increase in blood pressure when epinephrine is released during exercise or hypoglycemia.

Betaxolol, another cardioselective antagonist, has been approved for management of glaucoma. As used for glaucoma, it is reported to have minimal respiratory effect in asthmatics and less cardiac activity than timolol. **Levobunolol** is another recently introduced, long-acting β-blocker provided for treatment of glaucoma. It remains to be seen if these drugs will replace timolol in ophthalmology.[18]

REFERENCES

1. Avorn, J., Everitt, D.E., and Weiss, S.: Increased antidepressant use in patients prescribed β-blockers, J.A.M.A. **255:**357, 1986.

2. Benfield, P., Clissold, S.P., and Brodgen, R.N.: Metoprolol: an updated review of its pharmacodynamic and pharmacokinetic properties, and therapeutic efficacy, in hypertension, ischaemic heart disease and related cardiovascular disorders, Drugs **31:**376, 1986.

3. Brass, E.P.: Effects of antihypertensive drugs on endocrine function, Drugs **27:**447, 1984.

4. Cho, A.K., and Takimoto, G.S.: Irreversible inhibitors of adrenergic nerve terminal function, Trends Pharmacol. Sci. **6:**443, 1985.

5. Choice of a beta-blocker, Med. Lett. Drugs Ther. **28:**20, 1986.

6. Epstein, D.L.: Chandler and Grant's glaucoma, ed. 3, Philadelphia, 1986, Lea & Febiger.

7. Foerster, E.-C., Greminger, P., Siegenthaler, W., et al.: Atenolol versus pindolol: side-effects in hypertension, Eur. J. Clin. Pharmacol. **28**(suppl.):89, 1985.

8. ISIS-1 (First International Study of Infarct Survival) Collaborative Group: Randomized trial of intravenous atenolol among 16,027 cases of suspected acute myocardial infarction: ISIS-1, Lancet **2:**57, 1986.

9. Jackson, C.D., and Fishbein, L.: A toxicological review of beta-adrenergic blockers, Fundam. Appl. Toxicol. **6:**395, 1986.

10. Koella, W.P.: CNS-related (side-)effects of β-blockers with special reference to mechanisms of action, Eur. J. Clin. Pharmacol. **28**(suppl.):55, 1985.

11. Leopold, I.H., and Duzman, E.: Observations on the pharmacology of glaucoma, Annu. Rev. Pharmacol. Toxicol. **26:**401, 1986.

12. Man in 't Veld, A.J., van den Meiracker, A., and Schalekamp, M.A.D.H.: The effect of β blockers on total peripheral resistance, J. Cardiovasc. Pharmacol. **8**(suppl. 4):S49, 1986.

13. Prichard, B.N.C., and Tomlinson, B.: The additional properties of beta adrenoceptor blocking drugs, J. Cardiovasc. Pharmacol. **8**(suppl. 4):S1, 1986.

14. Reeves, R.A., Boer, W.H., DeLeve, L., and Leenen, F.H.H.: Nonselective beta-blockade enhances pressor responsiveness to epinephrine, norepinephrine, and angiotensin II in normal man, Clin. Pharmacol. Ther. **35:**461, 1984.

15. Singh, B.N., Thoden, W.R., and Ward, A.: Acebutolol: a review of its pharmacological properties and therapeutic efficacy in hypertension, angina pectoris and arrhythmia, Drugs **29:**531, 1985.

16. Stanaszek, W.F., Kellerman, D., Brogden, R.N., and Romankiewicz, J.A.: Prazosin update: a review of its pharmacological properties and therapeutic use in hypertension and congestive heart failure, Drugs **25:**339, 1983.

17. Tattersfield, A.E.: Beta adrenoceptor antagonists and respiratory disease, J. Cardiovasc. Pharmacol. **8**(suppl. 4):S35, 1986.

18. Two new beta-blockers for glaucoma, Med. Lett. Drugs Ther. **28:**45, 1986.

19. Wood, A.J.J.: β-Blocker withdrawal, Drugs **25**(suppl. 2):318, 1983.

20. Yusuf, S., Peto, R., Lewis, J., et al.: Beta blockade during and after myocardial infarction: an overview of the randomized trials, Prog. Cardiovasc. Dis. **27:**335, 1985.

Chapter 17

Drugs acting on the adrenergic neuron

GENERAL
CONCEPT

Certain drugs can influence sympathetic functions by affecting storage and re-lease of catecholamines,[4] thus providing an entirely new pharmacologic approach to the nervous system. Such drugs have found wide application as *antihypertensive agents* and in the field of *psychopharmacology*.

This field began with the discovery that reserpine, a *Rauwolfia* alkaloid, releases serotonin (5-hydroxytryptamine) from its binding sites in various tissues. Subse-quently, it was shown that reserpine also releases norepinephrine and dopamine. Decreased sympathetic function induced by reserpine, leading to hypotension and bradycardia, is now generally attributed to catecholamine depletion from adrenergic nerve endings.

Other drugs can influence catecholamine stores. Guanethidine, which does not reach the brain, depletes peripheral amine stores. In contrast, bretylium blocks adrenergic transmission without depleting neuronal catecholamine content.

The monoamine oxidase (MAO) inhibitors raise the catecholamine content of neural tissues in several species. Hypotension that occurs after use of MAO inhibitors may be related to the accumulation of a false transmitter such as octopamine in adrenergic fibers (see pp. 94 and 175).

MECHANISMS OF
CATECHOLAMINE
RELEASE

The *two basic* mechanisms of release and the drugs that illustrate them are as follows:

Interference with granular storage mechanism
  Reserpine
  Guanethidine
Displacement of catecholamines
  Tyramine
  Amphetamine
  Metaraminol
  Methyldopa (through its metabolite α-methylnorepinephrine)

Interference with granular storage mechanism. As depicted in Fig. 17-1, when the contents of a norepinephrine-containing granule are released into the neuroeffector junction, the amine can act on postsynaptic receptors. On the other hand, when storage of the amine is inhibited by drugs such as reserpine or guanethidine, the amine becomes free within the axoplasm, making it subject to attack by MAO. Instead of the active amine, mostly its inactivated products appear outside the nerve. This

Schematic representation of nerve ending and effector cell. (For details see text.)   *FIG. 17-1*

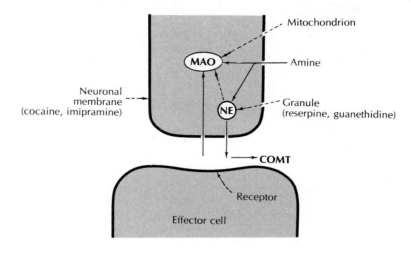

explains why ingestion of reserpine, though causing massive depletion of catechol-amines, does not elevate blood pressure.

Displacement of catecholamines. Like nerve stimulation, indirectly acting sympathomimetic agents, such as tyramine and amphetamine, release catecholamines from the neurons. Other amines not only displace catecholamines but also are incorporated as false transmitters into the granule.

These mechanisms of catecholamine release can be modified by at least four additional pharmacologic influences.

MAO inhibitors protect the intraneuronally released catecholamines from inactivation. Unlike reserpine alone, injection of reserpine in the presence of MAO inhibition will increase blood pressure.

Bretylium and some other agents, such as debrisoquin and guanethidine, can prevent catecholamine release by nerve stimulation in the absence of depletion. Conceptually these drugs appear to anesthetize the adrenergic fibers. Indeed, they do have local anesthetic properties and concentrate in adrenergic fibers.

Drugs that inhibit the membrane amine pump (Fig. 17-1), such as cocaine and tricyclic antidepressants, block the actions of tyramine, other indirectly acting amines, and *guanethidine* by preventing their uptake into neurons. In addition, they potentiate the neurotransmitter by allowing its extraneuronal accumulation in the neuroeffector junction in the vicinity of postsynaptic receptors. They do not affect the action of reserpine.

Finally, *drugs may act on presynaptic α- or β-receptors*, which modulate catecholamine release.[3]

Mechanism of decreased sympathetic activity induced by catecholamine depletion	When the catecholamine content of a nerve is decreased to below 50% of normal, nerve stimulation causes a lessened response. The rate of depletion varies in different organs. Cardiac catecholamines decline rapidly; adrenal stores are more resistant. The rate of depletion is a function not only of the dose of reserpine but also of the rate of turnover of the amine at the various sites. It has been estimated that the half-life of catecholamines in the heart is 4 to 8 hours, in contrast to their half-life of 7 days in the adrenal medulla. Depletion must be rapid in arterioles and venules. This is the reason reserpine is useful as an antihypertensive drug.
RESERPINE	Alkaloids of *Rauwolfia serpentina* have antihypertensive and antipsychotic properties. Reserpine and some other *Rauwolfia* alkaloids deplete norepinephrine, dopamine, and also serotonin from binding sites in the brain and peripheral nerves.[5] The drug not only releases amines into the cytoplasm but also blocks their granular uptake. It does not, however, block the action of catecholamines. It may have some inhibitory effect on norepinephrine synthesis by preventing uptake of dopamine into the storage granules, which contain dopamine-β-hydroxylase. Dosage forms and structures of these agents are given in the next chapter.
GUANETHIDINE	Guanethidine monosulfate (Ismelin) decreases sympathetic activity by a dual mechanism. Although both reserpine and guanethidine deplete catecholamine from nerves by acting on the granular storage mechanism, guanethidine also has a *bretylium-like* action to cause early sympathetic neuronal blockade before the catecholamine is depleted from nerves. Other differences between reserpine and guanethidine are of considerable importance. Intravenous injection of guanethidine regularly leads to a transient elevation of blood pressure, caused by a *tyramine-like* effect. For this reason guanethidine is not used parenterally for management of hypertensive emergencies. Also reserpine depletes catecholamines and serotonin from the central nervous system. Guanethidine fails to cross the blood-brain barrier and has no effect on brain amines. **Guanadrel sulfate** (Hylorel), a pharmacologically similar agent with a short duration of action, is also available for control of hypertension (see Chapter 18).
BRETYLIUM	Bretylium tosylate (Bretylol) produces a selective block in the peripheral sympathetic nervous system without opposing the action of injected or released catecholamines and without depleting the neurons of their catecholamine content. It appears to act as a local anesthetic that concentrates in adrenergic fibers. Although bretylium is an interesting drug, its clinical use has been attended by many toxic effects,[1] including muscular weakness and mental confusion. It is no longer approved as an antihypertensive drug but is used to control ventricular arrhythmias[2] (see p. 445).

Catecholamine metabolism in the adrenergic neuron, indicating the possible role of false   **FIG. 17-2**
transmitters.

From Kopin, I.J.: In Adrenergic neurotransmission, Ciba Foundation Study Group No. 33, Boston, 1968, Little, Brown & Co.

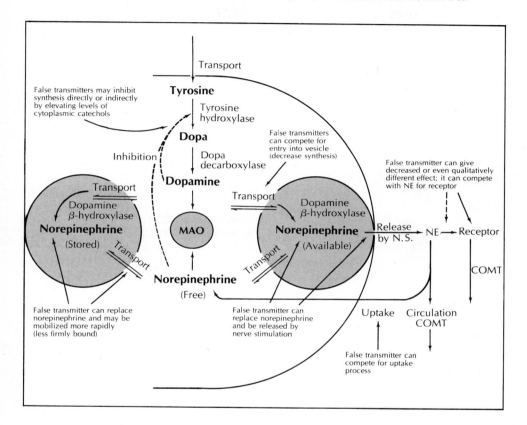

Methyldopa (Aldomet), an analog of dopa, competes with this precursor of nor-   **METHYLDOPA**
epinephrine for the enzyme that decarboxylates aromatic L-amino acids. Although
it inhibits the synthesis of both norepinephrine and serotonin, norepinephrine levels
in the brain remain low for a much longer time than serotonin levels. This and other
evidence indicates that much of the catecholamine depletion induced by methyldopa
may be caused by the drug's metabolism to α-methylnorepinephrine. α-Methylnorepinephrine replaces norepinephrine to act as a potent false transmitter that, like
clonidine, stimulates central α_2-receptors (Chapter 18). Various potential consequences of the presence of false transmitters are summarized in Fig. 17-2.

MAO INHIBITORS   MAO inhibitors were introduced as antidepressants (see Chapter 25). One of their surprising side effects was orthostatic hypotension, which indicated possible interference with sympathetic functions.

Experimentally, the MAO inhibitors elevate levels of norepinephrine and serotonin in the brain, ganglia, and other peripheral tissues. In addition, they prevent many of the actions of reserpine, including its ability to lower amine levels. One of the serious disadvantages of MAO inhibitors is the likelihood of adverse reactions to ingested foods and to drugs that release monoamines in the body (see p. 269).

Although MAO inhibitors are used primarily as antidepressants, one of them, pargyline (Eutonyl), is still used occasionally as an antihypertensive agent.

REFERENCES

1. Anderson, J.L., Popat, K.D., and Pitt, B.: Paradoxical ventricular tachycardia and fibrillation after intravenous bretylium therapy, Arch. Intern. Med. **141**:801, 1981.

2. Heissenbuttel, R.H., and Bigger, J.T., Jr.: Bretylium tosylate: a newly available antiarrhythmic drug for ventricular arrhythmias, Ann. Intern. Med. **91**:229, 1979.

3. Langer, S.Z., Duval, N., and Massingham, R.: Pharmacologic and therapeutic significance of α-adrenoceptor subtypes, J. Cardiovasc. Pharmacol. **7**(supp. 8):S1, 1985.

4. Maxwell, R.A., and Wastila, W.B.: Adrenergic neuron blocking drugs, Handb. Exp. Pharmacol. **39**:161, 1977.

5. Rand, M.J., and Jurevics, H.: The pharmacology of Rauwolfia alkaloids, Handb. Exp. Pharmacol. **39**:77, 1977.

Chapter 18

Antihypertensive drugs

Effective treatment of hypertension is one of the major developments in medicine. Beginning in 1949 when ganglionic blocking agents were introduced, a series of important discoveries has led to the availability of numerous drugs that can exert a favorable effect on life expectancy and ameliorate, if not prevent, the complications of hypertension.[16,34,35]

Among the most significant developments have been the introduction of hydralazine in 1952, reserpine in 1953, the thiazide diuretics in 1959, guanethidine in 1960, methyldopa and clonidine in 1967, β-adrenergic blocking drugs in 1968, and more recently prazosin, an α-adrenergic blocking drug, angiotensin-converting-enzyme inhibitors, and slow calcium-channel antagonists.

The antihypertensive drugs act by many different mechanisms, as summarized in Table 18-1. A diagram of blood pressure–regulating mechanisms is shown in Fig. 18-1. The agents listed in Table 18-1 act at one or more of the sites depicted. Delineation of their sites of action is important for optimal use of the antihypertensives, for understanding the pathophysiology of hypertension itself, and for development of new drugs.

In the clinical approach to treatment of hypertension, however, a more simple schema can be used, one that shows hypertension in terms of its cardiovascular hemodynamics. As such, blood pressure (BP) equals cardiac output (CO) times peripheral vascular resistance (PVR):

$$BP = CO \times PVR$$

In turn, CO and PVR can be subdivided into their determinants:

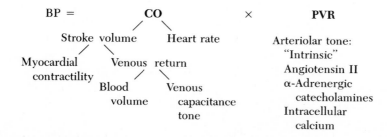

A fundamentally important concept inherent in the above schema is that an antihypertensive agent that acts on one component of the system can induce reflex

GENERAL CONCEPTS

177

TABLE 18-1   Site of action of antihypertensive drugs

Site of action	Mode of action	Drug	Trade name
Arteriolar smooth muscle	Direct vasodilatation	Hydralazine Minoxidil Diazoxide Nitroprusside Thiazide diuretics	Apresoline Loniten Hyperstat Nipride
Converting enzyme	Decreased angiotensin II formation	Captopril Enalapril	Capoten Vasotec
Sympathetic neurons	Blockade of norepinephrine release (also depletion)	Reserpine Guanethidine Guanadrel	 Ismelin Hylorel
	Inhibition of monoamine oxidase (MAO)	Pargyline	Eutonyl
α-Adrenergic receptors	Receptor blockade (vasodilatation)	Phentolamine Phenoxybenzamine Prazosin	Regitine Dibenzyline Minipress
Central α₂-receptors	Receptor stimulation (decreased peripheral sympathetic tone)	Methyldopa Clonidine Guanabenz	Aldomet Catapres Wytensin
Slow calcium channel	Vasodilatation	Verapamil Diltiazem Nifedipine	Calan, Isoptin Cardizem Adalat, Procardia
β-Adrenergic receptors	Decreased cardiac output Nonselective β-receptor blockade	 Propranolol Nadolol Timolol	 Inderal Corgard Blocadren
	Cardioselective (β₁-receptor) blockade	Metoprolol Atenolol	Lopressor Tenormin

	Decreased peripheral vascular resistance
	   Nonselective β-receptor blockade + ISA*
	   Cardioselective β-receptor blockade + ISA
		
		Pindolol
		Acebutolol
			
			Visken
			Sectral

β- and α-adrenergic receptors	Blockade (decreased cardiac output and peripheral vascular resistance)	Labetalol	Normodyne, Trandate
Kidney	Sodium excretion, volume depletion	Many diuretics	
Autonomic ganglia	Ganglionic blockade	Trimethaphan	Arfonad
Carotid sinus	Reflex sympathetic depression	*Veratrum* alkaloids	

*Intrinsic sympathomimetic activity.

changes in other components, the net effect of which may be maintenance of blood pressure at an elevated level despite therapy. For example, a drug that decreases peripheral vascular resistance may initially lower blood pressure; however, this effect can dissipate with time because reflex increases in heart rate and retention of sodium (increasing blood volume) together can increase cardiac output sufficiently to nullify the benefit from the vasodilator. This scenario was frequently observed with use of hydralazine (a direct vasodilator) as a single agent. Its efficacy was not optimized until β-adrenergic antagonists and diuretics were used concomitantly to block the reflex tachycardia and to prevent volume expansion respectively.[38] From a clinical perspective, the foregoing emphasizes that in patients with moderate and severe

Diagram of blood pressure–regulating mechanisms.

From Abrams, W.B.: Dis. Chest **55**:148, 1969.

FIG. 18-1

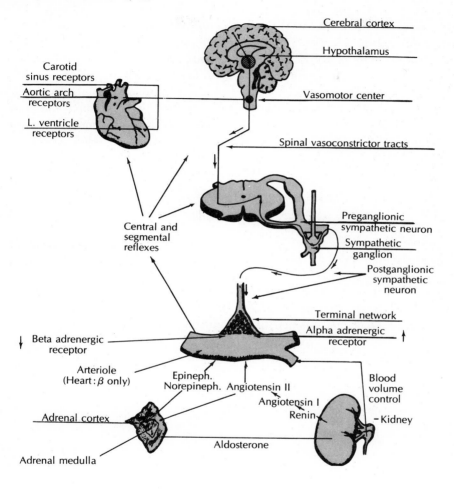

hypertension, who often require use of multiple agents, the drugs used should affect different components of the hemodynamic system schematized above. For example, if a patient requires three antihypertensives, it is far more logical to use a vasodilator, a β-blocker, and a diuretic than to use three different vasodilators.[38]

A second important consideration when one is using the hemodynamic schema is that peripheral vascular resistance is increased in most patients with hypertension. Hence the initial agents to be used (and the single agent for those patients who need only one drug) should lower peripheral vascular resistance.

A final consideration is that drugs that affect venous capacitance tone also cause orthostatic hypotension. In fact, effects on venous tone primarily diminish upright pressures and do not contribute to lowering of supine blood pressure. If such drugs also have an effect on supine blood pressure, it is by a concomitant decrease in arteriolar tone. Effects on capacitance tone are unwanted and constitute an adverse effect that limits their utility. The guanidinium antihypertensives (guanethidine and guanadrel) and the ganglionic blockers are the drugs of concern in this regard. The present availability of a variety of effective antihypertensives that do not affect capacitance tone has relegated those that do to historic interest.

RELATION OF ANGIOTENSIN AND ALDOSTERONE TO HYPERTENSION

The demonstration that renal ischemia leads to hypertension resulted in the discovery of a kidney enzyme, *renin*, in granules of the juxtaglomerular apparatus. When this enzyme is released, it acts on a substrate in blood and eventually yields angiotensin II, a potent vasopressor polypeptide. This sequence of events is shown in Table 18-2.

The amino acid composition of angiotensin I is as follows:

Asp-Arg-Val-Tyr-Ile-His-Pro-Phe-His-Leu

Converting enzyme removes the terminal histidyl-leucine to form angiotensin II. Angiotensin I has little biologic activity, though it may have some effect on aldosterone release, as angiotensin III does.

Saralasin (1-sarcosyl-8-alanyl-angiotensin II) is a specific angiotensin antagonist with essentially no other pharmacologic action. Given intravenously it serves as an investigational tool for assessment of the contribution of angiotensin to blood pressure elevation.

TABLE 18-2   Metabolism of angiotensin

Sequence	Inhibitors
Renin in kidney	
↓	β-Receptor blockers
Renin released	
+	
Angiotensinogen	
↓	
Angiotensin I (decapeptide)	
+	
Converting enzyme	Inhibitors (captopril)
↓	
Angiotensin II (octapeptide)	Antagonists (saralasin)
+	
Angiotensinases A, B, C	
↓ ↘ Split product	
Angiotensin III (heptapeptide)	

Lowering of blood pressure and renal perfusion pressure or a decrease in access of chloride to the macula densa of the juxtaglomerular apparatus promotes release of renin. Some of the effect of lowered blood pressure on renin release may be sympathetically mediated through β-receptors, since propranolol blocks catecholamine-induced renin release. Prostaglandins (presumably PGI_2) also induce renin release; the stimulus in this case is unclear. Some argue that prostaglandins are the final common pathway for all stimuli of renin release; others disagree, particularly with regard to participation of the macula densa.

Renin release

The pharmacologic effects of angiotensin II are as follows: (1) elevation of blood pressure, (2) contraction of isolated smooth muscle, (3) release of aldosterone, and (4) release of catecholamines from the adrenal medulla and adrenergic nerves. Not only does angiotensin release catecholamines, it also prevents their reuptake by adrenergic nerves.

Pharmacologic effects

The vasopressor actions of angiotensin are exerted primarily on peripheral resistance vessels in the skin, splanchnic area, and kidney. It has little cardiac stimulant action. The capacitance vessels are not greatly affected; they differ in this respect from their sensitivity to catecholamines.

Several features of the action of angiotensin have stimulated extensive investigation of the role of the renin-angiotensin-aldosterone system in hypertension, the nuances of which are still not understood. An action of this polypeptide on the vasomotor centers increases sympathetic activity. The peptide also potentiates the actions of catecholamines. It causes sodium retention by promoting release of aldosterone from the adrenal cortex. Angiotensin is also a potent central dipsogenic agent in animals and can alter vasopressin secretion. As one would predict, inhibition of the formation of angiotensin II is an effective means of lowering blood pressure. Two drugs that inhibit converting enzyme are currently available (and others are under development).

The various antihypertensive drugs may be grouped according to their actions on cardiovascular hemodynamics. They will be discussed under the headings of direct vasodilators, converting-enzyme inhibitors, agents that interfere with α-adrenergic mechanisms, calcium antagonists, β-adrenergic receptor blocking drugs, and diuretics. For a historic perspective, monoamine oxidase inhibitors, ganglionic blocking agents, and reflex inhibitors of central sympathetic function are discussed briefly.

CLASSIFICATION OF ANTIHYPER-TENSIVE DRUGS

Direct vasodilators act on vascular smooth muscle. They include hydralazine and minoxidil for chronic use. Diazoxide and sodium nitroprusside are reserved for hypertensive emergencies. Thiazide diuretics may also be considered in this group. When these diuretics are administered acutely to patients with hypertension, the initial decrease in blood pressure is attributable to the diuresis, which shrinks blood volume.[9] With chronic therapy, however, the vascular volume is restored, and the persistent antihypertensive effect is the result of a decrease in peripheral vascular

DIRECT VASODILATORS

resistance, the mechanism of which is unknown.[22] This vasodilating effect of thiazides is the rationale for their traditional use as a first step or single agent in patients with hypertension. The diuretic and natriuretic effects of these drugs are discussed in detail in Chapter 38; their use as antihypertensives is discussed in a separate section of this chapter.

Hydralazine

Hydralazine, a direct relaxant (mechanism unknown) of vascular smooth muscle, is used commonly in management of hypertension.[24] Although it is available in combination products advocated for use in mild hypertension, hydralazine is best reserved for patients with more severe hypertension (that is, with diastolic blood pressures above 105 mm Hg) who will probably require multiple medications to attain blood pressure control. Hydralazine is a sufficiently powerful vasodilator to routinely elicit reflex tachycardia and fluid retention; other drugs are therefore necessary to blunt these homeostatic responses.

ADVERSE EFFECTS

Headache, palpitations, and gastrointestinal disturbances are the most frequent adverse effects. With doses larger than 200 mg daily many patients develop a syndrome resembling systemic lupus erythematosus. This syndrome is reversible in most cases. Since the incidence of this effect is low if the dose is kept below 200 mg per day, this amount should not be exceeded.

Hydralazine

PREPARATIONS

Hydralazine hydrochloride is available in tablets of 20 to 100 mg. Twice-daily dosing is adequate. The drug is also available as a solution for injection, 20 mg/ml, in hypertensive emergencies. Currently, other drugs have more predictable blood pressure-lowering effects in this setting, and hydralazine is not a primary choice. Hydralazine in small amounts is also available in many combination preparations, the use of which we discourage.

Minoxidil

Minoxidil is indicated only for patients with severe hypertension who do not respond to other drugs.[3] It is such a powerful vasodilator that it causes considerable sodium retention and tachycardia, which necessitates concomitant use of large doses of potent diuretics and β-adrenergic receptor antagonists. Minoxidil also causes hirsutism, a side effect that has prompted its development as a solution or cream for baldness.

Minoxidil is available in tablets, 2.5 and 10 mg. The initial dose should be 5 mg;

the dosage is increased gradually to 40 mg a day in single or divided doses. Despite a half-life of 3 hours, the antihypertensive effect of the drug lasts at least 12 hours.

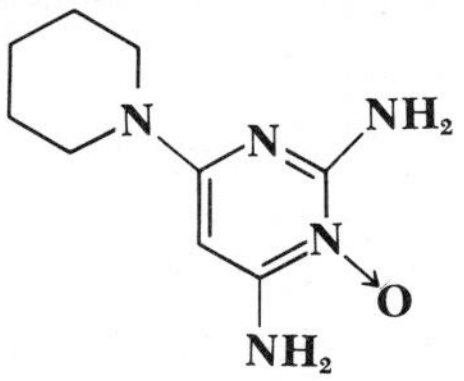

Minoxidil

Diazoxide

Diazoxide is a nondiuretic congener of the thiazide drugs.[19] Administered intravenously in hypertensive emergencies, it rapidly lowers blood pressure. The drug is supplied in a 20 ml ampule containing 300 mg. Initial guidelines for its use advocated bolus doses of 300 mg. Blood pressure decreases within 2 minutes to its lowest level. Then it increases fairly rapidly for 30 minutes and more slowly for the next 2 to 12 hours. Subsequent studies have shown that blood pressure can be lowered in a more controlled and predictable fashion by use of individual doses of 1 mg/kg every 10 minutes until the desired pressure is reached. Once this occurs the antihypertensive effect can last as long as 12 hours. Diazoxide can cause sufficient hyperglycemia, as a consequence of inhibition of insulin release, to require treatment with insulin. Whenever diazoxide is used, serum glucose concentrations should be monitored.

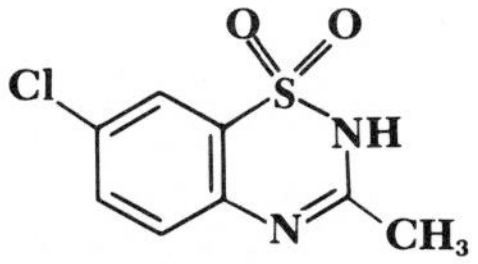

Diazoxide

Sodium nitroprusside

Sodium nitroprusside is the "gold standard" for use in hypertensive crises because it provides smooth and predictable blood pressure control.[29] The mechanism of its vasodilating effect is similar to that of the nitrates (Chapter 36); that is, in the vascular endothelium it forms an active nitrosothiol that increases cyclic GMP, thereby causing vasodilatation.

Adverse effects of nitroprusside include nausea, disorientation, and muscle spasms. A metabolic product of nitroprusside is cyanide, which is quickly metabolized to thiocyanate, which in turn is excreted by the kidney. When infused for prolonged periods in high doses or when given to patients with hepatic or renal disease, toxic concentrations of thiocyanate and cyanide may occur. Such patients should be monitored closely.

Sodium nitroprusside is available in 5 ml amber-colored vials containing the equivalent of 50 mg of sodium nitroprusside dihydrate for reconstitution with dextrose in water. A dose of 1 μg/kg/min is first administered by intravenous infusion. The infusion rate must then be adjusted by monitoring of the blood pressure, preferably by an intra-arterial cannula. The drug is very sensitive to light, and so the infusion system should be shielded.

CONVERTING-ENZYME INHIBITORS

As discussed previously, the multitude of mechanisms by which the renin-angiotensin system could influence blood pressure has stimulated the development of drugs that inhibit formation of angiotensin II.[21] Currently, captopril and enalapril are marketed, but many similar compounds are being developed.

Captopril

Captopril was the first converting-enzyme inhibitor available for clinical use.[13,28,36] Initially, dosing recommendations were too high, and therapy was associated with some alarming side effects, including neutropenia, proteinuria, and skin rash. It is now clear that total daily doses above 200 mg are superfluous and that lower doses are only infrequently associated with adverse effects. Consequently, the use of captopril has expanded. The initial indication for captopril was as therapy in patients who had not responded to other drugs. Because its therapeutic margin has widened with the use of lower doses, captopril is now frequently and effectively used as a single agent in patients with mild hypertension.

Captopril is supplied in tablets of 25 to 100 mg. Dosing should begin with 12.5 or 25 mg twice daily. This drug is eliminated by the kidney; therefore, in patients with decreased renal function, one should start with low doses and slowly titrate upwards.

Captopril

Enalapril

Enalapril

Enalapril is a prodrug that, after absorption, forms the active compound enalaprilat, which inhibits converting enzyme.[5,33] The active component has a half-life of about 11 hours and can be given once a day to most patients. Enalaprilat is excreted by the kidney, and dosage should be modified in patients with renal insufficiency. Enalapril, like smaller doses of captopril, has a low incidence of nonspecific adverse effects; it is therefore frequently used as a single agent in patients with mild hypertension as well as in multidrug regimens in patients with more severe disease.

Enalapril maleate is available in tablets, 5 to 20 mg. The initial dose is usually 10 mg; patients with decreased renal function and the elderly should begin with 5 mg. The maximal dose is usually 40 mg but may be as high as 80 mg in some patients.

α-Adrenergic functions can be inhibited by a variety of agents that can be grouped into those with predominant actions in the periphery and those for which the site of action is the central nervous system. The latter stimulate α_2-adrenergic receptors in the central nervous system and as a result diminish concentrations of circulating catecholamines; the net effect is diminished adrenergic activity.

AGENTS THAT INTERFERE WITH α-ADRENERGIC MECHANISMS

Reserpine is the prototype of several alkaloids present in *Rauwolfia serpentina*, an Indian snakeroot. Used in India for centuries, it was introduced into Western medicine in the 1950s. At first reserpine seemed as important for its tranquilizing properties as for its usefulness in the treatment of hypertension. It was gradually replaced as an antipsychotic drug by the phenothiazines. Newer antihypertensives have now relegated reserpine to historic interest because they are easier to use and have wider therapeutic margins.

Peripheral impairment of sympathetic neuronal function

RESERPINE

Basic action and effects. Reserpine causes depletion of catecholamines and serotonin in the central and peripheral nervous systems. Depletion is a consequence of amine release, followed by prevention of their reaccumulation. In addition, some interference by reserpine with catecholamine synthesis has been speculated.

Parasympathetic effects of reserpine are in part a result of decreased sympathetic activity. Bradycardia, aggravation of peptic ulcer, increased gastrointestinal motility, and miosis may be attributable to parasympathetic predominance when sympathetic effects are prevented.

The *central nervous system effects* of the drug are among its greatest disadvantages in treatment of hypertension. An unpleasant type of drowsiness and lethargy is particularly disliked by those who must be intellectually alert and creative. Depression and suicides have occurred during chronic reserpine administration. Central nervous system depression is a particular problem in patients also taking drugs such as barbiturates and alcohol. Reserpine also predisposes patients to severe hypotension during surgery and anesthesia.

Various derivatives of reserpine are similar to the parent compound. Syrosingopine produces fewer central effects in relation to its antihypertensive action. This selectivity has been attributed to the fact that its norepinephrine-depleting action is largely limited to the peripheral nervous system.

Reserpine

Preparations. The dried root of *Rauwolfia serpentina* Benth (Raudixin) is available in tablets containing 50 and 100 mg. *Reserpine* preparations include tablets of 0.1 to 1 mg, an elixir containing 0.25 mg/4 ml, and a solution for injection, 2.5 mg/ml. It is also available in combination preparations, the use of which should be discontinued. Syrosingopine (Singoserp) is available in tablets of 1 mg.

GUANETHIDINE AND GUANADREL

Several drugs, such as guanethidine, other guanidine compounds, and bretylium (Bretylol), can block the release of catecholamines from adrenergic nerve fibers.

Guanethidine is an adrenergic neuronal blocking agent that is a highly effective antihypertensive drug. In addition to blocking adrenergic neurons, guanethidine causes catecholamine release and depletion. In this respect it resembles reserpine. Guanadrel is a newer guanidine compound, which has a shorter duration of action than guanethidine.[7] Although these drugs produce adrenergic effects similar to those of reserpine, they share an important difference; they do not cross the blood-brain barrier, and so the adverse central nervous system effects associated with reserpine do not occur. Bretylium, another intraneuronal blocking agent, was first used as an antihypertensive drug but was abandoned for this purpose because of adverse side effects. Subsequently, it was noted to be effective treatment for refractory ventricular tachyarrhythmias, and it is now used for this purpose (see Chapter 35).

Mode of action. Guanethidine and guanadrel block adrenergic neurons selectively because they are concentrated within these neurons by the membrane transport system responsible for norepinephrine reuptake. For this reason, tricyclic antidepressants oppose the antihypertensive actions of these drugs by blocking their uptake into the adrenergic neurons.

In addition to their adrenergic neuron–blocking action, sometimes referred to as a *bretylium-like* action, guanethidine and guanadrel cause catecholamine depletion, a *reserpine-like* effect. Other less important actions are a *tyramine-like* action, meaning that the drug can cause release of catecholamines, and a *cocaine-like* action, which refers to competition for the membrane amine pump.

Clinical pharmacology. The onset of action of guanethidine is slow; that for guanadrel is more rapid. Maximum effects may not occur for 2 or 3 days after initiation of treatment with guanethidine, whereas effects of guanadrel maximize within 1 or 2 days. With guanethidine, then, patients are started on small doses, such as 10 mg once daily, which are maintained for 5 to 7 days before the dosage is increased. With guanadrel the dose can be titrated upward on a daily basis. The actions of guanethidine may persist for 7 days after its discontinuation, whereas those of guanadrel dissipate quickly. The delay of effect and long duration of action of guanethidine have made its use difficult.

Guanethidine

Guanadrel

Although guanethidine and guanadrel do not cause sedation and depression, both drugs cause substantial orthostatic hypotension, and they cause retrograde ejaculation (passage of ejaculate into the bladder) without affecting erection. These adverse effects are sufficiently limiting that these drugs should rarely be used today.

Preparations. Guanethidine sulfate is available in tablets containing 10 and 25 mg. Guanadrel sulfate is supplied in tablets, 10 and 25 mg.

The α-adrenergic receptor blocking drugs phenoxybenzamine and phentolamine (Chapter 16) have not been useful in management of hypertension because of their tendency to produce orthostatic hypotension and pronounced reflex tachycardia. Prazosin, a newer α-receptor blocking drug, causes the least tachycardia and is a useful antihypertensive agent.[10,37]

α-Adrenergic receptor antagonists

Prazosin produces its antihypertensive effect by blocking postsynaptic α_1-adrenergic receptors in blood vessels. Its superiority over other α-receptor blocking drugs is attributed to its greater affinity for postsynaptic receptors than for presynaptic α_2-adrenergic receptors. Blockade of presynaptic receptors by phenoxybenzamine or phentolamine increases release of norepinephrine. Since prazosin has little action on presynaptic receptors, norepinephrine concentrations do not increase and reflex sympathetic activity (for example, tachycardia) is less likely to occur.[10,37]

Prazosin

After oral administration, plasma concentrations of prazosin peak between 1 and 3 hours, followed by elimination with a half-life of about 4 hours. Prazosin is eliminated mainly through biliary excretion in the form of inactive metabolites.

Prazosin is particularly effective as a single agent in patients with mild hypertension. It has a low incidence of adverse effects and thereby a wide therapeutic margin. It was initially used to treat heart failure because it reduced both preload and afterload. Subsequent detailed studies showed that tolerance developed to the action on preload, and the drug is no longer used in patients with congestive heart failure. It is important to emphasize that tolerance does not develop to its antihypertensive action (on afterload), and its utility as an antihypertensive persists.

Untoward effects. A commonly encountered response to prazosin is called the *first-dose phenomenon;*[10,37] it is characterized by weakness and occasional syncope and occurs within 1 hour after the first dose is taken. This response, believed secondary to orthostatic hypotension, is aggravated by exercise and sodium depletion. The effect occurs by venodilatation (preload reduction) to which tolerance quickly develops, as mentioned above in regard to its use in congestive heart failure. One can avoid this response by having the patient take the first dose before going to bed. Prazosin hydrochloride is available in 1 to 5 mg tablets. The initial dosage should be 1 mg two times a day. The maximal daily dose is usually 20 mg, but some patients may require 40 mg.

Central α_2-adrenergic receptor agonists

METHYLDOPA

Methyldopa was introduced as an antihypertensive drug on the theory that being an inhibitor of aromatic amino acid decarboxylase it would lower catecholamine concentrations in the body by that mechanism. It was found, however, that the drug is taken up and metabolized to α-methylnorepinephrine. It was then postulated that this metabolite acted as an inactive or weak neurotransmitter, thereby diminishing overall sympathetic function. However, it is now apparent that α-methylnorepinephrine is an effective neurotransmitter and that the mode of action of methyldopa is through stimulation of central α_2-adrenergic receptors by this metabolite.[26] This effect in turn diminishes peripheral α-adrenergic activity.

$$\text{HO} \quad \text{HO} \diagdown \text{C}_6\text{H}_3 \diagup \text{CH}_2\text{—}\overset{\displaystyle \text{NH}_2}{\underset{\displaystyle \text{CH}_3}{\text{C}}}\text{—COOH}$$

Methyldopa

Methyldopa can be used for mild or more severe forms of hypertension. It causes much less orthostatic hypotension than guanethidine, ganglionic blocking drugs, or MAO inhibitors do.

Adverse reactions. Adverse reactions to methyldopa include pronounced drowsiness and dry mouth in many patients, depression, and nightmares. These side effects are clearly dose related. Early guidelines for use of methyldopa (and other central adrenergic stimulants) advocated doses that were associated with a high incidence of central nervous system side effects. Current recommendations are to use lower doses of methyldopa (for example, 250 mg twice daily) in which case central nervous system side effects are infrequent and, if they occur, usually dissipate with continued therapy. In some persons the administration of methyldopa for about a week causes an influenza-like reaction that may be attributed to sensitization to the drug. In some of these persons subsequent administration of small doses of methyldopa will elicit the same reaction. Methyldopa has also been associated with other immunologic phenomena. Twenty percent of patients develop a positive Coombs' test, but it is rare for the drug to cause hemolytic anemia. Rarely, cholestatic hepatitis occurs; this also may be immunologic in nature.

Pharmacokinetics. Methyldopa is absorbed well from the gastrointestinal tract. Its elimination half-life is 2 hours. Cumulation may occur when renal function is inadequate. The drug and its metabolites may give false-positive tests in the diagnosis of pheochromocytoma.

Preparations. Methyldopa is available in 250- and 500-mg tablets. Methyldopa hydrochloride (Aldomet ester hydrochloride) is available in solution for intravenous injection, 250 mg/5 ml, in patients with hypertensive emergencies. Other drugs are currently preferred in this setting however.

Intravenous administration of clonidine is followed by a transient pressor response attributable to stimulation of peripheral α-receptors; there is then a more sustained depressor effect accompanied by bradycardia. This antihypertensive effect is the result of stimulation of α_2-receptors within the central nervous system, which diminishes peripheral α-adrenergic receptor stimulation.[6,23] Clinically this can be quantified by measurement of the decrease in circulating norepinephrine that follows clonidine administration.

Clonidine

Adverse reactions and drug interactions. Drowsiness and dryness of the mouth are common dose-related responses, which can be avoided in most patients by use of low doses. Constipation occurs occasionally. Orthostatic hypotension is rare. Withdrawal symptoms on discontinuation of clonidine therapy include restlessness, tachycardia, and a rebound increase in blood pressure. These usually occur after abrupt withdrawal of large doses, particularly if β-receptor blockade is present. They can be reversed quickly by reinstitution of clonidine or another α_2-adrenergic stimulant and can be blocked by peripheral adrenergic antagonists; such withdrawal is not unique to clonidine. Desipramine and other tricyclic antidepressants may interfere with the antihypertensive activity of clonidine.

Pharmacokinetics. Clonidine is well absorbed after oral administration. Plasma concentrations reach their peak within 3 to 5 hours, and the half-life is 12 to 16 hours. Most of the drug is eliminated by hepatic metabolism, though sufficient renal excretion occurs to mandate changes in dosage in patients with renal dysfunction.

Preparations and dosages. Clonidine hydrochloride is available as tablets, 0.1 and 0.2 mg, and as a transdermal delivery system. The initial dose for adults is 0.1 mg two times daily. Dosage must be adjusted to the patient's requirement. Excessive doses increase the incidence of central nervous system side effects. If low doses of oral medication are effective, the transdermal system allows maintenance of stable plasma concentrations for a week. In noncompliant patients, its use may be helpful.

Guanabenz also stimulates central α_2-adrenergic receptors.[15] Its uses in hypertension are identical to those of clonidine and methyldopa. It is supplied as tablets, 4 to 16 mg. As with clonidine and methyldopa, low doses are advocated.

Guanabenz

<table>
<tr><td>

SLOW CALCIUM-
CHANNEL
BLOCKERS

</td><td>

Slow calcium-channel antagonists are discussed in more detail as antianginal agents (Chapter 36). These drugs are also effective vasodilators and can therefore be used as antihypertensives.[1,17] Although all block the slow calcium channel, these drugs differ in their pharmacologic profiles. *Nifedipine* is primarily a vasodilator.[18,32] At the other end of the spectrum, *verapamil* has less effect on peripheral vascular resistance and has a major action to slow cardiac conduction.[11] *Diltiazem* is intermediate in both effects.[4]

A drawback to use of currently available calcium antagonists is their short duration of action, which requires dosing three or four times a day. To circumvent this problem, sustained-release preparations have been released (verapamil) or are being developed, and other calcium antagonists with longer durations of action are under investigation. With availability of these newer preparations and agents, slow calcium-channel antagonists will be increasingly used both as single agents in mild hypertension and in combination regimens in patients with more severe disease.

In addition, nifedipine has proved to be effective in hypertensive emergencies.[18,32] Administration of 10 mg, either swallowed or sublingual, can promptly reduce blood pressure in this setting.

</td></tr>
</table>

β-ADRENERGIC *RECEPTOR* *BLOCKING DRUGS*	The β-adrenergic receptor blocking drugs have been widely used in treatment of hypertension.[14,30,35] For several years propranolol was the only β-blocker available in this country. The antihypertensive effect of this drug was quite unexpected and was discovered accidentally in England when patients with hypertension and angina were treated with β-blockers. With the recognition of the existence of β_1-, or cardiac, receptors efforts were made to develop specific β_1-receptor antagonists that would not affect the β_2-receptors mediating catecholamine effects on the bronchial tree and vasodilatation. Further development has lead to β-blockers that possess *intrinsic sympathomimetic activity* (ISA). These compounds act as partial agonists at β-receptors at low endogenous levels of sympathetic activity and function as antagonists when β-adrenergic activity increases. As such, these drugs do not affect resting heart rate but block exercise- or stress-induced increases in heart rate.

Mechanism of *action*	Despite extensive investigations, the mechanism of the antihypertensive action of the β-adrenergic receptor blocking drugs is not precisely known.[30] A single statement explaining the mechanism of action of *all* β-blockers in *all* hypertensive patients cannot be made. Main theories for this drug class center on (1) *central nervous system effects* (for example, propranolol), (2) *decreased renin release*, (3) *reduced cardiac output* (for example, propranolol), and (4) *diminished peripheral vascular resistance* (for example, β-blockers with intrinsic sympathomimetic activity). One or more of these actions is probably relevant in individual patients. The following issues illustrate the difficulty that exists when one is trying to make one of these theories encompass all patients. (1) *Central nervous system effects:* Some β-adrenergic receptor blockers are believed not to penetrate the central nervous system yet are fully effective. On the other hand, whether central nervous system

penetration occurs with chronic use or small amounts of such drugs reach a localized site in the central nervous system are unresolved possibilities. (2) *Decreased renin release:* Reductions in blood pressure can occur when plasma renin activity is unaffected by β-blockers; thus this action alone cannot be an *absolute* necessity for hypotension. There are reports that document no change in blood pressure control in patients switched from one β-blocker to another having intrinsic sympathomimetic activity. Plasma renin activity rose after the drug switch, but blood pressure control was unaffected. On the other hand, there are patients who respond to β-receptor blocking drugs with a clear fall in plasma renin activity. (3) *Reduced cardiac output:* Nonselective and cardioselective β-blockers reduce cardiac output in *essentially all subjects,* but only a portion will respond with a chronic hypotensive effect. (4) *Diminished peripheral vascular resistance:* β-blockers with intrinsic sympathomimetic activity tend to decrease peripheral vascular resistance, but on the average this effect is small in magnitude, and some patients who have a decrease in blood pressure exhibit a negligible effect on vascular resistance.

Propranolol has historically been the most widely used β-blocker in hypertension. Its mechanism of action is still poorly understood. Although the drug blocks renin release and reduces cardiac output, these effects cannot fully account for the usefulness of the drug as an antihypertensive agent.[14,30]

Nonselective β-adrenergic receptor blockers
PROPRANOLOL

Pharmacokinetics. Propranolol is well absorbed from the intestine, but 50% to 70% of an oral dose is extracted and metabolized by the liver during the first pass. The major metabolite, 4-hydroxypropranolol, is active, but its contribution to the overall pharmacologic effect is not clear. Propranolol has a half-life of 4 to 6 hours. Despite its short half-life, twice-daily dosage is sufficient in most patients. Patients with cirrhosis have both increased bioavailability of propranolol (diminished first-pass effect) and diminished clearance. Therefore they need much smaller doses of propranolol (on average one-fourth normal) or, preferably, use of a β-blocker eliminated by the kidney.

Effectiveness. It has been shown in a cooperative study that blood pressure was well controlled in only 52% of patients when propranolol was taken alone.[35] In combination with a diuretic this percentage increased to 81%, and the addition of hydralazine to the propranolol-diuretic combination produced good results in 92% of the patients. Propranolol therefore has a major role in combination therapy, particularly because it can counteract some of the adverse hemodynamic effects of other antihypertensive agents.[38] As a single drug in patients with mild hypertension, agents that lower peripheral vascular resistance are preferable to propranolol.

Adverse effects. β-Blockers including propranolol do not cause orthostatic hypotension. They may elicit congestive heart failure and asthmatic attacks in susceptible persons, with nonselective agents theoretically more prone to do so. Bradycardia is common but is not a contraindication to continued therapy. Gastrointestinal side effects, Raynaud's phenomenon, and worsening of claudication are rare. β-Blockers have a disadvantage in insulin-dependent diabetic patients, since they may mask the symptoms of hypoglycemia. Propranolol, in particular, has also been associated with central nervous system side effects, such as sleep disturbances, vivid dreams, and fatigue. This has been postulated to be related to propranolol's high lipid solubility, which allows greater access to the central nervous system. However, no data support a clear difference between propranolol and other, less lipid-soluble β-blockers.

Dosage. The initial dosage of propranolol is 40 mg twice daily. The usual effective dose range is 160 to 480 mg daily. See Table 16-2 for information regarding dosage forms of β-blockers.

| NADOLOL | Nadolol is characterized by slow elimination, having a plasma half-life of about 12 hours.[12] Thus it may be used once a day. The drug is excreted primarily by the kidney and thereby requires downward dose adjustment in patients with renal dysfunction. |

| TIMOLOL | Timolol is very similar to propranolol in its pharmacologic and pharmacokinetic profile, differing predominantly in its potency so that lower doses are used. Topical use of low doses of timolol for glaucoma (see p. 170) can occasionally cause systemic β-receptor blockade. |

| Cardioselective β-blockers METOPROLOL | Metoprolol is a cardioselective agent, since it blocks β-receptors in the heart preferentially.[2,20,27] The drug is therefore preferable to nonselective β-blockers in patients with asthma and in those having intermittent claudication, though β-blockers in general are still best avoided in these conditions. The plasma half-life of metoprolol is 3 to 6 hours, but the antihypertensive effect is longer, and the drug may be given twice daily in a total daily dose of 50 to 200 mg. The drug is eliminated by the liver, and patients with cirrhosis have both increased bioavailability and decreased clearance. Like propranolol and timolol in such patients, dosage should be decreased drastically or alternative agents should be used. |

| ATENOLOL | Atenolol is a cardioselective β-blocker, which has a half-life of 6 to 9 hours.[8] It can be administered once a day. It is eliminated by the kidney and requires dosage modification in patients with renal compromise. |

| β-Blockers with intrinsic sympathomimetic activity PINDOLOL | Pindolol is not cardioselective but has intrinsic sympathomimetic activity. By stimulating vascular β₂-receptors, the drug diminishes peripheral vascular resistance rather than decreasing cardiac output, and it does not suppress resting heart rate. Although its half-life is 3 to 4 hours, it is effective when given twice a day. |

| ACEBUTOLOL | Acebutolol has intrinsic sympathomimetic activity but differs from pindolol in having cardioselective β-blocking features.[31] It is metabolized to diacetolol, which is also active and cardioselective. The latter is eliminated by the kidney and accounts for the need to decrease the dose of acebutolol in patients with renal insufficiency. |

Acebutolol has an elimination half-life of 3 to 4 hours, whereas that for the active metabolite is 8 to 12 hours. The latter allows once a day dosing in most patients.

Combined β- and α-receptor blockade

Labetalol combines nonselective β- and α_1-adrenergic receptor blockade.[25] These exist in an approximate 7:1 ratio. The drug's hemodynamic actions decrease both cardiac output and peripheral vascular resistance. Labetalol has two asymmetric carbon atoms, and thus the racemate consists of four separate stereoisomers—one possesses the β-receptor blocking property, one is the α-blocker, and the other two forms are inert. Labetalol is eliminated by the liver with a half-life of 3 to 4 hours. Patients with cirrhosis exhibit both an increase in bioavailability and a decrease in clearance.

The usual starting dose of labetalol is 200 mg twice daily with upward titration to 2400 mg per day. The drug is also supplied as a solution for use in hypertensive emergencies. As such, it can be given as a continuous intravenous infusion at a rate of 2 mg/min or as successive intravenous bolus doses every 10 to 20 minutes. Twenty milligrams is administered first, followed by 40 mg and then repeated doses of 80 mg until the desired blood pressure or a maximum total dose of 300 mg is reached.

DIURETICS

Drugs that promote salt excretion, such as the thiazides, have been a mainstay in the treatment of hypertension. This implies that sodium is involved in some way in the pathogenesis of the disease.[9]

Rats on a high salt intake develop hypertension. Also, the hypertensive effect of deoxycorticosterone and aldosterone is probably attributable to salt retention. On the other hand, the antihypertensive action of a low salt diet is generally accepted. The mechanism whereby an excess of salt contributes to hypertension is not known. Expansion of extracellular fluid volume and alterations in the salt concentration in arteriolar walls, thereby increasing peripheral vascular resistance, have been suggested as important factors.

Thiazides and related drugs

Most investigators believe that thiazide diuretics initially exert their antihypertensive action through salt depletion. With chronic therapy they lower peripheral vascular resistance.

The most useful oral diuretics, discussed in detail in Chapter 38, are the thiazides and the related drugs chlorthalidone (Hygroton, others), quinethazone (Hydromox) and metolazone (Zaroxolyn, Diulo).[22] They are widely used for mild hypertension because of their safety and effectiveness and their ability to enhance the antihypertensive effect of other drugs. They differ only in their durations of action and potency, as discussed in Chapter 38.

The adverse effects of thiazide diuretics, such as hypokalemia, hyperuricemia, and aggravation of diabetes, are discussed in Chapter 38. A more recent concern that has limited their use as single agents in young patients with hypertension is their adverse effect on serum cholesterol. It appears that these drugs increase low-density lipoprotein cholesterol about 10% by unknown mechanisms. There is concern that over many years of treatment this may have an adverse effect on cardiovascular risk. As a result, many patients who would have heretofore been treated with thiazide diuretics as a single agent are now being treated with other drugs that lower peripheral vascular resistance.

Potassium-sparing diuretics	Spironolactone (Aldactone), triamterene (Dyrenium), and amiloride (Midamor) have only weak antihypertensive activity as single agents and should not be used as primary drugs in this disorder.[22] They have been promoted for use in combination with thiazides to prevent development of hypokalemia. However, hypokalemia is an infrequent adverse effect of thiazides used alone for hypertension; it occurs in only about 5% of patients. There is no good evidence that the combination formulations diminish this incidence, but it is clear that they entail a risk of hyperkalemia. Hence these products should not be used routinely and are indicated only in patients in whom potassium depletion develops while they are receiving thiazides alone.
Loop diuretics	Loop diuretics are less effective than thiazides in patients with uncomplicated essential hypertension, probably because they solely cause sodium depletion and lack an additional action on peripheral vascular resistance. They should be reserved for hypertensive patients with diminished renal function in whom thiazides are not effective.[22]
ANTIHYPERTEN-SIVE AGENTS OF HISTORICAL INTEREST *Monoamine oxidase inhibitors*	Historically, monoamine oxidase (MAO) inhibitors were used to treat hypertension, but drugs with greater effectiveness and safety were quickly developed. Probably the major disadvantage of the MAO inhibitors is their incompatibility with a large variety of drugs. Thus the indirectly acting sympathomimetics are contraindicated in patients receiving pargyline (Eutonyl). Such patients also exhibit a violent reaction to foods containing tyramine. Furthermore, combinations with tricyclic antidepressants are generally contraindicated (p. 270). Other side effects include orthostatic hypotension, gastrointestinal disturbances, insomnia, and headaches. This spectrum of risks obviates the use of MAO inhibitors for hypertension today.
Ganglionic blocking agents	Ganglionic blocking drugs (Chapter 13) such as hexamethonium, pentolinium, and mecamylamine have received extensive trial in hypertensive diseases. Reduction of blood pressure, particularly in the standing position, can be achieved, but the inevitable side effects of orthostatic hypotension and parasympathetic ganglionic blockade complicate this approach to management of hypertension. Trimethaphan continues to be used by some clinicians for hypertensive emergencies, particularly if associated with dissecting aortic aneurysm.

The *Veratrum* alkaloids protoveratrines A and B act by promoting the activity of afferent nerves from the carotid sinus and aortic arch; they thereby cause reflex inhibition of central sympathetic activity with subsequent parasympathetic predominance. If a small dose (less than 2 mg) of a mixture of protoveratrines A and B is injected intravenously, the characteristic response consists in bradycardia and a decrease in blood pressure. When proportionately larger doses are given to animals, temporary apnea is produced in addition to the circulatory effects. The protoveratrines cause considerable nausea in many patients, and their dosage must be carefully adjusted to obtain a good hypotensive effect. These disadvantages have limited the usefulness of these compounds, but their pharmacology has illustrated some unique mechanisms of drug action.

Reflex inhibitors of central sympathetic function

REFERENCES

1. Antman, E.M., Stone, P.H., Muller, J.E., and Braunwald, E.: Calcium channel blocking agents in the treatment of cardiovascular disorders, Ann. Intern. Med. **93**:875 and 886, 1980.
2. Benfield, P., Clissold, S.P., and Brogden, R.N.: Metoprolol: an updated review of its pharmacodynamic and pharmacokinetic properties, and therapeutic efficacy, in hypertension, ischaemic heart disease and related cardiovascular disorders, Drugs **31**:376, 1986.
3. Campese, V.M.: Minoxidil: a review of its pharmacological properties and therapeutic use, Drugs **22**:257, 1981.
4. Chaffman, M., and Brogden, R.N.: Diltiazem: a review of its pharmacological properties and therapeutic efficacy, Drugs **29**:387, 1985.
5. Davies, R.O., Gomez, H.J., Irvin, J.D., and Walker, J.F.: An overview of the clinical pharmacology of enalapril, Br. J. Clin. Pharmacol. **18**:215S, 1984.
6. Dollery, C.T., Davies, D.S., Draffan, G.H., et al.: Clinical pharmacology and pharmacokinetics of clonidine, Clin. Pharmacol. Ther. **19**:11, 1976.
7. Finnerty, F.A., Jr., and Brogden, R.N.: Guanadrel: a review of its pharmacodynamic and pharmacokinetic properties and therapeutic use in hypertension, Drugs **30**:22, 1985.
8. Fitzgerald, J.D., Ruffin, R., Smedstad, K.G., et al.: Studies on the pharmacokinetics and pharmacodynamics of atenolol in man, Eur. J. Clin. Pharmacol. **13**:81, 1978.
9. Freis, E.D.: Salt in hypertension and the effects of diuretics, Annu. Rev. Pharmacol. Toxicol. **19**:13, 1979.
10. Graham, R.M., and Pettinger, W.A.: Prazosin, N. Engl. J. Med. **300**:232, 1979.
11. Hamann, S.R., Blouin, R.A., and McAllister, R.G., Jr.: Clinical pharmacokinetics of verapamil, Clin. Pharmacokinet. **9**:26, 1984.
12. Heel, R.C., Brogden, R.N., Pakes, G.E., et al.: Nadolol: a review of its pharmacological properties and therapeutic efficacy in hypertension and angina pectoris, Drugs **20**:1, 1980.
13. Heel, R.C., Brogden, R.N., Speight, T.M., and Avery, G.S.: Captopril: a preliminary review of its pharmacological properties and therapeutic efficacy, Drugs **20**:409, 1980.
14. Holland, O.B., and Kaplan, N.M.: Propranolol in the treatment of hypertension, N. Engl. J. Med. **294**:930, 1976.
15. Holmes, B., Brogden, R.N., Heel, R.C., et al.: Guanabenz: a review of its pharmacodynamic properties and therapeutic efficacy in hypertension, Drugs **26**:212, 1983.

16. Hypertension Detection and Follow-up Program Cooperative Group: Five-year findings of the hypertension detection and follow-up program. I. Reduction in mortality of persons with high blood pressure, including mild hypertension, J.A.M.A. **242**:2562, 1979.

17. Kates, R.E.: Calcium antagonists: pharmacokinetic properties, Drugs **25**:113, 1983.

18. Kleinbloesem, C.H., van Brummelen, P., and Breimer, D.D.: Nifedipine: relationship between pharmacokinetics and pharmacodynamics, Clin. Pharmacokinet. **12**:12, 1987.

19. Koch-Weser, J.: Diazoxide, N. Engl. J. Med. **294**:1271, 1976.

20. Koch-Weser, J.: Metoprolol, N. Engl. J. Med. **301**:698, 1979.

21. Kubo, S.H., and Cody, R.J.: Clinical pharmacokinetics of the angiotensin converting enzyme inhibitors: a review, Clin. Pharmacokinet. **10**:377, 1985.

22. Lant, A.: Diuretics: clinical pharmacology and therapeutic use, Drugs **29**:57 and 162, 1985.

23. Lowenstein, J.: Clonidine, Ann. Intern. Med. **92**:74, 1980.

24. Ludden, T.M., McNay, J.L., Jr., Shepherd, A.M.M., and Lin, M.S.: Clinical pharmacokinetics of hydralazine, Clin. Pharmacokinet. **7**:185, 1982.

25. McNeil, J.J., and Louis, W.J.: Clinical pharmacokinetics of labetalol, Clin. Pharmacokinet. **9**:157, 1984.

26. Myhre, E., Rugstad, H.E., and Hansen, T.: Clinical pharmacokinetics of methyldopa, Clin. Pharmacokinet. **7**:221, 1982.

27. Regårdh, C.-G., and Johnsson, G.: Clinical pharmacokinetics of metoprolol, Clin. Pharmacokinet. **5**:557, 1980.

28. Romankiewicz, J.A., Brogden, R.N., Heel, R.C., et al.: Captopril: an update review of its pharmacological properties and therapeutic efficacy in congestive heart failure, Drugs **25**:6, 1983.

29. Schulz, V.: Clinical pharmacokinetics of nitroprusside, cyanide, thiosulphate and thiocyanate, Clin. Pharmacokinet. **9**:239, 1984.

30. Scriabine, A.: β-Adrenoceptor blocking drugs in hypertension, Annu. Rev. Pharmacol. Toxicol. **19**:269, 1979.

31. Singh, B.N., Thoden, W.R., and Ward, A.: Acebutolol: a review of its pharmacological properties and therapeutic efficacy in hypertension, angina pectoris and arrhythmia, Drugs **29**:531, 1985.

32. Sorkin, E.M., Clissold, S.P., and Brogden, R.N.: Nifedipine: a review of its pharmacodynamic and pharmacokinetic properties, and therapeutic efficacy, in ischaemic heart disease, hypertension and related cardiovascular disorders, Drugs **30**:182, 1985.

33. Todd, P.A., and Heel, R.C.: Enalapril: a review of its pharmacodynamic and pharmacokinetic properties, and therapeutic use in hypertension and congestive heart failure, Drugs **31**:198, 1986.

34. Veterans Administration Cooperative Study Group on Antihypertensive Agents: Effects of treatment on morbidity in hypertension. II. Results in patients with diastolic blood pressure averaging 90 through 114 mm Hg, J.A.M.A. **213**:1143, 1970.

35. Veterans Administration Cooperative Study Group on Antihypertensive Agents: Propranolol in the treatment of essential hypertension, J.A.M.A. **237**:2303, 1977.

36. Vidt, D.G., Bravo, E.L., and Fouad, F.M.: Captopril, N. Engl. J. Med. **306**:214, 1982.

37. Vincent, J., Meredith, P.A., Reid, J.L., et al.: Clinical pharmacokinetics of prazosin—1985, Clin. Pharmacokinet. **10**:144, 1985.

38. Zacest, R., Gilmore, E., and Koch-Weser, J.: Treatment of essential hypertension with combined vasodilation and beta-adrenergic blockade, N. Engl. J. Med. **286**:617, 1972.

Chapter 19

Histamine

Histamine was one of the first vasoactive materials to be identified in mammals. It is of particular interest in pharmacology and medicine not because of its usefulness as a drug but because of its potent pharmacologic activities. This potent amine is widely distributed in tissues and has actions on many organ systems. For example, histamine is probably a central neurotransmitter, and it is important in gastric secretion. There is good evidence that histamine participates in inflammation and in anaphylaxis, allergies, and reactions to drugs. When histamine is released, it can elicit pathologic reactions that range in intensity from mild itching to shock and death.

Histamine was first synthesized in 1906 by Windaus. It was later found in ergot, the rye fungus, as a product of bacterial contamination. The pharmacologic properties of histamine were studied extensively by Sir Henry Dale, who noted striking similarities between anaphylaxis and the effects of histamine injection in several animal species, including man. Sir Thomas Lewis suggested that injury releases a histamine-like, or "H substance" that mediates evanescent cutaneous inflammation. Once the wide distribution of histamine was appreciated, numerous additional roles were attributed to it, often uncritically. Research in the 1950s revealed a close association between the distribution of tissue mast cells and histamine, and many investigations focused on mechanisms of histamine release from mast cells. It was soon realized, however, that there are also physiologically important non–mast cell pools of histamine, as well.

HISTAMINE RECEPTORS

Histamine acts on two separate and distinct receptors, termed H_1- and H_2-receptors (Table 19-1). Contraction of smooth muscle of the bronchi and intestine is mediated by H_1-receptors and is antagonized by drugs that were called "antihistamines."[2] These drugs are actually H_1-receptor blocking agents. In addition to the classical H_1-receptors, H_2-receptors mediate the action of histamine on gastric secretion and on cardiac acceleration.[4] Stimulation of these receptors is inhibited by the H_2-receptor antagonists cimetidine, ranitidine, and famotidine.

Both H_1- and H_2-receptors mediate vasodilator actions of histamine.[12] The H_1-receptors are generally more important, except for specific vascular beds. For example, vasodilatation of the temporal artery in humans appears to be mediated by H_2-receptors.

TABLE 19-1   Distribution of histamine receptors in the body

Histamine receptor	Tissue	Antagonist
H_1	Smooth muscle of intestine, bronchi, blood vessels	Classical antihistamines (diphenhydramine)
H_2	Gastric parietal cell	Cimetidine
	Smooth muscle of some blood vessels	Ranitidine
	Guinea pig atria	Metiamide
	Rat uterus	Burimamide

TISSUE DISTRIBUTION AND FORMATION

Histamine is found in almost all tissues of the body. In humans the highest concentrations are in the lungs, skin, and stomach (Table 19-2). In most organs the concentration of histamine is related to the number of mast cells, which are associated with loose connective tissue and are distributed along small blood vessels.

Another source of histamine is the basophil. This blood cell, which closely resembles mast cells, contains very high concentrations. Like the mast cell, the basophil may participate in allergic and inflammatory reactions.[11] The non–mast cell pool of histamine includes the gastric mucosa and small amounts in brain, heart, and other organs.[9] Histamine is also associated with neural elements. The neural pool differs from mast cell histamine in having a more rapid turnover rate and resistance to agents that release histamine from mast cells.

HISTIDINE DECARBOXYLASES

Chemically, histamine is 2-(4-imidazolyl)ethylamine.

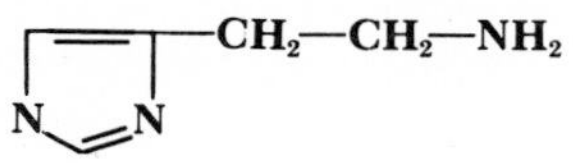

Histamine

Most of the histamine in tissues is formed by decarboxylation of the amino acid histidine. In man, synthesis of histamine is catalyzed by L-histidine decarboxylase. The enzyme aromatic L-amino acid decarboxylase, which acts on several different amino acid substrates, can also catalyze formation of histamine from histidine. Although this enzyme is more prevalent than L-histidine decarboxylase, it is less specific. Both enzymes require pyridoxal phosphate as a cofactor. Because histidine decarboxylase can be induced in some tissues, the enzyme may regulate blood flow within the microcirculation, or it may be involved in growth and repair of tissues.[7] Various foods contain histamine, and some intestinal bacteria can form it, but histamine from these sources is rapidly metabolized and is not stored in tissues.

TABLE 19-2 Histamine content of human tissues

Tissue	Histamine content
Lung	33 ± 10 µg/g*
Mucous membrane (nasal)	15.6 µg/g
Stomach	14 ± 4.0 µg/g*
Duodenum	14 ± 0.9 µg/g*
Skin	6.6 µg/g (abdomen) 30.4 µg/g (face)
Spleen	3.4 ± 0.97 µg/g*
Kidney	2.5 ± 1.2 µg/g*
Liver	2.2 ± 0.76 µg/g*
Heart	1.6 ± 0.07 µg/g*
Thyroid	1.0 ± 0.13 µg/g*
Skeletal muscle	0.97 ± 0.13 µg/g*
Central nervous tissue	0-0.2 µg/g
Plasma	2.6 µg/L
Basophils	1,080 µg/10^9 cells
Eosinophils	160 µg/10^9 cells
Neutrophils	3.0 µg/10^9 cells
Lymphocytes	0.6 µg/10^9 cells
Platelets	0.009 µg/10^9 platelets
Whole blood	16-89 µg/L

Based on data from Van Arsdel, P.P., Jr., and Beall, G.N.: Arch. Intern. Med. **106:**192, 1960.
*Mean ± Standard error.

Histamine is degraded through two main enzymatic pathways, with considerable species variation in their relative importance. In man, histamine is metabolized primarily to 1-methylhistamine by imidazole-*N*-methyltransferase. The methylated product is converted to 1-methylimidazole-4-acetic acid by monoamine oxidase. In the second pathway, histamine is oxidized by diamine oxidase to imidazole-4-acetic acid, much of which is conjugated with ribose and excreted as the riboside. These enzymatic pathways are shown in Fig. 19-1.

In addition to these metabolic products, some histamine is excreted as *N*-acetylhistamine. Acetylation occurs in bacteria in the intestine, and the acetylated product reflects metabolism of ingested histamine or histamine formed within the gut. It has been estimated that in a normal person 2 to 3 mg of histamine is released daily from tissues. Allergic or chemically induced release of histamine from mast cells or basophils greatly increases urinary excretion of histamine.

DEGRADATION OF HISTAMINE IN THE BODY

FIG. 19-1 *Known pathways of histamine metabolism. Relative importance of the different pathways in human males is indicated by figures at bottom, which are expressed as percent of the total ^{14}C excreted in the urine during 12 hours after intradermal injection of ^{14}C-histamine. Of the injected ^{14}C, 74% to 93% was excreted in 12 hours.*

From Nilsson, K., Lindell, S.-E., Schayer, R.W., and Westling, H.: Clin. Sci. **13**:313, 1959.

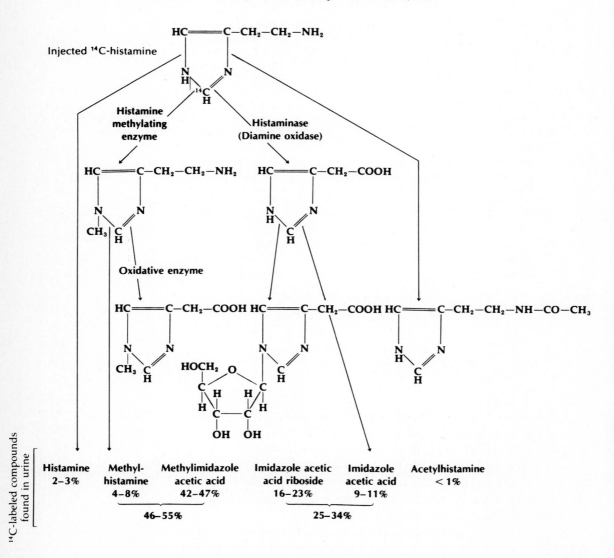

^{14}C-labeled compounds found in urine

Histamine	Methyl-histamine	Methylimidazole acetic acid	Imidazole acetic acid riboside	Imidazole acetic acid	Acetylhistamine
2–3%	4–8%	42–47%	16–23%	9–11%	<1%
	46–55%		25–34%		

Release of histamine and other mediators from mast cells is a prominent feature of immediate hypersensitivity reactions and also contributes to adverse effects of drugs and other chemical compounds. Histamine is concentrated within specific subcellular granules of the mast cell in association with a matrix of protein and heparin. Proteolytic enzymes and proinflammatory factors, such as eosinophil chemotactic factor, are also associated with mast cell granules.

BINDING AND RELEASE OF MAST CELL HISTAMINE

Histamine release involves at least two steps. First, a stimulus, such as antigen-IgE interaction, a drug, or a polypeptide, initiates extrusion of granular contents by exocytosis. In the second step, cations (sodium) from the extracellular environment displace cationic amines from anionic groups within the granular matrix and also displace cationic peptides, such as the eosinophil chemotactic factor. The appearance of granules within the mast cell is shown in Fig. 19-2.

Histamine is released from mast cells by various physical and chemical stimuli, including drugs and antigen-antibody reactions. Membrane stimulation evokes an influx of calcium, activation of membrane phospholipase, contraction of the cytostructure, and fusion of perigranular membranes in the process of exocytosis. Histamine release requires energy and is modulated by cyclic nucleotides. In addition, arachidonic acid metabolites may also regulate the release process.

Many early observations suggested that certain chemical compounds could release histamine within the body. Intracutaneous morphine injections in man produced localized erythema and edema. Curare alkaloids caused a similar response, and histamine was believed to cause episodes of bronchial constriction that accompanied intravenous injections of curare or polypeptide antibiotics, such as polymyxin.

Release by drugs and other chemicals

Many different chemical agents can release histamine from mast cells. These include certain large-molecule compounds, such as polysaccharides, lectins, and anaphylatoxins,[8] as well as small-molecule amines and a variety of organic bases, including some clinically useful drugs. The experimental histamine-releasing agent, compound 48/80 (Fig. 19-2), is a product of *p*-methoxyphenylethylmethylamine condensation with formaldehyde. This agent is a valuable tool for the study of histamine release from mast cells.

Histamine release can be caused by therapeutic administration of curare alkaloids, opioids such as morphine, and sometimes atropine, hydralazine, and sympathomimetic amines. Release, however, is significant only when these drugs are administered intravenously in fairly large doses.

Histamine release is clearly involved in the symptoms of anaphylactic shock in several species. In 1910 Dale and Laidlaw[5] observed that signs and symptoms elicited by histamine in experimental animals were very similar to the manifestations of anaphylactic shock. Similar reactions occur in man. The primary pathway for histamine release involves interaction of antigen with IgE bound to the mast cell surface. This reaction does not require complement, but it may be accentuated by concomitant

Release in anaphylaxis and allergy

FIG. 19-2 *Mast cells of rat mesentery 3 hours after intraperitoneal injection of compound 48/80.*

From Riley, J.F., and West, A.B.: J. Pathol. Bacteriol. **69:**269, 1955.

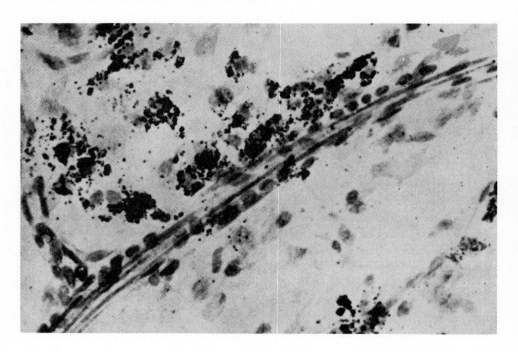

Compound 48/80

release of complement-derived peptides (anaphylatoxins), kinins, or other inflammatory mediators.

Histamine is a major mediator of acute allergic reactions in humans. Release of histamine from mast cells in the skin and mucosa can cause cutaneous and laryngeal edema, and bronchoconstriction and hypotension can occur if there is sufficient release into the systemic circulation.

Studies of histamine release from human leukocytes by ragweed extract[10] indicate that cyclic AMP and drugs that activate adenylate cyclase can inhibit release.

Similar studies on mast cells from human lungs support the concept of control by cyclic nucleotides. Catecholamines and theophylline, drugs widely used in allergic diseases, are believed to inhibit histamine release in addition to antagonizing many of its actions. Disodium cromoglycate (see Chapter 40) inhibits histamine release and also the release of SRS-A (see p. 204) by a mechanism independent of cyclic nucleotides.

Once liberated, histamine has potent actions on smooth muscles, blood vessels, and secretory glands. Histamine taken by mouth has no effect because it is rapidly metabolized by bacteria in the gastrointestinal tract, by the gastrointestinal mucosa, and by the liver.

If injected intravenously, however, as little as 0.1 mg of histamine causes systemic vasodilatation with a rapid fall in blood pressure, reflex acceleration of heart rate, elevation of cerebrospinal fluid pressure, flushing of the face, and headache. Gastric acid secretion is stimulated severalfold. These effects last only a few minutes.

PHARMACOLOGIC EFFECTS

There are both H_1- and H_2-receptors in the heart, but their distribution varies greatly with species, and their physiologic significance remains obscure. Histamine activates adenylate cyclase in the human heart, but this effect is not blocked by propranolol, in contrast to the activation by catecholamines. The autacoid increases the rate and force of contraction of the heart in several species.[13] In vivo most effects are probably mediated indirectly through changes in vasomotor tone.

The two major factors involved in the circulatory effects of histamine are arteriolar dilatation and increased capillary permeability. These factors act in concert to promote loss of plasma from the circulation and development of tissue edema.

Injection of very low concentrations of histamine intracutaneously in humans provides a striking demonstration of the action of histamine on capillaries. As little as 10 μg produces the "triple response of Lewis": localized erythema at the injection site, localized edema (or wheal), and diffuse erythema (or flare) at some distance from the injection site. The localized erythema and wheal are the consequences of vasodilatation and increased capillary permeability. The flare involves neural mechanisms, possibly a reflex vasodilatation, since it is prevented if the appropriate sensory nerves are cut. These phenomena are inhibited by antihistaminic drugs of the H_1 class.

Circulatory effects

Histamine also affects smooth muscle in many nonvascular structures. Its action on bronchiolar smooth muscle is the most important clinically. Humans and guinea pigs are particularly susceptible to its bronchoconstrictor action. Persons with a history of asthma may respond with an acute attack to a dose of histamine that would cause only a minor decrease in vital capacity in a normal person. Asthmatic persons are highly susceptible not only to histamine but also to methacholine, leukotrienes, and many airway irritants.

The limited benefit of antihistaminic therapy for asthmatic patients suggested

Other smooth muscle effects

that other mediators are involved. Slow-reacting substance of anaphylaxis (SRS-A) was found to be released along with histamine from IgE-sensitized fragments of human lung. This potent stimulant of human bronchial smooth muscle is actually a family of acidic lipids formed from arachidonic acid by the enzyme lipoxygenase (see Chapter 22). Leukotrienes C_4 and D_4, now known to be constituents of SRS-A, are believed to be the primary mediators of the bronchoconstrictive response in asthmatics. There is additional evidence that prostaglandin D_2, formed in mast cells during the histamine-release reaction, is also a potent bronchoconstrictor.[6]

Effect on secretions

Histamine is a potent stimulant of gastric acid and pepsin secretion. Subcutaneous injection of as little as 25 μg of the compound in humans will increase gastric secretion without causing other effects. This response is used as a test for complete achlorhydria, the lack of gastric hydrochloric acid production. Histamine-resistant achlorhydria has diagnostic importance in conditions such as pernicious anemia.

The concentration of histamine is particularly high in the acid-secreting part of the stomach. Histamine is believed to be localized both in mast cells in the submucosa and in mast cell–like cells in the lamina propria. Stimuli such as carbachol, gastrin, or food release histamine, primarily from the cells in the lamina propria, which can then stimulate secretion from parietal cells.

Histamine stimulates gastric secretion through H_2-receptors on parietal cells. The secretory response is accompanied by activation of adenylate cyclase. The precise relationship of histamine to the stimulus for gastric secretion is still being investigated. The polypeptide gastrin, an extremely potent stimulant of gastric acid secretion, is about 500 times more potent than histamine. Its effect is also inhibited by H_2-antagonists, an inhibition suggestive of a functional relationship between gastrin and histamine. A similar finding for cholinergic stimulation of gastric secretion further indicates that histamine may be the final common mediator of secretion.

Histamine stimulates the secretory activities of many other glandular cells to a slight extent. An increase in salivary and bronchial secretions by histamine can be demonstrated under experimental conditions, but these effects are not physiologically important.

ROLE IN HEALTH AND DISEASE

Physiologic roles for histamine in addition to gastric secretion are not yet firmly established, but several seem likely. Histamine is probably a neurotransmitter in the central nervous system. There are receptors for this amine in the brain as well as enzymes for its synthesis and inactivation. Histamine can stimulate autonomic ganglia, and it releases catecholamines from the adrenal medulla.

The large amount of histamine in mast cells, which are in intimate contact with blood vessels, is suggestive of a more general role than the production of allergic reactions. It has been proposed that certain types of vascular headaches are caused by histamine. Support for histamine as a mediator in migraine is provided by observations that injected histamine can reproduce symptoms of migraine and that repeated administration produces a certain amount of "desensitization" and symptomatic improvement.

Histamine has a firmly established place among mediators of inflammation, but it was only recently recognized that this amine also modifies immune and inflammatory responses. For example, histamine limits its own release from basophils and mast cells, inhibits chemotaxis of basophils and neutrophils, and reduces secretion of enzymes and oxidants from neutrophils. In addition, it inhibits lymphokine production and proliferation in T-lymphocytes. These phenomena are believed to be linked to elevation of cyclic AMP through interaction with H_2-receptors.[3]

Histamine also stimulates release of arachidonic acid in various types of cells; this effect is mediated through H_1-receptors.[1] Thus histamine released in an area of inflammation may also modify a local inflammatory response by generating prostaglandins or leukotrienes (see Chapter 22).

REFERENCES

1. Alhenc-Gelas, F., Tsai, S.J., Callahan, K.S., et al.: Stimulation of prostaglandin formation by vasoactive mediators in cultured human endothelial cells, Prostaglandins 24:723, 1982.
2. Beaven, M.A.: Histamine, N. Engl. J. Med. 294:30, 1976.
3. Beer, D.J., Matloff, S.M., and Rocklin, R.E.: The influence of histamine on immune and inflammatory responses, Adv. Immunol. 35:209, 1984.
4. Black, J.W., Duncan, W.A.M., Durant, C.J., et al.: Definition and antagonism of histamine H_2-receptors, Nature 236:385, 1972.
5. Dale, H.H., and Laidlaw, P.P.: The physiological action of β-iminazolylethylamine, J. Physiol. (Lond.) 41:318, 1910.
6. Hardy, C.C., Robinson, C., Tattersfield, A.E., and Holgate, S.T.: The bronchoconstrictor effect of inhaled prostaglandin D_2 in normal and asthmatic men, N. Engl. J. Med. 311:209, 1984.
7. Kahlson, G., and Rosengren, E.: Histamine: entering physiology, Experientia 28:993, 1972.
8. Lagunoff, D., Martin, T.W., and Read, G.: Agents that release histamine from mast cells, Annu. Rev. Pharmacol. Toxicol. 23:331, 1983.
9. Levine, R.J., Sato, T.L., and Sjoerdsma, A.: Inhibition of histamine synthesis in the rat by α-hydrazino analog of histidine and 4-bromo-3-hydroxy benzyloxyamine, Biochem. Pharmacol. 14:139, 1965.
10. Lichtenstein, L.M., and Margolis, S.: Histamine release in vitro: inhibition by catecholamines and methylxanthines, Science 161:902, 1968.
11. Osler, A.G., Lichtenstein, L.M., and Levy, D.A.: *In vitro* studies of human reaginic allergy, Adv. Immunol. 8:183, 1968.
12. Powell, J.R., and Brody, M.J.: Participation of H_1 and H_2 histamine receptors in physiological vasodilator responses, Am. J. Physiol. 231:1002, 1976.
13. Verma, S.C., and McNeill, J.H.: Cardiac histamine receptors and cyclic AMP, Life Sci. 19:1797, 1976.

Chapter 20

Antihistaminic drugs

Drugs that competitively block the actions of histamine at specific receptor sites are referred to as antihistaminic drugs. The effects of histamine on bronchial and intestinal smooth muscles can be prevented by the classical antihistamines, the H_1-receptor antagonists. However, the effects of histamine on gastric secretion are not blocked by these drugs. The gastric secretory effects and some vascular and other cellular responses are prevented by H_2-receptor antagonists.

Diphenhydramine and tripelennamine, the first H_1-antihistamines, were introduced many years ago in response to the discovery that histamine causes some of the effects of allergy and inflammation. Certain phenolic ethers were found to protect guinea pigs against both anaphylactic shock and exposure to histamine aerosols. It appeared that these antagonists would be useful both as therapeutic agents and as research tools. Thus the drugs were developed with specific goals in mind. It was not until many years later, when it was clear that the classical antagonists did not block all actions of histamine, that H_2-antagonists were developed.

The H_1-antihistamines are useful not only in allergic diseases but also for prevention of motion sickness. Selected compounds are also useful in parkinsonism. The sedative action of H_1-antihistamines is utilized in many over-the-counter hypnotic preparations. The H_2-antihistamines cimetidine, ranitidine, and famotidine are widely used to treat acid-peptic diseases.[2]

HISTAMINE
H_1-RECEPTOR
ANTAGONISTS
Chemistry

The basic structure of these antihistamines may be represented by a substituted ethylamine:

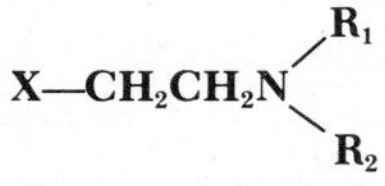

$$X-CH_2CH_2N\begin{matrix} R_1 \\ R_2 \end{matrix}$$

Since histamine is 2-(4-imidazolyl) ethylamine, it is likely that the ethylamine portion of histamine and the H_1-receptor antagonists is essential for interaction with the H_1-receptor. The R groups in the ethylamine structure are usually CH_3. If the X in the basic structure is nitrogen, the compound is a substituted ethylenediamine. Structural formulas of several H_1-receptor antagonists are shown on the next page.

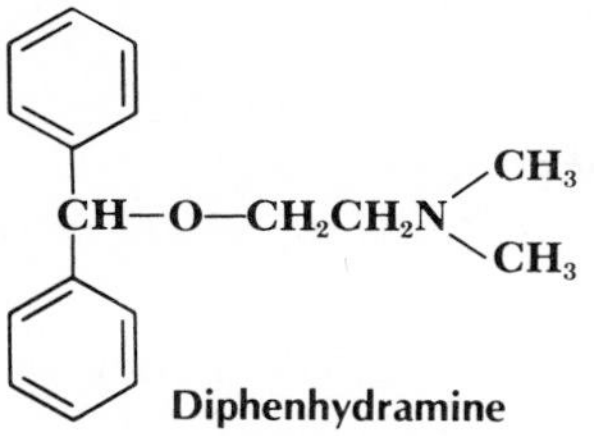

Diphenhydramine

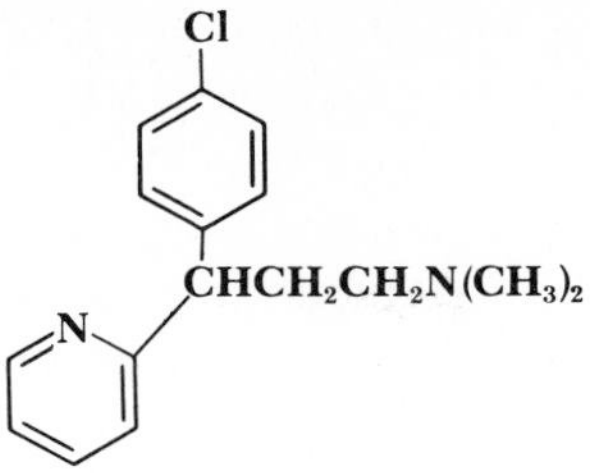

Chlorpheniramine

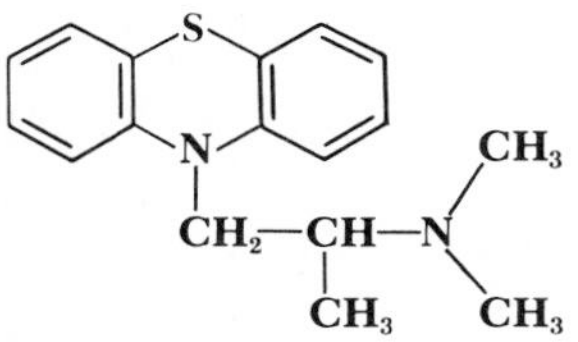

Promethazine

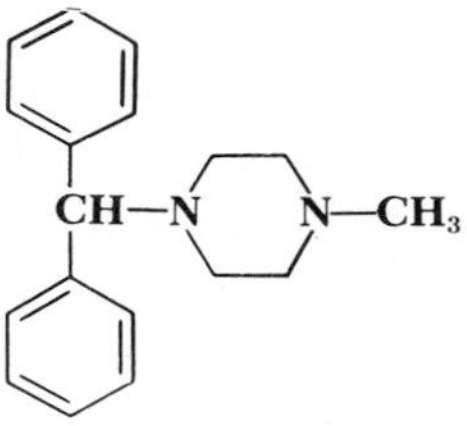

Cyclizine

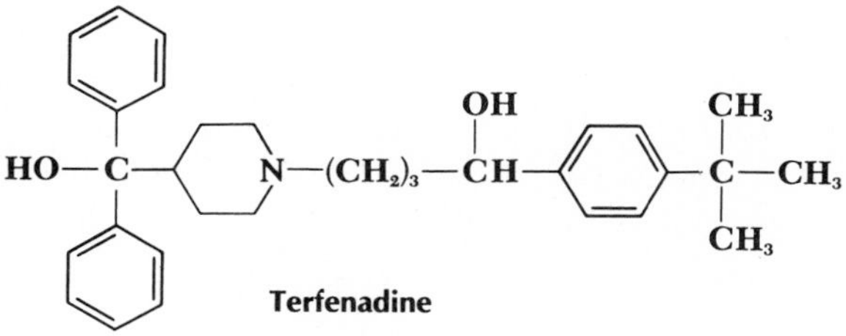

Terfenadine

All H_1-antihistamines are competitive antagonists; that is, they cause a parallel shift to the right of the log dose-response curve for a given histamine effect with no change in the maximal effect. None of the antihistamines in therapeutic doses affect metabolism of histamine, nor do they block its release.

Many H_1-antihistamines are marketed today. The variety of chemical structures indicates attempts to manufacture more selective drugs. Unfortunately, almost all H_1-receptor blocking drugs cause additional effects, such as sedation.

Clinical pharmacology

Therapeutic doses of common H_1-antagonists in a normal person often cause drowsiness, and other sedatives such as barbiturates or alcohol are at least additive; however, there is no relationship between the antihistaminic potency of these drugs and their central depressant action. If antihistamines are taken in excessive doses, sedation may be replaced by central nervous system stimulation manifested by irritability, convulsions, hyperthermia, and even death. These and other adverse central nervous system effects are probably related to an anticholinergic action. Not all H$_1$-antihistamines have the same central nervous system activity. Chlorpheniramine produces less sedation than diphenhydramine for an equivalent antihistaminic action. One recently marketed drug, *terfenadine*, appears promising for prevention of allergic rhinitis without impairment of the sensorium.[6] Another antihistamine, *phenindamine*, is unusual because it causes central nervous system stimulation in some persons, even at therapeutic doses.

Other properties attributed to H$_1$-antagonists include anti–motion sickness, anticholinergic, and local anesthetic activities. The *anticholinergic action* manifests itself primarily as drying of salivary and bronchial secretions. For this reason antihistaminic drugs may have an adverse effect in asthma; they can increase the viscosity of secretions in the respiratory tract. The anticholinergic action of antihistamines may also account for their usefulness in prevention of motion sickness. Dimenhydrinate, a widely used combination of diphenhydramine with 8-chlorotheophylline, owes its anti–motion sickness properties to the former component.

The prominence of the various actions depends, in part, on structure. For example, ethanolamines, such as diphenhydramine, have significant anticholinergic as well as sedative actions. Piperazines, such as cyclizine, are less sedative but are very effective in preventing motion sickness. Pyrilamine, an ethylenediamine, has a strong local anesthetic action. Alkylamines, such as chlorpheniramine, are the most potent anti-H$_1$ compounds, but they are also sedative, even at therapeutic doses.

The recognition of two distinct receptors for histamine and the development of H$_2$-receptor antagonists helped to explain many puzzling aspects of the pharmacologic properties of antihistamines. Gastric secretion is mediated by H$_2$-receptors and is not blocked by H$_1$-receptor antagonists.[1] Vasodilatation and increased capillary permeability are mediated by both receptor types and thus can be blocked completely only by a combination of H$_1$- and H$_2$-receptor antagonists.[1]

Therapeutic uses There are many conditions in which H$_1$-antihistamines are helpful. There are others in which they are used but perhaps should not be. Antihistaminic therapy may relieve or prevent allergic rhinitis, urticaria, insect envenomation, some types of asthma (of allergic origin), and motion sickness. Antihistamines alone are of little or no benefit in acute anaphylactic emergencies, in most types of asthma, in inflammatory disorders of the skin, eyes, and nose, and in the common cold. They are administered with epinephrine, however, to treat anaphylactic reactions, and they may be combined with other therapeutic modalities for reactions of the skin or airways in which there is clearly an allergic component.[5]

Selection of an antihistamine is usually based upon its other effects. The degree of sedation is a major consideration. Potency is of little importance, since it influences only the size of the tablets used. The duration of action of most antihistamines in therapeutic doses is about 4 hours. The usual adult dose and sedative activity of several antihistamines are indicated in Table 20-1.

TABLE 20-1	Doses and sedative property of various H_1-antihistamines		
Drug	Trade name	Usual adult dose (mg)	Degree of sedation
Phenindamine	Nolahist	25	+ *
Terfenadine	Seldane	60	±
Brompheniramine	Dimetane, others	4-8	+
Chlorpheniramine	Chlor-Trimeton, others	4	+
Cyproheptadine	Periactin	4	+
Dexchlorpheniramine	Polaramine, others	2	+
Diphenylpyraline	Hispril	5	+
Methdilazine	Tacaryl	8	+
Triprolidine	Actidil	2.5	+
Azatadine	Optimine	1-2	+ +
Clemastine	Tavist	1.34	+ +
Pyrilamine		25-50	+ +
Trimeprazine	Temaril	2.5	+ +
Tripelennamine	PBZ	25-50	+ +
Diphenhydramine	Benadryl, others	25-50	+ + +
Promethazine	Phenergan, others	12.5-25	+ + +

*Stimulation possible.

The H_1-receptor antagonists are absorbed rapidly and completely from the gastrointestinal tract. The onset of action is usually within 30 minutes, and absorption is complete in 4 hours. When diphenhydramine is administered orally, peak blood concentrations are achieved in 1 hour and are negligible by 6 hours. The H_1-receptor antagonists are metabolized in the liver by hydroxylation.

Absorption and metabolism

Antihistamines have a wide margin of safety, and several times the recommended dosage can be absorbed without danger of respiratory depression. Their widespread use, however, may contribute to automobile and other accidents because of their sedative activity, especially if combined with depressant drugs such as barbiturates, benzodiazepines, or alcohol.

Toxicity

Acute poisoning has occurred after ingestion of very large doses of antihistamines. The symptoms resemble those of atropine intoxication, including central nervous system excitation and convulsions. The management of acute poisoning is supportive.

Topical application of antihistamines was used in the past to obtain symptomatic relief from acute cutaneous allergic reactions. The local anesthetic action of some compounds was likely helpful, as well as the receptor-blocking action. Unfortunately, even though the antihistamines relieved some itching conditions, contact dermatitis often developed. This reaction was attributed to sensitization of the patient to the topically applied antihistamines. Currently, this route is seldom used.

Some antihistamines that were originally used to prevent motion sickness were later shown to be teratogenic in laboratory animals. For this reason meclizine (Antivert, Bonine) and cyclizine (Marezine) should not be given to pregnant women, and nonproprietary preparations that contain these agents must bear a warning to that effect. The teratogenic effect is not related to antihistaminic activity but seems to be related to the piperazine moiety.

Antihistamines with an antiserotonin action	Some antihistaminic drugs also block serotonin receptors. Promethazine has a potent antiserotonin action on isolated smooth muscle, but a related compound, the antipsychotic drug chlorpromazine, is only about half as active. Cyproheptadine is a potent antiserotonin drug as well. There is no reason to believe, however, that this activity offers any advantage over compounds that block only histamine receptors.

HISTAMINE H₂-RECEPTOR ANTAGONISTS	In 1972 Black and co-workers described the first agent, burimamide, that competitively antagonized the action of histamine on gastric parietal cells, guinea pig atria, and rat uteri.[1] These receptors were called H_2-receptors. The search for H_2-receptor blocking drugs was extensive, and more than 700 compounds were synthesized before burimamide was obtained. The realization that histamine stimulation of gastric acid and pepsin secretion might be involved in peptic ulcer disease led to the search for other compounds to block H_2-receptors. Further studies led to synthesis of metiamide, which was better absorbed from the gastrointestinal tract than burimamide. Unfortunately, after extensive clinical use, several patients treated with metiamide developed agranulocytosis, and the drug was withdrawn. Cimetidine, in which the thiourea in the side chain was changed to cyanoguanidine, was the next drug to be developed. Ranitidine and famotidine, closely related compounds, were introduced more recently.

Differences between H₁- and H₂-antihistamines	In addition to acting on different receptors, these two groups of drugs differ substantially in their chemistry, pharmacokinetics, and clinical uses. They differ from histamine in that the imidazole ring structure in the H_1-antihistamines is modified or replaced by other substituents. In the H_2-antagonists it is the side chain that is extensively modified.

Cimetidine

Ranitidine

$$CH_2S-(CH_2)_2-C-NH_2$$

Famotidine

In contrast to H_1-receptor antagonists, H_2-antihistamines are generally less lipid soluble. At therapeutic doses, they do not have prominent actions on the central nervous system or other organ systems and do not exhibit anticholinergic or local anesthetic activities. Thus, in comparison with H_1-receptor blocking drugs, the H_2-antagonists are far more selective for their histamine receptor.

The H_2-receptor antagonists inhibit gastric secretion caused by histamine, gastrin, and acetylcholine as well as by food.[7] There are several possible explanations for this apparent lack of specificity. Histamine may be the final mediator for the other stimuli. Alternatively, there could be separate receptors on the parietal cell for histamine, gastrin, and acetylcholine, linked so that blockade of the histamine receptor interferes with the activity of the others. Thus histamine may have a "permissive" effect on the actions of the other stimuli.

Mechanism of inhibition of gastric secretion

The H_2-antagonists have had a tremendous impact on the management of peptic ulcer disease. Cimetidine (Tagamet) reduces diurnal gastric acid secretion.[2] After 6 weeks of treatment with cimetidine, most ulcer patients are cured as compared with members of a placebo group. When the drug is administered in a dose of 200 or 300 mg four times a day (with meals and at bedtime), basal and food- or gastrin-stimulated gastric secretion is inhibited. A 300 mg dose of cimetidine at bedtime significantly reduces gastric acidity for at least 8 hours. Recent data indicate that 600 mg twice a day is also an adequate dosage, and in many patients a single 800 mg dose at bedtime may be sufficient. The newer drugs ranitidine and famotidine can be given in lower doses and less frequently. Cimetidine can be administered as tablets, 200 to 800 mg, or as the hydrochloride as a liquid, 300 mg in 5 ml, or by injection, 300 mg/2 ml.

Cimetidine

Cimetidine is well absorbed when taken orally, has a plasma half-life of 2 hours, and is excreted in the urine, 70% unchanged. Hence renal insufficiency impairs its elimination and requires dosage modification.

Approved indications for H_2-receptor antagonists include (1) hypersecretory states such as Zollinger-Ellison syndrome and mastocytosis, (2) short-term treatment of

CLINICAL PHARMACOLOGY, INDICATIONS, AND TOXICITY

active duodenal ulcer or benign gastric ulcer, which tends to be somewhat less responsive, and (3) prolonged therapy to prevent recurrence of duodenal ulcer. These agents are used widely in intensive care units to prevent "stress"-induced ulceration. Investigational uses include reflux esophagitis, pancreatic insufficiency, and upper gastrointestinal hemorrhage.

Cimetidine has been used by millions of patients for over 10 years. Serious adverse effects are unusual. Cimetidine has caused renal and hepatic damage in dogs, but the doses required were many times those necessary to suppress gastric acid secretion. As wide use of cimetidine continued, other adverse effects, such as dizziness, confusion (usually in elderly patients), leukopenia, rashes, or myalgias, were reported. In addition, a mild antiandrogenic action results in breast enlargement (gynecomastia) and tenderness in some persons. Impotence has also been reported, presumably caused by the same mechanism. Drug interactions are the primary limitation of cimetidine therapy. Cimetidine can decrease the metabolism of many other drugs (see Table 63-3). Those that may require a reduction in dosage when cimetidine is added include warfarin, phenytoin, and benzodiazepines. The dosage of propranolol, labetalol, and metoprolol should be reduced when cimetidine is added to treatment regimens since the H_2-receptor blocker reduces both the presystemic metabolism and systemic clearance of these drugs.

Ranitidine

Ranitidine is very similar to cimetidine in its actions and indications. It is more potent than cimetidine and has a longer duration of action so that twice daily dosage is sufficient. Single bedtime doses (300 mg) are also effective in most patients. Ranitidine is believed to cause fewer side effects than cimetidine, but it has not been so widely used. Early experience indicates that ranitidine does not consistently inhibit hepatic drug–metabolizing microsomal enzymes. As a consequence, the action of warfarin and other drugs is not prolonged. Ranitidine also probably does not inhibit the androgen receptor at usual doses.

Ranitidine hydrochloride (Zantac) is available in tablets, 150 and 300 mg, and in solution for injection, 25 mg/ml.

Famotidine

Famotidine (Pepcid) is a new, potent, long-acting H_2-receptor antagonist[4] containing a thiol ring that distinguishes it from the imidazole and furan structures of cimetidine and ranitidine. It is reported to be up to 100 times more potent than cimetidine and three times more potent than ranitidine, and it has a longer duration of action than either of these other antagonists.[3]

1. Black, J.W., Duncan, W.A.M., Durant, C.J., et al.: Definition and antagonism of histamine H_2-receptors, Nature **236**:385, 1972.

2. Bodemar, G., and Walan, A.: Cimetidine in the treatment of active duodenal and prepyloric ulcers, Lancet **2**:161, 1976.

3. Dammann, H.-G., Müller, P., and Simon, B.: 24 Hour intragastric acidity and single night-time dose of three H_2-blockers, Lancet **2**:1078, 1983.

4. Famotidine (Pepcid), Med. Lett. Drugs Ther. **29**:17, 1987.

5. Popa, V.: The classic antihistamines (H_1 blockers) in respiratory medicine, Clin. Chest Med. **7**:367, 1986.

6. Sorkin, E.M., and Heel, R.C.: Terfenadine: a review of its pharmacodynamic properties and therapeutic efficacy, Drugs **29**:34, 1985.

7. Schlippert, W.: Cimetidine: H_2-receptor blockade in gastrointestinal disease, Arch. Intern. Med. **138**:1257, 1978.

REFERENCES

Chapter 21

Serotonin, kinins, and miscellaneous autacoids

Many diverse, biologically active substances are formed, stored, and released within normal tissues. The agents are not hormones in the strict sense because they usually act at or very close to the site where they are generated. The collective term *autacoid*, or self-medicinal agent, is currently applied to these substances of disparate structure and function.[4] Autacoids include amines, such as histamine and serotonin, the polypeptide kinins, angiotensins, substance P, and VIP (vasoactive intestinal polypeptide). Some newly recognized immune mediators, such as the interleukins, are also considered autacoids. Prostaglandins and leukotrienes could likewise be classified as autacoids; they are discussed in the following chapter. The pharmacology of histamine is discussed in detail in Chapter 19, and angiotensins are discussed in Chapter 18.

SEROTONIN

Serotonin (5-hydroxytryptamine) occupies a prominent position in the medical literature, despite the ignorance that still surrounds its functions in the body. This endogenously produced amine is believed to be a central neurotransmitter, and it appears to have local (or autacoid) actions in various tissues. Serotonin has been implicated in various disease states ranging from mental disease to migraine, but its role in such conditions is still not established.

Studies of serotonin in the central nervous system have helped in understanding the biochemical basis of psychopharmacologic phenomena. Receptor relationships between serotonin and hallucinogens, such as lysergide (lysergic acid diethylamide, LSD), suggested that abnormalities in brain serotonin may cause abnormal brain function and aberrant behavior. The discovery that serotonin stores are depleted by reserpine focused additional attention on the role of this amine in the central nervous system.

Occurrence and distribution

Serotonin is widely distributed in the animal and plant kingdoms. It is found in various insect venoms and contributes to the inflammatory reaction to stings. Some fruits, such as bananas and pineapples, contain high concentrations of serotonin, but usually very little is absorbed from the gastrointestinal tract, and excretion of serotonin metabolites is normally very low. Enhanced concentrations of metabolites are used diagnostically as evidence for carcinoid tumor. This tumor is composed of *enterochromaffin* cells, and it can release large amounts of serotonin and other mediators.[14]

Approximately 90% of the total serotonin in mammalian tissues is in enterochromaffin cells in the intestine, about 8% is in platelets, and the remaining 2% is in the central nervous system, primarily in the pineal gland and the hypothalamus. In some animal species serotonin is also in granules of mast cells. Human mast cells probably do not contain serotonin, since mastocytosis is not associated with increased urinary excretion of 5-hydroxyindoleacetic acid (5-HIAA), the major serotonin metabolite.

Serotonin is synthesized in neurons and enterochromaffin cells by hydroxylation and decarboxylation of the amino acid tryptophan. Normally only a small fraction of dietary tryptophan is converted to serotonin. However, this fraction increases greatly in patients with carcinoid tumors. Platelets do not synthesize the amine, but they actively concentrate it in granules that are released during platelet aggregation. The mechanisms of storage and release appear similar to those for catecholamines, and drugs that affect catecholamine storage also affect the disposition of serotonin. There is rapid turnover of serotonin within neurons of the central nervous system and in the enterochromaffin cells of the intestine. In contrast, the amine stored in platelets has a very slow turnover rate. Most of the serotonin released into blood is metabolized by monoamine oxidase (MAO) in the liver; the lung is also an active site for metabolism. In addition, serotonin is converted in the pineal gland to *N*-acetylserotonin and its O-methylated derivative *melatonin*. Serotonin that escapes metabolism in these organs is taken up by platelets.[3] The steps in the biosynthesis and degradation of serotonin are shown below:

Biosynthesis and metabolism

Tryptophan → 5-Hydroxytryptophan → 5-Hydroxytryptamine → 5-Hydroxyindoleacetic acid

Tryptophan

5-Hydroxytryptophan

5-Hydroxytryptamine (serotonin)

5-Hydroxyindoleacetic acid (5-HIAA)

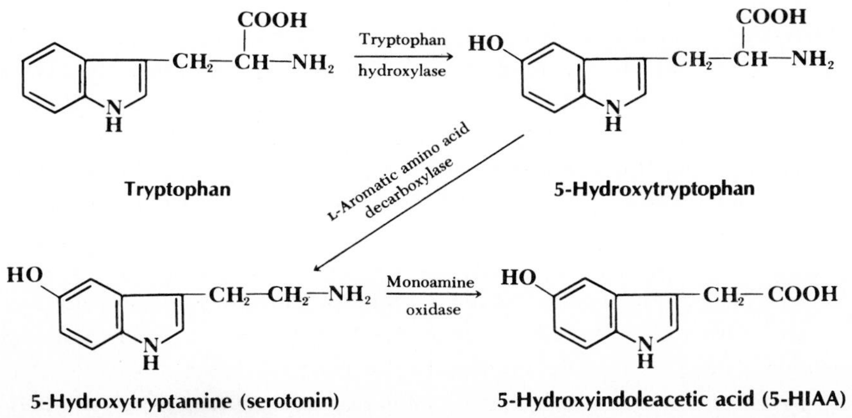

Several centrally acting drugs affect concentrations of free serotonin within the brain. The biosynthesis of serotonin is blocked by *p*-chlorophenylalanine, which inhibits tryptophan hydroxylase, the rate-limiting synthetic enzyme. Degradation of serotonin is blocked by MAO inhibitors, which can double the serotonin content of brain in less than 1 hour. Certain tricyclic antidepressants prevent membrane uptake and increase the amount of free synaptic serotonin within the central nervous system.

The daily excretion of 5-HIAA in the urine is from 3 to 10 mg in a normal adult. Excretion of this metabolite increases when there is endogenous production by a carcinoid tumor or after administration of drugs that inhibit granule uptake and storage. Excretion is decreased by MAO inhibitors.

Pharmacologic *effects*	The major actions of serotonin are on smooth muscle and nerve elements, including afferent nerve endings. The smooth muscle effects are most prominent in the cardiovascular system and in the gastrointestinal tract.

The actions on the cardiovascular system are complex. The effects include venoconstriction, arteriolar dilatation, contraction of isolated arterial and venous smooth muscle, and inhibition of peripheral adrenergic neurotransmission.[22] Effects of serotonin released within an isolated vascular bed may differ from those caused in vivo after injection of the amine. Intravenous injection of a few micrograms of serotonin typically causes a *triphasic* change in blood pressure: (1) a transient decrease, (2) a period of hypertension that lasts several minutes, and (3) a prolonged period of lowered pressure. The early depressor phase is probably attributable to reflex stimulation of chemoreceptors within the coronary arteries (Bezold-Jarisch reflex). The hypertensive phase is attributed to direct constriction of blood vessels in many regions, including splanchnic and renal vascular beds. The final depressor phase is attributed to vasodilatation of vessels in specific vascular beds, as in skeletal muscle. Continuous infusion of serotonin causes a prolonged reduction of peripheral resistance and blood pressure.

Serotonin stimulates gastrointestinal and bronchial smooth muscles. The gastrointestinal actions include both direct stimulation of intestinal muscle and indirect stimulation through excitation of ganglion cells within the intestinal wall. The action of serotonin on intestinal motility is blocked by serotonin antagonists. Elevation of the serotonin in circulation occurs after food or pentagastrin stimulation in both normal persons and those with carcinoid syndrome. The significance of this phenomenon is not known.[15] The bronchial stimulant action of serotonin is probably of little physiologic importance in humans, but asthmatic persons are particularly sensitive to this autacoid.

Serotonin can stimulate afferent nerve endings, ganglion cells, and adrenal medullary cells. Although it is a central neurotransmitter, serotonin does not cross the blood-brain barrier. Injection into the lateral cerebral ventricles of experimental animals causes many neurologic effects, including induction of sleep and disruption of temperature regulation.[10] A serotonin antagonist, quipazine, delays onset of rapid eye movement (REM) sleep in rats; this finding indicates that serotonin may also regulate neuronal activity during sleep.[6]

The participation of serotonin in determination of mood and behavior would be anticipated from its role as a central neurotransmitter. Changes in serotonin concentrations within the brain are believed to occur in various mental disorders, such as depression, but the mechanisms are still not established. In both the brain and the gastrointestinal tract, serotonin is found in cells that secrete polypeptides. Serotonin is believed to regulate release of peptide hormones within the anterior pituitary by an action on hypothalamic neuroendocrine pathways. It might influence intestinal motility, as well, through release of peptide hormones. Serotonin in enterochromaffin cells of the intestine is released by the mechanical stimulus of distention or by hypertonicity, but its relationship to gastrointestinal polypeptide hormones is still unclear.

Role in health and disease

Serotonin release probably causes some of the symptoms of the carcinoid syndrome, such as increased intestinal motility. However, catecholamines or kinins are the likely cause of the vascular phenomenon (flushing) that occurs with this condition.

Because serotonin is a potent constrictor of cerebral vessels, it has been implicated in migraine headaches. Although some serotonin antagonists may prevent migraine, there is no direct evidence that serotonin is a causal agent. The release of serotonin from aggregating platelets has suggested a role in coronary or cerebral ischemia. In addition, there is evidence from models of chronic hypertension that serotonin alters the responsiveness of blood vessels to vasoactive mediators.[21]

Drugs that compete with serotonin for tissue receptors have helped to define the actions of the amine in normal and pathologic conditions. Only a few have therapeutic use. The earliest recognized compounds include ergot alkaloids and derivatives of lysergic acid. Some antihistaminic compounds also block serotonin receptors on smooth muscles. Although many serotonin antagonists are relatively nonselective, they have aided in definition of two subclasses of serotonin receptors (5-HT$_1$ and 5-HT$_2$) in the central nervous system. In the periphery 5-HT$_2$-receptors appear to be associated with effects such as smooth muscle contraction.

SEROTONIN ANTAGONISTS

Methysergide, a congener of methylergonovine and LSD, is a potent antagonist of serotonin in various experimental preparations. It has been used to prevent migraine headache with some degree of success, but it is not effective in treatment of established migraine.

Individual agents

Methysergide

Methysergide may cause various adverse reactions, including nausea, dizziness, insomnia, and behavioral changes. A serious but infrequent complication after long-term use is development of an inflammatory fibrosis that may affect the lungs or other organs.

Methysergide maleate (Sansert) is available in tablets containing 2 mg.

Cyproheptadine is an antihistamine that also blocks serotonin receptors. It is structurally similar to the phenothiazine type of H_1-antagonists. Cyproheptadine has been used to relieve itching in a variety of skin disorders, and it is effective against the intestinal hypermotility of carcinoid syndrome. Adverse effects are similar to those of other antihistamines; drowsiness is the most prominent. In addition, cyproheptadine is reported to cause weight gain and increased growth in children, possibly by an effect on growth hormone secretion.

Preparations of cyproheptadine hydrochloride (Periactin) include tablets, 4 mg, and syrup, 2 mg/5 ml.

Ketanserin is a newly developed serotonin antagonist that appears to be selective for $5\text{-}HT_2$-receptors. It is of great interest for experimental studies and may have therapeutic application as an antihypertensive because of its vasodilator action.

The **ergot alkaloids** are products of fungi that grow on grains, particularly rye. This group includes several compounds that have partial agonist actions on adrenergic, dopaminergic, and serotonin receptors. They cause three major effects: (1) smooth muscle contraction, which is particularly evident on blood vessels and the uterus, (2) α-adrenergic blockade, and (3) various adverse central nervous system responses, including nausea, headache, dizziness, confusion, and even dementia. Although some ergot compounds affect serotonin receptors, their therapeutic effects are not obviously linked to serotonergic mechanisms.

The role of ergot in medicine has a long history. It was known for centuries that ingestion of grains contaminated with fungus caused a unique type of poisoning, characterized by abortions, a variety of central nervous system effects, and the development of gangrene. The subsequent isolation of *ergotamine* and *ergonovine* provided compounds that were used to stimulate uterine contractions and to inhibit α-adrenergic receptor–mediated vascular constriction. The ergot derivative LSD proved valuable for exploring the effects of serotonin within the central nervous system.

Lysergic acid

Ergonovine

Ergot alkaloids are no longer used to stimulate uterine contraction, and the centrally acting derivatives are primarily research tools, though they have limited application in the treatment of vascular headaches. Ergotamine is used in the diagnosis and initial treatment of migraine headache. It is believed that its vasoconstrictor action reduces the pain caused by dilatation and pulsation of cerebral arteries. Ergotamine is not indicated for long-term treatment or prevention of migraine because severe constriction of peripheral vessels and even gangrene can result from continued use.

The synthetic peptide-ergot derivative *bromocriptine mesylate* (Parlodel) is a dopaminergic agonist with many applications. It has been used in treatment of Parkinson's disease (see Chapter 12) and acromegaly and to inhibit secretion by prolactin-secreting tumors. Adverse effects of this agent include nausea, headache, and orthostatic hypotension as well as spasm of peripheral vessels and gastrointestinal distress.

The polypeptides *bradykinin* and *kallidin* (lysylbradykinin) are potent vasodilators that can increase vascular permeability and stimulate bronchial and gastrointestinal smooth muscle. In addition, they affect various organ systems through interactions with neural pathways and with other mediators. The recent recognition that kinins affect prostaglandin synthesis and metabolism emphasizes their potential for a wide range of activities. The effects of kinins on blood vessels and other smooth muscles are similar to those of histamine, but kinins do not interact with histamine receptors. Despite a large number of studies devoted to kinins and their effects on various organ systems, their role in normal physiology remains unknown.

KININS

Bradykinin is a nonapeptide cleaved from an α_2-globulin protein substrate (kininogen) by the enzymatic action of *kallikrein*. Both tissues and blood contain kallikrein, but the enzymes from blood and from tissues differ with respect to molecular structure and preferred substrates. Glandular tissues, such as salivary glands or pancreas, are the richest source of tissue kallikrein. Kallikrein is also found in urine. The active kallikrein is generated from a larger molecule, prekallikrein, in an activation sequence similar to that described for blood coagulation (Chapter 37). As depicted on the next page, contact activation of coagulation factor XII (Hageman factor) initiates kallikrein generation from prekallikrein. Kallikrein is inhibited by several protease inhibitors in blood and tissues, including C1-inactivator, α_2-macroglobulin, and antithrombin III. Kallikrein, as well as trypsin, plasmin, and similar enzymes, can release kinins from kininogen. Under some circumstances a decapeptide, kallidin, is the product. Kallidin is identical to bradykinin except for an additional N-terminal lysine residue.[13]

Formation and metabolism

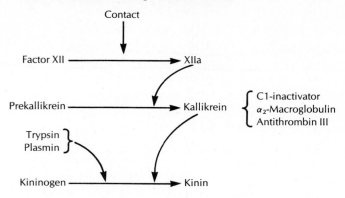

Activation of kallikrein and generation of kinins

The kinins are inactivated by peptidases in blood and tissues. Kininase I (carboxypeptidase N), the major inactivating enzyme in blood, cleaves a single arginine from the carboxyl terminal. Kininase II (angiotensin I converting enzyme) is found in blood and in tissues. It is concentrated on the luminal surface of endothelial cells and also on many epithelial surfaces, including the microvilli of the intestine, placenta, and renal tubules. Kininase II cleaves two carboxyl-terminal amino acids, just as it does to activate angiotension I to angiotensin II.[5] Other peptidases, such as enkephalinases from brain, lung, and kidney, can also inactive kinins by cleavage within the polypeptide chain.

INACTIVATION BY KININASES I AND II

Bradykinin: ARG_1—PRO_2—PRO_3—GLY_4—PHE_5—SER_6—PRO_7↑PHE_8↑ARG_9

II I

Kallidin: LYS_1—ARG_2—PRO_3—PRO_4—GLY_5—PHE_6—SER_7—PRO_8↑PHE_9↑ARG_{10}

II I

Actions on organ systems

Kinins have several potent biologic activities, including dilatation of blood vessels, contraction of smooth muscles, and enhancement of capillary permeability. Bradykinin injected into the skin causes pain, and it may be involved in initiation of nociceptive stimuli. Experimental evidence indicates that kinins may play a role in such diverse functions as vasodilatation after exercise, metabolic processing of glucose, ion and water transport, and sperm motility.

Kinins cause many effects similar to those of histamine. They are about 10 times more potent than histamine on blood vessels. Release or injection of bradykinin in humans causes arteriolar dilatation and a loss of fluid from capillaries and venules. Like histamine, bradykinin reduces blood pressure by shunting blood from large resistance vessels into mucosal and cutaneous capillary beds.

The observation that kinins constrict airway smooth muscle led to the suggestion that they are a cause of asthma. Although persons with asthma are particularly sensitive to them, kinins do not appear to be major mediators in asthma. They may exert indirect effects on lung, however, through release of arachidonic acid, which can be converted to leukotrienes and prostaglandins.

Kinins constrict uterine smooth muscle and most gastrointestinal smooth muscle in isolated tissue preparations. The gastrointestinal tract is rich in enzymes that form or inactive kinins; this finding indicates that kinins may have a regulatory role, perhaps through release of catecholamines or generation of prostaglandins.

Experimental evidence from human studies indicates that kinins may regulate uptake of glucose in skeletal muscle under conditions of hypoxia or during muscle work. Other studies suggest a role for kinins in functional hyperemia, but, as noted above, it is difficult to exclude indirect vasomotor effects caused by kinin-induced release of other mediators.

Many investigators have sought a role for the kallikrein-kinin system in reproduction. The enzymes and substrates for kinin generation and degradation are present in male and female genital tracts, and there is some evidence that kinins affect sperm maturation and motility. Vascular effects of kinins are evident during transformation of the fetal circulation to neonatal conditions. For example, kinins constrict the umbilical artery and promote closure of the ductus arteriosus. Many effects of kinins on the uterus and on blood flow in the fetal-maternal circulation are likely attributable to production of prostaglandins.[20]

In view of the ease with which plasma and tissue prekallikreins are activated, it is not surprising that numerous physiologic mechanisms have been attributed to kinin products. It is sometimes difficult to discriminate the singular effect of these peptides, however, as there is interregulation of the kinin-forming system with other mediators. Both coagulation and complement systems have control factors in common with the kinin system. For example, plasma prekallikrein can be activated by activated Hageman factor, antigen-antibody reactions, proteases, and endotoxins. In turn, kallikrein can activate Hageman factor.[13]

Clinical significance of kinins

Some clinical conditions in which kinin formation is implicated include endotoxin shock, carcinoid syndrome, hereditary angioneurotic edema, anaphylaxis, arthritis, and acute pancreatitis. A role for kinins in the early stages of inflammation is likely because they cause both vasodilatation and increased vascular permeability. Kinins may be responsible for the vascular flushing that occurs in the carcinoid syndrome. A deficiency of a kallikrein inhibitor, as in hereditary angioneurotic edema, permits kinin formation that would ordinarily be suppressed. Similarly, orthostatic hypotension associated with hyperbradykinemia[19] may reflect abnormal kinin concentrations. Interestingly, an earlier observation that some hypertensive patients excrete less kallikrein than normotensive controls was confirmed recently, suggestive of a role in regulation of blood pressure.

AUTACOIDS OF THE BRAIN AND GASTROINTESTINAL TRACT

Several peptides are found in both the gastrointestinal tract and in neural tissue. These include substance P, the enkephalins, neurotensin, vasoactive intestinal polypeptide (VIP), gastrin, and cholecystokinin. This coincidence provided evidence for a common origin of hormone-secreting gastrointestinal and neuroendocrine cells. In addition, there are secretory cells in the lung that have structural and cytochemical features similar to neuroendocrine cells. Thus it is possible that this array of biologically active peptide mediators arises from a progenitor cell type during embryonic development; these peptides may have similar functions despite their diverse tissue locations.

Substance P

Substance P is an undecapeptide (11 amino acids) that was originally discovered in extracts of brain and intestine when von Euler and Gaddum attempted to isolate acetylcholine.[11] It was named "substance P" because it was extracted and stored in powdered form.

ARG—PRO—LYS—PRO—GLN—GLN—PHE—PHE—GLY—LEU—MET—NH$_2$
Substance P

Substance P has several activities in common with kinins. Like bradykinin, it causes vasodilatation and lowers blood pressure. Thus hypotension can occur in patients with carcinoid tumors, from which substance P is released along with kinins and serotonin. Substance P can stimulate nerves, and it is very potent in evoking salivary secretion. These effects are not blocked by atropine.

Substance P is found in neurons throughout the body, including the autonomic nervous system. The highest concentrations are in the dorsal horn of the spinal cord, the trigeminal nucleus, and the substantia nigra. It is also found in nerves of tooth pulp, the myenteric plexus of the gut, and enterochromaffin cells. In the latter cells and in some neurons, substance P and serotonin are found together.[9] Substance P has also been found in various neuroendocrine cells, including those of the anterior pituitary.[1]

Several roles for substance P have been suggested. It is probably a neurotransmitter in the central and peripheral nervous systems. Substance P is believed to transmit nociceptive signals from small primary afferents entering the dorsal horn. Regulation of the actions of substance P by enkephalins is perhaps an important mechanism in neural control (Fig. 21-1).[9]

Because substance P is highly concentrated in the substantia nigra, a region concerned with movement, the peptide may be involved in movement disorders. Substance P in this region is reduced in Huntington's chorea, indicative of a causal link to the abnormal movement in that disease.

The localization of substance P in several different peptide hormone-secreting cells of the anterior pituitary indicates that it may play a role in regulation of neuroendocrine mechanisms.[1]

Hypothetical gating mechanism at first synaptic relay in spinal cord. Enkephalin released from interneuron inhibits release of substance P. ***FIG. 21-1***

From Iversen, L.L.: The chemistry of the brain, Sci. Am. ***241****:134, copyright 1979 by Scientific American, Inc.; all rights reserved.*

Enkephalins and endorphins

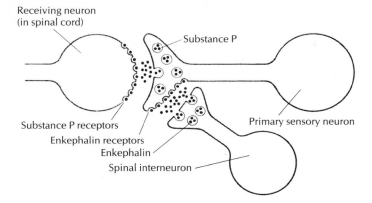

It was known for many years that opiates affect specific receptors in the brain and that electrical stimulation of certain brain regions could produce analgesia. Further, the fact that naloxone, a specific opiate antagonist, could prevent this analgesia indicated the possible release of naturally occurring opiate-like compounds in the brain. The enkephalins, two very similar pentapeptides, were subsequently isolated and found to mimic opiate activity. β-Endorphin, a larger molecule, was found to have opioid activity as well. This compound is a 31-residue peptide that contains the sequence of methionine enkephalin.

The endorphins are now recognized as a family of peptides whose sequences contain an enkephalin pentapeptide sequence. These peptides have common actions at opioid receptors as indicated by naloxone antagonism, and they are derived from a common precursor, pro-opiomelanocortin.[2] The common N-terminal sequence of Tyr-Gly-Gly-Phe conveys opioid activity, and the C-terminal extension affects potency and receptor specificity.[8]

The enkephalins are members of another family of peptides derived from a common proenkephalin precursor distinct from endorphins.[7, 12] The active sequence is released by proteolysis; the extent and sites at which proteolysis occurs can produce peptides with affinity for different opioid receptors.[7]

TYR—GLY—GLY—PHE—MET

[Met]Enkephalin

TYR—GLY—GLY—PHE—LEU

[Leu]Enkephalin

TYR—GLY—GLY—PHE—MET—THR—SER—GLU—LYS—SER—GLN—THR—PRO—LEU—VAL—
THR—LEU—PHE—LYS—ASN—ALA—ILE—ILE—LYS—ASN—ALA—TYR—LYS—LYS—GLY—GLU

β-Endorphin

The enkephalins and endorphins are found in separate and distinct regions of the central nervous system. β-Endorphin-containing cell bodies are localized primarily within the arcuate nucleus, whereas enkephalin-containing neurons are found throughout the brain. The neuroanatomy and distribution of enkephalin-containing neurons indicate that enkephalins may be neurotransmitters in many regions of the brain.[2]

Enkephalins are also found in the gastrointestinal tract, pancreas, and adrenal medulla. It is now accepted that they are endogenous opioid mediators that cause analgesia on electrical stimulation of certain regions of the brain; they may also be responsible for the analgesia from acupuncture. The precise mechanisms through which they relieve pain are still unknown, though interactions between enkephalins and substance P (see p. 222) are probably involved. Enkephalins are very rapidly degraded by proteolytic enzymes, which explains some of the difficulty in defining their physiologic role or roles.

Endorphins are less readily inactivated, and there is considerable speculation about their involvement in phenomena such as blood-pressure regulation, temperature regulation, and intake of food and water. It is still not clear, however, if endorphins mediate any of these functions or whether they act through peripheral or central mechanisms.[2]

VIP VIP (vasoactive intestinal polypeptide) is found in the intestine, brain, and lungs and in neuroendocrine tumors. It is structurally related to glucagon and secretin.[17] All three of these peptides stimulate adenylate cyclase in specific target cells. This action accounts for most if not all of the activities of VIP. It is a potent vasodilator and relaxes smooth muscle of both the gastrointestinal and respiratory tracts; it stimulates secretion of water and electrolytes from the intestine but blocks gastric acid secretion. VIP also releases hormones from the hypothalamus and pituitary. It is likely that VIP is a neurotransmitter or modulates neurotransmission, but the evidence is not so sound as for substance P. VIP is produced by cells in the pancreas and by pancreatic and other tumors. Patients with these tumors may have a high concentration of VIP in the circulation and excrete a profuse watery diarrhea.[18] This observation has led to the postulation that VIP causes the intestinal defect.

HIS—SER—ASP—ALA—VAL—PHE—THR—ASP—ASN—TYR—THR—ARG—LEU—ARG—LYS—
GLN—MET—ALA—VAL—LYS—LYS—TYR—LEU—ASN—SER—ILE—LEU—ASN

VIP

VIP may control secretion from other tissues as well. VIP-containing nerve fibers are found in the nasal mucosa and in the tracheobronchial wall. Stimulation of the vidian nerve dilates small vessels in the nasal mucosa and increases the amount of VIP in the venous effluent. Hence VIP may control vascular tone within the airways.

An additional role is suggested by the localization of VIP in esophageal smooth muscle and in sphincters of the digestive and urogenital tracts. Achalasia, which is characterized by defective peristalsis of the esophagus and a failure of the esophagus to relax with swallowing, is associated with reduced levels of VIP in the sphincter and in the esophageal smooth muscle.

These potential roles for VIP still require rigorous experimental proof, but the widespread distribution of VIP-containing nerves and tissues strongly indicates that this peptide is an integral component of physiologic and pathologic mechanisms. The coincidence of VIP with substance P and other autacoids in many tissues emphasizes the complex interrelationship among these peptides. There is currently considerable interest in the relationship of the VIP sequence to peptides that appear to block the infectivity of the AIDS virus.[16]

REFERENCES

1. Aronin, N., Coslovsky, R., and Leeman, S.E.: Substance P and neurotensin: their roles in the regulation of anterior pituitary function, Annu. Rev. Physiol. **48**:537, 1986.
2. Bloom, F.E.: The endorphins: a growing family of pharmacologically pertinent peptides, Annu. Rev. Pharmacol. Toxicol. **23**:151, 1983.
3. De Clerck, F.F., and Herman, A.G.: 5-Hydroxytryptamine and platelet aggregation, Fed. Proc. **42**:228, 1983.
4. Douglas, W.W.: Autacoids: introduction. In Gilman, A.G., Goodman, L.S., Rall, T.W., and Murad, F., editors: Goodman and Gilman's the pharmacological basis of therapeutics, New York, 1985, Macmillan Publishing Co., p. 604.
5. Erdös, E.G.: Kininases, Handb. Exp. Pharmacol. **25**(suppl.):427, 1979.
6. Fornal, C., and Radulovacki, M.: Sleep suppressant action of quipazine: relation to central serotonergic stimulation, Pharmacol. Biochem. Behav. **15**:937, 1981.
7. Höllt, V.: Opioid peptide processing and receptor selectivity, Annu. Rev. Pharmacol. Toxicol. **26**:59, 1986.
8. Howlett, T.A., and Rees, L.H.: Endogenous opioid peptides and hypothalamo-pituitary function, Annu. Rev. Physiol. **48**:527, 1986.
9. Iversen, L.L.: The chemistry of the brain, Sci. Am. **241**(3):134, 1979.
10. Jouvet, M.: Biogenic amines and the states of sleep, Science **163**:32, 1969.
11. Leeman, S.E., and Mroz, E.A.: Substance P, Life Sci. **15**:2033, 1974.
12. Lewis, R.V., and Stern, A.S.: Biosynthesis of the enkephalins and enkephalin-containing polypeptides, Annu. Rev. Pharmacol. Toxicol. **23**:353, 1983.
13. Movat, H.Z.: The plasma kallikrein-kinin system and its interrelationship with other components of blood, Handb. Exp. Pharmacol. **25**(suppl.):1, 1979.
14. Oates, J.A., and Butler, T.C.: Pharmacologic and endocrine aspects of carcinoid syndrome, Adv. Pharmacol. **5**:109, 1967.
15. Richter, G., Stöckmann, F., Conlon, J.M., and Creutzfeldt, W.: Serotonin release into blood after food and pentagastrin: studies in healthy subjects and in patients with metastatic carcinoid tumors, Gastroenterology **91**:612, 1986.

16. Ruff, M.R., Martin, B.M., Ginns, E.I., et al.: CD4 receptor binding peptides that block HIV infectivity cause human monocyte chemotaxis: relationship to vasoactive intestinal polypeptide, F.E.B.S. Lett. **211**:17, 1987.

17. Said, S.I.: Vasoactive intestinal polypeptide (VIP): current status. In Thompson, J.C., editor: Gastrointestinal hormones, Austin, 1975, University of Texas Press, p. 591.

18. Said, S.I., and Faloona, G.R.: Elevated plasma and tissue levels of vasoactive intestinal polypeptide in the watery-diarrhea syndrome due to pancreatic, bronchogenic and other tumors, N. Engl. J. Med. **293**:155, 1975.

19. Streeten, D.H.P., Kerr, L.P., Kerr, C.B., et al.: Hyperbradykininism: a new orthostatic syndrome, Lancet **2**:1048, 1972.

20. Terragno, N.A., and Terragno, A.: Release of vasoactive substances by kinins, Handb. Exp. Pharmacol. **25**(suppl.):401, 1979.

21. Vanhoutte, P.M.: 5-Hydroxytryptamine and vascular disease, Fed. Proc. **42**:233, 1983.

22. Van Nueten, J.M.: 5-Hydroxytryptamine and precapillary vessels, Fed. Proc. **42**:223, 1983.

Chapter 22

Prostaglandins and leukotrienes

The name "prostaglandin" was first applied to the potent hypotensive and spasmogenic activities recognized in human seminal fluid. Subsequent studies showed that these activities are caused by a family of *eicosanoid* compounds extracted from semen. Eicosanoids are derived from fatty acids in cell membrane phospholipids and include prostaglandins, thromboxanes, leukotrienes, and hydroperoxyeicosatetraenoic acids. Although eicosanoids affect many biologic processes, their importance as mediators and regulators of complex cellular functions has only recently been appreciated. The naturally occurring eicosanoids have only limited application in therapeutics, but the development of stable derivatives or otherwise modified compounds will likely produce valuable therapeutic agents.

The history of prostaglandins underscores many of their important properties. In the 1930s von Euler in Sweden and Goldblatt in England independently described the hypotensive and smooth muscle–stimulating properties of lipid extracts of seminal fluid. Von Euler soon recognized that these activities could not be attributed to any known substance. Because he believed that the active substance originated in the prostate gland, he named it *prostaglandin*. After a lapse of more than 10 years, another Swede, Sune Bergström, isolated a hydroxy fatty-acid fraction from lipid extracts of seminal vesicles. Almost 10 more years passed before he was able to purify from this fraction two components that had the biologic activities attributed to the original extracts; they were designated "prostaglandins E and F." Bergström's student, Bengt Samuelsson, subsequently isolated additional compounds from sheep vesicular gland extracts and identified the pathways for their formation. The active compounds are derived from oxygenation of arachidonic acid, a precursor released from membrane phospholipids.[18]

The development of sophisticated analytic techniques, such as gas-liquid chromatography, high-pressure liquid chromatography, and mass spectrometry, greatly facilitated research on these intriguing compounds. However, the classic work that led to a Nobel prize award to Drs. Bergström, Samuelsson, and the British pharmacologist John Vane depended heavily upon biologic assays of activity. In the late 1960s, 30 years after the original observations of von Euler, Vane and his colleagues described a potent "rabbit aorta–contracting substance" that was released when the lungs of experimental animals were perfused with arachidonic acid. The substance was originally believed to be an intermediate in prostaglandin synthesis, but it was

PROSTAGLANDINS AND THROMBOXANE *History*

eventually identified as *thromboxane* A_2 (see p. 230).[18] A signal achievement was the demonstration by Vane and his co-workers that aspirin and related drugs block formation of this mediator. Several years later it was established that aspirin also prevents synthesis of prostaglandins, and it was proposed that this might account for the anti-inflammatory and analgesic actions of aspirin.[23]

Through studies of the biosynthesis of arachidonic acid derivatives, the Swedish workers identified endoperoxide intermediates that are transformed enzymatically into prostaglandins and into a labile platelet-aggregating compound designated thromboxane A_2. The British group found that in vascular tissue the endoperoxides also evoke formation of a potent but transiently acting vasodilator. They recognized that its activity differed from that of known prostaglandins, and they called it "PGX."[17] PGX proved to be generated primarily from vascular endothelium. It also inhibits platelet aggregation, both in vivo and in vitro. When the structure of PGX was determined, it was renamed *prostacyclin*, or PGI_2. As with thromboxane and prostaglandins, pretreatment with aspirin and aspirin-like drugs greatly reduces synthesis of prostacyclin. Because prostacyclin and thromboxane are derived from common endoperoxide precursors, yet have opposing actions on blood vessels and platelets, a concept has emerged of a complex control system at the vascular level. The pharmacologic manipulation of these mediators is one approach to prevention of thrombosis (see Chapter 37).

Structures

The prostaglandins are 20-carbon carboxylic acids containing a five-membered ring (Fig. 22-1). Naturally occurring prostaglandins are classified according to their ring substituents as E and D (β-hydroxyketones), F (1,3-diols), or A, B, and C (α and β unsaturated ketones). They also have one, two, or three double bonds in the side chains. Biologic activity requires a carboxyl group at carbon position 1, a double bond at C-13, and a β-hydroxyl at C-15. When there are additional double bonds, they are at positions 5 and 17. The number of double bonds is indicated by the subscript, for example, PGE_1, PGE_2.

Synthesis and metabolism

The recognition that there are several enzymatic steps in the formation of prostaglandins and thromboxane stimulated interest in dissecting the synthesis of these mediators. It was learned that both glucocorticoids (Chapter 43) and nonsteroidal anti-inflammatory drugs (Chapter 31) block prostaglandin synthesis. The nonsteroidal compounds inhibit *cyclooxygenase*, the enzyme that converts precursor arachidonic acid to the endoperoxides PGG_2 and PGH_2. The steroids, including the naturally occurring hydrocortisone and synthetic analogs, inhibit release of arachidonic acid from membrane phospholipids. The basic scheme for prostaglandin synthesis is shown in Fig. 22-2.

The main precursor of prostaglandins and thromboxane is 5,8,11,14-eicosatetraenoic acid (arachidonic acid) (Fig. 22-3, *B*). The structurally related 8,11,14-eicosatrienoic acid is converted to prostaglandins with one double bond, for example, PGE_1. The polyunsaturated fatty acid 5,8,11,14,17-eicosapentaenoic acid (EPA) is converted to triene prostanoids, such as PGE_3.

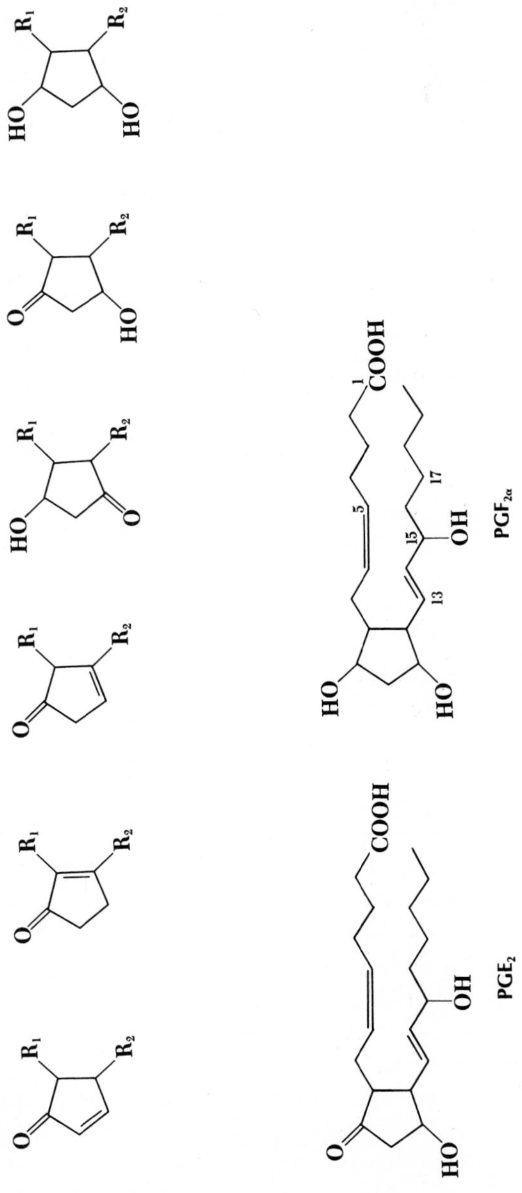

FIG. 22-1   Basic structures of prostaglandins.

FIG. 22-2 *Conversion of arachidonic acid to prostaglandins and intermediates. The enzymes at each synthetic step are designated as: 1, phospholipase A_2; 2, cyclooxygenase; 3, prostacyclin synthase; 4, thromboxane synthase; 5, endoperoxide isomerase; 6, endoperoxide reductase.*

Modified from Dunn, M.J., and Hood, V.L.: Am. J. Physiol. 233:F169, 1977.

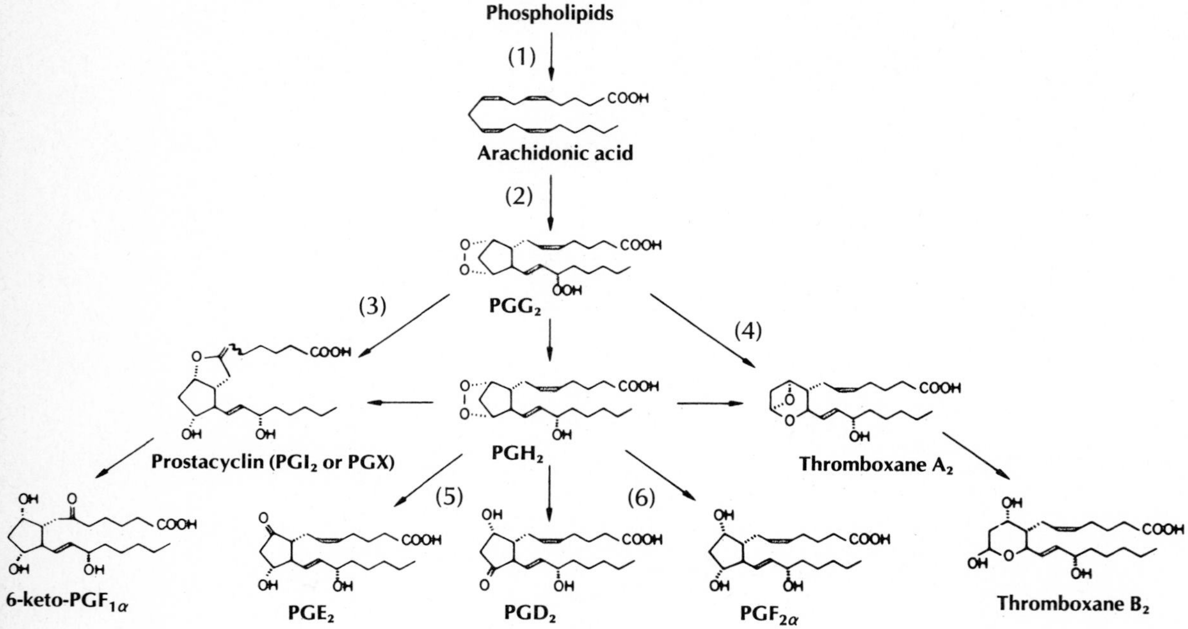

The precursor fatty acids are derived from the diet. They are not free within cells but are esterified in the form of phospholipids, triglycerides, or cholesterol esters. There is currently considerable interest in EPA, which is found in cold-water fish. Its conversion to triene prostanoids may account, in part, for the low incidence of cardiovascular disease among Eskimos. Although PGI_3 retains vasodilator and anti-platelet activity, TXA_3 is much less potent than TXA_2 as either a vasoconstrictor or a platelet aggregator.

The first step in prostaglandin synthesis is release of arachidonic acid by phospholipases within the cell membrane.[6] Various stimuli, including mechanical distortion of the membrane, changes in ion fluxes, ischemia, hormones, and drugs, can activate tissue phospholipases by a process that is dependent on calcium from extracellular and intracellular stores. The availability of arachidonic acid is limited by two opposing reactions: (1) its liberation from and (2) its reacylation back into membrane phospholipids.[9]

Precursors of prostaglandins.

FIG. 22-3

SUBSTRATE	PRODUCTS

A   8,11,14-Eicosatrienoic acid (dihomo-γ-linolenic acid) PGE_1, $PGF_{1\alpha}$

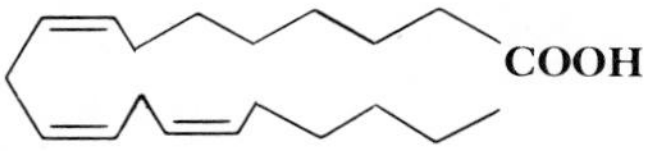

B   5,8,11,14-Eicosatetraenoic acid (arachidonic acid) PGE_2, $PGF_{2\alpha}$, PGI_2, TXA_2

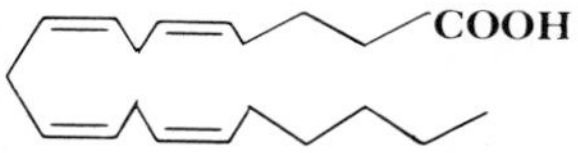

C   5,8,11,14,17-Eicosapentaenoic acid (EPA) PGE_3, $PGF_{3\alpha}$, PGI_3, TXA_3

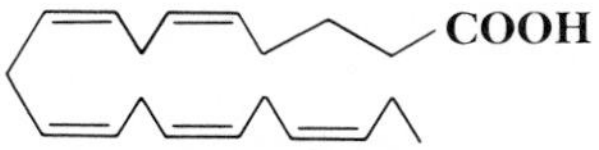

Once arachidonic acid is released, a portion that escapes reacylation is oxidized by either cyclooxygenase or lipoxygenases. Oxidation by cyclooxygenase forms labile prostaglandin endoperoxides (PGG_2 and PGH_2), which are further metabolized to prostaglandins and thromboxane. Lipoxygenation of arachidonic acid results in formation of hydroperoxyeicosatetraenoic acids and leukotrienes (see p. 235). The widespread distribution of arachidonic acid within cell membranes and the possibility of various regulatory steps within the enzymatic cascade implicate prostaglandins in many biologic activities.

Prostaglandins are not stored. They are synthesized in response to membrane stimuli and then act locally as mediators or regulators of biologic events. The newly formed prostaglandins affect target tissues through receptors distinct from adrenergic, cholinergic, histaminergic, or serotonergic receptors, but they may interact with other mediators to enhance or suppress cell functions. The particular arachidonate product formed in a given tissue depends on which endoperoxide-metabolizing enzymes are present (Fig. 22-2). For example, PGH_2 is converted to PGE_2 by endoperoxide isomerase or to $PGF_{2\alpha}$ by endoperoxide reductase. PGG_2 is converted to prostacyclin by prostacyclin synthase or to thromboxane by thromboxane synthase. Platelets produce thromboxane A_2 rather than prostacyclin because they have thromboxane synthase but lack prostacyclin synthase. Thromboxane is also produced in the lung, probably by cells in the interstitium. Endothelial cells in the lung produce primarily prostacyclin and also PGE_2 and $PGF_{2\alpha}$ but very little thromboxane.[13]

Prostaglandins are rapidly metabolized to inactive compounds by 15-hydroxy-prostaglandin dehydrogenase (PGDH); this accounts in part for their brief duration of action. This enzyme is found in most tissues, but the activity is greatest in lung, kidney cortex, and liver. The strategic location of this enzyme in the lung prevents the persistence of prostaglandins in the systemic circulation. PGE_2 and $PGF_{2\alpha}$ are almost entirely removed during one passage through the pulmonary circulation.[1] In contrast, circulating PGI_2 and TXA_2 are rapidly converted nonenzymatically to the inactive products 6-keto $PGF_{1\alpha}$ and TXB_2 respectively, which are further oxidized by PGDH.[18]

| Actions of prostaglandins and thromboxane | The cellular mechanisms of action of the prostaglandins are not completely known. They are believed to influence concentrations of cyclic nucleotides and calcium within cells.[10] Much information about the effects of eicosanoids on intracellular processes comes from studies on platelets. (The clinical application of nonsteroidal anti-inflammatory agents in prevention of platelet aggregation is discussed in Chapter 37.) An increase in free calcium within platelets promotes aggregation; conversely, decreased free calcium inhibits aggregation. Prostacyclin increases cyclic AMP by activation of adenylate cyclase. This in turn is linked to increased calcium binding within the platelet, which decreases the free calcium concentration and inhibits aggregation. Thromboxane has the opposite effect. It promotes aggregation by mobilizing intracellular calcium, though cyclic AMP concentration is not changed. The postreceptor events in other cells and with other eicosanoids are not as well defined, but there is evidence for modulation of cyclic nucleotides and intracellular calcium concentration by prostaglandin in several cell types. |

Thromboxane is best known for its potent platelet-aggregating activity. It can also cause contraction of vascular, gastrointestinal, and bronchial smooth muscle. It is synthesized by platelets and by cells in the lung. There are discrete thromboxane receptors in several tissues, and studies with receptor antagonists and inhibitors of synthesis indicate that this eicosanoid may be a physiologic regulator of airway and vascular tone. In addition, it may play a role in immune cell regulation.[20] Table 22-1 lists some of the prominent effects of the naturally occurring prostaglandins and thromboxane A_2.

TABLE 22-1   Major effects of prostanoids

Organ system	Prostaglandin	Effect
Blood vessels	PGD_2, PGE_2, PGI_2 $PGF_{2\alpha}$, TXA_2	Vasodilatation Vasoconstriction
Gastrointestinal tract	PGE_2 and PGI_2 PGE_2 and $PGF_{2\alpha}$	Inhibition of acid secretion (mucosal protective effect); smooth muscle contraction Increased motility
Kidney	PGE_2 and PGI_2	Vasodilatation, natriuresis, diuresis, renin release
Lung	PGE_2 and PGI_2 PGD_2, $PGF_{2\alpha}$, TXA_2	Bronchodilatation, vasodilatation Bronchoconstriction
Platelet	TXA_2 PGD_2 and PGI_2	Aggregation Inhibition of aggregation
Reproductive organs	PGE_2 and PGI_2 PGE_2 $PGF_{2\alpha}$	Relaxation of nonpregnant uterus Contraction of pregnant uterus Contraction of pregnant or nonpregnant uterus; lysis of corpus luteum

Role in disease

In general, the potent activity of prostaglandins on blood vessels, smooth muscles, and secretory glands indicates that any disarrangement of normal prostaglandin generation would alter physiologic function. There are several diseases in which prostaglandins and thromboxane clearly play a role. For example, vasodilatation induced by PGE_2 and PGI_2 helps maintain renal perfusion in clinical states of decreased cardiac output. The natriuretic effect of prostaglandins and the potential impact on renin release has led some investigators to speculate that some forms of hypertension result from altered prostaglandin production in the kidney.[3] Another important function of prostaglandins is on the prenatal circulation. The maintenance of a patent ductus arteriosus by the continued production of PGI_2 is necessary for circulation of oxygenated maternal blood through the fetal heart. PGE_1 has a similar effect, and alprostadil (PGE_1, Prostin VR Pediatric; 500 μg/ml) is available for administration, usually by intravenous infusion, to neonates in whom temporary maintenance of a patent ductus arteriosus is desirable. On the other hand, cyclooxygenase inhibitors are sometimes used to promote closure when the ductus remains patent after birth.

The effects of prostaglandins and thromboxane on coronary vessels are of particular interest. Studies in patients with unstable angina pectoris have revealed that local thromboxane release into the coronary circulation may contribute to anginal episodes by causing platelet aggregation and vasospasm.[12] These findings have stimulated interest in thromboxane synthase inhibitors and thromboxane receptor antagonists for use as therapeutic adjuncts in patients with coronary ischemia. PGI_2 is the major product of arachidonate metabolism in coronary vessels and in cells cultured from coronary arteries.[21] Inhibition of platelet aggregation and promotion of vasodilatation by PGI_2 may help prevent myocardial ischemia. Hence there is also considerable interest in developing stable analogs of PGI_2 for therapeutic use. Within the microcirculation of the heart, however, PGE_2 is generated to a greater extent than PGI_2 after stimulation by various hormones and mediators.[7] In addition to a direct vaso-dilatory action, PGE_2 may modulate vessel sensitivity to constrictors and may inhibit release of norepinephrine from nerve endings,[16] effects that are also potentially protective.

Prostaglandins E_2 and I_2 are 75 to 100 times more potent than isoproterenol as antagonists of bronchoconstriction caused by inhalation of a cholinergic agonist. These prostaglandins are not particularly useful in a clinical setting because their action is so brief. Stable derivatives of these agents may be more useful. In contrast, formation of $PGF_{2\alpha}$ or PGD_2 may contribute to acute airway constriction in asthma and allergic rhinitis. PGD_2, the primary prostanoid formed in mast cells, is the more potent bronchoconstrictor. It is synergistic with other mediators in contracting airway smooth muscle and promoting inflammatory changes. Thus PGD_2 is of considerable interest as a potential mediator of asthma.[11]

Prostaglandins are believed to have an important regulatory function in gastric secretion. PGE_2 and PGI_2 inhibit stimulation of gastric acid and pepsin secretion by foods, secretogogues, or irritants. Stimulation of prostaglandin formation by irritants, such as alcohol, is part of the "adaptive cytoprotective" response of the gastric mucosa.[22] Aspirin, other cyclooxygenase inhibitors and glucocorticoids are contraindicated in peptic ulcer disease because inhibition of prostaglandin synthesis leads to enhanced acid and pepsin secretion under conditions in which normal cytoprotective mechanisms are compromised. On the other hand, stable prostaglandin analogs are being developed as therapeutic agents for management of acid-peptic diseases.

High prostaglandin concentrations in seminal fluid indicate a probable role in sperm transport or motility, but there is, as yet, no proved role in male reproduction. In the female, effects of prostaglandins vary with the reproductive cycle and with pregnancy (Table 22-1). There is evidence that prostaglandins are intimately involved with ovulation. Prostaglandins synthesized by ovarian granulosa and theca cells are believed to control follicular hormone synthesis and vascularization.[4] Prostaglandins also have several activities that can interfere with pregnancy. The luteolytic effect and the enhanced uterine motility attributed to $PGF_{2\alpha}$ has led to use of prostaglandins to terminate pregnancy. PGE_2 has also been used to stimulate uterine motility at parturition. Available preparations include dinoprost tromethamine ($PGF_{2\alpha}$, Prostin F_2 alpha; 5 mg/ml) for injection and dinoprostone (PGE_2, Prostin E_2; 20 mg) suppositories.

Unfortunately, receptors for prostaglandins are ubiquitous, and systemic administration of any of these agents can cause several side effects in addition to the desired effect. For example, in studies in which $PGF_{2\alpha}$ was used to terminate an early pregnancy or to stimulate labor, it caused diarrhea, nausea, and changes in blood pressure as well as increased uterine motility. Similarly, analogs being developed for use in acid-peptic disorders are contraindicated in women of child-bearing age; they may induce miscarriage.

TABLE 22-2   Inhibitors of prostanoid synthesis

Enzyme inhibited	Inhibitor
Phospholipase A_2	Glucocorticoids Mepacrine*
Cyclooxygenase	Nonsteroidal anti-inflammatory agents, including aspirin
Prostacyclin synthase	Tranylcypromine*
Thromboxane synthase	Dazoxiben* Imidazole*

*Agents used experimentally.

Inhibitors

The enzymatic steps at which synthesis of prostaglandins or thromboxane can be inhibited include (1) the release of arachidonic acid, (2) the oxygenation to endoperoxides, and (3) the conversion to active prostanoids (Table 22-2). Finally, antagonism at the thromboxane receptor blocks the action of this mediator. Potential uses of such agents are discussed on p. 233.

LEUKOTRIENES AND HYDROPER-OXYEICOSATET-RAENOIC ACIDS
Formation and chemistry

Arachidonic acid is transformed by lipoxygenases to another family of highly active compounds, the leukotrienes. The intermediate products, the hydroperoxyeicosa-tetraenoic acids (HPETEs), are also active. The lipoxygenase reaction involves addition of a hydroperoxy group at a double bond of arachidonic acid (Fig. 22-4).

The position of the hydroperoxy group may vary with the particular tissue and will influence biologic activity. Activities that have been attributed to HPETEs include vasoconstriction, platelet aggregation, chemotaxis of neutrophils, inhibition of immune lymphocyte responses, and regulation of arachidonic acid metabolism; the physiologic importance of these is not yet established. The HPETEs are inactivated by conversion to the corresponding hydroxyeicosatetraenoic acids (HETEs) by a peroxidase.

5-HPETE, a precursor of leukotrienes, is also converted to the unstable epoxide leukotriene A_4 (LTA$_4$) by a dehydrase, leukotriene synthase (Fig. 22-5). A more stable derivative, leukotriene B_4 (LTB$_4$), has potent actions on neutrophils. Conjugation of LTA$_4$ to glutathione in a second enzymatic step forms the sulfidopeptide leukotriene C_4 (LTC$_4$). Active leukotrienes D_4 and E_4 (LTD$_4$ and LTE$_4$) are formed stepwise by hydrolysis of the glutathione peptide bonds.

Biologic activities

The actions of LTB$_4$ differ from those of the sulfidopeptide leukotrienes. LTB$_4$ is a prominent mediator of inflammation because of its chemotactic and phagocyte-activating actions. It is produced by neutrophils, macrophages, and to a lessor extent eosinophils. LTB$_4$ can be released in anaphylactic reactions, and it has been linked to bronchospasm in man and experimental animals, possibly through release of throm-

FIG. 22-4   *Oxygenation of arachidonic acid by lipoxygenase to form HPETE. A peroxidase converts HPETE to HETE.*

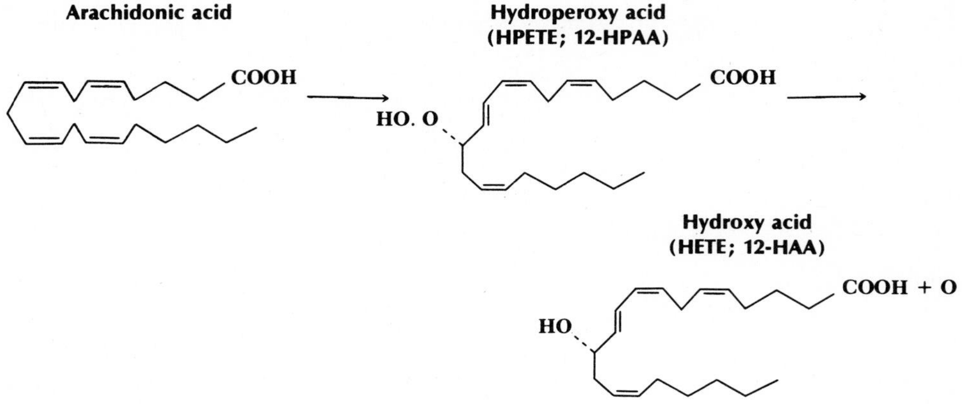

boxane.[19] LTB$_4$ also promotes attachment of neutrophils to vascular endothelium and may thus contribute to inflammation.[8]

Leukotrienes C$_4$ and D$_4$ are the active components of the slow-reacting substance of anaphylaxis (SRS-A).[15] These mediators are formed primarily by mast cells, monocytes, and eosinophils. They are recognized for their prominent bronchoconstrictive effect, which is probably involved in asthma. Furthermore, minute amounts of LTD$_4$ enhance bronchiolar sensitivity to histamine. In addition, LTC$_4$ and LTD$_4$ contract gastrointestinal and vascular smooth muscle and constrict coronary arteries and vessels of the skin. Both of these compounds have been reported to stimulate formation of prostacyclin in endothelial cells.[5] They are not chemotactic.

The sulfidopeptide leukotrienes are approximately 100 times more potent than histamine in increasing permeability within the microcirculation and may contribute to development of edema in inflammation. LTE$_4$ has actions similar to LTC$_4$ and LTD$_4$, but it is less potent in some tissues. These mediators presumably affect similar but distinct receptors.

Inhibitors   Although formation of lipoxygenase products can be decreased by inhibition of arachidonic acid release (glucocorticoids) or by a competing substance, such as eicosatetraynoic acid (ETYA), there is still no convenient means of inhibiting lipoxygenase as there is for cyclooxygenase. Many different compounds are being studied with the goal of inhibiting specific lipoxygenase mediators. There is some indication that analogs of prostacyclin might block conversion of LTA$_4$ to LTC$_4$.[2] Such analogs might be used to prevent the bronchoconstrictor actions of SRS-A.

Biosynthesis of leukotrienes from arachidonic acid.

FIG. 22-5

Modified from Lewis, R.A., and Austen, K.F.: J. Clin. Invest. **73**:889, 1984.

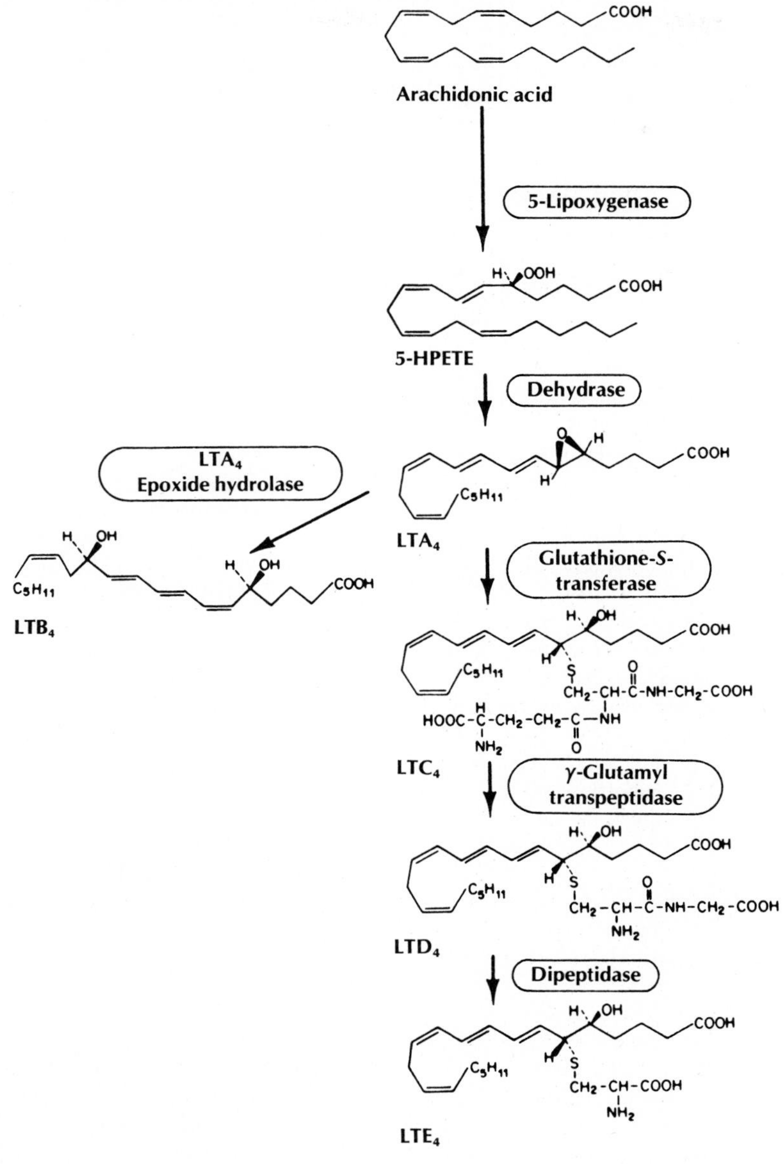

Another therapeutic approach is to modify the substrate available within membrane phospholipids. Eicosapentaenoic acid is a poor substrate for cyclooxygenase, but it is converted to the unsaturated leukotrienes, LTB$_5$ and LTC$_5$. Although LTC$_5$ has spasmogenic activity comparable to that of LTC$_4$, LTB$_5$ is much less potent as a chemotactic or aggregating agent than LTB$_4$ is.[14]

Antagonists of leukotriene receptors are not yet available for clinical use, but there is evidence that the effects of specific leukotrienes on target tissues can be blocked with synthetic compounds. Such agents will likely be applied to therapy of asthma and inflammatory disease in the near future.

REFERENCES

1. Anderson, M.W., and Eling, T.E.: Prostaglandin removal and metabolism by isolated perfused rat lung, Prostaglandins 11:645, 1976.
2. Bach, M.K., Brashler, J.R., Smith, H.W., et al.: 6,9-Deepoxy-6,9-(phenylimino)-$\Delta^{6,8}$-prostaglandin I$_1$, (U-60,257), a new inhibitor of leukotriene C and D synthesis: in vitro studies, Prostaglandins 23:759, 1982.
3. Baer, P.G., and McGiff, J.C.: Hormone systems and renal hemodynamics, Annu. Rev. Physiol. 42:589, 1980.
4. Carson, R., Trounson, A., and Mitchell, M.: Regulation of prostaglandin biosynthesis by human ovarian follicular fluid: a mechanism for ovulation? Prostaglandins 32:49, 1986.
5. Cramer, E.B., Pologe, L., Pawlowski, N.A., et al.: Leukotriene C promotes prostacyclin synthesis by human endothelial cells, Proc. Natl. Acad. Sci. U.S.A. 80:4109, 1983.
6. Flower, R.J., and Blackwell, G.J.: The importance of phospholipase-A$_2$ in prostaglandin biosynthesis, Biochem. Pharmacol. 25:285, 1976.
7. Gerritsen, M.E.: Eicosanoid production by the coronary microvascular endothelium, Fed. Proc. 46:47, 1987.
8. Gimbrone, M.A., Jr., Brock, A.F., and Schafer, A.I.: Leukotriene B$_4$ stimulates polymorphonuclear leukocyte adhesion to cultured vascular endothelial cells, J. Clin. Invest. 74:1552, 1984.
9. Goppelt-Struebe, M., Koerner, C.-F., Hausmann, G., et al.: Control of prostanoid synthesis: role of reincorporation of released precursor fatty acids, Prostaglandins 32:373, 1986.
10. Gorman, R.R.: Modulation of human platelet function by prostacyclin and thromboxane A$_2$, Fed. Proc. 38:83, 1979.
11. Hardy, C.C., Robinson, C., Tattersfield, A.E., and Holgate, S.T.: The bronchoconstrictor effect of inhaled prostaglandin D$_2$ in normal and asthmatic men, N. Engl. J. Med. 311:209, 1984.
12. Hirsh, P.D., Hillis, L.D., Campbell, W.B., et al.: Release of prostaglandins and thromboxane into the coronary circulation in patients with ischemic heart disease, N. Engl. J. Med. 304:685, 1981.
13. Johnson, A.R., Callahan, K.S., Tsai, S.C., and Campbell, W.B.: Prostacyclin and prostaglandin biosynthesis in human pulmonary endothelial cells, Bull. Eur. Physiopath. Respir. 17:531, 1981.
14. Lee, T.H., Mencia-Huerta, J.-M., Shih, C., et al.: Characterization and biologic properties of 5,12-dihydroxy derivatives of eicosapentaenoic acid, including leukotriene B$_5$ and the double lipoxygenase product, J. Biol. Chem. 259:2383, 1984.
15. Lewis, R.A., and Austen, K.F.: The biologically active leukotrienes: biosynthesis, metabolism, receptors, functions, and pharmacology, J. Clin. Invest. 73:889, 1984.
16. Messina, E.J., Weiner, R., and Kaley, G.:

Prostaglandins and local circulatory control, Fed. Proc. **35:**2367, 1976.

17. Moncada, S., Gryglewski, R., Bunting, S., and Vane, J.R.: An enzyme isolated from arteries transforms prostaglandin endoperoxides to an unstable substance that inhibits platelet aggregation, Nature **263:**663, 1976.

18. Moncada, S., and Vane, J.R.: Pharmacology and endogenous roles of prostaglandin endoperoxides, thromboxane A_2, and prostacyclin, Pharmacol. Rev. **30:**293, 1979.

19. O'Byrne, P.M., Leikauf, G.D., Aizawa, H., et al.: Leukotriene B_4 induces airway hyperresponsiveness in dogs, J. Appl. Physiol. **59:**1941, 1985.

20. Ogletree, M.L.: Overview of physiological and pathophysiological effects of thromboxane A_2, Fed. Proc. **46:**133, 1987.

21. Revtyak, G.E., Johnson, A.R., and Campbell, W.B.: Cultured coronary artery endothelial cells synthesize monohydroxyeicosatetraenoic acids and prostacyclin, Am. J. Physiol. **254:**Jan. 1988.

22. Robert, A., Nezamis, J.E., Lancaster, C., et al.: Mild irritants prevent gastric necrosis through "adaptive cytoprotection" mediated by prostaglandins, Am. J. Physiol. **245:**G113, 1983.

23. Vane, J.R.: The mode of action of aspirin and similar compounds, J. Allergy Clin. Immunol. **58:**691, 1976.

section three

Psychopharmacology

23 General concepts of psychopharmacology, 242

24 Antipsychotic and antianxiety drugs, 250

25 Antidepressant and psychotomimetic drugs, 268

Chapter 23

General concepts of psychopharmacology

Before the 1950s there were no effective drugs for treatment of the major mental illnesses.[10] Large doses of barbiturates were used to calm agitated psychotic patients, and amphetamine was used to combat acute depression. In the early 1950s reserpine and chlorpromazine were introduced for management of psychotic patients. These drugs have since been major investigational tools for assessment of the roles of central neurotransmitters and neuronal circuits in the antipsychotic effects of drugs and in the pathophysiology of the disease process itself. There is now a large number of agents (see Chapters 24 and 25) for specific management of schizophrenia, manic-depressive psychoses, anxiety states, and depression.

MONOAMINE BASIS OF PSYCHOPHARMA-COLOGY
Antipsychotic agents

Reserpine, the major active substance of *Rauwolfia serpentina* and related plants, provided the earliest insights into possible roles of specific brain amines in mental disease. It was initially found that this drug depletes stores of serotonin in the brain and peripheral organs and that only the psychoactive alkaloids of *Rauwolfia* share this activity. It was later discovered that reserpine likewise depletes stores of nor-epinephrine and epinephrine. After identification of dopamine stores in the brain, it was established that reserpine depletes these as well. These findings, coupled with observations that monoamine oxidase (MAO) inhibitors interfere with metabolism of these amines and also alter behavioral effects of reserpine in animals, implicated one or more of the amines in the central actions of reserpine.

The inability of chlorpromazine, a phenothiazine antipsychotic, to affect brain amine concentrations was at first an obstacle to further advances. However, it was soon demonstrated that chlorpromazine and related drugs are antagonists at dopamine receptors in various brain regions.[5] It now appears that the major antipsychotic action of phenothiazines and related drugs is blockade of dopamine receptors (specifically the D_2 subtype) in mesolimbic and mesocortical pathways, whereas blockade of D_2 receptors in the corpus striatum is responsible for major motor side effects of these drugs.[11,17]

Some of the evidence for involvement of dopamine in the therapeutic action of antischizophrenic drugs may be summarized as follows:

1. Ligand-binding studies have shown a close association between clinical potency and the affinity of antipsychotic drugs for dopamine receptors on brain membrane fractions (Fig. 23-1).

Concentrations of various antipsychotic drugs that produce 50% inhibition of binding of   **FIG. 23-1**
*haloperidol to a preparation of caudate nucleus are plotted against the average clinical
dose in humans to control schizophrenic symptoms.*

From Seeman, P., Lee, T., Chau-Wong, M., and Wong, K. Reprinted by permission from Nature **261**:717, copyright 1976, Macmillan
Journals Ltd.

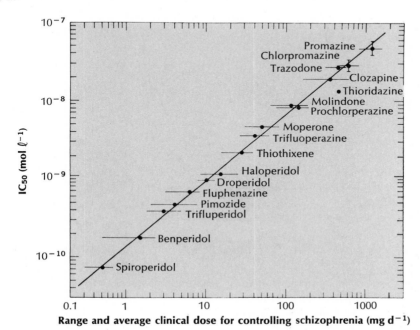

2. The potencies of antipsychotic drugs for enhancing brain concentrations of the
dopamine metabolites homovanillic acid and dihydroxyphenylacetic acid (Fig. 23-2)
in dopamine neuronal brain regions, in general, correlate well with their clinical
potencies. Thus blockade of dopamine receptors appears to cause a compensatory
increase in dopamine synthesis, though alternative explanations are possible.[6] This
compensation has been attributed (1) to a reduction of normal inhibitory feedback
to presynaptic dopaminergic neurons through collaterals from the postsynaptic neurons or (2) to blockade of presynaptic dopamine autoreceptors.[2]

3. Similarly, electrophysiologic studies on dopamine neurons demonstrate a correlation between clinical antipsychotic potency and the ability of the drugs to increase
neuronal firing rate. Some examples are given in Fig. 23-3.

4. Of less specific evidence, inhibition of tyrosine hydroxylase, the rate-limiting
enzyme in the biosynthesis of catecholamines, allows a major reduction in the dose
of antipsychotic drug required to control symptoms in schizophrenic patients (Fig.
23-4).

5. Drugs, such as the amphetamines, that release dopamine in the brain can
exacerbate schizophrenic symptoms or even initiate symptoms of paranoid schizo-

FIG. 23-2 *Metabolism of dopamine in the brain. MAO, Monoamine oxidase; COMT, catechol-O-methyltransferase.*

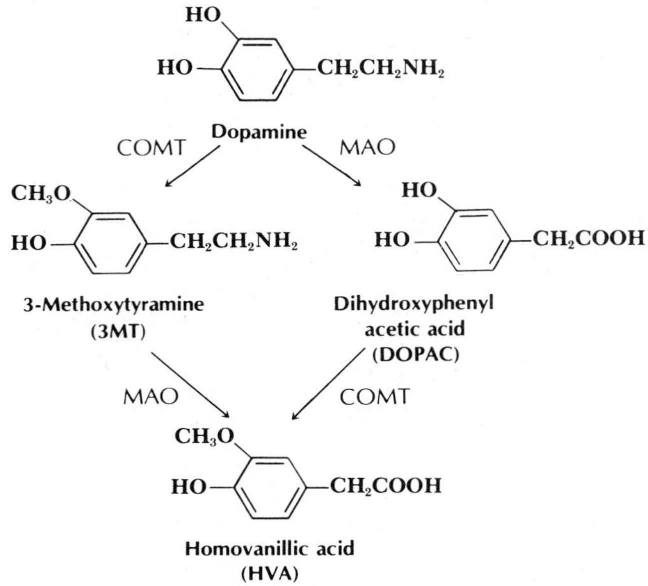

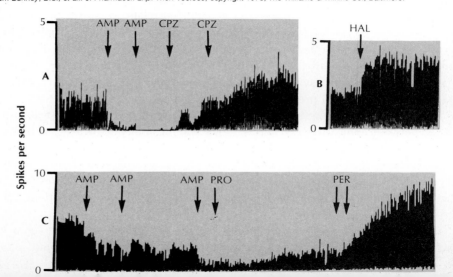

3-Methoxytyramine (3MT)

Dihydroxyphenyl acetic acid (DOPAC)

Homovanillic acid (HVA)

FIG. 23-3 *A, Antagonism by chlorpromazine (CPZ) of d-amphetamine (AMP)–induced slowing of dopaminergic cell activity in a nonanesthetized animal. AMP significantly decreased firing rate. After CPZ, cell firing resumed and increased. B, Effect of haloperidol on a dopaminergic cell in a nonanesthetized animal. Haloperidol increased basal activity. C, Lack of effect of promethazine (PRO) on cell firing rate subsequent to AMP-induced depression in an anesthetized animal. Promethazine, which is not antipsychotic, failed to increase the rate, whereas perphenazine (PER) rapidly increased rate to above baseline values.*

From Bunney, B.S., et al.: J. Pharmacol. Exp. Ther. **185**:560, copyright 1973, The Williams & Wilkins Co., Baltimore.

Social behavior (solid lines) *and mental symptoms* (dashed lines) *in a patient with chronic*   **FIG. 23-4**
schizophrenia. Patient had been receiving 1000 mg of chlorpromazine daily. The patient's
condition worsened when this dosage was reduced but improved when α-methyltyrosine
was given with a small dose of chlorpromazine.

From Carlsson, A., Persson, T., Roos, B.-E., and Walinder, J.: J. Neural Transm. **33**:83, 1972.

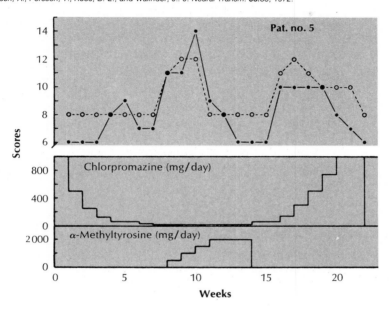

phrenia (see Chapter 30). These effects are blocked by dopamine antagonists such as chlorpromazine.

Although this brief summary is not a complete citation, there is an impressive array of evidence for a role of dopamine in therapeutic actions of antipsychotic drugs. It must be pointed out, however, that these findings do not, in themselves, constitute evidence that dopamine neuronal abnormalities *cause* schizophrenia.

Antidepressant drugs

Basic and clinical investigations have led to development of drugs for treatment of depression and have improved understanding of their basic actions. The MAO inhibitors were tried because they altered central depressant effects evoked in animals by reserpine and because of their unusual effect on mood in patients with tuberculosis. Their beneficial effect in depression is now believed to result from downregulation of adrenergic or serotonergic receptors, secondary to chronic inhibition of MAO subtype A in mitochondria of the terminals of monoamine neurons.[12]

MAO inhibitors have largely been replaced in clinical practice by the safer tricyclic and second-generation antidepressants, such as imipramine and trazodone respectively. The latter drugs are not MAO inhibitors; rather they inhibit amine reuptake into neurons. In vitro some inhibit reuptake of both norepinephrine and serotonin, whereas others preferentially affect one or the other of the pumps. Mianserin, however, is nearly devoid of uptake-blocking activity. Interestingly, antidepressants have

FIG. 23-5   *Synaptic effects of different types of antidepressant or stimulant drugs as conceptualized in the biogenic amine hypothesis of mental illness. Four aminergic axon varicosities are in synaptic contact with a target cell. Depicted is an association between intraneuronal and extraneuronal transmitter (stippling) as governed by incorporation into vesicles (shading), release by exocytosis, and uptake via the amine pump (arrows). Compared with the normal, drug-free condition, the terminal altered by a tricyclic antidepressant has a greater proportion of transmitter in the synaptic cleft because of inhibition of uptake mechanisms. The terminal subjected to an MAO inhibitor has a greater accumulation of transmitter outside and inside the terminal as a result of decreased breakdown of the amine. Psychomotor stimulants of the amphetamine type increase the amount of transmitter in the cleft mainly by enhancing release mechanisms. Reuptake may be partially blocked. With repeated administration of amphetamine, amine synthesis and vesicular incorporation may not keep pace with release; therefore some vesicles are shown empty.*

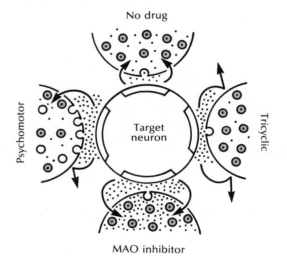

little effect on dopamine reuptake. One explanation for depression has been that it is attributable to a deficiency of functional amines, which can be corrected by slowing removal of amine from the synaptic cleft. However, the diversity of their effects on reuptake, among agents that provide similar therapeutic benefit, coupled with the long delay before therapeutic response, even though their effects on amine uptake are immediate, have evoked a change in this monoamine hypothesis of depression.[7,8,14,18] The more recent idea is that depression arises from supersensitivity of amine pathways and that prolonged exposure to antidepressants, acting either directly on adrenergic neurons or less directly through serotonergic neurons, desensitizes (downregulates) postsynaptic β-receptors. Downregulation of presynaptic α_2-receptors as well as sensitization (upregulation) of α_1-receptors have also been reported. Furthermore, antidepressants have a variety of effects on serotonergic pathways. Thus different antidepressants may act at a variety of points in complex pathways that modulate mood.[7] Future refinement of theories on their modes of action will, one would hope, further integrate their seemingly selective actions at various syn-

Sites of action of several neuronal depressants and stimulants as hypothesized for the   **FIG. 23-6**
GABA receptor/chloride ionophore. The complex is depicted as it might appear on the
outer surface of a membrane. Except for GABA, endogenous ligands (in italics) are iden-
tified only tentatively, and the effects of their binding on cellular responsiveness are un-
known. Drugs that tend to close the chloride channel are stimulants and convulsants.
Drugs that open or facilitate opening of the channel are depressants. BDZ, Benzodiazepine;
PICRO, picrotoxinin.

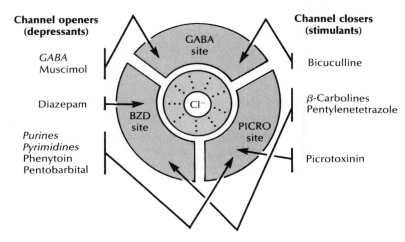

apses. Fig. 23-5 illustrates the modes of action of different types of antidepressants as these relate to acute changes in amine distribution at the synaptic level.

Side effects of these agents often appear more immediately from their actions as antagonists at muscarinic (dry mouth), histaminic (sedation), and α-adrenergic (orthostatic hypotension) receptors.

ANTIANXIETY
AGENTS

Unlike the agents discussed above, the mode of action of benzodiazepines, the primary agents used today to relieve anxiety and alleviate insomnia, is related to the inhibitory amino acid γ-aminobutyric acid (GABA)[3,9] rather than to monoamines. Interactions between benzodiazepines, the convulsant picrotoxin, and this amino acid have been observed at receptors widespread within the brain. High-affinity binding sites for GABA and benzodiazepines have been demonstrated in vitro.[13] GABA increases the affinity of benzodiazepine receptors for benzodiazepines, and electrophysiologic effects of GABA are enhanced in the presence of benzodiazepines.

Some current ideas about the action of benzodiazepines are illustrated in Fig. 23-6. The final common path at the GABA/benzodiazepine/picrotoxinin receptor complex is the chloride channel. Most commonly, influx of chloride from the extraneuronal to the intraneuronal compartment causes hyperpolarization and stabilization of the membrane. In the absence of GABA, benzodiazepines will not open the chloride channel. In the presence of GABA, however, they increase the *frequency* of channel opening. In contrast, the more generally depressant barbiturates (see Chapter 26) act on the so-called *picrotoxinin* site to *prolong* the period that the channels are open. In high enough concentrations they may affect the calcium channel independently of GABA. It has been proposed that the anticonvulsant and sedative effects of benzodiazepines are mediated through benzodiazepine receptors linked to GABA as described on the previous page, whereas anxiolytic and muscle-relaxant effects are mediated by benzodiazepine receptors linked to glycine-mediated neurotransmission in the brainstem and spinal cord respectively.[15]

The ability of various benzodiazepines to displace labeled, bound diazepam parallels their clinical potency. An unusual feature of the benzodiazepine complex is that two types of agonist have been discovered.[4] The benzodiazepines relieve anxiety and are anticonvulsant, whereas certain β-carboline derivatives that also bind to benzodiazepine receptors cause seizures and appear to elicit "anxiety" in animals. The latter compounds have been called *inverse* agonists, or *contragonists*. There are also competitive antagonists that produce little or no effect alone but prevent the actions of both benzodiazepines and these β-carbolines. Presently efforts are also being made to identify possible endogenous ligands, for the benzodiazepine-binding sites especially. Evidence for both an anxiolytic ligand[16] and an anxiogenic ligand termed *diazepam-binding inhibitor*[1] has been presented recently.

REFERENCES

1. Alho, H., Costa, E., Ferrero, P., et al.: Diazepam-binding inhibitor: a neuropeptide located in selected neuronal populations of rat brain, Science **229**:179, 1985.

2. Bannon, M.J., and Roth, R.H.: Pharmacology of mesocortical dopamine neurons, Pharmacol. Rev. **35**:53, 1983.

3. Braestrup, C., and Nielsen, M.: Benzodiazepine receptors, Handb. Psychopharmacol. **17**:285, 1983.

4. Braestrup, C., Nielsen, M., Honoré, T., et al.: Benzodiazepine receptor ligands with positive and negative efficacy, Neuropharmacology **22**:1451, 1983.

5. Carlsson, A.: Does dopamine have a role in schizophrenia? Biol. Psychiatry **13**:3, 1978.

6. Commissiong, J.W.: Monoamine metabolites: their relationship and lack of relationship to monoaminergic neuronal activity, Biochem. Pharmacol. **34**:1127, 1985.

7. Costa, E., Chuang, D.M., Barbaccia, M.L., and Gandolfi, O.: Molecular mechanisms in the action of imipramine, Experientia **39**:855, 1983.

8. Goodman, W.K., and Charney, D.S.: Therapeutic applications and mechanisms of action of monoamine oxidase inhibitor and heterocyclic antidepressant drugs, J. Clin. Psychiatry **46**(10, sec. 2):6, 1985.

9. Guidotti, A., Corda, M.G., Wise, B.C., et al.: GABAergic synapses: supramolecular organization and biochemical regulation, Neuropharmacology **22**:1471, 1983.

10. Jacobsen, E.: The early history of psychotherapeutic drugs, Psychopharmacology **89**:138, 1986.

11. Joyce, J.N.: Multiple dopamine receptors

and behavior, Neurosci. Biobehav. Rev. 7:227, 1983.

12. McDaniel, K.D.: Clinical pharmacology of monoamine oxidase inhibitors, Clin. Neuropharmacol. 9:207, 1986.

13. Olsen, R.W.: Drug interactions at the GABA receptor–ionophore complex, Annu. Rev. Pharmacol. Toxicol. 22:245, 1982.

14. Peroutka, S.J., and Snyder, S.H.: Relationship of neuroleptic drug effects at brain dopamine, serotonin, α-adrenergic, and histamine receptors to clinical potency, Am. J. Psychiatry 137:1518, 1980.

15. Richter, J.J.: Current theories about the mechanisms of benzodiazepines and neuroleptic drugs, Anesthesiology 54:66, 1981.

16. Sangameswaran, L., and de Blas, A.L.: Demonstration of benzodiazepine-like molecules in the mammalian brain with a monoclonal antibody to benzodiazepines, Proc. Natl. Acad. Sci. U.S.A. 82:5560, 1985.

17. Snyder, S.H.: Drug and neurotransmitter receptors in the brain, Science 224:22, 1984.

18. Sugrue, M.F.: Do antidepressants possess a common mechanism of action? Biochem. Pharmacol. 32:1811, 1983.

Chapter 24

Antipsychotic and antianxiety drugs

Antipsychotic and antianxiety (anxiolytic) drugs were previously termed "major and minor tranquilizers" respectively. The antipsychotic drugs, represented by *phenothiazines, thioxanthenes,* and *butyrophenones,* improve the mood and behavior of psychotic patients without excessive sedation and without causing drug dependence. Psychoses are not cured by antipsychotic agents, but the drugs relieve signs and symptoms in a large percentage of affected persons. The relapse rate for schizophrenics maintained on antipsychotic agents during remission is much lower than the rate for patients given placebo.

The antianxiety drugs include the *benzodiazepines* and *meprobamate.* Anxiety can be a disabling medical problem. Whether any drugs have selective anxiolytic activity is a matter of discussion, mainly because "anxiety," like the labels "mental stress" or "psychosomatic illness," is an amorphous culture-laden diagnosis. Although controlled clinical trials may show one or more antianxiety agents to be superior to placebo, the differences are often small. Not infrequently, no differences emerge. Despite the difficulties in proving efficacy, prescribing patterns strongly indicate that a large percentage of physicians believe that these drugs are useful. In general, antianxiety drugs have a spectrum of activity in humans and animals that resembles the spectra of barbiturates and ethanol: they are sedatives, anticonvulsants, and muscle relaxants and can induce drug dependency. The notable popularity of benzodiazepines derives from three differences between them and meprobamate or a barbiturate: they are less likely to induce tolerance or physical dependence; they are much safer when overdoses are taken accidentally or intentionally; and the gap between doses that depress nonspecifically and doses that appear more selectively anxiolytic is larger.

ANTIPSYCHOTIC DRUGS
Development

Greatly improved pharmacologic management of psychotic patients, which enables most of them to function outside a hospital environment, began with the almost simultaneous introduction of two powerful drugs, chlorpromazine and reserpine. Preparations of *Rauwolfia serpentina,* a wild shrub, have been used in India for centuries for the treatment of various illnesses. **Reserpine,** one of its alkaloids, was isolated in 1952. Reserpine depletes neuronal stores of the monoamines, serotonin, norepinephrine, and dopamine by interfering with their transport into the intraneuronal storage granules.[29] For example, norepinephrine concentrations may be reduced more than 90%. Consequently, there is loss of transmitter function, loss of

Brain nuclei and pathways especially relevant to the actions of antipsychotic drugs. The **FIG. 24-1**
diagram depicts the base of the midbrain as viewed sagittally. Three cell bodies (un-
shaded) *signify neurons of the three main pathways that synthesize dopamine (DA)* *and*
use it to communicate with target cells (shaded). Large arrows designate brain activities
influenced by dopamine and altered by antipsychotic drugs.

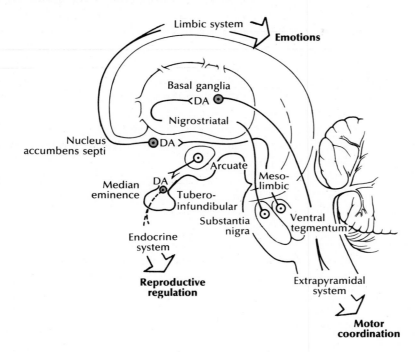

formalin fluorescence in cells and terminal fields that are normally rich in amines, and degranulation of vesicles (fewer electron-dense cores) in autonomic terminals.

Chlorpromazine, the prototype phenothiazine antipsychotic drug, originated in France from a search for new antihistamines having a phenothiazine structure. Chlorpromazine and related drugs bind to adrenergic, muscarinic, serotonergic, and histaminic (H_1) receptors to varying degrees, and their relative antagonistic activities at these receptors may influence the choice of neuroleptic for a particular patient.[4] However, their antipsychotic potencies correlate best with antagonism of dopamine.[23,26] Blockade of dopamine, in particular D_2, receptors in pathways that lead into the limbic system via the nucleus accumbens septi (Fig. 24-1) appears important.[31] On the other hand, interference with regulation of endocrine and motor pathways normally mediated by dopamine is responsible for some of their undesirable effects.

Calming of wild animals and disturbed patients by reserpine and chlorpromazine can be quite striking. Once the unusually beneficial effect of chlorpromazine in psychotic patients was recognized, many related compounds were introduced. Considered as a group, these drugs calm psychotic persons without sedating them excessively and lack propensity for inducing drug dependence, though unfortunately they can cause extrapyramidal effects. Several of these compounds are also used as antiemetics, and some are antipruritic.

From a chemical standpoint the available antipyschotic drugs include the *phenothiazines, thioxanthenes, butyrophenones*, and individual agents from other classes. The properties of these drugs are quite similar so that emphasis in this discussion is placed primarily on the phenothiazines. Reserpine was once used as a "major tranquilizer" but has been essentially abandoned in psychiatric practice. Its use as an antihypertensive is discussed in Chapter 18.

The term *neuroleptic* is often used synonymously with *antipsychotic* because all antischizophrenic drugs used at the present time are neuroleptics; that is, they cause psychomotor slowing, emotional quieting, and in higher doses psychic indifference to the environment. It is likely that drugs will be developed that control the symptoms of schizophrenia without being neuroleptic.

Phenothiazine derivatives

Several phenothiazines are in current use. They resemble chlorpromazine in action but differ from it in potency, special clinical indications, and incidence of side effects.

The antipsychotic phenothiazines can be classified on the basis of their structures and pharmacology into three groups (Table 24-1). Notice that all these compounds have a *three*-carbon link between the nitrogen on the ring and the nitrogen on the side chain.

The piperazines are more potent than other phenothiazines, cause significant extrapyramidal effects, and are not very sedative. The piperidines are less potent, induce fewer extrapyramidal effects, and cause sedation and weight gain. The aliphatic compounds are somewhat intermediate but tend to resemble the piperidines.

CHLORPROMAZINE

Chlorpromazine, an aliphatic phenothiazine, is a sedative antipsychotic drug. In addition to usefulness in agitated psychotic patients, it has other applications such as prevention of nausea and vomiting and relief of intractable hiccups. The structural formulas of chlorpromazine and the antihistaminic drug promethazine are quite similar. However, promethazine and other phenothiazines that have only a *two*-carbon link between the nitrogens lack antipsychotic activity.

Promethazine   **Chlorpromazine**

TABLE 24-1 Classification of phenothiazines used as antipsychotic agents

Phenothiazine nucleus

	Substitution in (2)	Substitution in (10)	Equivalent average daily dose (mg)*	Daily dose range[12] (mg)	Summary of effects by groups
Piperazine					
Acetophenazine (Tindal)	C—CH₃ ‖ O	CH₂—CH₂—CH₂—N⟨piperazine⟩N—CH₂—CH₂—OH	169	60-600	Most potent antipsychotic and antiemetic; highest incidence of extrapyramidal effects and catalepsy; least sedative
Fluphenazine (Prolixin, Permitil)	CF₃	CH₂—CH₂—CH₂—N⟨piperazine⟩N—CH₂—CH₂—OH	9	0.5-40	
Perphenazine (Trilafon)	Cl	CH₂—CH₂—CH₂—N⟨piperazine⟩N—CH₂—CH₂—OH	66	12-64	
Prochlorperazine (Compazine)	Cl	CH₂—CH₂—CH₂—N⟨piperazine⟩N—CH₃	103	15-150	
Trifluoperazine (Stelazine)	CF₃	CH₂—CH₂—CH₂—N⟨piperazine⟩N—CH₃	20	2-40	
Aliphatic					
Chlorpromazine (Thorazine)	Cl	CH₂—CH₂—CH₂—N—(CH₃)₂	734	30-800	Less antipsychotic and antiemetic potency; notable parkinsonian side effects; hypotension, sedation, and antihistaminic activity
Promazine (Sparine)	—	CH₂—CH₂—CH₂—N—(CH₃)₂	—	40-1000	
Trifluopromazine (Vesprin)	CF₃	CH₂—CH₂—CH₂—N—(CH₃)₂	205	100	
Piperidine					
Mesoridazine (Serentil)	SCH₃ ↓ O	CH₂—CH₂—⟨piperidine N—CH₃⟩	411	150-400	Less potent antiemetic and antipsychotic but lower incidence of extrapyramidal effects; most anticholinergic; most electrocardiographic changes
Piperacetazine (Quide)	C—CH₃ ‖ O	CH₂—CH₂—CH₂—N⟨piperazine⟩N—CH₂—CH₂—OH	80	20-160	
Thioridazine (Mellaril)	SCH₃	CH₂—CH₂—⟨piperidine N—CH₃⟩	712	150-800	

*Calculated from analysis of double-blind trials.[9]

Pharmacologic effects. The original French proprietary name for chlorpromazine, Largactil, reflects the fact that it has a great many actions.

Antipsychotic effects. Phenothiazines produce emotional quieting, psychomotor slowing, and affective indifference. They tend to decrease paranoid ideation, fear, hostility, and agitation. They lessen the intensity of delusions and hallucinations of schizophrenia. However, improvement may not be apparent for 3 or more weeks after initiation of therapy, especially in chronic schizophrenia. On the other hand, acute mania can be brought under control more quickly by neuroleptics than by lithium. In normal subjects phenothiazines induce dysphoria and impair intellectual functions.

Changes in extrapyramidal motor function. Phenothiazines precipitate an unusual variety of motor disorders,[30] presumably as a result of acute and chronic blockade of dopamine receptors in the basal ganglia. Akathisia (restless pacing) and painful dystonic spasticities of the face, neck, and tongue may occur very early in therapy, especially in young patients. Parkinsonian signs (tremor, rigidity, and bradykinesia) may be encountered after continuous administration of phenothiazines for several weeks or more. They can be a limiting factor in dose escalation. These "early" motor abnormalities are reversible, dose dependent (that is, severity decreases if daily phenothiazine intake is reduced), and at least partially controlled by drugs that are used to manage true Parkinson's disease (benztropine, diphenhydramine, and amantadine).

Tardive dyskinesia is increasingly recognized as a major medical problem in long-term use of antipsychotic drugs. It has been estimated that up to 40% of the patients receiving such drugs for 1 year or more develop some form of this syndrome, which is most often seen as grossly abnormal orofacial movements though other body regions may be involved. Tardive dyskinesia is often "uncovered" or exacerbated, when the dose of phenothiazine is reduced or the drug is eliminated.

Unlike the other neuroleptic-induced motor symptoms, anticholinergic drugs do not reverse tardive dyskinesia nor do compounds that may increase the availability of acetylcholine for synaptic transmission in the brain. Although increasing the dose of neuroleptic may suppress the clinical signs, this approach is likely to worsen the problem eventually. It is preferable to minimize the hazard from the beginning by using the lowest effective dose, if possible in short courses or with periodic drug "holidays." The elderly exhibit increased susceptibility to parkinsonian signs and tardive dyskinesia but are less susceptible to dystonias.[32] Dopamine receptor supersensitivity, as a consequence of persistent receptor blockade, is believed to contribute to dyskinetic responses.[3] Fig. 24-2 summarizes current perceptions of the complex relationships between transmitter activities and motor abnormalities in response to antipsychotic drugs and in true Parkinson's disease.

Anticholinergic and antiadrenergic effects. The atropine-like activity of chlorpromazine may cause dry mouth, constipation, urinary retention, and paralysis of accommodation. Thioridazine, a more potent muscarinic antagonist, is likely to dilate

---

Consequences of perturbations in the balance between dopamine and acetylcholine in   **FIG. 24-2**
the basal ganglia (neostriatum). Imbalances are depicted as results of aberrant amounts
of dopamine (DA) relative to unchanging concentrations of acetylcholine (ACh).

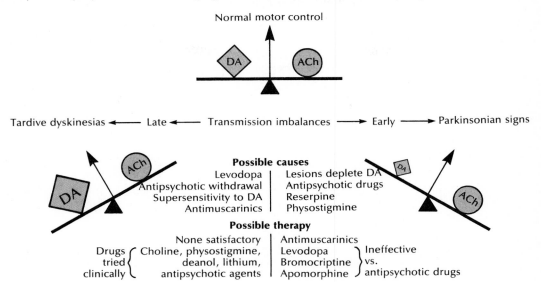

the pupils, whereas α-adrenergic blockade by chlorpromazine contributes to miosis
and also to orthostatic hypotension. Pronounced hypotension and reflex tachycardia
may occur after parenteral administration of phenothiazines.

Temperature regulation. Chlorpromazine depresses thermoregulation and has
been used to prevent shivering to facilitate development of a deeply hypothermic
state for surgery. On the other hand, neuroleptics are probably the leading cause of
drug-related heatstroke.[8] In hot environments, they impair heat-loss mechanisms,
in particular sweating, so that dangerous elevations in body temperature can occur.
In ordinary thermal environments life-threatening hyperthermias may also develop,
especially in the context of the *neuroleptic malignant syndrome* in which excessive
motor tone or activity is apparently responsible for the increase in body temperature.
Treatment with dantrolene or bromocriptine may be beneficial in such cases.

Antiemetic effect. Chlorpromazine blocks the emetic action of apomorphine and
certain other agents at the chemoreceptor trigger zone (CTZ) in the area postrema
on the floor of the fourth cerebral ventricle. The blood-brain barrier is weak in this
region, and stimulation of these chemoreceptors by circulating toxins and emetic
drugs initiates the complex vomiting reflex. Trimethobenzamide, though not a phenothiazine, may have similar antiemetic activity. Two other nonphenothiazine dopamine antagonists may also be useful antiemetics. The antiemetic properties of

FIG. 24-3   *Survey of mechanisms for emesis and the sites of action for several drugs or chemicals that initiate or control vomiting.*

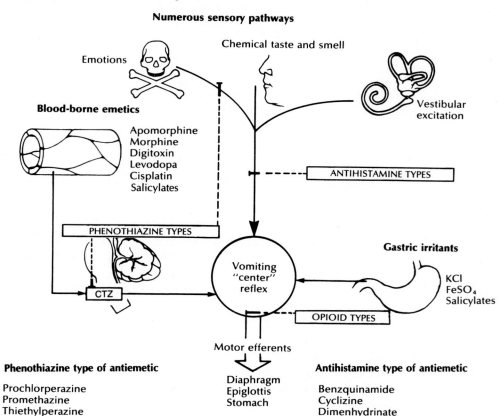

metoclopromide hydrochloride (Reglan) (see p. 522) are believed to result from blockade of dopamine receptors in the CTZ and in the enteric nervous system.[1] The drug is reported to be effective against the nausea and vomiting induced by cisplatin, a chemotherapeutic agent and powerful emetic that is resistant to antagonism by phenothiazines. Results of clinical trials with **domperidone,** which blocks enteric dopamine receptors but does not enter the brain, indicate that it too may be an effective antiemetic.[27] Phenothiazines are not useful for preventing motion sickness, for which muscarinic antagonists and antihistamines that have strong atropine-like activity are more beneficial (see p. 118). Fig. 24-3 summarizes the sites of action of commonly prescribed antiemetics along the various avenues that evoke emesis.

Endocrine effects. Chlorpromazine may cause galactorrhea, delayed menstruation, amenorrhea, and weight gain. It is generally believed that these effects are caused by disruption of hypothalamic control over the pituitary gland. For example, dopamine release at synapses in the tuberoinfundibular pathway (Fig. 24-1) normally inhibits prolactin secretion. Prolonged blockade of these receptors by chlorpromazine can lead to inappropriate lactation in women and gynecomastia in men.

Miscellaneous adverse effects and drug interactions. In addition to the adverse effects just discussed, chlorpromazine may lower the convulsive threshold and cause skin reactions and photosensitivity, electrocardiographic changes, cholestatic jaundice, agranulocytosis, skin pigmentation, and deposition of pigments in the cornea and lens. Phenothiazines can also intensify the effects of alcohol, barbiturates, and other hypnotics, morphine-like analgesics, anesthetics, and antihypertensive and anticholinergic drugs. The patient and close relatives should be made aware of potential problems, especially the extrapyramidal disorders, that may arise with continued therapy.

Pharmacokinetics. Chlorpromazine is absorbed somewhat erratically when given by mouth. Peak plasma concentrations occur in 2 to 4 hours. The plasma half-life is extremely variable but averages about 30 hours. Blood concentrations have not proved to be useful as guides to therapy. In a particular patient the optimum dose is the smallest that relieves psychotic symptoms without causing intolerable side effects. In general, a single dose of neuroleptic can be given at bedtime.

The distribution of chlorpromazine in various tissues is quite uneven. The brain contains about four times more of it than the plasma does. Chlorpromazine has numerous dealkylated, hydroxylated, and conjugated metabolites. Chlorpromazine is also excreted in milk.

Some phenothiazines with powerful antihistaminic activity are used to relieve the pruritus of various skin diseases. Examples are **promethazine** hydrochloride (Phenergan), **trimeprazine** tartrate (Temaril) and **methdilazine** (Tacaryl). In general, these phenothiazines can cause drowsiness and all the toxic effects described above so that precautions applicable to the other phenothiazines should be observed. *ANTIHISTAMINIC ACTIVITY*

The phenothiazines (Table 24-1), as well as the thioxanthenes and butyrophenones, are available in a variety of dosage forms including tablets, capsules, syrups, elixirs, injectables, and rectal suppositories.[9] Fluphenazine, as the decanoate and enanthate esters, has an extended duration of action after intramuscular or subcutaneous injection.[19] These dosage forms are useful for managing combative or noncompliant patients, since the effects of a single injection persist for 1 to 3 weeks. *PREPARATIONS*

The thioxanthene derivatives **chlorprothixene** and **thiothixene** are structurally and pharmacologically similar to the phenothiazines. The side chain on the carbon atom that takes the place of the nitrogen in the phenothiazine nucleus influences *Thioxanthene derivatives* activity in a similar way. Since thiothixene has a piperazine side chain whereas chlorprothixene is an aliphatic thioxanthene, the former is the more potent neuroleptic.

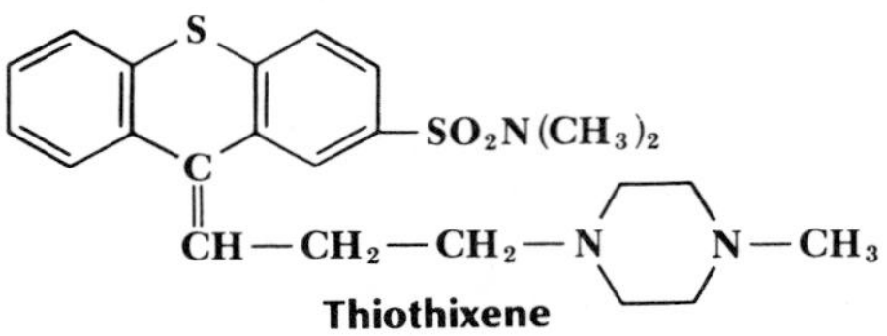

Thiothixene

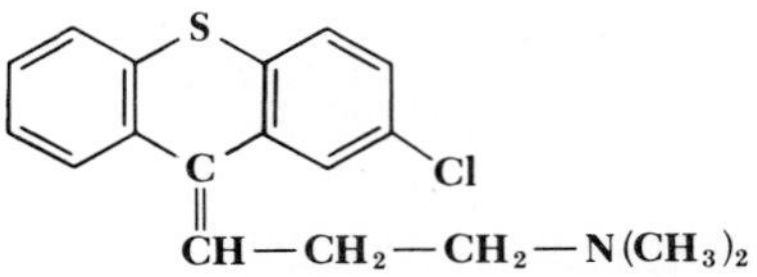

Chlorprothixene

Chlorprothixene (Taractan) may be effective in psychotic conditions in which agitation and anxiety are prominent symptoms. It is available in tablets of 10 to 100 mg, in a concentrate containing 20 mg/ml, and as the hydrochloride in solutions for injection containing 12.5 mg/ml. Thiothixene (Navane) is useful in treatment of schizophrenic patients who are apathetic. This drug is available in capsules containing 1 to 20 mg and as the hydrochloride in a concentrate containing 5 mg/ml and in vials for injection.

Butyrophenones

Substituted butyrophenones have been used increasingly as antipsychotic agents and in anesthesiology. **Haloperidol** (Haldol), the prototype of this series, is a potent antipsychotic and antiemetic, available in tablets, 0.5 to 20 mg, in an oral concentrate of 2 mg/ml, and for intramuscular injection as the lactate, 5 mg/ml, or the long-acting decanoate, 50 mg/ml. Although there is no obvious chemical similarity, pharmacologically haloperidol resembles piperazine phenothiazines; it can cause extrapyramidal reactions and has been associated with several cases of neuroleptic malignant syndrome. Haloperidol is often prescribed for depressed patients because it is less sedating than many other antipsychotics, and it is useful for temporary management of acute mania. Haloperidol is also the first-line drug in the control of the neurologic tics of Gilles de la Tourette's syndrome. **Pimozide** (Orap), a structurally unrelated neuroleptic, can be used for this indication in patients in whom haloperidol is intolerable or ineffective. Pimozide commonly causes drowsiness as well as the more serious side effects of neuroleptics in general. It is taken as tablets containing 2 mg. Pimozide has also caused sudden death in some patients taking doses well in excess of the recommended maximum of 20 mg daily.

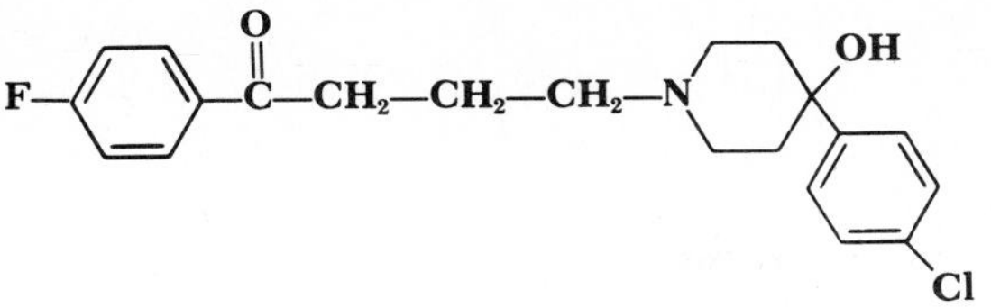

Haloperidol

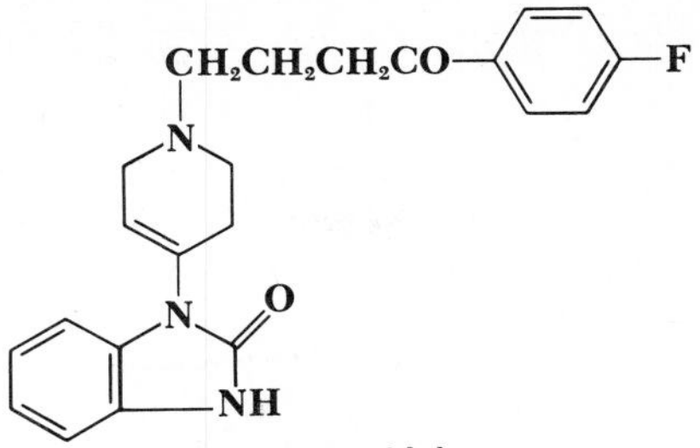

Droperidol

The butyrophenone **droperidol** (Inapsine) in combination with fentanyl, a meperidine-like analgesic, is often employed in *neuroleptanalgesia* and with the addition of nitrous oxide in *neuroleptanesthesia*. Although the fixed-ratio combination is available under the trade name Innovar, for repeated administration droperidol and fentanyl are usually administered separately because droperidol has a much longer duration of action.

Two recently introduced drugs are **loxapine** hydrochloride or succinate (Loxitane) and **molindone** hydrochloride (Moban). Although structurally different, their pharmacology in general resembles the other antipsychotic drugs. They have antischizophrenic and antiemetic actions and cause extrapyramidal effects. Molindone may occasionally cause weight loss. **Clozapine,** which is not available in the United States, is an antipsychotic drug that appears not to elicit extrapyramidal side effects, perhaps not even tardive dyskinesia.

Other antipsychotic drugs

From results of several clinical trials it has been concluded that although the many antipsychotic drugs differ considerably in their potencies, relative propensities for particular side effects, and duration of action there is little or no difference in therapeutic benefit when they are used in optimal dosage regimens.[9] Thus it is generally accepted that the best medical practice is to become familiar with a few drugs representative of the various structural classes, rather than to use a great number of them.

Choosing antipsychotic drugs

Lithium carbonate, a simple inorganic compound, lessens the intensity of the manic phase of manic-depressive (bipolar) psychosis. In 1949 Cade[20] of Australia studied its effect on psychotic behavior after the observation that lithium carbonate caused lethargy in guinea pigs. Lithium may also be of benefit when given with a tricyclic antidepressant to depressed (unipolar) patients who respond poorly to the antidepressant alone.[11,18]

LITHIUM CARBONATE IN MANIC PSYCHOSIS

Patients in an acute manic phase usually require about 600 mg three times a day, which should produce a serum lithium-ion concentration of 1.0 to 1.5 mEq/L. Continuous therapy for a week or more may be needed before the manic signs abate, and more rapid control may be achieved by temporary coadministration of a neuroleptic. As soon as a good response is achieved, the dosage of lithium should be reduced to 300 mg three or four times a day to maintain a concentration of 0.6 to 1.2 mEq/L. Because of its low margin of safety, steady-state lithium-ion concentrations, determined 8 to 12 hours after the previous dose, ordinarily should not exceed 1.2 to 1.5 mEq/L. Lithium is distributed in the total body water, and its renal clearance is proportional to its concentration in plasma. By interfering with sodium reabsorption, lithium may promote sodium depletion, but more importantly sodium depletion may cause significant lithium retention.

The dose-related adverse effects of lithium administration may progress from *mild* symptoms such as drowsiness, nausea, vomiting, diarrhea, ataxia, and tremor to *moderately severe* symptoms that include hyperactive reflexes and spasticity, leading finally to peripheral circulatory collapse, convulsions, coma, and death. The very severe reactions are associated with serum lithium-ion concentrations of 2.5 mEq/L or more. One can hasten excretion by forcing fluids while increasing sodium intake, but hemodialysis is the most effective method for removing the ion.

Therapeutic concentrations of lithium frequently cause nephrogenic diabetes insipidus. In most patients this manifests as increased thirst. However, if patients do not have access to fluids, dangerous hypernatremia can occur. It also appears that long-term therapy with lithium can diminish renal function by unknown mechanisms. Thyroid involvement in the form of goiter may also occur.

The mechanism of action of lithium ion in manic psychosis is not understood, but it competes with sodium, potassium, calcium, and magnesium ions at a variety of sites and also inhibits adenylate cyclase. Actions on adrenergic, cholinergic, and serotonergic neurotransmission have all been studied.[6]

Lithium carbonate is available in capsules (Eskalith, Lithonate) and tablets (Eskalith, Lithane, Lithotabs), all containing 300 mg of the drug, and in controlled-release tablets containing 300 mg (Lithobid) or 450 mg (Eskalith-CR). A syrup (Cibalith-S) of lithium citrate is also available; it provides the equivalent of 300 mg of lithium carbonate in 5 ml.

ANTIANXIETY DRUGS

Although drugs for relief of anxiety were once called "minor tranquilizers," this term is misleading. It implies that these are simply less efficacious versions of phenothiazines. In fact, antipsychotic and antianxiety drugs differ greatly in their mechanisms of action, in the beneficial and untoward effects they induce, and in indications for their use.

Anxiety in one form or another is a familiar disorder that is ordinarily a productive force. It merits medical attention only when it becomes so counterproductive that it is psychologically paralyzing. Administration of antianxiety drugs is the most common means for reducing anxiety to a level with which patients can cope. However, certain forms of anxiety, such as panic disorder or agoraphobia (with or without panic attacks), respond better to administration of drugs considered to be primarily anti-depressants.[2,5,28] Anxieties that are prominent components of painful or paroxysmal organic diseases, such as angina pectoris or thyrotoxicosis, often vanish with treatment directed at the underlying condition. Injudicious overprescribing of antianxiety drugs has been a matter of justifiable concern.

Benzodiazepine derivatives are currently the dominant drugs for management of *generalized anxiety disorder*.[17] The structures of several of the benzodiazepines currently available in the United States are summarized below. Diazepam, the most often prescribed of these agents, is now available as a generic product.

	R_1	R_2	R_3	R_4	R_5	R_6
Chlordiazepoxide		Cl		NHCH$_3$		→O
Clonazepam*	Cl	NO$_2$		O		
Clorazepate		Cl		(OH)$_2$	COOH	
Diazepam		Cl	CH$_3$	O		
Halazepam		Cl	CH$_2$CF$_3$	O		
Lorazepam	Cl	Cl		O	OH	
Oxazepam		Cl		O	OH	
Prazepam		Cl	CH$_2$—◁	O		
Alprazolam		Cl				

*Main use as anticonvulsant.

Numerous nonbenzodiazepine antianxiety agents have been withdrawn by their manufacturers in recent years. Drugs in this category that remain available are **meprobamate, chlormezanone** (Trancopal), and **hydroxyzine** (Atarax, Hy-Pam, Vistaril).

Benzodiazepine drugs

The clinical effects of biologically active benzodiazepines are qualitatively similar,[17] even though certain benzodiazepines are approved and marketed specifically for purposes other than relief of anxiety. For instance, flurazepam, temazepam, and triazolam are promoted as hypnotics (see Chapter 26), whereas clonazepam is offered as an anticonvulsant (see p. 315).

In animal models of epilepsy, convulsions evoked by central nervous system stimulants such as strychnine, picrotoxin, or pentylenetetrazol are antagonized by benzodiazepines. In this respect benzodiazepines are similar to phenobarbital but are quite different from phenothiazines or reserpine, which may promote seizures. Intravenous diazepam is a primary treatment for status epilepticus and seizures induced by drugs or toxins. Lorazepam also shows promise for this indication.[33] Although much of the benefit may be secondary to its sedative or anxiolytic effects, diazepam, which experimentally can relax skeletal muscle by depressing reflex pathways, is often prescribed to relieve spontaneous muscle spasms and those associated with procedures such as endoscopy.[17] Alprazolam, unlike other benzodiazepines, has clinically useful antidepressant activity[13] and appears beneficial in alleviating agoraphobia and panic disorder.[7]

Kinetics. Blood concentrations of benzodiazepines peak between 1 and 4 hours after oral administration. Absorption of diazepam is particularly rapid. Chlordiazepoxide is poorly absorbed after intramuscular injection, whereas diazepam is well absorbed from the deltoid but less well absorbed from gluteal sites. Lorazepam is well absorbed by the intramuscular route. Benzodiazepines readily cross the placenta and, with chronic administration, tend to accumulate in the fetus.[21] Many of these drugs, including chlordiazepoxide, diazepam, clorazepate, halazepam, and prazepam, are converted in the stomach or by the hepatic microsomal system to one or more metabolites, often *N*-desmethyldiazepam, which is active and has an elimination half-life of 50 (range 30 to 200) hours. This metabolite is responsible for most if not all of the activity of the latter three compounds.[17] Factors such as age, liver disease, or concurrent therapy with cimetidine can decrease the clearance of such benzodiazepines though this latter result may not always have major clinical import.[15] Lorazepam and oxazepam, both short acting, are excreted as glucuronide conjugates, and their metabolism is relatively unaffected by these factors. Doses and dosage forms are summarized in Table 24-2.

TABLE 24-2   Antianxiety benzodiazepines

Names and durations	Daily oral dose (mg)	Dosage forms* (mg)
Short acting (3-20 hours)†		
Alprazolam (Xanax)	1-4	T: 0.25-1
Halazepam (Paxipam)	60-160	T: 20, 40
Lorazepam (Ativan)	2-6	T: 0.5-2; I: 2, 4/ml
Oxazepam (Serax)	30-120	C: 10-30; T: 15
Long acting (>24 hours)†		
Chlordiazepoxide (Librium, others)	15-100	C: 5-25: T: 5-25; P: 100
Clorazepate (Tranxene)	15-60	C: 3.75-15; T: 11.25-15
Diazepam (Valium, others)	4-40	C: 15; T: 2-10; I: 5/ml
Prazepam (Centrax)	10-60	C: 5-20; T: 10

*C, Capsule; T, tablet; I, injection; P, powder for reconstitution.
†T$_{1/2}$ of β phase of elimination from plasma; it pertains to parent compound and any active metabolites.

Adverse effects. Benzodiazepines cause drowsiness, ataxia, paradoxical excitement, skin reactions, nausea, and altered libido. Even with massive overdose the victim can often be aroused, but caution should be exercised in using them with other central nervous system depressants (barbiturates, ethanol, opiates, antihypertensives, anticonvulsants, and so forth).[16] Diminished alertness from benzodiazepines in elderly patients may be mistaken for signs of senility. Apparently, with continued therapy, tolerance develops to the most common unwanted effect, drowsiness, whereas anxiolytic effectiveness is retained.[24]

Anterograde amnesia from a benzodiazepine is not uncommon, especially after parenteral administration. This response can be beneficial, as well as adverse, and is one of the reasons for including a benzodiazepine in the presurgical regimen of balanced anesthesia.

Life-threatening reactions like agranulocytosis are very rare, and deaths from benzodiazepines alone seldom occur.[14] Considering the extent to which benzodiazepines are used worldwide, the incidence of true toxicity must be very low indeed.

Physical and psychologic dependence is a proper area for concern when benzodiazepines are taken for long periods of time. However, regular long-term use of therapeutic doses is usually associated with chronic physical (cardiovascular, arthritic) and emotional problems rather than with abuse of the drugs for pleasurable mental effects.[22] In such patients abstinence signs such as sleep and gastrointestinal disturbances, anxiety, irritability, tremor, sweating, headache, and hypersensitivity to various sensory stimuli have been reported and may be severe.[24,25] Seizures have occurred in dependent persons who had taken larger than therapeutic doses for several months or longer. The addictive liability of benzodiazepines is lower than that of meprobamate or barbiturates. Nevertheless, a prudent prescriber takes these precautions with benzodiazepines: (1) they are not normally given to persons with a history of drug or alcohol abuse; (2) the dosage should be titrated for each patient's need so that daily intake is not needlessly large; (3) an expected duration of treatment should be identified at the outset so that drug taking does not become prolonged through lack of planning.

Buspirone   Buspirone, a nonbenzodiazepine compound, was introduced as an anxiolytic in 1986. Advantages appear to include minimal drowsiness and abuse potential, but a week or two of therapy may be required for full benefit. Buspirone hydrochloride (BuSpar) is available in tablets, 5 and 10 mg, for daily administration of 15 to 30 mg.

Buspirone

Meprobamate   Meprobamate was developed as a result of studies on mephenesin-like drugs (see p. 138). Clinical trials of mephenesin indicated that related compounds have sedative and anxiolytic properties.

Mephenesin   **Meprobamate**

Meprobamate is available in 200 to 600 mg tablets (Equanil, Miltown, others) and in capsules (Meprospan) containing 200 or 400 mg. Oral administration of 400 mg causes only mild sedation. Larger doses tend to produce drowsiness and reduction of muscle spasm without interference with normal proprioception.

Mode of action. It is believed that meprobamate has a blocking action on spinal interneurons, since it has no effect on knee jerk but diminishes flexor and crossed extensor reflexes. The central muscle relaxant effect of meprobamate is also illustrated by its reduction of experimental tremors induced by strychnine.

Meprobamate, though offered as an antianxiety agent, is better regarded as a nonspecific sedative similar to the barbiturates. In addition to somnolence, addiction resembling that caused by barbiturates can develop in patients who take large doses for a long time. Serious withdrawal symptoms characterized by muscle twitching and convulsions may result when meprobamate is discontinued abruptly. The drug should be withdrawn slowly.

Metabolism. Meprobamate is largely metabolized; only about 10% is excreted unchanged in the urine. Conjugation with glucuronic acid appears to be important though meprobamate is first converted to hydroxymeprobamate.

Side effects and toxicity. Drowsiness and ataxia occur when fairly large doses of meprobamate are used. Rash, purpura, and gastrointestinal disturbances may be caused by the drug. Coma, hypotension, hypothermia, and pulmonary edema have been observed after the ingestion of large doses.[10]

REFERENCES

1. Albibi, R., and McCallum, R.W.: Metoclopramide: pharmacology and clinical application, Ann. Intern. Med. **98**:86, 1983.

2. Altesman, R.I., and Cole, J.O.: Psychopharmacologic treatment of anxiety, J. Clin. Psychiatry **44**(8, sec. 2):12, 1983.

3. Baldessarini, R.J., and Tarsy, D.: The pathophysiologic basis of tardive dyskinesia. In Fann, W.E., Smith, R.C., Davis, J.M., and Domino, E.F., editors: Tardive dyskinesia: research and treatment, Jamaica, N.Y., 1980, Spectrum Publications, p. 181.

4. Black, J.L., Richelson, E., and Richardson, J.W.: Antipsychotic agents: a clinical update, Mayo Clin. Proc. **60**:777, 1985.

5. Breier, A., Charney, D.S., and Heninger, G.R.: The diagnostic validity of anxiety disorders and their relationship to depressive illness, Am. J. Psychiatry **142**:787, 1985.

6. Bunney, W.E., Jr., and Garland, B.L.: Possible receptor effects of chronic lithium administration, Neuropharmacology **22**:367, 1983.

7. Charney, D.S., and Heninger, G.R.: Noradrenergic function and the mechanism of action of antianxiety treatment. I. The effect of long-term alprazolam treatment, Arch. Gen. Psychiatry **42**:458, 1985.

8. Clark, W.G., and Lipton, J.M.: Drug-related heatstroke, Pharmacol. Ther. **26**:345, 1984.

9. Davis, J.M.: Antipsychotic drugs. In Kaplan, H.I., and Sadock, B.J., editors: Comprehensive textbook of psychiatry, vol. 2, ed. 4, 1985, Williams & Wilkins, p. 1481.

10. Davis, J.M., Bartlett, E., and Termini, B.A.: Overdosage of psychotropic drugs: a review. Part I: Major and minor tranquilizers, Dis. Nerv. Syst. **29**:157, 1968.

11. De Montigny, C., Cournoyer, G., Morissette, R., et al.: Lithium carbonate addition in tricyclic antidepressant–resistant unipolar depression: correlations with the neurobiologic actions of tricyclic antidepressant drugs and lithium ion on the serotonin system, Arch. Gen. Psychiatry **40**:1327, 1983.

12. Drug Information 1986: Bethesda, Md., 1986, American Society of Hospital Pharmacists, Inc.

13. Feighner, J.P., Aden, G.C., Fabre, L.F., et al.: Comparison of alprazolam, imipramine, and placebo in the treatment of depression, J.A.M.A. **249**:3057, 1983.

14. Finkle, B.S., McCloskey, K.L., and Goodman, L.S.: Diazepam and drug-associated deaths: a survey in the United States and Canada, J.A.M.A. **242**:429, 1979.

15. Greenblatt, D.J., Abernethy, D.R., Morse, D.S., et al.: Clinical importance of the interaction of diazepam and cimetidine, N. Engl. J. Med. **310**:1639, 1984.

16. Greenblatt, D.J., Allen, M.D., Noel, B.J., and Shader, R.I.: Acute overdosage with benzodiazepine derivatives, Clin. Pharmacol. Ther. **21**:497, 1977.

17. Greenblatt, D.J., Shader, R.I., and Abernethy, D.R.: Current status of benzodiazepines, N. Engl. J. Med. **309**:354 and 410, 1983.

18. Heninger, G.R., Charney D.S., and Sternberg, D.E.: Lithium carbonate augmentation of antidepressant treatment: an effective prescription for treatment-refractory depression, Arch. Gen. Psychiatry **40**:1335, 1983.

19. Jann, M.W., Ereshefsky, L., and Saklad, S.R.: Clinical pharmacokinetics of the depot antipsychotics, Clin. Pharmacokinet. **10**:315, 1985.

20. Johnson, F.N.: The history of lithium therapy, London, 1984, The Macmillan Press Ltd.

21. Kanto, J.H.: Use of benzodiazepines during pregnancy, labour and lactation, with particular reference to pharmacokinetic considerations, Drugs 23:354, 1982.
22. Mellinger, G.D., Balter, M.B., and Uhlenhuth, E.H.: Prevalence and correlates of the long-term regular use of anxiolytics, J.A.M.A. 251:375, 1984.
23. Peroutka, S.J., and Snyder, S.H.: Relationship of neuroleptic drug effects at brain dopamine, serotonin, α-adrenergic, and histamine receptors to clinical potency, Am. J. Psychiatry 137:1518, 1980.
24. Rickels, K., Case, W.G., Downing, R.W., and Winokur, A.: Long-term diazepam therapy and clinical outcome, J.A.M.A. 250:767, 1983.
25. Schöpf, J.: Withdrawal phenomena after long-term administration of benzodiazepines: a review of recent investigations, Pharmacopsychiatria 16:1, 1983.
26. Seeman, P.: Anti-schizophrenic drugs: membrane receptor sites of action, Biochem. Pharmacol. 26:1741, 1977.
27. Seigel, L.J., and Longo, D.L.: The control of chemotherapy-induced emesis, Ann. Intern. Med. 95:352, 1981.
28. Sheehan, D.V.: Panic attacks and phobias, N. Engl. J. Med. 307:156, 1982.
29. Shore, P.A., and Giachetti, A.: Reserpine: basic and clinical pharmacology, Handb. Psychopharmacol. 10:197, 1978.
30. Simpson, G.M., Pi, E.H., and Sramek, J.J., Jr.: Adverse effects of antipsychotic agents, Drugs 21:138, 1981.
31. Snyder, S.H.: Schizophrenia, Lancet 2:970, 1982.
32. Thompson, T.L., II, Moran, M.G., and Nies, A.S.: Psychotropic drug use in the elderly, N. Engl. J. Med. 308:134 and 194, 1983.
33. Walker, J.E., Homan, R.W., Vasko, M.R., et al.: Lorazepam in status epilepticus, Ann. Neurol. 6:207, 1979.

Chapter 25

Antidepressant and psychotomimetic drugs

GENERAL CONCEPT   Affective disorders (mental depression in its various forms) are the most frequent of the serious psychiatric illnesses. Most depressed persons are treated as outpatients by physicians who are not psychiatrists. The greatest danger to the patient is suicide, though the disease may also be characterized by severe physical and psychiatric debilitation.

A simple definition of severe depression is that it is sadness of duration and intensity that makes it incapacitating. Emotional complaints, which may not surface without probing, include apathy, hopelessness, guilt, disinterest in work or family, and preoccupation with tragedy or death. Physical complaints voiced frequently include abnormal eating and sleeping patterns, fatigue, headache, decreased libido, and vague gastrointestinal disturbances. There may be either psychomotor agitation or retardation.

According to the third edition of *Diagnostic and Statistical Manual of Mental Disorders*,[7] affective disorders have two major divisions: *major depression*, often referred to as unipolar, and *bipolar disorder*, in which episodes of both mania and depression occur. The use of lithium carbonate in the latter condition is discussed in Chapter 24. There have been many other classifications,[10] including *reactive depression* for lingering reactions to an identifiable personal disaster or setback and *endogenous depression*, which occurs without an established cause. Although an episode of major depression may include psychotic symptoms, depression associated with schizophrenia is just one of the numerous signs of psychosis. In the latter case, neuroleptics, especially those that are the least sedating, are the drugs of choice. Benzodiazepines may initially relieve some of the symptoms of depression[11] but, except for alprazolam, are not likely to be of benefit for long-term relief.

Some depressed persons, especially those who have a reactive type, may respond to simple reassurance from family, friends, and physician. At the other extreme, profoundly depressed, catatonic, or suicidal persons may benefit from a course of electroconvulsive therapy. Antidepressant drugs are indicated for many of the rest.

Cyclic shifts between depression and normal affect tend to occur, even without medical intervention. Some patients need therapy only during episodes of depression. Others may benefit from maintenance treatment to decrease the incidence of relapse.[5] It is essential that patients be closely monitored initially and that they understand that drug-induced relief of depression is not immediate.

Monoamine oxidase (MAO) inhibitors were introduced as the first antidepressants. *Iproniazid,* a chemical relative of a tuberculostatic drug and the first MAO inhibitor used clinically, has since been replaced by somewhat less toxic drugs. The MAO inhibitors are generally reserved for depressed patients not responding to other antidepressants.

The *tricyclic antidepressant* imipramine was discovered accidentally during clinical testing for antipsychotic drugs. It was soon followed by a series of related drugs, including two (desipramine and nortriptyline) that were identified as active metabolites of other tricyclics. Current ideas about the mechanisms of action of these drugs are discussed in Chapter 23.

A *central stimulant,* such as methylphenidate, can be useful in narcolepsy, in *attention deficit disorder* in children, and perhaps briefly in relief from depression.

On the basis of chemical structure, MAO inhibitors are characterized as hydrazines or nonhydrazines. Hydrazine drugs in current but limited use are **phenelzine** and **isocarboxazid.** In addition to being antidepressant, phenelzine also appears effective in management of panic disorders,[2,14] which are classified as a form of anxiety. These drugs cause a variety of side effects including orthostatic hypotension, hypomania, insomnia, and hypertensive crises.[13] The last response, which may be fatal, is generally associated with the ingestion of foods and drinks that have gone through a fermentation process so that they contain a high concentration of tyramine or possibly another amine. Such foods include aged cheeses and some wines and beer. Dietary monoamines are normally inactivated by MAO in the intestine and liver. If this enzyme is inhibited, amines may enter the circulation in sufficient concentrations to release norepinephrine from adrenergic neurons, which have increased stores of transmitter because of MAO inhibition.

MAO INHIBITORS
Types and actions

Phenelzine

Isocarboxazid

Tranylcypromine is a potent *nonhydrazine* MAO inhibitor, closely related structurally to amphetamine, that also has a direct amphetamine-like stimulant action that may account for a somewhat more rapid behavioral improvement. The faster onset of tranylcypromine action may be advantageous, but like other MAO inhibitors it can cause orthostatic hypotension or, after ingestion of certain foods, hypertensive crisis. If the sense of euphoria produced by tranylcypromine progresses into unwanted excitement, the signs may be controlled with a phenothiazine. The use of this drug should be restricted to hospitalized or closely supervised patients.

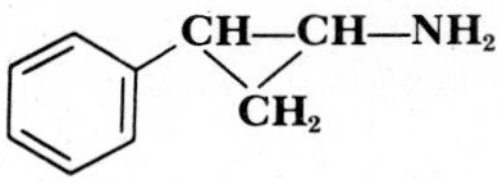

$$\text{Tranylcypromine}$$

(chemical structure: benzene ring attached to CH—CH—NH$_2$ with CH$_2$)

Tranylcypromine

Pargyline (Eutonyl), another nonhydrazine MAO inhibitor, is mentioned with the antihypertensive drugs in Chapter 18.

Interactions with other drugs	Combination with vasoconstrictors, just as with tyramine in food, can cause a hypertensive crisis, whereas concurrent administration with agents that depress the central nervous system can greatly lower blood pressure. The use of an MAO inhibitor with a tricyclic antidepressant or with the opioid meperidine may cause a dangerous interaction characterized by hyperthermia, delirium, convulsions, and coma.[22] The inhibition of MAO is irreversible and will last until new enzyme is synthesized. It is recommended that a withdrawal period of about 2 weeks be allowed for either MAO inhibitors or tricyclics before elective surgery or before initiating therapy with the other class of drugs. The same is true when shifting from one MAO inhibitor to another or before administration of meperidine. Nevertheless, results of a recent clinical trial indicate that tranylcypromine and amitriptyline can be safely taken together if the drugs are introduced concurrently.[17]
TRICYCLIC ANTI-DEPRESSANTS	The tricyclic antidepressants, which have in common two benzene rings separated by a seven-membered ring, have become the most widely used medications in the treatment of depression. Fig. 25-1 is a summary of the chemical structures of the tricyclic drugs available in the United States. Major effects of the tricyclic antidepressants derive from their ability to impair amine reuptake into neurons, to block transmission at cholinergic, adrenergic, and histaminic receptors, and to mimic quinidine in the heart.
Antidepressant effect	After a delay of 1 to 3 weeks, the tricyclic compounds elevate mood, increase alertness, and improve appetite in about 80% of depressed patients. Unsatisfactory responses are usually attributable to inadequate dosage, administration for too short a period, or lack of compliance, which may be related to development of unacceptable side effects or to lack of perceived improvement.

Dosage forms and some clinical comparisons of antidepressant drugs are summarized in Table 25-1. Imipramine pamoate is intended for once daily ingestion. The daily oral dosages are for otherwise healthy, adult outpatients. It has recently been suggested that larger doses are likely to be necessary for many patients.[16] In general, lower dosages are indicated for adolescents, the elderly, or other patients with disorders that would be exacerbated by the anticholinergic, quinidine-like, or sedative actions of tricyclic antidepressants. Use in preadolescents has not been approved except for the use of imipramine in management of enuresis.

Structural formulas in the tricyclic antidepressant series.   **FIG. 25-1**

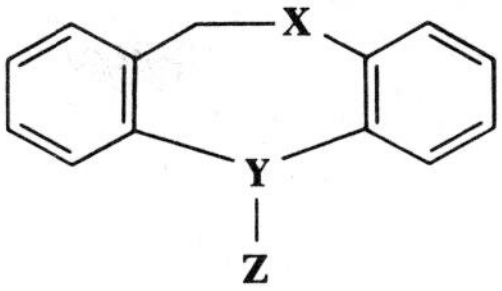

	X	**Y**	**Z**
Amitriptyline	C	C	$=CH(CH_2)_2N(CH_3)_2$
Desipramine	C	N	$(CH_2)_3NHCH_3$
Doxepin	O	C	$=CH(CH_2)_2N(CH_3)_2$
Imipramine	C	N	$(CH_2)_3N(CH_3)_2$
Nortriptyline	C	C	$=CH(CH_2)_2NHCH_3$
Protriptyline	$=C$	C	$(CH_2)_3NHCH_3$
Trimipramine	C	N	$CH_2CHCH_2N(CH_3)_2$ $\quad\quad\;\vert$ $\quad\quad CH_3$

Amoxapine

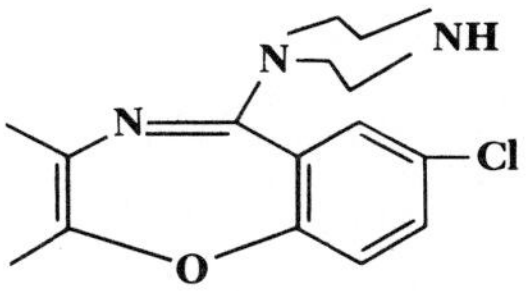

Other effects and uses

In children 6 years of age or older, tricyclic antidepressants are used in management of enuresis (bed wetting), which responds rapidly in contrast to the delay in antidepressant effect. Imipramine, in particular, has been found to alleviate agoraphobia and to decrease the frequency of attacks in panic disorder.[2,14] Tricyclics may also prove to be of benefit in a variety of other situations, as in certain types of chronic pain, attention deficit disorder in children,[9] alleviation of laughing or weeping spells in patients with multiple sclerosis,[19] and control of bulimia.[1]

The anticholinergic action of the tricyclic compounds causes symptoms such as dry mouth, blurred vision, constipation, and urinary retention. Disorientation, confusion, and motor disturbances are apparently related to a central anticholinergic action, since they can be counteracted with physostigmine.

Sedation may be considerable, and there is an increasing tendency to prescribe tricyclic drugs for maintenance in a single dose at bedtime, once a satisfactory response has developed. Most persons become tolerant to the sedative effects during continuous therapy. Excessive weight gain can occur. The frequency of extrapyramidal side effects is much lower than with phenothiazines. It is not yet clear if the risk of extrapyramidal effects, such as tardive dyskinesia, is greater with amoxapine, a demethylated congener of the neuroleptic loxapine.

The cardiovascular side effect that occurs most often in healthy patients receiving therapeutic doses of tricyclic antidepressants is orthostatic hypotension.[8] Among the

TABLE 25-1   Antidepressants: synopsis of clinical responses and doses

Compound	Adverse effects*			Usual daily oral dose (mg)	Dosage forms‡ (mg)
	Cardiovascular†	Anticholinergic	Sedative		
MAO inhibitors					
Isocarboxazid (Marplan)	H	L	0	10-30	T: 10
Phenelzine sulfate (Nardil)	H	L	0	15-60	T: 15
Tranylcypromine sulfate (Parnate)	H	L	0	20-30	T: 10
Tricyclics					
Amitriptyline hydrochloride (Elavil, others)	H	H	H	75-150	T: 10-150 V: 100/10 ml
Amoxapine (Asendin)	L	L	M	200-300	T: 25-150
Desipramine hydrochloride (Norpramin, Pertofrane)	M	L	L	75-200	C: 25, 50 T: 10-150
Doxepin hydrochloride (Adapin, Sinequan)	H	M	H	75-150	C: 10-150 S: 1200/120 ml
Imipramine hydrochloride (Tofranil, others)	H	H	M	75-200	T: 10-50 A: 25/2 ml
Imipramine pamoate (Tofranil-PM)	H	H	M	75-200	C: 75-150
Nortriptyline hydrochloride (Aventyl, Pamelor)	M	M	L	75-150	C: 10-75 S: 10/5 ml
Protriptyline hydrochloride (Vivactil)	H	L	L	15-40	T: 5, 10
Trimipramine maleate (Surmontil)	H	H	H	50-150	C: 25-100
Miscellaneous					
Maprotiline hydrochloride (Ludiomil)	M	M	M	75-150	T: 25-75
Trazodone hydrochloride (Desyrel)	L	0	M	150-400	T: 50, 100

*H, High; M, moderate; L, low; 0, none.
†Labile blood pressure or abnormal electrocardiographic tracing.
‡A, Ampule; C, capsule; S, oral solution; T, tablet; V, vial.

tricyclic antidepressants, nortriptyline seems to be the safest in this regard. Sinus tachycardia is also common and is partially attributable to muscarinic blockade. At plasma concentrations slightly above therapeutic, slowing of atrioventricular conduction can occur and can culminate in heart block if the patient already has a conduction disorder. A quinidine-like action of these antidepressants may actually be beneficial in depressed patients with ventricular arrhythmias, but intoxication is characterized by arrhythmias typical of quinidine. Extra caution and initiation of therapy with lower doses is important in the elderly and in patients with preexisting cardiovascular disease.

Intoxication

Based on reports from poison control centers, acute tricyclic antidepressant poisoning carries a high risk of death relative to most other types of drug intoxication.[21] As one would expect, acute intoxication may be characterized by anticholinergic effects and in severe cases by quinidine-like disturbances in cardiac rhythm, such as a prolonged Q-T interval and widened QRS complex.[4] When these electrocardiographic changes are recorded in the emergency room, the patient should be admitted and observed closely. Extrapyramidal motor disturbances, respiratory depression, acidosis, hyperthermia, seizures, and coma can also occur. Symptomatic and supportive treatment includes gastric aspiration and lavage, support of respiration, correction of acid-base and fluid imbalances, and possibly administration of a β-adrenergic agonist to counteract myocardial depression and hypotension. Activated charcoal may reduce absorption of the drug. Physostigmine can reverse central nervous system and peripheral manifestations of anticholinergic activity, but it should be used carefully, if at all, because of its short duration of action and to avoid bradycardia and hypotension. It has not been established that physostigmine reduces morbidity or mortality. Diazepam can be given to control seizures.

Interactions with other drugs

Tricyclic antidepressants prevent the antihypertensive actions of guanethidine by blocking the amine pump that transports guanethidine into the adrenergic fiber. Anticholinergic drugs and central nervous system depressants should be used cautiously in patients taking a tricyclic antidepressant because of additive effects. The interaction with MAO inhibitors is discussed on p. 270.

SECOND-GENERATION ANTIDEPRESSANTS

Many new drugs, known collectively as *second-generation antidepressants,* are now available or are in clinical trials. Compounds that have been approved recently for use in the United States are **trazodone, maprotiline,** and the tricyclic **amoxapine.** Others still under investigation include mianserin and viloxazine. In addition, the benzodiazepine **alprazolam** (Zanax) apparently differs from many other members of its class in having antidepressant activity[18] and in being useful in panic disorder.[2,20] In treatment of the latter, it has the advantage of fewer side effects and perhaps a more rapid response than the classical antidepressants have. The structures of these drugs are quite diverse.

Maprotiline **Trazodone**

It seems unlikely that any of the newer compounds will displace the tricyclics because of remarkably greater efficacy or lower cost for a course of therapy. However, the tricyclics are vulnerable on the issues of safety, patient acceptance, and slow onset. Initial trials with the second-generation drugs[3] indicate that trazodone, for example, may have little anticholinergic activity and is relatively less toxic to the heart. The primary serious effects of intoxication with this drug have been hypotension and central nervous system depression. Other adverse responses to these newer drugs include a high incidence of seizures in maprotiline and amoxapine intoxication,[6] neuroleptic type of side effects with amoxapine, and priapism, which may require surgery, with trazodone. A few of the newer agents have been claimed to have a somewhat faster onset of action. It remains to be seen, however, if such claims will survive the scrutiny that comes with widespread clinical experience.

PSYCHOTOMI-METIC DRUGS
Psychomotor stimulants

Some central nervous system stimulants, the amphetamines and methylphenidate, have been used for rapid elevation of mood in depressed patients without convincing evidence of benefit.[12] Unlike the antidepressants discussed above, these stimulants increase the general level of central nervous system excitability and lack a selective effect on psychologic depression. Hence the terms *antidepressant* and *stimulant* indicate quite different effects. Psychomotor stimulants may be divided into two general types: amphetamine and nonamphetamine. Examples of the first are amphetamine and methamphetamine; examples of the latter are methylphenidate and cocaine.

This differentiation is based on mechanism of action as well as on structure. An important action of amphetamine is to promote release of monoamines from presynaptic terminals. Its central stimulant action is dependent on rapid turnover of a small pool of catecholamines and is blocked by metyrosine, a catecholamine synthesis inhibitor.

Cocaine does not release amines. Rather, its psychomotor stimulant activity is probably related to its local anesthetic action on central inhibitory pathways. Its euphoric effect is believed related to inhibition of dopamine reuptake. It has been proposed that such inhibition results in intraneuronal translocation of stored dopamine so as to make readily mobilized transmitter more available for impulse-induced release. The mechanism of stimulant action of methylphenidate is not well characterized.

Both types of stimulants can exacerbate or, in high doses, induce paranoid schizo-phrenic symptoms. These and other central actions of the drugs can be blocked by dopamine receptor–blocking agents such as chlorpromazine or haloperidol.

Major disadvantages of **amphetamine,** particularly the more potent *dextro* form (dextroamphetamine), include its cardiovascular effects, the letdown that follows the short period of stimulation, and its potential for abuse (see Chapter 30). Amphetamine and the less potent stimulants discussed below are used orally in children 6 years of age or older in management of hyperactivity and other symptoms of attention deficit disorder.

Methylphenidate is primarily useful in management of attention deficit disorder and narcolepsy. Methylphenidate in the usual adult dose of 10 mg taken orally two or three times daily is unlikely to elevate blood pressure. However, it should be used cautiously, if at all, in hypertensive persons or in any patients in whom sympathetic stimulation may be hazardous, such as a patient taking an MAO inhibitor.

Methylphenidate

Preparations of methylphenidate (Ritalin) hydrochloride include tablets containing 5 to 20 mg as well as a sustained-release 20 mg tablet. **Pemoline** (Cylert) is available in tablets of 18.75 to 75 mg and as a chewable tablet of 37.5 mg.

Hallucinogens

Unlike psychomotor stimulants that induce psychosis if taken in excessive amounts, only small doses of certain other chemicals are needed to evoke toxic psychosis. Interest in the latter compounds has been great, partly because of their usefulness in experimental psychiatry and partly because their actions suggest a chemical basis for mental illness. There is a significant difference between the central effects of hallucinogens and the mental responses to high doses of stimulants such as amphetamine. In the case of hallucinogens, human subjects generally retain insight into their experience and realize that their reaction is drug induced. Thus these hallucinations have been termed *pseudohallucinations*. Amphetamines are more truly psychotomimetic and may cause symptoms of paranoid schizophrenia indistinguishable from the actual disease. Among the more interesting hallucinogens are lysergic acid diethylamide, mescaline, and psilocybin.

Lysergic acid diethylamide (lysergide, LSD, Delysid) is closely related to the ergot alkaloids. Discovery of its hallucinogenic properties was made by the chemist who synthesized the drug and noted the reactions in himself. Subjects who ingest a few milligrams of LSD develop visual, or rarely auditory, hallucinations. The body may be perceived as distorted, so that the arms, for example, appear to extend a great distance. The subject may become fearful and irrational. Sympathomimetic effects, such as tachycardia and mydriasis, also occur. In animal experiments, LSD may cause excitement and hyperthermia. With repeated administration, tolerance rapidly develops.

Lysergide (LSD)   Mescaline

LSD is a potent antagonist of the action of serotonin on smooth muscles. The association of antiserotonin activity with psychic effects was once the basis for speculations concerning the role of serotonin in behavior. However, there is now evidence that LSD is an agonist at serotonin receptors in the brain. How an interaction between LSD and serotonin may be related to hallucinations is an unresolved question. Bromolysergide has no hallucinogenic properties but, like LSD, can antagonize serotonin peripherally.

Mescaline is obtained from the cactus known as peyote or mescal (*Lophophora williamsii*) that grows in the southwestern United States. This cactus is used by certain Indians in religious ceremonies. Persons who have ingested dried peyote "buttons" report that they experience stupor with visual hallucinations. Colored lights, reported to be extremely beautiful, are the most striking feature of these hallucinations. Interestingly, some volunteers report that they have seen colors they did not know existed.

Mescaline is 3,4,5-trimethoxyphenethylamine, a structure resembling the sympathomimetic amines. It has been given in doses of 300 to 500 mg in experimental psychiatry. Trace amounts of β-phenethylamine are present in normal human brain. Moreover, urinary concentrations of β-phenethylamine have been reported as much higher in paranoid schizophrenics than in other mental patients or in normal persons.[15]

Psilocybin (*O*-phosphoryl-4-hydroxy-*N*,*N*-dimethyltryptamine) has been isolated from Mexican mushrooms that have hallucinogenic activity. Chemically it is closely related to serotonin.

It is of great interest that compounds related to endogenously occurring amines have hallucinogenic properties. Further research is needed to clarify the relevant relationships.

The abuse of psychotomimetic drugs is discussed in detail in Chapter 30.

1. Bond, W.S., Crabbe, S., and Sanders, M.C.: Pharmacotherapy of eating disorders: a critical review, Drug Intell. Clin. Pharm. **20**:659, 1986.
2. Breier, A., Charney, D.S., and Heninger, G.R.: The diagnostic validity of anxiety disorders and their relationship to depressive illness, Am. J. Psychiatry **142**:787, 1985.
3. Coccaro, E.F., and Siever, L.J.: Second generation antidepressants: a comparative review, J. Clin. Pharmacol. **25**:241, 1985.
4. Crome, P.: Antidepressant overdosage, Drugs **23**:431, 1982.
5. Davis, J.M.: Antidepressant drugs. In Kaplan, H.I., and Sadock, B.J., editors: Comprehensive textbook of psychiatry, vol. 2, ed. 4, Baltimore, 1985, Williams & Wilkins, p. 1513.
6. Dessain, E.C., Schatzberg, A.F., Woods, B.T., and Cole, J.O.: Maprotiline treatment in depression: a perspective on seizures, Arch. Gen. Psychiatry **43**:86, 1986.
7. Diagnostic and statistical manual of mental disorders, ed. 3, Washington, 1980, The American Psychiatric Association.
8. Glassman, A.H.: Cardiovascular effects of tricyclic antidepressants, Annu. Rev. Med. **35**:503, 1984.
9. Goodman, W.K., and Charney, D.S.: Therapeutic applications and mechanisms of action of monoamine oxidase inhibitor and heterocyclic antidepressant drugs, J. Clin. Psychiatry **46**(10, sec. 2):6, 1985.
10. Lehmann, H.E.: Clinical evaluation and natural course of depression, J. Clin. Psychiatry **44**(5, sec. 2):5, 1983.
11. Lipman, R.S., Covi, L., Rickels, K., et al.: Imipramine and chlordiazepoxide in depressive and anxiety disorders. I. Efficacy in depressed outpatients, Arch. Gen. Psychiatry **43**:68, 1986.

12. Mattes, J.A.: Methylphenidate in mild depression: a double-blind controlled trial, J. Clin. Psychiatry **46**:525, 1985.
13. McDaniel, K.D.: Clinical pharmacology of monoamine oxidase inhibitors, Clin. Neuropharmacol. **9**:207, 1986.
14. Pohl, R., Rainey, J.M., Jr., and Gershon, S.: Changes in the drug treatment of anxiety disorders, Psychopathology **17** (suppl. 1):6, 1984.
15. Potkin, S.G., Karoum, F., Chuang, L.-W., et al.: Phenylethylamine in paranoid chronic schizophrenia, Science **206**:470, 1979.
16. Quitkin, F.M.: The importance of dosage in prescribing antidepressants, Br. J. Psychiatry **147**:593, 1985.
17. Razani, J., White, K.L., White, J., et al.: The safety and efficacy of combined amitriptyline and tranylcypromine antidepressant treatment: a controlled trial, Arch. Gen. Psychiatry **40**:657, 1983.
18. Rickels, K., Feighner, J.P., and Smith, W.T.: Alprazolam, amitriptyline, doxepin, and placebo in the treatment of depression, Arch. Gen. Psychiatry **42**: 134, 1985.
19. Schiffer, R.B., Herndon, R.M., and Rudick, R.A.: Treatment of pathologic laughing and weeping with amitriptyline, N. Engl. J. Med. **312**:1480, 1985.
20. Sheehan, D.V., Coleman, J.H., Greenblatt, D.J., et al.: Some biochemical correlates of panic attacks with agoraphobia and their response to a new treatment, J. Clin. Psychopharmacol. **4**:66, 1984.
21. Veltri, J.C., and Litovitz, T.L.: 1983 annual report of the American Association of Poison Control Centers National Data Collection System, Am. J. Emerg. Med. **2**:420, 1984.
22. White, K., and Simpson, G.: The combined use of MAOIs and tricyclics, J. Clin. Psychiatry **45**(7, sec. 2):67, 1984.

section four

Depressants and stimulants of the central nervous system

26 Hypnotic drugs and alcohol, 280

27 Central nervous system stimulants of the convulsant type, 302

28 Antiepileptic drugs, 308

29 Narcotic (opioid) analgesic drugs, 319

30 Contemporary drug abuse, 337

31 Nonsteroidal anti-inflammatory antipyretic analgesics, 364

Chapter 26

Hypnotic drugs and alcohol

GENERAL
CONSIDERATIONS

By definition, hypnotic drugs are used to promote sleep. These agents were previously called "sedative-hypnotics" because of their general sedating properties. For about 100 years drugs of this class (first the bromides and after the turn of the century the barbiturates and chloral hydrate) were the only medications available to calm agitated patients, from the anxious neurotic to the most disturbed psychotic. However, with the advent of modern psychopharmacology, after the discovery of the antipsychotic properties of chlorpromazine, more specific compounds have been developed for sedation as well as for overall treatment of patients with different psychiatric disorders (for example, neuroleptics for the manic or schizophrenic patient). Thus hypnotics are now used strictly in adjunctive treatment of patients with the complaint of insomnia.

Before the introduction of benzodiazepines, barbiturates and, to a lesser extent, nonbarbiturates such as chloral hydrate dominated among drugs used as hypnotics. However, tolerance to these develops fairly rapidly[15] and may lead to use of higher doses. This in turn increases the likelihood that an abstinence syndrome will occur after abrupt drug withdrawal and will create a greater potential for drug dependence. Another concern with these substances is their rather narrow margin of safety.

Currently the most commonly used hypnotics are benzodiazepines. Flurazepam, the first of these marketed specifically as a hypnotic, was introduced in 1970. The benzodiazepines are safer drugs and have a relatively low dependence liability. Nevertheless, barbiturates and a few other nonbenzodiazepine drugs are still used as hypnotics, albeit to a much lesser extent.

BENZODIAZEPINES
USED PRIMARILY
AS HYPNOTICS

The general characteristics of benzodiazepines are discussed in Chapter 24. This chapter focuses more specifically on the three benzodiazepines promoted mainly as hypnotics, each with different elimination half-lives: flurazepam (long), temazepam (intermediate), and triazolam (short). Midazolam, a benzodiazepine approved in 1986 for perioperative use, is also discussed.

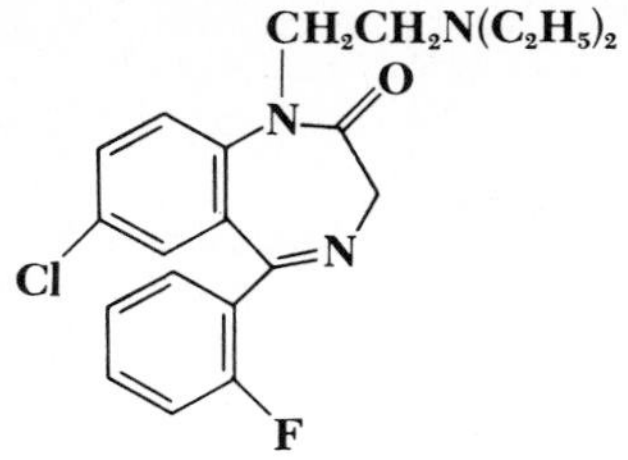

Flurazepam

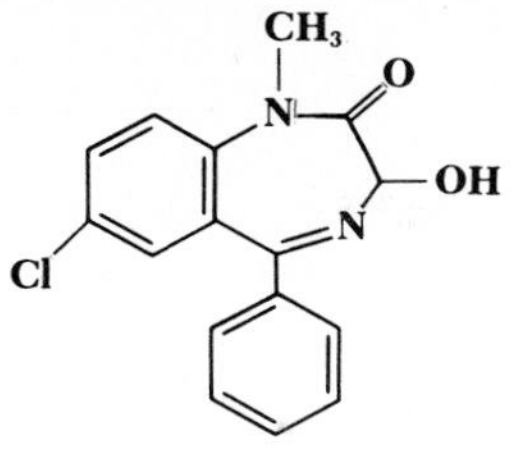

Temazepam

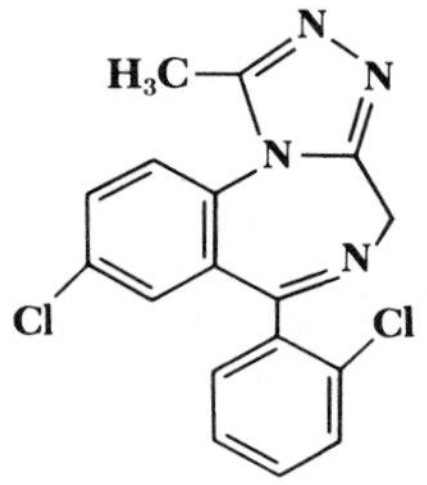

Triazolam

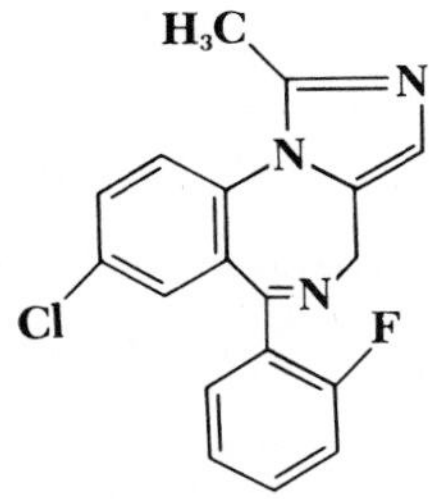

Midazolam

Kinetics

Diazepam is the most rapidly absorbed benzodiazepine; flurazepam is intermediate, followed by triazolam, and the U.S. formulation of temazepam has a very slow rate of absorption.[11] Accordingly, diazepam, flurazepam, and triazolam are useful for inducing sleep, whereas temazepam is primarily useful for maintaining sleep.

An important characteristic of benzodiazepine metabolism is the formation of active metabolites.[11] Flurazepam is converted to two rapidly eliminated metabolites (hydroxyethylflurazepam and flurazepam aldehyde) and one that is slowly eliminated (desalkylflurazepam with a half-life of 40 to 150 hours). Triazolam, like oxazepam and lorazepam, is metabolized directly to inactive substances and has a short elimination half-life. The half-lives of these drugs range from 2 hours or less for triazolam up to 200 hours for a diazepam metabolite (Table 26-1).

Mechanism of action

The ratio between anxiolytic and sedative potencies for benzodiazepines is greater than for barbiturates. In animals benzodiazepines cause calming and taming effects similar to those of barbiturates; however, in contrast to barbiturates, these effects occur at doses greatly lower than those that decrease activity or induce sleepiness. Benzodiazepines consistently attenuate the effects of punishment or lack of reward on animal behavior; again, sedation is not a necessary component. In general, benzodiazepines also reduce both evoked and spontaneous hostility and aggressive behavior, but the disinhibitory effects of these drugs may also produce paradoxical increases in aggression.

TABLE 26-1   Benzodiazepines used primarily for hypnosis or perioperatively

Drug	Elimination half-life* (hr)	Oral dose (mg)	Dosage forms† (mg)
Diazepam (Valium)	20-200	2-10	C: 15; T: 2-10; I: 5/ml
Flurazepam hydrochloride (Dalmane)	50-100	15-30	C: 15, 30
Midazolam hydrochloride (Versed)	2-4	10-15‡	I: 5/ml
Temazepam (Restoril, Somaz)	5-11	10-30	C: 15, 30
Triazolam (Halcion)	2-5	0.25-0.5	T: 0.125-0.5

*Pertains to parent compound and any active metabolites.
†*C*, Capsule; *I*, injection; *T*, tablet.
‡Not available for oral administration.

Recently the presence of high-affinity binding sites for benzodiazepines has been demonstrated in various brain regions, including the cerebral cortex, midbrain, and hippocampus.[25] Although the physiologic importance of benzodiazepine receptors is not well understood, there appears to be a relationship between their presence in certain regions and their pharmacologic effects. Anxiolytic activity may relate to receptors in the limbic system (amygdala, hippocampus, and olfactory bulb) and frontal cortex. High concentrations of receptors in the cerebral cortex, hippocampus, and amygdala may account for anticonvulsant activity, whereas receptors in the reticular formation and other structures of the pons and medulla oblongata are more likely related to the sedative action of benzodiazepines. The interaction between benzodiazepines and GABA regulation of chloride channels is discussed in Chapter 23.

Rebound insomnia and *rebound anxiety* (noticeable increases in wakefulness and in daytime anxiety, respectively, compared with baseline levels) appear related to the rates of elimination of benzodiazepines and to the rate of change in occupancy of benzodiazepine receptors.[19] Thus, after abrupt withdrawal of a benzodiazepine with a short elimination half-life, these symptoms usually occur and may be severe, possibly because of a lag in replacement by an endogenous benzodiazepine-like compound, the synthesis of which decreases during the continuous presence of the drug.[16,19] With benzodiazepines that have an intermediate half-life, rebound insomnia and anxiety frequently occur and are moderately intense. When benzodiazepines with long elimination half-lives are withdrawn, such effects occur infrequently and are relatively mild, presumably because the postulated endogenous benzodiazepine-like compound is partially restored before active drug metabolites are completely eliminated. Patients experiencing insomnia at night because of withdrawal of a short-acting benzodiazepine, taken nightly as a hypnotic, may also experience rebound anxiety during the day. Part of this anxiety may be caused by psychologic reactions to the sleep disturbance itself. On the other hand, patients experiencing rebound anxiety after withdrawal of a rapidly inactivated benzodiazepine taken chronically as an anxiolytic may also experience rebound insomnia at night.

Comparison of effectiveness of temazepam, triazolam, and flurazepam. The percentage   
of change in total wake time from baseline is illustrated for each of the three drugs (tem-
azepam [clear bar], triazolam [diagonally hatched bar], and flurazepam [stippled bar])
during short- (STD), intermediate- (ITD), and long-term (LTD) drug use. Data for triazolam
with long-term use were not included in the figure, since the drug was not studied beyond
2 weeks of continuous nightly usage. Statistically significant reductions in total wake time
were obtained with flurazepam on STD, ITD, and LTD and with triazolam on STD.

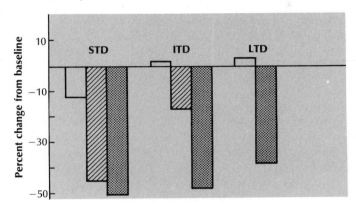

Flurazepam

    Flurazepam has been studied more extensively than any other hypnotic agent. With short-term administration of 30 mg of flurazepam, there is an appreciable improvement in sleep, both in terms of induction and maintenance.[15,16] Although sleep is significantly improved on the first night of drug administration, peak effectiveness of the drug occurs on the second and third consecutive drug nights. These data indicate that the short elimination half-life metabolites of the drug, hydroxyethylflurazepam and flurazepam aldehyde, account for much of its activity because the long half-life metabolite desalkylflurazepam is not available to affect sleep induction on the first night and is present only to a limited extent to affect sleep maintenance.[11,16]

    An important consideration is that the effectiveness of flurazepam, in contrast to that of most nonbenzodiazepine hypnotics and the more rapidly eliminated benzodiazepine hypnotics, is maintained with consecutive nightly administration of the drug over a 2-week period.[15,16] Even with long-term use of the drug (1 month), sleep is still greatly and significantly improved; there is only a slight loss of efficacy over this lengthy period of drug administration[24] (Fig. 26-1). This apparent lack of tolerance may reflect accumulation of desalkylflurazepam, which should require 10 to 20 days to reach steady state.

    During the first 2 to 3 nights after withdrawal of flurazepam, there is clear-cut evidence of carry-over effectiveness; that is, levels of total wake time remain somewhat below the baseline values.[16,19] The carry-over effect for flurazepam is an advantage not only in enhancing effectiveness but also in facilitating withdrawal. Serious rebound insomnia has not been demonstrated after withdrawal of the drug; the sleep disturbances have been mild in intensity and delayed in appearance.[24]

The incidence of adverse effects with flurazepam administration is generally low. Because of its carry-over, however, daytime sedation and performance decrements have been found to be greater with flurazepam than with more rapidly eliminated benzodiazepines.[13,24] These problems generally peak after the first several nights of drug administration and decrease as drug administration continues.[11,24] Short-term efficacy, effectiveness with continued use, and an absence of rebound phenomena after withdrawal have also been demonstrated with the 15 mg dose of flurazepam.[16] Since daytime sedation and performance decrement are much less frequent with the 15 mg dose, therapy should be initiated with this dose in the majority of patients, particularly the elderly.

Temazepam

The usefulness of temazepam is severely restricted by its ineffectiveness for inducing sleep, since difficulty in falling asleep is the most frequent complaint of insomniac subjects.[11,16] In the hard gelatin capsule formulation available in the United States, temazepam is slowly absorbed from the gastrointestinal tract; peak concentrations are reached an average of 2.5 hours after oral ingestion. The drug is moderately effective for maintaining sleep, but even so its effect on total wake time is limited (Fig. 26-1).

Since it takes so long for the drug to reach peak blood concentration and because it has an intermediate elimination half-life, there may be excessive drowsiness the next morning.[16] The U.S. formulation of temazepam should produce greater morning drowsiness and, possibly, performance decrements than the European preparation, since the latter is absorbed more quickly and lower doses are often used. Rebound insomnia often occurs after withdrawal, is moderate in intensity, and may be somewhat delayed. Increases in total time awake of greater than 50% over baseline levels have been reported.

Triazolam

Triazolam is absorbed rapidly, even after sublingual administration,[30] and is also inactivated rapidly so that there is little or no accumulation.[11] This drug therefore is the least likely to cause daytime drowsiness and performance decrements.[24] It may even be useful for overcoming "jet lag."[31] However, triazolam has several disadvantages, including relatively rapid development of tolerance, a strong potential for producing sleep disturbances, both during administration and after withdrawal, and the occurrence of serious behavioral side effects, particularly at higher doses.

With short-term use, triazolam is effective both for inducing and maintaining sleep.[16] However, sustained effectiveness with long-term nightly administration has not been clearly demonstrated. In one study[24] the drug appeared to maintain effectiveness for 5 weeks of therapy, but the sleep duration of the control group steadily increased over the same period. Data from some studies in which efficacy is claimed actually show that total sleep time increased by only 5 to 15 minutes, a rather small and clinically insignificant degree of change. Also, triazolam administration, partic-

Efficacy and withdrawal of triazolam. Changes in total wake time with administration and after withdrawal of triazolam, 0.5 mg. The ± standard error of the minutes of total wake time is represented by the vertical bars. Values are plotted for the following conditions: baseline (nights 2-4), initial (nights 5-7) and continued (nights 16-18) drug administration, and drug withdrawal (nights 19-21). The baseline mean is indicated by the broken line. The mean degree of worsening of sleep after withdrawal is considerably greater than even the maximum degree of improvement of sleep with drug administration. **FIG. 26-2**

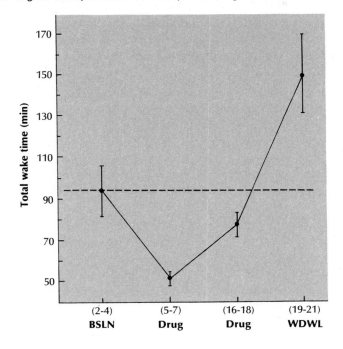

ularly when tolerance has developed, can produce significant increases in wakefulness during the final hours of drug nights (early morning insomnia) and in daytime anxiety or tension the next day.[18]

Since triazolam is rapidly eliminated, its withdrawal is usually accompanied by an immediate and intense degree of rebound insomnia.[16,19,24] Total awake time may increase two to three times over the level of the predrug nights. Early morning insomnia, daytime anxiety, and rebound insomnia are all factors that may reinforce drug-taking behavior and contribute to development of dependence (Fig. 26-2).

Memory impairment and even prolonged anterograde amnesia have been reported during administration of 0.5 mg of triazolam.[16] The occurrence of serious behavioral side effects (confusional states, depersonalization, severe anxiety, or hallucinations) during triazolam administration, reported from the Netherlands, has been attributed by others to patients taking doses higher than those clinically recommended. However, these doses were only 1 to 2 mg, and it is quite possible that the short half-life of triazolam, its high potency, and the occurrence of amnesia, early morning insomnia, daytime anxiety, and rebound insomnia all contribute to the development of adverse behavioral effects in susceptible persons.[16,19]

Midazolam

Midazolam is a short-acting compound that has the advantage of being more water soluble and less irritating than other injected benzodiazepines.[6] It is available in 2 ml disposable syringes and in 1 to 10 ml vials containing the drug in a solution so that reconstitution is unnecessary. Midazolam is used intravenously or intramuscularly to facilitate short diagnostic procedures and in anesthesia for preoperative sedation, for induction, and along with other agents for balanced anesthesia.[29]

BARBITURATES
Chemistry and
pharmacokinetics

Barbituric acid, the parent compound of the barbiturate series, is synthesized through the combination of urea and malonic acid.

Urea   **Malonic acid**   **Barbituric acid**

Barbituric acid has no hypnotic activity. Clinically useful barbiturates are synthesized by replacing the hydrogens at carbon position 5 of the molecule with alkyl or aryl groups. The resulting substances are weak acids that are at least 50% unionized in the body, except possibly in an alkaline urine. Pharmacokinetic variables such as absorption, distribution, protein-binding, metabolism, duration of action, and excretion of the barbiturates are influenced strongly by their lipid solubility and to a lesser extent by their degree of ionization. Substitution of sulfur for the oxygen at position 2 of pentobarbital and secobarbital yields thiopental and thiamylal respectively. The latter *ultrashort-acting* barbiturates are highly lipid-soluble, reach the brain very rapidly, and are used as anesthetics. In contrast, the long-acting barbiturates are much less lipid-soluble and reach the brain more slowly. In Table 26-2 the barbiturates are classified as ultrashort-, intermediate-, and long-acting drugs.

Central nervous system depression caused by barbiturates depends primarily on their general concentration in the brain, since they do not selectively concentrate in specific brain regions. Unlike with most drugs, the duration of action of a single dose of the ultrashort-acting drugs is not determined by metabolism or excretion. Because of their extreme lipid solubility, there is virtually no barrier to their passage into tissues. Therefore the major factor affecting uptake is blood flow to each organ. After administration of an intravenous bolus of thiopental, its concentration in the brain, which is well perfused, almost immediately equilibrates with the plasma

Generic name	Trade name	Elimination half-life (hr)	Clinical use	Dosage (mg)	Route of administration
Long acting					
Barbital			Hypnotic	300-500	Oral
Butabarbital	Butisol	34-42	Hypnotic	100-200	Oral
Phenobarbital	Luminal	24-140	Hypnotic	100-200	Oral
Intermediate acting					
Amobarbital	Amytal	8-42	Hypnotic	100-200	Oral
Aprobarbital	Alurate	14-34	Hypnotic	120	Oral
Pentobarbital	Nembutal	15-48	Hypnotic	100	Oral
Secobarbital	Seconal	19-34	Hypnotic	100	Oral
Talbutal	Lotusate	15	Hypnotic	120	Oral
Ultrashort acting					
Thiopental	Pentothal	3-6	Anesthetic	2.5%*; 0.3%†	Intravenous
Thiamylal	Surital		Anesthetic	2.5%*; 0.3%†	Intravenous
Methohexital	Brevital	1-2	Anesthetic	1.0%*; 0.2%†	Intravenous

TABLE 26-2 Barbiturates: elimination half-life and clinical data

*Concentration of intravenous solution for induction of anesthesia.
†Concentration of a continuous intravenous drip when used as a sole anesthetic.

concentration of free drug, and anesthesia occurs. As other, less well vascularized tissues continue to take up thiopental from the blood, plasma and brain concentrations decrease. Within a few minutes the brain concentration drops to below the threshold for anesthesia and consciousness returns. Thus rapid *redistribution* from the brain to other tissues is responsible for the brief period of anesthesia.

The barbiturates are metabolized by liver microsomal enzymes to more water-soluble compounds, which are then more readily excreted in urine. This accounts for the eventual removal of the ultrashort-acting agents as well. The long-acting barbiturate phenobarbital is metabolized slowly, and as a consequence a significant amount is excreted unchanged in the urine. Excretion of phenobarbital is enhanced by an alkaline urinary pH, a fact that is important in management of intoxication with this drug. Because of the roles of the liver and kidney in the metabolism and excretion of barbiturates, diseases of these organs may significantly prolong the actions of these agents.

Barbiturates depress the activity of all brain cells; however, the diffuse pathways in the brainstem known as the "reticular activating system" are especially sensitive.[22] Low doses of the drugs appear to enhance the effects of the inhibitory neurotransmitter GABA or to have GABA-like activity, presumably by acting at the *picrotoxinin* receptor (see Chapter 23).

Sites and mechanism of action

Clinical and miscellaneous effects

Ultrashort-acting barbiturates are used in anesthesia for induction as well as for supplementation of inhalation agents. Their main advantage is that rapid onset and redistribution in the body allows minute-to-minute adjustment of their effect during intravenous infusion. The intermediate-acting barbiturates have been extensively used as hypnotics and have been shown in both sleep laboratory and clinical trials to be effective initially for inducing and maintaining sleep. However, much of their effectiveness is lost with continued administration over a 2-week period.[15] Such tolerance may explain why some patients take excessive doses of the drug; they can then become dependent and experience an abstinence syndrome when attempting to discontinue the drug.[7,12]

The available barbiturates, in general, inhibit development of seizures. They can abolish convulsions secondary to tetanus and eclampsia and are effective antidotes for convulsant drugs. Phenobarbital is more selectively antiepileptic, however, in that it is often useful for chronic management of grand mal and jacksonian epilepsy without excessive drowsiness.

Paradoxically, in certain persons or if pain is present, barbiturates may produce restlessness, excitement, and delirium. Elderly people are generally more prone to carry-over effects and to become confused or agitated.

Intoxication

The most serious drawback of barbiturates as hypnotics relates to their narrow margin of safety; only 10 times the therapeutic dose may be lethal. As an example, barbiturates were implicated in over 21% of all drug-related (not including carbon monoxide) deaths in Maryland from 1975 through 1980.[4] Since insomnia may be a symptom of depression with suicidal potential, safety is an important issue in prescribing barbiturates as hypnotics.

Large doses of barbiturates depress the respiratory center and especially decrease its responsiveness to carbon dioxide. Low blood pressure in barbiturate poisoning may be secondary to hypoxia or, in very severe cases, may result from direct depression of central and peripheral elements of the autonomic nervous system. Such effects on respiration and circulation are commonly the cause of early death from barbiturate overdosage. As with opiate intoxication, miosis and coma also occur, but barbiturate poisoning is not dramatically reversed by naloxone. A flat electroencephalographic tracing in this setting does not denote brain death. Treatment of intoxication is symptomatic and supportive, with particular attention to maintenace of patent airways along with oxygen administration and mechanical ventilation, if necessary. Additional measures are directed toward removal (emesis, lavage) and inactivation (activated charcoal) of residual drug in the stomach, restoration of blood pressure, if improved ventilation does not reverse hypotension, and maintenance of urine flow, body temperature, and so on. There is no specific chemical antidote, and the use of analeptic drugs (see Chapter 27) is not recommended and may be harmful. A clinically beneficial increase in excretion can be achieved for *long-acting barbiturates only* by alkalinization of the urine and forced diuresis. Hemodialysis and particularly hemoperfusion increase clearance of any barbiturate, though again it is easier to remove the longer-acting agents.

Whenever other drugs are administered in combination with barbiturates, potential interactions should be carefully considered, since the effects of these drugs may be additive to those of the barbiturates, thereby creating potential clinical hazards. Alcohol, reserpine, and neuroleptics, as well as sedative-hypnotics belonging to other drug classes, may enhance the depressant effect of barbiturates. Such interactions can lead to serious impairment of daytime performance or to respiratory depression with relatively low doses of barbiturates.

Other significant drug interactions encountered with barbiturates arise from their ability to induce hepatic microsomal enzymes. Chronic administration of barbiturates can increase the metabolism of drugs such as phenytoin and coumarin anticoagulants. Moreover, if the dosage of a drug is then increased to compensate for enhanced metabolism, discontinuation of barbiturate administration may result in an exaggerated response to this other drug as its rate of metabolism reverts toward normal.

Barbiturates may also induce a mitochondrial enzyme, δ-aminolevulinic acid synthetase, and for this reason are contraindicated in patients with *acute intermittent*[36] or *variegate prophyrias* in whom they can precipitate neuronal demyelination.

Barbiturates can produce both psychologic and physiologic dependence.[7,12] The abstinence syndrome after abrupt withdrawal of barbiturates from a drug-dependent person is characterized by anxiety, irritability, insomnia, restlessness, and tremors. If dependence is pronounced, even convulsions can occur, and withdrawal may be more dangerous than withdrawal from an opiate. (See Chapter 30 for further discussion of abuse of this type of drug.)

Before development of benzodiazepine hypnotics, which currently dominate among prescribed sleeping pills, several agents besides barbiturates were used as hypnotics. Ethchlorvynol (Placidyl) and ethinamate (Valmid) are short-acting drugs that are less effective than most of the commonly used hypnotics. Glutethimide (Doriden) and methyprylon (Noludar) are intermediate-acting drugs. Poisoning with glutethimide presents a particular hazard because the drug is more prone to depress the cardiovascular system and is not effectively removed by hemodialysis or hemoperfusion. Methaqualone (Quaalude) is a fast-acting hypnotic that is frequently abused. It was recently reclassified as a Schedule I drug and is no longer manufactured legally in this country. These agents have as great a potential for tolerance and dependence as the barbiturates, and there appears to be little indication for their use. Two of the older hypnotics, chloral hydrate and paraldehyde, can still be useful on rare occasions.

Chloral hydrate

Chloral hydrate was introduced in 1869 and is still used occasionally. It is rapidly reduced in vivo to trichloroethanol, CCl_3CH_2OH, the active form of the drug. Chloral hydrate is short acting and has been especially useful in pediatric and geriatric patients in whom it is less likely than barbiturates to cause excitation. The recommended dose is 0.5 to 1 g, but 2 g may be required. Preparations for oral (Noctec, Oradrate) and rectal (Aquachloral) administration are available. Tolerance to its hypnotic effect occurs after about 2 weeks of continued use. In its concentrated form, chloral hydrate can cause gastric irritation. **Triclofos** (Triclos), an ester of trichloroethanol that shares the properties of chloral hydrate, is somewhat less potent; the usual dose is 1.5 g.

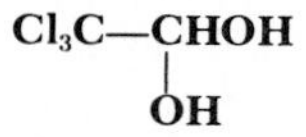

$$Cl_3C—CHOH$$
$$|$$
$$OH$$

Chloral hydrate

The toxicity of chloral hydrate is generally low. The lethal dose may range between 3 and 30 g. Although usual hypnotic doses have no detectable effect on the heart, overdosage may adversely affect cardiac muscle. Thus chloral hydrate should be avoided in patients suffering from heart disease. Finally, administration of chloral hydrate can acutely potentiate other protein-bound drugs, such as warfarin, phenytoin, or tolbutamide, since trichloroethanol is partially metabolized to trichloroacetic acid, which is tightly bound to serum albumin and displaces other drugs from their binding sites.

Paraldehyde

Paraldehyde (Paral) is a cyclic ether, a trimer of acetaldehyde to which it decomposes on exposure to light and oxygen. In the liver both paraldehyde and ethanol are transformed initially to acetaldehyde, and paraldehyde should not be given to patients taking disulfiram (see p. 297).

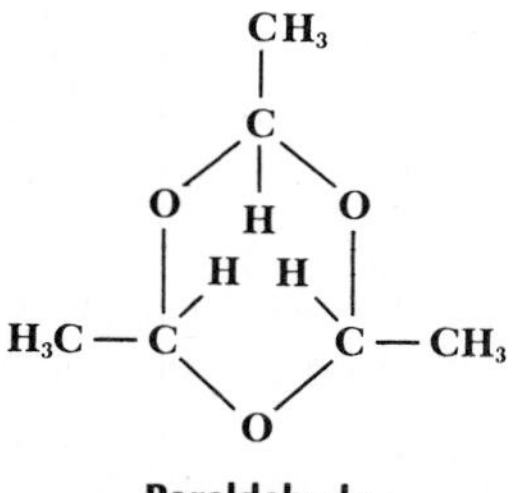

Paraldehyde

The drug is a liquid that has a strong odor and a characteristic, disagreeable taste. It is usually administered in a cold beverage to disguise its taste. An effective hypnotic dose is 10 to 30 ml at bedtime. Currently, paraldehyde is almost exclusively used in management of hospitalized patients undergoing alcohol withdrawal, though a double-blind, controlled comparison has proved benzodiazepines to be superior.

Paraldehyde has also been used in patients with convulsive states such as eclampsia or tetanus in whom intravenous (well diluted) or intramuscular administration may be necessary. It is also used for patients with renal shutdown, since up to a third of the drug is eliminated through the lungs, and the remainder is metabolized ultimately to carbon dioxide and water.

Because of its irritant effect, paraldehyde should not be administered orally to patients suffering from inflammatory conditions or ulcers in the esophageal, gastric, or duodenal regions. Similarly, rectal administration should be avoided in patients with inflammatory conditions in this region.

Over-the-counter hypnotics

Nowadays nonprescription sleep medications contain an antihistamine, usually diphenhydramine or pyrilamine. The manufacturers' intent is to use the sedative side effect of the antihistamine to facilitate sleep. In the past scopolamine and bromide were common ingredients. The widespread availability of such over-the-counter (OTC) medications might be justified if they are indeed effective in relieving insomnia. As with many prescription drugs, however, claims of efficacy of OTC preparations in inducing or maintaining sleep have not been verified.

Many insomniacs, fearing addiction to prescription hypnotics, may turn to nonprescription medications in the belief that they are safer. However, clinical disturbances have been reported with varied dosages of these drugs. Because of the antimuscarinic activity of antihistamines, even recommended doses of these drugs may precipitate glaucoma, especially in elderly patients prone to narrow-angle glaucoma. Two to three times the recommended dosage can cause transient disorientation or even hallucinations, especially in emotionally unstable persons. With a considerable overdose of these drugs (15 to 30 tablets), a stuporous state, confusion, extreme psychiatric disturbance, coma, and even death have been reported.

TREATMENT OF INSOMNIA

Hypnotics are only an adjunctive component of the overall therapy of insomnia.[5,17,33] Effective evaluation and management of this condition is dependent on a thorough knowledge of its multifaceted nature. Insomnia is by far the most prevalent sleep disorder; over 40% of the population report a current or past problem. The complaint of insomnia is more frequent with increasing age, in women, and in persons with high levels of psychologic distress.

Transient sleep disturbances are extremely prevalent and may relate to situational problems at home or at work or involving finances. Jet travel or changes in work shift may disrupt circadian rhythms and disturb sleep. Medical conditions with significant pain, physical discomfort, anxiety, or depression are likely to produce complaints of insomnia.

Pharmacologic agents themselves can disrupt sleep. Insomnia can result from stimulant drugs, steroids, antidepressants, or β-adrenergic receptor blockers, particularly when these drugs are taken near bedtime. Coffee or cola drinks as well as cigarette smoking may delay sleep, whereas alcohol consumption can lead to early morning awakenings. Abrupt withdrawal of high doses of nonbenzodiazepine or benzodiazepine hypnotics can cause an abstinence syndrome that may include both insomnia and nightmares. Benzodiazepines with a rapid elimination rate may produce early morning insomnia. Aging is also a factor contributing to disturbed sleep; the elderly sleep less and have very little of the deeper sleep at stages 3 and 4.

Although medical conditions and aging may often contribute to the problem of chronic insomnia, psychopathology is by far the predominant etiologic factor. Personality patterns of most patients with chronic insomnia are characterized by an internalization of emotions. Retrospective studies indicate that chronic insomnia may develop in persons who are predisposed to having inadequate coping mechanisms when life-stress factors are prevalent.

A thorough evaluation of patients with chronic insomnia includes taking sleep, drug, and psychiatric histories. The sleep history should include determination of the specific sleep problem and assessment of its clinical course, exclusion of other sleep disorders, evaluation of sleep/wakefulness patterns, questioning of close family members, and evaluation of the impact of the sleep problem on the patient's life.

The drug history should include information on current use of prescribed and nonprescribed medication and the timing of its administration, particularly in relation to bedtime. In terms of past drug use, the focus is on dosage and length of administration of any sedative-hypnotics recently discontinued. Also included is a review of current or past use of substances such as alcohol, caffeine, and nicotine.

Since transient insomnia usually develops in reaction to some immediate stress, it can be expected to subside when the person adapts through his or her own coping mechanisms. If the stress-generating situation cannot be eliminated, the physician is best able to help by identifying adaptive coping mechanisms and by aiding the patient to strengthen them.

Treatment of chronic insomnia is more complex, since chronic insomnia is multifaceted; any approach directed to only one of the factors involved will usually be inadequate. In general, the most effective treatment for the patient with chronic insomnia combines the following elements: (1) nonpharmacologic treatment, including improvement of sleep hygiene (regularizing schedules including time for bed, gradually increasing levels of physical exercise during the day, restricting the use of caffeinated beverages, and avoiding the use of alcohol as a sedative), supportive counseling, behavioral therapy, and psychotherapy and (2) pharmacologic treatment consisting in adjunctive use of hypnotic medication or the use of antidepressant medication. A hypnotic with an intermediate elimination half-life of 8 to 10 hours may be the best choice.[27]

ALCOHOL   As a medicinal agent, **ethanol** (ethyl alcohol) is only of moderate importance. It has great toxicologic interest, however, and chronic alcoholism is one of the great social problems of humankind.

The main action of alcohol is exerted on the central nervous system. It may be regarded as an unusual hypnotic and as an anesthetic with a very low margin of safety. There is general agreement that the apparent stimulant action of the drug is a consequence of primary depression of higher centers, resulting in uninhibited behavior. A variety of mechanisms, including changes in membrane fluidity[34] and interactions with the GABA system,[20] have been proposed to account for its effects and for central tolerance. In addition to actions on behavior and consciousness, alcohol influences cardiovascular, gastrointestinal, and renal functions.

Pharmacologic effects

Cutaneous vasodilatation and a feeling of warmth are generally observed after ingestion of an alcoholic beverage. This vasodilatation is attributable, at least partially, to central nervous system actions affecting thermoregulation,[14] though a direct action of the drug on blood vessels may contribute as well.[1] There is a popular impression that alcohol dilates coronary vessels, but it does not prevent electrocardiographic evidence of coronary insufficiency after exercise. Adverse myocardial responses, in particular congestive cardiomyopathy, are commonly associated with chronic alcoholism.

Although evidence is lacking in humans, ingestion of alcohol is generally believed to promote secretion of acid gastric juice. Small doses of alcohol are said to improve appetite, whereas excessive concentrations, either acutely or chronically, can impair the mucosal barrier to acid diffusion and cause gastritis.[3] Alcohol also has adverse effects on the esophagus and on lower esophageal sphincter pressure that contribute to reflux and esophagitis.

The diuresis observed in persons who drink alcoholic beverages is partly caused by ingestion of water. Alcohol also inhibits release of antidiuretic hormone (ADH) from the posterior pituitary. On the other hand, liver disease associated with chronic abuse may cause an elevated ADH level and water retention.

The influence of alcohol on carbohydrate and lipid metabolism has received much attention. Alcoholism is a common cause of hypoglycemia,[23] which can be induced in humans by ingestion of 35 to 50 ml of ethanol after a 2-day fast. Such persons must have low liver glycogen because they do not respond to glucagon with the characteristic increase in blood glucose. Animal studies indicate that alcohol inhibits gluconeogenesis.

It is quite likely that acute hyperlipemia after alcohol ingestion and the hyperlipemia of the chronic alcoholic develop through different mechanisms. The acute hyperlipemia is probably mediated by sympathetic activation, with subsequent lipolysis from fat depots, since it can be prevented by β-adrenergic receptor blocking agents. In contrast, hyperlipemia in the chronic alcoholic may depend largely on deficient removal of lipid from the blood. Evidence for decreased lipoprotein lipase activity in alcoholic patients has been presented.

Fatty livers are commonly observed in alcoholic patients. The most likely explanations would appear to be (1) increased mobilization from fat deposits, (2) increased

TABLE 26-3	Relative concentration of alcohol in various body fluids, tissues, and alveolar air (concentration in blood is 1.0)
Serum	1.15
Urine	1.3
Saliva	1.3
Spinal fluid	1.15
Brain or liver	0.85 to 0.90
Kidney	0.83
Alveolar air	0.0005 of blood concentration

esterification to triglycerides rather than to phospholipids and cholesterol esters, and (3) decreased triglyceride release from the liver.

Local injection of alcohol can destroy neuronal pathways and is used to provide permanent or, at least, prolonged nerve block in such conditions as trigeminal neuralgia and terminal cancer. The sponging of alcohol on the skin to enhance heat loss in fever has led to acute intoxication in children, and it is now recommended that tepid water be used instead. Alcohol is also used as a disinfectant and as a solvent for many drugs.

Kinetics   Alcohol is absorbed rapidly from the stomach and small intestine. The rate of absorption is influenced by the concentration of the alcohol ingested and most importantly by the presence of food in the stomach. On an empty stomach the drinking of an alcoholic beverage produces peak blood concentration in less than 1 hour. There may be a considerable delay if the stomach is filled with food.

Once absorbed, alcohol is distributed in total body water. Its concentration in different tissues and body fluids correlates well with the concentration of water at these sites. If the concentration of alcohol in blood is assigned the value of 1.0, the relative values given in Table 26-3 may be expected in the various body fluids, tissues, and alveolar air.

The concentration of alcohol in blood has great medicolegal importance, since it is generally accepted that a blood alcohol concentration of 100 mg/100 ml (0.10%) indicates intoxication. It is of some importance to know also the relationship between the quantity of alcohol ingested and the blood concentration that may be expected. The concentration of alcohol in blood will depend on (1) the quantity of alcohol ingested and the rate at which it was drunk, (2) the speed of absorption, (3) the body weight and the percentage of total body water, and (4) the rate of alcohol metabolism.

Approximate blood concentrations of alcohol after ingestion of various alcoholic beverages can be calculated. If intoxication occurs at a concentration of 0.10%, it can be calculated that this will occur if approximately 6 fluid ounces of a distilled spirit containing 45% alcohol is drunk rapidly. If a distilled spirit is drunk over a

Concentration of alcohol in blood of an automobile driver relative to his being "under the   FIG. 26-3
influence."

From Harger, R.N. In Economos, J.P., and Kreml, F.M., editors: Judge and prosecutor in traffic court, Chicago, 1951, American Bar
Association and The Traffic Institute, Northwestern University.

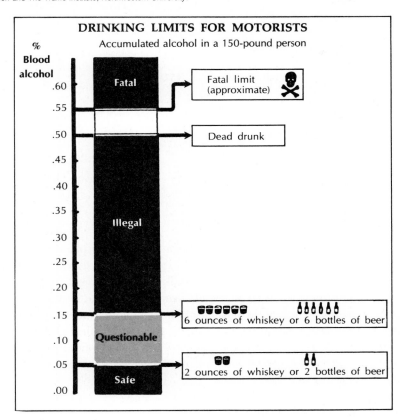

period of several hours, the number of ounces required to produce a blood level of
0.15% may be calculated by the following formula:

$8 + H$ = Number of ounces of distilled spirits required to cause intoxication

where H is the number of hours during which the beverage is drunk.

The corresponding formula for fortified wine (containing 20% alcohol) is $18 + 2H$;
for ordinary wine (containing 10% alcohol) it is $36 + 4H$; for beer (containing 4.5%
alcohol) the figure would be $80 + 10H$.

Relationships between ingestion of whiskey and beer, blood concentrations of
alcohol, and ability to drive an automobile are depicted in Fig. 26-3.

The quantity of alcohol excreted in the urine, exhaled through the lungs, and
lost in perspiration ordinarily represents less than 10% of the total ingested. The

remainder is metabolized; the end products are carbon dioxide and water. The steps in hepatic transformation of alcohol are indicated below:

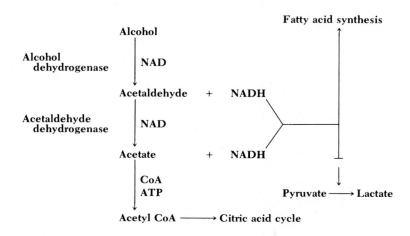

The first step occurs in the cytosol, whereas the second takes place mainly in mitochondria. Alcohol is also broken down to some extent by the microsomal system and can affect metabolism of many drugs that are handled by this system. In general, acute ingestion of alcohol tends to decrease metabolism of other drugs, and chronic alcoholism tends to increase their metabolism (until hepatic impairment supervenes).[21,26]

The average person metabolizes 6 to 8 g (7.5 to 10 ml) of alcohol per hour. This figure is fairly constant for a given individual and is independent of the quantity present in the body (a *zero-order reaction*). Habitual drinkers may metabolize alcohol slightly more rapidly than abstainers.

Metabolism of 1 g of alcohol yields 7 calories. Since the maximal amount that can be metabolized in 24 hours is approximately 170 g, alcohol can contribute up to 1200 calories per day to the metabolic requirement of a person.

Tolerance and acute intoxication   It is well known that the experienced drinker shows fewer and less noticeable responses to moderate amounts of alcohol than the abstainer does. This "tolerance" cannot be explained on the basis of what is known about absorption, distribution, and metabolism in the chronic alcoholic. It is concluded therefore that the experienced drinker has learned to behave and to perform habitual tasks at blood alcohol concentrations that would seriously disturb the unaccustomed person. This apparent tolerance does not appear to extend to the lethal effects of alcohol, and blood concentrations exceeding 550 mg/100 ml may produce death in the chronic alcoholic. If the person has taken some other central nervous system depressant such as a barbiturate, even lower alcohol concentrations may result in a lethal outcome. Acute intoxication with alcohol alone was implicated in 14% of drug- and chemical-related deaths (not including carbon monoxide) in Maryland from 1975 through 1980, and alcohol was present in over a third of the intoxications overall.[4]

The severely intoxicated patient represents a medical emergency and should be managed according to the following recommendations[28]:

1. Respiratory support should be given if necessary.
2. Aspiration of vomitus should be prevented by placement of the patient in the semilateral decubitus position with head forward and mouth down.
3. Fluid needs should be assessed. The patient may be fluid overloaded or may have a fluid deficit.
4. Gastric lavage can be helpful provided that airways are protected.
5. Hypoglycemia is suspected on the basis of unusual neurologic findings, such as convulsions or coma. Intravenous glucose and thiamine are recommended.
6. Metabolic acidosis, if severe, may require use of sodium bicarbonate.
7. Hemodialysis may be useful in patients with greatly excessive blood concentrations of alcohol.
8. Fructose and other measures that supposedly increase the rate of metabolism of alcohol are not recommended.

Chronic alcoholism

A variety of pathologic changes occur in alcoholics with much greater frequency than in the general population. Chronic gastritis, cirrhosis of the liver, peripheral polyneuropathy, and the neuropsychiatric condition known as Korsakoff's syndrome have received considerable attention. The mechanisms responsible for these abnormalities are not always clear because the alcoholic often suffers from nutritional deficiencies as well. Thiamine deficiency results in Wernicke's encephalopathy, for example. When aided by psychiatric treatment or the organization known as Alcoholics Anonymous, about 50% of alcoholics may be able to abstain from drinking.

Another approach to the problem, which may facilitate abstinence in the well-motivated patient, has been the administration of drugs that make the effects of alcohol extremely unpleasant or even dangerous. The best known of these is disulfiram. Several factors that complicate design of clinical trials of the efficacy of disulfiram have been discussed,[9] and there are many contraindications to its use.[32] A recent trial using outpatients found that although it reduced the mean number of drinking days disulfiram did not affect the incidence of total abstinence over a 1-year period relative to control groups.[8] Those subjects, regardless of their treatment group, who were judged to be compliant were more likely to have been abstinent as well. Other drugs that create intolerance to alcohol and may elicit a similar reaction include citrated calcium cyanamide, hypoglycemic sulfonylureas, chloramphenicol, furazolidone, griseofulvin, metronidazole, quinacrine,[32] isoniazid, and cephalosporins with a tetrazolethiomethyl group, such as cefoperazone.

DISULFIRAM

The development of the disulfiram approach to chronic alcoholism was the consequence of a chance observation. While certain new drugs were being tested as potential anthelmintics, it was observed that after ingestion of disulfiram even a few bottles of beer caused very unpleasant side effects. Careful study of this unusual occurrence led to discovery of the mechanism and to the introduction of disulfiram into therapeutics.

Disulfiram (Antabuse) is tetraethylthiuram disulfide. Certain other disulfides have similar properties with respect to alcohol intolerance. If alcohol is ingested several hours after disulfiram is taken in doses of 1 to 2 g, the person develops a typical reaction characterized by nausea, vomiting, flushing, palpitation, and headache. There may be a fall in blood pressure and occasionally shock. These symptoms are sufficiently unpleasant that the patient is unlikely to drink alcohol while maintained on disulfiram. When drug administration is stopped, it may take a week or more for intolerance to alcohol to disappear. Disulfiram by itself can cause drowsiness, a metallic taste, diminished libido, and skin reactions.

Disulfiram

When a patient ingests alcohol while maintained on disulfiram, the blood concentration of acetaldehyde increases. Acetaldehyde levels in this condition may be of the order of 1 mg/100 ml. Intravenous infusion of acetaldehyde, to produce comparable blood concentrations, reproduces the manifestations of the *Antabuse reaction*. Disulfiram, likewise, delays metabolism of acetaldehyde given to experimental animals. From such results it has been concluded that disulfiram inhibits the second step in alcohol metabolism, the oxidation of acetaldehyde. This intermediate has both vasoconstrictor and vasodilator actions,[2] but hypotension characterizes the Antabuse reaction. Acetaldehyde also releases catecholamines to increase heart rate and cardiac output and may affect the pharmacokinetics of other amines that contribute to symptoms of the reaction.

Initially, after a patient is alcohol free, disulfiram is usually administered as a single morning dose of 500 mg. After a week or two, the dose is reduced to 250 or even 125 mg.

OTHER ALCOHOLS

Aliphatic alcohols other than ethanol are of interest in medicine largely because they are sometimes involved in cases of poisoning.

Methanol

Generally the toxicity of the alcohols increases with chain length, an exception being methanol, which is unique in producing pronounced acidosis and blindness in primates but not in lower animals. Intoxication with methanol usually occurs from drinking "denatured" alcohol, that is, ethanol to which methanol (wood alcohol, methyl alcohol) has been added expressly to prevent its use as a beverage. Methanol is slowly converted by alcohol dehydrogenase to formaldehyde, which is rapidly oxidized to formic acid. The presence of ethanol slows the metabolism of methanol so that poisoning may be obscured until the ethanol is largely inactivated. As little as 30 ml of methanol has caused serious poisoning, and even death has been attributed to this quantity or less. In addition to acidosis, methanol intoxication involves the central nervous system, with the production of headache, dizziness, delirium, and coma. Blindness appears to be a consequence of formic acid toxicity on the retina.

Treatment of the life-threatening acidosis is based primarily on its correction with sodium bicarbonate. Therapeutic administration of ethanol, based on the competition between the alcohols for metabolism, can be lifesaving and is likely to provide protection from blindness. Ethanol concentrations of 0.1% or higher may need to be maintained for several days.[35] Hemodialysis can be instituted to efficiently remove the methanol while ethanol is used to block methanol metabolism. In so doing, ethanol administration must be increased because it too is removed by the dialysis.

Ethylene glycol is another alcohol metabolized by alcohol dehydrogenase. Intoxication results in formation of glyoxylic, formic, and oxalic acids.[37] These cause central nervous system depression, systemic acidosis, and oxalate crystalluria, which may contribute to acute renal failure. Treatment is the same as for methanol intoxication, including administration of ethanol.

Isopropyl alcohol (isopropanol) is of some toxicologic interest also. It is metabolized to acetone in the body. Severe renal damage is found in patients who have recovered from ingestion of a few ounces of isopropyl alcohol. The fatal dose is estimated as 120 to 240 ml.

A variety of adverse central nervous system effects and death in 10 premature infants was attributed to benzyl alcohol used as a preservative in solutions given intravenously.[10]

Miscellaneous alcohols or glycols

REFERENCES

1. Altura, B.M., and Altura, B.T.: Microvascular and vascular smooth muscle actions of ethanol, acetaldehyde, and acetate, Fed. Proc. 41:2447, 1982.
2. Brien, J.F., and Loomis, C.W.: Pharmacology of acetaldehyde, Can. J. Physiol. Pharmacol. 61:1, 1983.
3. Burbige, E.J., Lewis, D.R., Jr., and Halsted, C.H.: Alcohol and the gastrointestinal tract, Med. Clin. North. Am. 68:77, 1984.
4. Caplan, Y.H., Ottinger, W.E., Park, J., and Smith, T.D.: Drug and chemical related deaths: incidence in the state of Maryland—1975 to 1980, J. Forens. Sci. 30:1012, 1985.
5. Consensus Development Conference Summary: Drugs and insomnia, Bethesda, Md., 1984, National Institutes of Health.
6. Davis, P.J., and Cook, D.R.: Clinical pharmacokinetics of the newer intravenous anaesthetic agents, Clin. Pharmacokinet. 11:18, 1986.
7. Essig, C.F.: Addiction to nonbarbiturate sedative and tranquilizing drugs, Clin. Pharmacol. Ther. 5:334, 1964.
8. Fuller, R.K., Branchey, L., Brightwell, D.R., et al.: Disulfiram treatment of alcoholism: a Veterans Administration cooperative study, J.A.M.A. 256:1449, 1986.
9. Fuller, R.K., Williford, W.O., Lee, K.K., and Derman, R.: Veterans Administration Cooperative Study of disulfiram in the treatment of alcoholism: study design and methodological considerations, Controlled Clin. Trials 5:263, 1984.
10. Gershanik, J., Boecler, B., Ensley, H., et al.: The gasping syndrome and benzyl alcohol poisoning, N. Engl. J. Med. 307:1384, 1982.

11. Greenblatt, D.J., Divoll, M., Abernethy, D.R., and Shader, R.I.: Benzodiazepine hypnotics: kinetic and therapeutic options, Sleep 5:S18, 1982.

12. Isbell, H., and Fraser, H.F.: Addiction to analgesics and barbiturates, Pharmacol. Rev. 2:355, 1950.

13. Johnson, L.C., and Chernik, D.A.: Sedative-hypnotics and human performance, Psychopharmacology 76:101, 1982.

14. Kalant, H., and Lê, A.D.: Effects of ethanol on thermoregulation, Pharmacol. Ther. 23:313, 1984.

15. Kales, A., Bixler, E.O., Kales, J.D., and Scharf, M.B.: Comparative effectiveness of nine hypnotic drugs: sleep laboratory studies, J. Clin. Pharmacol. 17:207, 1977.

16. Kales, A., and Kales, J.D.: Sleep laboratory studies of hypnotic drugs: efficacy and withdrawal effects, J. Clin. Psychopharmacol. 3:140, 1983.

17. Kales, A., Kales, J.D., and Soldatos, C.R.: Insomnia and other sleep disorders, Med. Clin. North Am. 66:971, 1982.

18. Kales, A., Soldatos, C.R., Bixler, E.O., and Kales, J.D.: Early morning insomnia with rapidly eliminated benzodiazepines, Science 220:95, 1983.

19. Kales, A., Soldatos, C.R., Bixler, E.O., and Kales, J.D.: Rebound insomnia and rebound anxiety: a review, Pharmacology 26:121, 1983.

20. Kulonen, E.: Ethanol and GABA, Med. Biol. 61:147, 1983.

21. Lieber, C.S.: Metabolism and metabolic effects of alcohol, Med. Clin. North Am. 68:3, 1984.

22. Magoun, H.W.: The waking brain, ed. 2, Springfield, Ill., 1963, Charles C Thomas, Publisher.

23. Malouf, R., and Brust, J.C.M.: Hypoglycemia: causes, neurological manifestations, and outcome, Ann. Neurol. 17:421, 1985.

24. Mitler, M.M., Seidel, W.F., van den Hoed, J., et al.: Comparative hypnotic effects of flurazepam, triazolam, and placebo: a long-term simultaneous nighttime and daytime study, J. Clin. Psychopharmacol, 4:2, 1984.

25. Möhler, H., and Richards, J.G.: Receptors for anxiolytic drugs. In Malick, J.B., Enna, S.J., and Yamamura, H.I., editors: Anxiolytics: neurochemical, behavioral, and clinical perspectives, New York, 1983, Raven Press, p. 15.

26. Muhoberac, B.B., Roberts, R.K., Hoyumpa, A.M., Jr., and Schenker, S.: Mechanism(s) of ethanol-drug interaction, Alcoholism Clin. Exp. Res. 8:583, 1984.

27. Oswald, I.: Hypnotic drugs for 1984. In Hindmarch, I., Ott, H., and Roth, T., editors: Sleep, benzodiazepines and performance: experimental methodologies and research prospects, Berlin, 1984, Springer-Verlag, p. 84.

28. Redetzki, H.M.: Treatment of ethanol intoxication, Hosp. Formulary, p. 934, Oct. 1979.

29. Reves, J.G., Fragen, R.J., Vinik, H.R., and Greenblatt, D.J.: Midazolam: pharmacology and uses, Anesthesiology 62:310, 1985.

30. Scavone, J.M., Greenblatt, D.J., Friedman, H., and Shader, R.I.: Enhanced bioavailability of triazolam following sublingual versus oral administration, J. Clin. Pharmacol. 26:208, 1986.

31. Seidel, W.F., Roth, T., Roehrs, T., et al.: Treatment of a 12-hour shift of sleep

schedule with benzodiazepines, Science **224**:1262, 1984.

32. Sellers, E.M., Naranjo, C.A., and Peachey, J.E.: Drugs to decrease alcohol consumption, N. Engl. J. Med. **305**:1255, 1981.

33. Soldatos, C.R., Kales, A., and Kales, J.D.: Management of insomnia, Annu. Rev. Med. **30**:301, 1979.

34. Taraschi, T.F., and Rubin, E.: Biology of disease: effects of ethanol on the chemical and structural properties of biologic membranes, Lab. Invest. **52**:120, 1985.

35. Tephly, T.R., Makar, A.B., McMartin, K.E., et al.: Methanol: its metabolism and toxicity. In Majchrowicz, E., and Noble, E.P., editors: Biochemistry and pharmacology of ethanol, vol. 1, New York, 1979, Plenum Press, p. 145.

36. Tschudy, D.P., Valsamis, M., and Magnussen, C.R.: Acute intermittent porphyria: clinical and selected research aspects, Ann. Intern. Med. **83**:851, 1975.

37. Turk, J., Morell, L., and Avioli, L.V.: Ethylene glycol intoxication, Arch. Intern. Med. **146**:1601, 1986.

Chapter 27

Central nervous system stimulants of the convulsant type

GENERAL CONCEPT

Analeptic agents cause two potentially beneficial effects: they promote generalized arousal, and they increase the rate and depth of respiration. Important sites of action to elicit these effects are the reticular activating system and the vital centers in the medulla. Unfortunately, analeptics also work in corticospinal pathways to raise levels of reflex excitability, which can lead to convulsions.[14] Analeptics are of toxicologic interest (strychnine), are tools for basic research on neurotransmission (bicuculline, pentylenetetrazol, picrotoxin), or may be used as respiratory stimulants (doxapram, nikethamide). They may excite neurons directly (doxapram), block presynaptic inhibition (picrotoxin), or block postsynaptic inhibition (strychnine). The methylxanthines, which are caffeine, theophylline, and theobromine, generally cause more mild central nervous system stimulation though toxic doses can elicit seizures. Theobromine is the least potent of these and is not used medicinally. Theophylline is used primarily for its peripheral action to dilate bronchi and is discussed in Chapter 40.

CENTRAL NERVOUS SYSTEM STIMULANTS

The older analeptics pentylenetetrazol, picrotoxin, and nikethamide have a low margin of safety between their analeptic and convulsant doses and have been replaced by agents with a more favorable margin, such as doxapram.

Pentylenetetrazol

There is much experience with the convulsant action of pentylenetetrazol (once available as Metrazol) in humans because the drug was used in shock treatment for mental disease and, in lower doses, in diagnosis of epilepsy. When approximately 5 ml of a 10% solution of pentylenetetrazol is injected rapidly by the intravenous route, the person becomes apprehensive and in a few seconds convulses and becomes unconscious. The major convulsive phase may last only a minute, to be followed by exhaustion and sleep. Muscular contractions may be so powerful that fractures of vertebrae and other bones may occur. For this reason, it was customary to administer a muscle relaxant such as succinylcholine before the convulsant.

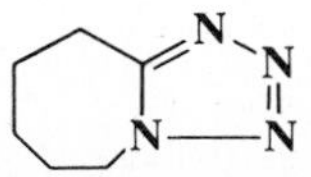

Pentylenetetrazol

Picrotoxin is a mixture of nonnitrogenous substances obtained from an East Indian *Picrotoxin*
shrub. The more active component is picrotoxinin. It is available in injectable solutions containing 3 mg/ml.

Picrotoxin is a typical convulsant of the pentylenetetrazol rather than the strychnine type. In normal animals it stimulates respiration only in doses near the convulsant dose. Barbiturate-anesthetized animals may show significant respiratory stimulation without a convulsant effect because the barbiturates antagonize the convulsive
tendency.

Picrotoxin, once recommended for barbiturate poisoning, is virtually obsolete as
a clinical drug. However, it has been an important research tool in the recent
elucidation in vitro of GABA-receptor mechanisms.[10,13] See Chapter 23 for discussion
of relationships between picrotoxinin receptors and GABA-regulated chloride channels.

Nikethamide (Coramine) is closely related to niacinamide (nicotinamide) and is *Nikethamide*
converted to the vitamin in the body. The structural relationships are as follows:

Niacinamide   Nikethamide

Nikethamide is available in ampules (1.5 ml) or bottles (90 ml) containing 250
mg/ml. The drug is not a cardiac stimulant and is seldom used today.

Doxapram (Dopram) is a powerful respiratory stimulant. Lower doses stimulate *Doxapram*
the carotid chemoreceptors; higher doses also stimulate brainstem respiratory centers. The drug increases respiratory volume more than rate. Its therapeutic index,
determined in animals and expressed as "convulsant dose$_{50}$/respiratory stimulant
dose$_{50}$," is considerably higher than that of the older analeptics. For improvement
of postanesthetic respiration, doxapram is given as a single intravenous bolus of 0.5
to 1 mg/kg of body weight, as divided doses at 5-minute intervals, totaling up to 2
mg/kg, or as an infusion of 5 mg/minute, tapered to 1 to 3 mg/minute for maintenance. Doxapram has a duration of activity as short as 3 or 4 minutes. It has
sympathomimetic side effects such as hypertension and may be considered a very
short-acting sympathomimetic stimulant.

Doxapram

Strychnine

Strychnine is a complex alkaloid obtained from the seed of the plant *Strychnos nux vomica*. It affects all levels of the neuraxis, but its action on the spinal cord predominates. By competitively blocking glycine receptors, strychnine opposes the inhibitory influence of Renshaw cells, thereby lowering the threshold of excitability of motoneurons. Strychnine convulsions differ from pentylenetetrazol seizures in humans by the predominance of the tonic extensor phase, *opisthotonos* being characteristic of both this type of poisoning and of tetanus. The person becomes highly susceptible to various stimuli, so that a sudden noise, light, or other stimulus can precipitate a seizure.

Strychnine

Toxicologic interest arises from uses of strychnine as a rodenticide and a contaminant in "street drugs." Death by strychnine poisoning is secondary to asphyxia associated with prolonged spasms of the respiratory musculature. Barbiturates and more recently diazepam have been effective antagonists against the convulsant and lethal actions of strychnine. Other measures that may be necessary include mechanical ventilation, physical cooling, correction of acidosis, and paralysis with a nondepolarizing neuromuscular blocking agent.[3] Intoxication may be lessened by gastric lavage with activated charcoal.

Caffeine

Caffeine (1,3,7-trimethylxanthine) is the stimulant most widely consumed by the lay public, and it also has some medical uses. A cup of coffee may contain from 50 to 150 mg of the alkaloid, whereas cola drinks have from 35 to 55 mg. A clinical dose for adults is 100 to 200 mg. Although coffee is believed to account for 90% of caffeine consumption in the United States, about 2 million pounds of caffeine is added yearly to other foodstuffs, most of it to soft drinks.[4]

Caffeine stimulates the cerebral cortex and medullary centers. In ordinary doses it causes wakefulness, increases mental alertness, and decreases response times for simple motor tasks. These effects of caffeine are considered pleasant by most persons. It is not surprising that wherever a caffeine-containing plant grows, the inhabitants have usually learned to utilize the drug. Some habituation to the use of caffeine occurs, but physical dependence does not develop. Many "look-alike" drugs, which counterfeit the physical appearance of controlled substances, contain caffeine. In large doses, caffeine stimulates respiration and can precipitate convulsions. The respiratory stimulant activity may be beneficial in apneic, preterm infants.[2,5]

Caffeine also has actions on the gastrointestinal tract and the cardiovascular system

TABLE 27-1   Chemical structures and relative activities of methylxanthines

Xanthine

Alkaloid	Source	Methyl	Analepsis and gastric secretion	Cardiac stimulation, bronchodilatation, and diuresis
Caffeine	Coffee, tea, cocoa, cola	1,3,7	+ + +[*]	+
Theophylline	Tea	1,3	+ +	+ + +
Theobromine	Cocoa	3,7	+	+ +

[*] +, Least potent; + + +, most potent.

and is a diuretic (Table 27-1). Even though it stimulates gastric secretion of acid, pepsin, and gastrin, the drug is not the only active ingredient in coffee because decaffeinated coffee may be a more potent stimulus to secretion than regular coffee or the alkaloid alone.[5,9] In naïve subjects, caffeine may evoke acute changes in the cardiovascular system, such as modest increases in blood pressure, heart rate, and stroke volume, but tolerance develops within a few days of chronic intake. High daily consumption of coffee or acute intoxication may induce ventricular premature contractions or tachyarrhythmias.[4] Increased coronary blood flow is probably a consequence of increased myocardial work and is not likely to be beneficial. Cerebral vessels are constricted by caffeine.

The end products of caffeine metabolism in the body are 1-methyluric acid primarily and other methyl derivatives of xanthine and uric acid.[1] Caffeine does not increase the miscible pool or urinary excretion of uric acid itself and is not contraindicated in gout.

For therapeutic use, caffeine is available as caffeine (125 mg/ml) with sodium benzoate in 2 ml ampules for intramuscular or intravenous injection. For oral administration, citrated caffeine is available in 65 mg tablets. Plain caffeine is also available over the counter as capsules (100 and 250 mg), prolonged-release capsules (200 and 250 mg) and tablets (100 and 200 mg). In addition, caffeine is often added to analgesic remedies containing salicylates and acetaminophen and, for the treatment of migraine, to ergotamine (Cafergot). In the latter combination constriction of cerebral vessels by both alkaloids is believed to account for pain relief. A recent assessment of the contribution of caffeine to the clinical effectiveness of over-the-counter analgesic mixtures[7] indicates that addition of 130 mg of caffeine to such mixtures (in two tablets) is equivalent to a 30% to 40% increase in the dose of analgesic. However, even this modest increment in activity is unlikely with most presently available mixtures, which provide half or less of this dose of caffeine.

Visceral smooth muscle relaxation, such as bronchodilatation, is accomplished better by theophylline or by aminophylline, a soluble complex of theophylline with ethylenediamine. For many years the methylxanthines were believed to act primarily by inhibition of phosphodiesterase, the enzyme that inactivates cyclic adenosine 3',5'-monophosphate (cyclic AMP). This would account nicely for the benefit in asthma from combinations with β-adrenergic receptor agonists, which promote the formation of this cyclic nucleotide. However, theophylline dilates bronchi at concentrations that are insufficient to inhibit phosphodiesterase so that some as yet unknown mechanism must be responsible for the therapeutic effect.[11] Methylxanthines are also potent competitive antagonists of adenosine, and this mechanism may account for many of their effects, including central nervous system and cardiac stimulation and diuresis.[8,11,12]

PENTOXIFYLLINE   Pentoxifylline (Trental) is a synthetic methylxanthine with a longer side chain in place of the methyl group in carbon position 1 of caffeine. It was approved in 1984 to prevent *intermittent claudication,* in which inadequate blood flow to skeletal muscle results in pain or fatigue in the legs. Mechanisms believed to contribute include an increase in red blood cell flexibility and a decrease in the viscosity of blood secondary to decreased plasma fibrinogen.[6] This drug is given as a controlled release tablet of 400 mg, usually three times daily. Benefit may not be apparent until 2 to 8 weeks after initiation of therapy.

Pentoxifylline

REFERENCES

1. Bonati, M., Latini, R., Galletti, F., et al.: Caffeine disposition after oral doses, Clin. Pharmacol. Ther. **32**:98, 1982.

2. Brouard, C., Moriette, G., Murat, I., et al.: Comparative efficacy of theophylline and caffeine in the treatment of idiopathic apnea in premature infants, Am. J. Dis. Child. **139**:698, 1985.

3. Boyd, R.E., Brennan, P.T., Deng, J.-F., et al.: Strychnine poisoning: recovery from profound lactic acidosis, hyperthermia, and rhabdomyolysis, Am. J. Med. **74**:507, 1983.

4. Council on Scientific Affairs: Caffeine labeling, J.A.M.A. **252**:803, 1984.

5. Curatolo, P.W., and Robertson, D.: The health consequences of caffeine, Ann. Intern. Med. **98**:641, 1983.

6. Dettelbach, H.R., and Aviado, D.M.: Clinical pharmacology of pentoxifylline with special reference to its hemorrheologic effect for the treatment of intermittent claudication, J. Clin. Pharmacol. **25**:8, 1985.

7. Laska, E.M., Sunshine, A., Mueller, F., et al.: Caffeine as an analgesic adjuvant, J.A.M.A. **251**:1711, 1984.

8. Marangos, P.J., and Boulenger, J.P.: Basic and clinical aspects of adenosinergic neuromodulation, Neurosci. Biobehav. Rev. **9**:421, 1985.

9. McArthur, K., Hogan, D., and Isenberg, J.I.: Relative stimulatory effects of commonly ingested beverages on gastric acid secretion in humans, Gastroenterology **83**:199, 1982.

10. Olsen, R.W.: Drug interactions at the GABA receptor–ionophore complex, Annu. Rev. Pharmacol. Toxicol. **22**:245, 1982.

11. Persson, C.G.A., Andersson, K.-E., and Kjellin, G.: Effects of enprofylline and theophylline may show the role of adenosine, Life Sci. **38**:1057, 1986.

12. Rall, T.W.: Evolution of the mechanism of action of methylxanthines: from calcium mobilizers to antagonists of adenosine receptors, Pharmacologist **24**:277, 1982.

13. Ticku, M.K.: Benzodiazepine–GABA receptor–ionophore complex, Neuropharmacology **22**:1459, 1983.

14. Wang, S.C., and Ward, J.W.: Analeptics, Pharmacol. Ther. [B] **3**:123, 1977.

Chapter 28

Antiepileptic drugs

GENERAL CONCEPT Convulsions are involuntary skeletal muscular contractions that are often a feature of epileptic seizures. Unconsciousness may or may not occur. Convulsions can arise from pathologic processes within or outside the brain, toxins, acute drug intoxication, or withdrawal from drug dependence. A frequent cause of convulsions is the assortment of neuronal deficits grouped under the term *epilepsy*. Epileptic seizures, however, take many forms and are not necessarily convulsive. For instance, in *absence* the victim exhibits a 5- to 30-second period of staring without motor manifestations.

Epilepsies are categorized for purposes of treatment, yet epilepsy is a symptom more than a specific disease. Diagnosis is based mainly on the clinical patterns of the seizure. Electroencephalography can be helpful. For instance, regular, symmetric, three-per-second spike-wave complexes are characteristic of absence seizures. A brief, annotated classification of epilepsies is given below. More detailed classifications and descriptions are offered elsewhere.[5,8,13]

1. *Generalized seizures* (abrupt bilateral involvement of both hemispheres)
   a. *Tonic-clonic,* or grand mal (unconsciousness, convulsions)
   b. *Absence,* or petit mal (impairment of consciousness, staring, often no motor signs, prepubertal or adolescent)
   c. *Myoclonic* (brief shocklike jerks or contractions)
   d. *Atonic* (sudden loss of muscle tone, *drop attacks*)
   e. *Infantile spasms* (short flexion spasms without loss of consciousness, infants, retarded development, *hypsarrhythmia* EEG pattern; may respond to ACTH or anti-inflammatory steroids if usual anticonvulsants fail)
2. *Partial,* or focal, *seizures* (spread contained within limits)
   a. *Simple* includes jacksonian (consciousness not impaired; motor, somatosensory, autonomic, or psychic symptoms)
   b. *Complex,* or psychomotor (consciousness impaired; may be preceded by prodromal sensation or aura [simple partial]; automatisms may occur)
   c. *Partial becoming generalized* (focal EEG discharge before generalized seizure occurs; focal behavioral events before or after tonic-clonic seizures)

A focal region is an essential feature in the origin of partial epileptic seizures. This focus may be *functional* (arising from proximity to a tumor, hypoxic tissue, a cyst) or *cryptogenic* (abnormal synaptic connections or a biochemical lesion). Within the focus, neurons discharge rapidly in bursts that coincide with periodic waves of depolarization. A seizure arises when discharges from focal neurons invade extrafocal

Diagram of neuronal connections believed to be important in the genesis of tonic-clonic   **FIG. 28-1**
convulsions. Excitation spreads from focal neuron (asterisk) *through excitatory synapses*
(e) *to form an aggregate of excited cells* (shaded). *Involvement of motor pathways leads*
to skeletal muscle contractions. Some neurons (unshaded), *when activated, feed back*
inhibitory signals through synapses (i) *on focal and other neurons in the chain to terminate*
the seizure episode. Intracellular recordings depicted are typical for cells in a focal region
during interictal periods: bursts of action potentials on waves of depolarization. Such bursts
are often coincident with spikes in electroencephalographic spike/wave combinations
(three combinations are shown). A paroxysm of exaggerated amplitude, slow (3 to 5/sec)
waves appears in the EEG during spread. These paroxysms can occur in the absence of
clinical convulsions if spread is not extensive. The time calibration is 200 msec for the
intracellular record and 1 sec for the electroencephalograms.

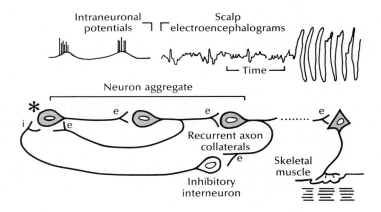

regions, recruiting neurons into a synchronously discharging aggregate of excited cells.[20] Reasons for spread of excitation in individual patients include changes in blood glucose, plasma pH, osmotic pressure, electrolytes, and circulating hormones. Fatigue, physical or mental stress, and nutritional deficiencies may also trigger spread. Generalized seizures ensue if excitation becomes sufficiently extensive to involve both cerebral hemispheres, or they may be the first manifestation of epilepsy without evidence of a specific focus. As part of the excitation process, certain neurons feed back inhibitory information to the neuronal aggregate (Fig. 28-1). Inhibitory synaptic potentials summate with time, gradually hyperpolarizing and desynchronizing the aggregate. This latter process terminates the motor or sensory manifestations (ictus) and may be partially responsible for the usual period of postictal lethargy.

The mechanisms of action of antiepileptic drugs are for the most part unknown.   **MODES OF**
Actions limited to focal neurons would be desirable; however, none of the present   **ACTION**
drugs have this degree of specificity. At the neurophysiologic level, the spread of
seizure discharge is decreased by phenytoin and carbamazepine, probably by a
reduction in posttetanic potentiation.[14] Convulsive threshold, as indicated by elec-

troshock- or pentylenetetrazol-induced convulsions, is elevated by most drugs in this class.

Working hypotheses for the actions of anticonvulsants stem from the idea of membrane stabilization. Drug-induced changes in permeability to specific ions may account for some of their effects. Phenytoin reduces sodium influx and calcium passage through membranes. These effects would tend to stabilize membranes and interfere with calcium-mediated release of neurotransmitters, hormones, and so forth.

Interest in "active inhibition" has emerged with recent descriptions of binding of anticonvulsants within the GABA-receptor complex (see Fig. 23-6). Receptors for a variety of drugs are located in the vicinity of chloride channels. Phenytoin and phenobarbital act at the so-called picrotoxinin site. Benzodiazepine anticonvulsants have a separate binding site in the complex. Valproic acid also facilitates GABA-mediated inhibition, but the specific mechanism is less clear.[14] The potential use of calcium channel blockers and GABA-receptor agonists for management of epilepsy are areas of current interest.

ADVERSE EFFECTS AND DRUG INTERACTIONS

The adverse effects of antiepileptic drugs tend to be gastrointestinal, neurologic, cutaneous, mental, hematopoietic, and renal. Gastrointestinal side effects, usually seen at the initiation of treatment, respond to reduction in dosage. Drugs that control tonic-clonic seizures may exacerbate or unmask other types of seizures and vice versa.[23] Skin eruptions are produced by many antiepileptic drugs. Rarely, they can become major medical problems. Personality, mood, and mental changes in patients treated with antiepileptic drugs are not uncommon, especially behavioral problems in children given sedative anticonvulsants. Clinically significant interactions among antiepileptics and with other drugs are numerous (Chapter 63) and frequently necessitate monitoring of serum concentrations.[10]

ANTIEPILEPTIC DRUG CLASSES

From a structural standpoint the various drugs used in epilepsy may be categorized as follows:

Barbiturates and related drugs
    Phenobarbital (Solfoton, others)
    Mephobarbital (Mebaral)
    Metharbital (Gemonil)
    Primidone (Mysoline, Myidone)
Hydantoins
    Phenytoin (Dilantin, Diphenylan)
    Mephenytoin (Mesantoin)
    Ethotoin (Peganone)
Succinimides
    Ethosuximide (Zarontin)
    Methsuximide (Celontin)
    Phensuximide (Milontin)

Oxazolidinediones
    Trimethadione (Tridione)
    Paramethadione (Paradione)
Benzodiazepines
    Clonazepam (Klonopin)
    Diazepam (Valium)
    Clorazepate (Tranxene)
Miscellaneous anticonvulsants
    Carbamazepine (Tegretol)
    Valproic acid (Depakene)
    Divalproex sodium (Depakote)
    Phenacemide (Phenurone)
    Acetazolamide (Diamox, others)
    ACTH, corticosteroids

TABLE 28-1   Primary antiepileptic drugs: summary of dosage, pharmacokinetics, and clinical activity

Drug	Daily maintenance dose[10] Adult (mg) Child (mg/kg)	Therapeutic serum concentration[10] (μg/ml)	Days to reach steady state	Partial[10] Simple, complex	Generalized Tonic-clonic[10]	Absence[10]	Myoclonic, atonic[10]	Infantile spasms†	Oral dosage forms‡ (mg)
Carbamazepine	600-1200 20-30	6-12	3-6	1	1				CT: 100; T: 200
Phenytoin	300-400 4-7	10-20	Variable	1	1				C: 30, 100; CT: 50; S: 30, 125
Phenobarbital	120-250 3-5	15-35	16-21	2	2				C: 16, 65; S: 15, 20; T: 8-100
Primidone	750-1500 10-25	6-12	1-5	2	2				S: 250; T: 50, 250
Ethosuximide	750-2000 15-60	40-100	5-12			1	3		C: 250; S: 250
Valproic acid	1000-3000 15-60	50-100	2-4	1§	1	1§		3	C: 250; S: 250
Clonazepam	1.5-20 0.01-0.2	0.013-0.072	4-5			2	2	2	T: 0.5-2
Trimethadione	900-2400 15-30	10-30	3			3			C: 300; CT: 150; S: 200

Preferred drugs for control of seizures*

Seizure type

*The numbers listed for each seizure type indicate a relative order of choice for seizure management. However, the order of preference by individual clinicians varies, and definite evidence of the superiority of one drug over another is often unavailable.[4]
†ACTH and glucocorticoids are first choice.
‡C, Capsules; CT, chewable tablets; S, liquid preparation (in 5 ml); T, tablets.
§Approved only with concurrent absence.

The formulas of barbiturates, hydantoins, succinimides, and oxazolidinediones have many similarities. Whereas barbituric acid is malonylurea, hydantoins have a five-membered ring formed by condensation of acetic acid and urea. In the oxazolidinedione and succinimide series, one of the nitrogens in the hydantoin ring is replaced by oxygen or carbon respectively. Bromides were the earliest antiepileptic drugs, followed by phenobarbital in 1912 and phenytoin in 1938. Information regarding dosage, pharmacokinetics, and therapeutic spectra of the major antiepileptic agents is summarized in Table 28-1.

Carbamazepine

Carbamazepine is related structurally to the tricyclic antidepressants. It is quite useful in management of generalized tonic-clonic seizures and partial seizures,[17] in the prophylaxis of childhood febrile seizures, and in trigeminal and glossopharyngeal neuralgias.[6] Its beneficial action in partial complex epilepsy, which is often refractory to drug therapy, is particularly important.

Carbamazepine   Imipramine

Carbamazepine is absorbed slowly from the gastrointestinal tract. It is oxidized partially to an active epoxide metabolite.[3] The drug induces its own metabolism so that its elimination half-life with chronic administration ranges from 10 to 25 hours, whereas the half-life of a single dose may be twice as long. This change and also induction by concurrent exposure to other anticonvulsant drugs are likely to require gradual increases in dosage. Whenever possible it is preferable to avoid the concurrent use of carbamazepine with other antiepileptic drugs. Adverse effects of carbamazepine include ataxia, dizziness, headache, drowsiness, diplopia, dyskinetic movements, and rarely hepatic damage and cardiotoxicity.[11] Carbamazepine also has potential for bone-marrow depression, and so initial and periodic blood counts are indicated. Patients should be alert for such signs as fever, sore throat, ulcers in the mouth, easy bruising, and petechial or purpuric hemorrhage.

Hydantoins **Phenytoin** is still one of the most valuable antiepileptic drugs.[17] Its main advantage in management of tonic-clonic and partial epilepsy is that it exerts little sedative action at effective dose levels. It may be given intravenously in status epilepticus; 30 to 50 mg/min (adults) or 0.5 to 1.5 mg/kg/min (children) for a loading dose of 15 to 20 mg/kg.[10]

Adverse effects of phenytoin. Chronic intoxication is characterized by nystagmus, ataxia, lethargy, and a paradoxical increase in seizures. These manifestations are dose related and appear at plasma concentrations of 20 to 40 μg/ml. Severe and prolonged intoxication may cause degeneration of cerebellar Purkinje cells. Acute intoxication can also induce cardiac arrhythmias and hypotension.

Osteomalacia and hypocalcemia are probably attributable to interference with vitamin D metabolism by unknown mechanisms. Long-term use of phenytoin may impair utilization of folic acid to result in megaloblastic anemia. Hypertrophy of the gums (gingival hyperplasia) occurs in approximately 20% of patients, is generally attributed to a disorder of fibroblastic activity, and is exacerbated by poor dental hygiene.

Although increased risk of teratogenesis may be associated with use of phenytoin during pregnancy, other antiepileptic drugs and perhaps epilepsy itself may contribute to the teratogenesis.[7] Current thinking is that anticonvulsant medication should be withdrawn from a pregnant woman who has had no seizures for "many years" but that otherwise seizures during pregnancy pose a greater risk to the developing fetus than antiepileptic drugs do.[2]

Drugs of the hydantoin group may produce blood dyscrasias and rarely a clinical picture resembling malignant lymphoma. Skin rash is an indication for immediate withdrawal to avoid rare but serious exfoliative dermatitis. The use of phenytoin as an antiarrhythmic drug is discussed in Chapter 35.

Pharmacokinetics of phenytoin. Phenytoin is slowly absorbed from the intestinal tract and is about 90% protein bound. Like salicylic acid, it shows an unusual pharmacokinetic feature. An increase in dosage beyond that needed for a steady-state plasma concentration of 10 μg/ml produces a disproportionate rise in concentration as pathways for inactivation of the drug become saturated. As a consequence, the half-life of phenytoin increases as plasma concentration increases. Even at low doses the half-life averages about a day, and so at least 4 to 5 days will be necessary to reach steady state at a given dose. Since the therapeutic plasma concentration is usually between 10 and 20 μg/ml, monitoring of the concentration is quite important. Minor increases in dosage can result in greatly elevated, toxic concentrations. Concurrent therapy with cimetidine and several other drugs can impair metabolism of phenytoin (see Table 63-3). Phenobarbital has the opposite effect, though this interaction seldom creates a serious problem.

Ethylphenylhydantoin, an active anticonvulsant, was withdrawn from the market because it produced an extraordinarily high incidence of drug fever, skin sensitization, and eosinophilia. Interestingly, replacement of the ethyl radical by a phenyl group yielded phenytoin. **Mephenytoin,** the N-methyl derivative of ethylphenylhydantoin, is partially demethylated in the body to the latter drug. It is not surprising therefore that a high incidence of reactions has been reported for mephenytoin. Clearly it should be used only if safer agents are ineffective. The antiepileptic effectiveness of **ethotoin,** the newest hydantoin available, has not been well established.

| Phenytoin | Phenobarbital | Primidone |

Phenobarbital is one of the oldest and least expensive antiepileptic drugs. It differs from most barbiturates in possessing significant antiepileptic activity at doses that do not cause excessive sedation in many patients. Care must be taken never to withdraw phenobarbital suddenly because this can precipitate a generalized seizure or even status epilepticus.

Barbiturates and related drugs

The major usefulness of phenobarbital is in prevention of tonic-clonic and simple partial seizures. It has little effect on absence seizures but may be combined with ethosuximide in patients who have mixed types of generalized epilepsy. Phenobarbital has a long half-life of up to 140 hours, and so a single daily dose at bedtime is effective.[25] Blood concentrations above 25 µg/ml may be associated with perceptual/ motor impairment. Drowsiness and, in children, irritability and hyperactivity are its main side effects, but patients tend to become tolerant to the sedative action. Phenobarbital is the drug of choice for prophylaxis of febrile convulsions in young children at high risk.[12]

Mephobarbital is *N*-methylphenobarbital. Its indications and uses are similar to those of phenobarbital. The compound is demethylated to phenobarbital to a significant extent in the body; thus its antiepileptic action is attributable at least in part to phenobarbital. The dosage of mephobarbital is 300 to 600 mg/day.

Metharbital is *N*-methylbarbital and is probably demethylated in the body to barbital. It is seldom used today, and convincing evidence of its antiepileptic effectiveness is lacking. Its dosage is 100 mg two or three times a day.

Primidone, though not a true barbiturate, is similar in structure to phenobarbital. Because sedation and ataxia can be pronounced, it should be started in small doses, about 50 mg, with a gradual increase to as much as 250 mg three times daily. The drug is converted to two active metabolites: phenobarbital and phenylethylmalonamide. If primidone is used during pregnancy, vitamin K should be given prophylactically before delivery, since maternal and neonatal problems with hemorrhage have been ascribed to the drug.

Succinimides
Ethosuximide, methsuximide, and **phensuximide** are useful in the order listed for management of typical and atypical absence seizures. They are less toxic than the oxazolidinediones below, though nausea, drowsiness, anorexia, and headache may occur. Rare cases of rash, leukopenia, and lupus-like syndromes have been reported. Their mechanism of action is unknown.

Usual dosages of these drugs are 500 mg of ethosuximide two to four times daily, 300 to 600 mg of methsuximide three times a day, and 0.5 to 1 g of phensuximide three times a day. Ethosuximide and valproic acid are now considered the drugs of choice for management of absence seizures; the former if hepatotoxicity is a particular concern, the latter if the patient also has tonic-clonic seizures. Monthly blood counts are recommended.

Ethosuximide   Methsuximide

Oxazolidinediones
Trimethadione and **paramethadione,** once primary agents for control of absence seizures, are now seldom used. Toxic effects include drowsiness, ataxia, photophobia and white halos around objects in the visual field (hemeralopia), rashes, and alopecia. Bone-marrow depression and kidney damage have been described after prolonged

use. A fetal teratogenic trimethadione syndrome has resulted in facial abnormalities, growth retardation, cardiac and ocular problems, and microcephaly.[2,7] Trimethadione is used mainly in patients with absence seizures that have not responded to other therapy and should not be taken by pregnant women.

Trimethadione

Clonazepam, diazepam, and **clorazepate dipotassium** are the benzodiazepines used as antiepileptic drugs. Clonazepam is useful for management of drug-resistant absence seizures and progressive myoclonic epilepsy. Tolerance may slowly diminish its effectiveness in some patients. Adverse side effects include drowsiness, ataxia, and, in children, personality changes. Diazepam is indicated for status epilepticus. It is highly lipophilic and readily enters the central nervous system. Like thiopental, its duration of action after a single intravenous bolus is relatively short because it rapidly redistributes from the brain to peripheral tissues. Accordingly, an infusion of diazepam is more useful for control of status epilepticus. Diazepam for intravenous use is available in ampules containing 10 mg/2 ml. Lorazepam undergoes less rapid redistribution from the brain than diazepam and may prove to be a longer-acting alternative in control of status epilepticus.[15] Clorazepate has been approved as an adjunct in control of partial seizures.

Benzodiazepines

Valproic acid, dipropylacetic acid, is one of the more recently introduced antiepileptics. It is absorbed rapidly from the gastrointestinal tract and has a short half-life. Thus it must be administered three or four times daily. **Divalproex sodium,** a prodrug converted to valproic acid in the gastrointestinal tract, is available as 125 to 500 mg equivalents of the active drug.

Valproic acid is highly effective in therapy of generalized seizures, both tonic-clonic and absence, and is indicated also in myoclonic seizures. Thus it has a remarkably wide range of applications.

Adverse effects of valproic acid include nausea, transient hair loss, and weight gain. Serum transaminase levels are elevated in many patients but usually without clinical manifestations. However, fatal hepatotoxicity may occur within 6 months of initiation of therapy, and patients should be monitored regularly during this period, especially for clinical indications of liver damage, such as loss of seizure control, malaise, weakness, lethargy, anorexia, and vomiting. Valproic acid may also cause neural-tube defects and is best avoided in pregnancy.[7] The drug may interact with other antiepileptic agents.[16] For instance, it inhibits the metabolism of phenobarbital, and it alters phenytoin plasma concentrations by competition for protein binding.

Miscellaneous anticonvulsants

$$CH_3—CH_2—CH_2$$
$$HC—COOH$$
$$CH_3—CH_2—CH_2$$

Valproic acid

Phenacemide, a quite toxic anticonvulsant, may cause severe bone-marrow depression, hepatocellular damage, and toxic psychoses. It is used, mostly for partial complex seizures, only after all other measures fail. Tablets of 500 mg are taken three times a day.

Metabolic acidosis induced by a ketogenic diet is occasionally used for infantile spasms and other refractory seizures. **Acetazolamide,** a carbonic anhydrase inhibitor (see Chapter 38), is likewise used adjunctively as an anticonvulsant. Its effectiveness may be attributable to inhibition of carbonic anhydrase in the central nervous system rather than to systemic acidosis. The activity of the enzyme is high in the choroid plexus, which regulates the composition of cerebrospinal fluid. Acetazolamide is given in doses of 250 to 500 mg two or three times a day.

Bromides are now rarely used for control of seizures. Their use is associated with mental depression, toxic psychoses, and skin rashes.

---

*CLINICAL
PHARMACOLOGY*

The relative usefulness of the major antiepileptic drugs in management of various types of seizures is indicated in Table 28-1. Specific guidelines for their use in children have recently been published.[18]

The clearance of many of these drugs is greater in children than in adults, and so the effective dose per kilogram of body weight is usually higher in children (Table 28-1). The general incidence of side effects is less if anticonvulsant doses are low initially and then increased slowly. Complete seizure control is a desirable goal but may not be attainable because of side effects. Sufficient time to reach steady state must be allowed between increments in dosage.

Patient compliance is a major problem. More often than not "nonresponders" are either not taking their medication at all or are not taking it as prescribed. Periodic monitoring of serum concentrations of these drugs is useful both for ensuring adequate but not toxic dosage and as an indication of compliance.

Management of epilepsy solely with the nonsedative (or at least less sedative) agents (phenytoin, carbamazepine, valproic acid, and ethosuximide) whenever possible has been advocated to reduce problems with daytime drowsiness, behavior, and withdrawal.[19,24] It is also advantageous if seizures can be controlled by a single drug because drug interactions and the potential for side effects are then minimized.[1] Unfortunately, these goals are not always possible. After prolonged drug therapy some patients are candidates for cautious drug withdrawal to determine if anticonvulsants are still needed.[21] The usual criteria for slowly decreasing the dose are no seizures in the previous 3 to 4 years, no overt neurologic deficits, and normal electroencephalograms.

Status epilepticus is the occurrence of a prolonged seizure or a series of seizures, most often generalized tonic-clonic but possibly absence or even partial complex, without full recovery between episodes. Tonic-clonic status is life threatening and causes hyperthermia, metabolic acidosis, catecholamine release, and often pulmonary edema.[22] A treatment protocol proceeding as necessary from (1) intravenous infusion of diazepam *and* phenytoin to (2) diazepam *or* phenobarbital drip to (3) general anesthesia with halothane *and* neuromuscular blockade has been detailed elsewhere.[9] Paraldehyde infusion *or* intravenous lidocaine push is recommended at the third stage if an anesthesiologist is not yet present.

Status epilepticus

REFERENCES

1. Albright, P., and Bruni, J.: Reduction of polypharmacy in epileptic patients, Arch. Neurol. **42:**797, 1985.
2. American Academy of Pediatrics Committee on Drugs: Anticonvulsants and pregnancy, Pediatrics **63:**331, 1979.
3. Bertilsson, L., and Tomson, T.: Clinical pharmacokinetics and pharmacological effects of carbamazepine and carbamazepine-10,11-epoxide: an update, Clin. Pharmacokinet. **11:**177, 1986.
4. Chadwick, D., and Turnbull, D.M.: The comparative efficacy of antiepileptic drugs for partial and tonic-clonic seizures, J. Neurol. Neurosurg. Psychiatry **48:**1073, 1985.
5. Commission on Classification and Terminology of the International League against Epilepsy: Proposal for revised clinical and electroencephalographic classification of epileptic seizures, Epilepsia **22:**489, 1981.
6. Dalessio, D.J.: Trigeminal neuralgia: a practical approach to treatment, Drugs **24:**248, 1982.
7. Dalessio, D.J.: Seizure disorders and pregnancy, N. Engl. J. Med. **312:**559, 1985.
8. Delgado-Escueta, A.V., Treiman, D.M., and Walsh, G.O.: The treatable epilepsies, N. Engl. J. Med. **308:**1508 and 1576, 1983.

9. Delgado-Escueta, A.V., Wasterlain, C., Treiman, D.M., and Porter, R.J.: Management of status epilepticus, N. Engl. J. Med. **306:**1337, 1982.
10. Drugs for epilepsy, Med. Lett. Drugs Ther. **28:**91, 1986.
11. Evans, R.W., and Gualtieri, C.T.: Carbamazepine: a neuropsychological and psychiatric profile, Clin. Neuropharmacol. **8:**221, 1985.
12. Fishman, M.A.: Febrile seizures: the treatment controversy, J. Pediatr. **94:**177, 1979.
13. Janz, D.: Epilepsy: seizures and syndromes, Handb. Exp. Pharmacol. **74:**3, 1985.
14. Jurna, I.: Electrophysiological effects of antiepileptic drugs, Handb. Exp. Pharmacol. **74:**611, 1985.
15. Leppik, L.E., Derivan, A.T., Homan, R.W., et al.: Double-blind study of lorazepam and diazepam in status epilepticus, J.A.M.A. **249:**1452, 1983.
16. Levy, R.H., and Koch, K.M.: Drug interactions with valproic acid, Drugs **24:**543, 1982.
17. Mattson, R.H., Cramer, J.A., Collins, J.F., et al.: Comparison of carbamazepine, phenobarbital, phenytoin, and primidone in partial and secondarily generalized tonic-clonic seizures, N. Engl. J. Med. **313:**145, 1985.

18. Morselli, P.L., Pippenger, C.E., and Penry, J.K., editors: Antiepileptic drug therapy in pediatrics, New York, 1983, Raven Press.

19. Porter, R.J., and Theodore, W.H.: Nonsedative regimens in the treatment of epilepsy, Arch. Intern. Med. **143**:945, 1983.

20. Schwartzkroin, P.A., and Wyler, A.R.: Mechanisms underlying epileptiform burst discharge, Ann. Neurol. **7**:95, 1980.

21. Shinnar, S., Vining, E.P.G., Mellits, E.D., et al.: Discontinuing antiepileptic medication in children with epilepsy after two years without seizures: a prospective study, N. Engl. J. Med. **313**:976, 1985.

22. Simon, R.P.: Physiologic consequences of status epilepticus, Epilepsia **26**(suppl. 1):S58, 1985.

23. Snead, O.C., III, and Hosey, L.C.: Exacerbation of seizures in children by carbamazepine, N. Engl. J. Med. **313**:916, 1985.

24. Theodore, W.H., and Porter, R.J.: Removal of sedative-hypnotic antiepileptic drugs from the regimens of patients with intractable epilepsy, Ann. Neurol. **13**:320, 1983.

25. Wroblewski, B.A., and Garvin, W.H., Jr.: Once-daily administration of phenobarbital in adults: clinical efficacy and benefit, Arch. Neurol. **42**:699, 1985.

Chapter 29

Narcotic (opioid) analgesic drugs

Suffering and disability caused by unrelieved pain lower the quality of life for vast numbers of persons, and alleviation of pain is a major objective in medicine. Drugs with a prominent pain-relieving action are called *analgesics*. The two types, *narcotic* (opioid) and *nonnarcotic* (see Chapter 31), differ in several respects that greatly affect the ways they are used: (1) Perhaps the most important distinctions are that only the narcotics have potential for abuse and that tolerance to their actions can develop. Accordingly, narcotics are usually administered for short periods, and precautions are taken to avoid their diversion to illicit use. (2) Narcotics are the more powerful analgesics, but they do not reduce inflammation. In an individual patient with severe pain a narcotic is likely to provide greater relief than a nonnarcotic. When groups of patients are treated, narcotics are generally analgesic in a higher percentage. (3) Narcotics undergo sufficient first-pass metabolism that a given dose is more effective by injection than after oral administration, as reflected by the differences between equianalgesic oral and parenteral doses tabulated in Table 29-1. Nonnarcotic analgesics are very seldom injected. Another difference is that narcotics act mainly within the central nervous system, whereas the primary *analgesic* action of nonnarcotics is peripheral.

The narcotic class includes alkaloids found in opium and their semisynthetic derivatives (opiates) as well as synthetic compounds (opioids) that resemble the alkaloids in their pharmacology if less so in their structures. Their use is regulated by the Federal Controlled Substances Act of 1970. Morphine, the prototype opiate, has been available for nearly 200 years, but opium has been used for thousands of years. The opioid antagonist nalorphine was introduced in 1941. Recent characterizations of opioid receptors and discoveries of endogenous opioid peptides have given new perspective to the topics of pain and analgesia. It must be remembered, however, that use of narcotic analgesics is only one approach to pain alleviation (Fig. 29-1).

OPIOID RECEPTORS

For some time the existence of opioid receptors in the brain was suspected, based on several different observations: (1) some analgesics are extremely potent, etorphine being up to 10,000 times more potent than morphine; (2) opioids are stereospecific with activity residing in the *levo* isomers; (3) there are selective competitive opioid antagonists, such as naloxone, that are not analgesic.

In the early 1970s, the concept of specific opioid receptors was supported by demonstrations that opioid agonists and antagonists bind stereospecifically in vitro

FIG. 29-1   *Correlation of neural projections and chemical mediators in pain perception with some of the different types of drugs that alleviate pain.*

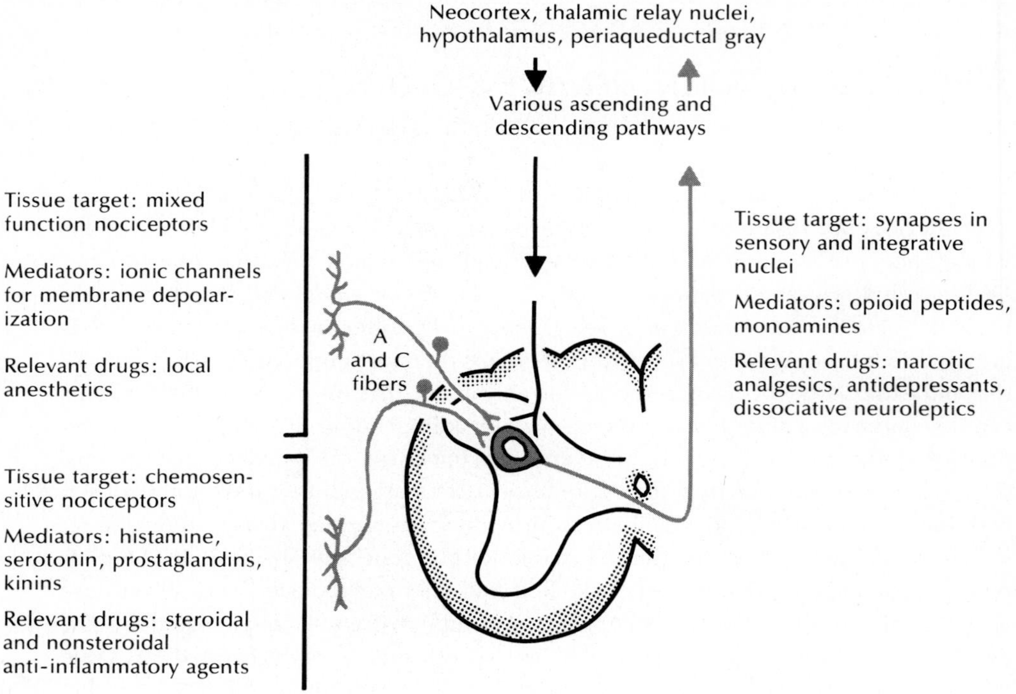

Neocortex, thalamic relay nuclei, hypothalamus, periaqueductal gray

Various ascending and descending pathways

Tissue target: mixed function nociceptors

Mediators: ionic channels for membrane depolarization

Relevant drugs: local anesthetics

A and C fibers

Tissue target: synapses in sensory and integrative nuclei

Mediators: opioid peptides, monoamines

Relevant drugs: narcotic analgesics, antidepressants, dissociative neuroleptics

Tissue target: chemosensitive nociceptors

Mediators: histamine, serotonin, prostaglandins, kinins

Relevant drugs: steroidal and nonsteroidal anti-inflammatory agents

to membranes of pinched-off nerve terminals. The affinities of the agonists for binding sites parallel closely their relative clinical potencies.

Receptors (stereospecific binding sites) for opioids are concentrated in the limbic system, spinoreticular tracts, medial thalamic nuclei, hypothalamus, and other regions involved in pain perception,[29] such as the *substantia gelatinosa* of the spinal cord and spinal trigeminal nucleus. Receptors are also found in the *nucleus tractus solitarii* and related nuclei concerned with vagal reflexes. High receptor densities in these latter regions indicate possible contributions to the cough reflex, gastric secretion, and orthostatic hypotension. Of several types of opioid receptors (see p. 332), the one most responsible for the analgesic activity of morphine has been designated the μ (mu, for *morphine*) receptor.

ENDOGENOUS OPIOID PEPTIDES   The demonstration of opioid receptors suggested the existence of endogenous morphine-like compounds.[11,21] Isolation from brain tissue of pentapeptides with opiate-like activity, [Met]enkephalin (Tyr-Gly-Gly-Phe-Met) and [Leu]enkephalin (Tyr-Gly-Gly-Phe-Leu), was reported in 1975. β-Lipotropin, a 91 amino-acid peptide isolated from the pituitary some years before, contains another opioid peptide, β-endorphin, in residues 61 to 91 (see p. 223). Although residues 61 to 65 are the same as [Met]enkephalin, β-endorphin is not the precursor of the enkephalin, and their brain distributions are quite different.[9,17] Determination of physiologic functions of these and other endogenous opioid peptides is now a topic of major interest.[9]

Beecher[2] had a major impact on concepts of pain and analgesia when he emphasized that two major factors contribute to pain or, perhaps more accurately, suffering. One factor is the *perception* of a noxious stimulus, which involves classic neuroanatomic pathways that ascend in the spinal cord to the reticular substance, the thalamus, and eventually the cortex. The other factor, the *reaction component*, was invoked to account for the wide variation in suffering among persons who have comparable tissue damage and in whom afferent input should be about the same. Since patients given morphine may indicate that even though they still feel pain it no longer bothers them, Beecher attributed the analgesic effect of morphine principally to a beneficial action on the reaction component. Patients given opioids may also be indifferent to other stimuli, such as urges to urinate or defecate. The benefit of morphine, a respiratory depressant, in patients with dyspnea secondary to acute left ventricular failure and pulmonary edema may also be, at least partially, attributable to diminished reaction and anxiety. Presumably opioid receptors in the limbic system are involved in effects on reaction, whereas stimulation of receptors in the spinal cord and brainstem might affect perception of stimuli. Recent research on opioid-induced analgesia has focused on perception rather than on reaction. Morphine, given by the usual routes, appears to act primarily at the *supraspinal* level to activate pathways that descend in the dorsolateral funiculus to influence afferent input from Aδ and C fibers.[7,10] However, when the spinal cord is directly exposed to opioids, given intrathecally or extradurally, a sufficient local concentration can provide analgesia by stimulating opioid receptors in the dorsal horn.

Clinical comparisons of analgesics are difficult because of the complex interplay between perception and reaction, neither of which can be objectively measured. The most useful approach has been to administer analgesics to patients with pain of pathologic origin. Typically the patient is asked to rank the pain, as severe, moderate, or slight, before and at intervals after treatment to arrive at a subjective estimate of pain relief. The pain-relieving efficacy of the agent in question is compared in comparable groups of subjects with that of a placebo or an established analgesic, such as morphine or aspirin. Positive placebo responses often occur, overall in about 30% of patients tested in acute situations.

Potent narcotic analgesics alleviate severe pain and are antagonized by drugs such as naloxone. Pure agonists exhibit cross-tolerance and (in contrast to mixed agonist-antagonists, see p. 332) can be substituted for each other in the addict. It could be anticipated that these analgesics would have some basic structural similarity, and examination of their formulas reveals the presence of a common moiety, γ-

CURRENT CONCEPTS OF ANALGESIC ACTION

phenyl-*N*-methylpiperidine. The chair form of piperidine is believed to be the more realistic representation, with heavy lines indicating projection from the plane of the paper. Substituent R is often quite bulky.

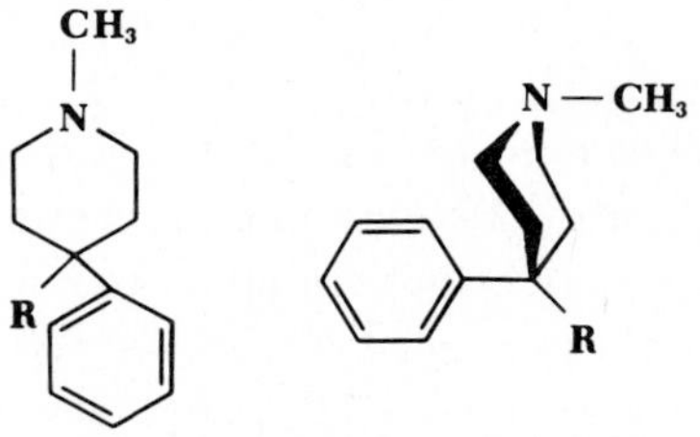

Disubstituted *N*-methylpiperidine

Narcotic analgesics and antagonists can be divided into several structural categories, as in Table 29-1, which also summarizes information regarding administration of these agents. Of more practical importance, however, is their division into agonists, antagonists, and agents with both of these activities. The agonists are discussed first.

NATURAL OPIATES
AND
SEMISYNTHETIC
DERIVATIVES
Morphine
CHEMISTRY

Morphine remains the most important narcotic analgesic. It is obtained from opium, the dried juice of the poppy plant, *Papaver somniferum*. Alkaloids in opium are of two types, called *phenanthrenes* and *benzylisoquinolines*. Of the latter, noscapine is used to relieve cough, and papaverine has been used as an antispasmotic and vasodilator, though its effectiveness has never been satisfactorily established. Neither agent is analgesic. Morphine and codeine in the phenanthrene group are the important narcotics. Opium contains about 10% morphine and 0.5% codeine. Thebaine, another phenanthrene, evokes strychnine-like convulsions and has no medical uses, but it is manufactured into the opioid antagonist naloxone. In the poppy thebaine is demethylated to codeine, which in turn is demethylated to morphine.

Morphine was isolated in the first decade of the nineteenth century by Serturner. Its total synthesis in 1952 confirmed a structure proposed by Gulland and Robinson in 1925. The two hydroxyls, one phenolic and the other alcoholic, are important because certain semisynthetic alkaloids are prepared by modifications of these groups. Codeine, for instance, is 3-methylmorphine, and heroin is 3,6-diacetylmorphine. On the other hand, the narcotic antagonist nalorphine is prepared by replacement of the methyl group on the nitrogen with an allyl radical $-CH_2CH=CH_2$.

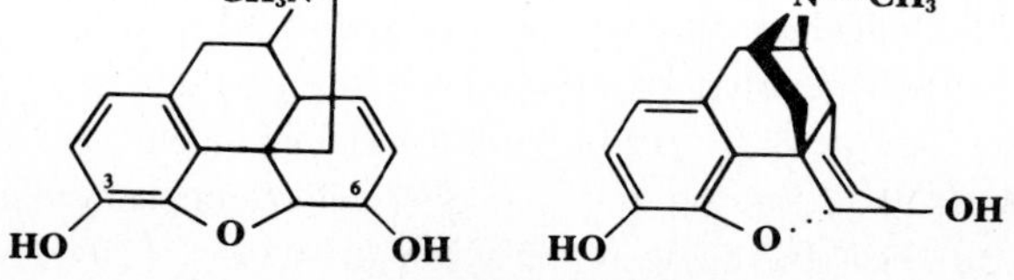

Morphine

Morphine sulfate is available in many forms (Table 29-1), including 30 mg tablets for prolonged-release and preservative-free solutions for spinal administration. The subcutaneous dose range is usually 8 to 15 mg.

When a therapeutic dose of morphine is administered to normal persons, it induces drowsiness (stupor, or *narcosis*) and euphoria in some, but dysphoria and other unpleasant reactions such as nausea are not uncommon. The person may sleep, respiration may slow, and pupils may constrict. Dysphoria is less common in patients with pain.

Analgesia. Subcutaneous or intramuscular injection of 10 mg of morphine relieves moderate to severe postoperative pain in 70% to 80% of adult patients. Interestingly a placebo is effective in about 30%, whereas oral aspirin may benefit just 40%. Because of pronounced first-pass inactivation, the oral dose of morphine for comparable peak analgesia is about 60 mg. Consequently morphine is usually injected for relief of acute pain. In contrast is its oral use for chronic analgesia in patients with terminal cancer. The best approach to this problem is to provide the opiate at regular intervals in a dose sufficient to *prevent* pain, rather than to wait for pain to develop.[8,14] The doses required in such regimens may be surprisingly low, and the need to increase the dosage does not necessarily indicate tolerance; it may reflect progression of the disease.[28] For relief of pain by a direct action on the spinal cord, extradural administration of morphine appears much less likely than intrathecal administration to induce dangerous respiratory depression.[13] Elderly people tend to receive more prolonged pain relief from morphine, and so their daily opiate requirement may be less.

Respiration. The sensitivity of respiratory centers to carbon dioxide is reduced by morphine, and cessation of respiration is the usual cause of death in morphine poisoning. Therapeutic doses of morphine moderately decrease respiratory minute volume. The tendency to reduce respiratory rate may be obscured as carbon dioxide retention increases, but larger doses will clearly lower the rate. Carbon dioxide retention is responsible for cerebral vasodilatation and increased intracranial pressure after administration of morphine. As tolerance develops to the analgesic and euphoric actions of morphine, the respiratory center becomes tolerant also. For this reason an addict may tolerate otherwise lethal doses of morphine.

Excitation. Morphine is not a uniform depressant of neural structures. It does not oppose the action of stimulants such as strychnine or picrotoxin. Morphine alone may actually be excitatory in susceptible persons. Some animals, such as cats and horses, are consistently stimulated by morphine.

Emesis. The emetic action of morphine is exerted on the chemoreceptor trigger zone (CTZ) in the medulla. However, morphine also depresses the vomiting center, which is located nearby, and so subsequent doses are less likely to induce nausea and vomiting. Apomorphine, used as an emetic to minimize some types of poisoning, is manufactured from morphine and is a potent stimulant of the CTZ.

Miscellaneous effects

Pupils. The pupils are constricted by morphine, and this effect is inhibited by atropine. The response is most likely attributable to enhanced parasympathetic input from the Edinger-Westphal nucleus. Tolerance can be demonstrated, but addicts usually exhibit miosis. Their pupils maximally dilate during withdrawal. Animals, such as cats, that are excited by morphine develop mydriasis upon acute administration.

Gastrointestinal tract. Morphine is constipating, and opiates are time-honored remedies in the management of diarrhea.[1] Paregoric, a preparation of opium, has been used for centuries for this purpose. The amount of morphine (2 to 4 mg) in a typical adult dose of paregoric is much less than the oral dose of morphine needed acutely for analgesia. The dose of paregoric for children is 0.1 to 0.2 mg of morphine per kilogram of body weight.

In general, morphine increases the tone of intestinal smooth muscle and decreases propulsive peristalsis. Morphine delays gastric emptying through decreased gastric motility and contraction of the pylorus and duodenum. Atropine can partially oppose the spasmogenic action of morphine. Reduction in fluid and electrolyte secretion and failure to perceive sensory stimuli that would otherwise elicit defecation also may contribute to constipation.

Biliary tract. Morphine can increase intrabiliary pressure by contracting smooth muscle in the biliary tract. Pain relief in biliary colic therefore must be caused by the central analgesic action of morphine. Meperidine and pentazocine, which cause less increase in pressure, are preferred narcotics for analgesia in this circumstance.

Cardiovascular system. Morphine reduces arterial resistance and venous tone. These effects may lead to orthostatic hypotension, but they can be beneficial in reducing ventricular work, pulmonary congestion, and edema. Histamine release by intravenous morphine administration may contribute to the hypotensive reaction. The hemodynamic effects of morphine are unfavorable in hemorrhagic shock.

Bronchial smooth muscle. Contraction of bronchial smooth muscle by large doses of morphine may decrease the diameter of the airway. Many investigators have attributed deaths in asthmatic patients to the bronchoconstrictor action of morphine. It is possible, however, that mortality in asthmatics is caused by reduction of the stimulant action of carbon dioxide on the respiratory center. According to this view, carbon dioxide narcosis, rather than bronchial constriction, is the cause of death. The question is not settled.

Genitourinary tract. Opiates contract the smooth muscle of the ureter and the detrusor muscle of the bladder and increase the tone of the vesicle sphincter. The latter along with decreased attention to the stimulus for urination may result in urinary retention. In addition, morphine may release antidiuretic hormone, and its hemodynamic actions also contribute to antidiuresis. Despite its spasmogenic action, morphine is used for the relief of ureteral colic, where its effectiveness must be attributable to its analgesic action. Uterine contractions during labor may be slowed somewhat by a therapeutic dose of morphine.

Depending on the route of administration, several factors may delay absorption of morphine and other opioids. These include delayed gastric emptying, reduced cutaneous circulation, hypothermia, and shock. Because first-pass hepatic inactivation can be considerable, parenteral routes are preferred for relief of acute pain.

Morphine partitions from blood into most tissues, but very little actually reaches the central nervous system. The plasma half-life is about 3 hours, and the period of effective analgesia is 4 to 5 hours. Morphine is conjugated to a glucuronide that is excreted in the urine; a small percentage can be recovered from the feces.

PHARMACOKINETICS

A striking feature of the pharmacology of opioids is the tolerance that develops to their actions. However, tolerance does not develop rapidly to all its actions, and addicts typically exhibit constricted pupils and constipation.

TOLERANCE

Chronic abuse (see Chapter 30) will require progressively larger doses of morphine to obtain the same subjective effects. Tolerance can reach incredible proportions. Addicts have been known to take 4 g of the drug in 24 hours, and a patient with terminal cancer received over 8 grams on the seventh day of a continuous intravenous infusion.[5] These quantities are far greater than the lethal dose, about 100 to 200 mg, in a nontolerant person. After 1 to 2 weeks of abstinence the person is again sensitive to a small dose of the drug.

The mechanism or mechanisms of tolerance may be clarified as a consequence of the discovery of the enkephalins. If enkephalins are neurotransmitters or neuromodulators, the continued presence of morphine at the opioid receptor could inhibit peptide production or release (Fig. 29-2). Thus larger doses of morphine would be required in the face of steadily decreasing peptide availability. When the supply of morphine is withdrawn abruptly, insufficient concentrations of analgesic compounds (endogenous and exogenous) may cause abstinence signs.

In severe *acute* morphine poisoning the person is comatose and cyanotic, respiration is very slow or absent, and the pupils are of pinpoint size, unless hypoxia is appreciable. As in barbiturate intoxication, central stimulant drugs such as picrotoxin or pentylenetetrazol should not be used.

INTOXICATION

The major development in treatment of acute morphine poisoning has been the discovery of specific antidotes. Naloxone is the antagonist of choice, since it has virtually no adverse effects if used properly. Intravenous injection of naloxone improves respiration and circulation promptly in acutely poisoned persons. Opioid antagonists are not of benefit in overdoses with barbiturates or general anesthetics. If a course of naloxone therapy does not dramatically reverse respiratory depression, the initial diagnosis must be questioned. In narcotic-dependent persons, whether abusers or patients in chronic pain, naloxone can precipitate a severe abstinence syndrome.

Codeine is a very important oral analgesic and antitussive drug. In the usual doses of 30 to 60 mg it is equally or slightly more analgesic than aspirin. Tolerance

Codeine

Possible servomechanisms in morphine tolerance and abstinence. Opioid peptides are assumed to act as neruotransmitters or neuromodulators. Peptide binding to μ receptors initiates effects on target neurons compatible with normal function. Synthesis and release of peptide commensurate with need is under feedback control. Morphine competes with the peptide either directly or indirectly. Continuously available morphine is responsible for persistent feedback signals to decrease peptide production. With time, higher concentrations of morphine are required to maintain a specified level of responsiveness in the target neuron (tolerance). If morphine is withdrawn or blocked abruptly with naloxone, the available level of "analgesia" (opioid plus morphine) is grossly inadequate to meet need. In response to the deficit, target cells enter into activities that lead to withdrawal signs. The abstinence syndrome subsides as peptide stores are replenished.

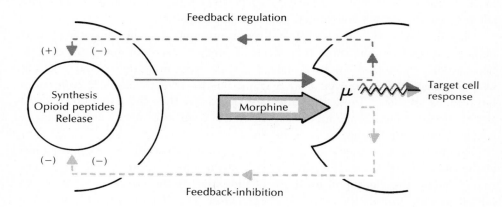

to codeine develops more slowly, and the drug is less likely to be abused than morphine. As used clinically, codeine also has less activity on the gastrointestinal and urinary tracts and on the pupil, and it causes less nausea and constipation. It is the opiate most frequently prescribed, often in combinations with aspirin or acetaminophen and miscellaneous other agents. Codeine is widely used to relieve moderate pain and may be injected if necessary.

Codeine is partly demethylated to morphine in the body and is partly changed to norcodeine. The conjugated forms of these compounds are excreted in the urine.

Semisynthetic opiates and other phenanthrene derivatives

None of the semisynthetic opiate agonists (Table 29-1) are commonly used in the United States. **Hydrocodone** and **oxycodone** resemble codeine structurally. **Oxymorphone** is a more potent analgesic than morphine but causes more side effects. **Hydromorphone** is also more potent than morphine in producing analgesia and respiratory depression but may be less nauseating and constipating. The **hydrochlorides of opium alkaloids** product is a concentrated preparation that contains the alkaloids of opium in the same proportion as they exist naturally. It contains about 50% morphine.

TABLE 29-1   Dosage information for opioids

Drug	Route*	Equieffective doses†‡ (mg) Oral	Equieffective doses†‡ (mg) Injection	Duration[8,22] (hours)	Available preparations§ (mg)
Agonists:					
Naturally-occurring alkaloids					
Morphine sulfate	1-4	60	10	4-5	S: 10, 20/5 ml; 20/ml; T: 15, 30; R: 5-20; I: 2-15/ml; I°: 10-30; PF: 0.5, 1/ml
Codeine phosphate	1, 2	200	130	4-6	S: 15/5 ml; T: 15-60; I: 15-60/ml; I°: 15-60
Codeine sulfate	1, 2	200	130	4-6	T: 15-60; I°: 15-60
Hydrochlorides of opium alkaloids (Pantopon)	2		20	4-5	I: 20/ml
Semisynthetic opiates and other phenanthrene derivatives					
Hydrocodone bitartrate	1				Combinations only
Hydromorphone hydrochloride (Dilaudid)	1-3	7.5	1.5	4-5	T: 1-4; R: 3; I: 1-10/ml
Heroin hydrochloride	1, 2	60	5	3-4	Not available in U.S.A.
Levorphanol tartrate (Levo-Dromoran)	1, 2	4	2	4-7	T: 2; I: 2/ml
Nalbuphine hydrochloride‖ (Nubain)	2		10	4-6	I: 10, 20/ml
Oxycodone hydrochloride	1	30		4-5	S: 5/5 ml; T: 5
Oxymorphone hydrochloride (Numorphan)	2, 3		1	4-6	R: 5; I: 1, 1.5/ml
Butorphanol tartrate‖ (Stadol)	2		2	4-6	I: 1, 2/ml
Buprenorphine‖ (Buprenex)	2		0.4	4-6	I: 0.3/ml
Phenylpiperidines					
Meperidine hydrochloride (Demerol, Pethadol)	1, 2	300	80	2-4	S: 50/5 ml; T: 50, 100; I: 25-100/ml
Alphaprodine hydrochloride (Nisentil)	2		45		I: 40, 60/ml
Diphenoxylate hydrochloride (Lomotil, others)	1	5-10		3-4	T: 2.5; S: 2.5/5 ml (with atropine)
Loperamide hydrochloride (Imodium)	1	2-4		8-12	C: 2; S: 1/5 ml
Fentanyl (citrate) (Sublimaze)	2		0.1	0.5-2	I: 0.05/ml
Sufentanil (citrate) (Sufenta)	2		0.02	2-4	I: 0.05/ml
Alfentanil (Alfenta)	2		0.5	0.5-1	I: 0.5/ml
Diphenylheptanes					
Methadone hydrochloride (Dolophine, Methadose)	1, 2	20	10	3-6	S: 5, 10/5 ml, 10/ml; T: 5-40; I: 10/ml
Propoxyphene hydrochloride (Darvon)	1	130		4-6	C: 32, 65
Propoxyphene napsylate (Darvon-N)	1	130		4-6	S: 50/5 ml; T: 100
Miscellaneous					
Pentazocine hydrochloride‖ (Talwin Nx)	1	180		4-7	T: 50
Pentazocine (lactate)‖ (Talwin)	2		60	4-6	I: 30/ml
Antagonists:					
Naloxone hydrochloride (Narcan)	2		0.4		I: 0.02-1/ml
Naltrexone (Trexan)	1	50/day			T: 50

*1, Oral; 2, parenteral; 3, rectal; 4, extradural.
†Primary source.[8]
‡Agonists: acute analgesia or antidiarrheal (diphenoxylate, loperamide); antagonists: initial doses for acute opioid intoxication or maintenance dose (naltrexone).
§C, Capsules; I, solution for injection; I°, soluble tablets to be dissolved for injection; PF, preservative-free for spinal administration; R, rectal suppositories; S, solution, syrup for ingestion; T, tablets.
‖Agonist-antagonist.

Heroin is a highly euphoriant and analgesic drug. It is much preferred by addicts, who may take it intravenously to obtain a peculiar orgastic sensation. Heroin may not be legally manufactured in or imported into the United States, though it is used clinically elsewhere for its analgesic properties. Its acetyl groups reduce its polarity, relative to morphine, so that heroin penetrates the blood-brain barrier more quickly. However, in the body heroin is rapidly hydrolyzed to 6-acetylmorphine and then to morphine,[15] which is believed primarily responsible for the effects. Although its use in the United States for relief of chronic pain has been advocated, there is no evidence that heroin can provide better analgesia than morphine.[16] The greater solubility of heroin would be advantageous in reducing the volume injected in patients whose pain is not adequately relieved by oral morphine, but other opioids that share this attribute, such as hydromorphone, are already available.

MEPERIDINE AND RELATED COMPOUNDS

Meperidine, introduced originally as an antispasmotic of the atropine type, is probably the opioid most frequently used for parenteral inpatient analgesia, despite local irritation. Its action is relatively short, and intermittent intramuscular administration may inadequately sustain analgesia. Intravenous infusion and oral administration at frequent intervals have been recommended for more consistent relief of acute pain.[6]

Despite early claims, meperidine is just as depressant to respiration and as addictive as morphine when compared in equianalgesic doses, though at birth neonates may exhibit somewhat less respiratory depression if the mother receives meperidine rather than morphine. It is generally believed that meperidine has relatively less activity on the gastrointestinal and biliary tracts and on bronchial smooth muscle. Meperidine lacks useful antitussive or antidiarrheal activity but may cause mydriasis in addicts and tachycardia because of muscarinic blockade.

The liver plays an important role in the metabolism of meperidine, and so usual doses of the drug may be toxic to persons with liver disease. Meperidine is not useful for management of chronic pain because normeperidine, a metabolite that can cause seizures, tends to accumulate, particularly in the elderly and patients with diminished renal function. Ordinary doses of meperidine have caused severe untoward reactions and death in patients taking MAO inhibitors.

Meperidine

Fentanyl

Diphenoxylate

Alphaprodine has a prompt but short analgesic action. It is not given intramuscularly because of unpredictable absorption and adverse reactions.

Fentanyl is a very potent opioid used as an intramuscular or intravenous analgesic in *balanced anesthesia* with nitrous oxide and oxygen, in *neuroleptanalgesia* with a neuroleptic, such as droperidol (in Innovar), or even as the primary anesthetic with oxygen alone. Such combinations maintain a relatively stable cardiovascular system and constitute a common anesthetic regimen for cardiac surgery.[3] The doses of opioid used, for instance 1 to 3 mg/kg in the case of morphine, are much higher than those ordinarily used for analgesia, and residual respiratory depression may require prolonged postoperative ventilation. Alternatively, postoperative depression can be reversed by the antagonist naloxone, provided that the patient is watched carefully to ensure that the antagonist outlasts the agonist. With such doses there is a high incidence of skeletal muscle rigidity, especially in the thorax and abdomen, that responds to neuromuscular blocking drugs. Anesthesia has sometimes been inadequate, as indicated by autonomic stimulation and postoperative reports of patient awareness. Bradycardia or hypotension may also occur. In another context, fentanyl has formed a starting point for manufacture of so-called *designer drugs* (see Chapter 30). **Sufentanil** is about five times more potent than fentanyl and provides somewhat faster recovery. Unlike morphine, these agents do not release histamine in man.[23] **Alfentanil,** another agent in this class, is less potent but also shorter acting and may become especially useful for short procedures.

Diphenoxylate (with atropine) and **loperamide** are used only as antidiarrheal drugs.[1] Atropine is combined with diphenoxylate to discourage overzealous self-medication. Although its central nervous system effects are usually minimal, intoxication with this mixture can be characterized by typical symptoms of both opioid and anticholinergic intoxication. Loperamide undergoes extensive enterohepatic circulation and has minimal, if any, abuse potential or central nervous system activity. If central nervous system depression should occur, it can be antagonized by naloxone. Neither agent is recommended for children under 2 years of age, and they should not be used if the diarrhea is attributable to organisms, such as *Salmonella*, that penetrate the intestinal mucosa.

METHADONE AND RELATED COMPOUNDS

Methadone was developed in Germany during World War II as a substitute for morphine. The two-dimensional structural formula of methadone does not resemble that of morphine; however a disubstituted *pseudo*piperidine ring is evident in three-dimensional representation. The analgesic potency and other properties of methadone are quite similar to those of morphine, but methadone is more suitable for oral administration since it undergoes less first-pass inactivation. Although a single dose of methadone has about the same duration of analgesic action as morphine, when given chronically methadone accumulates and can be given at longer intervals.

Tolerance to and dependence on methadone occur, but the abstinence syndrome is less severe, though more prolonged, than that after morphine withdrawal. Several favorable properties have led to unique applications of methadone in the withdrawal or maintenance of opioid addicts, discussed in Chapter 30. Methadone is also employed for relief of severe chronic pain. Methadyl acetate (*l*-α-acetylmethadol, LAAM) is under investigation as a long-acting methadone substitute for maintenance therapy. An oral dose has a duration of action of 2 to 4 days.

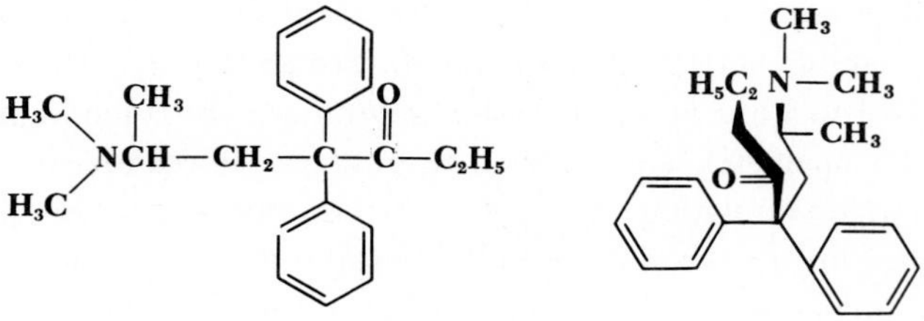

Methadone

Propoxyphene is a widely prescribed drug despite serious reservations about its efficacy. It is a weak narcotic analgesic that is available only for oral administration and is commonly used in combinations with aspirin or acetaminophen. Occasional doses of less than 100 mg of propoxyphene alone probably have placebo value only and are certainly no more analgesic than aspirin. The *dextro* isomer of propoxyphene is used for analgesia. The *levo* isomer has been used as an antitussive.

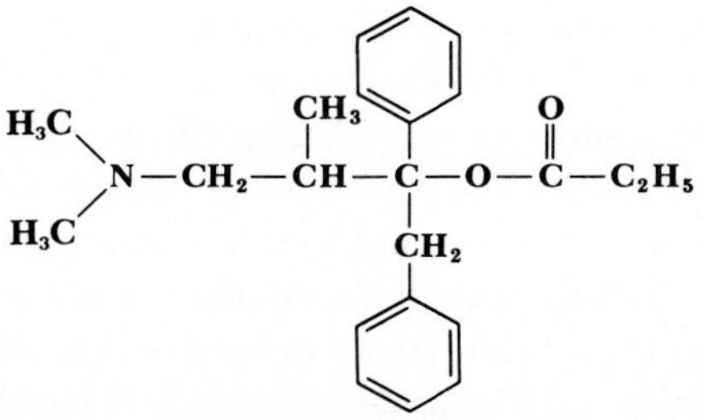

Propoxyphene

Propoxyphene overdose was once responsible for many deaths each year in the United States, partly because the drug is so readily available. Signs of serious overdose resemble those of morphine[26]—respiratory depression, cardiovascular abnormalities, stupor, and constricted pupils. Convulsions are not uncommon. Respiratory depression responds to naloxone. The presence of aspirin or acetaminophen in the mixtures complicates management of toxicity as does concomitant ingestion of alcohol or other depressants. When its widespread use is taken into consideration, the number of persons addicted to propoxyphene is low, though tolerance and dependence are known to occur. The prudent physician, however, will exercise caution in prescribing propoxyphene for persons with a history of substance abuse.

An allyl ($-CH_2CH=CH_2$) substitution on the nitrogen atom of opioids yields compounds that antagonize narcotic actions. Allyl-substituted morphine (*N*-allylnormorphine), or **nalorphine,** once clinically important in reversing narcotic intoxication, has been replaced by naloxone. Nalorphine precipitates acute withdrawal in dependent persons. In contrast, in a person who is neither intoxicated nor dependent nalorphine behaves as an agonist and can be analgesic and dysphoric or depress respiration. The latter action can worsen ventilation in someone intoxicated with general central nervous system depressants or mildly intoxicated with an opioid.

NARCOTIC ANTAGONISTS

Nalorphine

Naloxone

Naloxone, the *N*-allyl derivative of oxymorphone, is now the most important antagonist. It differs from nalorphine primarily in lacking agonist activity and hence does not depress respiration. The usual adult dosage of naloxone is 0.4 to 2 mg intravenously, at 2- to 3-minute intervals if necessary. If a cumulative dose of 10 mg of naloxone has not improved respiration, an opioid is unlikely to have contributed to the central depression. Although the initial dose for children is 0.01 mg/kg, 10 times that much may be necessary.[19] Naloxone has a nearly immediate action that lasts 45 minutes or more. Since some agonists, such as methadone, may depress respiration for a day or two, additional injections or an infusion of naloxone may be necessary. A difficult therapeutic problem is the treatment of opioid intoxication in an addict. When naloxone precipitates abstinence in such patients, the syndrome is short but may be very severe.

Naltrexone, a longer-acting pure antagonist, has been approved to facilitate maintenance of abusers in an opioid-free state after withdrawal (detoxification). After an opioid-free period of 7 to 10 days, a naloxone challenge should be given before naltrexone therapy to be certain that detoxification is complete. Naltrexone doses of 50 to 150 mg given daily to every third day, respectively, can then prevent physical dependence as well as the pleasurable effects of opioid agonists. Liver damage is a potential problem, and periodic tests of hepatic function are recommended.

Classification of opioid receptors

Until recently, the explanation for the pattern of effects of nalorphine was that it is a *partial agonist* at opioid receptors. Hence nalorphine would mimic opiates in a person previously unexposed to an opioid, whereas in severe intoxication replacement of morphine by nalorphine would lessen depression. In 1976 Martin and his co-workers presented evidence of three types of opioid receptors, which they termed μ (for morphine), κ (for ketocyclazocine), and σ (for SKF 10,047). A δ-receptor has since been widely accepted, and several other receptor types and approaches to nomenclature have been proposed.[18,20] Opioids and endogenous opioid peptides have different degrees of selectivity for the various receptors.[20] Although morphine and ketocyclazocine seem to act on different receptors, they induce many of the same effects. Responses to nalorphine can also be accounted for if it is an antagonist at the μ receptor and an agonist at the κ receptor. Dysphoria, hallucinations, and other adverse mental effects of nalorphine are attributed to stimulation of the σ receptor, which may be a receptor for phencyclidine as well. Clinically, naloxone is a useful antagonist of narcotic analgesics regardless of the type of receptor involved. Somewhat larger doses of naloxone, however, are needed to antagonize agonist-antagonist opioids (see below) than to antagonize morphine. Naloxone is a major tool in studies to ascertain physiologic roles of the endogenous opioid peptides. An understanding of such roles may lead to new therapeutic uses for opioid antagonists.

MIXED AGONIST-ANTAGONISTS

Although a high incidence of dysphoria precluded clinical use of nalorphine itself as an analgesic, its minimal abuse potential led to the search for analgesic drugs that were similar but lacked dysphoric activity. Such agents, like nalorphine, are currently classified as *agonist-antagonist* drugs regardless of their precise interactions with various receptors. As a group, the newer agents are much less likely than nalorphine to elicit dysphoria or hallucinations. They have relatively low potential for abuse but can induce dependence. They cause less severe maximal respiratory depression than pure agonists and are potent enough antagonists to precipitate withdrawal in dependent abusers.

Pentazocine lactate was the first of these agents to be used clinically.[12] It may be useful in prolonged but not terminal illnesses in which more readily addictive drugs would constitute a hazard. However, because of abuse of pentazocine in combination with the antihistamine tripelennamine, so-called *Ts and blues*, naloxone has recently been added to the oral preparation of **pentazocine hydrochloride.** The dose of naloxone (0.5 mg) is too small to have an effect after oral administration, but if the tablets are dissolved for injection, the naloxone can precipitate withdrawal in a dependent user. Pentazocine is more likely to precipitate psychotomimetic effects than pure agonists, and it tends to increase cardiac work, a disadvantage in patients with myocardial infarction.

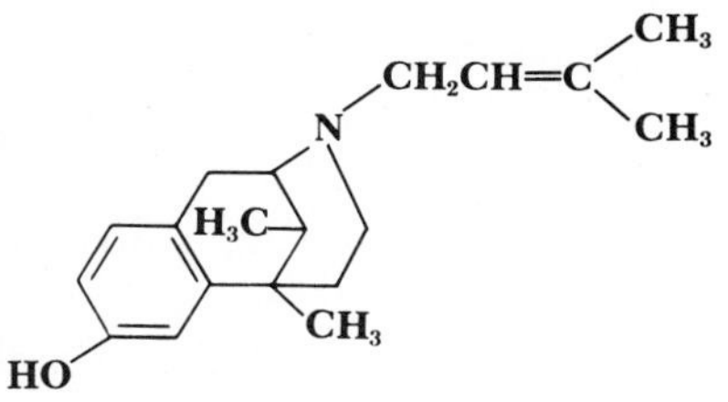

Pentazocine 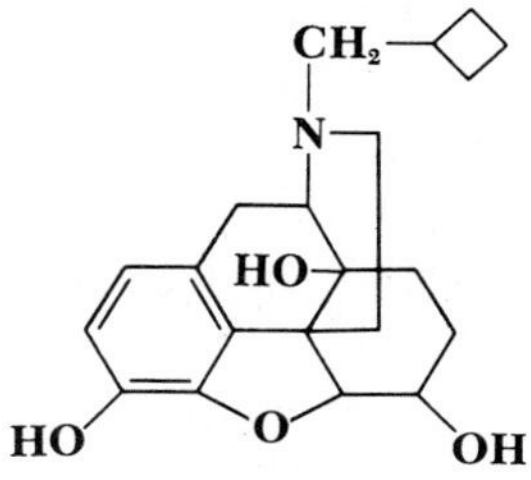 **Nalbuphine** 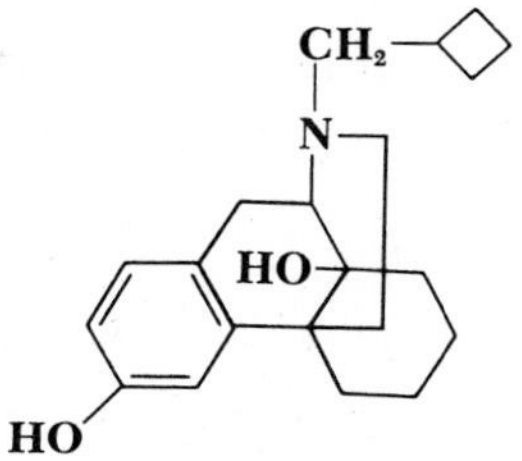 **Butorphanol**

Nalbuphine is equivalent to morphine in analgesic potency.[24] As an antagonist, it has about one hundredth the potency of naloxone. The incidence of dysphoric reactions seems the least of agents in this group. **Butorphanol** has about five times the analgesic potency of morphine and one fortieth the antagonist potency of naloxone. Its clinical applications and abuse potential appear to be roughly comparable to those of pentazocine. **Buprenorphine** is about 30 times more potent than morphine with an analgesic action lasting perhaps 6 to 8 hours. Drowsiness is a very common side effect.

In the following medical conditions morphine and related drugs should be avoided entirely or used with extreme caution:

Head injuries and after craniotomy
Bronchial asthma and other hypoxic states
Acute alcohol intoxication
Convulsive disorders
Undiagnosed acute abdominal conditions

CONTRAINDICATIONS TO THE USE OF MORPHINE AND RELATED AGENTS

Relief of pain may be considered in at least five clinical contexts. (1) Pharmacologic relief of *mild to moderate acute pain,* such as muscle aches or simple headache, is provided by ingestion of aspirin-like drugs discussed in detail in Chapter 31. Neither tolerance nor physical dependence is a problem with these analgesics. (2) More *severe acute pain* after surgery is typically treated initially by injections of morphine or meperidine. The goals in this case are to provide adequate pain relief but at the same time to minimize exposure to the narcotic. Unfortunately, excessive concern with abuse potential can lead to prescription or administration of insufficient analgesic for optimal relief of symptoms.[27] Although a mild degree of physical dependence may develop within a matter of days or a week, such patients seldom if ever become "addicted" to opioids secondary to therapeutic usage. Within a few days, as the pain

CURRENT CLINICAL APPROACHES TO PAIN RELIEF

lessens, injections may be replaced by orally administered codeine or codeine-containing combinations and then by aspirin-like agents alone. (3) *Chronic pain associated with inflammation*, as in rheumatoid arthritis, can be managed for years, without tolerance or physical dependence, by nonsteroidal anti-inflammatory drugs. Aspirin is the least expensive agent, but, if the daily doses required for the anti-inflammatory effect cause intolerable side effects, a large number of alternatives are available. Eventually, as the disease progresses, other modalities of treatment, such as gold salts or other disease-modifying agents may become necessary. (4) One need not be overly concerned about dependence when opioids are used to relieve the *pain of terminal disease*. Here the objective is to extend for as long as possible the period of adequate pain relief.[8,14] The progression of analgesic use is therefore somewhat the reverse of that for postoperative pain, progressing from aspirin to oral codeine to oral morphine to parenteral morphine, eventually perhaps by intravenous infusion or epidural administration.[25] Transcutaneous nerve stimulation, local anesthetics, surgical interruption of afferent neuronal pathways, and so forth may ultimately be required. (5) Finally there are patients who experience pain, which may be very severe and debilitating, for which no organic cause can be found. There is no justification in such cases for opioid therapy, and one of the first goals in pain clinics is to stop analgesic use. Further considerations in management of this type of pain are detailed elsewhere.[22]

CLINICAL PHARMACOLOGY OF ANTITUSSIVE DRUGS	Coughing is usually considered a defense mechanism for clearing the respiratory tract. However, some coughs indicate cardiac dyspnea, pleurisy, hiatal hernia, or other conditions not directly related to tracheobronchial irritation. In many instances coughs should not be restrained lest their prevention lead to pneumonia or other infections. Medical intervention is indicated if coughing serves no useful purpose and interferes with sleep or other normal activities.

Antitussives may suppress the neural component of the cough reflex or may influence the quantity or viscosity of respiratory tract fluid. Drugs that act on the neural component may act in the central nervous system or on sensory endings in the mucous membrane of the respiratory tract. The specific effectiveness of antitussives is difficult to determine because nonspecific sedation and placebos can be of benefit. Furthermore, in many cough mixtures, the demulcent action of the vehicle may play a significant part in the effects claimed.

There is little doubt that morphine and synthetic opioid-like drugs are potent cough suppressants. **Codeine** is the traditional suppressant to which nonaddictive antitussives should be compared in controlled clinical trials. In contrast to morphine, excessive doses of codeine may cause convulsions, especially in children. These convulsions are attributed to disinhibitory effects on spinal neurons. The usual adult antitussive dose of codeine is 15 to 20 mg every 4 to 6 hours. For cough suppression it is usually dispensed in a demulcent syrup or suspension. Mixtures of codeine with an assortment of antihistamines, antipyretics, and other drugs are common; however, these would seem to have little advantage over codeine alone.

Hydrocodone bitartrate (Dicodid) is a more potent antitussive than codeine, but its addiction liability is greater. It is available in 5 mg tablets.

Dextromethorphan hydrobromide (Romilar) is a substituted *dextro* isomer of the narcotic levomethorphan. Dextromethorphan is not analgesic and is not addictive, but toxic doses can depress the central nervous system. It equals codeine in antitussive potency but appears to act on a different receptor.[4] The usual dose is 10 to 30 mg every 4 to 8 hours. Dextromethorphan is available in lozenges with or without benzocaine, in syrups, and in controlled-release liquids.

Noscapine (Tusscapine) is narcotine, an isoquinoline alkaloid found in opium. It is not addictive or analgesic but is claimed to be antitussive. The dose is one or two 15 mg chewable tablets every 4 to 6 hours.

As a general statement, antitussive drugs may be valuable in reducing a useless cough. They are purely symptomatic medications, and their use should not obviate the necessity for treating the cause of the cough if possible.

REFERENCES

1. Awouters, F., Niemegeers, C.J.E., and Janssen, P.A.J.: Pharmacology of antidiarrheal drugs, Annu. Rev. Pharmacol. Toxicol. **23**:279, 1983.
2. Beecher, H.K.: Measurement of subjective responses: quantitative effects of drugs, New York, 1959, Oxford University Press.
3. Bovill, J.G., Sebel, P.S., and Stanley, T.H.: Opioid analgesics in anesthesia: with special reference to their use in cardiovascular anesthesia, Anesthesiology **61**:731, 1984.
4. Chau, T.T., Carter, F.E., and Harris, L.S.: Antitussive effect of the optical isomers of *mu, kappa* and *sigma* opiate agonists/antagonists in the cat, J. Pharmacol. Exp. Ther. **226**:108, 1983.
5. Citron, M.L., Johnston-Early, A., Fossieck, B.E., Jr., et al.: Safety and efficacy of continuous intravenous morphine for severe cancer pain, Am. J. Med. **77**:199, 1984.
6. Edwards, D.J., Svensson, C.K., Visco, J.P., and Lalka, D.: Clinical pharmacokinetics of pethidine: 1982, Clin. Pharmacokinet. **7**:421, 1982.
7. Fields, H.L., and Basbaum, A.I.: Endogenous pain control mechanisms. In Wall, P.D., and Melzack, R., editors: Textbook of pain, Edinburgh, 1984, Churchill Livingstone, p. 142.
8. Foley, K.M.: The treatment of cancer pain, N. Engl. J. Med. **313**:84, 1985.
9. Frederickson, R.C.A., and Geary, L.E.: Endogenous opioid peptides: review of physiological, pharmacological and clinical aspects, Prog. Neurobiol. **19**:19, 1982.
10. Gebhart, G.F.: Opiate and opioid peptide effects on brainstem neurons: relevance to nociception and antinociceptive mechanisms, Pain **12**:93, 1982.
11. Goldstein, A.: Opioid peptides (endorphins) in pituitary and brain: studies on opiate receptors have led to identification of endogenous peptides with morphinelike actions, Science **193**:1081, 1976.
12. Goldstein, G.: Pentazocine, Drug Alcohol Depend. **14**:313, 1985.
13. Gustafsson, L.L., Schildt, B., and Jacobsen, K.: Adverse effects of extradural and intrathecal opiates: report of a nationwide survey in Sweden, Br. J. Anaesth. **54**:479, 1982.
14. Health and Public Policy Committee: Drug therapy for severe, chronic pain in terminal illness, Ann. Intern. Med. **99**:870, 1983.
15. Inturrisi, C.E., Max, M.B., Foley, K.M., et al.: The pharmacokinetics of heroin in patients with chronic pain, N. Engl. J. Med. **310**:1213, 1984.
16. Kaiko, R.F., Wallenstein, S.L., Rogers, A.G., et al.: Analgesic and mood effects

of heroin and morphine in cancer patients with postoperative pain, N. Engl. J. Med. **304**:1501, 1981.

17. Khachaturian, H., Lewis, M.E., Schäfer, M.K.-H., and Watson, S.J.: Anatomy of the CNS opioid systems, Trends NeuroSci. **8**:111, 1985.

18. Martin, W.R.: Pharmacology of opioids, Pharmacol. Rev. **35**:283, 1984.

19. Moore, R.A., Rumack, B.H., Conner, C.S., and Peterson, R.G.: Naloxone: underdosage after narcotic poisoning, Am. J. Dis. Child. **134**:156, 1980.

20. Paterson, S.J., Robson, L.E., and Kosterlitz, H.W.: Classification of opioid receptors, Br. Med. Bull. **39**:31, 1983.

21. Pert, A.: Mechanisms of opiate analgesia and the role of endorphins in pain suppression, Adv. Neurol. **33**:107, 1982.

22. Reuler, J.B., Girard, D.E., and Nardone, D.A.: The chronic pain syndrome: misconceptions and management, Ann. Intern. Med. **93**:588, 1980.

23. Rosow, C.E., Moss, J., Philbin, D.M., and Savarese, J.J.: Histamine release during morphine and fentanyl anesthesia, Anesthesiology **56**:93, 1982.

24. Schmidt, W.K., Tam, S.W., Shotzberger, G.S., et al.: Nalbuphine, Drug Alcohol Depend. **14**:339, 1985.

25. Slattery, P.J., and Boas, R.A.: Newer methods of delivery of opiates for relief of pain, Drugs **30**:539, 1985.

26. Sloth Madsen, P., Strøm, J., Reiz, S., and Sørensen, M.B.: Acute propoxyphene self-poisoning in 222 consecutive patients, Acta Anaesthesiol. Scand. **28**:661, 1984.

27. Sriwatanakul, K., Weis, O.F., Alloza, J.L., et al.: Analysis of narcotic analgesic usage in the treatment of postoperative pain, J.A.M.A. **250**:926, 1983.

28. Twycross, R.G.: The Brompton cocktail. In Bonica, J.J., and Ventafridda, V., editors: Advances in pain research and therapy, vol. 2, New York, 1979, Raven Press, p. 291.

29. Wamsley, J.K.: Opioid receptors: autoradiography, Pharmacol. Rev. **35**:69, 1983.

Chapter 30

Contemporary drug abuse

Most abused drugs are neuropharmacologic agents for an obvious reason: the user wishes to modify his mental state. Abuse of other drugs is encountered less commonly but is seen, for example, in administration of thyroid hormones, cardiac glycosides, and diuretics in weight-reduction programs.

Drug abuse may exist with or without drug dependence, and dependence may occur without abuse. Initial experimentation with heroin represents abuse without dependence though dependence may soon follow; the maintenance of a diabetic on insulin represents dependence without abuse.

Drug dependence has traditionally been conceptualized in terms of a rigid duality: *psychologic dependence* and *physical dependence*. This paradigm may originate in the ancient distinction between mind and body. This approach is still prevalent today and is incorporated into discussions in this chapter. If a physiologically disruptive withdrawal illness occurs after abrupt discontinuation of a drug that has been taken over a prolonged period of time, the drug is said to be physically addicting. Physically addicting drugs include opiates, barbiturates, antianxiety agents, ethanol, and some nonbarbiturate sedatives (Table 30-1). Psychologic drug dependence, on the other hand, has been described as a craving for a drug that produces a desired effect and to which one has become accustomed by habit; the habit has become a "crutch" and may assume enormous importance to the person. It is said that psychologic dependence, not physical dependence, drives opiate addicts back to their drug after months or years of successful abstinence.

The strict dichotomy between psychologic and physical dependence is now being reevaluated. Although there are instances in which one or the other is clearly dominant, there are other cases in which neither is exactly separate from the other. We may find that psychologic dependence is accompanied by alterations in cell-surface receptor sites and is fundamentally structural after all. It may nevertheless be useful to conceptualize the seizures of barbiturate withdrawal as an expression of physical dependence and the yearning for another marijuana "joint" as psychologic, until we show, for example, that marijuana use has actually altered the neural substrate.

Drug abuse has radically altered the face of today's society. With the ever-growing skills of undercover chemists producing "designer" drugs and ready and willing customers from all cultural levels, the trend is strong and growing. New expressions of morbidity crop up almost daily, from the induction of a parkinsonian-like syndrome by a contaminant in the "new heroin" to fatal ventricular arrhythmias in cocaine users. Parenteral drug abusers constitute a major category of victims of acquired

TABLE 30-1	Comparison of commonly abused centrally acting drugs		
Drug category	Physical dependence*	Tolerance	Psychotogenic in high doses
Opiates	X	X	
Marijuana		X	X
Ethanol	X	X	
Barbiturates	X	X	
Amphetamines		X	X
Cocaine			X
Psychotomimetics		X	X
Antianxiety agents	X	X	
Inhalants†		?	X

*An abstinence syndrome results from abrupt discontinuation of any drug producing physical dependence.
†See text for details.

immunodeficiency syndrome (AIDS) in the United States; public health authorities in some communities are considering the advantages of providing free sterile needles to drug users, to reduce the probability of transmission of human immunodeficiency virus.

Epidemiologic research has become an important tool in drug abuse research.[13] Epidemiologists use statistical methods to detect and analyze variations in patterns of health and illness; unexpected associations are found through exhaustive analysis of the data, and causative factors may emerge with greater clarity. In some cases the spread of an abused drug resembles an epidemic. It has even been suggested that drug abuse may be considered a communicable disease; the drug is the infectious agent, humans are the host and reservoir, and the drug user is the vector.

The major categories of abused neuropharmacologic agents will be considered separately, followed by discussion of the multifaceted clinical picture of drug abuse.

OPIATES AND OPIATE-LIKE DRUGS

In some state statutes the legal category "narcotics" embraces the opiates, opiate-like drugs, marijuana, and cocaine. Medically defined, however, the term "narcotic" refers only to drugs having both a sedative and an analgesic action and is essentially restricted to the opiates and opiate-like drugs. These drugs are classified in Table 29-1, p. 327.

Physical dependence and tolerance

Pronounced physical dependence develops rapidly during continued administration of the narcotic drugs. A striking tolerance also develops to all but the constipating and miotic actions; the addict continues to have constricted pupils, even after low doses. A high degree of cross-tolerance exists among opiates and opiate-like drugs despite chemical dissimilarities.

Since the 1960s opiate abuse has spread to all socioeconomic groups and consists largely in intravenous heroin use. Heroin is believed by most users to be more euphoric than other opiates. The user seeks a mood state commonly described as "relief," consisting in a dreamy state of drive satiation and a feeling of well-being; he also seeks avoidance of the withdrawal illness, and his desperation after the onset of withdrawal symptoms may provoke aggressive and risk-taking behavior.

There is no evidence that opiates produce organic central nervous system damage or other organ pathosis, even after years of continuous use. An 84-year-old physician morphine addict showed no evidence of mental or physical deterioration after continuous use for 62 years.[5] Complications of unsterile parenteral administration, however, are legion and include AIDS, viral hepatitis, bacterial and fungal endocarditis, nephropathy with massive proteinuria, systemic and pulmonary mycoses, lung abscess, pulmonary fibrosis or granulomatosis, pneumonia, chronic liver disease (of obscure type), transverse myelitis, osteomyelitis (frequently by *Pseudomonas*), acute and chronic polyneuropathy, acute and chronic myopathy, acute rhabdomyolysis with myoglobinuria, tetanus, tuberculosis (including tuberculous vertebral osteomyelitis), malaria (now rare in the United States), thrombophlebitis, cellulitis, local abscesses, and sclerosis and occlusion of veins. In addition, there is a constant risk of overdose and death from an unexpectedly concentrated sample of heroin; the triad of coma (or stupor), respiratory depression, and pinpoint pupils is stongly suggestive of opiate overdose. Death from overdose results from respiratory depression or acute pulmonary edema or both; the mechanism of production of pulmonary edema is obscure. Still another hazard is the masking of pain, which may delay awareness of a serious medical condition; cigarette burns between the fingers of opiate addicts are a common finding. Since 1955 most cases of tetanus in New York City have occurred in heroin addicts.

Additional dangers arise from foreign substances intentionally or accidentally added to the sample by the supplier. Heroin is commonly "cut" (diluted) with lactose or quinine; other adulterants include barbiturates, procaine, mannitol, aminopyrine, methapyrilene, and baking soda.

One ever-present danger of street drugs, of course, is that the actual chemical at hand is not the one it is supposed to be. The recent "designer" drugs are so-named because they are new, at least temporarily legal creations designed to circumvent the law, yet produce effects similar to their illegal counterparts. "New heroin" is such a creation and was found to contain 1-methyl-4-phenyl-1,2,3,6-tetrahydropyridine (MPTP), which is believed to have induced a syndrome similar to Parkinson's disease in several victims[3] (see p. 122).

The social consequences of narcotic addiction include crime, interruption of employment, and personal and family neglect. Criminal activity is usually restricted to property offenses and peddling, which may become necessary, in the absence of employment, to support the habit. Some addicts become functionally disabled, spending much of the 24-hour period "nodding" (remaining inactive in a semistuporous state) or suffering withdrawal symptoms; other addicts who have an uninter-rupted drug supply and are careful with dosage may lead a seemingly normal life at work and at home. The concept of the opiate addict as a dangerous dope fiend is not justified; in contrast to alcohol, the opiates tend to quell aggressive drives. When an addict's supply of drugs is exhausted, however, violence may be used to obtain a continuing supply.

Pentazocine, a synthetic opioid with both agonist and weak antagonist properties, has become increasingly popular as a street drug since its introduction as an analgesic of low addiction liability in 1967. The combination, called "Ts and blues," of pen-tazocine with the antihistamine tripelennamine is currently widely abused in the United States; serious medical complications including seizures and acute psychotic episodes have resulted. In addition, severe skin ulcerations, subcutaneous abscesses, and muscle necrosis have occurred after parenteral administration of this combina-tion.

Abstinence syndromes MORPHINE AND HEROIN	Symptoms first appear about 8 hours after the last dose, reaching peak intensity between 36 and 72 hours. Lacrimation, rhinorrhea, yawning, and diaphoresis appear between 8 and 12 hours. Shortly thereafter, at about 13 hours, a restless sleep (the "yen") may intervene. At about 20 hours, gooseflesh, dilated pupils, agitation, and tremors may appear. During the second and third day, when the illness is at its peak, symptoms and signs include weakness, insomnia, chills, intestinal cramps, nausea, vomiting, diarrhea, violent yawning, muscle aches in the legs, severe low back pain, elevation of blood pressure and pulse rate, diaphoresis, and waves of gooseflesh. The skin may have the appearance of a cold plucked turkey, hence the expression "cold turkey," denoting abrupt withdrawal. Fluid depletion during the withdrawal period has at times resulted in cardiovascular collapse and death. At any point during the course of withdrawal, administration of an opioid in adequate dosage will dramatically eliminate the symptoms and restore a state of apparent normalcy. The duration of the syndrome is roughly 7 to 10 days.
OTHER NARCOTIC DRUGS	Most narcotic abstinence syndromes are similar to that of morphine or heroin. Narcotics with a shorter duration of action tend to produce a shorter and more severe abstinence syndrome; those with a longer duration of action, such as methadone, usually produce a milder but more prolonged syndrome.
Treatment approaches to opioid dependence	An opiate user must first be withdrawn, or "detoxified" from his physical depen-dence on the drug. Withdrawal may be accomplished simply by administration of smaller and smaller doses of the same opiate over a period of days, under close supervision in a hospital. Recently, however, the drug clonidine, a centrally acting antihypertensive agent, has been found effective in reducing the severity of opiate withdrawal. Like opiates, clonidine produces sedation, but it is not an opiate and is not antagonized by naloxone. The discovery that clonidine, like opiates, decreases the excitability of noradrenergic locus ceruleus neurons indicated that clonidine might

be effective in opiate withdrawal. It was subsequently found that both clonidine and opiates depress preganglionic sympathetic activity; the effectiveness of clonidine in opiate withdrawal may be related in part to this action on nonopiate receptors.[6] Clonidine has been found to be a safe and effective nonopiate method of opiate detoxification.[9,31]

After detoxification, a far more difficult task confronts the clinician: rehabilitation. The craving for opiates is probably "remembered" longer than that for other drugs of abuse and results in exceedingly high rates of recidivism. The first major advance in rehabilitation programs for opiate abusers was made in 1964, when Drs. Dole and Nyswander reported that if heroin addicts were maintained on methadone given orally they could give up heroin and engage in an active rehabilitation program.[2] Methadone, a synthetic opiate-like drug, substitutes for most other opiates and is well absorbed from the gastrointestinal tract, unlike morphine or heroin; parenteral administration is thereby avoided. In addition, methadone has a longer duration of action than other opioids, permitting administration only once in a 24-hour period.

In the early 1970s methadone maintenance was attempted with federal support on a nationwide scale. It was found to be less effective on a large scale than on the smaller personal scale initiated by Dole and Nyswander, but it was more effective than any other known approach. One-year retention rates were found to be about 50% at best. After a period of 12 to 36 months of methadone maintenance, withdrawal of methadone (methadone detoxification) is attempted. One study has shown a 58% return to narcotic use 6 years after methadone detoxification.[29] The highest recidivism rates appear to be associated with premature detoxification from methadone maintenance.

A synthetic congener of methadone, l-α-acetylmethadol hydrochloride (methadylacetate), can prevent withdrawal symptoms for more than 72 hours. Because of this relative advantage, methadylacetate is currently being evaluated as a substitute for methadone. It appears that the two drugs are equivalent in rehabilitative efficacy but that one or the other may be more effective with different subsets of the addict population.[15,26]

Narcotic antagonists

The search continues for the "ideal" narcotic antagonist, that is, a pharmacologic agent that blocks the effects of opiates, has few or no side effects of its own, requires relatively infrequent administration, and is not prohibitively expensive. No drug has yet met these criteria, but some have come close. The earliest known narcotic antagonists were nalorphine and levallorphan. However, these antagonists also have some agonist activity. Their administration in the presence of nonnarcotic respiratory depressants like alcohol or barbiturates caused additive central nervous system depression. On the other hand, naloxone abolishes the euphoria, respiratory depression, nausea, and gastrointestinal disturbances produced by opiates and causes virtually no side effects; it is expensive, however, and its limited duration of action requires frequent dosing for treatment or prevention of addiction. Another narcotic antagonist, naltrexone, has been used with some success. It possesses a much greater affinity for opiate receptors than the opiates themselves and therefore effectively abolishes the action of opiates. Treatment with naltrexone is begun after a drug-free interval of 7 to 10 days; this delay constitutes a disadvantage in the treatment program because of the difficulty of remaining abstinent for that period of time. However, the delay is necessary to avoid precipitating withdrawal when the antagonist is first administered.

ETHANOL

The intemperate use of ethanol probably represents the most serious form of drug abuse in Western society, if not in all civilized countries. Ethanol is a significant contributing factor in 35% to 50% of cases of marital violence and 10% of occupational injuries. Some 18,000 or more traffic deaths annually (about 40%) in the United States are alcohol related. Such accidents and injuries are estimated to have cost Americans $117 billion in 1983.[14]

Alcohol has recently been shown to exert a potentiating effect on motor vehicle injury.[30] Data on more than one million drivers involved in highway crashes indicate that the drinking driver is more likely to suffer serious injury or death in comparison with the nondrinking driver. The intoxicated passenger is also at greater risk of injury in any given crash. These findings are consistent with earlier evidence from animal research that alcohol renders a victim more vulnerable, all else being equal, to trauma.

Physical dependence and tolerance

A great degree of physical dependence and a moderate degree of tolerance develop when ethanol is ingested regularly and in large amounts. Tolerance may be explained in part by induced hypertrophy of hepatic smooth endoplasmic reticulum with stimulation of ethanol metabolism.

Characteristics of abuse

Alcohol is a primary and continuous depressant of the central nervous system. Even a small amount decreases mental acuity and impairs motor coordination; at times, however, this deficit may be more than compensated for by improved performance accompanying the induced state of euphoria and disinhibition.

In chronic alcoholism one may observe organ pathoses and clinical syndromes not usually associated with other types of drug abuse, including fatty metamorphosis and cirrhosis of the liver, peripheral polyneuropathy, alcoholic gastritis, Korsakoff's psychosis, Wernicke's encephalopathy, and complications of portal hypertension. Some of these changes are believed to result from nutritional deficiency rather than the direct action of alcohol; unlike other commonly abused drugs, alcohol supplies calories, depressing the appetite and encouraging a dietary deficit in the face of a deceptive maintenance of body weight. It is believed that alcohol is directly incriminated, however, in the pathogenesis of alcoholic fatty liver. Chronic consumption leads to hypertrophy of hepatic smooth endoplasmic reticulum, with consequent stimulation of drug metabolism. This may explain in part the tolerance of alcoholics, *when sober*, to other drugs such as barbiturates.

Genetic factors appear to be highly significant in the predisposition to alcoholism.[19] Familial occurrence of alcoholism has been well documented, and the risk to an individual increases with the proximity of relationships and the number of affected relatives. A higher concordance rate occurs in identical as compared to fraternal twins. Children from families of alcoholics, when adopted by other families, show a fourfold higher risk of alcoholism than controls, whereas children of nonalcoholics reared by alcoholics are at no greater risk than controls.[24]

Developmental defects of the central nervous system occur with prenatal exposure to ethanol and may result in motor dysfunction, hypotonia, cognitive deficiencies, and microcephaly. As many as 2% of all babies born in the Western world may suffer to some extent from this *fetal alcohol syndrome*. A recent study provides evidence that cortical neuronal proliferation and migration are impaired by prenatal exposure to ethanol in the earliest stages of neuronal ontogeny.[20]

There is compelling evidence that alcoholism interferes with immune defense and thereby predisposes to infection.[1,14] Chronic alcohol intake depresses both development and expression of cell-mediated immunity. Persons using alcohol to excess should therefore be considered as being immunosuppressed.

Abstinence syndrome

After prolonged, heavy intake of alcohol, withdrawal symptoms may appear within a few hours after the last dose; these include tremulousness, weakness, anxiety, intestinal cramps, and hyperreflexia. Between 12 and 24 hours the state of "acute alcoholic hallucinosis" may appear, in which visual hallucinations are reported, at first only with the eyes closed. By 48 hours an acute neurologic syndrome may become apparent, with confusion, disorientation, and delusional thinking. When this syndrome is accompanied by gross tremulousness, it is called "delirium tremens." Major convulsive seizures ("rum fits") may occur but are less common than in barbiturate withdrawal. The chronic alcoholic may be in too poor a condition to withstand the stress of withdrawal; if death is not the price, recovery occurs by the fifth to the seventh day.

Treatment

The treatment of acute and chronic alcoholism, like that of other types of drug abuse, often requires in-hospital detoxification and intensive psychiatric treatment. Alcoholics Anonymous represents a unique and often pivotal source of help for alcoholics, with no parallel in other forms of drug abuse, though AA groups may offer help to any drug abuser. The only pharmacologic agent used specifically for treatment of alcoholism is disulfiram (see p. 297). There is some question as to the effectiveness of disulfiram in promoting abstinence. For a certain subset of more reliable patients who can be counted on to take the drug regularly, disulfiram may help sustain abstinence; like most treatment methods in any form of drug abuse, its usefulness is limited.[7]

MARIJUANA   SLANG EQUIVALENTS:

Grass, weed, pot, dope, hemp
Marijuana cigarette = joint, "j," number, reefer, root
Cigarette butt = roach

Marijuana (Mexican Spanish *marihuana*) is inadequately described by any one drug category because it possesses properties of a sedative, euphoriant, and hallucinogen.

The source of marijuana is the Indian hemp plant *Cannabis sativa*, a herbaceous annual growing wild in temperate climates all over the world. The plant is dioecious; that is, male and female flowers are borne on separate plants. The active compounds are most concentrated in the resinous exudate of the female flower clusters.

In the United States the term *marijuana* refers to any part or extract of the plant. The smoking mixture termed "bhang" consists only of the cut tops of uncultivated female plants. The most concentrated natural supply of cannabinols is found in preparations called "hashish" and "charas," which consist largely of the actual resin from the flower clusters of cultivated female plants. The potency of any marijuana preparation varies with plant strain and growth conditions.

The principal psychoactive compound in marijuana is *l*-Δ^9-*trans*-tetrahydrocannabinol (hereafter referred to as Δ^9-THC; Δ^1-THC and Δ^9-THC represent different systems of nomenclature for the same compound). A varying, usually small, amount of $\Delta^{8(9)}$-THC may also be present.

Δ^9-THC

$\Delta^{8(9)}$-THC ($\Delta^{1(6)}$-THC)

Physical dependence and tolerance

Physical dependence is not known to develop; tolerance has been observed in most animal species studied. One study has demonstrated a dose-related cross-tolerance between Δ^9-THC and ethanol, and the cross-tolerance is symmetric (either drug inducing cross-tolerance to the other).

Characteristics of intoxication
ANECDOTAL REPORTS

Most users report that marijuana induces a dreamy, euphoric state of altered consciousness, with feelings of detachment, gaiety, jocularity, and preoccupation with simple and familiar things. In the company of others there is a tendency toward laughter and loquaciousness. Perceptual distortion of space and time is regularly reported; distances may be judged inaccurately, and things may seem to be happening very slowly or very rapidly.

Dissociative phenomena such as partial amnesia or a feeling of being outside of oneself are frequently reported. Libido is variably affected; since sexual desire may be enhanced, marijuana has gained a reputation as an aphrodisiac. There may be an unusually vivid remembrance or reliving of experiences or mood states of the past. The continuity of a story or movie may be lost, to be replaced by an intense experiencing of individual segments or scenes. Users are sometimes recognized by the characteristic hilarity of their mutual laughter, which may become prolonged and uncontrolled. Appetite and appreciation of the flavor of food are usually enhanced, and weight gain may accompany regular smoking.

A paranoid state is sometimes reported, in which the smoker is keenly aware of others watching him; some forsake marijuana for this reason. Antisocial behavior under the influence of marijuana appears to be rare; users ordinarily withdraw from company that they find unpleasant.

Adverse reactions to unadulterated preparations of marijuana are relatively rare but may be serious when they do occur. Such reactions include acute paranoid states, dissociative states, and, less commonly, acute psychotic reactions. Adverse reactions to marijuana appear to be dose related (they are more frequent with hashish) and highly individualized (some users regularly have adverse reactions and some never do). Evaluation of reports of adverse reactions is complicated by the fact that marijuana is frequently adulterated with other drugs; some reports have failed to consider this possibility.

CLINICAL FINDINGS

Regular use of marijuana may result in a pervasive feeling of apathy, the so-called *amotivational syndrome*. The user discovers that "things just don't seem important to me any more." This development may be especially damaging to the psychologic maturation of the adolescent. Such a syndrome is undoubtedly multidetermined, but in many adolescents undergoing psychotherapy, its development has been observed to coincide temporally with regular use of marijuana.

A study of marijuana-induced temporal disintegration was conducted at the Stanford University School of Medicine,[17,18] using doses of 20, 40, and 60 mg of THC (the higher two doses were admittedly larger than the dose to be expected from ordinary social smoking). All three doses significantly impaired serial operations in performing a task requiring sequential cognitive functions. Progressively more errors were made with increasing dose. The subjects reported a feeling of timelessness and uncertainty of how much time had elapsed; the time line extending from past to future seemed discontinuous, and past and future seemed unrelated to the present. One person said, "I . . . can't stay on the same subject . . . I can't remember what I just said or what I want to say . . . because there are just so many thoughts that are broken in time, one chunk there and one chunk here." Impairment of short-term memory with emergence of loose associations was noted, and the latter was considered to have its probable origin in the former. The serious implications of such an effect over a prolonged period of time are clear.

Apparent overestimation of the passage of time was also observed in chimpanzees to whom Δ^9-THC was administered orally. Temporally spaced responses of the chimps came to be made closer and closer together as the dose of THC was increased, an indication that the chimps preceived shorter and shorter intervals of time as being of the original familiar duration.

In a study of aggression in mice, rats, and squirrel monkeys, THC was shown to decrease species-specific attack behavior. Comparatively low doses of THC were administered and did not appear to induce a general depression or incapacitation; other social interactions, such as allogrooming, actually increased in frequency.

It appears that a serious hazard of marijuana smoking is enhancement of a paranoid thought disorder and exacerbation of psychosis in schizophrenic patients.

In contrast to anecdotal reports that marijuana smoking increased interpersonal communication, experimental studies have demonstrated an overall decrease in affective exchange and interpersonal skills during marijuana use.

Marijuana appears to have a detrimental effect on driving ability. This effect is dose related and not uniform for all persons. Marijuana and alcohol are commonly used together; driving performance deteriorates rapidly with simultaneous use of both. A striking deterioration of aircraft handling by pilots was demonstrated 24 hours after smoking marijuana.[32] Aileron changes, elevator operation, landing skills, and vertical and lateral maneuvering were all significantly impaired; the pilots reported no awareness of performance deterioration! These results bear disturbing implications for driving, flying, or performing any other complex tasks even as long as a day after smoking marijuana.

Both smoked marijuana and orally administered Δ^9-THC produce significant bronchodilatation of relatively long duration (6 hours for the 20 mg dose). Results of a pulmonary function study indicate that occasional social smoking of marijuana may not cause functional respiratory impairment in healthy young men whereas heavy marijuana use for 6 to 8 weeks produces mild but definite *narrowing* of large, medium, and small airways, despite the acute bronchodilator action of THC.

THC has been shown to impair spermatogenesis, inhibit synthesis of testosterone, and, in females, decrease serum concentrations of follicle-stimulating hormone (FSH), luteinizing hormone (LH), and prolactin. Oral administration of cannabinoids to female mice late in pregnancy and during early lactation produces a permanent alteration in body weight regulation, pituitary-gonadal function, and adult copulatory activity in male offspring. Clearly cannabinoids exert profound effects on reproductive function, though the mechanisms are unknown. Dose-related fetal resorptions are produced by cannabinoids in rats and mice; the mechanism may involve disruption of placental function.

In several species of animals THC induces hypothermia at room temperature.[4] In human subjects marijuana smoking results in little or no change in temperature in a cool environment, but in a hot environment it can inhibit sweating and predispose to hyperthermia. The mechanism by which THC interferes with thermoregulation is unknown.

$[^{14}C]\Delta^9$-THC administered to rats has been shown to accumulate in tenfold greater concentrations in fat than in other tissues; 11-hydroxy-THC, an active metabolite of Δ^9-THC, showed a similar distribution. The importance of fat localization in prolonging pharmacologic activity of drugs is well known; slow release from fat stores may help explain the phenomenon of "reverse tolerance," in which regular users of marijuana achieve a "high" more quickly and easily than sporadic users. Plasma concentrations of THC fall rapidly to a low value that is maintained for days. One study has demonstrated a half-life in tissues of 7 days; after 5 days, 15% of the THC is found as metabolites excreted by the kidney and 40% to 50% is excreted by the intestines.

Urinary tests for detection of marijuana metabolites are now effective and specific; metabolites reach detectable concentrations within an hour after smoking marijuana.[25]

FURTHER CONSIDERATIONS

Cannabinol derivatives may prove to be useful drugs in the near future. THC reduces intraocular pressure, has a bronchodilator action, may be an effective antiemetic, and has properties of a sedative and an antianxiety agent.

Long-term use of marijuana has been directly related to subsequent abuse of other illicit drugs.[13] Marijuana use in adolescence has been found to be the most reliable predictor of cocaine use.

Marijuana is often compared with alcohol. Unlike alcohol, marijuana is not known to be physically addicting, and tolerance does not develop to the effects of ordinary marijuana preparations. When inebriated, the alcoholic usually suffers a greater temporary loss of judgment and control than the marijuana user, whose "highs" are usually characterized by mild alterations in perception and mood without a great loss of behavioral control. Hostility and aggression are commonly released by alcohol but rarely by marijuana. Appetite is stimulated by marijuana, whereas calories are provided by alcohol; nutritional deficiency commonly complicates chronic alcoholism. Psychologic dependence may develop on either drug, and both may impair the physical performance essential to safe automobile driving. Acute paranoid states, dissociative reactions, and near-psychotic reactions are occasionally seen with marijuana use; moderate drinking rarely if ever induces such reactions. There is strong suggestive evidence that chronic marijuana use interferes with motivational and goal-directed thinking; chronic alcoholism may do the same and ultimately result in brain damage and general physical deterioration.

In summary, the known medical risks of marijuana use are (1) the occasional adverse reaction, characterized by paranoid thinking and extreme anxiety, sometimes with an acute psychotic reaction; (2) enhancement of preexisting paranoid thought disorders and exacerbation of psychosis in schizophrenic patients; (3) alteration of time and space perception, with significant impairment of driving and other motor skills; (4) impairment of learning and short-term memory; (5) loss of motivation and drive, associated with regular and frequent use; (6) probable impairment of vascular reflex responses; (7) possible impairment of immune response; (8) disturbance of the hypothalamopituitary axis with impairment of reproductive functions; and (9) interference with temperature regulation.

AMPHETAMINES   SLANG EQUIVALENTS:

Methamphetamine = meth, speed, crystal, crank, white cross

It appears that little if any physical dependence develops to amphetamines. A change in sleep pattern on abrupt withdrawal has been reported in association with minimal EEG changes, but there is no physiologically disruptive abstinence syndrome. Abrupt withdrawal is characterized by lethargy, somnolence, and often a precipitous depressive reaction; the possibility of suicide should be kept in mind. Some consider the period of lethargy and somnolence an abstinence syndrome in itself.

Tolerance to amphetamines develops slowly and becomes pronounced. At any level of tolerance the margin between euphoria and toxic psychosis remains narrow.

Characteristics of abuse   Amphetamines are direct central nervous system stimulants and in ordinary therapeutic doses produce (1) euphoria, with an increased sense of well-being; (2) heightened mental acuity, until fatigue sets in from lack of sleep; (3) nervousness, with insomnia; and (4) anorexia. Amphetamines are commonly abused by students, housewives, truck drivers, and all-night workers who self-administer the drugs for extended periods of time. Liberal dispensing by physicians of amphetamines for dietary management has contributed to the abuse of these agents.

Undesirable and potentially hazardous effects accompany prolonged use of amphetamines. Fatigue eventually supervenes and blocks coherent thought at inopportune times. In addition, brief lapses of alertness, with sudden drooping of the head ("nodding"), may occur without warning as fatigue "breaks through"; this may result in catastrophic loss of control in dangerous circumstances.

High doses of amphetamines reduce mental acuity and impair performance of complex acts, even in the absence of fatigue. Behavior may become irrational. A peculiar phenomenon observed among amphetamine users is a condition described as being "hung up." The user may get stuck in a repetitious behavioral sequence, repeating an act ritually for hours; this perseverative behavior may become progressively more irrational.

"Amphetamine psychosis" may develop during long- or short-term abuse of amphetamines and is characterized by visual and auditory hallucinations and paranoid delusions in the setting of a clear sensorium and full orientation. The psychosis clears within a few days after the drug is discontinued. It has been compared to a severe paranoid state closely resembling paranoid schizophrenia, with fixed, systematized delusions aggravated by attempts at intervention.

Tolerance develops to such a degree that the habitual user may eventually inject several hundred milligrams of an amphetamine every few hours. A total 24-hour dose of methamphetamine estimated at over 10 g has been reported. Some users report that the subjective effects of intravenous amphetamines are similar to those of intravenous cocaine except for the longer action of the former.

Physiologic effects of high doses of amphetamines include mydriasis, elevation of blood pressure, hyperreflexia, and hyperthermia. Hypertensive crisis with intracranial hemorrhage has been reported after oral and intravenous administration of methamphetamine. It is important to recall that amphetamine is an indirectly acting adrenergic drug, promoting central dopamine release and peripheral norepinephrine release.

Other sympathomimetic agents that are chemically related to the amphetamines and commonly abused include ephedrine, phenmetrazine, mephentermine inhalers, and methylphenidate. These drugs all produce central stimulation, generally less pronounced than with amphetamines.

SLANG EQUIVALENTS: *COCAINE*

Coke, crack, base, free base, rock, coca, snow, toot

Cocaine is a local anesthetic, vasoconstrictor, and powerful central nervous system stimulant. It occurs naturally in the leaves of the coca plant *Erythroxylon coca* and in other species of *Erythroxylon*, which are indigenous to Peru and Bolivia. Coca chewing has been a way of life for centuries for Quechua Indians living in the Andean highlands. Cocaine usage has become the fastest growing serious drug abuse problem in the world.

Although an acute withdrawal illness like those associated with opiate or sedative dependence does not follow cocaine withdrawal, serious depression and hypersomnolence occur after termination of high dosage or continuous administration, and these symptoms constitute a dangerous abstinence syndrome. Tolerance is not known to develop.

Physical dependence and tolerance

Euphoric excitement is rapidly produced even when cocaine is sniffed ("snorted" or "horned"). Grandiose feelings of mental and physical prowess may cause users to overestimate their capabilities. Sexual desire may be enhanced. After intravenous injection, male users have reported spontaneous ejaculation in the absence of genital stimulation. The recent practice of smoking the highly purified preparation known as "crack" produces a virtually instantaneous rush.

Characteristics of abuse

Acute toxicity from an excessive dose, regardless of the route of administration, is characterized by extreme agitation, restlessness, confusion, blurred vision, and tremors. Cocaine overdose is extremely dangerous[21] and may rapidly induce paranoid thinking, hallucinations, cardiac arrhythmias, and convulsions. Reports of acute myocardial infarction after cocaine use have appeared over the past few years, even in patients with normal coronary arteries.[11] In addition, cardiac arrhythmias may result from mobilization of epinephrine and blockade of norepinephrine reuptake. Death has resulted from ventricular fibrillation. Central stimulation is followed by depression; higher centers are the first to become depressed, making this transition while lower centers are still excited. Death may result from medullary paralysis and respiratory failure.

Paranoid delusions may be so compelling as to provoke assaultive behavior directed toward innocent people. The paranoid state is similar to the amphetamine psychosis except that it is shorter lived, at least in cases of parenteral injection. Experienced users may inject an opiate to "come down" from a toxic state.

Overdose deaths have resulted from the "body packer syndrome," in which packages of cocaine, ingested for purposes of transport, rupture in the gastrointestinal tract.[16] It was once assumed that orally administered cocaine is hydrolyzed and rendered ineffective in the gastrointestinal tract. In reality cocaine is well absorbed after ingestion, with peak plasma levels occurring 50 to 90 minutes after ingestion.

With intravenous injection the effects are short lived, in contrast to the longer action of amphetamines. The intravenous user often leaves the needle in place in order to repeat injections every 5 or 10 minutes.

One complication among cocaine sniffers is perforation of the nasal septum, a result of ischemic necrosis caused by intense and prolonged vasoconstriction. Plasma concentrations peak between 15 and 60 minutes after intranasal application, and the drug persists in plasma for 4 to 6 hours. This persistence may result from continous absorption secondary to its vasoconstrictor action and brings about a far more enduring toxic state than parenteral injection does. Cocaine remains on the nasal mucosa for about 3 hours after application. Adulterants found in cocaine include amphetamines, procaine, caffeine, ephedrine, nicotine, mannitol, and lactose.

BARBITURATES

SLANG EQUIVALENTS:

> *Short acting:* secobarbital = red birds, red devils, reds; pentobarbital = yellow jackets
> *Intermediate acting:* amobarbital = blue heavens
> *Long acting:* phenobarbital = purple hearts
> *Combinations:* secobarbital + amobarbital (Tuinal) = tooies, Christmas trees, rainbows

---

Physical dependence and tolerance

A pronounced degree of both physical dependence and tolerance can develop to all barbiturates. There is a sharp upper border to the tolerance, so that a slight increase in dosage may evoke toxicity.

Characteristics of abuse

The effects of ordinary doses of barbiturates include sedation (without analgesia), decreased mental acuity, slowed speech, and emotional lability. Symptoms resulting from overdose include ataxia, diplopia, nystagmus, difficulty in accommodation, vertigo, and a positive Romberg sign. There is risk of overdose as a result of the delayed onset of action of longer acting barbiturates and also as a result of perceptual time distortion, which induces users to ingest more than they intended in a short period of time. Death from overdose, as with the opiates, results from respiratory depression, which in this case is not reversed by narcotic antagonists. Use of most barbiturates in modern medicine has greatly declined because of their disadvantages and hazards (see Chapter 26).

The barbiturate abstinence syndrome is one of the most dangerous withdrawal syndromes. Symptoms progress from weakness, restlessness, tremulousness, and insomnia to abdominal cramps, nausea, vomiting, hyperthermia, blepharoclonus (clonic blink reflex), orthostatic hypotension, confusion, disorientation, and eventually major convulsive seizures. The syndrome is sometimes mistaken for the delirium tremens of alcohol withdrawal. Seizures may be prolonged. Agitation and hyperthermia may lead to exhaustion and cardiovascular collapse. With short-acting barbiturates, convulsions are most likely to appear during the second or third day of abstinence; with the longer-acting barbiturates, convulsions are less likely to occur or appear usually between the third and the eighth day.

The barbiturate type of abstinence syndrome is occasionally observed in an addict being withdrawn from heroin who insists that he or she has used no other drug. In such cases one should suspect that the heroin recently used by the patient had been diluted with barbiturates. A barbiturate withdrawal regimen is then instituted immediately.

Abstinence syndrome

Hospitalization is advisable for the duration of the withdrawal period. Instead of accepting the addict's word for the level of barbiturate usage, an objective test is made to determine the level of tolerance to barbiturates. An ordinary therapeutic dose of pentobarbital is administered, and the patient is observed for clinical signs of drug effect. If the sedative action of the drug is not soon apparent, it is concluded that the patient's level of tolerance is higher and that he or she has become accustomed to higher individual doses. Additional increments of pentobarbital are administered until a drug effect is evident; at this point the total dose of drug administered is considered the base line from which subsequent doses are tapered over the ensuing 7 to 14 days. The long withdrawal period is advisable to minimize the likelihood of convulsions.

Withdrawal from barbiturates

Once called "minor tranquilizers," the **benzodiazepine** antianxiety agents have a significant abuse potential and can produce physical dependence of the barbiturate type. There is even risk of major convulsive seizures after abrupt withdrawal from high doses.

Methaqualone (Quaalude: "quaas" or "ludes"). Methaqualone in large doses may produce serious and even fatal complications, including convulsive seizures, pulmonary edema, and respiratory arrest. Physical dependence develops after prolonged use. "Street" methaqualone may be adulterated with or may consist entirely of diazepam or phencyclidine.

Glutethimide. Pronounced physical dependence develops, resulting in a severe abstinence syndrome characterized by nausea, vomiting, abdominal cramps, tachycardia, hyperthermia, hyperesthesia, dysphagia, and major convulsive seizures.

Chloral hydrate. Moderate physical dependence develops, as manifested by a "chloral delirium" on abrupt withdrawal, characterized by agitation, confusion, disorientation, and hallucinations. Slight to moderate tolerance develops; a "break in

NONBARBITURATE SEDATIVES

tolerance" may result from abrupt impairment of hepatic detoxification, with resulting overdose and death.

Methyprylon. Abrupt withdrawal has resulted in confusion, agitation, hallucinations, and generalized convulsions.

Paraldehyde. Moderate physical dependence develops, as seen by withdrawal symptoms of tremulousness, visual and auditory hallucinations, and a state of agitation and disorientation similar to delirium tremens.

Bromides. Physical dependence has not been demonstrated. In low doses bromides act as sedatives; in toxic doses they produce a "bromide psychosis" characterized by confusion, disorientation, vivid hallucinations, and eventually coma. Slow elimination of bromide from the body may lead to chronic accumulation when it is administered over a period of time, with a subtle onset of the toxic syndrome.

Antipsychotic agents	A remarkable feature of the antipsychotic drugs is the absence of a disruptive withdrawal illness after discontinuation. A mild to moderate degree of anxiety and insomnia follow abrupt withdrawal, and psychotic symptoms may recur after an interval of time, but there is no disruptive or dangerous abstinence syndrome comparable to those after opiate or sedative-hypnotic withdrawal.

Moderate tolerance develops to sedative effects of all antipsychotic agents; it is not known that tolerance develops to the antipsychotic action. These drugs have low abuse potential, as they do not produce euphoria. On the few occasions when they have been abused, the sought-after reactions were atropine-like side effects.

PSYCHOTO-MIMETIC DRUGS	Considered in this category are drugs with stimulant and hallucinogenic activity that are taken to achieve either a euphoric or hallucinogenic state. Many other drugs, such as amphetamines and cocaine, are also psychotogenic in high doses, and many of the drugs considered here are derivatives of amphetamines.

These are among the most dangerous of abused drugs, since many can disorganize cognitive and affective functions and create panic and frenzied confusion. Some, such as phencyclidine and LSD, are more dangerous than others, such as peyote. The milder effects of the less dangerous agents include mystical, euphoric states appreciated (and often greatly valued) by many primitive as well as modern cultures.

Phencyclidine	SLANG EQUIVALENTS:

PCP, angel dust, DOA, peace pill, hog

Phencyclidine hydrochloride[27,28] (*l*-phenylcyclohexylpiperidine), a veterinary anesthetic agent, has become increasingly popular since the late 1970s as a psychotomimetic drug, in part because it is easily synthesized from readily available precursors. It is taken by ingestion, inhalation (sprinkled on smoking preparations or inhaled directly), and injection.

In low doses of 1 to 5 mg phencyclidine may induce euphoria and disinhibition, with release from social inhibitory attitudes and increased emotional lability. Many use the drug for this effect alone. In higher doses a variable clinical picture is produced, with excitement, somatic perceptual distortions, impairment of pain and touch perception, confusion, disorientation, and difficulty speaking. The user may appear agitated or quiet and withdrawn. The clinical syndrome may resemble schizophrenia in many respects and can persist for days or weeks. Posturing, catatonic states and mutism have been reported. Attack behavior, directed or chaotic, has also been observed after large doses.

Phencyclidine produces both sympathomimetic (tachycardia, hypertension) and cholinergic effects (flushing, diaphoresis, drooling, miosis). Increased deep tendon reflexes, clonic movements, nystagmus, ataxia, and dysarthria are common effects. Paresthesias and analgesia can develop. At higher doses convulsions, status epilepticus, hypertensive crisis, and cardiac or respiratory arrest may occur. Coma may be the presenting clinical picture, mimicking head injury.

Treatment measures include emesis (if early after ingestion), control of hypertension, ventilatory support, and control of behavioral disturbances.

Phencyclidine is one of the most dangerous drugs ever to appear on the street. Like most other street drugs, it is commonly misrepresented by sellers as THC, mescaline, peyote, or other drugs. It is produced as a powder, tablet, or capsule of almost any color. Phencyclidine is inexpensive to produce and may bring spectacular profits (1 pound costs $100 to produce and may bring $20,000).

At least five phencyclidine analogs have been widely distributed in the United States and marketed as PCP. Their structures vary from a piperidine to a phenyl-cyclohexylamine.

SLANG EQUIVALENT: *Lysergide, or LSD*

    Acid; many different local names

LSD (LSD-25; D-lysergic acid diethylamide) was first synthesized from alkaloids of ergot *(Claviceps purpurea)*, a fungus that parasitizes rye and other grains in Europe and North America. Ergot alkaloids, which include ergotamine and ergonovine, are active oxytocics and vasoconstrictors. The chance synthesis of LSD was accomplished in 1938 by a research chemist working for Sandoz, Ltd., who attached a diethylamide radical to lysergic acid, the skeletal structure common to ergot alkaloids. The sample was set aside until 1943, when it was found by the researcher to cause strange and pronounced central effects.

Physical dependence is not known to develop. Tolerance, however, develops rapidly and is lost as rapidly after discontinuance of LSD. The usual dose of 200 to 400 μg is often raised to several milligrams after a few days of continuous use. Cross-tolerance between LSD, mescaline, and psilocybin has been shown; it appears that cross-tolerance between LSD and DMT (dimethyltryptamine) or between LSD and Δ^9-THC does not develop.

PHYSICAL DEPENDENCE

AND TOLERANCE

The nature of the "trip" taken with LSD is not predictable but is influenced to some degree by the state of mind, mood, and expectations when the drug is taken. The usual trip with LSD is characterized by exhilarating feelings of strangeness and newness of experience, vividly colored and changing hallucinations, reveries, "free thinking," and "new insight." Colors become alive and may seem to glow; the space between objects may take on greater subjective importance as a thing in itself; there is dazed wonderment at the beauty in common things. The introspective experience may be intense and sobering; it has been described as an intellectual earthquake in which conditioned attitudes and feelings are reevaluated and values are reshuffled. To some degree there appears to be a regression to primary process thinking.

Unpleasant experiences with LSD are relatively frequent and may involve an uncontrollable drift into confusion, dissociative reactions, acute panic reactions, a reliving of earlier traumatic experiences, or an acute psychotic hospitalization. Prolonged nonpsychotic reactions have included dissociative reactions, time and space distortion, body-image changes, and a residue of fear or depression stemming from morbid or terrifying experiences under the drug.

Catastrophic reactions to LSD are better understood when one conceptualizes the disruption by the drug of psychologic defense mechanisms such as repression and denial in a person precariously defended against psychologic stress. With the failure of the usual defenses, the onslaught of repressed feelings overwhelms the integrative capacity of the ego, and a psychotic reaction results. After heavy use of LSD this disruption of ego functions may persist for years and perhaps indefinitely.

It also appears that LSD removes the usual intrinsic restraints on the intensity of affective response. It is well known to LSD users that a specific emotional response, whether it be fear, dread, delight, or sadness, may become rapidly more intense under the influence of the drug until it reaches overwhelming proportions. The user is then virtually in the grip of the reaction; he may indeed derive insight from the introspective experience, as many users report, but he may also become so disturbed that he is not in control of his behavior. Deaths under the influence of LSD have occurred by drowning, falling from a window, and walking into the path of a car.

Disturbing implications are inherent in the finding of many "acid heads" that after 25 to 50 trips the frequency of taking LSD may be reduced progressively without sacrificing the desired state of mind. Users may discover that between trips they begin to feel as they did while under the influence of the drug, until they eventually find themselves on a continuous trip with no further ingestion of the drug. They state that their thinking has become different, and they no longer "need" the drug. Indeed, their changed behavior is apparent to others; with no further drug ingestion, they remain preoccupied with any trivial thing at hand, feel "at one" with all living things, and act as they often did while under the influence of the drug.

Symptoms occurring during an LSD trip can recur unpredictably days, weeks, or months after a single dose. Strangest of drug effects, these "flashback" reactions may occur at intervals after administration of many drugs with central nervous system activity, but they most commonly follow an LSD reaction. Flashback symptoms vary from gentle mood states to severely disruptive changes in thought and feeling and may occur with or without further administration of the drug. The reaction can be initiated voluntarily in some cases. The mechanism remains unknown, but the existence of the phenomenon suggests a residual impairment of psychologic defense mechanisms, with periodic emergence of repressed feelings. Flashback reactions may also be triggered by strong affective states or by administration of a drug with central nervous system activity.

The physiologic effects of LSD are few and include mydriasis, hyperreflexia, and muscular incoordination. Grand mal seizures have been observed after ingestion of LSD. It has been demonstrated that injections of LSD in rats decrease the turnover rate of serotonin (5-hydroxytryptamine). Some investigators suggest that this may in part explain the psychotomimetic action.

LSD is usually taken by mouth. It is occasionally "mainlined," however, alone or in combination with other drugs. It is also absorbed through the lungs when marijuana soaked in an LSD solution is smoked.

It was once believed that a transient "model psychosis" resembling schizophrenia could be experimentally induced with LSD. It was soon recognized, however, that the psychotic reacton to LSD differs substantially from most types of schizophrenic reactions. In schizophrenia one usually finds a disordered thought pattern characterized by subtle or flagrant delusions that are systematized and integrated into the personality structure of the person. The LSD psychosis, on the contrary, is characterized by a chaotic and unpredictable thought disturbance with little or no organization or integration. It resembles an acute brain syndrome more closely than it does most schizophrenic reactions, though it differs somewhat from a brain syndrome in the wide range of affective disturbance and in the complex nature of the hallucinatory experiences.

Antipsychotic agents are usually the most effective drugs for treating the agitation and confusion of LSD intoxication or flashback reactions. If moderate to large doses are needed, it is preferable to chose an antipsychotic agent with minimal anticholinergic action so that atropine-like central stimulation is avoided. For mild agitation, antianxiety agents may suffice, but these are subject to abuse if a large supply is provided.

Other psychotomimetic agents

Numerous amphetamine derivatives have been synthesized and widely distributed over the last decade. The most recent is **3,4-methylenedioxymethamphetamine** (MDMA), or "ecstasy," which has spread rapidly throughout the United States. It appears to be a mild hallucinogen in low doses and to produce overt psychotic episodes in larger doses. As with LSD, some mental health professionals are pressing for trials of MDMA as a therapeutic agent that might facilitate exploration of repressed feelings. A similar amphetamine derivative is **3-methoxy-4,5-methylenedioxyamphetamine** (MDA), or the "love pill," which appears to produce similar effects; both amphetamine derivatives induce a sense of euphoria in addition to mild hallucinations in low doses. Death has been reported from overdose after uncontrolled hyperthermia, hypertension, seizures, hyperreflexia, and coma. MDA has also been found to be toxic to serotonergic neurons in rat brain.[23] A third amphetamine derivative, **2,5-dimethoxy-4-methylamphetamine** (DOM or STP), is reported to induce a serious LSD-like reaction lasting 72 hours or longer.

These three amphetamine congeners are surely not the only ones synthesized in underground laboratories; on the contrary, probably dozens or hundreds have or will be created, and some may be more dangerous than others. Reports of clinical effects are often difficult to evaluate because the causative street drugs are not available for laboratory identification.

p-**Chlorophenylalanine** (PCPA), a particularly dangerous psychotomimetic agent, is unrelated to amphetamines and has been found to induce long-lasting sexual excitation in male rats. Nicknamed "steam" by drug users, it has gained a reputation as a dangerous drug capable of inducing a prolonged psychotic reaction.

Three tryptamine derivatives, less commonly abused than the above psychotomimetic agents, produce a syndrome resembling an LSD reaction. These are **dimethyltryptamine** (DMT), **diethyltryptamine** (DET), and **dipropyltryptamine** (DPT). This syndrome, however, differs from an LSD reaction in that (1) the onset is more rapid, increasing the likelihood of panic reaction, and (2) the duration of action is only 1 to 2 hours. The effects, consisting in pupillary dilatation and elevation of blood pressure, are more pronounced than with LSD. DMT is present in several South American snuffs, including cohoba snuff.

Morning glory seeds VARIETIES:

1. *Rivea corymbosa:* ololiuqui, Mexican morning glory, "heavenly blue" (used in ceremonies by the Aztec Indians of Mexico)
2. *Ipomoea versicolor* (alternate names: *I. violacea, I. tricolor):* "pearly gates"

Morning glory seeds, readily purchasable in stores, contain compounds similar to LSD—D-lysergic acid amide among others. Up to several hundred seeds are ingested at a time to produce effects; less commonly an extract is injected intravenously.

Symptoms include drowsiness, perceptual distortion, confusion, lability of affect, and hallucinations; giddiness and euphoria may alternate with intense anxiety. Common side effects of oral ingestion include nausea, vomiting, and diarrhea.

Mescaline The dumpling (peyote) cactus, *Lophophora williamsii*, is indigenous to the Rio Grande Valley. Protuberances atop the plant are cut off and dried in the sun to form the peyote, or mescal "buttons"; these contain the active drug mescaline (peyote, peyotl), 3,4,5-trimethoxyphenethylamine). The buttons are prepared into cakes, tablets, or powder; the powder is water soluble and may be administered orally or parenterally. Peyote is used in ceremonies by indians of northern Mexico and by the Navahos, Apaches, Comanches, and other tribes of the southwestern United States.

Mescaline produces effects similar to those of LSD, but it is less potent. Vivid and colorful hallucinations are reported. Flagrant psychotic reactions are far less common than with LSD.

Mescaline has been found in smaller quantities in another North American cactus, *Pelecyphora aselliformis*, and is also known to occur in some species of South American cactuses.

The hallucinogenic agents psilocybin and psilocin, available in powder and liquid form, are extracted from the mushrooms *Stropharia* spp. and *Psilocybe* spp., which occur principally in Mexico. A native religious cult in which these mushrooms are consumed as a sacrament has deep roots in Mexican tradition.

Psilocybin and psilocin

Commonly abused anticholinergic agents include atropine, scopolamine, synthetic atropine substitutes, and preparations or plants containing these agents such as the over-the-counter preparation Asthmador and the plants jimsonweed and angel's trumpet (both *Datura* spp.). In high doses these agents produce a central anticholinergic syndrome characterized by hyperthermia, agitation, veridical hallucinations (bugs, spiders, and so on), and confusion. Severe intoxication may result in convulsions, flaccid paralysis, coma, and death. Other indications of anticholinergic intoxication are present, such as mydriasis, tachycardia, decreased salivary secretion, anhidrosis, urinary retention, and warm, flushed skin. Anticholinergic agents abused for their psychotomimetic effects are sometimes falsely marketed as LSD.

Anticholinergics

Nutmeg *(Myristica)*, a spice used throughout the world, is the powdered seed kernel of the East Indian tree *Myristica fragrans*. Unknown to many, it contains a hallucinogen believed to be myristicin. Ingestion of large amounts of nutmeg produces euphoria, hallucinations, and an acute psychotic reaction. Side effects, which may be confused with atropine poisoning, include flushing of the skin, tachycardia, and decreased salivary secretion. Unlike atropine, nutmeg may produce early pupillary constriction.

Nutmeg

The term *inhalant*, as used here, includes gases and highly volatile organic compounds and excludes liquids sprayed into the nasopharynx (droplet-transport required) and substances that must be ignited before inhalation (such as marijuana).

INHALANTS

This category of drug abuse attracts the youngest customers. Not infrequently one learns of elementary school children who have experimented dangerously with inhalants for weeks or months before being discovered.

Currently among the most popular inhalants are the volatile nitrites, principally amyl nitrite and isobutyl nitrite. They are nicknamed "poppers" and "snappers" because of the sound produced by breaking open the thin glass ampule in which amyl nitrite is marketed. Isobutyl nitrite has been marketed in various containers with trade names such as Bolt, Heart-On, Rush, and Locker Room. The effects of inhalation of volatile nitrites are immediate but fleeting and include light-headedness, euphoria (variable), headache, and enhancement of sexual orgasm. The last effect accounts for the most common usage of the drugs. The basic pharmacologic effect is relaxation of vascular smooth muscle; complaints of users include a prolonged pulsatile headache and symptoms of orthostatic hypotension and glaucoma. If inhalation is prolonged or practiced regularly, hemoglobin may be converted to methemoglobin; this should be kept in mind in the evaluation of the regular user.

Other popular inhalants include model airplane glues, plastic cements, gasoline, brake and lighter fluids, paint and lacquer thinners, varnish remover, cleaning fluid (spot remover) and nail polish remover. These household agents contain a variety of volative aliphatic and aromatic hydrocarbons, including toluene, xylene, carbon tetrachloride, chloroform, acetone, amyl acetate, trichloroethane, naphtha, ethanol, and isopropanol (isopropyl alcohol). Some of these compounds are central nervous system depressants and may produce anesthesia and death in high concentrations. Some have known toxic effects. Chloroform and carbon tetrachloride, for example, may produce hepatic or renal failure or cardiac arrhythmias with severe hypotension; mild poisoning with either agent may produce reversible oliguria for a few days. Exposure to high concentrations of toluene can cause renal tubular acidosis, acute hepatic failure, bone-marrow suppression, and permanent encephalopathy. Lead poisoning has resulted from gasoline sniffing. Chronic toluene abuse has produced severe brain damage characterized by cognitive impairment, defective modulation of affect, scanning speech, tremors, and ataxia. A case of fatal aplastic anemia secondary to glue sniffing has been reported.[22]

Symptoms produced by inhalation of the agents listed above are essentially similar for all. A sense of exhilaration and light-headedness is usually reported, progressing to hallucinations. Judgment and perception of reality are impaired. Transient ataxia, slurred speech, diplopia, and vomiting have occurred in cases of glue sniffing. If inhalation is not interrupted, coma and death may result. The development of tolerance has been reported. Physical dependence is not known to develop.

Inhalation anesthetics such as nitrous oxide (N_2O, laughing gas), diethyl ether, cyclopropane, trichloroethylene, and halothane are also abused, most often by medical personnel. Cardiac arrhythmias associated with light-plane anesthesia may account for many deaths from inhalation anesthetics.

Nitrous oxide is an exception to the general rule that inhalants are organic compounds. It is a popular inhalant among young drug users who acquire a large tank of the gas and share the hose, often in the privacy of a closed car! (Even with the windows partly down, air is soon expelled, and deaths have occurred.) Long-term abuse of nitrous oxide is associated with myelopathy and peripheral neuropathy.

"Sudden sniffing death" has been reported in association with inhalant abuse. Four adolescents died suddenly, for example, after inhaling the vapors of typewriter correction fluid, which contains trichloroethane and trichloroethylene.[12] Inhalation of a volatile hydrocarbon, usually a fluorocarbon, is followed by an agitated state in which the user may decide to run; after sprinting a short distance he falls to the ground dead. The cause of death appears to be a cardiac arrhythmia induced by the inhaled agent and intensified by exercise and hypercapnia. Most reported cases have occurred after inhalation of fluoroalkane gases such as the pressurized propellants of aerosol sprays. Once believed to be inert, fluoroalkane gases sensitize the hearts of mice to asphyxia-induced sinus bradycardia, atrioventricular block, and ventricular T-wave depression. Inhalation of airplane glue or toluene likewise sensitizes mouse hearts to asphyxia-induced atrioventricular block. Fatal cardiac arrhythmias have been produced in dogs by inhalation of fluorinated hydrocarbons even with careful maintenance of normal arterial blood gases; this implies direct, potentially lethal cardiac effects.

MISCELLANEOUS DRUGS
Propoxyphene

There is no evidence that significant physical dependence or tolerance develops when propoxyphene is administered in ordinary therapeutic doses. In very large doses, however, both physical dependence and tolerance have developed. Evidence that propoxyphene is pharmacologically related to the opiates is provided by the finding that it can suppress the morphine abstinence syndrome to a slight degree. Perhaps the most convincing evidence of a relationship is the finding that toxic effects of an overdose of propoxyphene are antagonized by narcotic antagonists.

In a study at the Addiction Research Center in Lexington, Kentucky, comparison of propoxyphene with codeine was made on the basis of the occurrence of an abstinence syndrome after abrupt withdrawal, suppression of a morphine abstinence syndrome, and precipitation of an abstinence syndrome on administration of nalorphine. It was concluded that propoxyphene induces considerably less physical dependence and has substantially less addiction liability than codeine. The investigators found that a toxic psychosis was induced by single doses of propoxyphene in excess of 900 mg. Propoxyphene overdosage may rapidly be fatal. Respiratory depression, convulsions, and pulmonary edema are common terminal events.

Nicotine

Nicotine is produced by the tobacco plant *Nicotiana tabacum*, which has been cultivated from antiquity and in every country of the world where the climate permits. It has never been found in the wild and fails to survive without cultivation. The plant has therefore been altered by domestication and maintained throughout recorded history. Cigarette smoke delivers hundreds of distinct products to the smoker, one of which is nicotine. The stimulus properties of nicotine have not been clearly identified in either animal or human studies, but the molecule is known to be very active physiologically and one of the most toxic of all drugs. It elevates blood pressure, increases bowel motility, and exerts an antidiuretic action. The dosage encountered in cigarettes is very small but adequate to produce immediate physiologic effects that could serve as a reinforcing stimulus for the smoking habit. When nicotine is withdrawn, its physiologic effects rebound in the opposite direction. In addition, chronic nicotine intake produces mild tolerance to its physiologic actions.[10]

Clonidine has been found to diminish cigarette withdrawal symptoms more effectively than alprazolam or placebo, a finding suggestive of central noradrenergic activity as a feature in the pathophysiology of withdrawal.[8]

The consideration of cigarette smoking as another form of drug abuse provides a rational basis for developing treatment and prevention programs based on approaches developed for other forms of substance abuse.

Caffeine	Caffeine and related methylxanthines occur naturally in the coffee bean (seeds of *Coffea arabica* and related species), the leaves of the tea plant *(Thea sinensis)*, and the seeds of the chocolate tree *(Theobroma cacao)*. Physical dependence on caffeine has not been demonstrated. It appears that a mild degree of tolerance develops during continued use. Caffeine is probably the most widely consumed psychoactive drug in the world. It has recently been shown to elevate plasma catecholamine concentration when ingested in doses encountered in beverages; a hyperadrenergic syndrome has been reported from overdose of caffeine, from either coffee or caffeine tablets, that is characterized by agitation, psychosis, hyperventilation, tachycardia, and dilated, reactive pupils. Metabolic acidosis may also result from generation of lactate. Caffeine poisoning should be considered along with salicylate poisoning and diabetes in the differential diagnosis of metabolic acidosis, hyperglycemia, and hyperventilation.

Cantharidin

Cantharidin (Spanish fly) is erroneously reputed to have a specific aphrodisiac effect, presumably because priapism may result from irritation of the male urethra when the drug is excreted in the urine. In addition, ingestion of cantharidin may be followed by stomatitis, abdominal cramps, vomiting, bloody diarrhea, urinary urgency, dysuria, and hematuria. Cantharidin is directly toxic to the kidneys; deaths from renal damage and cardiorespiratory collapse have been reported.

Catnip

The dried leaves of the catnip plant *(Nepeta cataria)* are smoked like marijuana or an extract is sprayed over ordinary tobacco. Effects are said to include euphoria and enhanced appreciation of sensory experiences. No definite pharmacologic activity has yet been demonstrated.

DRUG MIXING

Users are aware that drug combinations may provide a dimension of feeling unobtainable with a single drug alone. A second drug may be taken to enhance the effects of the first drug, to prevent undesired effects of the first drug or to reduce the discomfort of discontinuing the first drug. As mentioned, inadvertent administration of a mixture of drugs is virtually unavoidable when using street drugs, in which a single sample is almost always adulterated with a second or third unknown substance.

CLINICAL EVALUATION OF THE DRUG USER

It is often forgotten that most drugs of abuse are black-market samples and that each and every sample is characterized by three unknowns—purity, dose, and actual identity—any one of which constitutes a serious danger.

Fundamental to diagnostic evaluation of the suspected drug user is an attempt to place the apparent drug-related symptoms into one or more of four categories: (1) symptoms occurring during intoxication, (2) symptoms of withdrawal, (3) flashback symptoms, and (4) the masking of symptoms of illness or injury by a drug.

The lack of symptom specificity in cases of intoxication makes evaluation tricky even for an experienced observer; manic excitement, panic reaction, dissociative reaction, paranoid reaction, and overt psychotic reactions may occur during a "bad trip" with most of the drugs discussed. Furthermore, a patient under the influence of or in withdrawal from almost any drug may show no obvious symptoms or signs referable to recent drug use. An etiologic diagnosis is best reached through laboratory analysis of drug sample, gastric aspirate, blood, or urine; even this may be difficult, however, because of introduction of new chemical entities in an evolving drug scene. To complicate matters, a patient can be simultaneously in withdrawal from one drug and intoxicated with another. Contrary to earlier thinking, it is now apparent that discontinuing almost any drug after heavy use is likely to result in serious abstinence symptoms.

Symptoms of coincident illness or injury may not be reported by the intoxicated user because of the analgesic action of the drug or because of a mental state in which the patient is only vaguely aware of the symptoms; even if aware of the symptoms, the patient may lack the incentive to report them.

A syndrome of necrotizing angiitis associated with drug abuse has been described. It appears to be pathologically indistinguishable from periarteritis nodosa and is manifest clinically by few or no symptoms in some patients and multiple-system involvement, with pulmonary edema, hypertension, pancreatitis, and renal failure, in others. Although the cause is unclear, a frequent associated finding has been the intravenous injection of methamphetamine.

Injection of oral drug preparations may release a shower of vascular emboli, in the form of tablet-filler material, that deposit in capillary beds of the retina, lung, endocardium, liver, spleen, and kidney. Pulmonary angiothrombotic granulomatosis has been reported, with consequent pulmonary hypertension and fatal cor pulmonale, from deposition of talc (magnesium trisilicate) in pulmonary vessels. Ophthalmologic examination may reveal crystals of talc and cornstarch clustered in the macular region. Retinopathy and retinal detachment have resulted. The list of tablet-filler materials is endless but includes lactose, colloidal silica, microcrystalline cellulose, magnesium stearate, and dibasic calcium phosphate.

Gangrene of an extremity is a common result of inadvertent arterial injection of a drug. The mechanism of vascular injury in not known, but chemical damage to the intima by the concentrated drug may play an important role. Tissue ischemia after intra-arterial injection of drug preparations manufactured for *oral* administration appears to be more severe than that after injection of parenteral preparations, perhaps because of the presence of the many additives of the filler.

REFERENCES

1. Adams, H.G., and Jordan, C.: Infections in the alcoholic, Med. Clin. North Am. **68**:179, 1984.

2. Ausubel, D.P.: The Dole-Nyswander treatment of heroin addiction, J.A.M.A. **195**:949, 1966.

3. Burns, R.S., LeWitt, P.A., Ebert, M.H., et al.: The clinical syndrome of striatal dopamine deficiency: parkinsonism induced by 1-methyl-4-phenyl-1,2,3,6-tetrahydropyridine (MPTP), N. Engl. J. Med. **312**:1418, 1985.

4. Clark, W.G., and Clark, Y.L.: Changes in body temperature after administration of antipyretics, LSD, Δ^9-THC, CNS depressants and stimulants, hormones, inorganic ions, gases, 2,4-DNP and miscellaneous agents, Neurosci. Biobehav. Rev. **5**:1, 1981.

5. Cutting, W.C.: Morphine addiction for 62 years: a case report, Stanford Med. Bull. **1**:39, 1942.

6. Franz, D.N., Hare, B.D., and McCloskey, K.L.: Spinal sympathetic neurons: possible sites of opiate-withdrawal suppression by clonidine, Science **215**:1643, 1982.

7. Fuller, R.K., Branchey, L., Brightwell, D.R., et al.: Disulfiram treatment of alcoholism: a Veterans Administration cooperative study, J.A.M.A. **256**:1449, 1986.

8. Glassman, A.H., Jackson, W.K., Walsh, B.T., et al.: Cigarette craving, smoking withdrawal, and clonidine, Science **226**:864, 1984.

9. Gold, M.S., Pottash, A.C., Sweeney, D.R., and Kleber, H.D.: Opiate withdrawal using clonidine: a safe, effective, and rapid nonopiate treatment, J.A.M.A. **243**:343, 1980.

10. Henningfield, J.E.: Behavioral pharmacology of cigarette smoking. In Thompson, T., Dews, P.B., and Barrett, J.E., editors: Advances in behavioral pharmacology, vol. 4, Orlando, Florida, 1984, Academic Press, Inc., p. 131.

11. Howard, R.E., Hueter, D.C., and Davis, G.J.: Acute myocardial infarction following cocaine abuse in a young woman with normal coronary arteries, J.A.M.A. **254**:95, 1985.

12. King, G.S., Smialek, J.E., and Troutman, W.G.: Sudden death in adolescents resulting from the inhalation of typewriter correction fluid, J.A.M.A. **253**:1604, 1985.

13. Kozel, N.J., and Adams, E.H.: Epidemiology of drug abuse: an overview, Science **234**:970, 1986.

14. MacGregor, R.R,: Alcohol and immune defense, J.A.M.A. **256**:1474, 1986.

15. Marcovici, M., O'Brien, C.P., Mclellan, A.T., and Kacian, J.: A clinical, controlled study of *l*-α-acetylmethadol in the treatment of narcotic addiction, Am. J. Psychiatry **138**:234, 1981.

16. McCarron, M.M., and Wood, J.D.: The cocaine 'body packer' syndrome: diagnosis and treatment, J.A.M.A. **250**:1417, 1983.

17. Melges, F.T., Tinklenberg, J.R., Hollister, L.E., and Gillespie, H.K.: Marihuana and the temporal disintegration, Science **168**:1118, 1970.

18. Melges, F.T., Tinklenberg, J.R., Hollister, L.E., and Gillespie, H.K.: Marihuana and the temporal span of awareness, Arch. Gen. Psychiatry **24**:564, 1971.

19. Mendelson, J.H., and Mello, N.K.: Biologic concomitants of alcoholism, N. Engl. J. Med. **301**:912, 1979.

20. Miller, M.W.: Effects of alcohol on the generation and migration of cerebral cortical neurons, Science **233**:1308, 1986.

21. Mittleman, R.E., and Wetli, C.V.: Death caused by recreational cocaine use: an update, J.A.M.A. **252**:1889, 1984.

22. Powars, D.: Aplastic anemia secondary to glue sniffing, N. Engl. J. Med. **273**:700, 1965.

23. Ricaurte, G., Bryan, G., Strauss, L., et al.: Hallucinogenic amphetamine selectively destroys brain serotonin nerve terminals, Science **229**:986, 1985.

24. Schuckit, M.A.: Genetics and the risk for alcoholism, J.A.M.A. **254:**2614, 1985.

25. Schwartz, R.H., and Hawks, R.L.: Laboratory detection of marijuana use, J.A.M.A. **254:**788, 1985.

26. Senay, E.C., Dorus, W., and Renault, P.F.: Methadyl acetate and methadone: an open comparison, J.A.M.A. **237:**138, 1977.

27. Showalter, C.V., and Thornton, W.E.: Clinical pharmacology of phencyclidine toxicity, Am. J. Psychiatry **134:**1234, 1977.

28. Snyder, S.H.: Phencyclidine, Nature **285:** 355, 1980.

29. Stimmel, B., Goldberg, J., Rotkopf, E., and Cohen, M.: Ability to remain abstinent after methadone detoxification: a six-year study, J.A.M.A. **237:**1216, 1977.

30. Waller, P.F., Stewart, J.R., Hansen, A.R., et al.: The potentiating effects of alcohol on driver injury, J.A.M.A. **256:** 1461, 1986.

31. Washton, A.M., and Resnick, R.B.: Clonidine for opiate detoxification: outpatient clinical trials, Am. J. Psychiatry **137:**1121, 1980.

32. Yesavage, J.A., Leirer, V.O., Denari, M., and Hollister, L.E.: Carry-over effects of marijuana intoxication on aircraft pilot performance: a preliminary report, Am. J. Psychiatry **142:**1325, 1985.

Chapter 31

Nonsteroidal anti-inflammatory antipyretic analgesics

GENERAL CONCEPT

Several drugs from diverse structural classes share analgesic, antipyretic, and anti-inflammatory activity. Collectively they have been termed *nonsteroidal anti-inflammatory drugs* (NSAIDs) to distinguish them from anti-inflammatory glucocorticoids (Chapter 43), *nonnarcotic analgesics* to distinguish them from opioid analgesics (Chapter 29), *antipyretic analgesics, aspirin-like agents*, and so forth. A widely accepted mechanism for many of their actions is their ability to inhibit the enzyme *cyclooxygenase* and thereby decrease the conversion of arachidonic acid to prostaglandins, thromboxane A_2, or prostacyclin (see Chapter 22). In general, adverse gastrointestinal effects may limit their use as anti-inflammatory agents. They may also elevate serum concentrations of hepatic enzymes, promote water and electrolyte retention, or cause acute renal insufficiency. They can displace oral anticoagulants, sulfonylureas, hydantoins, and sulfonamides from binding to plasma proteins. NSAIDs should be used with caution in pregnant women and in patients with cardiac, hepatic, or renal disease. They should be avoided in patients with bleeding disorders, gastrointestinal ulcers, renal disease, or an intolerance to aspirin. The prototypical salicylates, in particular aspirin, are considered in detail. Acetaminophen, a widely used antipyretic analgesic, differs in that it lacks useful anti-inflammatory activity, and its mechanism of action is less well established.

DRUG CLASSIFICATION

The NSAIDs and other nonnarcotic analgesics are classified on the next page according to their therapeutic uses and structural classes.

SALICYLATES

Salicylic acid (2-hydroxybenzoic acid) is closely related to compounds that occur naturally in willow bark and oil of wintergreen. Since most compounds related to salicylic acid act by conversion to this acid or by similar mechanisms, they are referred to as *salicylates*. The most commonly employed is aspirin (acetylsalicylic acid). Salicylamide is not converted to salicylic acid in the body and is not a useful antipyretic or analgesic though it is included in several combination products. Diflunisal is a long-acting salicylate that, likewise, is not metabolized to salicylic acid. Oil of wintergreen is methyl salicylate.

COONa   COOH   COOCH₃

Sodium salicylate   **Aspirin**   **Methyl salicylate**

Salicylates—anti-inflammatory antipyretic analgesics
  Acetylsalicylic acid (aspirin)
  Sodium salicylate (Uracel, Double-Sal)
  Magnesium salicylate (Magan, others)
  Choline salicylate (Arthropan)
  Choline magnesium trisalicylate (Trilisate)
  Diflunisal (Dolobid)
  Salsalate (Disalcid)
  Salicylamide (Uromide)
  Sodium thiosalicylate (Arthrolate, Rexolate)
  Trolamine salicylate (Aspercreme, others)
  Never ingest
  Salicylic acid, used topically for wart and corn removal
  Methyl salicylate, used as a counterirritant in ointments
Salicylate-like anti-inflammatory agents
  Propionic acid derivatives
    Ibuprofen (Motrin, Rufen, others)
    Naproxen (Anaprox, Naprosyn)
    Fenoprofen (Nalfon)
    Ketoprofen (Orudis)
    Suprofen (Suprol)
  Tolmetin (Tolectin)
  Piroxicam (Feldene)
  Indole derivatives
    Indomethacin (Indocin, others)
    Sulindac (Clinoril)
  Pyrazolone derivatives
    Phenylbutazone (Butazolidin, others)
    Oxyphenbutazone
  Fenamates
    Meclophenamate sodium (Meclomen)
    Mefenamic acid (Ponstel)
Antipyretic analgesics
  p-Aminophenol derivatives
    Acetaminophen (Tylenol, others)
    Phenacetin
Sedative analgesic
  Methotrimeprazine (Levoprome)
Combinations with other analgesics, caffeine, sedatives, and so forth

Mechanisms and sites of action

When 600 mg of aspirin is taken orally by a healthy adult, the effects are negligible, though some may complain of gastric irritation. In disease states or in painful conditions, however, the therapeutic effects of salicylates can be quite prominent.

Most if not all mammalian cells contain microsomal enzymes for synthesis of prostaglandins. Aspirin inhibits cyclooxygenase activity without antagonizing the action of any of the end products (Fig. 22-2). Since prostaglandins are not stored, their release during inflammation is dependent on repeated synthesis. Thus inhibition of cyclooxygenase reduces the influence of prostaglandins at sites of inflammation, tissue damage, and so forth. One obstacle to acceptance of cyclooxygenase inhibition as the major action of NSAIDs has been an inability to demonstrate that sodium salicylate, which has analgesic, antipyretic, and anti-inflammatory activity, is an effective inhibitor of cyclooxygenase in vitro.

CLASSICAL THERAPEUTIC USES

Analgesia. Prostaglandins alone induce pain only in concentrations that are unlikely to occur physiologically. Rather they seem to enhance the potency of *algesic* (pain-inducing) substances,[4,10] such as bradykinin, that stimulate nerve endings of unmyelinated C fibers and small-diameter Aδ fibers to elicit noxious afferent input. Furthermore, bradykinin stimulates the formation and release of prostaglandins, a positive feedback of sorts. Thus, unlike the narcotic analgesics which act centrally, the primary *analgesic* action of NSAIDs is peripheral, apparently to reduce potentiation of algesic activity by prostaglandins. NSAIDs are most effective in alleviating pain of mild to moderate intensity, though they may be more effective than narcotic analgesics in alleviating pain associated with prostaglandin-stimulated smooth muscle contractions, as in primary dysmenorrhea.

Antipyresis. In contrast to analgesia, the site of antipyretic action of NSAIDs is central[5] and presumed to be in the hypothalamus. In fever the temperature-regulating system maintains temperature at a higher level than normal. The stimulus for the shift to a higher level is the action of an *endogenous pyrogen* (quite likely the same as interleukin 1) on neurons of the thermoregulatory system in the preoptic hypothalamus[16] (Fig. 31-1). Aspirin does not act directly on the thermoregulatory system and does not affect pyrogen release; rather it reduces the effect of the pyrogen. Although the antipyretic action of NSAIDs is commonly attributed to inhibition of prostaglandin synthesis,[20] there are observations inconsistent with this explanation.[5,16] Therapeutic doses of aspirin affect neither normal body temperature nor elevated temperatures (hyperthermias), associated with exercise, drugs, or hypothalamic lesions, to which pyrogen does not contribute.[16,31] Although the role of fever in combating infection is not clear, antipyretic agents are best utilized when body temperature is dangerously high or when significant relief is experienced by the patient when temperature is lowered. Temperatures to 39° C (102° F) or somewhat higher are often well tolerated, and body temperature provides an indication of the progression of a disease. Salicylates, acetaminophen, and ibuprofen are the only drugs approved as antipyretics, though indomethacin has been recommended to lower fever of Hodgkins' disease that is uncontrolled by other antipyretics.

Fever production.   *FIG. 31-1*

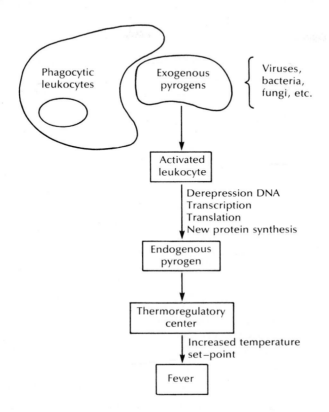

Anti-inflammatory effect. Since prostaglandins induce symptoms of inflammation and potentiate bradykinin and histamine, a reduction of prostaglandins at sites of inflammation should be beneficial. In rheumatic fever administration of large daily doses of salicylates lowers fever, relieves joint symptoms, and normalizes sedimentation rate but has no effect on rheumatic carditis. In arthritic diseases NSAIDs reduce inflammation, swelling, and so on and provide considerable relief. Although they are not usually considered to alter the progression of disease, this concept and the role of cyclooxygenase inhibition as the sole or primary mechanism for their beneficial effects have been challenged.[14,18]

There is considerable individual variability in therapeutic response and adverse reactions to NSAIDs, and so treatment of arthritic patients must be individualized. Aspirin is often tried first,[21] since it is least expensive and an excellent drug if tolerated. If it is ineffective or cannot be tolerated, usually a propionic acid derivative or tolmetin, sulindac, or piroxicam is tried. Some persons will require treatment with more toxic drugs such as gold salts, penicillamine, or glucocorticoids. In children only drugs such as aspirin, ibuprofen, or tolmetin, which have been tested extensively in children, should be prescribed. Low doses of aspirin are probably the safest in pregnant women. However, the drug should be discontinued before parturition to minimize bleeding in both the mother and neonate.

Proposed clinical uses. NSAIDs have been used to treat ocular inflammation, acute and chronic glomerulonephritis, Bartter's syndrome, and traveler's diarrhea. Aspirin is recommended as prophylactic therapy in the treatment of migraine. Uses based on the "antiplatelet" action of aspirin are discussed in Chapter 37. Treatment of dysmenorrhea and patent ductus arteriosus with NSAIDs, usually not aspirin, is discussed below (pp. 376 and 378 respectively).

ADVERSE AND SIDE EFFECTS	*Uric acid retention and excretion.* The effect of salicylic acid on uric acid excretion is dose related and varies from a decrease (low dose) to an increase (high dose). Salicylates given chronically in high daily doses inhibit uric acid reabsorption from the proximal tubule of the nephron. This property was used before the advent of better tolerated uricosuric agents, such as probenecid (see Chapter 48), to promote uric acid excretion in patients with gout. However, when aspirin is given acutely, its metabolite salicylic acid competes with uric acid and probenecid for secretion into tubular fluid. This can cause uric acid retention and perhaps precipitate an attack of gouty arthritis. Salicylates should be avoided by patients taking other uricosuric drugs.

Intolerance. Intolerance to aspirin develops in approximately 0.3% of the normal population. Aspirin intolerance, which does not extend to sodium salicylate, has been defined as "acute urticaria-angioedema, bronchospasm, severe rhinitis, or shock occurring within three hours of aspirin ingestion."[28] The specific manifestation of intolerance is usually an exacerbation of the patient's preexisting problem, such as bronchoconstriction in an asthmatic, but may also present as an anaphylactic reaction. Aspirin should be avoided by patients with severe asthma, nasal polyps, chronic urticaria, or recurrent rhinitis. Since no specific antibodies for aspirin have been found in sera of such patients, the term "intolerance" is preferable to the term "hypersensitivity." Aspirin may directly release autacoids or perhaps shift metabolism of arachidonic acid to favor synthesis of leukotrienes. Patients show cross-intolerance to varying degrees to other NSAIDs and to tartrazine, a yellow dye used in food and many pharmaceutical preparations. Such agents should not be used by patients intolerant to aspirin.

Gastrointestinal irritation and bleeding. Therapeutic doses of aspirin may cause gastric irritation and increase blood loss in a majority of persons. Many patients cannot tolerate the large daily doses needed for chronic management of arthritic conditions. Gastric ulceration has been produced by aspirin in experimental animals. Salicylates are contraindicated in patients with a history of gastrointestinal ulcers and should not be used concurrently with other agents that promote ulcer formation, such as alcohol.

The mechanism of gastrointestinal bleeding induced by aspirin may be quite complex.[15] Lesions of the gastric mucosa are more common after aspirin ingestion when intragastric pH is low. This finding indicates that hydrochloric acid may contribute to the condition. Aspirin-induced bleeding can be reduced by use of enteric-coated preparations or by administration of bicarbonate to neutralize much of the acid. Inhibition of prostaglandin synthesis should reduce cytoprotection (see Chapter 22). It is likely also that bleeding is aggravated by effects of aspirin on platelet aggregation.

Reye's syndrome. Reye's syndrome is primarily a childhood illness, with a death rate of about 35%,[24] that develops after apparent recovery from influenza or chicken pox and is characterized by vomiting, liver abnormalities, and encephalopathy progressing from drowsiness to combative behavior and delirium to coma. Nearly all victims had received salicylates for management of the viral illness. "Case-control" studies have supported an association between salicylate use and Reye's syndrome. The earlier reports were criticized on a number of grounds,[9] but a more recent study by the Centers for Disease Control[17] has also supported a link between salicylate use and the disease. Since there is no evidence of an association between acetaminophen and Reye's syndrome, it would appear prudent, if an analgesic-antipyretic is needed, to use acetaminophen in acute viral illness in children.

Miscellaneous side effects

Renal toxicity. Although drugs in this class are regarded as nonaddicting, some people become chronic users of combination analgesics. In particular, combinations of aspirin, phenacetin, and caffeine (APC tablets) have been abused. Chronic toxicity begins as medullary ischemia, leading to papillary necrosis followed by chronic interstitial nephritis and ultimately to renal failure. Although phenacetin was initially believed responsible, it appears to be the use of such drugs in combinations that is dangerous.[22] The prognosis is best if all the analgesics are discontinued, rather than just phenacetin. Kidney damage appears to result from both a reduction in prostaglandin influence on renal function and a direct toxic action of the drugs on tubular cells. Such analgesic abuse may also be associated with development of uroepithelial tumors, most commonly transitional cell carcinoma.[22]

On an acute basis, prostaglandins become important for maintenance of renal function in many situations, including congestive heart failure, cirrhosis with ascites, nephrotic syndrome, and dehydration,[6] and acute renal failure may develop if NSAIDs are administered. Fluid and electrolyte retention can also occur.[2] By inhibiting prostaglandin-mediated renin release, NSAIDs can cause the hyporenin-hypoaldosterone syndrome manifesting as hyperkalemia. Patients with renal insufficiency are particularly susceptible.

Liver. Anti-inflammatory therapy with aspirin, especially if the serum salicylate concentration exceeds 250 µg/ml, may be associated with elevations in serum transaminases. This has been observed primarily in patients with juvenile or adult rheumatoid arthritis, rheumatic fever, or systemic lupus erythematosus.[36]

Metabolic effects. Salicylates uncouple oxidative phosphorylation. This accounts for the hyperthermia that develops during intoxication. Disturbances in acid-base balance after toxic doses of salicylates are discussed on p. 372.

Interference with thyroid function is more apparent than real. The salicylates

FIG. 31-2   *Absorption of aspirin.*

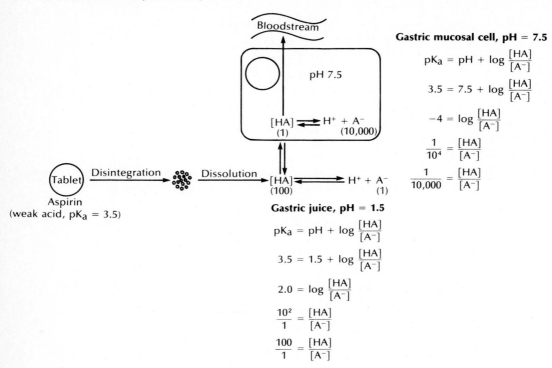

interfere with binding of thyroxin to plasma proteins. Consequently, certain tests of thyroid function, such as the protein-bound iodine test, are altered.

Pharmacokinetics

ABSORPTION

Aspirin, a weak acid with a pK_a of 3.5, is rapidly absorbed from the upper gastrointestinal tract.[23] Of the factors affecting its absorption, dissolution of tablets, which is favored by higher pH, is the rate-limiting step. Dosage forms in which aspirin is already dissolved (for example, an effervescent preparation) speed absorption. Buffered tablets undergo more rapid dissolution, but the buffering neither prevents gastric irritation nor significantly enhances therapeutic effectiveness.[1] Several preparations (enteric coated or timed release, magnesium or choline salicylates, and salsalate) have been developed in attempts to minimize irritation.

Once aspirin is dissolved, the nonionized fraction diffuses into mucosal cells where the equilibrium is shifted in favor of the ionized moiety (Fig. 31-2). Although aspirin is absorbed from the stomach, more is absorbed in the duodenum and upper small intestine, despite the higher pH, because of greater surface area. Thus faster gastric emptying hastens absorption of aspirin. Absorption of enteric-coated aspirin will reflect gastric emptying, and sustained-release preparations do not appreciably prolong the therapeutic action.

Salicylate metabolism. SAG, *Salicyl acyl glucuronide;* SPG, *salicyl phenolic glucuronide;* **FIG. 31-3**
SU, *salicyluric acid;* GA, *gentisic acid;* GU, *gentisuric acid.*

From Needs, C.J., and Brooks, P.M.: Clin. Pharmacokinet. 10:164, 1985.

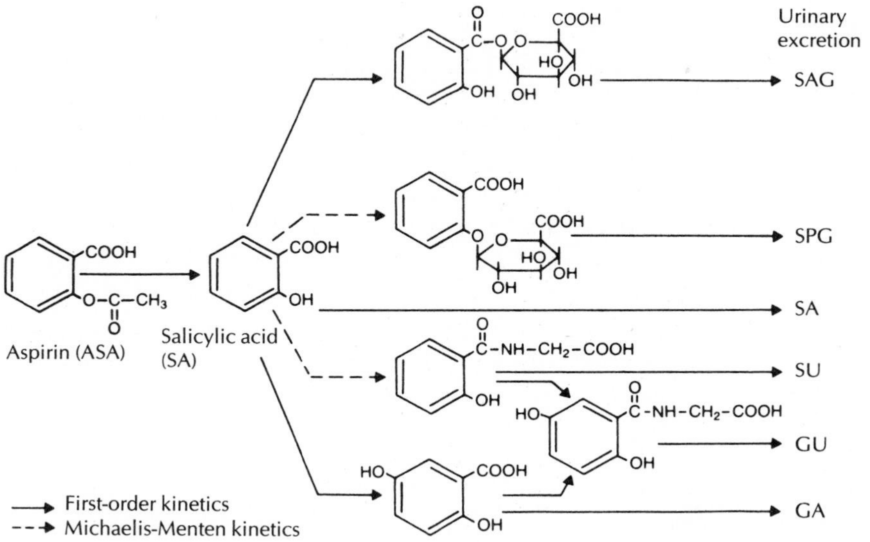

Approximately 80% to 90% of salicylate in plasma is bound to protein, primarily **DISTRIBUTION** to albumin. The unbound fraction distributes throughout body fluids by passive, pH-dependent processes. Aspirin and its active metabolite salicylate are found in saliva and in cerebrospinal, peritoneal, and synovial fluids.[23] Salicylic acid crosses the placental barrier to reach the developing fetus and can be ingested during breast feeding.

Aspirin is rapidly deacetylated to salicylic acid, a pharmacologically active me- **METABOLISM** tabolite. The half-life of aspirin in plasma is short, only 15 to 20 minutes. Salicylic acid is then oxidized to gentisic acid and conjugated with glycine to form salicyluric acid and with glucuronide to form ester and ether conjugates (Fig. 31-3).[23] Of salicylate, 90% (after an aspirin dose of 300 mg) to 50% (after 3 g of aspirin) is excreted as salicyluric acid. The half-life of salicylate (3 to 6 hours with acute administration) increases to a range of 15 to 30 hours after chronic administration of the amounts needed to manage arthritis. The prolonged half-life results from saturation of the enzymes for conjugation of salicylate with glycine and glucuronide (ether formation). These metabolic changes become important with daily doses exceeding 2.5 to 3 g of aspirin in adults and contribute to salicylate intoxication during therapeutic administration to children.

EXCRETION   Salicylates are excreted mainly by the kidney. The clearance of salicylate is increased approximately fourfold when the pH of urine is ≥8.0. At this pH, it is highly ionized and cannot readily diffuse from the tubular fluid. A high rate of urine flow decreases reabsorption, whereas oliguria increases reabsorption of salicylate from the renal tubule. The glucuronide conjugates of salicylic and gentisic acids do not readily backdiffuse from the tubules regardless of urinary pH.

DOSAGE   The usual analgesic or antipyretic dose of aspirin for adults is 650 mg (range 325 mg to 1 g) and for children is about 10 to 15 mg/kg every 4 to 6 hours. Single doses are not anti-inflammatory, but when 4 to 6 g is taken daily by adults, salicylate accumulates, the plasma salicylate concentration and half-life increase for reasons discussed on p. 371, and the anti-inflammatory effect is achieved when the plasma concentration is 150 to 250 μg/ml. With anti-inflammatory regimens, a small change in dosage causes a much greater change in plasma concentration,[23] though several days are required to reach the new steady state. Accordingly, if the anti-inflammatory effect is inadequate, a small increase in daily dosage may be sufficient, whereas a large increase in dosage is likely to become toxic.

Intoxication   Mild salicylate intoxication *(salicylism)* is characterized by ringing in the ears (tinnitus), dizziness, headache, and mental confusion. The picture is similar to *cinchonism* after large doses of quinine. Severe intoxication is characterized by hyperpnea, nausea and vomiting, acid-base disturbances, petechial hemorrhage, hyperthermia, delirium, convulsions, and coma. The lethal dose of aspirin for adults is usually over 10 g. As little as a teaspoonful of methyl salicylate may kill a child. Since the introduction of "child-proof" caps for medicine bottles, the incidence of pediatric intoxication has declined dramatically. It is likely that the majority of such intoxications now occur because therapeutic administration leads to accumulation.[11] Vomiting and hyperthermia caused by overdosage may be interpreted by a parent as manifestations of the original illness that require still more aspirin.

Disturbances in acid-base balance are quite complex. Salicylates increase the sensitivity of medullary chemoreceptors to carbon dioxide, and hyperventilation leads to respiratory alkalosis. Enhanced production of carbon dioxide also increases respiratory drive. Respiratory alkalosis is usually present in older children and adults and early in acute intoxication in infants. Secondarily, in infants, in severe acute intoxication in older children, and in chronic intoxication formation of lactic acid and ketone bodies contributes to metabolic acidosis. As intoxication increases central nervous system depression, respiratory depression, and respiratory acidosis occur. Infants usually arrive at the emergency room in an acidotic state. Dehydration is produced by several mechanisms: sweating, vomiting, hyperpnea, and failure to drink.

Treatment includes correction of fluid and electrolyte disturbances, replacement of potassium, glucose administration, and so forth.[34] The severity of acute intoxication can be predicted with the Done nomogram[11] if serum salicylate concentration is known at a given time after ingestion. Correction of acidosis has two beneficial consequences. More salicylate is then ionized in plasma so that it less readily enters the central nervous system. If sufficient bicarbonate can be given to alkalinize the urine, reabsorption from the renal tubules is reduced. Although dialysis is efficient, a forced diuresis along with alkalinization of the urine can greatly shorten the period of dangerous intoxication. Other measures are directed toward removal of residual salicylate from the stomach (lavage or emesis followed by activated charcoal) and counteracting hyperthermia by physical methods (sponging with tepid water, cooling blanket, and so on).

ACETAMINOPHEN

Acetaminophen is a metabolic product of phenacetin (acetophenetidin). It is an effective analgesic and antipyretic without the anti-inflammatory, antirheumatic, or uric acid excretory effects of aspirin. Acetaminophen is given in the same doses[35] and is equipotent to aspirin as an antipyretic or for simple analgesia, and it can be especially useful in patients (1) with peptic ulcer, (2) with gout taking a uricosuric agent, (3) taking oral anticoagulants, (4) with clotting disorders, (5) at risk of Reye's syndrome, or (6) intolerant to aspirin. In the last case there is still about a 6% chance of cross-intolerance to acetaminophen.[28] Like salicylates, acetaminophen acts centrally to cause antipyresis. It is not a cyclooxygenase inhibitor in the periphery, and the mechanism of its analgesic action is totally unknown. Like aspirin, acetaminophen is available in a wide variety of over-the-counter and prescription combinations.

Phenacetin   Acetaminophen

Intoxication and metabolism

Partially because of concern with salicylate toxicity, in about the mid-1960s the use of acetaminophen, especially in England, increased greatly. Liver damage from acetaminophen intoxication, which was virtually unknown before, then became apparent. Necrosis is localized to hepatocytes in the centrolobular region of the liver. These cells contain the highest activity of the cytochrome P-450 mixed-function oxidase system. At recommended doses acetaminophen is conjugated to glucuronide (especially in adults) and sulfate (especially in children).[12] A small percentage is oxidized to a highly reactive, toxic metabolite (Fig. 31-4). This metabolite, suggested to be either acetimidoquinone or the semiquinone, is normally inactivated by conjugation with glutathione. However, when the dose of acetaminophen is above about 10 g, the enzymes catalyzing glucuronide and sulfate conjugation become saturated, and a greater proportion of drug is converted to the reactive metabolite. Hepatic

FIG. 31-4   *Metabolism of acetaminophen.*

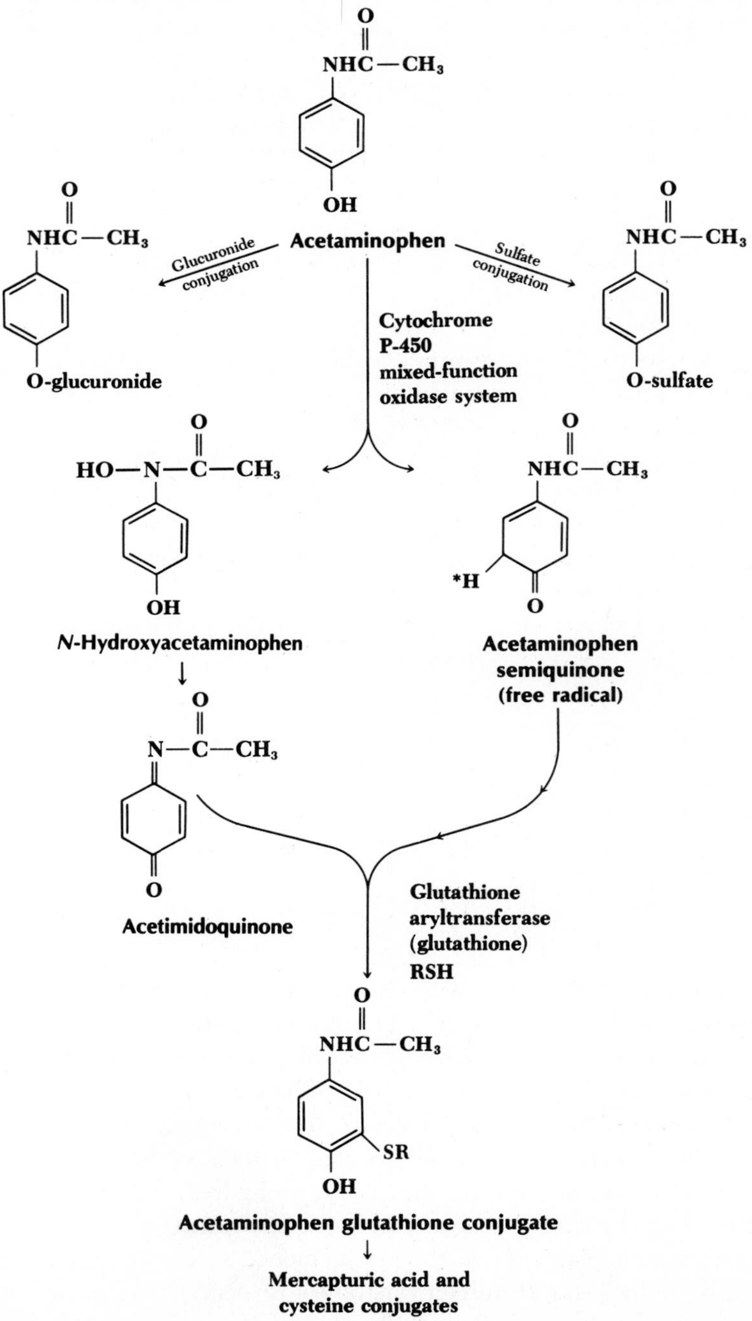

TABLE 31-1   Dosages, dosage forms, and indications for nonsteroidal anti-inflammatory drugs (NSAIDs) and other analgesics

Drug	Usual single dose* (mg)	Usual daily dose range† (mg)	Dosage interval (hours)	Dosage forms‡ (mg)	AN	AP	RA	OA	AS	PS	Dys	GA	MI
Aspirin||	650	4000-6000	4	C: 325, 500; T: 65-975; R: 60-1200	X	X	X	X	X	X	X		X
Diflunisal	500	500-1000	12	T: 250, 500	X		X	X					
Acetaminophen||¶	650		4-6	C: 325, 500; T: 325, 500	X	X							
Ibuprofen	200	900-2400	6-8	T: 200-800	X	X	X	X			X		
Naproxen	250	500-750	12	T: 250-500	X		X	X	X	X	X	X	
Fenoprofen	200	900-2400	6-8	C: 200, 300; T: 600	X		X	X					
Ketoprofen		150-300	6-8	C: 50, 75			X	X					
Suprofen	200		4-6	C: 200	X						X		
Tolmetin		1200-1600	6-8	C: 400; T: 200			X	X					
Piroxicam		10-20	24	C: 10, 20			X	X					
Indomethacin		50-200	8-12	C: 25-75; R: 50; I:1#			X	X	X	X		X	
Sulindac		300-400	12	T: 150, 200			X	X	X	X		X	
Phenylbutazone		100-600	6-8	C: 100; T: 100			X	X	X			X	
Meclofenamate		200-400	6-8	C: 50, 100			X	X					
Mefenamic acid	250		6	C: 250	X						X		
Methotrimeprazine¶	15		4-6	I: 20/ml	X								

*For short-term simple analgesia, antipyresis (adults).
†For chronic anti-inflammatory effect (adults).
‡C, Capsule; I, injection; R, rectal suppository; T, tablet.
§AN, Simple analgesia; AP, antipyresis; RA, rheumatoid arthritis, rheumatic fever; OA, osteoarthritis; AS, ankylosing spondylitis; PS, (acute) painful shoulder; Dys, dysmenorrhea; GA, (acute) gouty arthritis; MI, prophylaxis after myocardial infarction.
||Children's strength (65 mg) also available.
¶Lacks anti-inflammatory activity.
#Powder for reconstitution.

damage results when glutathione stores are depleted. Necrosis is likely if the concentration of drug in plasma exceeds, respectively, 200 and 50 µg/ml at 4 and 12 hours after ingestion.[26] Treatment includes gastric lavage or emesis followed by administration within 24 hours of a substance that enhances glutathione synthesis. The current choice in the United States is *N*-acetylcysteine (Mucomyst), diluted in a soft drink or fruit juice, 140 mg/kg by mouth as a loading dose followed by 70 mg/kg by mouth every 4 hours for 17 doses.[26] Charcoal is not used in this regimen, since it will absorb acetylcysteine. Children under 6 years of age appear less susceptible to hepatic damage, even with plasma concentrations in the range toxic to older victims.[25] In contrast, alcoholics taking therapeutic doses of acetaminophen may exhibit hepatic effects.[27]

These NSAIDs along with tolmetin, piroxicam, and sulindac (Table 31-1) have been introduced into therapy since 1975 and present an improvement in safety over aspirin, indomethacin, and phenylbutazone. In general gastrointestinal distress is

PROPIONIC ACID DERIVATIVES

less of a problem. Acute intoxication is apparently less of a hazard than with aspirin and acetaminophen.[8] In contrast, two other recently marketed agents, benoxaprofen and zomepirac, were withdrawn shortly after introduction because of fatalities associated with their use. The newer agents are more expensive than aspirin and acetaminophen, an important consideration in chronic diseases.

Ibuprofen is useful in dysmenorrhea and as a substitute for aspirin in patients with rheumatoid arthritis and osteoarthritis. It is also available over the counter in 200 mg tablets (Advil, Nuprin, others) as an analgesic and, for children over 12 years of age, as an antipyretic. Drug interactions with oral anticoagulants may be anticipated. After a survey of clinical trials, it was concluded that variability was such that no statistical differences in adverse effects could be demonstrated among six of the newer agents.[7] Ibuprofen, naproxen, fenoprofen, tolmetin, sulindac, and meclofenamate were all associated with, in roughly descending order of frequency: gastrointestinal disturbances > headache ≥ tinnitus = rash.

Ibuprofen

Naproxen

Naproxen has the advantage of a relatively long half-life, and so twice daily administration is sufficient for chronic antiarthritic therapy. Administration every 8 hours is recommended for acute relief of gouty arthritis.

Primary dysmenorrhea results from excessive uterine production of prostaglandins, which cause muscle contractions and ischemia in the uterus and can also reach other organs to induce diarrhea, vomiting, and other symptoms.[3] Oral contraceptives (see Chapter 47), which decrease prostaglandin synthesis by actions on the endometrium, are highly effective therapy of primary dysmenorrhea, provided that contraception is desired. Otherwise, naproxen and ibuprofen appear as effective as and better tolerated than other NSAIDs, and they are consistently more effective than aspirin, which has usually been no better than placebo in clinical trials.[3] Treatment with NSAIDs beginning a few days before menstruation may be most effective. However, if there is any likelihood of pregnancy, the drug should be administered after menstrual flow has begun so that exposure of a developing fetus is avoided.

Fenoprofen exhibits greater potential for acute nephrotoxicity than some other NSAIDs.[2] **Suprofen** and **ketoprofen** were released in 1986, the former as an analgesic and the latter as an anti-inflammatory drug. Suprofen has been associated with acute flank pain of uncertain cause.

Tolmetin differs structurally from the propionic acid derivatives but is similar pharmacologically. Aside from aspirin it is the only drug approved for therapy of juvenile rheumatoid arthritis. Several anaphylactoid reactions to this agent have been reported.

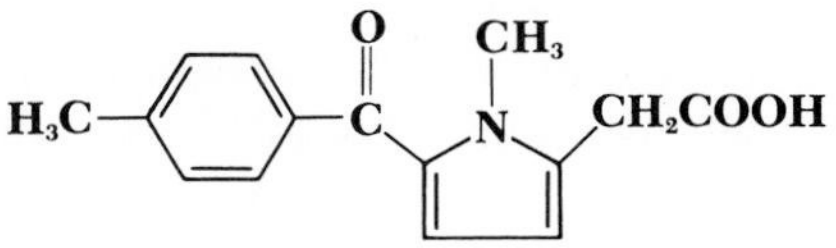

TOLMETIN

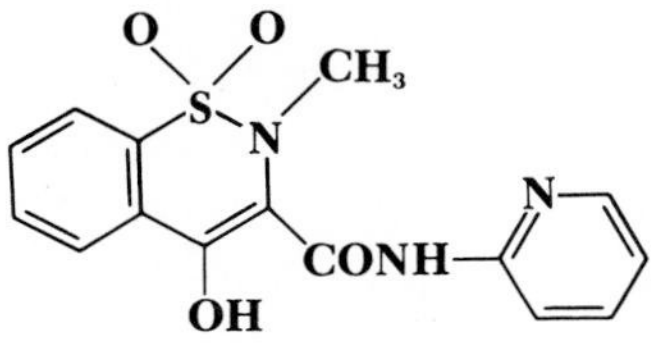

Tolmetin

Piroxicam

Piroxicam has a long half-life and can be taken once a day. Seven to 12 days are required to reach steady state. It can cause cutaneous reactions including photosensitivity.[30] Although a relatively high incidence of gastrointestinal bleeding and ulceration has been noted, recent evidence indicates that the risk with piroxicam is less than that with aspirin and no greater than that with other newer NSAIDs.[32]

PIROXICAM

In many experimental studies, indomethacin has been the prototypic NSAID for comparison with other such drugs. In treatment of arthritis adverse effects are more common than with many newer agents and include headache, gastrointestinal symptoms, blood dyscrasias, acute renal failure, and tubular and papillary necrosis.[2]

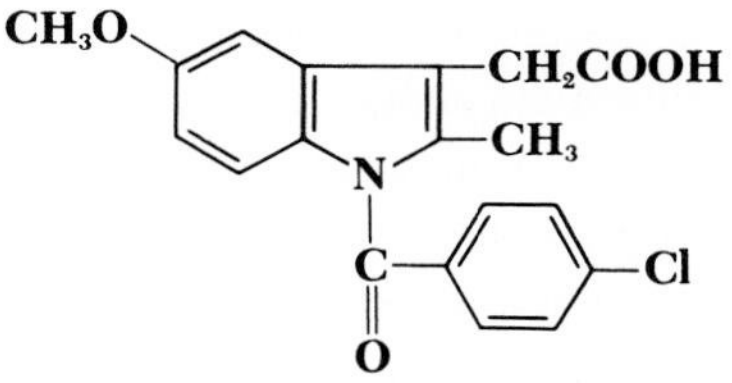

INDOMETHACIN AND SULINDAC

Indomethacin

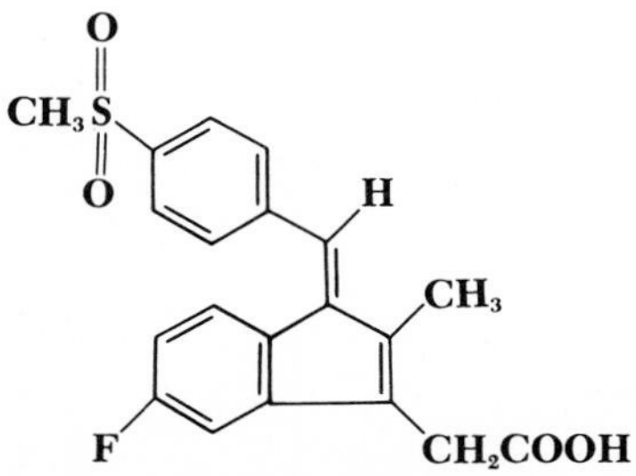

Sulindac sulfone
(inactive)

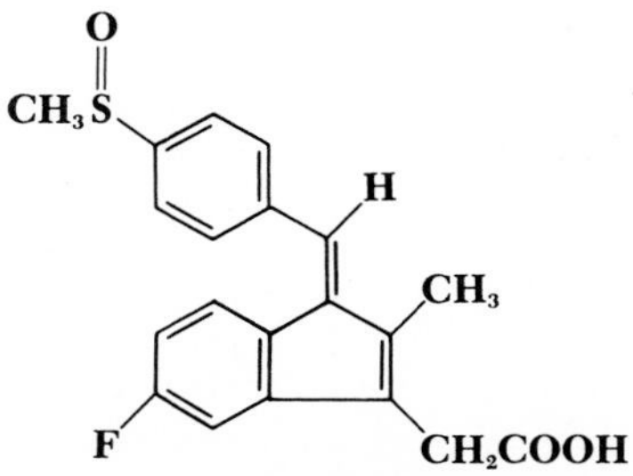

Sulindac
(inactive)

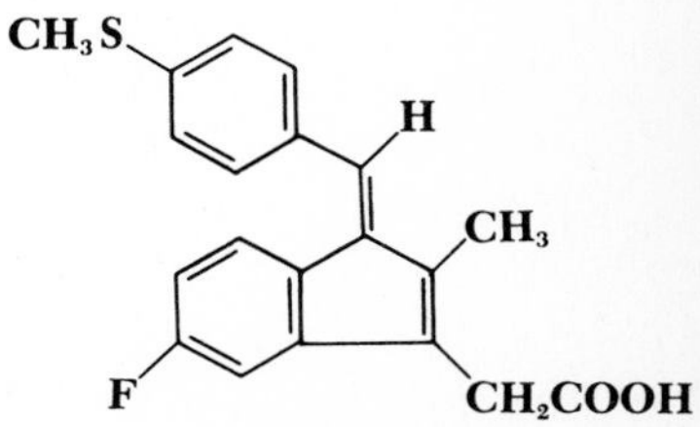

Sulindac sulfide
(active)

Sulindac is a sulfoxide that has some structural similarity to indomethacin with similar anti-inflammatory properties but less gastrointestinal and renal toxicity.[2] Sulindac itself is an inactive *prodrug* that is oxidized irreversibly to a sulfone that is also inactive and is reversibly reduced to an active anti-inflammatory sulfide.

Patent ductus arteriosus

The ductus arteriosus is the distal segment of the sixth aortic arch, which connects the pulmonary artery to the descending aorta so that blood can bypass the lungs in the developing fetus. Its patency is believed to be mediated by prostaglandins (see Chapter 22). This vessel normally constricts during the first day of life, resulting in functional closure.[13] In some neonates, particularly in premature infants of low body weight, it remains patent after birth. Although surgical closure is an established therapy, cyclooxygenase inhibitors can also be effective. Indomethacin promotes closure of the patent ductus arteriosus and alleviates the associated symptoms of cardiac failure in the neonate. Transient renal insufficiency and fluid retention are the most common adverse effects. Early diagnosis and treatment of the patent ductus arteriosus is important, since sensitivity to closure by indomethacin decreases with time after birth.

MISCELLANEOUS AGENTS

Pyrazolone derivatives

The two pyrazolones used as anti-inflammatory drugs are **phenylbutazone** and **oxyphenbutazone.** Sulfinpyrazone is used as a uricosuric agent (Chapter 48). Phenylbutazone is intermediate in effectiveness for treatment of rheumatoid arthritis, ankylosing spondylitis, and osteoarthritis between salicylates and anti-inflammatory steroids and is used for acute relief of gouty arthritis. It is uricosuric but is not used for this effect.

Metabolism. The metabolic alteration of phenylbutazone leads to two active compounds. Oxyphenbutazone has activity and toxicity similar to those of the parent compound. The other product is strongly uricosuric and is similar to sulfinpyrazone.

Toxic effects. Phenylbutazone should be used only when safer medications do not suffice. Some toxicity may appear in 25% of patients receiving the drug. These include sodium and water retention, visual disturbances, gastrointestinal symptoms, generalized hypersensitivity reactions that are unrelated to aspirin intolerance,[33] bone-marrow depression, jaundice, acute renal failure, and tubular necrosis.[2] When these drugs are used, particularly in the elderly, patients should be closely monitored for indications of toxicity.

Mefenamic acid is not more effective than aspirin and may produce serious adverse effects such as diarrhea, gastrointestinal bleeding, and impairment of renal function. **Meclofenamate sodium** is the most recent derivative of this class approved for chronic management of arthritis.

Fenamates

This phenothiazine derivative is a novel nonaddictive and non–anti-inflammatory analgesic. It is approximately equivalent to 10 mg of morphine by the intramuscular route. Special advantages claimed for methotrimeprazine are an antiemetic action and a lack of respiratory-depressant action. On the other hand, pronounced sedation and possible orthostatic hypotension limit its use to hospitalized patients.

Methotrimeprazine

In addition to the NSAIDs, several other agents are used to treat rheumatic diseases. Adrenal corticosteroids and chloroquine are discussed in Chapters 43 and 58 respectively. In contrast to NSAIDs, which control only inflammatory symptoms, antimalarials, gold salts, and penicillamine are believed to induce remission, though the mechanisms are unknown.[29]

MISCELLANEOUS DRUGS USED IN RHEUMATIC DISEASES

Gold salts such as **aurothioglucose** (Solganal) and **gold sodium thiomalate** (Myochrysine) are given initially at weekly intervals (progressively from 10 to 50 mg) by intramuscular injection. In one series of over 1000 patients given the latter drug, therapy was discontinued in about 38% within the first 2 years because of toxicity, most frequently rash, pruritus, or buccal irritation.[19] An oral preparation of gold, **auranofin** (Ridaura), which is taken daily, is now available. Diarrhea, cramping, pruritus, and rashes are common side effects of this agent.

Penicillamine (Cuprimine) is also used to treat rheumatoid arthritis. It causes rash, thrombocytopenia, and proteinuria in a high percentage of patients.

REFERENCES

1. Aspirin products, Med. Lett. Drugs Ther. **23**:65, 1981.

2. Carmichael, J., and Shankel, S.W.: Effects of nonsteroidal anti-inflammatory drugs on prostaglandins and renal function, Am. J. Med. **78**:992, 1985.

3. Chan, W.Y.: Prostaglandins and nonsteroidal antiinflammatory drugs in dysmenorrhea, Annu. Rev. Pharmacol. Toxicol. **23**:131, 1983.

4. Clark, W.G.: Kinins and the peripheral and central nervous systems, Handb. Exp. Pharmacol. **25**(suppl.):311, 1979.

5. Clark, W.G.: Mechanisms of antipyretic action, Gen. Pharmacol. **10**:71, 1979.

6. Clive, D.M., and Stoff, J.S.: Renal syndromes associated with nonsteroidal antiinflammatory drugs, N. Engl. J. Med. **310**:563, 1984.

7. Coles, L.S., Fries, J.F., Kraines, R.G., and Roth, S.H.: From experiment to experience: side effects of nonsteroidal antiinflammatory drugs, Am. J. Med. **74**:820, 1983.

8. Court, H., and Volans, G.N.: Poisoning after overdose with non-steroidal antiinflammatory drugs, Adv. Drug React. Ac. Pois. Rev. **3**:1, 1984.

9. Daniels, S.R., Greenberg, R.S., and Ibrahim, M.A.: Scientific uncertainties in the studies of salicylate use and Reye's syndrome, J.A.M.A. **249**:1311, 1983.

10. Davies, P., Bailey, P.J., Goldenberg, M., and Ford-Hutchison, A.W.: The role of arachidonic acid oxygenation products in pain and inflammation, Annu. Rev. Immunol. **2**:335, 1984.

11. Done, A.K.: Aspirin overdosage: incidence, diagnosis, and management, Pediatrics **62**(5, suppl.):890, 1978.

12. Forrest, J.A.H., Clements, J.A., and Prescott, L.F.: Clinical pharmacokinetics of paracetamol, Clin. Pharmacokinet. **7**:93, 1982.

13. Gersony, W.M.: Patent ductus arteriosus in the neonate, Pediatr. Clin. North Am. **33**:545, 1986.

14. Goodwin, J.S.: Mechanism of action of nonsteroidal anti-inflammatory agents, Am. J. Med., p. 57, July 13, 1984.

15. Graham, D.Y., and Smith, J.L.: Aspirin and the stomach, Ann. Intern Med. **104**:390, 1986.

16. Hellon, R., and Townsend, Y.: Mechanisms of fever, Pharmacol. Ther. **19**:211, 1983.

17. Hurwitz, E.S., Barrett, M.J., Bregman, D., et al.: Public Health Service study of Reye's syndrome and medications: report of the main study, J.A.M.A. **257**:1905, 1987.

18. Huskisson, E.C.: How to choose a nonsteroidal anti-inflammatory drug, Clin. Rheum. Dis. **10**:313, 1984.

19. Lockie, L.M., and Smith, D.M.: Fortyseven years experience with gold therapy in 1,019 rheumatoid arthritis patients, Semin. Arthritis Rheum. **14**:238, 1985.

20. Milton, A.S.: Evidence for the involvement of prostaglandins in pyrogen fever. In Lipton, J.M., editor: Fever, New York, 1980, Raven Press, p. 141.

21. Moskowitz, R.W.: Use of nonsteroidal anti-inflammatory drugs in rheumatology: a review, Semin. Arthritis Rheum. **15**(suppl 2):1, 1986.

22. Nanra, R.S.: Renal effects of antipyretic analgesics, Am. J. Med., p. 70, Nov. 14, 1983.

23. Needs, C.J., and Brooks, P.M.: Clinical pharmacokinetics of the salicylates, Clin. Pharmacokinet. **10**:164, 1985.

24. Rogers, M.F., Schonberger, L.B., Hurwitz, E.S., and Rowley, D.L.: National Reye syndrome surveillance, 1982, Pediatrics **75**:260, 1985.

25. Rumack, B.H.: Acetaminophen overdose in young children: treatment and effects of alcohol and other additional ingestants in 417 cases, Am. J. Dis. Child. **138**:428, 1984.

26. Rumack, B.H.: Acetaminophen overdose in children and adolescents, Pediatr. Clin. North Am. **33**:691, 1986.

27. Seeff, L.B., Cuccherini, B.A., Zimmerman, H.J., et al.: Acetaminophen hepatotoxicity in alcoholics: a therapeutic misadventure, Ann. Intern. Med. **104:**399, 1986.

28. Settipane, G.A.: Aspirin and allergic diseases: a review, Am. J. Med., p. 102, June 14, 1983.

29. Stecher, V.J., Carlson, J.A., Connolly, K.M., and Bailey, D.M.: Disease-modifying antirheumatic drugs, Med. Res. Rev. **5:**371, 1985.

30. Stern, R.S., and Bigby, M.: An expanded profile of cutaneous reactions to nonsteroidal anti-inflammatory drugs: reports to a specialty-based system for spontaneous reporting of adverse reactions to drugs, J.A.M.A. **252:**1433, 1984.

31. Stitt, J.T.: Fever versus hyperthermia, Fed. Proc. **38:**39, 1979.

32. Symposium: Piroxicam: a clinical perspective, Am. J. Med. **81**(5B), 1986.

33. Szczeklik, A.: Analgesics, allergy and asthma, Br. J. Clin. Pharmacol. **10:**401S, 1980.

34. Temple, A.R.: Acute and chronic effects of aspirin toxicity and their treatment, Arch. Intern. Med. **141:**364, 1981.

35. Temple, A.R.: Pediatric dosing of acetaminophen, Pediatr. Pharmacol. **3:**321, 1983.

36. Zimmerman, H.J.: Effects of aspirin and acetaminophen on the liver, Arch. Intern. Med. **141:**333, 1981.

section five

Anesthetics

32   Pharmacology of general anesthesia, 384

33   Pharmacology of local anesthesia, 407

Chapter 32

Pharmacology of general anesthesia

GENERAL CONCEPT   The scope of anesthesiology touches nearly every specialty of medicine. Drugs that allow painless, controlled surgical, obstetrical, and diagnostic procedures constitute one of the cornerstones of modern pharmacologic therapy. It is estimated that 20 million anesthetics are administered annually in the United States alone.

The hallmark of anesthetic drugs is *controllability*. For this reason, most of the potent anesthetics are gases or vapors. Such drugs can be administered through the lungs with consequent rapid uptake into the systemic circulation. Elimination of these drugs is also primarily by the pulmonary route. Unlike nonvolatile drugs, elimination and termination of pharmacologic activity therefore do not depend on intrinsic hepatic biotransformation or renal excretion; rather they depend on a pulmonary process that can be actively controlled by the anesthesiologist. The lungs possess a large surface area, which can be utilized for precise dosage administration or elimination.

Inhalation anesthetics are nonspecific; that is, they do not function by interacting with specific receptors. As a corollary to this generalization, there are no specific antagonists to anesthetics. Inhalation anesthetics should produce all the following effects (though there may be quantitative differences among various drugs): (1) hypnosis, (2) analgesia, that is, freedom from pain, (3) skeletal muscle relaxation, and (4) reduction of certain autonomic reflexes. General anesthesia has been defined as a condition characterized by these four attributes.

Selection of a particular anesthetic or combination of anesthetics is predicated on the patient's pathophysiologic state and the nature of the anticipated surgical procedure. Anesthetics differ in their abilities to depress various organ systems, in potency, in speed of induction and awakening, in degree of skeletal muscle relaxation, and so forth. Thus one anesthetic may be superior to another depending on the clinical circumstances. Final selection of an anesthetic or anesthetic sequence is based on three factors in the following order: (1) those drugs and anesthetic techniques judged safest for the patient, (2) drugs and techniques that facilitate performance of the surgical procedure, and (3) techniques most acceptable to the patient. The last factor is generally a judgment between general and regional (for example, spinal) anesthesia.

Popular potent organohalogen inhalation anesthetics include enflurane, isoflurane, and halothane. Isoflurane is the newest halogenated anesthetic in clinical practice. Nitrous oxide, a weak gaseous anesthetic, is frequently used in combination with these volatile compounds or with intermittent doses of intravenous drugs such as barbiturates (for hypnosis), narcotics (for analgesia), and neuromuscular blockers (for skeletal muscle relaxation). Use of nitrous oxide in this latter circumstance is termed *balanced anesthesia*. The older anesthetics cyclopropane and diethyl ether are used infrequently because of their flammability, which is incompatible with the cautery and electronic monitoring equipment of modern operating suites.

Intravenous anesthetics are used for specific purposes or to supplement inhalation anesthetics, but they lack controllability and other salutary features of the inhalation anesthetics. Thiobarbiturates such as thiopental are still the preferred induction agents because they rapidly and pleasantly produce hypnosis. Lack of analgesic or muscle-relaxant properties and slow elimination limit both usefulness and dosage. Benzodiazepines are occasionally used for induction. Narcotics such as morphine and the more rapidly eliminated fentanyl are frequently used to supplement nitrous oxide anesthesia. Combinations of narcotics and neuroleptics, such as fentanyl with droperidol, are employed commonly with nitrous oxide. The sobriquet *dissociative anesthesia* has been given to the effect of the drug ketamine, which is related to phencyclidine. This drug has limited scope, however, as it does not allow for other than superficial procedures and often produces prolonged effects including abnormal psychic reactions.

POTENCY AND EFFICACY

Because volatile and gaseous anesthetics distribute and reach equilibrium in the body by virtue of their partial pressures, it is convenient to establish potency in terms of this physical characteristic rather than the more conventional ED_{50}. Equilibrium is the state in which net transfer of anesthetic is zero, and it can occur regardless of inspired concentration. The minimum alveolar concentration (MAC) is defined as *that concentration of anesthetic (in v/v percent or mm Hg) measured in end-tidal gas that prevents response to a standard painful stimulus in 50% of humans or test animals*.[4] In the clinical setting anesthetics are usually given in multiples of MAC (1.5 to 2.5 × MAC). Several factors change MAC. These include circadian (1) rhythm, body temperature (direct proportional decrease), age (direct proportional decrease), and other drugs (sedatives, hypnotics, anesthetics, and other central nervous system depressants decrease MAC). Factors that do not influence MAC include sex, species, state of oxygenation, acid-base changes, and arterial blood pressure. A response to a painful stimulus is different from awareness; "MAC aware" is a measure of awareness. At this partial pressure of anesthetic, 50% of subjects are aware; 50% are not. "MAC aware" is generally about 40% of the MAC value of any anesthetic.

SOLUBILITY

Anesthetic gases and vapors are soluble in blood, tissue fluids, and tissues and are quite lipophilic. Various tissues and fluids differ in their lipid content; nevertheless, any particular gas or vapor, depending on its lipid solubility, will eventually reach equilibrium at different concentrations in the various biophases. Table 32-1 illustrates this concept with a hypothetical inhalation anesthetic at equilibrium for a

TABLE 32-1	Distribution of inhalation anesthetic concentrations in various biophases after partial pressure equilibrium		
	Biophase		
Anesthetic	Blood	Lean tissue	Fat
Concentration at equilibrium	3 mM ⇌	6 mM ⇌	660 mM
Partial pressure at equilibrium	8 mm Hg ⇌	8 mm Hg ⇌	8 mm Hg

given inspired concentration. Notice that although the partial pressure of the anesthetic is the same in all phases, the concentrations in those tissues differ over a hundredfold. This is attributable to differences in solubility of the drug in the various tissues. Table 32-1 also illustrates the large capacity for storage in fat of an anesthetic that is highly lipophilic.

There are three solubility coefficients germane to anesthetic distribution. All are based on Henry's law and are temperature dependent. For clinical purposes these coefficients are measured at 37° C.

1. *Blood-gas partition coefficient* (λ). This is the most important solubility parameter for understanding uptake of inhaled gases and vapors. Fig. 32-1 illustrates how this coefficient is derived. Notice in this figure that when equilibrium is reached (right side), the end-tidal concentration of the anesthetic in the alveoli is proportional to the pulmonary blood concentration. Thus end-tidal concentration or partial pressure (abbreviated F_E) can be used as a measure of degree of equilibrium at steady-state. The partial pressure of anesthetics being administered to the lungs for uptake by the blood is the inspired alveolar partial pressure (F_I). When

$$F_E/F_I = 1$$

blood-gas equilibrium with the inspired gas concentration has been reached.

2. *Tissue solubility*. In the lungs anesthetics enter pulmonary arterial blood and then are distributed to peripheral tissues. Obviously, those organs with the most blood flow per unit time will receive more anesthetic than organs with lower flow. Richly perfused organs include brain, heart, liver, and kidney; skeletal muscle perfusion is intermediate; the lowest perfusion is in bone, ligaments, and fat. The tissue:blood partition coefficient is between 1 and 2 for most anesthetics. Fat is an exception in that solubility is much higher; at times this exceeds solubility in blood several hundredfold. However, as a result of the low blood flow, even though solubility is high, a long time is required before the anesthetic partial pressure in body fat achieves equilibrium with other tissues. In Fig. 32-2 transfer of anesthetics from the anesthesia machine to peripheral tissues is illustrated.

Schema illustrating derivation of blood-gas partition coefficient (λ). Gas or vapor is inhaled **FIG. 32-1**
into lungs perfused with pulmonary arterial blood. Anesthetic partial pressure in lungs is
high initially and absent in blood, A. Anesthetic molecules diffuse into blood and reach
partial pressure equilibrium, B. Because of partition coefficient, partial pressure equilibrium
results in concentration differences in anesthetic. Anesthetic of low blood-gas coefficient
will have fewer molecules in blood than in gas phase; high coefficient produces fewer
molecules in gas than in blood at equilibrium.

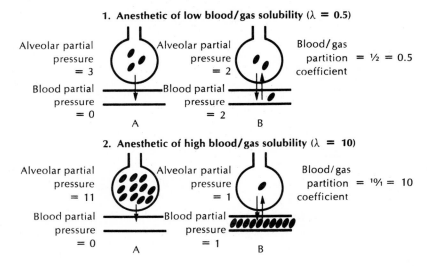

Flow of anesthetic gases and vapors from anesthesia machine to peripheral tissues. **FIG. 32-2**

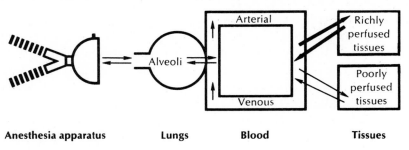

3. *Oil-gas partition coefficient.* The oil-gas partition coefficient is an artificial one
   in certain respects because the oil commonly used, olive oil, is not a biologic
   constituent of the body. However, olive oil has solubility characteristics similar
   to body fat. The lipid solubility of anesthetics is proportional to their potency.
   This is the basis of the direct Meyer-Overton correlation, which demonstrates
   proportionality between fat solubility and anesthetic potency. Thus a high oil-
   gas partition coefficient indicates a potent anesthetic (that is, one with a low

TABLE 32-2 MAC with blood-gas and oil-gas partition coefficients for six general anesthetics

Anesthetic	MAC in humans (v/v%)	Blood-gas (λ)	Oil-gas
Halothane	0.78	2.3	224
Enflurane	1.7	1.8	98
Diethyl ether	2.0	12.1	65
Isoflurane	1.3	1.4	99
Nitrous oxide	188*	0.5	1.4
Methoxyflurane	0.16	12.0	970

MAC, Minimum alveolar concentration.
*Extrapolated.

MAC and low partial pressure required for anesthesia). This correlation does not explain the mechanism of anesthesia, but it can be used to predict MAC. In fact, the correlation between MAC and the oil-gas partition of inhalation anesthetics is essentially linear.

Importance of blood-gas partition coefficient to speed of induction. A low blood-gas partition coefficient indicates that the anesthetic's partial pressure in the alveoli will rapidly approach equilibrium with the partial pressure in blood; that is, an F_E/F_I equaling 1 will be approached quickly because such a gas or vapor is relatively insoluble in blood. Thus clinical induction of anesthesia is rapid with such an agent. On the other hand, a high blood-gas coefficient correlates with a relatively long interval before blood-gas equilibrium is attained and thus a slower induction. Because of the higher solubility, it takes more time for the blood to take up enough anesthetic to reach the partial pressure required for anesthesia. Table 32-2 lists the MAC and the blood-gas and oil-gas partition coefficients for six inhalation anesthetics.

UPTAKE OF AN ANESTHETIC

Ventilation with an inhaled anesthetic causes a rapid rise in alveolar anesthetic partial pressure or concentration (F_I). However, this increase in F_I slows as uptake into pulmonary arterial blood removes the gas or vapor from the lungs. Arterial blood containing anesthetic in turn distributes the anesthetic throughout the body. Uptake of the anesthetic by a specific tissue is a function of anesthetic solubility, blood flow to that tissue, and the arterial blood to tissue anesthetic partial pressure difference. The partial pressure difference is the driving force. When the partial pressure difference becomes zero, equilibrium has been achieved; no further net uptake occurs.

Uptake from the lungs as from any tissue is directly related to three variables: (1) the blood-gas partition coefficient of the anesthetic, (2) cardiac output ($\dot{Q}$), and (3) the alveolar to venous anesthetic partial pressure difference. The time to equilibrium depends on the non–lung tissue capacity, which is related to the volume and capacity of the tissues concerned. In summary:

$$Uptake = \lambda \cdot \dot{Q} \cdot (P_A - P_V)/BP$$

where

$(P_A - P_V)$ = (Alveolar − Venous partial pressure of anesthetic)
$\dot{Q}$ = Cardiac output
λ = Blood-gas partition coefficient
BP = Barometric pressure

An increase in any of these factors will increase uptake. It is worthwhile noting that if uptake of an anesthetic is plotted graphically, the resulting curve is the inverse of the equilibrium curve.

There are several variables that prevent or slow attainment of the $F_E/F_I = 1$ state of equilibrium.

1. *Fat solubility*. Because of its poor perfusion but large storage capacity for general anesthetics, hours or even days may be required before body fat achieves equilibrium with alveolar anesthetic partial pressure.

2. *Biotransformation of anesthetics*. Inhalation anesthetics are metabolized by hepatic microsomal enzyme systems. Actually the degree of metabolism is small compared with the overabundance of drug given during the course of anesthesia. Nevertheless, metabolism limits attainment of equilibrium. However, unlike the case with nonvolatile drugs, such degradation has little if any effect on the conduct of anesthesia or dosage requirements of the anesthetic drug. On the other hand, biotransformation may convert a halogenated anesthetic to a toxic metabolite.

3. *Diffusion through skin or into bowel or into other air spaces*. Diffusion of an anesthetic through the skin into the atmosphere is another type of loss that delays equilibrium. Typical losses include nitrous oxide ($F_I = 70\%$) at 2.5 ml/min/m² and halothane ($F_I = 0.9\%$) at 0.006 ml/min/m². Anesthetics with a high F_I (nitrous oxide) replace nitrogen in the bowel and other air spaces, such as the middle ear. Since nitrous oxide is more soluble than nitrogen at the same partial pressure, when it passes from a dissolved state in blood into such an air space, it expands to a larger volume than the nitrogen it replaces. In this manner nitrous oxide anesthesia produces variable increases in bowel volume. Enlargement of a preexisting pneumothorax can occur by the same mechanism.

Factors that prevent attainment of equilibrium

Basically the *concentration effect* denotes that the higher the inspired concentration of an anesthetic, the faster the rate of rise toward equilibrium. In theory, the equilibrium curves in Fig. 32-3 should be independent of the concentration or partial pressure of the anesthetic inspired. In practice, this is not so. High concentrations give a more rapid initial rise toward the equilibrium state than low concentrations. Actually the concentration effect is seen only with nitrous oxide given in relatively high concentrations. To understand this effect, first imagine an inspired concentration of an anesthetic to be 100% ($F_I = 1.0$). If this 100% concentration fills the alveoli,

Concentration effect

FIG. 32-3   *Equilibrium curves for two anesthetics. Notice that the anesthetic with the lower blood-gas partition coefficient approaches equilibrium much faster than the anesthetic with the higher coefficient. The anesthetic with the lower solubility in blood will induce a state of anesthesia more rapidly.*

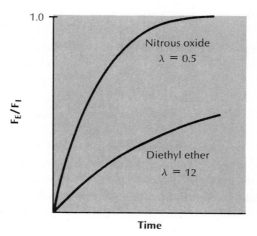

regardless of uptake into blood, the end-tidal alveolar concentration will remain 100% (F_E = 1.0) even though total lung volume is reduced. In this circumstance there is rapid uptake of a significant portion of the anesthetic into the blood. To maintain lung volume there is literal sucking of the anesthetic mixture from the reservoir of the anesthesia machine into the lungs. With a high concentration of nitrous oxide (F_I = 0.5 to 0.7), the nitrous oxide sucked from the machine mixes with residual alveolar nitrous oxide to increase the partial pressure of the anesthetic at end-tidal ventilation. Thus this mixing produces a higher F_E than would be expected, and the F_E/F_I ratio approaches 1.0 more quickly.

Second gas effect   Uptake of a large volume of a *first*, or primary, gas given in high concentration (the concentration effect) accelerates the alveolar rate of rise of a *second* gas given simultaneously. Thus the second gas, given in a low concentration, approaches equilibrium faster than if it were given in the absence of the primary, high-concentration gas. Clinically, nitrous oxide (the primary gas) is given with low concentrations of a potent anesthetic such as halothane or enflurane (F_I = 0.005 to 0.02). Uptake of a large volume of nitrous oxide appears to sweep along a higher volume of the second gas. Attainment of anesthesia will be hastened somewhat by this effect.

Effects of ventilation   An increase in minute alveolar ventilation ($\dot{V}_A$) obviously causes a more rapid rise in F_E regardless of partition coefficients because more anesthetic is presented to the alveoli per unit time. However, uptake of anesthetics of high solubility is altered relatively more by changes in ventilation than is uptake of anesthetics of low solubility.

1. *High-solubility anesthetics ($\lambda > 1.0$).* Increasing $\dot{V}A$ causes a large increase in FE per unit time. The reason is that the blood has a large capacity for soluble anesthetics. When blood is exposed to more molecules of higher solubility anesthetics, more of these can be absorbed. This increases the partial pressure of the anesthetic in the blood, manifested as an increase in FE partial pressure.

2. *Low-solubility drugs ($\lambda < 1.0$).* In contrast, an increase in amount of low-solubility anesthetic presented to pulmonary arterial blood per unit time does not increase uptake (or arterial blood partial pressure and FE) to a great extent. The insoluble anesthetic reaches equilibrium with blood rapidly. Being near saturation because of its low capacity for such drugs, the blood can pick up only a few of the extra molecules presented to it by an increase in $\dot{V}A$.

The clinical corollary of uptake changes produced by increases in $\dot{V}A$ are obvious. Higher solubility anesthetics are taken up more rapidly with forced mechanical ventilation. They may quickly reach dangerous concentrations in tissues. On the other hand, it is generally safe to hyperventilate patients with anesthetics of low solubility, since any change in uptake is minimal.

Effects of cardiac output

An increase in cardiac output ($\dot{Q}$) lowers FE because there is more pulmonary arterial blood available for uptake of the anesthetic per unit time. Similarly to the reasoning above, one would predict that low-solubility anesthetics are altered to a lesser extent than those with high solubility. Clinical corollaries of these relationships are that (1) depression of cardiac output by an anesthetic can alter its own uptake because the alveolar end-tidal rate of rise (FE) is rapid with decreased cardiac output and (2) highly soluble anesthetics more rapidly approach equilibrium when cardiac output is depressed. Use of soluble anesthetics in shock can thus excessively depress an already compromised circulation.

In summary of the salient features of uptake and distribution of inhaled gases and vapors, the blood-gas partition coefficient is the most important physical constant determining speed of induction of an anesthetic. The lower this coefficient, the faster the pulmonary blood reaches equilibrium with a given anesthetic partial pressure and hence the faster the induction of anesthesia. Awakening from anesthesia is similar. The lower the solubility, the faster the awakening as the anesthetic rapidly passes from pulmonary venous blood into alveoli and is exhaled. The concentration and second gas effects can be used to hasten induction with an inhalation anesthetic. Changes in ventilation and cardiac output have opposite effects—increasing ventilation causes an increase in the rise to equilibrium (more prominent with soluble anesthetics), and increased cardiac output delays equilibrium. In clinical practice these and factors such as ventilation/perfusion inequalities, alterations of regional blood flow, volume status, the degree of circulatory depression, and the pathophysiologic status of the patient are taken into account during the conduct of general anesthesia.

STAGES AND SIGNS OF ANESTHESIA

Early pioneers in the field of anesthesia such as W.T.G. Morton, John Snow, and Arthur Guedel recognized that there is a progression of predictable physiologic changes during anesthesia. The signs and stages of increasing depth of anesthesia with diethyl ether were characterized by Guedel as follows:

Stage I Analgesia
Stage II Delirium
Stage III Surgical anesthesia

Phase 1. Sleep and analgesia. Patient unresponsive to surgical stimulation. Pupils constricted and eyes moist. Intercostal ventilation. (Arterial blood concentration of diethyl ether = 1.1 mg/ml)

Phase 2. Pupils dilate and eyes dry. Beginning of intercostal paralysis with increased diaphragmatic ventilation. (Arterial blood concentration = 1.2 mg/ml)

Phase 3. Increasing skeletal muscle relaxation. Intercostal activity greatly decreased, diaphragmatic ventilation predominates. Tidal volume falls. Corneal reflexes absent with dilated pupils. (Arterial blood concentration = 1.3 mg/ml)

Phase 4. Onset of complete intercostal paralysis, ending with diaphragmatic paralysis. Circulatory depression. Pupils maximally dilate. (Arterial blood concentration = 1.4 to 1.6 mg/ml)

Stage IV Medullary paralysis; failure of ventilation and circulation.

Although evaluation of the patient anesthetized with diethyl ether is rather straightforward, newer more potent anesthetics with lower solubilities pass through these phases more quickly. In addition, the overall pharmacologic effects are somewhat different, though the result is similar. Basically, anesthesia with the newer, more rapid agents can be categorized into two stages: (1) the stage of analgesia and delirium and (2) the stage of surgical anesthesia. The latter is divided into light, moderate, and deep. With progressive deepening of surgical anesthesia there are parallel diminutions in ventilation and circulatory integrity. With overdosage of potent anesthetics, death can occur from medullary paralysis and circulatory arrest in the absence of hypoxia. As a general rule, deepening the level of anesthesia with the newer halogenated agents produces the following effects in a dose-dependent fashion:

1. Decreased blood pressure caused by peripheral vasodilatation or a direct decrease in cardiac contractility, or both.
2. Decreased alveolar minute ventilation because of reduced tidal volume. (Ventilation becomes more diaphragmatic in nature as anesthesia deepens.)
3. Constriction and centering of the pupils in medium levels of surgical anesthesia that proceeds to pupillary dilatation with onset of deep anesthesia. (Increased lacrimation is observed in light surgical levels of anesthesia, but the eyes are dry during deep anesthesia.)

Schema of, **A,** closed anesthesia system and, **B,** pediatric valveless system. **A,** 1, Vaporizer   FIG. 32-4
for volatile liquid anesthetics; 2, compressed gas source; 3, inhalation unidirectional valve;
4, mask; 5, unidirectional exhalation valve; 6, rebreathing bag; and 7, carbon dioxide
absorption chamber. **B,** 1, Vaporizer for volatile liquid anesthetics; 2, compressed gas
source; 3, mask; 4, rebreathing bag; and 5, gas exhaust port.

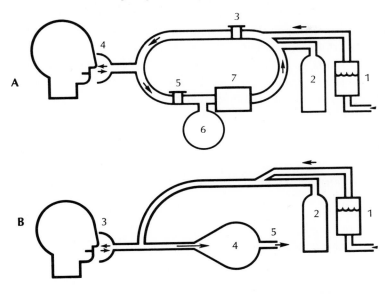

The anesthetic gases and vapors are customarily administered through an anes-   **METHODS OF**
thesia machine, basic components of which include the following: **ADMINISTRATION**

1. Steel cylinders containing anesthetic gases and oxygen under pressure. Re-   **OF GENERAL**
   duction valves lower the extremely high pressures of the cylinders to usable   **ANESTHETICS**
   pressures conducive to flow gradients.
2. Flowmeters that accurately measure minute flow of gases.
3. Calibrated vaporizers. These are containers of a high heat capacity metal such
   as copper, filled with liquid anesthetic. A sintered bronze disk in the bottom
   of the vaporizer disperses in-flowing oxygen into small bubbles that vaporize
   the liquid anesthetic in a precise fashion. Volatile anesthetics such as halothane
   and enflurane are vaporized to permit administration of precise amounts.
4. A carbon dioxide absorber.
5. A rebreathing bag.
6. Connecting tubing.
7. Unidirectional valves.

Although open-drop and insufflation techniques were used in the past, they are
only of historic interest. The closed and semiclosed systems are used commonly for
adult patients at present; the nonrebreathing, nonvalvular systems are used for

pediatric patients. A description, including the advantages and disadvantages of these systems, follows:

1. *Closed system:* Economical; prevents excess anesthetics from polluting operating room; conserves heat and respiratory moisture; more difficult to calibrate anesthetic dosage.
2. *Semiclosed system:* Easy to calibrate anesthetic dose; not economical because gases are expelled into the environment; the system loses heat and moisture.
3. *Nonrebreathing, nonvalvular system:* Low resistance highly suitable for pediatric patients; loses heat and contributes to operating room pollution with trace anesthetic concentrations. Despite the term "nonrebreathing," some rebreathing may occur depending on flow rate.

Fig. 32-4 illustrates the schemes of each of these systems. Administration of gases and vapors from the anesthesia machine is accomplished either by face mask or endotracheal tube.

THEORIES OF GENERAL ANESTHESIA

The mechanism or mechanisms by which anesthetics exert their effects are not known. Inhaled anesthetics possess no unique molecular configuration that can be associated with a particular structure-activity relationship. Interaction with cellular components is by means of van der Waals forces only. The anesthetics are nonspecific and can affect the function of all cellular constituents.

Effects of anesthetics have been attributed to blockade of ionic channels and alterations of neurotransmitter release, but these do not correlate well enough with potency to allow a unitary hypothesis of mechanism of action. Several theories of anesthesia have been postulated, but each is deficient in certain respects.

1. *Biochemical hypothesis.* Quastel theorized that anesthetics depress cellular respiration. This theory was based on the finding that certain anesthetics decrease adenosine triphosphate (ATP) production and cellular oxygen utilization in vitro. However, brain ATP concentration is not reduced by anesthetics in vivo.
2. *Hydrate theory.* Pauling and Miller postulated that anesthetic molecules form gas hydrates or structured water, which inhibit brain function at crucial sites. However, recent studies have demonstrated little correlation between hydrate formation and potency of inhalation anesthetics.
3. *Ionic pore theory.* Another hypothesis attributes the anesthetic state to blockade of ionic channels by interaction of anesthetic molecules with membranes. In many cases, high pressures can reverse anesthesia, perhaps by changing membrane structure so that the anesthetics no longer interact at such sites.

The Meyer-Overton correlation relating fat solubility to anesthetic potency has stood the test of time. In general, the more lipid soluble an anesthetic, the more potent it is. However, this correlation does not explain the anesthesic state. It is difficult to imagine that anesthetics act on lipids only, and many fat-soluble organic solvents lack anesthetic properties.

Several classes of drugs are frequently given before induction of anesthesia. The primary objective is to produce an anxiety-free, sedated patient. Additional reasons for such medications are to depress vagal tone and to supplement the anesthetic drugs. Individual drugs used for preanesthetic medication are described in the following categories:

1. *Anticholinergic agents:* Atropine, scopolamine, and glycopyrrolate are frequently given intramuscularly before anesthesia to decrease vagal cardiac tone and to inhibit bronchial secretion. The value of such muscarinic blockers is less now than when cyclopropane and diethyl ether were used, the irritant effects of which stimulated secretion.
2. *Narcotics:* Analgesics such as meperidine, morphine, and fentanyl are given to decrease anxiety and as a supplement to anesthesia. These drugs cause respiratory depression, which is increased when combined with anesthetics.
3. *Sedatives:* Barbiturates, primarily the short-acting drugs secobarbital and pentobarbital, are given to allay anxiety and to produce a drowsy patient.
4. *Benzodiazepines:* Diazepam given orally or intravenously produces sedation and some amnesia without significant effects on circulation or ventilation. For this reason, drugs of this class are now quite frequently employed as preanesthetic medications. **Midazolam** is a water-soluble, rapidly acting benzodiazepine that is replacing diazepam because of its shorter half-life and lack of venous irritation (see p. 286).

All preanesthetic drugs possess certain disadvantages, for example, respiratory depression. Thus their proper use necessitates intimate pharmacologic and pathologic knowledge and clinical judgment. As important as the premedicant drugs are in allaying the patient's anxiety, of equal importance is psychologic rapport with the anesthesiologist.

PREANESTHETIC MEDICATION

Because of the ubiquitous nature of anesthetic distribution and their nonspecific action on all cellular functions, discussion of their specific effects on various organs is frequently incomplete. Although anesthetics in general are depressants of function, there are many quantitative differences in their activities. To add complexity, the anesthetics also differ qualitatively in their effects.

PHARMACOLOGIC EFFECTS OF ANESTHETICS

Anesthetics depress all portions of the central nervous system. There is no single site or focus of action; however, there are considerable regional differences. It is believed that the higher cortical centers and the ascending reticular activating system are the most susceptible portions of the brain. However, as anesthetic concentration in the brain increases, lower centers also become depressed. This eventually leads to respiratory and circulatory arrest, the mechanism of death with overdosage. The neurons of the reticular activating system are depressed in a differential manner. For example, in very light planes of anesthesia, one commonly encounters clonus, hyperreflexia, and other neurologic signs because of suppression of inhibitory neurons of the reticular activating system. At higher dosages overall depression occurs.

Nervous system
CENTRAL NERVOUS SYSTEM

PERIPHERAL NERVOUS
SYSTEM

Recent studies have indicated that profound effects on the spinal cord are produced by general anesthetics. The gating region for pain impulses, the substantia gelatinosa of Rolando, is depressed such that nociceptive input ascending by pathways such as the spinothalamic tract is reduced. Thus fewer pain impulses reach the brain during anesthesia. Many general anesthetics also produce skeletal muscle relaxation by effects on the internuncial pool of neurons in the spinal cord. Although there are discernible effects of general anesthetics in the region of the myoneural junction, it is believed that actions on the cord are responsible for most of the skeletal muscle relaxation seen with administration of these drugs.

AUTONOMIC NERVOUS
SYSTEM

In the autonomic nervous system there are wide differences in the range of effects produced by general anesthetics, which are made more complex by the dose-response relationships involved. Some of the inhalation anesthetics, particularly the older ones diethyl ether and cyclopropane, appear to stimulate the sympathetic nervous system. Actually, this phenomenon may be attributable to quantitative differences in action on excitatory and inhibitory neurons controlling sympathetic nervous activity, rather than to direct stimulation. The concentration of plasma norepinephrine may increase three- to tenfold during anesthesia with an agent such as cyclopropane. This is one of the primary reasons that, until a decade or so ago, cyclopropane was considered the anesthetic of choice in shock. Because of release of norepinephrine, blood pressure was maintained with this anesthetic, though flow to organs was diminished because of arteriolar constriction. Another sympathomimetic effect is the increased glycogenolysis seen with diethyl ether. Blood glucose may reach concentrations as high as 200 to 250 mg/100 ml with this anesthetic. Nitrous oxide is the only presently employed anesthetic with sympathetic excitatory actions. In contrast, modern halogenated anesthetics such as halothane inhibit the sympathetic nervous system and reduce plasma catecholamine concentration. These agents also do not induce glycogenolysis.

Effects of inhalation general anesthetics on parasympathetic activity are quite variable. Some anesthetics such as cyclopropane and halothane have been adjudged to be vagal stimulants, particularly in lighter planes of anesthesia. The evidence for this is scanty, but both anesthetics seem to produce a mild degree of bradycardia that can be overcome by atropine. Further evidence for enhanced vagal activity comes from clinical reports implicating cyclopropane as a trigger for bronchial constriction in asthmatics. On the other hand, halothane and the other halogenated hydrocarbon anesthetics do not have this effect on bronchial smooth muscle and are therefore considered drugs of choice for the patient with lung disease.

Respiration

With deep levels of anesthesia, respiratory depression is common with all potent volatile general anesthetics. Diethyl ether clearly depresses tidal volume because of intercostal muscle and finally diaphragmatic paralysis. With other anesthetics, such as halothane, this effect on muscle activity is less clear. Certainly, at all planes of anesthesia there is a graded depression of medullary activity. Classically, ventilation during anesthesia is characterized by lowered tidal volume and increased frequency of breathing with a net reduction of alveolar minute ventilation. The response to arterial and alveolar carbon dioxide tensions is decreased, and so there is a classic rightward shift and decreased slope of the carbon dioxide–response curve. This is a dose-dependent phenomenon. In higher planes of surgical anesthesia, some anesthetics, such as diethyl ether, have less effect on respiration, such that normal or near normal carbon dioxide tension is maintained. However, with most of the halogenated anesthetics, the drop in alveolar ventilation and alveolar minute ventilation ($\dot{V}A$) will increase $PaCO_2$. For this reason the administration of a general anesthetic is frequently performed with assisted or controlled ventilation. This may be done by manipulation of the rebreathing bag of the anesthesia machine or by insertion of a mechanical ventilator into the circuit.

Circulation

Anesthetics affect both the heart and the peripheral circulation. They all produce a dose-related, negative inotropic effect, least with nitrous oxide. This can be seen as depression of twitch height in isolated animal papillary muscles and in intact humans as a fall in cardiac output. Anesthetics differ quantitatively in this activity. Halothane, for example, depresses the myocardium to a greater extent than diethyl ether does in equally anesthetic dosages. With those anesthetics that stimulate norepinephrine release, there is less negative inotropic effect because increased sympathetic tone stimulates the myocardium. Anesthetics, particularly the halogenated ones, by affecting ganglia depress peripheral sympathetic nerve activity and thereby result in vasodilatation. For this reason, peripheral vasodilatation usually occurs during anesthesia. The negative inotropic effect combined with the peripheral effects results in a dose-dependent decrease in blood pressure. Systolic blood pressure seems to be affected to a greater extent than diastolic blood pressure, and so during anesthesia there is a tendency for the pulse pressure to narrow.

Changes in cardiac rhythm and conduction are not uncommon during anesthesia. The most common arrhythmias involve the pacemaker, with progression from a wandering pacemaker to nodal rhythms. These arrhythmias are usually benign. The second most common form of arrhythmia is premature ventricular contractions. Many anesthetics can interact with an elevation in plasma epinephrine or norepinephrine concentration. Since the straight chain hydrocarbons, namely, cyclopropane and halothane, are most likely to cause this effect, these arrhythmias are often called "hydrocarbon anesthetic arrhythmias." The ether series of anesthetics, halogenated or not, seems to present far fewer problems in this regard.

Probably as a result of changes in automaticity, the threshold for premature ventricular contractions is lowered by many anesthetics. In light planes of anesthesia, if there is sympathetic stimulation or if exogenous sympathomimetic amines are administered, troublesome ventricular arrhythmias can develop. For example, sequential administration of cyclopropane and epinephrine is used in pharmacology for testing cardiac antifibrillatory drugs. Hypercapnia can increase release of catecholamines, which interact with the myocardium "sensitized" by hydrocarbon anesthetics to a lower arrhythmia threshold to produce ventricular arrhythmias. These arrhythmias are frequently clues to the clinician that ventilation is not adequate. Administration of catecholamines during anesthesia with certain of these anesthetics should be done with caution, if at all. Recommendations of minimal doses of drugs such as epinephrine that can be safely injected during the course of halothane anesthesia are available, but caution should still be exercised.[5]

Uterus	The halogenated anesthetics inhibit the contractile response of the gravid uterus to administration of oxytocic drugs. Thus they may produce or allow uterine relaxation, which may be advantageous for version extractions or other intrauterine manipulations. This effect is a two-edged sword, however, because these anesthetics will also permit sufficient degrees of uterine relaxation to increase postpartum bleeding. The gaseous and vapor anesthetics readily cross the placenta into the fetus. These effects must be taken into consideration during obstetrical anesthesia.

Hepatic and metabolic actions	Anesthetics have several actions on the liver. They depress mitochondrial function such that total body oxygen consumption is reduced. Actually, this has a certain advantage, since reduction in hepatic blood flow with impaired oxygen delivery will have fewer adverse effects if oxygen need is diminished. The anesthetics also seem to have an "anti-insulin action" that decreases the ability of the liver to take up glucose and incorporate it into glucose-6-phosphate. If an exogenous glucose load is administered during the course of general anesthesia, a diabetic type of prolonged glucose-tolerance curve will result. This effect coupled with the enhanced glycogenolysis that occurs with some anesthetics can increase blood glucose. The activity of hepatic microsomal enzymes responsible for biotransformation of various drugs is diminished during clinical anesthesia. This effect combined with decreased hepatic blood flow, which limits access of drugs to the liver, will decrease the clearances of some drugs. Recent evidence indicates that during deep anesthesia there is also impairment of certain synthetic pathways, such as the urea cycle and bilirubin conjugation. These effects quickly dissipate as the anesthetic is terminated.

Biotransformation and toxicity	Until 1965 it was believed that the general inhalation anesthetics were inert and were not extensively metabolized in the body. This concept has proved to be incorrect.[9,12] The anesthetics are metabolized to various degrees, depending on their molecular structure and partition coefficient. A low partition coefficient limits the time that an anesthetic is in contact with metabolic enzymes. Thus an anesthetic of rather low partition coefficient would not be expected to undergo as much biotransformation as one that persists in the body for a long time. The extremes occur in the case of isoflurane, which is less than 1% metabolized, as compared to methoxyflurane of which over 50% is metabolized. Biotransformation of certain anesthetics may be responsible for cases of toxicity reported after anesthesia. For example, methoxyflurane metabolism releases free fluoride ion. Fluoride concentrations greater than 80 μM may cause nephrotoxicity, which often manifests as a so-called

high-output renal failure syndrome.[7,10] Metabolism of chloroform, an older anesthetic no longer clinically employed, causes hepatic toxicity. Free radicals or other reactive intermediates that combine covalently with liver macromolecules are formed. The altered proteins and lipoproteins no longer function, and tissue necrosis can occur.[8] Halothane, ordinarily a very safe anesthetic, has been implicated in unpredictable hepatic toxicity. This is a rare event that probably occurs no more often than 1:10,000 administrations.[2] The injury is believed to be caused by biotransformation of the anesthetic to reactive metabolites that bind covalently to hepatic macromolecules to produce a hapten. This hapten then induces an immunologic inflammatory response that causes hepatitis and centrolobular necrosis. Repeated exposure to halothane anesthesia over short periods of time seem more likely to produce this event, particularly in obese, middle-aged women. Although this effect is rare, it is unpredictable and has a lethality approaching 50%.

A reduction in renal function is commonly seen during the course of anesthesia.[3] This is primarily caused by decreased renal blood flow with consequently reduced glomerular filtration rate. Nausea and vomiting may occur after administration of general anesthetics. Although these effects may have a central nervous system cause, one must keep in mind that surgical pain and stimulation probably also play a role. Cyclopropane and diethyl ether seem to cause postoperative nausea and vomiting to a greater degree than some of the newer anesthetics such as halothane. Because of hypothalamic depression, patients' temperatures generally decrease slightly during anesthesia. Certain anesthetics, such as halothane, may trigger a catastrophic syndrome known as *malignant hyperthermia* in genetically susceptible persons. This sudden and often lethal event can increase temperatures to 42° C or higher with severe metabolic acidosis. It can be treated or even prevented in susceptible patients with dantrolene (see p. 140). If ventilation is unassisted, many anesthetics can increase intracranial pressure.[11]

Miscellaneous effects

The inhalation anesthetics (Table 32-3) are divided into two major categories: gaseous and volatile liquid. Gaseous anesthetics are those with boiling points below room temperature and critical pressures greater than 760 torr. They are usually marketed as compressed gases, in the liquid or gaseous state, under high pressure in steel cylinders. The cylinders are colored differently for each gas, such as blue for nitrous oxide and orange for cyclopropane. The volatile anesthetics are liquids at room temperature, are usually more potent than the gases, and are ethers or halogenated hydrocarbons. Gaseous anesthetics generally possess blood-air and oil-gas partition coefficients lower than those of the volatile anesthetics, are consequently faster for induction and recovery, and are less potent. Selection of a particular anesthetic for an individual patient is predicated on pathophysiology and the type of surgical procedure involved. Selection of the appropriate anesthetic(s) is one of the critical factors to be resolved in the presurgical rounds of the anesthesiologist.

CLINICAL PHARMACOLOGY OF INDIVIDUAL ANESTHETICS

TABLE 32-3   Clinical characteristics of general anesthetics

Anesthetic	Analgesia	Hypnosis	Skeletal muscle relaxation	Depression of reflexes	Flammability	Compatibility with epinephrine
Nitrous oxide	+	+	0	+	No	Yes
Cyclopropane	+ +	+ + + +	+	+ +	Yes	No
Diethyl ether	+ + + +	+ + + +	+ + + +	+ + + +	Yes	Yes
Methoxyflurane	+ + + +	+ + + +	+ + + +	+ + + +	No	Yes
Halothane	+ +	+ + + +	+ +	+ + + +	No	No
Enflurane	+ + +	+ + + +	+ + +	+ + + +	No	Yes
Isoflurane	+ + +	+ + + +	+ + +	+ + + +	No	Yes

+ + + +, Maximum effect, +, minimum effect.

Gaseous anesthetics
NITROUS OXIDE

Nitrous oxide (N_2O) is a colorless, odorless, tasteless gas that is not metabolized. It is carried in the body in physical solution. Nitrous oxide is a weak anesthetic. It is usually supplemented in balanced anesthesia with hypnotics (barbiturate or benzodiazepine), analgesics (intravenous narcotic), and muscle relaxants (curariform drug). Nitrous oxide is not flammable and is compatible with all other drugs, including catecholamines. Analgesia occurs with inspired concentrations greater than 20% and hypnosis at concentrations of about 40% at sea level. However, because of its low potency, it is impossible to achieve complete surgical anesthesia with nitrous oxide without depriving the patient of oxygen.

Nitrous oxide has no significant effects on the respiratory, hepatic, renal, or autonomic nervous systems, except for slight myocardial depression and sympathomimetic effects. Because of this supposed lack of depressant effects, nitrous oxide has been called an ideal anesthetic. However, recent investigations indicate that it may not be totally benign. Nitrous oxide inhalation for only 2 hours can drastically lower levels of methionine synthetase used in vitamin B_{12} synthesis.[6] Although surgical patients given nitrous oxide do not develop pernicious anemia, persons abusing the drug chronically for long periods have demonstrated neurologic manifestations of vitamin B_{12} deficiency.

In addition to use in the balanced technique, nitrous oxide is commonly administered with the more powerful anesthetics such as halothane. This is done to hasten the uptake of the more powerful agent and to add the analgesic activity of nitrous oxide without harmful systemic effects. For example, halothane depresses myocardial contractility. The MAC for halothane in oxygen alone is 0.8%. If halothane is administered in 70% nitrous oxide with 30% oxygen, the MAC of halothane is reduced to 0.35%. Hence anesthesia can be accomplished with less adverse cardiac effects.

CYCLOPROPANE

Cyclopropane (C_3H_6) is a potent gas that can produce complete anesthesia without supplementation by intravenous anesthetics. The usual anesthetic dose at equilibrium is 10% to 20% inspired. Cyclopropane is no longer a popular anesthetic because of its flammability and tendency to explode. It stimulates the sympathoadrenal system so that blood pressure is well sustained. However, maintenance of pressure is obtained at the expense of alternations in peripheral blood flow distribution. Cyclopropane is the classic drug that is incompatible with catecholamines. It is rarely used at present.

Diethyl ether ($[C_2H_5]_2O$) is a pungent, volatile liquid that is irritating to respiratory mucosa and may reflexly stimulate ventilation. Diethyl ether was the first general anesthetic to be employed clinically. It is rarely used now, primarily because of its flammability. The hallmark of diethyl ether is that it is more benign to the cardiovascular system than any other complete anesthetic. Although it causes a certain degree of negative inotropic effect, this is countered in humans by a reflex release of catecholamines. The net effect is only a slight fall in cardiac output. Ether does not lower the threshold of the ventricular myocardium to catecholamines. It produces good skeletal muscle and uterine relaxation. Because of its high partition coefficient and the clear clinical signs of depth of anesthesia, following the planes of anesthesia with this drug is easier than with many anesthetics of lower solubility. For this reason, ether has often been termed the safest complete anesthetic.

Volatile liquid anesthetics

DIETHYL ETHER

The major disadvantages of diethyl ether, in addition to its flammability, are a high incidence of nausea and vomiting during recovery and its slow induction and emergence.

Halothane ($CF_3CHBrCl$, Fluothane) was the first of the truly modern, nonflammable halogenated inhalation anesthetics. It is rapid in onset and pleasant for patients and possesses a proved record of safety. The unresolved problem of hepatotoxicity has caused a decline in its use.

HALOTHANE

Halothane greatly depresses alveolar minute ventilation with the classical decrease in tidal volume but with increased inspiratory rate. Therefore assisted or controlled ventilation is commonly employed when halothane is administered. It is nonirritating to the respiratory tract and does not cause increased pulmonary secretions.

Halothane is an example of an anesthetic with depressant effects on the heart[1] with no increase in sympathetic nervous activity to secondarily augment contractility. Cardiac output, contractile force, and blood pressure all fall during its administration. Part of the blood-pressure decline results from a decrease in sympathetic nervous activity with a consequent reduction in peripheral vascular resistance. Some degree of bradycardia is frequently seen during anesthesia with halothane. Halothane also lowers the threshold of ventricular muscle to catecholamine-induced arrhythmias. This effect is not so great as with cyclopropane, though it still warrants extreme caution when epinephrine or other sympathomimetic amines are to be administered during the course of halothane anesthesia. Uterine relaxation is good with halothane anesthesia.

Because of its low-solubility, halothane is considered a rapid anesthetic. It is commonly used with nitrous oxide, though it may be given alone in oxygen. At the present time, it is regarded as the primary anesthetic for pediatric patients because of the ease of induction and rapid awakening. Although there is the specter of hepatic damage, which is occasionally reported after its use, this effect is diminishingly rare in infants and children.

METHOXYFLURANE

Methoxyflurane ($CCl_2HCF_2OCH_3$, Penthrane), a potent, nonflammable anesthetic, is one of the first of a series of halogenated ethers. Its hallmark is that it produces excellent skeletal muscle relaxation. A drawback, however, is the rather high solubility which results in slow induction and awakening. Unlike halothane, methoxyflurane does not sensitize the myocardium to catecholamines. This may be related to the ether link of the anesthetic. It is a rather pleasant-smelling liquid of low volatility and is only slightly irritating to the respiratory tract. Although it depresses ventilation, depression of cardiac contractility is probably less than that with halothane at equally effective dosages.

The great drawback to methoxyflurane, which has decreased its clinical use, is its biotransformation with release of free fluoride ions that contribute to high output renal failure. To reduce the amount of free fluoride released, it has been recommended that methoxyflurane anesthesia be limited to 2 MAC hours.

ENFLURANE

Enflurane (CF_2HOCF_2CFClH, Ethrane) is one of the most popular anesthetics in clinical use at this time. It is a halogenated ether that possesses many of the virtues of halothane and methoxyflurane without some of their disadvantages. It is usually administered in oxygen or with nitrous oxide. Enflurane depresses myocardial contractility comparably to halothane. However, because of its ether link, it does not sensitize the myocardium to endogenous and exogenous catecholamines to the degree that halothane does. The ether link also gives enflurane its excellent skeletal muscle–relaxant properties.

Because of lower solubility parameters, no more than 2% to 3% of an absorbed dose of enflurane is metabolized. Even though free fluoride ion is a metabolic product, it does not achieve blood concentrations sufficient to produce renal disease. An exception is in patients taking the antitubercular drug isoniazid, which can specifically induce defluorination enzymes. High free fluoride concentrations may then develop. The incidence of hepatic damage with enflurane seems to be far less than with halothane so that repeated doses are not contraindicated. Clinically the drug may be a little more difficult to use than halothane, which it seems to be replacing in adult anesthesia.

A major problem associated with enflurane is that the combination of high anesthetic concentrations and hypocapnia fosters grand mal seizures. In this setting, the EEG exhibits classical spike and dome traces. This effect does not seem to be a deleterious one, and one can avoid it by maintaining normocapnia and employing just that concentration necessary for the surgery.

Isoflurane ($CF_3CHClOCHF_2$, Forane) is an isomer of enflurane. It is the newest of the halogenated ether compounds, and clinical experience with it is not so extensive as with halothane and enflurane. Less than 1% of the total absorbed dose is metabolized. Therefore it may cause less renal and hepatic toxicity than any other commonly employed anesthetic. Many of its features are similar to those of enflurane. However, there is evidence that its respiratory depressant effect may be slightly greater than that of enflurane, whereas its cardiovascular depressant effect is less. Although it lacks a significant negative inotropic action, the anesthetic does produce rather profound peripheral vasodilatation with concomitant decreases in blood pressure. A resulting tachycardia can occur, and it may be bothersome in patients with coronary artery disease. Isoflurane does not foster convulsive activity. The drug is nonflammable and is compatible to a certain degree with catecholamines, similarly to enflurane. Skeletal muscle and uterine relaxant properties are good. Because of a somewhat pungent odor, inductions are often not so smooth as with halothane.

Some nonvolatile drugs are classified as anesthetics though they do not have all four attributes ascribed to general anesthetics and lack the ready controllability of the inhaled drugs.

Highly lipid-soluble barbiturates are used intravenously to produce or supplement hypnosis during anesthesia. They exhibit many of the distribution characteristics of inhaled anesthetics. One must remember that barbiturates are hypnotics only and do not possess analgesic or muscle-relaxant activity except with gross overdosage. Two barbiturates, thiopental and methohexital, are commonly employed.

Thiopental sodium (Pentothal), a potent ultrashort-acting thiobarbiturate, is the sulfur analog of pentobarbital. The thio group gives the drug greater lipid solubility and hence facilitates entry into the brain. Although barbiturates are organic acids, the pH has to be increased to 10 (as the sodium salt) to produce aqueous solubility.

Thiopental sodium

Thiopental is commonly used to produce a smooth, pleasant induction of anesthesia. It has no adverse effects on the viscera; overdosage is characterized by pronounced circulatory and ventilatory depression with upper airway obstruction.

Termination of the action of thiopental, and other intravenously administered barbiturates, is attributable primarily to redistribution. Plasma concentration initially falls rapidly as the drug is taken up by richly perfused organs, including the brain. The drug then redistributes out of these tissues and into muscle and eventually to fatty tissues. Awakening after normal therapeutic doses occurs within 15 minutes, which corresponds to the time drug concentration in skeletal muscle becomes maximal. Metabolism of the barbiturate is extensive; less than 5% is excreted unchanged by the kidney. Although metabolism begins as soon as the drug is administered, the rate, compared to redistribution, is not sufficient to be important in terminating the activity of a single bolus of thiopental. **Thiamylal** (Surital) is a thiobarbiturate similar to thiopental.

Methohexital (Brevital) is an ultrashort-acting oxybarbiturate. It was designed to have a slightly shorter duration of hypnosis than thiopental, but clinically this difference is not always apparent.

Contraindications to the use of intravenous barbiturates include shock and asthma. Barbiturates exacerbate acute intermittent porphyria, a metabolic disease, and should not be used in affected patients. Inadvertent intra-arterial injection of barbiturates can induce severe arterial spasm and thrombosis followed by gangrene of the extremities. Barbiturates are given intravenously in 1.0% to 2.5% solutions.

Innovar   Innovar is the trade name for a combination of fentanyl, a narcotic analgesic, and droperidol, a butyrophenone neuroleptic. Each milliliter contains 0.05 mg of fentanyl and 2.5 mg of droperidol. The anesthetic-like state produced by Innovar has been termed "neuroleptanesthesia" This combination given intravenously is a useful adjuvant in balanced anesthesia as a supplement to nitrous oxide. Innovar, given by the intramuscular route, is also used for preoperative medication in certain patients.

Because the action of fentanyl is relatively brief compared to that of droperidol, supplements with fentanyl (Sublimaze) alone may be necessary. Fentanyl is also used as an analgesic during anesthesia. Conventional doses of fentanyl for routine surgery vary from 3 to 5 μg/kg. Fentanyl is now used extensively as a narcotic-analgesic for open-heart procedures because it lacks some of the cardiac depressant actions of other anesthetics. For this purpose large doses of fentanyl, approximately 50 μg/kg or higher, are administered.

Fentanyl, like all narcotics, severely depresses ventilation. A peculiar increase in chest wall muscle tone, termed "wooden rigidity," is occasionally observed if the narcotic is injected rapidly. Rarely, droperidol produces a parkinsonian type of extrapyramidal reaction.

Ketamine is a phencyclidine derivative capable of producing a trancelike state *Ketamine* with freedom from pain, termed "dissociative anesthesia." Ketamine produces little or no muscular relaxation. Patients will respond to visceral pain but not to superficial pain under the influence of ketamine. It frequently produces psychic problems in adults, described as terrifying dreams and severe distortions of reality. For this reason ketamine use is usually limited to anesthesia for superficial procedures in infants and children. The drug stimulates the sympathetic nervous system and may increase blood pressure. It frequently increases salivation. Ketamine increases intracranial pressure and is relatively contraindicated in the presence of central nervous system tumors or space-occupying lesions. Ketamine hydrochloride (Ketalar) is available in solutions of 10 mg/ml for intravenous use and 50 mg/ml for intramuscular administration.

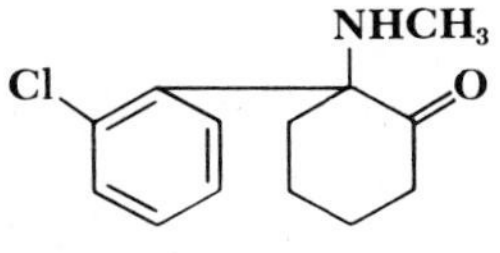

Ketamine

Etomidate (Amidate) was recently introduced into clinical practice in the United *Etomidate* States for anesthetic induction. It is an imidazole congener and is quite distinct from other induction agents. Etomidate is hypnotic only and possesses no analgesic properties. The dose is 0.3 to 0.4 mg/kg.

Hallmarks of the drug include rapid biotransformation, by liver and kidney, contributing to a very brief duration of action. Clinically there is essentially no depression of cardiovascular or ventilatory function. Animal studies have demonstrated that the drug has a wider margin of safety than thiopental or methohexital. Thus etomidate may have desirable characteristics for induction in certain poor-risk patients. Adverse reactions of involuntary skeletal muscle contractions and pain on injection, with secondary thrombophlebitis, limit the use of etomidate for routine anesthetic induction. The venous irritant action is believed to be caused by the propylene glycol vehicle that is employed for solubility. Inhibition of adrenal steroid production has also seriously limited the usefulness of this drug.

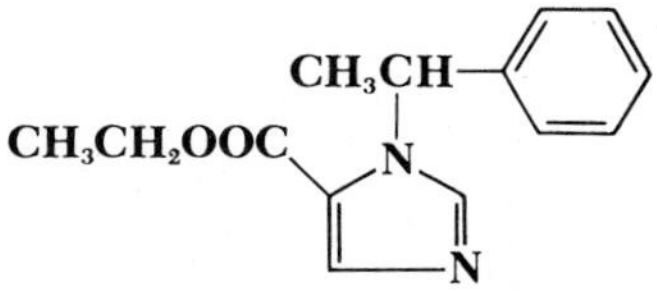

Etomidate

REFERENCES

1. Brown, B.R., Jr., and Crout, J.R.: A comparative study of the effects of five general anesthetics on myocardial contractility: I. Isometric conditions, Anesthesiology 34:236, 1971.
2. Bunker, J.P., Forrest, W.H., Jr., Mosteller, F., and Vandam, L.D., editors: The National Halothane Study, Bethesda Md., 1969, NIH, NIGMS.
3. Deutsch, S., Goldberg, M., Stephen, G.W., and Wu, W.-H.: Effects of halothane anesthesia on renal function in normal man, Anesthesiology 27:793, 1966.
4. Eger, E.I., II, Saidman, L.J., and Brandstater, B.: Minimum alveolar anesthetic concentration: a standard of anesthetic potency, Anesthesiology 26:756, 1965.
5. Johnston, R.R., Eger, E.I., II, and Wilson, C.: A comparative interaction of epinephrine with enflurane, isoflurane, and halothane in man, Anesth. Analg. 55:709, 1976.
6. Layzer, R.B.: Myeloneuropathy after prolonged exposure to nitrous oxide, Lancet 2:1227, 1978.
7. Mazze, R.I., Trudell, J.R., and Cousins, M.J.: Methoxyflurane metabolism and renal dysfunction: clinical correlation in man, Anesthesiology 36:247, 1971.
8. McLain, G.E., Sipes, I.G., and Brown, B.R., Jr.: An animal model of halothane hepatotoxicity: role of enzyme induction and hypoxia, Anesthesiology 51:321, 1979.
9. Rehder, K., Forbes, J., Alter, H., et al.: Halothane biotransformation in man: a quantitative study, Anesthesiology 28:711, 1967.
10. Sakai, T., and Takaori, M.: Biodegradation of halothane, enflurane and methoxyflurane, Br. J. Anaesthesiol. 50:785, 1978.
11. Shapiro, H.M.: Intracranial hypertension: therapeutic and anesthetic considerations, Anesthesiology 43:445, 1975.
12. Van Dyke, R.A., Chenoweth, M.B., and Van Poznak, A.: Metabolism of volatile anesthetics: I. Conversion *in vivo* of several anesthetics to $^{14}CO_2$ and chloride, Biochem. Pharmacol. 13:1239, 1964.

ADDITIONAL READINGS

Brown, B.R., Jr., Blitt, C.D., and Vaughan, R.W.: Clinical anesthesiology, St. Louis, 1985, The C.V. Mosby Co.

Eger, E.I., II: Anesthetic uptake and action, Baltimore, 1974, The Williams & Wilkins Co.

Eger, E.I., II: Isoflurane (Forane), Madison, Wis., 1981, Airco.

Miller, R.D., editor: Anesthesia, ed. 2, New York, 1986, Churchill-Livingstone.

Chapter 33

Pharmacology of local anesthesia

Local anesthetics are drugs employed to produce a transient and reversible loss of sensation in a circumscribed region of the body. They achieve this effect by interfering with nerve conduction.

In 1884 Koller, who had studied *cocaine* with Sigmund Freud, introduced the drug as a topical anesthetic in ophthalmology. This was the beginning of the first era in the history of local anesthesia.

The second era began in 1904 with the introduction of *procaine* by Einhorn. This was the first safe local anesthetic suitable for injection. Procaine remained the most widely used local anesthetic until the introduction of *lidocaine*, which is now considered the agent of choice for infiltration. Other local anesthetics of importance are tetracaine, mepivacaine, prilocaine, and bupivacaine. These drugs differ from each other in their toxicity, metabolism, and onset and duration of action. Lidocaine, in addition to being an important local anesthetic, has important uses as an antiarrhythmic agent (p. 441).

Electrophysiologic studies indicate that the local anesthetics interfere with the rate of rise of the depolarization phase of the action potential. As a consequence the cell does not depolarize sufficiently after excitation to fire, and the propagated action potential is blocked.

Local anesthetics may be classified according to their chemistry or on the basis of their clinical usage.

Local anesthetics are either esters or amides (Table 33-1). They consist of an aromatic portion, an intermediate chain, and an amine portion. The aromatic portion confers lipophilic properties to the molecule, whereas the amine portion is hydrophilic. The ester or amide components of the molecule determine the characteristics of metabolic degradation in that the esters are mostly hydrolyzed in plasma by pseudocholinesterase, whereas the amides are destroyed largely in the liver.

Local anesthetics have several types of clinical application, and their suitability for these varies with their pharmacologic properties. These applications and preferred agents for each are also indicated in Table 33-1.

Marginal notes:

GENERAL CONCEPT

CLASSIFICATION

According to chemistry

According to clinical usage

TABLE 33-1   Local anesthetics and their uses

Drug	Infiltration and block	Surface	Spinal	Epidural and caudal	Intravenous
Esters					
Butacaine (Butyn)					
Chloroprocaine (Nesacaine)	1			2	
Cocaine		1			
Cyclomethycaine (Surfacaine)					
Ethyl aminobenzoate (benzocaine, Hurricaine, others)		1			
Hexylcaine (Cyclaine)					
Procaine (Novocain)	1		2		
Proparacaine (Ophthaine, others)					
Propoxycaine (Ravocaine)	3				
Tetracaine (Pontocaine)	2	2	1	2	
Amides					
Bupivacaine (Marcaine, Sensorcaine)	1		2	2	
Dibucaine (Nupercaine)		2			
Etidocaine (Duranest)					
Lidocaine (Xylocaine, others)	1	2	2	1	1
Mepivacaine (Carbocaine)	2			1	
Prilocaine (Citanest)					

1, Primary agent; *2*, secondary agent; *3*, primarily dental use.

MODE OF ACTION   Electrophysiologic studies indicate that the local anesthetics do not alter the resting membrane potential or threshold potential of nerves. They decrease the rate of the depolarization phase of the action potential so that threshold (the point at which firing occurs) is not reached; therefore a propagated action potential fails to occur.[1]

The effects of local anesthetics on ionic fluxes are of great interest, and recent studies emphasize the relationships between these drugs and the calcium ion, with secondary effects on sodium flux. Although no detailed discussions are given here, local anesthetic agents appear to compete with calcium for a site in the nerve membrane that controls the passage of sodium across the membrane. It is believed at present that calcium is bound to phospholipids in the cell membrane. There is a correlation between the potencies of local anesthetics and their ability to prevent binding of calcium by phosphatidylserine in artificial membranes. The implication is that a potent local anesthetic blocks calcium binding in the membrane, thereby diminishing sodium flux with its resultant effect on the action potential. Consistent with this scenario are experimental studies that indicate that an increase in calcium concentration is able to overcome the nerve block produced by local anesthetics.[4]

PROBLEM 33-1. *When the hydrochloride of a local anesthetic is injected, which is the active* | *Active form*
form, the uncharged base or the charged cation? When one is dealing with an intact isolated nerve,
the local anesthetics such as lidocaine are more potent in an alkaline solution, an indication that the
uncharged base is the active form. On the other hand, when a desheathed nerve is used, the less
alkaline preparations are more efficacious. It is believed at present that the uncharged base penetrates
better across the nerve sheath but that the charged cation exerts the pharmacologic action. The
problem is complicated by the fact that the results are not applicable to all members of the series of
local anesthetics.

According to diameter, myelination, and conduction velocities, nerve fibers can *Action on various* be classified into three types—A, B, and C fibers. The A fibers have a diameter of *nerve fibers* 1 to 20 μm, are myelinated, and have conduction velocities up to 100 m/sec. Somatic motor and some sensory fibers fall into this classification. Blockade of these fibers results in skeletal muscle relaxation, loss of thermal and tactile sensation, proprioceptive loss, and loss of the sensation of sharp pain. B fibers vary in diameter from 1 to 3 μm, are also myelinated, and conduct at intermediate velocities. Preganglionic fibers fall into this group, and their blockade results in autonomic paralysis. C fibers are usually under 1 μm in diameter, are not myelinated, and conduct at approximately 1 m/sec. Postganglionic fibers as well as some somatic sensory fibers fall into this classification. Blockade results in autonomic paralysis; loss of the sensations of itch, tickle, and dull pain; and loss of much of the thermal sensation.

Clinically the general order of loss of function (upon exposure to a local anesthetic) is as follows: (1) pain, (2) temperature, (3) touch, (4) proprioception, and (5) skeletal muscle tone. If pressure is exerted on a mixed nerve, the fibers are depressed in somewhat the reverse order.

In summary, local anesthetic drugs depress the small, unmyelinated fibers first and the larger, myelinated fibers last. The time for the onset of action is shorter for the smaller fibers, and the concentration of drug required is less.[2]

Absorption of the various local anesthetics depends on the site of injection, the **ABSORPTION,** degree of vasodilatation caused by the agent itself, the dose, and the presence or **FATE, AND** absence of a vasoconstrictor. Epinephrine is frequently added to the solution to **EXCRETION** greatly increase the duration of action of procaine as an infiltration agent. The vasoconstriction caused by the sympathomimetic diminishes blood flow at the site of injection and allows the local anesthetic to persist at that site for a longer period of time.

The onset and duration of action of various local anesthetics are listed in Table 33-2.

Local anesthetics of the ester type (procaine) are hydrolyzed by plasma pseudocholinesterase (Table 33-3). Those having the amide linkage (lidocaine) are largely destroyed in the liver.

TABLE 33-2   Onset and duration of action of various local anesthetics, as determined by a standardized ulnar block technique

Drug	Concentration	Relative potency	Onset in minutes	Duration of action in minutes
Procaine	1	1	7	19
Lidocaine	1	4	5	40
Mepivacaine	1	4	4	99
Prilocaine	1	4	3	98
Tetracaine*	0.25	16	7	135
Bupivacaine*	0.25	16	8	415

Modified from Covino, B.G.: N. Engl. J. Med. **286**:975, 1035, 1972; based on data from Albért, J., and Löfström, B.: Acta Anaesth. Scand. **5**:99, 1961.
*Solutions contain epinephrine 1:200,000.

TABLE 33-3   Relative hydrolysis rates of local anesthetics by plasma esterase

Local anesthetic	Rate of hydrolysis
Piperocaine	6.5
Chloroprocaine	5.0
Procaine	1.0
Tetracaine	0.2
Dibucaine	0

In humans, procaine is cleaved to *p*-aminobenzoic acid, 80% of which is excreted in the urine, and diethylaminoethanol, 30% of which is excreted in the urine. Only 2% of the drug is excreted unchanged. Procaine is hydrolyzed in spinal fluid, in which there is very little esterase, 150 times more slowly than in plasma. Hydrolysis results from the alkalinity of the spinal fluid and is approximately the same in a buffered solution of the same pH.

About 10% to 20% of lidocaine is excreted intact. The rest is metabolized in the liver by removal of one or both ethyl groups. The resulting metabolites still have pharmacologic activity and may contribute to central nervous system toxicity.

METHODS OF ADMINISTRATION

Local anesthetics may be administered by topical application, by infiltration of tissues to bathe fine nerve elements, by injection adjacent to nerves and their branches, and by injection into the epidural or subarachnoid spaces. In certain situations intravenous injections are utilized to control pain. The details of subarachnoid and epidural anesthesia are outside the scope of this discussion.

Local anesthetics largely exert their action on a circumscribed region. Nevertheless, they are absorbed from the site of injection and may cause systemic effects, particularly in the cardiovascular and central nervous systems and especially when an excessive dose is utilized. *SYSTEMIC ACTIONS*

Since lidocaine is widely used as an antiarrhythmic drug (see Chapter 35), much has been learned about its effects on the heart. The same effects are generally also produced by other local anesthetics. At nontoxic concentrations lidocaine alters or abolishes slow diastolic depolarization in Purkinje fibers and may shorten the effective refractory period as well as the duration of the action potential. In toxic doses lidocaine decreases the maximal depolarization of Purkinje fibers and reduces conduction velocity. Toxic doses may also have a direct negative inotropic effect. Before such doses are reached, however, patients usually manifest central nervous system toxicity, such as restlessness, irritability, or seizures. *Cardiovascular effects*

Local anesthetics tend to relax vascular smooth muscle, but cocaine can cause vasoconstriction by blocking reuptake of norepinephrine.

Although local anesthesia usually produces no central effects, excessive absorption can cause excitation, convulsions, and eventually respiratory depression. It is believed on the basis of animal experiments that the local anesthetics block inhibitory cortical synapses. This leads to excitation. Larger doses that depress both inhibitory and facilitatory neurons produce general central nervous system depression. *Central nervous system effects*

Other than their effects on the cardiovascular and central nervous systems, the local anesthetics cause few systemic responses. They may depress ganglionic and neuromuscular transmission. These actions are unimportant unless another agent that affects these systems is used concomitantly. For example, lidocaine may enhance the action of neuromuscular blocking agents. *Miscellaneous effects*

Vasoconstrictors, particularly epinephrine, are commonly added to local anesthetic solutions that are to be used for infiltration or nerve block. One purpose is to slow absorption of the drug, thereby prolonging the anesthetic action locally. The concentrations of epinephrine used for this purpose vary from 2 to 10 µg/ml, also referred to as 1:500,000 to 1:100,000. Vasoconstrictors can also enhance safety; delayed absorption depresses peak plasma concentration, thereby decreasing anesthetic toxicity. However, epinephrine used in this fashion may itself cause systemic effects such as anxiety, tachycardia, and hypertension. Although the addition of epinephrine to a drug such as procaine is useful, agents such as lidocaine, prilocaine, mepivacaine, and bupivacaine may be used without the addition of vasoconstrictors. *Vasoconstrictors and local anesthetics*

The ester type of local anesthetics, such as procaine and tetracaine, may produce allergic reactions manifested as skin rashes or bronchospasm. Allergic reactions to *TOXICITY*

TABLE 33-4	Maximum safe dosages of local anesthetics administered to healthy adults	
Anesthetic	mg/kg of body weight	
4% cocaine	1 (topical)	
1% procaine	10 (injection)	
0.15% tetracaine	1 (injection)	
1% lidocaine	1 (injection)	
0.5% bupivacaine	2.5 (injection)	

the amides, such as lidocaine, are very rare if they occur at all, and there is no cross-reactivity with the esters. Consequently, allergy to an ester does not preclude use of an amide local anesthetic.

The majority of toxic reactions are a result of overdosage. The figures given in Table 33-4 refer to maximum dosages that can be administered safely to healthy adults, provided that inadvertent intravascular or subarachnoid injection is avoided.

In general the pharmacologic signs of toxicity from local anesthetics are central nervous system stimulation followed by depression and peripheral cardiovascular depression. Salivation, tremor, and convulsions, associated with hypertension and tachycardia followed by coma and hypotension, all occurring within a few minutes, characterize a full-blown episode.[3]

Treatment is symptomatic and essentially involves restoration of normal ventilation and circulation. Succinylcholine is useful for allowing oxygenation, abolishing the muscle spasm of tonic seizures. Diazepam is used both for treatment and prevention of seizures.

CLINICAL CHARACTERISTICS

Cocaine

Cocaine is too toxic to be injected into tissues and is therefore used only topically. It produces excellent topical anesthesia and vasoconstriction, which shrinks mucous membranes. Absorption from the urinary mucous membranes is rapid, and cocaine should not be used in this area. Some clinicians believe that vasoconstriction with 10% cocaine is better than with a 4% solution and that toxicity will be less with the stronger preparation because the cocaine will be more slowly absorbed. This may be dangerous, however. The vasoconstrictor effect of cocaine and potentiation by this local anesthetic of the actions of catecholamines are most likely consequences of inhibition of catecholamine uptake by adrenergic nerve terminals. Cocaine abuse is discussed in Chapter 30. Acute cocaine poisoning is probably best treated with chlorpromazine.

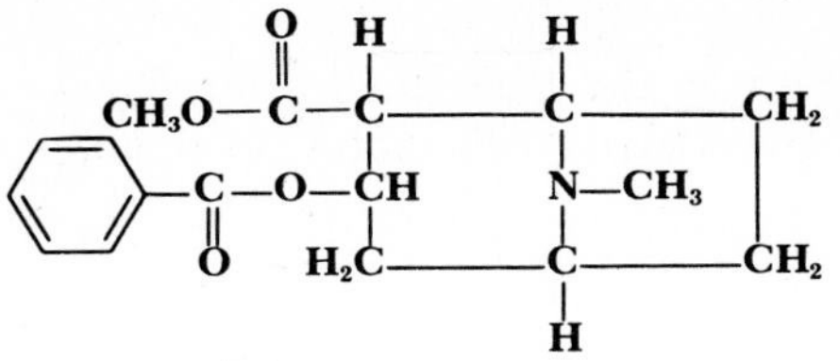

Cocaine

Ethyl aminobenzoate (benzocaine) is so poorly soluble that it is not absorbed from mucous membranes. Ointments containing 5% to 10% concentrations of the drug provide potent, safe topical anesthesia.

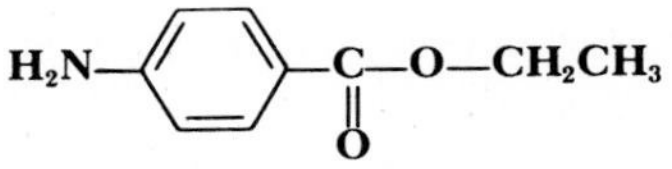

Ethyl aminobenzoate

Ethyl aminobenzoate

Procaine was once the standard to which all local anesthetics were compared. However, it is a poor topical anesthetic. Its duration of action is approximately 1 hour but can be significantly prolonged by the presence of epinephrine. Onset of anesthesia occurs rapidly. Afterward the patient often notes only the soreness produced by the needle used for injection. Procaine will block small to large nerve fibers in concentrations of 0.5% to 2%.

Procaine

Chloroprocaine is a derivative of procaine that has a much shorter duration of action because of its more rapid hydrolysis.

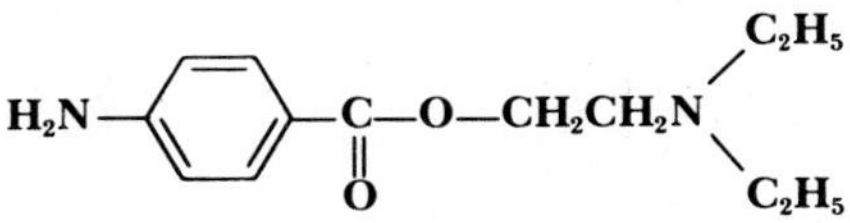

Procaine

Lidocaine, in concentrations of 0.5% to 2%, has supplanted procaine as the standard of comparison for local anesthetics. It is twice as potent as procaine and is more versatile, being suitable not only for infiltration and nerve block but for surface anesthesia as well. It also has a rapid anesthetic action. Lidocaine has one other characteristic that distinguishes it from procaine and other local anesthetics—it very

Lidocaine

often produces sedation along with the anesthesia. Lidocaine is an amide rather than an ester. It is metabolized in the liver by N-dealkylation. Two of its metabolites retain activity and may contribute to toxic central nervous system reactions in patients with altered metabolism.

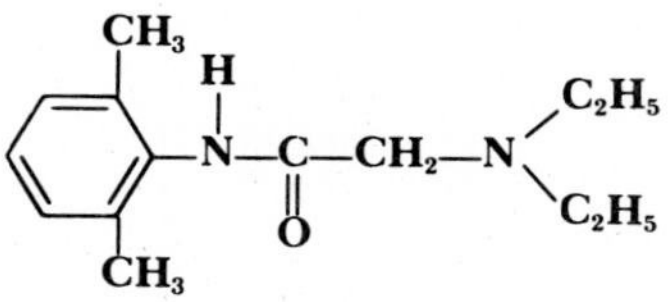

Lidocaine

Tetracaine   The chief differences between tetracaine and procaine or lidocaine are tetracaine's slower onset of maximal effect (10 minutes or more), approximately 50% longer duration of action, and greater potency. Tetracaine is available for injection in a 0.15% solution. For topical anesthesia it is used in 1% and 2% concentrations. Tetracaine should not be sprayed into the airway in concentrations greater than 2%. The total dose should be carefully calculated and probably should not, in this situation, exceed 0.5 mg/kg of body weight. The drug is rapidly absorbed topically and has resulted in several fatalities from topical misuse. The chief disadvantage of tetracaine is slowness in onset of action.

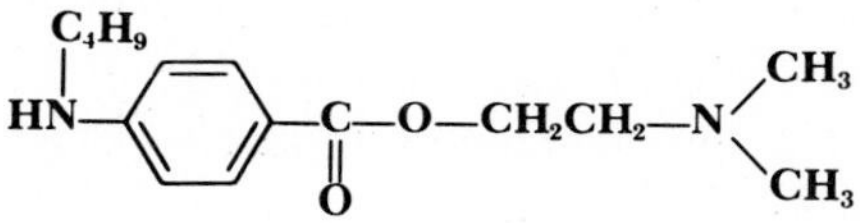

Tetracaine

Mepivacaine   Mepivacaine has essentially the same clinical activity as lidocaine, but it does not spread in the tissues quite so well, and its duration of action is longer.

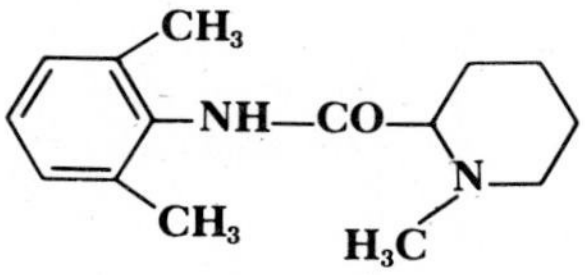

Mepivacaine

Bupivacaine   Bupivacaine is an amide chemically related to mepivacaine. It has a long duration of action, and its potency is four times greater than that of mepivacaine. Bupivacaine is used for infiltration, nerve block, and peridural anesthesia. Its adverse effects are similar to those produced by other local anesthetics. Bupivacaine is available in solutions containing 0.25% to 0.75% of the drug.

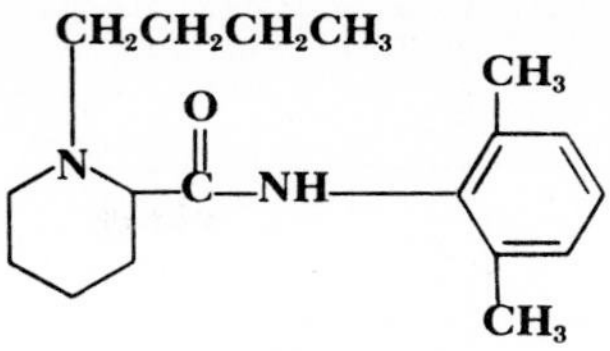

$$CH_2CH_2CH_2CH_3$$

Bupivacaine

Dibucaine is a very potent local anesthetic with a long duration of action. It is from 10 to 20 times more potent than procaine. As a consequence, it is employed in more dilute solutions (0.05% to 0.1%). Dibucaine is suitable for topical use and also for spinal anesthesia.

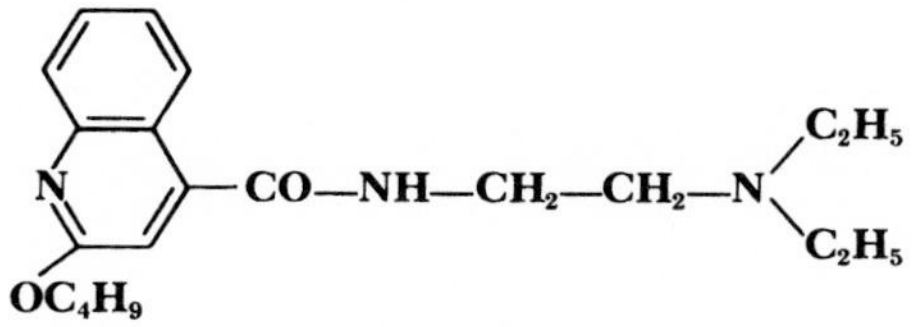

$$N \quad CO-NH-CH_2-CH_2-N \quad {C_2H_5 \atop C_2H_5}$$

$$OC_4H_9$$

Dibucaine

The needs of most physicians can be met by a few of the available local anesthetics. For infiltration lidocaine and bupivacaine are preferred. For spinal anesthesia tetracaine appears to be best. It has a duration of action of 2 hours or more and is hydrolyzed by plasma cholinesterase. For epidural anesthesia lidocaine (short duration) or bupivacaine (long duration) are often employed. Cocaine still has some use for topical anesthesia.

1. Covino, B.G., and Vassallo, H.G.: Local anesthetics: mechanisms of action and clinical use, New York, 1976, Grune & Stratton.
2. Gissen, A.J., Covino, B.G., and Gregus, J.: Differential sensitivities of mammalian nerve fibers to local anesthetic agents, Anesthesiology **53**:467, 1980.
3. Scott, D.B.: Toxicity caused by local anaesthetic drugs, Br. J. Anaesth. **53**:553, 1981.
4. Skou, J.C.: The effect of drugs in cell membranes with special reference to local anaesthetics, J. Pharm. Pharmacol. **13**:204, 1961.

Cousins, M.J., and Brindenbaugh, P.O.: Neural blockade in clinical anesthesia and management of pain, Philadelphia, 1980, J.B. Lippincott Co.

section six

Drugs used in cardiovascular disease

Although many drugs exert an effect on the heart, five groups of agents are discussed in this section either because they act selectively on the heart or because they are particularly useful in the treatment of cardiac disease: digitalis glycosides, antiarrhythmic drugs, vasodilator drugs, anticoagulant drugs, and diuretic drugs. In addition, the hypocholesterolemic agents are discussed. Antihypertensive drugs are considered in Chapter 18.

34 Digitalis, 418

35 Antiarrhythmic drugs, 433

36 Antianginal drugs, 450

37 Drugs that affect hemostasis, 459

38 Diuretic drugs, 477

39 Pharmacologic approaches to atherosclerosis, 493

Chapter 34

Digitalis

WILLIAM WITHERING, 1785 *. . . it has a power over the motion of the heart, to a degree yet unobserved in any other medicine, and . . . this power may be converted to salutary ends.*

GENERAL CONCEPT

Certain steroids and their glycosides have characteristic actions on contractility and electrophysiology of the heart. Most of these glycosides are obtained from leaves of the foxglove, *Digitalis purpurea* or *Digitalis lanata,* or from the seeds of *Strophanthus gratus*. These cardioactive steroids are widely used in treatment of heart failure and management of certain arrhythmias. They are collectively referred to as digitalis glycosides. Although catecholamines, methylxanthines and glucagon also increase the contractility of the myocardium, digitalis accomplishes its effect by a unique mechanism.

At the molecular level digitalis is a powerful inhibitor of sodium-potassium-adenosine triphosphatase (Na^+, K^+-ATPase). It is probable that the cardiac effects of the glycosides are a consequence of ATPase inhibition. The resultant increase in sodium concentration within the cell is believed to enhance calcium availability to the contractile apparatus.

Digitalis exerts striking actions on the *electrophysiology* of the heart. The effects are not the same in all portions of the organ. Most significant are more rapid repolarization of the ventricles (shortened electric systole) and, in higher concentrations, increased automaticity or increased rate of diastolic depolarization with appearance of ectopic activity. The atrioventricular (AV) node is greatly affected by the glycosides; digitalis slows conduction and prolongs the refractory period.

Digitalis toxicity is common in clinical practice.[2] However, with the development of assays to monitor serum concentrations, and as special problems with the drug in specific disease states have been noted,[16] management has improved, and the occurrence of intoxication has decreased.[12] The therapeutic index of the drug is small, and it is dangerous in certain circumstances. For example, hypokalemia, hypomagnesemia, or hypercalcemia increase the possibility of fatal arrhythmias during digitalis administration.

HISTORY

The history of digitalis is an example of the discovery of an important drug in a folk remedy. William Withering,[23] having heard of a mixture of herbs that an old woman of Shropshire used successfully to treat dropsy (congestive heart failure), suspected that the beneficial properties of the mixture were attributable to the foxglove. In testing digitalis leaf, Withering was greatly impressed with its diuretic

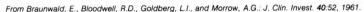

Contractile force and arterial pressure recordings immediately and 20 minutes after injec-   **FIG. 34-1**
tion of 1.4 mg of acetylstrophanthidin in a 28-year-old woman with an atrial septal defect.
The lower tracings show contractile force recordings before injection and at intervals after
acetylstrophanthidin. Notice that the drug augments the contractile force of the nonfailing
human heart and constricts the systemic vascular bed as manifested by an increase in
arterial pressure.

From Braunwald, E., Bloodwell, R.D., Goldberg, L.I., and Morrow, A.G.: J. Clin. Invest. **40**:52, 1961.

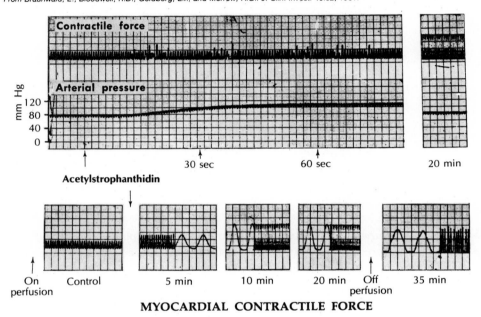

MYOCARDIAL CONTRACTILE FORCE

effect and believed that it probably acted on the kidney. On the other hand, he also
stated that the preparation had a remarkable "power over the . . . heart."

Over the years digitalis has become the most important drug in treatment of
congestive failure and atrial flutter and fibrillation. Although its position is being
challenged by more intensive use of diuretics, by reduction of afterload and preload,
and by newer inotropic agents, digitalis is still a mainstay in medicine.

The usefulness of digitalis in treatment of congestive failure is a consequence of   *EFFECTS ON*
its positive inotropic effect. In addition, some of its electrophysiologic actions make   *THE HEART*
the drug highly useful for treatment of a variety of arrhythmias.

Contractility is influenced by digitalis in both the normal and the failing heart.
In a now classic study (Fig. 34-1), Braunwald and his co-workers demonstrated this
effect in humans by attaching a Walton-Brodie strain gage to the right ventricular
myocardium of patients undergoing cardiac surgery. The effect of digitalis on contractility has also been shown in the isolated heart (Fig. 34-2).

Digitalis increases both the force and the velocity of myocardial contraction, and

FIG. 34-2 *Effect of digitalis on left ventricular function curves. Left ventricular stroke work is a measure of ventricular performance. Notice that digitalis shifts the ventricular function curve upward and to the left; that is, myocardial contractility is increased. CHF, Congestive heart failure.*

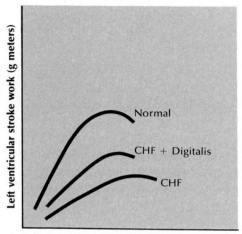

it shortens the duration of systole. It promotes more complete emptying of the ventricles and decreases the size of the failed heart. This reduction in heart size decreases cardiac wall tension, thereby lowering the energy requirement and rate of oxygen consumption by cardiac muscle. The final result, overall, is a beneficial decrease in myocardial oxygen need.

PROBLEM 34-1. Although digitalis increases the contractility of the normal as well as the failing heart, its effect on cardiac output is much greater in congestive failure. In fact, its ability to increase cardiac output in normal persons was questioned for many years.

The explanation of this paradox is related to hemodynamic adjustments. In the normal person, digitalis not only increases cardiac contractility but also causes constriction of peripheral vessels. It may also decrease venous pressure and may slow the sinus rate. Under these circumstances no increase in cardiac output can be demonstrated despite the positive inotropic effect.

The situation is different in the failing heart. In patients with congestive failure, the peripheral resistance is already high because falling cardiac output increases sympathetic tone. Under these circumstances the positive inotropic effect of digitalis increases cardiac output because the tone of peripheral vessels is lowered as a result of decreased sympathetic tone.

PROBLEM 34-2. Does digitalis increase the efficiency of the failing heart? It has been observed that digitalis will increase cardiac output in the failing heart without a corresponding increase in oxygen consumption. At first glance this could be interpreted as an increase in efficiency, since more work is performed by the heart per unit of oxygen consumed.

The problem is much more complicated, however. Myocardial oxygen requirement is determined by heart rate, myocardial contractility, and wall tension, which is a function of ventricular size. In a patient with heart failure and a dilated heart, by improving cardiac function digitalis decreases sympathetic tone and heart rate. Similarly, the diuresis that occurs will decrease ventricular size. Hence overall there is a reduction in myocardial oxygen need. In contrast, in a normal or nondilated heart there is no change in heart rate or ventricular size. In this setting the net result is an increase in oxygen need because of greater contractility.

FIG. 34-3

Diagram of the effect of digitalis on isolated Purkinje fibers. Notice that digitalis decreases the duration of the action potential as it shortens the plateau. Refractory period is shortened. Increased rate of diastolic depolarization can result in the development of ectopic pacemaker activity.

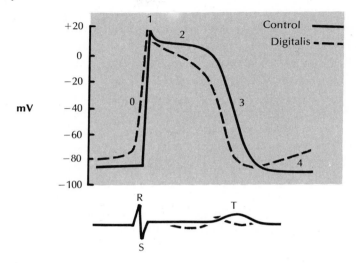

The electrophysiologic effects of digitalis account for its actions on *conductivity*, *refractory period*, and *automaticity*. These effects differ in conducting tissue and ventricular and atrial muscle cells. The outcome is made complex by the existence of both *autonomic* and *direct* actions of the glycosides and by differences in the sensitivity of normal and diseased heart to the electrophysiologic effects.

Electrophysiologic effects

At low doses, digitalis slows AV conduction. Since this action is reversed by atropine, it is commonly referred to as a "vagal effect." The direct effect of the drug that is not reversed by atropine becomes evident with higher doses.

Conducting tissue

AV nodal conduction is prolonged by digitalis. Prolongation of the P-R interval and varying degrees of heart block are electrocardiographic manifestations of this action.

AV refractory period is also prolonged by digitalis. This action becomes important when the supraventricular rate is rapid, as in atrial flutter and fibrillation, when the purpose in using digitalis is to decrease the number of impulses reaching the ventricles.

Purkinje fibers and to a lesser extent ventricular muscle respond to digitalis with a shortening of the action potential, decreased refractory period, and the appearance of pacemaker activity as a result of increased rate of diastolic depolarization (phase 4) (Fig. 34-3).

Ventricular and atrial muscle	In the ventricle, digitalis shortens the refractory period and the duration of the action potential. Thus the Q-T interval shortens. Isolated tissue studies imply that this effect may be dissociated from inotropy because low concentrations of digitalis increase contractility before a significant change in action potential.

In the atrium, the actions of digitalis are complicated by vagal effects. Digitalis may increase release of acetylcholine and may also increase the sensitivity of the fibers to the released mediator.[18] In a normally innervated atrium, digitalis decreases the refractory period. On the other hand, in a denervated or atropine-treated atrium, digitalis may increase the refractory period. |
| **EFFECT ON HEART RATE** | In normal persons, digitalis has little effect on heart rate. In congestive failure, digitalis slows the rapid sinus rhythm primarily by an indirect mechanism. The tachycardia in this case is a consequence of increased sympathetic activity brought about by decreased cardiac output. As digitalis increases cardiac output, the sympathetic drive to the sinoatrial node is reduced. Digitalis is not useful in treatment of sinus tachycardia caused by fever and other conditions.

Depending on the clinical condition, other factors play a role in cardiac slowing caused by digitalis: (1) prolongation of the refractory period of the AV node when atrial rate is rapid; (2) slowing of AV conduction (a partial block may be converted to complete block); (3) reflex vagal stimulation elicited by digitalis. These mechanisms are discussed in Chapter 35. |
| *Electro-cardiographic effects* | Electrocardiographic manifestations of the electrophysiologic effects are characterized by S-T segment depression, inversion of the T wave, shortened Q-T interval, and prolongation of the P-R interval. In toxic concentrations AV dissociation and ventricular arrhythmias such as premature ventricular contractions, bigeminal rhythm, and ventricular fibrillation occur. |
| **FUNDAMENTAL CELLULAR EFFECTS** | Inhibition of Na^+,K^+-ATPase by digitalis increases intracellular sodium. This sodium in turn may exchange with extracellular calcium.[1] It is also possible that inhibition of the enzyme decreases outward pumping of both sodium and calcium, thus increasing the calcium pool available for excitation-contraction coupling. This linkage of digitalis's effect with increased availability of intracellular calcium explains interactions observed clinically between the two. They are synergistic,[15] and calcium administration can be dangerous in digitalized patients. On the other hand, hypocalcemia has been shown to result in insensitivity to digoxin.[5] |
| **EXTRACARDIAC EFFECTS** | Digitalis also has extracardiac effects that may be helpful in recognizing impending digitalis-induced cardiac toxicity.

Gastrointestinal effects manifest themselves as nausea and anorexia. These effects are central in origin when purified glycosides or intravenous preparations are used. With powdered digitalis or digitalis tincture, a local effect also contributes. *Neurologic effects* consist in blurred vision, paresthesias, and toxic psychosis. Classically, patients |

may see objects with a yellow hue or see a yellow halo around objects. Although classic, this manifestation is rare. These symptoms are often misdiagnosed in elderly patients. *Endocrinologic changes* such as gynecomastia occur rarely. Allergic reactions are extremely uncommon.

Some experiments indicate that an action of digitalis on the central nervous system may contribute to arrhythmias and ventricular fibrillation.[10,21] In definitive experiments, electrical activity was monitored in sympathetic, parasympathetic, and phrenic nerves before and after ouabain administration to cats.[10] Ouabain increased traffic in these nerves. Spinal transection prevented these effects and increased the dose of ouabain needed to produce ventricular arrhythmias. It appears then that neural activation, probably at the level of the brainstem, plays a role in the development of ouabain-induced arrhythmias.

SOURCES AND CHEMISTRY

The cardioactive steroids and their glycosides are widely distributed in nature. Since their effects on the heart are qualitatively the same, it is sufficient to utilize only a few of these in therapeutics. Their sources and chemistry will be briefly summarized. The most important glycosides obtained from these plants are as follows:

Digitalis purpurea	*Digitalis lanata*	*Strophanthus gratus*
Digitoxin	Digoxin	Ouabain
Digoxin	Lanatoside C	
Digitalis leaf	Deslanoside	

The structure of digitoxin is characterized by a steroid nucleus with an unsaturated lactone attached at the C-17 position. The three sugars attached to the C-3 position are unusual deoxyhexoses. The molecule without the sugars is called an *aglycone*, or *genin*. The steroidal structure and the unsaturated lactone are essential for characteristic cardioactivity. Removal of the sugars results in generally weaker and more evanescent activity.

Digitoxin

Ouabain

Digoxin differs from digitoxin only in the presence of an OH at the C-12 position. Lanatoside C (Cedilanid) is the parent compound of digoxin and differs from the latter only in having an additional glucose molecule and an acetyl group on the oligosaccharide side chain. Removal of the acetyl group by alkaline hydrolysis yields the deslanoside, and further removal of glucose by enzymatic hydrolysis gives digoxin.

TABLE 34-1   Properties of digitalis preparations

Preparation	Gastro-intestinal absorption	Onset of action* (min)	Half-life†	Peak effect	Excretion or metabolism	Digitalizing dose (mg)		Oral maintenance dose (mg)
						Oral	Intravenous	
Digoxin	75%	15-30	36 hr	1½-5 hr	Renal; some GI	1.25-1.5	0.75-1.0	0.25-0.5
Digitoxin	95%	25-120	5 days	4-6 days	Hepatic‡	0.7-1.2	1.0	0.1
Ouabain	Unreliable	5-10	21 hr	½-2 hr	Renal; some GI	—	0.3-0.5	—
Deslanoside	Unreliable	10-30	33 hr	1-2 hr	Renal	—	0.8	—

Modified from Smith, T.W.: N. Engl. J. Med. **288**:721, 1973.
*Intravenous administration.
†For normal subjects.
‡Enterohepatic circulation exists.
GI, Gastrointestinal.

Ouabain differs somewhat in its steroidal portion from the previously discussed compounds. Its aglycone is known as G-strophanthidin, and the sugar to which it is attached in the glycoside is rhamnose.

PHARMACOKI-NETICS AND DOSING

The clinically useful glycosides and genins differ mainly in their pharmacokinetic characteristics, which are a reflection of their water or lipid solubility, gastrointestinal absorption, metabolism, and excretion. Digitoxin is highly lipid soluble; digoxin is less so, and ouabain is water soluble. As expected from their solubilities, digitoxin is completely absorbed from the gastrointestinal tract and persists in the body for a long time (Table 34-1). Ouabain, a highly polar compound, is not well absorbed from the gastrointestinal tract and has a short duration of action. Digoxin is intermediate.

Digitoxin is highly bound to plasma proteins and is metabolized in the liver; experimental hepatectomy decreases its clearance. In contrast, digoxin is eliminated mainly by the kidney, and renal insufficiency reduces its clearance. Thereby patients with diminished renal function require lower maintenance doses.

The elimination of various digitalis compounds is first order. In a patient with normal renal function, the half-life of digoxin is 1.5 days. Therefore, in such a patient, about two thirds of a dose will still be in the body 1 day later. In some settings a *loading dose* is administered to quickly attain a therapeutic concentration. The loading dose is usually 0.75 to 1.5 mg divided into three doses several hours apart. Since the purpose of subsequent *maintenance doses* is to replace losses, the daily maintenance dose will be one third of the loading dose.

If no loading dose is given and the patient is placed on a fixed daily maintenance dose, body stores of the glycoside will accumulate until steady state is reached, that is, when the amount lost daily equals the maintenance dose. This will occur in approximately 5 half-lives. Ninety percent of maximum will be reached in 3.3 half-lives (Fig. 34-4).

Serum digoxin concentrations related in general to effects.   *FIG. 34-5*

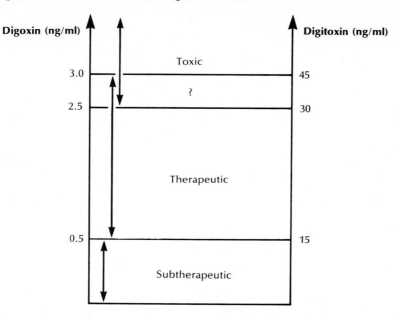

In addition to the potassium-losing diuretics that predispose to digitalis toxicity, there are other drug interactions of clinical significance (Table 34-2). Calcium (parenteral) and catecholamines or sympathomimetic drugs may promote ectopic pacemaker activity in digitalized patients. Barbiturates such as phenobarbital may accelerate metabolism of digitoxin. Cholestyramine, colestipol, and some antacids bind digitoxin in the intestine and interfere with its enterohepatic circulation. Digitalis can be used in reserpinized patients, since the glycosides still exert their characteristic cardiotonic effect. On the other hand, administration of parenteral reserpine to a digitalized patient may cause arrhythmias, probably as a consequence of sudden catecholamine release.

Digoxin toxicity is enhanced by quinidine.[11] When therapeutic doses of quinidine are administered to patients maintained on digoxin, there is on average a doubling of the serum digoxin concentration. The exact mechanism of this interaction remains controversial. However, in most of these patients renal clearance of digoxin decreases, and many exhibit a reduced volume of distribution.[3,7] If it is judged clinically necessary to administer digoxin and quinidine concomitantly, serum digoxin concentrations should be monitored closely so that appropriate dosage adjustments can be made. Physicians should anticipate this interaction and halve the digoxin dose to maintain the same serum concentration.

Drug interactions and digitalis intoxication

TABLE 34-2	Drug interactions with digoxin	
Drug	Effect	Mechanism
Amphotericin B	↑	Induces hypokalemia
Cholestyramine, colestipol	↓	Binds digoxin in gastrointestinal tract; interferes with enterohepatic circulation
Quinidine	↑	Decreases renal clearance of digoxin
Reserpine	↑	See text
Spironolactone	↑	Inhibits tubular secretion of digoxin
Thiazides, furosemide, bumetanide	↑	Diuretic-induced hypokalemia potentiates digitalis action
Verapamil	↑	Decreases renal clearance of digoxin

↑, Enhances digitalis effect; ↓, impairs digitalis effect.

Treatment of digitalis poisoning

The most important measure in the treatment of digitalis poisoning is discontinuation of the drug. Potassium chloride by mouth or by slow intravenous infusion may be helpful in stopping ventricular arrhythmias. It should be remembered, however, that elevated potassium concentrations may aggravate AV block, though potassium may lessen the block if serum potassium is low. It is believed by many investigators that infusion of potassium in a digitalized patient may produce abnormally high serum concentrations because of the effect of the glycosides on the membrane ATPase in various tissues. Other drugs that are used occasionally in digitalis poisoning are antiarrhythmic drugs such as phenytoin and lidocaine. Purified Fab fragments of digoxin-specific antibodies (digoxin immune Fab [ovine], Digibind) have been used successfully to treat digitalis intoxication in animals and in patients with advanced, life-threatening toxicity.[20] Hemoperfusion, a technique that passes the patient's blood over an absorbing substance such as charcoal, has been used to accelerate digitalis elimination in patients poisoned with digoxin[19] and digitoxin.[9]

DIGITALIZATION AND MAINTENANCE

The principles behind the loading dose and the maintenance dose have already been discussed in relation to pharmacokinetics of digitalis (p. 424). For practical purposes, initial digitalization is accomplished by either a *rapid method* or a *cumulative (slow) method*.

In the rapid method, the estimated loading dose is administered in a single dose or in two or three partial doses given a few hours apart. In the cumulative method, smaller doses are employed at frequent intervals until full digitalization takes place. For example, digoxin may be given for initial digitalization as a single dose of 0.75 to 1.0 mg or as 0.25 mg every 6 to 8 hours for 3 or 4 days. This initial digitalization is followed in subsequent days by the maintenance dose, which in the case of digoxin is about 0.25 mg daily (Table 34-1).

Dobutamine hydrochloride (Dobutrex) is a derivative of isoproterenol. It increases myocardial contractility but causes less tachycardia or peripheral arterial effects.[22] Available in vials of 250 mg for reconstitution and administration by intravenous infusion, the drug may be useful in heart failure without severe hypotension. In cardiogenic shock with severe hypotension, dobutamine is not sufficient to elevate blood pressure adequately, since it does not increase peripheral resistance. Since the electrophysiologic effects of dobutamine are similar to those of isoproterenol, the drug may increase heart rate. In the presence of coronary artery disease ischemia may be aggravated.

NEWER
INOTROPIC
AGENTS

Dobutamine

Amrinone

Amrinone lactate (Inocor) is the first of a new series of inotropic agents that differ in mode of action from digitalis and β-adrenergic receptor agonists.[14] These drugs appear to inhibit cardiac phosphodiesterase selectively.[6] They are bipyridine derivatives that cause strong positive inotropic effects in a variety of experimental preparations. In patients with congestive heart failure that did not respond well to digitalization, amrinone and milrinone further increased resting cardiac output while decreasing left ventricular end-diastolic, pulmonary capillary wedge, and right atrial pressures as well as systemic vascular resistance. The exact mechanism of action of these drugs remains unclear, though they are believed to influence excitation-contraction coupling in cardiac muscle. Whether the increased inotropy in patients is direct or indirect as a result of decreased afterload is unclear.

Amrinone, though efficacious, has been found to have considerable toxicity with chronic administration. As a result, only the intravenous formulation (5 mg/ml) has been marketed, to be used for short-term treatment of severe refractory heart failure. When used in this fashion, a loading dose of 0.75 mg/kg is administered, followed by a maintenance infusion of 5 to 10 μg/kg/min.[6]

Milrinone is closely related to amrinone but is approximately 15 times more potent and has fewer side effects. It has a half-life of about 2 hours and is eliminated for the most part by the kidney.[6] The drug may be suitable for chronic administration but has not yet been approved by the FDA.

REFERENCES

1. Akera, T., and Brody, T.M.: The role of Na+,K+-ATPase in the inotropic action of digitalis, Pharmacol. Rev. **29**:187, 1977.
2. Beller, G.A., Smith, T.W., Abelmann, W.H., et al.: Digitalis intoxication: a prospective clinical study with serum level correlations, N. Engl. J. Med. **284**:989, 1971.
3. Bigger, J.T., Jr., and Leahey, E.B., Jr.: Quinidine and digoxin: an important interaction, Drugs **24**:229, 1982.
4. Brown, D.D., and Juhl, R.P.: Decreased bioavailability of digoxin due to antacids and kaolin-pectin, N. Engl. J. Med. **295**:1034, 1976.
5. Chopra, D., Janson, P., and Sawin, C.T.: Insensitivity to digoxin associated with hypocalcemia, N. Engl. J. Med. **296**:917, 1977.
6. Colucci, W.S., Wright, R.F., and Braunwald, E.: New positive inotropic agents in the treatment of congestive heart failure: mechanisms of action and recent clinical developments, N. Engl. J. Med. **314**:290 and 349, 1986.
7. Doering, W.: Quinidine-digoxin interaction: pharmacokinetics, underlying mechanism and clinical implications, N. Engl. J. Med. **301**:400, 1979.
8. Doherty, J.E., de Soyza, N., Kane, J.J., et al.: Clinical pharmacokinetics of digitalis glycosides, Prog. Cardiovasc. Dis. **21**:141, 1978.
9. Gilfrich, H.-J., Kasper, W., Meinertz, T., et al.: Treatment of massive digitoxin overdose by charcoal haemoperfusion and cholestyramine, Lancet **1**:505, 1978.
10. Gillis, R.A., Raines, A., Sohn, Y.J., et al: Neuroexcitatory effects of digitalis and their role in the development of cardiac arrhythmias, J. Pharmacol. Exp. Ther. **183**:154, 1972.
11. Hager, W.D., Fenster, P., Mayersohn, M., et al.: Digoxin-quinidine interaction: pharmacokinetic evaluation, N. Engl. J. Med. **300**:1238, 1979.
12. Henry, D.A., Lowe, J.M., Lawson, D.H., and Whiting, B.: The changing pattern of toxicity to digoxin, Postgrad. Med. J. **57**:358, 1981.
13. Huffman, D.H., and Azarnoff, D.L.: Absorption of orally given digoxin preparations, J.A.M.A. **222**:957, 1972.
14. Katz, A.M.: A new inotropic drug: its promise and a caution, N. Engl. J. Med. **299**:1409, 1978.
15. Nola, G.T., Pope, S., and Harrison, D.C.: Assessment of the synergistic relationship between serum calcium and digitalis, Am. Heart J. **79**:499, 1970.
16. Ochs, H.R., Greenblatt, D.J., Bodem, G., and Dengler, H.J.: Disease-related alterations in cardiac glycoside disposition, Clin. Pharmacokinet. **7**:434, 1982.
17. Ogilive, R.I., and Ruedy, J.: An educational program in digitalis therapy, J.A.M.A. **222**:50, 1972.
18. Rosen, M.R., Wit, A.L., and Hoffman, B.F.: Electrophysiology and pharmacology of cardiac arrhythmias. IV. Cardiac antiarrhythmic and toxic effects of digitalis, Am. Heart J. **89**:391, 1975.
19. Smiley, J.W., March, N.M., and Del Guercio, E.T.: Hemoperfusion in the management of digoxin toxicity, J.A.M.A. **240**:2736, 1978.
20. Smith, T.W., Butler, V.P., Jr., Haber, E., et al.: Treatment of life-threatening digitalis intoxication with digoxin-specific Fab antibody fragments: experience in 26 cases, N. Engl. J. Med. **307**:1357, 1982.
21. Somberg, J.C., and Smith, T.W.: Localization of the neurally mediated arrhythmogenic properties of digitalis, Science **204**:321, 1979.
22. Sonnenblick, E.H., Frishman, W.H., and LeJemtel, T.H.: Dobutamine: a new synthetic cardioactive sympathetic amine, N. Engl. J. Med. **300**:17, 1979.
23. Withering, W.: An account of the foxglove, and some of its medicinal uses: with practical remarks on dropsy, and other diseases, London, 1785, C.G.J. and J. Robinson; reprinted in Medical Classics **2**:305, 1937.

Chapter 35

Antiarrhythmic drugs

Antiarrhythmic drugs are useful in prevention and treatment of disorders of cardiac rhythm that have high morbidity and mortality. Major advances have taken place in our understanding of cardiac electrophysiology and of the mode of action of drugs used in treatment of arrhythmias. In general, cardiac arrhythmias can be considered to arise from abnormal conduction, abnormal impulse initiation, or both.[17]

Antiarrhythmic agents have been placed into four groups on the basis of their electrophysiologic effects (Table 35-1). *Class I* drugs depress the fast inward sodium current in cardiac muscle, thereby prolonging the effective refractory period and reducing phase 4 depolarization. *Class II* drugs, the β-adrenergic blocking agents, reduce sympathetic stimulation of the heart and inhibit phase 4 depolarization, especially that augmented by catecholamines. *Class III* agents prolong the action potential and refractory period. Finally, *Class IV* drugs selectively block the slow calcium channel.

GENERAL CONCEPTS

An understanding of the pharmacology of antiarrhythmic drugs requires some knowledge of cardiac electrophysiology. Fig. 35-1 depicts a normal cardiac action potential from a Purkinje fiber. The resting cell membrane potential is approximately -90 mV, with the inside of the cell electronegative relative to the outside. This negative potential results primarily from a transmembrane potassium-ion gradient maintained by Na^+,K^+-ATPase. If the cell is adequately stimulated, there is rapid influx of sodium through specific membrane channels. This rapid depolarization (phase 0) of ventricular tissue corresponds to the QRS complex of the surface electrocardiogram. As sodium influx decreases, the cell membrane starts to repolarize (that is, becomes more negative), resulting in phase 1 of the action potential. In addition, a second inward current, arising primarily from movement of calcium, begins. This calcium influx maintains a depolarized state and is primarily responsible for phase 2 (the plateau) of the action potential. Finally, both inward sodium and calcium currents decline, and rapid repolarization (phase 3) occurs as a result of potassium efflux. In essence, the action potential is a coordinated sequence of ion movements; initially sodium rapidly enters the cell, followed by calcium influx and finally potassium efflux, which returns the cell to its resting state. Several antiarrhythmic drugs exert their effects by altering these ion fluxes.

CARDIAC ELECTRO-PHYSIOLOGY

FIG. 35-1   *Cardiac action potential as recorded from a Purkinje fiber and a ventricular fiber electrogram. Phases of the action potential are indicated by 0, 1, 2, 3, and 4. g, Transmembrane conductance of an ion.*

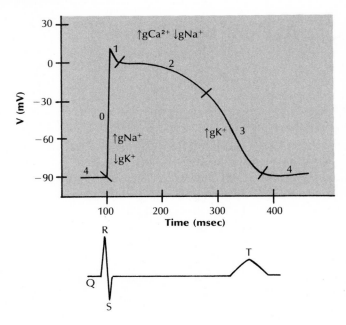

TABLE 35-1   Classification of antiarrhythmic drugs

Class I: blockade of fast sodium channel
   Quinidine-like: quinidine, procainamide, disopyramide
   Lidocaine-like: lidocaine, mexiletine, tocainide
   Flecainide-like: flecainide, encainide, lorcainide,* aprindine*
   Phenytoin

Class II: β-adrenergic antagonists

Class III: repolarization prolonging
   Bretylium, Amiodarone, *N*-acetylprocainamide

Class IV: calcium-channel blockade
   Verapamil

*Investigational drug.

ELECTRO-PHYSIOLOGIC BASIS OF ANTIARRHYTHMIC ACTION

Most tachyarrhythmias are consequences of two basic mechanisms:[17,24] ectopic focal activity and reentry. With ectopic focal activity a potential pacemaker fires independently because of an increase in the slope of diastolic depolarization, the threshold potential being more negative, or because of a decrease in the maximum diastolic potential.[22] Myocardial ischemia, excessive myocardial catecholamine release, stretching of the myocardium, and cardiac glycoside toxicity can be causal.

FIG. 35-2

Schema of reentry in the Purkinje system. Purkinje fiber (P) in the distal ventricular conducting system divides into two branches (a and b) before making contact with ventricular muscle (VM) to form a loop. Panel A shows the sequence of activation under normal conditions; the sinus impulse descends via the main Purkinje bundle leading to the loop, conducts through both branches (a and b) into ventricular muscle, collides, and terminates. Panel B shows the pattern of activation when an area of unidirectional conduction block is present (shaded area in branch b). Conduction is blocked in the antegrade direction in b but not in the retrograde direction (from VM to b). The impulse in limb a conducts slowly around the loop and returns to the site of antegrade block in limb b. Because of slowed conduction, this impulse arrives at the site of antegrade block in b after the refractory period has passed and is able to conduct in a retrograde manner. In panel C the impulse traveling retrogradely past the site of antegrade block into b conducts into P, activating the ventricle giving rise to a reciprocal beat. It may also continue the "circus" via limb a, producing repetitive reciprocal beats. The rate of this reciprocal beating will be determined by the total conduction time around the loop.

From Vera, Z., and Mason, D.T.: Am. Heart J. 101:329, 1981.

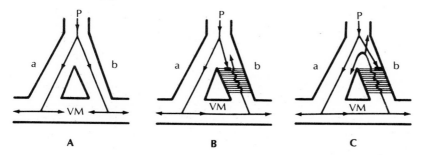

The conditions necessary for reentry to occur are as follows:[24] (1) the conduction pathway must be blocked, (2) there must be slow conduction over an alternate route to a point beyond the block, and (3) there must be delayed excitation beyond the block. With a sufficient delay in excitation beyond the block, the tissue proximal to the block can be excited from the opposite direction and a circular (reentry) circuit is then established. These principles are illustrated in Fig. 35-2.

The various classes of antiarrhythmic drugs have characteristic electrophysiologic effects on the myocardium, modified in some instances by extracardiac effects.

Class I antiarrhythmic drugs have local anesthetic properties. They block the fast inward sodium current and, by so doing, reduce the maximum rate of depolarization, increase the threshold of excitability, depress conduction velocity, prolong the effective refractory period, and reduce spontaneous diastolic depolarization in pacemaker cells. These effects of quinidine are shown in Fig. 35-3. The decrease in diastolic depolarization tends to suppress ectopic focal activity. Prolongation of the refractory period tends to abolish reentry. These drugs generally increase the duration of the action potential, but lidocaine, its derivatives, and phenytoin differ from other members of the class in shortening the action potential. Quinidine, procainamide, and disopyramide also have anticholinergic activity.

FIG. 35-3 *Diagram of the effect of quinidine on the transmembrane electrical potential of a spontaneously depolarizing conductive fiber in the ventricular myocardium.*

Modified from Mason, D.T., et al.: Clin. Pharmacol. Ther. 11:460, 1970.

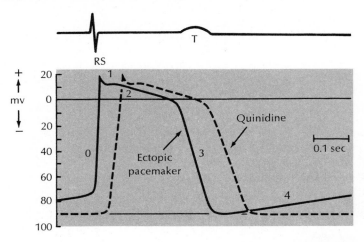

Class II antiarrhythmic drugs are the β-adrenergic receptor blocking agents such as propranolol. Their β-blocking effect is much more important than any local anesthetic activity they may have. Their mode of action is related to depression of the slope of spontaneous diastolic depolarization (phase 4).

Class III antiarrhythmic drugs appear to act by prolonging the action potential, an effect associated with prolongation of the effective refractory period.

Class IV antiarrhythmic drugs selectively block the slow inward current (slow response) carried primarily by calcium.[1,13] Verapamil reduces the action potential amplitude in the upper– and mid–AV nodal regions and prolongs the time-dependent recovery of excitability and the effective refractory period of AV nodal fibers. These effects block conduction of premature impulses in the AV node and thereby prevent the conduction delay necessary to allow AV nodal reentry and tachycardia. The ability of verapamil to prevent atrial arrhythmias may result from abolition of slow response activity in diseased atrial muscle or from suppression of propagation of the impulse through the AV node.

ANTIARRHYTHMIC
DRUGS
Quinidine

Quinidine is the dextrorotatory isomer of quinine.

Quinidine

The introduction of quinidine into therapeutics is one of the classical stories of medical history. In 1914 the Viennese cardiologist Wenckebach[26] had a Dutch sea captain as a patient. The captain had an irregular pulse as a consequence of atrial fibrillation. Wenckebach described the situation in this way:

> He did not feel great discomfort during the attack but, as he said, being a Dutch merchant, used to good order in his affairs, he would like to have good order in his heart business also and asked why there were heart specialists if they could not abolish this very disagreeable phenomenon. On my telling him that I could promise him nothing, he told me that he knew himself how to get rid of his attacks, and as I did not believe him he promised to come back the next morning with a regular pulse, and he did. It happens that quinine in many countries, especially in countries where there is a good deal of malaria, is a sort of drug for everything, just as one takes acetylsalicylic acid today if one does not feel well or is afraid of having taken cold. Occasionally, taking the drug during an attack of fibrillation, the patient found that the attack was stopped within from twenty to twenty-five minutes, and later he found that a gram of quinine regularly abolished his irregularity.*

In 1918 Frey[4] tested drugs related to quinine in patients with atrial fibrillation and introduced quinidine into cardiac therapy. During the succeeding years the antifibrillatory action of quinidine was confirmed, but its widespread use led to several sudden deaths. Eventually it was recognized that there are definite contraindications to the use of the drug. In the presence of conduction defects it may produce cardiac standstill and should be avoided. Once the mode of action of the drug was understood and contraindications to its use were recognized, quinidine reached its present position in cardiac therapy.

As a Class I antiarrhythmic drug quinidine is useful in both supraventricular and ventricular tachyarrhythmias. In many patients it can convert atrial tachyarrhythmias to normal sinus rhythm.

CARDIAC EFFECTS

A complicating factor in the action of quinidine is its "vagolytic" or anticholinergic effect. This effect tends to predominate at low plasma quinidine concentrations and may increase conduction velocity in the AV node. This may counteract its direct effect and explains the acceleration of heart rate that may be caused by the drug. The anticholinergic effect may also explain the paradoxical tachycardia seen in some patients during treatment of atrial flutter with block. At therapeutic plasma concentrations the direct electrophysiologic actions of quinidine predominate.

Electrocardiographic effects. Quinidine in higher doses prolongs the P-R, QRS, and Q-T intervals (Fig. 35-4). Widening of the QRS complex is related to slowed conduction in the His-Purkinje system and in the ventricular muscle. Changes in the Q-T interval and alterations in T waves are related to changes in repolarization. The direct effect of the drug on AV conduction and refractoriness of the AV system explains the prolongation of the P-R interval.

---

*From Beckman, H.: Treatment in general practice, ed. 2, Philadelphia, 1934, W.B. Saunders Co.

FIG. 35-4 *Effect of quinidine on electrocardiogram. Notice changes in P wave, QRS complex, and T wave at varying dose levels.*

From Burch, G.E., and Winsor, T.: A primer of electrocardiography, Philadelphia, 1960, Lea & Febiger.

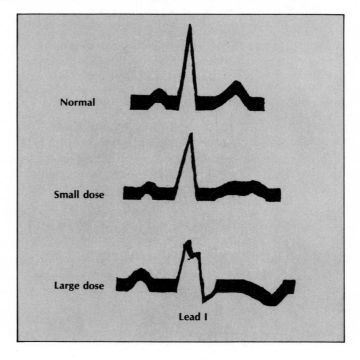

EXTRACARDIAC AND
ADVERSE EFFECTS

Quinidine tends to depress all muscle tissue, including vascular smooth muscle and skeletal muscle. When it is rapidly injected intravenously, sufficient vasodilatation can develop to cause profound hypotension and shock. Its effect on skeletal muscle becomes particularly evident in patients with myasthenia gravis, in whom it exacerbates weakness.

Cinchonism induced by quinidine is characterized by ringing of the ears and dizziness and is the same syndrome produced by quinine or salicylates. Quinidine commonly causes adverse gastrointestinal effects, particularly diarrhea, which is probably the most common reason patients cannot tolerate the drug.

Quinidine-induced thrombocytopenia appears to occur on an immune basis. In a typical case, a patient taking quinidine for several weeks notices the development of petechial hemorrhages in the buccal mucous membranes. The symptoms disappear when the drug is discontinued and reappear after reinstitution of therapy. This disorder is believed to be caused by formation of a plasma protein-quinidine complex that evokes a circulating antibody; platelet destruction is the result.[6]

Quinidine may cause ventricular arrhythmias and even ventricular fibrillation. So-called quinidine syncope is probably a consequence of the latter.[25] It may seem paradoxical that an antiarrhythmic drug can cause ventricular arrhythmias. Since quinidine depresses automaticity, ventricular arrhythmias from quinidine are probably caused by reentry mechanisms rather than by increased automaticity.

CARDIOTOXICITY

Quinidine is particularly dangerous in patients with conduction defects. In such patients, when conduction is further impaired and automaticity of the Purkinje system is depressed, the ventricles may not take over when AV conduction fails and so cardiac standstill ensues. The administration of the drug should be stopped when significant QRS widening or Q-T prolongation supervene during treatment.

When given orally, quinidine sulfate is rapidly absorbed, with peak levels in about 1.5 hours. In contrast, quinidine gluconate is absorbed more slowly, with peak levels about 4 hours after a dose.[5] The more prolonged absorption of the gluconate results in lower peak concentrations but allows it to be administered less frequently than the sulfate.

PHARMACOKINETICS

About 10% to 50% of administered quinidine is excreted unchanged in the urine. The amount is influenced by the pH of the urine, though at physiologic ranges of urinary pH this effect is unlikely to be clinically important. The rest is hydroxylated in the liver. Drug interactions with quinidine are discussed in Chapter 63.

The usual initial adult dosage of quinidine is 600 to 900 mg daily. The actual dose and dosage interval vary depending on the formulation, the effects of disease, and individual variations in kinetics. Optimum therapy requires monitoring of serum concentrations.

ADMINISTRATION AND DOSAGE

Quinidine gluconate is available for intramuscular injection. Intravenous administration can be dangerous. If given by this route, the infusion should be very slow and careful monitoring must be employed. Additional information on the pharmacokinetics and preparations of antiarrhythmic drugs is given in Table 35-2.

The commonly used local anesthetic procaine was shown by Mautz[12] in 1936 to elevate the threshold to electrical stimulation when applied to the myocardium of animals. In subsequent years thoracic surgeons and anesthesiologists frequently used topical procaine to reduce premature ventricular and atrial contractions during surgery. Procaine was even administered intravenously for this purpose.

Procainamide
DEVELOPMENT AS CARDIAC DRUG

Procaine   Procainamide

TABLE 35-2 Pharmacokinetics and preparations of antiarrhythmic drugs

Drug	Half-life (hours)	Therapeutic plasma concentration (μg/ml)	Dosage forms* (mg)
Quinidine sulfate (Cin-Quin, Quinora, Quinidex)	4-6	2-5	T: 100-300; I: 200/ml
Quinidine gluconate (Quinaglute, Duraquin, others)			T: 324, 330; I: 80/ml
Quinidine polygalacturonate (Cardioquin)			T: 275
Procainamide hydrochloride (Pronestyl, Procan, Promine)	2.5-4.5	4-10	T: 250-1000; I: 100, 500/ml
Disopyramide phosphate (Norpace)	4-5	2-5	C: 100, 150
Lidocaine hydrochloride (Xylocaine)	1.5-2	1.5-5	I: 2-8/ml†, 10-200/ml
Mexiletine hydrochloride (Mexitil)	11	0.8-2	C: 150-250
Tocainide hydrochloride (Tonocard)	14	3-10	T: 400, 600
Flecainide acetate (Tambocor)	15	0.2-1	T: 100
Encainide hydrochloride (Enkaid)	2-3		T: 25-50
Phenytoin (Dilantin)	18-24	10-20	C: 30, 100; I: 50/ml; S: 30, 125/5 ml; T: 50
Bretylium tosylate (Bretylol)	5-10		I: 50/ml
Amiodarone hydrochloride (Cordarone)	100 days	1-2.5	T: 200
Verapamil hydrochloride (Calan, Isoptin)	3-7		T: 80, 120; I: 2.5/ml

*C, Capsules; I, injection; S, suspension; T, tablets.
†For infusion.

Encouraged by these studies, investigators studied the antifibrillatory activities of compounds related to procaine, including the two hydrolysis products *p*-aminobenzoic acid and diethylaminoethanol. The most fruitful consequence was the finding that if the ester linkage in procaine was replaced by an amide linkage, the resulting compound had distinct advantages as an antiarrhythmic drug, that is, greater stability in the body and fewer central nervous system effects.

CARDIAC EFFECTS   Procainamide is so similar in its actions to quinidine that the two drugs can be used interchangeably. Quinidine is preferred by some physicians for prolonged oral use because procainamide can cause a lupus erythematosus–like syndrome characterized by rheumatic symptoms, pleuropericardial inflammation, and antinuclear antibodies.[3] On the other hand, procainamide is safer than quinidine when used intravenously and has fewer gastrointestinal side effects.

Procainamide is absorbed well from the gastrointestinal tract and is 15% protein bound. It is metabolized in the liver to *N*-acetylprocainamide (NAPA), which has a different type of antiarrhythmic activity (Table 35-1) but does not appear to induce lupus erythematosus.[9] The rate of acetylation is genetically determined, and patients may be fast or slow acetylators. It has been demonstrated that genetically slow acetylators of procainamide have an earlier onset of and a higher prevalence of drug-induced lupus compared to rapid acetylators.[28] Renal disease decreases the clearance of procainamide to some degree but has a major effect on NAPA, which is predominately eliminated by the kidney. Regular and sustained-release preparations of procainamide are available.

PHARMACOKINETICS

Large intravenous doses of procainamide may decrease blood pressure. This is probably a consequence of vascular smooth muscle relaxation and depressed myocardial contractility. Although the drug has local anesthetic properties, it is not useful for nerve block.

EXTRACARDIAC EFFECTS AND TOXICITY

Nausea, anorexia, mental confusion, hallucinations, skin rashes, agranulocytosis, chills, and fever have been reported after the use of procainamide, in addition to the lupus-like syndrome.

Disopyramide is a Class I antiarrhythmic drug that resembles quinidine and procainamide in its action. However, this drug has considerable anticholinergic activity, which limits its use. Disopyramide is absorbed well from the gastrointestinal tract. Renal impairment decreases its clearance.

Disopyramide

Disopyramide may cause or worsen congestive heart failure or produce severe hypotension as a consequence of its negative inotropic properties. This is most likely to occur in patients with marginally compensated underlying cardiac failure.[16] Because of its anticholinergic action disopyramide should not be given to patients with glaucoma, myasthenia gravis, or urinary retention. Disopyramide is administered every 6 hours to patients with normal renal function.

Disopyramide

Lidocaine is a Class I antiarrhythmic drug that has become the most widely used agent for treatment and prevention of ventricular ectopic activity associated with myocardial infarction. Lidocaine and its derivatives differ in important aspects from most other members of the Class I antiarrhythmic drugs. Although it depresses

Lidocaine

automaticity and diastolic depolarization, lidocaine does not slow conduction and has little effect on atrial function. It does not prolong the action potential or refractory period. Lidocaine must be injected intravenously or intramuscularly because when given orally the first-pass effect is so extensive that therapeutic systemic concentrations are not attained.

PHARMACOKINETICS

The distribution half-life of lidocaine is about 10 minutes. Its elimination half-life is 1.5 to 2 hours. The volume of distribution is about 500 ml/kg, and its clearance is 10 ml/kg/min. Clearance of lidocaine is reduced in patients with chronic liver disease or congestive heart failure (because of decreased hepatic blood flow), and dosage must be reduced to prevent toxicity.

Lidocaine is given as a loading dose (1 mg/kg) followed by a continuous infusion (1 to 4 mg/min). There is significant variability among patients in the plasma concentration resulting from a given dose.[29] In many instances this variation can be accounted for by changes in α_1-acid glycoprotein (AAG), the plasma protein to which lidocaine binds.[21] For example, the AAG concentration rises after myocardial infarction, increasing total plasma lidocaine concentration while the free (non–protein bound) fraction remains unchanged. Rapid, clinically useful methods for measuring free (and presumably active) lidocaine concentration are needed to monitor therapy most effectively.

Adverse effects of lidocaine include agitation, drowsiness, convulsions, and coma. Very large doses have adverse effects on the heart, manifested by depression of AV conduction and a negative inotropic effect.

An intravenous loading dose of 50 to 100 mg of lidocaine hydrochloride is recommended, given over a period of 2 to 5 minutes. The dose may be repeated after 5 minutes, not to exceed 300 mg/hour.

Mexiletine

Mexiletine is very similar to lidocaine in its electrophysiologic effects, chemical structure, and clinical spectrum of antiarrhythmic actions.[14,15] It differs from lidocaine in its suitability for oral administration and its pharmacokinetics and side effects. Unlike lidocaine, mexiletine has high systemic availability after ingestion. Peak plasma concentration is obtained 2 to 4 hours after the dose is taken, and the drug is eliminated by hepatic metabolism.

Mexiletine has minimal hemodynamic effects and only a mild negative inotropic action. However, its myocardial depressant action can be more pronounced in patients with poorly compensated congestive heart failure. The major therapeutic indication for mexiletine is in long-term treatment of ventricular arrhythmias, particularly those associated with previous myocardial infarction.

The major adverse effects of mexiletine are neurologic and include tremors, nystagmus, diplopia, ataxia, and confusion. Nausea and vomiting may also occur; the incidence of these diminishes when the medication is taken with food. The usual dose of mexiletine is 600 to 1000 mg every 8 to 12 hours.

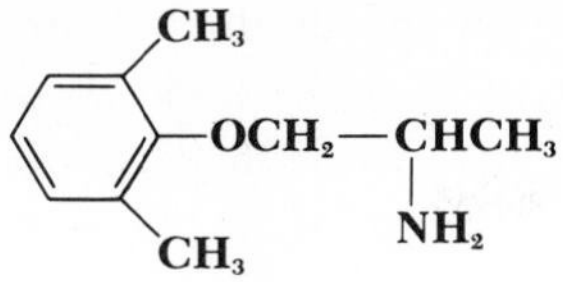

Mexiletine 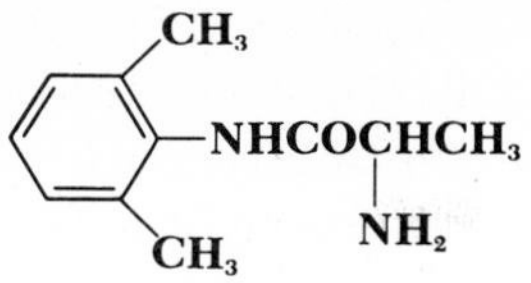   Tocainide

Tocainide

Tocainide is another lidocaine congener, similar to mexiletine in its electrophysiologic properties and antiarrhythmic action.[14,20] Tocainide is active after oral ingestion, with peak serum concentrations occurring within 60 to 90 minutes. Effective plasma concentrations can usually be achieved with a total oral daily dose between 400 and 1200 mg of the hydrochloride given in two or three divided doses. The major clinical indication for tocainide is in treatment of ventricular tachyarrhythmias.[27] Tocainide can produce the same neurologic and gastrointestinal side effects as mexiletine.

Flecainide

Flecainide is representative of a newer group of type I antiarrhythmic drugs, which also includes encainide and lorcainide.[7,19] These drugs are characterized by a lack of effect on the duration of the action potential. They are effective in patients with ventricular tachyarrhythmias and are being used predominately in those in whom other drugs have failed or were poorly tolerated. Their use has not (and probably will not) become more widespread because of their proarrhythmic actions; they can also cause ventricular tachyarrhythmias. Whether this tendency is greater than that of traditional Class I drugs like quinidine and procainamide is not clear. Other side effects include dizziness, visual disturbances, headache, and nausea.

Flecainide has a bioavailability of 90% to 95%. Approximately 40% of a dose is eliminated in the urine, and the dose must be reduced in patients with renal insufficiency. It can be administered twice a day. At therapeutic concentrations, P-R intervals and QRS durations are increased approximately 25%.

Flecainide is available for oral or intravenous administration. In emergent settings, 1 to 2 mg/kg can be given by slow intravenous injection. Oral dosing usually begins at 100 mg twice daily with average daily maintenance doses from 200 to 600 mg.

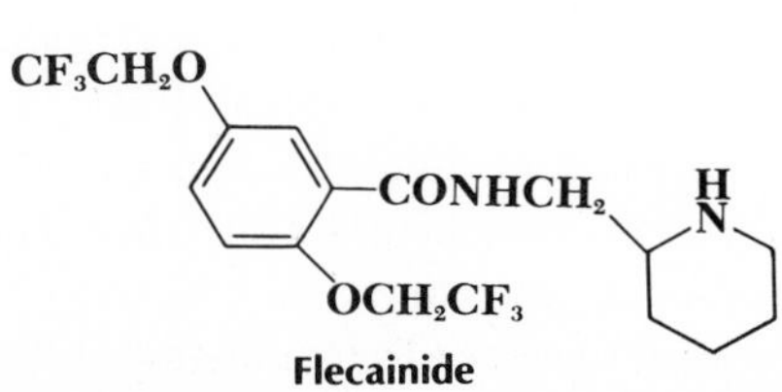

Flecainide 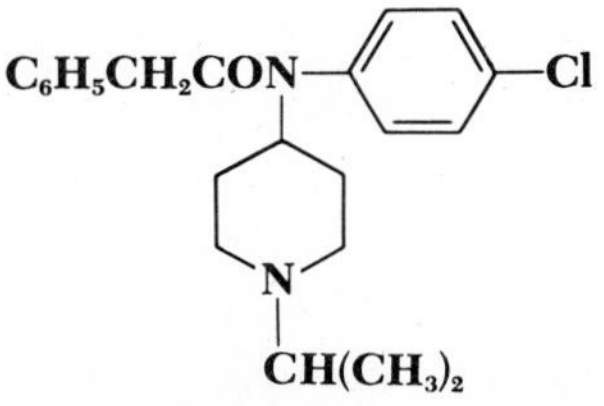   Lorcainide

Encainide

Encainide appears similar pharmacologically to flecainide. Of interest, however, is that much of the activity of encainide is attributable to the *O*-desmethyl metabolite, the formation of which is genetically controlled.[18] As with flecainide, therapeutic doses of encainide prolong P-R intervals and QRS durations (40% or more).

Lorcainide

Lorcainide is also similar to flecainide pharmacologically. Interestingly, it appears to cause a syndrome of inappropriate secretion of antidiuretic hormone, which results in hyponatremia in some patients.[23] The mechanism is unknown.

Aprindine

Aprindine (Fibocil) is a powerful Class I antiarrhythmic drug that may reverse both supraventricular and ventricular arrhythmias. It is orally active and has a very long half-life but may cause neurologic side effects in a small percentage of patients.[14]

$$N-(CH_2)_3N(C_2H_5)_2$$
$$C_6H_5$$

Aprindine

Phenytoin

The antiepileptic drug phenytoin was found in 1950 to decrease ventricular arrhythmias after coronary ligation in dogs. More recently it has also been used as an antiarrhythmic drug, especially in digitalis-induced tachyarrhythmias, which may be its only indication.

Phenytoin depresses automaticity in ventricular and atrial tissues and may actually improve AV conduction. Generally it is not a useful antiarrhythmic drug, and even in digitalis toxicity lidocaine is usually preferred.

PHARMACOKINETICS

Phenytoin is absorbed slowly when given by mouth, and peak concentrations are not obtained for several hours. The drug should not be given intramuscularly, since its absorption is erratic.[25] It is parahydroxylated by liver microsomal enzymes. The disappearance of phenytoin does not follow first-order kinetics because of saturation of the microsomal enzymes at therapeutic serum concentrations. With this reservation, it is useful to know that within the usual therapeutically effective range serum concentrations fall by one half in 18 to 24 hours.

DOSAGE

To obtain a prompt effect, one may administer phenytoin as an oral or intravenous loading dose of 1 g the first day, usually in three or four divided doses spread several hours apart, after which a maintenance oral dose of 300 to 400 mg per day is appropriate, guided by measurement of serum concentration.

Intravenous phenytoin should be given by infusion only to severely ill patients. The infusion rate should be 25 to 50 mg/min. A total dose of 500 mg to 1 g should not be exceeded.

Propranolol and other β-receptor antagonists exert their antiarrhythmic activity by blocking β-adrenergic receptors. The membrane-stabilizing effect of propranolol and some of the other β-blockers is not clinically important because plasma concentrations are not high enough to achieve this effect.

β-Adrenergic receptor antagonists

β-Blockers depress automaticity, prolong AV conduction, reduce heart rate (unless they have intrinsic sympathomimetic activity), and also decrease contractility. These drugs are primarily effective in treatment of tachyarrhythmias caused by increased sympathetic activity. They prevent the reflex tachycardia caused by vasodilator antihypertensive drugs. As with digitalis they slow ventricular rate in atrial flutter and fibrillation. They have been used in digitalis toxicity, but lidocaine and phenytoin are preferred.

Adverse effects of β-blockers include bronchospasm and arteriolar vasoconstriction (less prevalent with cardioselective agents and those with intrinsic sympathomimetic activity) and congestive heart failure. Sudden withdrawal of β-blockers may lead to a recurrence of angina and even sudden death.

Available preparations of β-blockers are listed in Table 16-2, and specific information on dosage is given in Chapter 18. With their administration, patients should be monitored for myocardial depression and bradycardia. Atropine or isoproterenol will reverse the latter. One should remember that relatively large doses of isoproterenol by intravenous infusion may be needed to counteract the bradycardia, since the β-receptors are blocked.

Dosage

Bretylium is an adrenergic neuronal blocking drug that was originally developed as an antihypertensive agent. Troublesome side effects made it useless as an antihypertensive drug, but its antiarrhythmic properties brought it back into clinical use.

Bretylium tosylate

Bretylium prolongs the action potential and the effective refractory period simultaneously. The drug is used to treat severe ventricular tachyarrhythmias that are unresponsive to other drugs. Even after intravenous injection, its effect may be delayed for several minutes or even hours. Initially, the drug causes norepinephrine release and an increase in blood pressure. This is followed by a fall in pressure. In addition to these changes in blood pressure, adverse effects of bretylium include nausea, bradycardia, angina, diarrhea, and skin rash.

Bretylium, a quaternary ammonium compound, is eliminated unchanged by the kidney. It is administered intramuscularly or by slow intravenous infusion.

Bretylium tosylate

Amiodarone   Amiodarone is a Class III antiarrhythmic agent useful for both supraventricular and ventricular tachyarrhythmias. Despite its proved efficacy, because of its extremely prolonged action and its profile of adverse effects, it has been reserved for patients refractory to other modes of therapy.[10] As many as 90% of patients receiving amiodarone will develop side effects. Photosensitivity is frequent. Some patients develop a gray skin discoloration ("gray man syndrome"). Most patients develop corneal microdeposits during prolonged therapy. Thyroid disorders, either hyperthyroidism or hypothyroidism, are related by unknown mechanisms to the iodine contained in the drug (0.375 µg of organic iodine per milligram of drug). Other toxicities include neuropathies, pulmonary fibrosis, and hepatotoxicity.

Bioavailability of amiodarone shows great variability, ranging from 22% to 86%. The drug is eliminated by metabolism with negligible amounts excreted by the kidney. Amiodarone can inhibit the metabolism of other drugs, such as oral anticoagulants. Its half-life, as long as 100 days, makes dosing difficult. Most authorities agree on an average daily maintenance dose of 400 mg alternating with 600 mg. However, various loading regimens have been promulgated, the simplest of which may be 1200 mg daily for approximately 2 weeks.

Amiodarone

Verapamil   Verapamil is a *papaverine* derivative that is of value in certain atrial tachyarrhythmias and also in management of angina pectoris[1] (see Chapter 36). The drug is the first of a new type of antiarrhythmic agent. Verapamil inhibits transmembrane fluxes of calcium.[22] Verapamil suppresses firing of the sinoatrial (SA) node, prolongs AV refractoriness, and depresses the potential of latent pacemaker cells. It also produces vasodilatation.

Intravenous verapamil is effective in converting reentrant paroxysmal supraventricular tachycardia (PSVT) to normal sinus rhythm.[13] Long-term oral therapy with verapamil decreases the frequency and duration of PSVT and the severity of symptoms.[11] Because of its ability to slow AV conduction and hence ventricular responses, verapamil is also useful for patients with atrial fibrillation. The slower heart rate is maintained with exercise (in contrast to use of cardiac glycosides for this same purpose), and many patients experience subjective improvement as manifested by increased effort tolerance and decreased palpitations during exertion.[8]

There are certain principles that should be remembered before one selects a drug for the treatment of a cardiac arrhythmia: (1) many arrhythmias do not require drug treatment; (2) most antiarrhythmic drugs can be dangerous; (3) cardioversion (DC countershock) has lessened many of the indications for use of antiarrhythmic medications.

With these limitations, the use of antiarrhythmic drugs in various arrhythmias are briefly summarized below.

SELECTION OF
DRUGS

Paroxysmal atrial tachycardia can occur in otherwise normal persons. Spontaneous termination, but with recurrences, is common. It may also be a manifestation of digitalis toxicity.

Vagal maneuvers, such as carotid massage or administration of the anticholinesterase drugs edrophonium and neostigmine, can be used to end attacks. Vasoconstrictors, such as methoxamine or phenylephrine, may terminate an attack by eliciting reflex vagal activity as a consequence of blood pressure elevation. However, verapamil has become the agent of choice for most supraventricular tachyarrhythmias and successfully converts at least 90% to normal sinus rhythm. Hence previous strategies are for the most part of historic interest.

Digitalis can also be effective and is commonly used in atrial tachycardias in children. β-Blockers, usually propranolol, may be of benefit.

Supraventricular
arrhythmias
PAROXYSMAL ATRIAL
TACHYCARDIA

Digitalis is the most important drug in treatment of atrial flutter. It acts primarily by increasing the degree of AV block, thereby decreasing ventricular rate. As for the flutter itself, digitalis tends to convert it to fibrillation by shortening the refractory period in the atrial muscle. Occasionally quinidine is used for conversion of flutter to normal sinus rhythm. In this case digitalis should be employed first to prevent excessive tachycardia, a consequence of the vagolytic action of quinidine. When quinidine is added to digoxin treatment, the plasma concentration of the glycoside doubles and thereby may rise to dangerous levels.[2] If digitalis is not effective, the addition of a β-blocker may be helpful. Cardioversion finds increasing usefulness in the treatment of flutter.

Intravenous verapamil converts atrial flutter to normal sinus rhythm in about 30% of cases.[13] As with digitalis, verapamil often converts flutter to atrial fibrillation, which, in turn, may convert to sinus rhythm.

ATRIAL FLUTTER

Digitalis is also the most important drug in management of atrial fibrillation. It does not convert atrial fibrillation to normal sinus rhythm, but it slows ventricular rate, and it treats cardiac failure. Quinidine can convert atrial fibrillation to normal sinus rhythm. Cardioversion can also be employed. Even when DC countershock is employed, chronic therapy with quinidine may be helpful in preventing the recurrence of atrial fibrillation. Administration of quinidine is often started before car-

ATRIAL FIBRILLATION

dioversion, and it may terminate the fibrillation by itself. Disopyramide may be used in the same manner.

Verapamil can also be used in atrial fibrillation because of its ability to slow ventricular response by blocking AV conduction. It has the advantage of controlling the ventricular response during exercise, a setting in which cardiac glycosides often fail.

Ventricular arrhythmias	Occasional premature ventricular contractions generally do not require drug treatment. On the other hand, ventricular tachycardia may be a serious condition that requires intensive treatment. Although DC countershock is commonly used for stopping ventricular tachycardia, it should not be employed if the arrhythmia is caused by digitalis.

For acute treatment of ventricular tachyarrhythmias, lidocaine is the drug of choice, but procainamide may also be tried. For chronic treatment, quinidine, procainamide, or disopyramide are suitable. If they fail or toxicity supervenes, mexiletine or tocainide may be effective. If these drugs also fail, flecainide and finally amiodarone may be beneficial. Lastly, combinations may be successfully used. Guiding the choice of antiarrhythmic agent by electrophysiologic testing is often helpful in difficult cases.

Digitalis-induced arrhythmias may be treated with lidocaine, phenytoin, or β-blockers. Antibody fractions to digitalis have also recently become available (see Chapter 34). |

REFERENCES

1. Antman, E.M., Stone, P.H., Muller, J.E., and Braunwald, E.: Calcium channel blocking agents in the treatment of cardiovascular disorders: Part I, Basic and clinical electrophysiologic effects, Ann. Intern. Med. **93**:875, 1980.

2. Bigger, J.T., Jr., and Leahey, E.B., Jr.: Quinidine and digoxin: an important interaction, Drugs **24**:229, 1982.

3. Blomgren, S.E., Condemi, J.J., and Vaughan, J.H.: Procainamide-induced lupus erythematosus: clinical and laboratory observations, Am. J. Med. **52**:338, 1972.

4. Frey, W.: Weitere Erfahrungen mit Chinidin bei absoluter Herzunregelmässigkeit, Klin. Wochenschr. **55**:849, 1918.

5. Greenblatt, D.J., Pfeifer, H.J., Oches, H.R., et al.: Pharmacokinetics of quinidine in humans after intravenous, intramuscular and oral administration, J. Pharmacol. Exp. Ther. **202**:365, 1977.

6. Hackett, T., Kelton, J.G., and Powers, P.: Drug-induced platelet destruction, Semin. Thromb. Hemostas. **8**:116, 1982.

7. Holmes, B., and Heel, R.C.: Flecainide: a preliminary review of its pharmacodynamic properties and therapeutic efficacy, Drugs **29**:1-33, 1985.

8. Klein, H.O., Pauzner, H., Di Segni, E., et al.: The beneficial effects of verapamil on chronic atrial fibrillation, Arch. Intern. Med. **139**:747, 1979.

9. Kluger, J., Drayer, D.E., Reidenberg, M.M., and Lahita, R.: Acetylprocainamide therapy in patients with previous procainamide-induced lupus syndrome, Ann. Intern. Med. **95**:18, 1981.

10. Latini, R., Tognoni, G., and Kates, R.E.: Clinical pharmacokinetics of amiodarone, Clin. Pharmacokinet. **9**:136, 1984.

11. Mauritson, D.R., Winniford, M.D., Walker, W.S., et al.: Oral verapamil for paroxysmal supraventricular tachycardia: a long-term, double-blind randomized trial, Ann. Intern. Med. **96**:409, 1982.

12. Mautz, F.R.: Reduction of cardiac irritability by the epicardial and systemic administration of drugs as a protection in cardiac surgery, J. Thorac. Surg. **5**:612, 1936.

13. McGoon, M.D., Vlietstra, R.E., Holmes, D.R., Jr. and Osborn, J.E.: The clinical use of verapamil, Mayo Clin. Proc. **57**:495, 1982.

14. Nademanee, K., and Singh, B.N.: Advances in antiarrhythmic therapy: the role of newer antiarrhythmic drugs, J.A.M.A. **247**:217, 1982.

15. Podrid, P.J., and Lown, B.: Mexiletine for ventricular arrhythmias, Am. J. Cardiol. **47**:895, 1981.

16. Podrid, P.J., Schoeneberger, A., and Lown, B.: Congestive heart failure caused by oral disopyramide, N. Engl. J. Med. **302**:614, 1980.

17. Reder, R.F., and Rosen, M.R.: Mechanisms of cardiac arrhythmias, Cardiovasc. Rev. Rep. **2**:1007, 1981.

18. Roden, D.M., Reele, S.B., Higgins, S.B., et al.: Total suppression of ventricular arrhythmias by encainide: pharmacokinetic and electrocardiographic characteristics, N. Engl. J. Med. **302**:877, 1980.

19. Roden, D.M., and Woosley, R.L.: Flecainide, N. Engl. J. Med. **315**:36, 1986.

20. Roden, D.M., and Woosley, R.L.: Tocainide, N. Engl. J. Med. **315**:41, 1986.

21. Routledge, P.A., Stargel, W.W., Wagner, G.S., and Shand, D.G.: Increased alpha-1-acid glycoprotein and lidocaine disposition in myocardial infarction, Ann. Intern. Med. **93**:701, 1980.

22. Singh, B.N., Collett, J.T., and Chew, C.Y.C.: New perspectives in the pharmacologic therapy of cardiac arrhythmias, Prog. Cardiovasc. Dis. **22**:243, 1980.

23. Somani, P., Temesy-Armos, P.N., Leighton, R.F., et al.: Hyponatremia in patients treated with lorcainide, a new antiarrhythmic drug, Am. Heart J. **108**: 1443, 1984.

24. Vera, Z., and Mason, D.T.: Reentry versus automaticity: role of tachyarrhythmia genesis and antiarrhythmic therapy, Am. Heart J. **101**:329, 1981.

25. Wasserman, A.J., and Proctor, J.D.: Pharmacology of antiarrhythmics: quinidine, beta-blockers, diphenylhydantoin, bretylium, Med. Coll. Va. Q. **9**:53, 1973.

26. Wenckebach, K.F.: Die unregelmässige Herztätigkeit und ihre klinische Bedeutung, Leipzig, 1914, W. Englemann.

27. Winkle, R.A., Mason, J.W., and Harrison, D.C.: Tocainide for drug-resistant ventricular arrhythmias: efficacy, side effects, and lidocaine responsiveness for predicting tocainide success, Am. Heart J. **100**:1031, 1980.

28. Woosley, R.L., Drayer, D.E., Reidenberg, M.M., et al.: Effect of acetylator phenotype on the rate at which procainamide induces antinuclear antibodies and the lupus syndrome, N. Engl. J. Med. **298**:1157, 1978.

29. Zito, R.A., Reid, P.R., and Longstreth, J.A.: Variability of early lidocaine levels in patients, Am. Heart J. **94**:292, 1977.

Chapter 36

Antianginal drugs

GENERAL CONCEPT   It is an old empiric observation that amyl nitrite (1867) and nitroglycerin (1879) relieve the pain of angina pectoris. Since nitrates and nitrites dilate blood vessels, including the coronary arteries, the role of coronary vasodilatation in relief of angina has been generally assumed.

The problem is much more complex, however. Angina results from an imbalance between oxygen demand and supply in ischemic regions of the myocardium. Drugs may improve angina theoretically by reducing the demand for or by increasing the supply of oxygen. There is increasing evidence that nitrates reduce demand by a peripheral action to cause venodilatation, thereby decreasing cardiac preload and reducing myocardial wall tension, a major determinant of oxygen demand.[1] In addition to its use in angina pectoris, this same effect of nitrates has been of benefit in management of some patients with congestive heart failure. The use of nitrates has expanded because of recent availability of intravenous formulations and longer acting oral and topical preparations.

β-Adrenergic receptor blocking agents, such as propranolol, are also used extensively in treatment of angina. Drugs of this class illustrate the importance of reduction of cardiac work in relief of angina.[5]

Calcium-channel blocking drugs, such as verapamil, nifedipine, and diltiazem, are also effective antianginal agents. They dilate coronary arteries and are particularly useful in patients with Prinzmetal's variant angina resulting from coronary artery spasm. It has become increasingly evident that coronary spasm is an important component of unstable angina, acute myocardial infarction, and even stable, effort-induced angina.[2,3,7] Calcium antagonists can therefore be of benefit in most myocardial ischemia syndromes. The effectiveness of these agents in exercise-induced angina is probably also a consequence of systemic vasodilatation, which reduces cardiac afterload and thereby myocardial oxygen requirement.

NITRATES AND NITRITES
Chemistry   The effects of nitrates, calcium blockers, and β-blockers on myocardial oxygen requirements and oxygen supply are shown in Table 36-1. The clinically useful nitrates and nitrites cause qualitatively similar effects. The most interesting compounds in the group and their formulas are as follows:

Nitrates

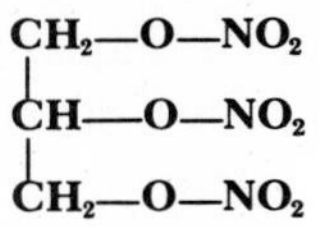

CH₂—O—NO₂
CH—O—NO₂
CH₂—O—NO₂

Nitroglycerin

$$CH_2-O-NO_2$$
$$O_2N-O-CH_2-C-CH_2-O-NO_2$$
$$CH_2-O-NO_2$$

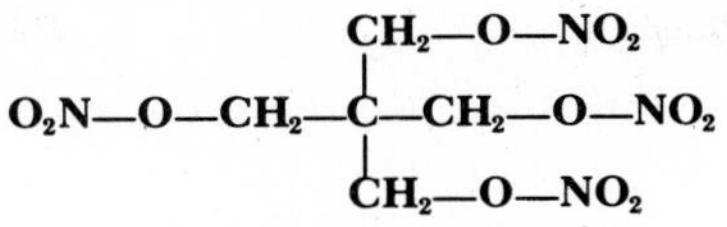

Pentaerythritol tetranitrate

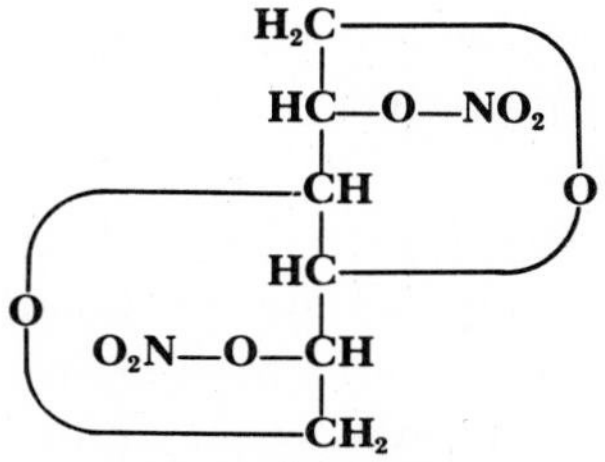

Isosorbide dinitrate

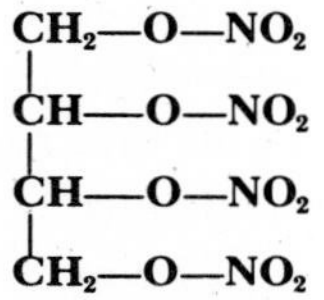

CH₂—O—NO₂
CH—O—NO₂
CH—O—NO₂
CH₂—O—NO₂

Erythrityl tetranitrate

Nitrites

NaNO₂

Sodium nitrite

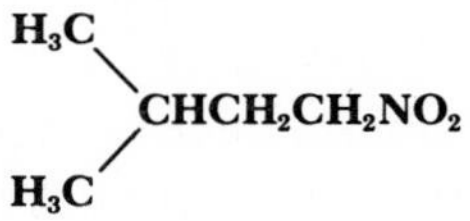

H₃C
⟩CHCH₂CH₂NO₂
H₃C

Amyl nitrite

TABLE 36-1 Effects of nitrates, calcium blockers, and β-blockers on myocardial oxygen requirements and supply

	Nitrates	Calcium blockers			β-blockers
		NF	DZ	VP	
Determinants of myocardial oxygen requirements					
Heart rate	↑	↑	↓ —	↓ —	↓ *
Left ventricular pressure	↓	↓	↓ —	↓	↓ *
Left ventricular volume/radius	↓ *	↓	↓	↑ —	↑
Velocity of contraction	↑	↑	—	↓	↓
Systolic ejection period	↓	↓	↑ —	—	↑
Determinants of myocardial oxygen supply					
Coronary vasodilatation	↑ *	↑ *	↑ *	↑ *	↓
Aortic diastolic pressure	↓	↓	↓	↓	↓
Diastolic perfusion time	↓	↓	↑	↑	↑

*Most significant effects.
—, No change; *NF*, nifedipine; *DZ*, diltiazem; *VP*, verapamil.

Effects of
nitroglycerin

If a patient suffering from an attack of angina pectoris places a tablet of nitroglycerin (glyceryl trinitrate) under the tongue, the attack frequently subsides in a matter of minutes. Furthermore, the drug is often effective if taken prophylactically before performance of a task that ordinarily induces angina.

This is not a placebo effect. If a patient with stable angina performs an exercise tolerance test, precordial pain and T-wave inversion on the electrocardiogram will develop as a consequence of myocardial ischemia. After receiving prophylactic nitroglycerin, the same patient is often protected against both pain and the electrocardiographic alterations during exercise.

The simplest interpretation of this effect of nitroglycerin would be that it improves blood flow to ischemic regions in the myocardium by dilating coronary vessels. However, the antianginal effect of nitroglycerin is now believed to result primarily from reduction of venous tone with diminished venous return, decreased cardiac preload, decreased myocardial wall tension, and subsequently decreased oxygen demand.[1] In addition, some benefit is derived from peripheral arterial dilatation and from dilatation of coronary arteries. All nitrate esters produce the same effects as nitroglycerin.

In addition to coronary vessels, other vascular areas are susceptible to the action of nitrates. Cutaneous vessels of the face and neck, the so-called blush area, may be greatly dilated. Meningeal vessels are dilated also, and this dilatation is the likely cause of the headache that may be produced by nitrates.

Effects of nitrates
on other smooth
muscles

Probably all smooth muscles can be made to relax by nitrates, with some minor therapeutic applications of this effect. Sublingual nitroglycerin can decrease biliary pressure. The nitrates can also relax the ureter and the lower esophageal sphincter. Occasionally, relief of pain by nitrates is assumed to indicate a myocardial ischemic cause when, in fact, the salutary effect has occurred elsewhere. Although nitrates relax bronchial smooth muscle, more effective medications are available for this purpose. The action of nitrates on smooth muscle involves a nitrosothiol intermediate formed within the smooth muscle itself by the reaction of the nitrate with glutathione. This intermediate, in turn, increases cyclic guanine nucleotides, which cause smooth muscle relaxation. Tolerance to nitrates occurs when glutathione becomes depleted, precluding the formation of the intermediate.

Nitrites

Amyl nitrite is a volatile liquid available in small glass pearls containing 0.2 ml. These are crushed in a handkerchief by the patient, and the vapor is inhaled. Amyl nitrite has a short onset of action (less than 1 minute), but its duration of action is also short (not exceeding 10 minutes). It is particularly prone to cause cutaneous vasodilatation, pronounced lowering of systemic pressure, and even syncope and tachycardia. In addition, its odor is objectionable. Thus nitroglycerin is preferred.

Sodium nitrite has more toxicologic than therapeutic importance. Although its effects on smooth muscle are similar to those of other nitrites, its irritant action on the gastric mucosa and its tendency to produce methemoglobin make it unsuitable as a coronary vasodilator.

TABLE 36-2   Long-acting nitrates: recommended dosage and duration of action

Drug	Dosage	Duration of action (hr)
Oral nitroglycerin	6.5-19.5 mg every 4-6 hr*	4-6
2% nitroglycerin ointment	½-2 in (1.3-5 cm; 7.5-30 mg) every 4-6 hr	3-6
Isosorbide dinitrate		
Sublingual	2.5-10 mg every 2-4 hr	1.5-3†
Oral	10-60 mg every 4-6 hr*	4-6
Chewable	5-10 mg every 2-4 hr	2-3
Oral pentaerythritol tetranitrate	40-80 mg every 4-6 hr*	3-5
Patch preparations	1-2 patches every 24 hr	24

Modified from Abrams, J.: N. Engl. J. Med. **302**:1234, 1980. Reprinted by permission of the New England Journal of Medicine.
*Large doses, often greater than manufacturers recommend, may be necessary to produce a therapeutic effect.
†Most studies indicate a duration of action for sublingual isosorbide dinitrate of 90 to 120 minutes; some indicate activity for 4 hours.

Preparations

Nitroglycerin is available in oral, sublingual, topical, and intravenous formulations.[8] To achieve a longer action, a variety of oral sustained-release preparations, nitroglycerin ointment, and synthetic nitrate esters have been marketed (Table 36-2). The oral preparations often must be given in large doses to overcome extensive first-pass hepatic metabolism.

In addition to nitroglycerin ointment, a variety of transdermal nitroglycerin preparations are available. These adhesive bandages contain nitroglycerin on lactose in a viscous silicone fluid (Transderm) or nitroglycerin microsealed in a solid silicone polymer (Nitrodisc). These delivery systems are intended to release nitroglycerin continuously over a 24-hour period. Pharmacokinetic studies show that in most patients once-a-day dosage is sufficient.

Metabolism of organic nitrates

Organic nitrates are changed in the body to nitrites. Blood concentrations of nitrites, however, do not correlate well with antianginal activity. It has been suggested that coronary dilator activity depends on the intact organic nitrate and not on its reduction to nitrite.

Degradation of nitroglycerin occurs primarily in the liver by means of a glutathione-dependent organic nitrate reductase. The activity of the liver is responsible for the need for larger doses of orally administered nitrates compared with sublingual tablets.

Tolerance to vascular actions of nitrites and nitrates

Tolerance develops to the headache produced by nitrates. Thus munitions workers when first exposed to nitrates complain of headaches, but they become tolerant in a few days. They may also develop nitrate dependence, since some workers develop anginal attacks when they terminate their exposure to the chemical. Tolerance to the antianginal effects of nitrates and nitrites was not documented until transdermal delivery systems became available. Efficacy can be demonstrated up to 6 hours after placement of a patch on the skin but not at 24 hours even though a constant serum concentration of nitroglycerin is maintained. It is speculated that the peak and valley pattern of serum concentrations that occurs with intermittent dosing with other nitrate formulations allows sufficient time for glutathione to recover and thereby prevent development of tolerance.

Toxic effects of nitrites and nitrates

A severe decrease in blood pressure with syncope, headache, glaucoma, and elevated intracranial pressure can result from excessive dosage or unusual susceptibility of the patient. In addition, nitrites can produce methemoglobinemia by oxidizing the iron of hemoglobin from the ferrous to the ferric state. This ability is used to advantage in treatment of cyanide poisoning.

Nitrite poisoning may be acute or chronic. It can result from therapeutic or accidental intake of nitrites or from ingestion of a nitrate that is converted to a nitrite by intestinal bacteria. This has occurred after ingestion of bismuth subnitrate. Increasing attention is paid to the fact that well water in some rural areas may contain enough nitrate to cause chronic methemoglobinemia. Chronic poisoning from nitrates and nitrites is an industrial hazard, particularly in the explosives industry.

There is increasing concern also about the addition of nitrites and nitrates to meat products. The nitrites may be converted in the stomach to nitrosamines, which are carcinogenic.

Therapeutic aims in use of nitrites and nitrates

The most important indication for use of these compounds is management of angina pectoris. If necessary, nitrates can be used in combination with β-adrenergic receptor blocking agents or calcium-channel antagonists.

Nitrates are also used in management of congestive heart failure. Their benefit in this setting is derived primarily from venodilatation (which decreases preload) and to a lesser extent from arteriolar dilatation (which decreases afterload).

Continuous intravenous nitroglycerin infusions have been used for unstable angina, congestive heart failure complicating acute myocardial infarction, perioperative control of blood pressure in patients undergoing coronary artery bypass surgery, and controlled hypotension during noncardiac surgery.[8] Because nitroglycerin can be absorbed into various plastics, care must be taken to use approved infusion sets when nitroglycerin is given intravenously. The infusion is generally begun at a rate of 5 μg/min, and the dose is titrated to the clinically desired end point (that is, the desired blood pressure, cessation of chest pain, or the appropriate reduction in the pulmonary capillary wedge pressure).

β-ADRENERGIC RECEPTOR BLOCKING AGENTS

β-Receptor antagonists are widely used in management of angina pectoris.[5] The general pharmacology of this class of drugs is discussed in Chapter 16. They are effective in angina because they reduce myocardial oxygen demand as a result of their negative chronotropic and inotropic effects, secondary to their ability to reduce blood pressure and to block increments in heart rate induced by circulating catecholamines. These agents must be used cautiously because of their ability to precipitate congestive heart failure or bronchospasm in susceptible patients.

Variant, or Prinzmetal's, angina is characterized by chest pain at rest rather than during exercise. Coronary artery spasm appears to be the cause of the pain and S-T segment elevation.

Attacks may be precipitated by administration of epinephrine, norepinephrine, and sympathomimetic drugs in general. Ergonovine maleate, a constrictor of vascular smooth muscle, has been used as a diagnostic agent for variant angina. However, this drug is not without danger, since it can cause prolonged spasm of coronary arteries. Coronary artery spasm can be treated effectively with calcium-channel blocking agents.[2,3,7,9,10,12] These drugs interfere with calcium entry into vascular smooth muscle and cause coronary vasodilatation and relief of spasm. Spasm has recently been recognized to be important in other anginal syndromes. In unstable angina and acute myocardial infarction, coronary spasm is prevalent and may be caused by platelet plugging at sites of atheromatous lesions, associated with release of vasoconstrictors such as thromboxane and serotonin. Although calcium antagonists do not affect platelet aggregation, they can blunt or block the secondary spasm. Spasm may also play a role in stable angina and in silent ischemia—painless and therefore asymptomatic ischemic episodes in patients with coronary artery disease. Vasodilatation also occurs in the vasculature and decreases afterload. This is an additional mechanism that contributes to the antianginal effect of calcium blockers and to their efficacy in chronic effort-induced angina. Because of this latter action, these drugs have proved effective in treatment of hypertension as well.

The use of verapamil as an antiarrhythmic agent is discussed in Chapter 35. Despite these drugs being classified together as calcium antagonists, there are considerable differences in their pharmacology as indicated in Table 36-3. Their side effects and dosages are summarized in Tables 36-4 and 36-5 respectively. It should be noted that these agents, particularly verapamil, can induce left ventricular dysfunction. For this reason the calcium blockers should be used cautiously in patients with myocardial disease, especially if given in combination with β-blocking agents.

SLOW CALCIUM-CHANNEL ANTAGONISTS

Verapamil is used most frequently for its ability to slow conduction through the AV node and, as such, has become the agent of choice in most cases of supraventricular tachyarrhythmias. In addition, it has been used successfully in all forms of angina and can be an effective antihypertensive drug. For use in this latter setting, the effects on cardiac conduction may be unwanted.

Verapamil

TABLE 36-3	Pharmacologic activities of calcium antagonists			
	Coronary vasodilatation	Peripheral vasodilatation	Negative inotropy	Slowed AV conduction
Verapamil	+ + +	+ +	+	+ +
Nifedipine	+ + +	+ + +	−	−
Diltiazem	+ + +	+	+	+

+, Mild; + +, moderate; + + +, pronounced; −, negligible.

TABLE 36-4   Side effects of antianginal drugs*

	Hypotension, flushing, headache	Left ventricular dysfunction	Decreased heart rate, atrioventricular block†	Gastrointestinal symptoms	Broncho-constriction‡
β-Blockers	0	+ +	+ + +	+	+ + +
Nitrates	+ + +	0	0	0	0
Diltiazem	+	+	+	0	0
Nifedipine	+ + +	0	0	0	0
Verapamil	+	+	+ +	+ +	0

From Braunwald, E.: N. Engl. J. Med. **307**:1618, 1982. Reprinted by permission of the New England Journal of Medicine.
*0, Absent; +, mild; + +, moderate; + + +, sometimes severe.
†In patients with sick-sinus-node syndrome or conduction-system disease.
‡In patients with obstructive lung disease.

TABLE 36-5   Preparations and dosages of calcium antagonists

Drug	Initial dosage* (mg)	Maximum daily dosage (mg)	Oral dosage forms† (mg)
Verapamil hydrochloride (Calan, Isoptin)	80	480	T: 80, 120, 240
Nifedipine (Adalat, Procardia)	10	120	C: 10, 20
Diltiazem hydrochloride (Cardizem)	30	240	T: 30, 60

*Given three times daily.
†C, Capsules; T, tablets.

Verapamil is eliminated by the liver and has a substantial first-pass effect; bioavailability is only about 20%.[6] Its half-life of 3 to 5 hours mandates dosing 3 to 4 times per day. Interestingly, the stereoisomers of verapamil have different efficacies. After oral dosing the more active isomer is selectively metabolized during the first pass through the liver; therefore, of the verapamil in blood, the active isomer is relatively less in proportion, compared to intravenous dosing. The result is that after ingestion a *total* serum concentration three times higher than after intravenous dosing is needed to cause the same effect.

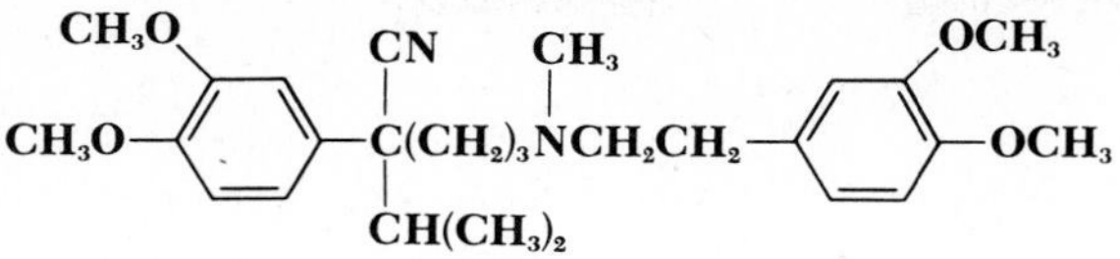

Verapamil

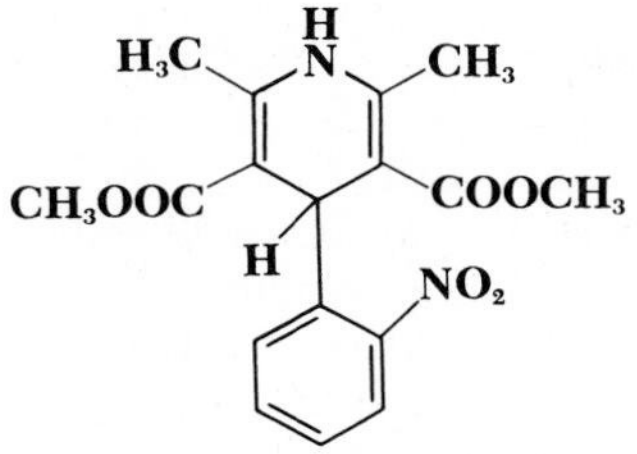

Nifedipine

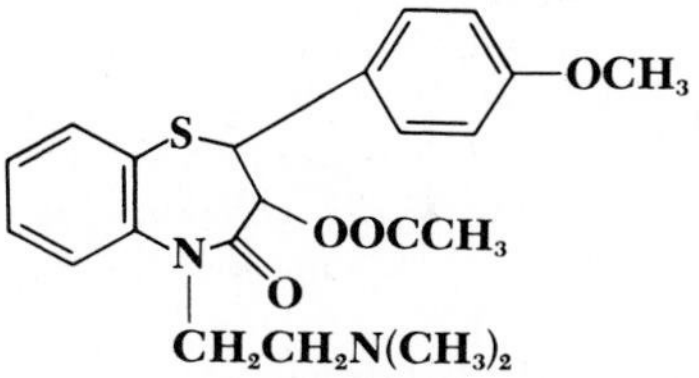

Diltiazem

Nifedipine

In contrast to verapamil, nifedipine has negligible effects on cardiac conduction and a major action to lower peripheral vascular resistance. Hence, in addition to decreasing coronary spasm, it may be used to decrease afterload and to lower blood pressure. Because of the pronounced vasodilating effect, its use is associated with side effects of headache, reflex tachycardia, and fluid retention.

Like verapamil, nifedipine is eliminated by the liver, but it has a bioavailability approaching 90%.[11] Its half-life is 3 to 4 hours.

Diltiazem

Diltiazem has pharmacologic properties essentially intermediate between those of verapamil and nifedipine, that is, less effect on cardiac conduction than verapamil and less vasodilatation than nifedipine.

Similarly to the other calcium antagonists, diltiazem is eliminated by the liver, with a half-life of about 4 hours.[4] It has an active metabolite that probably contributes little to its activity.

REFERENCES

1. Abrams, J.: Nitroglycerin and long-acting nitrates, N. Engl. J. Med. **302**:1234, 1980.
2. Antman, E.M., Stone, P.H., Muller, J.E., and Braunwald, E.: Calcium channel blocking agents in the treatment of cardiovascular disorders: Part I, Basic and clinical electrophysiologic effects, Ann. Intern. Med. **93**:875, 1980.
3. Braunwald, E.: Mechanisms of action of calcium-channel-blocking agents, N. Engl. J. Med. **307**:1618, 1982.
4. Chaffman, M., and Brogden, R.N.: Diltiazem: a review of its pharmacological properties and therapeutic efficacy, Drugs **29**:387, 1985.
5. Frishman, W.H.: β-Adrenoceptor antagonists: new drugs and new indications, N. Engl. J. Med. **305**:500, 1981.
6. Hamann, S.R., Blouin, R.A., and McAllister, R.G., Jr.: Clinical pharmacokinetics of verapamil, Clin. Pharmacokinet. **9**:26, 1984.
7. Henry, P.D.: Comparative pharmacology of calcium antagonists: nifedipine, verapamil, and diltiazem, Am. J. Cardiol. **46**:1047, 1980.
8. Hill, N.S., Antman, E.M., Green, L.H., and Alpert, J.S.: Intravenous nitroglycerin: a review of pharmacology, indications, therapeutic effects and complications, Chest **79**:69, 1981.
9. Kates, R.E.: Calcium antagonists: pharmacokinetic properties, Drugs **25**:113, 1983.
10. McAllister, R.G., Jr., Hamann, S.R., and Blouin, R.A.: Pharmacokinetics of calcium-entry blockers, Am. J. Cardiol. **55**:30B, 1985.
11. Sorkin, E.M., Clissold, S.P., and Brogden, R.N.: Nifedipine: a review of its pharmacodynamic and pharmacokinetic properties, and therapeutic efficacy, in ischaemic heart disease, hypertension and related cardiovascular disorders, Drugs **30**:182, 1985.
12. Stone, P.H., Antman, E.M., Muller, J.E., and Braunwald, E.: Calcium channel blocking agents in the treatment of cardiovascular disorders: Part II, Hemodynamic effects and clinical applications, Ann. Intern. Med. **93**:886, 1980.

Chapter 37

Drugs that affect hemostasis

Hemostatic mechanisms that prevent excessive bleeding are normally activated by tissue injury. Hemostasis involves a carefully regulated cascade of biochemical reactions that promote aggregation of platelets within damaged vessels, blood coagulation, and the eventual resolution of the clot by fibrinolysis. Inappropriate stimulation of coagulation may occur as a complication of cardiovascular disease, vascular injury, neoplasms, sickle cell anemia, or tissue trauma. The resulting thrombosis can cause significant morbidity and mortality, particularly in patients who must remain immobilized for extended periods of time, because immobilization increases the possibility that an embolus may lodge in the brain or lungs. An exaggerated platelet response is believed to contribute to the pathogenesis of stroke, myocardial infarction, and atherosclerosis.

GENERAL CONCEPT

Drugs that are used to prevent or to treat thromboembolic disease are classified according to their major actions as *anticoagulants*, *platelet inhibitors*, and *thrombolytic agents*. The judicious use of these drugs requires an understanding of how they affect key reactions in primary hemostasis, blood coagulation, and thrombolysis, which involve a complex integration of reactions on cellular surfaces and in the fluid phase of blood. For example, generation of thrombin usually occurs on the surface of activated platelets, whereas the conversion of fibrinogen to fibrin occurs within the fluid phase. The vascular endothelium also participates both as a surface for binding of coagulation proteins and as a source of various regulator molecules, such as prostacyclin.[13]

Anticoagulant drugs prevent the progression of coagulation by interference with one or more clotting factors or their controlling proteins. For example, binding of heparin to the plasma protein antithrombin III enhances the affinity of this inhibitor for thrombin (factor II) and for factor X, a pivotal protein in the coagulation cascade. The anticoagulant drug warfarin decreases hepatic synthesis of several vitamin K–dependent protein coagulation factors and thereby lowers the rate of coagulation.

Platelet inhibitors interfere with platelet adhesion and aggregation and with release of platelet-derived vasoactive mediators. This group of drugs includes nonsteroidal anti-inflammatory drugs, such as aspirin and indomethacin, which block platelet cyclooxygenase and prevent conversion of arachidonic acid to the potent platelet aggregator, thromboxane A_2. Other platelet inhibitory drugs, such as dipyridamole and sulfinpyrazone, may have additional actions, on platelets or on the vessel wall, that modulate activation of platelets or prolong their survival in the circulation.

Thrombolytic agents include activators of plasmin, a fibrinolytic enzyme that stimulates the lysis and removal of an existing clot. Streptokinase causes a nonenzymatic alteration of the conformation of plasminogen to generate plasmin; urokinase and tissue plasminogen activator activate plasmin through an enzymatic mechanism. Activation of the fibrinolytic system by these agents enhances digestion of fibrin and other components of the formed clot.

THE CLOTTING PROCESS AND DRUG ACTION

A complex integration of control mechanisms maintains fluidity of the blood or promotes coagulation in response to imbalances within the system. Various factors, including diet, hormones, or the presence of disease, influence the normal balance. Although the classic concept of blood coagulation is that of a cascade of enzymatic reactions, it is currently believed that coagulation is a surface-oriented phenomenon that integrates interaction of enzymes, cofactors, and substrates within a specific environment. An important feature is that the process is limited by specific inhibitors and inactivators. These include antithrombin III, an inhibitor of serine proteases, and protein C, a protease that inactivates factors V and VIII. Deficiencies of the regulatory proteins are reflected by recurrent thromboses, pulmonary emboli, and occlusive arterial complications.[1]

Coagulation and clot resolution proceed through discrete stages, each of which may involve several enzymatic steps. These are outlined in simplified form below.

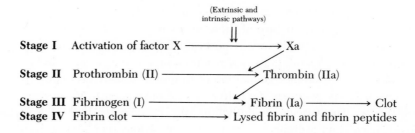

In stage I factor X is activated by a series of enzymatic steps and formation of complexes. In stage II thrombin is formed by a series of reactions involving activated factor X (Xa) and additional coagulation factors. In stage III fibrin (Ia), the basic component of a clot, is generated from fibrinogen, a soluble plasma protein, by the proteolytic action of thrombin (IIa). Fibrin is an insoluble protein that forms a mechanical barrier to blood flow, and it also provides the surface upon which additional coagulation and platelet activation reactions can occur. Finally, the lysis of fibrin by plasmin results in dissolution of the clot and restoration of flow.

There are two converging pathways of thrombin formation, designated as the *intrinsic* and *extrinsic* pathways (Fig. 37-1). In both pathways a complex is formed between coagulation factors, cofactors, and calcium on a phospholipid surface, as in cell membranes. Both pathways require vitamin K–dependent coagulation factors, and activation of either pathway results in formation of activated factor X (Xa).[14]

The intrinsic pathway is triggered when Hageman factor (XII) in blood is activated

Compartmentalization of blood coagulation into the intrinsic and extrinsic system is useful   **FIG. 37-1**
in the diagnostic laboratory. The intrinsic system is evaluated with the activated partial
thromboplastin time and the extrinsic system with the prothrombin time. HMK, *High mo-*
lecular weight kininogen; KAL, *kallikrein;* PF₃, *platelet factor 3*.

From Triplett, D.A.: Clin. Lab. Med. 4:221, 1984.

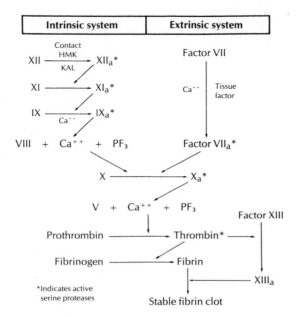

by contact with a negatively charged surface. In vitro this reaction can be initiated by contact with glass, and in vivo contact with subendothelial surface components, such as collagen, may promote it. Hageman factor can be activated by proteases, such as kallikrein, as well. Intrinsic pathway activation requires activated factor IX (IXa), which complexes with factor VIII. This complex, in association with cell-membrane phospholipids, or a similar surface, forms an enzyme that activates factor X. Factor Xa may be derived from either intrinsic or extrinsic pathways (by activation by factor VIIa). Thus both pathways are normally involved in coagulation.

The extrinsic pathway bypasses several steps of the intrinsic pathway but depends on the proteolytic action of factors from the intrinsic pathway. The interactions of factor VII with the cell membrane–associated tissue factor (thromboplastin) and calcium on a phospholipid-containing surface is probably the most important physiologic mechanism for initiation of coagulation. With injury to the endothelium or other components of the vessel wall, tissue-factor activity is expressed on damaged cell membranes. Its reaction with factor VII results in formation of an enzymatically active complex that activates factor X and thereby proceeds to the formation of thrombin.

In addition to generation of fibrin from fibrinogen, thrombin has several other important enzymatic actions that can amplify or attenuate coagulation. Thrombin can activate factor XIII to XIIIa, which promotes cross-linking and stabilization of the fibrin clot. Thrombin also activates platelets to enhance aggregation, and it activates factors V and VIII to further enhance coagulation. In addition, thrombin appears to be part of a mechanism to limit coagulation. It interacts with thrombomodulin from the vessel wall, phospholipid, and calcium to form an enzymatically active complex that converts a zymogen, protein C, to an active protease. The activated protein C can then inactivate factors Va and VIIIa, which are the major cofactors of the coagulation cascade, to limit the coagulation process.[8]

ANTICOAGULANTS

Anticoagulant drugs are used to prevent or reduce thromboembolic sequelae of vascular damage attributable to cardiac disease, surgery, neoplasm, or trauma. Extended inhibition of coagulation is desirable in patients who must remain immobilized for long periods of time, particularly if tissue injury has occurred, as in postsurgical patients, in patients with prosthetic heart valves, and in patients with documented pulmonary embolism.[3] Thrombus formation within the deep leg veins can lead to pulmonary embolism, sometimes with fatal consequences because a single large embolus can occlude as much as 5% of the pulmonary vascular bed. Anticoagulant drugs do not dissolve clots but are used to reduce formation of new clots and extension of old clots and thus the possibility of embolism to the lung and other organs.

Blood coagulation is vulnerable to drug action at several points. Binding of free calcium by oxalate, citrate, or edetate (ethylenediaminetetraacetic acid, EDTA) will prevent coagulation, and these agents are widely used in laboratory procedures. Because lowering the ionized calcium concentration sufficiently to prevent coagulation is incompatible with life, however, these agents are useful only in vitro. Heparin can interfere with coagulation both in vitro and in vivo by a physical interaction with coagulation components and their controlling proteins. Finally, compounds that interfere with the synthesis of coagulation factors will prevent clotting in vivo but not in a test tube.

Heparin

The anticoagulant action of heparin depends on its unique structure. Heparin is a negatively charged mucopolysaccharide composed of repeating units of sulfated glucosamine and glucuronic acid. The numerous sulfate and carboxyl groups enable heparin to interact with several different blood proteins, including certain coagulation proteins and control factors.[5] Commercial heparin from bovine lung or porcine intestinal mucosa is a heterogeneous mixture of polymers ranging from 6,000 to approximately 25,000 daltons. The different size molecules vary in anticoagulant activity, probably because of differences in affinity for the coagulant proteins.

Configuration of disaccharides in heparin

Heparin is believed to cause anticoagulation by accelerating formation of complexes between antithrombin III and several proteases involved with the coagulation cascade.[9] These include factors IXa, Xa, XIa, and XIIa as well as thrombin (IIa). Antithrombin III, an α_2-globulin normally present in blood, is an important control protein. It forms a complex with active serine proteases (including coagulation factors), which interact with its arginine-containing site (Fig. 37-2). In the absence of heparin, this complex forms slowly, permitting a limited expression of enzyme activity. Heparin binds to lysyl residues on antithrombin III and, through a conformational change in the molecule, accelerates the rate of complex formation approximately a thousandfold.[11] The heterogeneity of heparin is important because high and low molecular weight species have different spectra of activity. Low molecular weight heparin has the most potent action on factor Xa binding, whereas the high molecular weight heparin is most active on thrombin binding.[1]

In addition, heparin has an action that is unrelated to its effect on antithrombin III. Because of its concentrated anionic charge, heparin can directly inhibit the actions of factors II and X on their substrates by disrupting the protein complexes formed between the coagulation protein and proactivator. This contribution, however, to the overall anticoagulant activity of heparin is small.

Heparin-like proteoglycans are normally present on the surface of the vascular endothelium. These molecules function like heparin in accelerating complex formation between activated serine proteases and antithrombin III. The formation of these complexes is probably one of the mechanisms through which the endothelium maintains its antithrombotic surface. In addition, circulating heparin is taken up by the endothelium where it increases the electronegative potential of the vessel wall.[5]

Heparin is not absorbed from the gastrointestinal tract. Because its action depends on the large number of anionic groups, enteric sulfatases, which remove these groups, inactivate it. Heparin administered parenterally is readily absorbed and retains its activity.

Commercial heparin preparations, as supplied for hospital use, are standardized by their activity, which is expressed in units rather than by weight. One hundred USP units corresponds to approximately 1 mg of heparin.

ADMINISTRATION AND DOSAGE

FIG. 37-2   *Effect of heparin on antithrombin III. Heparin will accelerate the inactivation of active serine proteases by antithrombin III.*

From McGann, M.A., and Triplett, D.A.: Lab. Med. **13**:742, 1982.

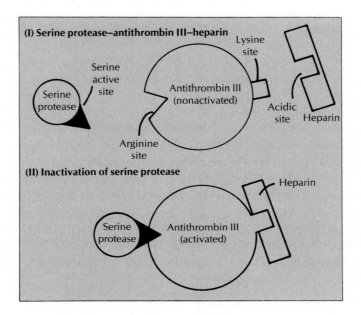

Heparin is usually the first drug administered when anticoagulation is desired. It is immediately effective after intravenous administration and is very rapidly effective after subcutaneous injection. Heparin has few if any other actions to complicate the anticoagulant effect. Its duration of action is short, however, and it must be administered by continuous infusion or by frequent intermittent (4 to 6 hours) injection. Approximately 80% of the heparin in circulation is inactivated by the liver, and the metabolites and residual heparin are excreted by the kidneys.

USE   Heparin is administered to patients with an acute need for anticoagulation, such as those with suspected or verified pulmonary emboli. Doses on the order of 30,000 units per day are usually required. The objective is to prevent extension of already formed clots, thus lessening chances for embolization from the legs to the lungs or from the heart to the brain. Low-dose heparin (1000 units) may be administered subcutaneously every 12 hours to patients at risk for thromboembolism just before various surgical procedures. This approach may prevent postoperative venous thrombosis, and it does not impose a risk of excessive bleeding because the anticoagulant effect is slight.

Heparin is also used in vitro to prevent coagulation, and it is used in solutions for extracorporeal circulation and dialysis to maintain fluidity of blood circulating through artificial environments. The technique of regional heparinization adds heparin to the patient's blood before it enters the extracorporeal device, and the antagonist protamine is added to neutralize the anticoagulant action before the blood is returned to the patient. As a result, the blood is anticoagulated only within the extracorporeal circulation, and the patient avoids the risk of systemic anticoagulation.

Monitoring of anticoagulant activity after heparin administration was traditionally by the Lee-White clotting time. This procedure has been abandoned in recent years because of poor reproducibility. The activated partial thromboplastin time (APTT or PTT) is now generally used to monitor anticoagulation. When heparin is used to treat or prevent thrombosis, plasma concentrations of about 0.3 to 0.4 units/ml will extend the APTT to approximately twice control values, which will usually prevent extension of a thrombus. Laboratory monitoring is very important because the response to heparin varies from one patient to another and sometimes even within the same patient over time. Furthermore, close control of the heparin action can achieve a greater antithrombotic effect while also preventing hemorrhagic episodes.

Except for anticoagulation, heparin causes few important effects. It has been reported to antagonize the vascular actions of inflammatory mediators, such as histamine, bradykinin, and prostaglandins, in experimental animals, and it can change the activity of several different enzymes,[5] probably because of its strong anionic charge.

The major complication of heparin therapy is hemorrhage. Even with standard anticoagulant dosage, heparin may promote bleeding from open wounds and mucous membranes. Cerebral hemorrhage or retroperitoneal bleeding can be catastrophic. Fortunately, these complications are rare. Several types of patients are considered to be at high risk while undergoing heparin anticoagulation. These include alcoholics, the elderly (over 60 years of age), and persons with coagulopathies.

The acute effects of heparin are relatively short lived because the drug is rapidly metabolized. Its half-life is on the order of 1 hour; overdosage can be rapidly corrected by cessation of administration and waiting. **Protamine sulfate,** a positively charged polymer, will block the action of heparin both in vivo and in vitro by chemical antagonism.

Although it is usually assumed that heparin does not affect platelet function, a mild thrombocytopenia sometimes occurs after onset of anticoagulation. This phenomenon affects 5% to 30% of patients, usually within 2 to 3 days of treatment. The effect is slight, and platelet count generally returns to normal even with continued therapy. An immune-mediated thrombocytopenia associated with intravascular thrombosis is a rare complication of heparin therapy. Since commercial heparin contains some impurities, allergic reactions may also occur, particularly at the site of subcutaneous injection.

Prolonged administration of heparin (more than 6 months) has been linked to osteoporosis. This phenomenon, which likely results from inhibition of osteoblasts, is of little importance for short-term anticoagulation in most patients. For patients at particular risk of osteoporosis or those with bone disorders, it may be more significant.

TOXICITY AND COMPLICATIONS OF THERAPY

Orally effective anticoagulant drugs

One of the major drawbacks to anticoagulant therapy with heparin is the drug's short duration of action. Furthermore, heparin is effective only if administered parenterally, and its effect must be consistently and rigorously monitored in the laboratory. Thus heparin is not suitable for extended control of coagulation or for therapy outside the hospital setting.

The recognition and development of orally effective agents for anticoagulation is an interesting story. It had been known for years that cattle develop a hemorrhagic disorder after consumption of spoiled sweet clover hay and that the bleeding is caused by a lowered prothrombin concentration. In 1941 Link and his associates at the University of Wisconsin showed that a *coumarin* compound from the spoiled clover is responsible for the hemorrhagic condition.[7]

The synthesis of **dicumarol** (bishydroxycoumarin) led to its use in clinical medicine. Other anticoagulants were synthesized by structural modification of the dicumarol molecule. Interestingly, **warfarin** was originally used as a rodent poison because it was believed too toxic for use in man. Warfarin is still the active ingredient in various rodenticides, but it is also the drug of choice for maintaining an extended anticoagulated state in humans. Coumarin anticoagulants are widely used to manage thromboembolic vascular disease. Although the compounds vary in structure, potency, and duration of action, they all act by the same basic mechanism.

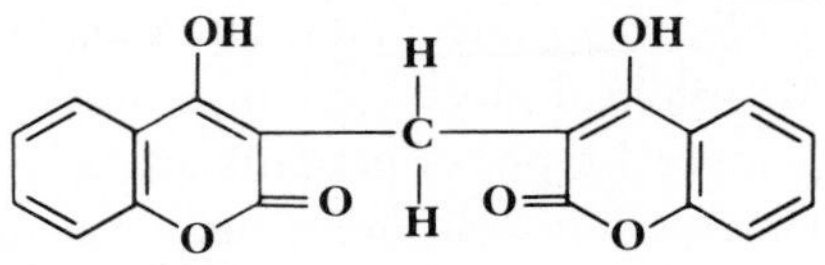

Dicumarol

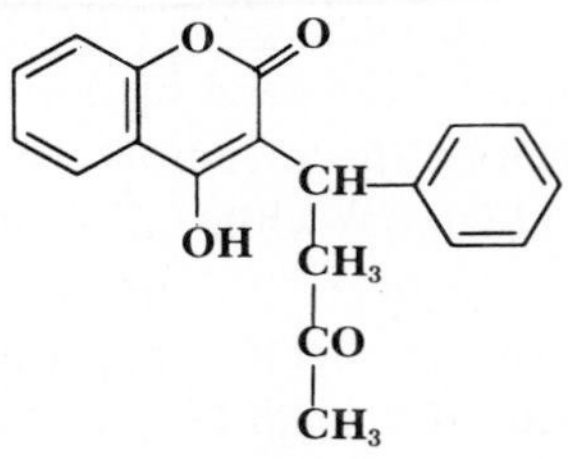

Warfarin

MECHANISM OF ACTION

The coumarin anticoagulants are effective *only* in vivo. They interfere with the vitamin K–dependent synthesis of factors II, VII, IX, and X by blocking a carboxylation step required to produce the active factors. Each of the vitamin K–dependent factors has 10 to 12 γ-carboxyglutamic acid residues at the amino terminus. This structure is necessary for binding of the proteins to charged phospholipid membranes during the coagulation process; with inadequate binding the factors cannot function either as enzymes or substrates within the assembled complex. Coumarin anticoagulants prevent postribosomal incorporation of the γ-carboxyglutamate residues and thus prevent synthesis of functional factors (Fig. 37-3). Factor VII, the first protein affected, decreases to less than 10% of its original activity within 12 hours. However, there remain active factors, circulating at the onset of medication, that must be

Mechanism of coumarin action. Drugs of the coumarin type interfere with the vitamin K cycle by blocking the enzyme that reduces vitamin K epoxide to vitamin K. Carboxylation of the glutamic acid residues of factors II, VII, IX, and X (left) is prevented, thereby inhibiting the activation of these factors.   FIG. 37-3

Modified from Walsh, P.N.: Hosp. Pract. 18(1):101, 1983.

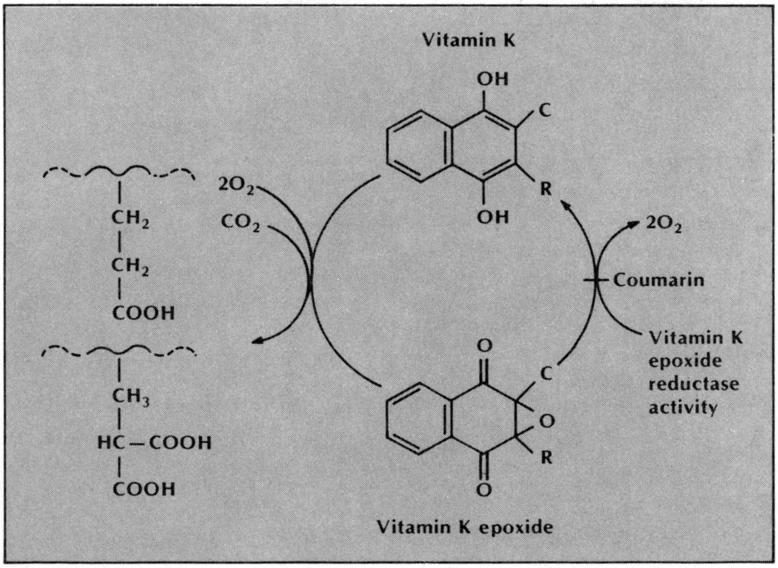

metabolized and eliminated before the anticoagulant effect is apparent, a process that may require up to 48 hours.

The great individual variability in response to coumarin anticoagulants is caused by many different factors, including the rate of absorption and metabolic transformation, diet, and genetically determined resistance to the drugs. Because the coumarin drugs are highly bound to plasma proteins, other drugs or clinical conditions that affect plasma protein concentration (particularly albumin) or binding capacity will influence the efficacy of therapy. Warfarin, the prototype of the coumarin anticoagulants, exerts a peak effect within 36 to 72 hours, and the effect lasts for 2 to 5 days. As Table 37-1 indicates, a much higher dose is required to initiate anticoagulation than to maintain it. Warfarin is the agent most commonly used because it is readily absorbed from the gastrointestinal tract.

USE

Warfarin and related drugs are used in states such as pulmonary embolism and deep venous thrombosis and in patients with artificial heart valves or those who must remain immobilized for long periods.[3] Because of their delayed onset of action, coumarin drugs may be administered simultaneously with heparin at first, so that there is a continued inhibition of coagulation. Heparin, which is usually administered only in a hospital setting, may be continued in gradually decreasing doses for several

TABLE 37-1	Daily doses of various coumarin and indanedione anticoagulants		
Preparation	Initial (mg)	Maintenance (mg)	Oral tablet forms (mg)
Dicumarol	200-300	25-200	25-100
Warfarin sodium (Coumadin, others)	10-15	2-10	2-10
Warfarin potassium (Athrombin-K)	40-60	2.5-10	5
Anisindione (Miradon)	300	25-250	50
Phenprocoumon (Liquamar)	24	0.75-6	3

days while the anticoagulant effect of warfarin develops. Once the desired degree of inhibition is achieved, warfarin may be continued for as long as 3 to 6 months in ambulatory patients.

The use of anticoagulants in acute myocardial infarction remains controversial. Long-term anticoagulation after infarction offers little benefit, but the judicious use of heparin or coumarin drugs for the hospitalized, immobile patient may prevent thrombotic sequelae. Anticoagulant drugs are often contraindicated in stroke victims, however, because of the potential danger associated with cerebrovascular damage and uncontrolled bleeding into the brain.

LABORATORY CONTROL
Control of the anticoagulant effect is very important to prevent bleeding complications. The effect of warfarin is monitored at regular intervals during therapy by the one-stage *prothrombin time*, which is the time required for clotting in the presence of standardized tissue thromboplastin. The desired end point is a prothrombin time between one and a half to twice that of normal plasma, and dosage is adjusted to achieve this aim. Control of coagulation requires accurate and frequent testing under standardized laboratory conditions, particularly when therapy is first initiated. Severe depression of prothrombin concentration may result in bleeding, which may be manifest as microscopic hematuria, or gastrointestinal or cerebral hemorrhage.

If serious bleeding does occur, withdrawal of the drug is insufficient to reverse its action because of the long time required to synthesize new coagulation factors. The factors can be supplied immediately by transfusion of fresh plasma or whole blood, and administration of vitamin K facilitates synthesis of new factors. A water-soluble form of vitamin K, phytonadione (vitamin K_1, AquaMEPHYTON), can be administered intravenously when rapid reversal of the anticoagulant effect is necessary, but because anaphylactic reactions have occurred with phytonadione this route is used only in the event of severe bleeding. Vitamin K preparations used as coumarin antidotes may interfere with further use of coumarin anticoagulants for as long as 2 weeks.

TABLE 37-2 Interactions of warfarin with other drugs	
Drugs that potentiate warfarin action	**Probable mechanism**
Antibiotics (some)	Decreased production of vitamin K
Cholestyramine	Decreased absorption of vitamin K
Anabolic steroids	Increased synthesis of coagulation factors; enhanced receptor affinity for warfarin
Aspirin, clofibrate, diazoxide, mefenamic acid, nalidixic acid, phenylbutazone	Competition with warfarin for binding to plasma proteins (transient)
Cimetidine, clofibrate, disulfiram, phenylbutazone	Inhibition of warfarin degradation
Drugs that inhibit warfarin action	
Barbiturates, carbamazepine, ethanol, griseofulvin, haloperidol, rifampin	Enhanced metabolism of warfarin by liver microsomal enzymes
Potentiation of other drugs by warfarin	
Phenytoin, tolbutamide	Competition with warfarin for binding to plasma proteins (transient)

As with heparin, the contraindications to warfarin therapy relate to the possibility of severe bleeding. Major contraindications include a history of a recent bleeding episode, a known hemorrhagic disease, gastrointestinal pathosis that increases the risk of hemorrhage, unexplained anemia or gastrointestinal bleeding, central nervous system trauma or surgery, malignant hypertension, and pregnancy. In addition, anticoagulant therapy should be avoided in unreliable persons or when adequate laboratory facilities for continued monitoring are lacking.

CONTRAINDICATIONS

In the circulation warfarin and other coumarin drugs are primarily complexed with albumin and other plasma proteins. Factors that alter the amount of binding can have a dramatic effect on the anticoagulant activity. The coumarin agents are inactivated by hepatic microsomal enzymes.

CLINICAL PHARMACOLOGY AND DRUG INTERACTIONS

Drug interactions are an important consideration in anticoagulant therapy. One reason is that anticoagulants are usually administered to patients with diseases that require other medication. Another is that patients who need anticoagulants must usually continue therapy for several months. Although interactions with the short-lived heparin are few, the orally effective anticoagulants can interact with many other agents. Table 37-2 lists some prominent interactions and probable mechanisms.

Drug interactions involving anticoagulants can result from several mechanisms. Because warfarin interferes with vitamin K–dependent synthesis of coagulation factors, its action is enhanced by drugs or conditions that interfere with absorption of vitamin K. Some antibiotics affect the normal flora of the intestine and thereby the endogenous production of vitamin K. Drugs that alter hepatic synthesis of coagulation proteins or affect their catabolism will interact with warfarin. Agents that affect hepatic microsomal enzymes will alter the metabolism and thus the activity of warfarin and related drugs. For example, induction of these enzymes by barbiturates increases metabolism of warfarin, and larger doses are required to achieve the desired anticoagulant effect. Drugs that inhibit enzymatic degradation, such as cimetidine, obviously will prolong the anticoagulant action. Since cimetidine is widely used in clinical practice, the clinician should be particularly alert to this interaction.

Because of the potential for such interactions and their possible major consequences, continued laboratory monitoring of prothrombin time is necessary for patients taking coumarin drugs. Disruption of the stabilized anticoagulated state by drug interactions is both dangerous and costly to the patient because it may take some time to stabilize the warfarin dose again.

ANTIPLATELET DRUGS

Platelet activation is essential to hemostasis. When tissue is damaged, vasoconstriction initially decreases blood flow from severed vessels and reduces the area that must be occluded by a hemostatic plug. Adherence of platelets to damaged cell surfaces or to collagen and basement membrane components initiates activation and stimulates release of substances, such as ADP, thromboxane A_2, and serotonin, that promote aggregation and vasoconstriction. As platelets aggregate at the wound site, they form a plug that eventually occludes the severed vessel. Thrombi that occur within small arterioles are primarily from platelet activation. Tissue factor (thromboplastin) from injured tissues activates coagulation and results in production of thrombin. Venous thrombi result primarily from activation of coagulation within vessels. Thrombin stimulates further platelet aggregation and produces a network of fibrin to stabilize the plug.[4] Although essential for hemostasis, these reactions are sometimes undesirable. The reactions between platelets, coagulation factors, and the vessel are shown in Fig. 37-4.

The rationale for use of drugs that interfere with the platelet component of hemostasis is that anticoagulants do not prevent formation of arterial thrombi. In addition, platelet activation may promote atherogenesis through release of a growth factor for smooth muscle cells. Because smooth muscle proliferation occurs early in the atherosclerotic process, platelet activation may play a pivotal role in the pathogenesis of stroke, myocardial infarction, and atherosclerosis.

Antiplatelet drugs have been used, with varying degrees of success, in patients at risk for myocardial infarction or stroke. One common finding is that platelets from persons with these disease states appear more sensitive to activation by physiologic stimuli. Platelet hyperreactivity has been associated with cigarette smoking, elevated plasma catecholamines, hypertension, atherosclerotic heart disease, and the presence of artificial surfaces, as in heart valve replacement.

Drugs can affect platelet activation and response by several different mechanisms. Some decrease adherence of platelets to the vascular wall; others prevent production of thromboxane A_2 and block aggregation. Still other agents affect platelet survival in the circulation through mechanisms that remain obscure.[4] Table 37-3 lists some platelet-inhibitory agents and their general mechanisms of action.

In arterial thrombus formation, platelet adhesion is initiated by exposure of collagen fibers on injured endothelial surface, and platelets spread by pseudopodia (top). Platelets aggregate; discharge of ADP and generation of thromboxane A₂ enhance aggregation (middle). Last, the clotting mechanism is activated, generating thrombin, and the action of thrombin on fibrinogen yields fibrin polymers, which stabilize the thrombus.

FIG. 37-4

<small>From Frishman, W.H.: Hosp. Pract. 17(5):73, 1982; this illustration drawn by Nancy Lou Makris, Wilton, Conn.</small>

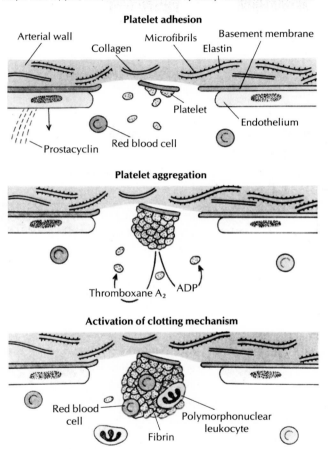

Platelet adhesion

Arterial wall — Microfibrils — Basement membrane
Collagen — Elastin
Platelet
Endothelium
Prostacyclin — Red blood cell

Platelet aggregation

Thromboxane A₂ — ADP

Activation of clotting mechanism

Red blood cell — Polymorphonuclear leukocyte
Fibrin

Drugs that affect metabolism of arachidonic acid are discussed in detail in Chapter 31. Nonsteroidal anti-inflammatory agents, such as aspirin and indomethacin, inhibit platelet function by blocking formation of thromboxane A₂. Aspirin is the agent most commonly used to prevent platelet activation. It is inexpensive, effective, and usually well tolerated in low doses. It irreversibly inhibits platelet cyclooxygenase through acetylation. (Salicylates that lack an acetyl group do not act by this mechanism.) Since the platelet is unable to synthesize new cyclooxygenase, the effect persists for

Aspirin and other nonsteroidal anti-inflammatory agents

TABLE 37-3 Platelet-inhibiting agents	
Mechanism	Examples
Inhibition of thromboxane formation	Glucocorticoids, aspirin, indomethacin, sulfinpyrazone
Increased cyclic AMP with inhibition of activation and aggregation	Prostacyclin, propranolol, dipyridamole
Inhibition of thrombin formation	Heparin, oral anticoagulants
Surfaces coated to block interactions	Dextran

the life of the cell. Thus the effect of aspirin is cumulative, and even small doses of aspirin, as low as 1 mg per day, can inhibit platelet activation. Indomethacin, ibuprofen, and other nonsteroidal anti-inflammatory drugs are reversible inhibitors of cyclooxygenase.

Dipyridamole   Platelet activation and aggregation are associated with a decrease in their content of cyclic AMP, and agents that increase platelet cyclic AMP inhibit activation and the release reaction. When circulating platelets contact the vascular endothelium, prostacyclin, produced by the endothelium, stimulates adenylate cyclase of the platelet membranes and enhances formation of cyclic AMP. The very brief action of prostacyclin renders it ineffective as a drug for prevention of platelet thrombi, but its continuous production by the endothelium is doubtless important for maintaining fluidity of flowing blood.

Dipyridamole inhibits platelet phosphodiesterase, the enzyme that breaks down cyclic AMP. Inhibition of this enzyme, coupled with enhancement of adenylate cyclase activity by endogenous prostacyclin, increases platelet cyclic AMP and decreases activation. Dipyridamole also inhibits adhesion of platelets to damaged endothelium or to artificial surfaces. It has been used to prevent emboli in patients with artificial heart valves.

Sulfinpyrazone   Sulfinpyrazone can inhibit platelet cyclooxygenase, but it is a competitive and reversible inhibitor. Unlike aspirin, sulfinpyrazone neither prolongs bleeding time nor affects platelet aggregation in normal persons. Furthermore, sulfinpyrazone increases platelet survival within the circulation, whereas aspirin does not. The mechanism of this effect is unknown.

Some studies indicate that certain subgroups of patients may be at risk for thrombosis, even when aspirin is administered to inhibit platelet thromboxane formation. These persons have chronically elevated concentrations of catecholamines, and there is some indication that they may be better protected with sulfinpyrazone or agents that affect catecholamine-induced aggregation.

Antiplatelet drugs are currently used to prevent recurrent cerebral ischemic events and stroke, coronary heart disease, and systemic arterial embolism in persons with prosthetic heart valves. They are also used in patients who have arteriovenous shunts and in those with peripheral arterial disease. As platelet aggregation may contribute to the vasospasm of unstable angina, antiplatelet drugs are a rational choice for treatment of this condition as well. Platelets contribute to cardiovascular disease in two ways: by acute occlusion of a vessel through aggregation and by release of vasoactive agents, such as thromboxane, that cause spasm of cerebral and coronary arteries.

The possibility of intervention through inhibition of the platelet response aroused considerable interest and led to several clinical studies. Aspirin, sulfinpyrazone, and dipyridamole in various combinations were evaluated in several large-scale clinical trials to determine if they could prevent myocardial infarction in patients with established heart disease or if they could prevent stroke or transient ischemic attacks in patients with cerebrovascular disease.[2] The results were not sufficiently encouraging to justify a general recommendation for antiplatelet therapy in myocardial infarction, but aspirin is currently approved for prevention of reinfarction. A recent study of patients with unstable angina suggested that low-dose aspirin reduced the incidence of myocardial infarction and death by 50%.[6] There is some indication that a combination of aspirin and dipyridamole is beneficial after bypass grafting. At least one study indicated that aspirin offers some protection against transient ischemic attacks or stroke in patients at significant risk.[10]

The fibrinolytic system is normally activated simultaneously with coagulation, and the subsequent dissolution of a formed clot provides the basis for repair of damaged tissues. The continual availability of the fibrinolytic system is clearly important for removal of fibrin deposits that form within small vessels. *Plasmin*, or fibrinolysin, is a proteolytic enzyme that is generated from plasminogen, a larger, precursor molecule. Plasmin can cleave various proteins, but it has a particular affinity for fibrin. Plasmin degrades fibrin and dissolves the clot.

```
          Plasminogen activators      Inactivators
                   |                        |
                   ↓                        ↓
Plasminogen ────────────→ Plasmin ────────────→ Inactive enzyme
                                      |
                                      ↓
            Fibrin ────────────→ Fibrin split products
                                 Fibrin peptides
```

Control mechanisms for fibrinolysis are important for both limitation of clot formation and for removal of formed clots. One control mechanism is the expression of plasminogen activator on the surface of the endothelium and on circulating blood cells (Fig. 37-5). Plasminogen activator is normally inhibited by a control protein but becomes effective when it contacts fibrin within a clot or along the vessel wall.

FIG. 37-5 *Fibrinolysis is localized in consolidating thrombus. There plasminogen, bound to fibrin and to platelets, is activated by fibrin-bound tissue plasminogen activator, with local release of plasmin.*

From Del Zoppo, G.J., and Harker, L.A.: Hosp. Pract. **19**(5):163, 1984.

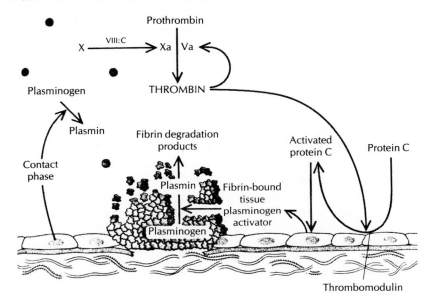

Plasmin is usually activated within a thrombus in which concentrations of inhibitors are low. Thus endogenous plasmin is responsible for restoration of patency in occluded vessels. There are several naturally occurring inhibitors of plasminogen activator in blood and tissues that prevent inappropriate action of plasminogen. Plasmin released in circulation is neutralized immediately by circulating inactivators.

Thrombolytic therapy is based on the need for rapid dissolution of clots that can cause significant morbidity or mortality. Administration of either streptokinase or urokinase can activate the fibrinolytic system by stimulating conversion of plasminogen to plasmin.[12] In addition, endogenous tissue plasminogen activator is important for continuous control of fibrinolysis in normal blood.

Streptokinase   Streptokinase (Kabikinase, Streptase) is an enzyme produced by certain strains of streptococci. It activates plasminogen by a nonenzymatic alteration in the conformation of the molecule. It is a foreign protein, and most problems with this agent, other than bleeding, result from its antigenicity. Many people have antibodies to streptokinase from previous infections with streptococci. These antibodies can cause hypersensitivity reactions, and they can also neutralize infused streptokinase to decrease its fibrinolytic effect.

Urokinase (Abbokinase) was originally isolated from human urine. It is produced *Urokinase*
by the human kidney and is thus not antigenic in man, but some preparations may
be pyrogenic because of contaminating substances. Urokinase activates plasminogen
directly through an enzymatic mechanism. It is highly effective but very expensive.
Urokinase is now obtained from cultures of human kidney cells, but the cost of a
course of therapy remains high.

TPA is the most recent thrombolytic agent. It has been used as an alternative to *Tissue plasminogen*
streptokinase in evolving myocardial infarction. TPA forms a complex with fibrin, *activator (TPA)*
and the complex converts inactive plasminogen into plasmin within the confines of
the clot. In contrast, streptokinase is less selective. It activates plasminogen in the
circulation as well as at the clot, and the active plasmin degrades fibrinogen and
other proteins in addition to fibrin. Theoretically, this distinction may result in less
risk of bleeding with TPA.

TPA has been isolated from blood and various tissues, including blood vessels.
The amounts that could be purified were too sparse, however, for use as a thrombolytic agent. TPA is now produced through genetically engineered cells in culture,
and its efficacy in arresting an evolving myocardial infarction is under investigation.

The decision to use a thrombolytic agent is based on the definitive diagnosis of *Use*
thromboembolic disease and a careful determination of its severity. Venography or
angiography is required to establish the position of the clot and to estimate its size.
Clinical indications for thrombolytic therapy include acute pulmonary embolism with
hemodynamic instability, extensive deep venous thrombosis, arterial thrombosis,
acute myocardial infarction, and occlusion of access shunts and catheters. Although
the need for clot dissolution is acute, fibrinolytic agents should be used in suspected
pulmonary embolism only after embolism is confirmed by angiography. Since they
act only on newly formed clots, therapy must be prompt. The use of thrombolytic
agents in myocardial infarction is limited to the first 24 to 48 hours. It is believed
that most thrombus dissolution occurs within the first 12 hours of therapy. After that,
the remaining thrombus is resistant to further thrombolysis.

Contraindications to use of thrombolytic agents include the presence of active
internal bleeding, cerebrovascular injury or disease, recent surgery, the need for
further invasive procedures, and bleeding disorders or severe coagulation defects.
In addition, these agents should be avoided during pregnancy and the postpartum
period.

Adverse effects and complications. Bleeding and allergic reactions may occur as
complications of streptokinase and urokinase therapy. Fever and skin reactions occur
in a small percentage of patients receiving streptokinase but are less frequent in
those receiving urokinase. The use of purified TPA may avoid such complications.

REFERENCES

1. Brandt, J.T.: The role of natural coagulation inhibitors in hemostasis, Clin. Lab. Med. 4:245, 1984.
2. Del Zoppo, G.J., and Harker, L.A.: Blood/vessel interaction in coronary disease, Hosp. Pract. 19(5):163, 1984.
3. Deykin, D.: Current status of anticoagulant therapy, Am. J. Med. 72:659, 1982.
4. Frishman, W.H.: Antiplatelet therapy in coronary heart disease, Hosp. Pract. 17(5):73, 1982.
5. Jaques, L.B.: Heparin: an old drug with a new paradigm, Science 206:528, 1979.
6. Lewis, H.D., Jr., Davis, J.W., Archibald, D.G., et al.: Protective effects of aspirin against acute myocardial infarction and death in men with unstable angina, N. Engl. J. Med. 309:396, 1983.
7. Link, K.P.: The anticoagulant from spoiled sweet clover hay, Harvey Lect. 39:162, 1944.
8. Mann, K.G.: The biochemistry of coagulation, Clin. Lab. Med. 4:207, 1984.
9. McGann, M.A., and Triplett, D.A.: Interpretation of antithrombin III activity, Lab. Med. 13:742, 1982.
10. Ramirez-Lassepas, M.: Platelet inhibitors for TIAs: a review of prospective drug trial results, Postgrad. Med. 75(5):52, 1984.
11. Rosenberg, R.D.: The heparin-antithrombin mechanism, Triangle 23:43, 1984.
12. Sharma, G.V.R.K., Cella, G., Parisi, A.F., and Sasahara, A.A.: Thrombolytic therapy, N. Engl. J. Med. 306:1268, 1982.
13. Silver, M.J.: Mechanisms of hemostasis and therapy of thrombosis: new concepts based on the metabolism of arachidonic acid by platelets and endothelial cells, Adv. Pharmacol. Chemother. 18:1, 1981.
14. Triplett, D.A.: The extrinsic system, Clin. Lab. Med. 4:221, 1984.

Chapter 38

Diuretic drugs

Diuretic agents increase renal excretion of solute and water, for the most part by decreasing renal tubular reabsorption of Na^+, Cl^-, and water. Excretion of K^+ and HCO_3^- and to a much lesser extent divalent cations such as Ca^{++} and Mg^{++} may also be increased. Diuretics do not directly affect either glomerular filtration or the action of antidiuretic hormone (ADH) on the distal portion of the nephron.

Reduction in water reabsorption by diuretic drugs is dependent on their ability to increase solute excretion. This reduction in water reabsorption can be accomplished by glomerular ultrafiltration of a substance that the tubules have limited or no ability to reabsorb (an osmotic diuretic) or by a drug that decreases reabsorption of Na^+ and preferably Cl^- (a saluretic agent). The electrolyte more or less carries with it an osmotic equivalent of water, depending on how and where the drug acts. The types of diuretics that will be considered in some detail include (1) osmotic diuretics, (2) organomercurial diuretics, (3) carbonic anhydrase inhibitors that act predominantly in the proximal segment, (4) diuretics that act on the loop of Henle, including those that affect the cortical segment and those that act at both medullary and cortical sites, and (5) antikaliuretic diuretics, which decrease exchange of Na^+ (reabsorption) for K^+ (secretion) in the distal segment of the nephron.

To use a diuretic drug effectively, the status of both renal and extrarenal factors involved in diuresis must be understood.[6] For instance, if glomerular filtration is decreased by disease or a reduction in systemic blood pressure, the amount of filtered sodium may be limiting, and the less diuresis an agent will cause. On the other hand, a diuretic agent may induce only limited diuresis even by normal kidneys if the patient's disease results in avid reabsorption of solute by the tubules as occurs with hypoalbuminemia or heart failure.

GENERAL CONCEPT

The use of diuretic drugs for relief of edema (extravascular accumulation of fluid in tissues) requires an understanding of the factors that influence movement of plasma water from the vascular system to the extravascular space and its return. Salient features of these factors follow:

1. Extracellular-extravascular fluid, plasma, and glomerular ultrafiltrate have essentially the same electrolyte composition (Fig. 38-1). The site of action of a diuretic agent on the renal tubules may seem remote to the site at which edema is evident. However, as the drug inhibits the reabsorption of salt and water, it reduces commensurately the volume of extracellular fluid and ultimately total body water. In

EXTRARENAL ASPECTS

FIG. 38-1 *The concentration of electrolytes essential to water balance is essentially the same in extracellular fluid, plasma, and glomerular ultrafiltrate.*

From Beyer, Karl H., Jr.: *Discovery, development and delivery of new drugs*, Jamaica, N.Y., copyright 1978, Spectrum Publications, Inc., Fig. 2, p. 73; reprinted by permission.

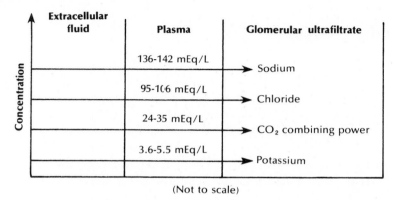

(Not to scale)

other words, the diuresis derives from the intravascular and then the extracellular fluid space.

2. Even seemingly slight changes in hemodynamic forces relating cardiac output to peripheral vascular resistance can profoundly alter the action of diuretics. For instance, simple bed rest and salt restriction in an edematous patient may be sufficient to cause an impressive loss of edema fluid as reflected by a decline in body weight (Fig. 38-2).

3. Either an improvement in the function of a failing heart induced by a cardiotonic agent such as digitalis or inhibition of electrolyte and water reabsorption by a diuretic may increase urine volume and reduce edema. Employed together, the therapeutic efficacy of these two mechanisms is enhanced to an extent neither can cause alone.

4. Diuresis may be unsatisfactory unless the concentration, hence osmotic force, of plasma protein is adequate to return extravascular fluid to the vascular space, thereby sustaining plasma volume and favorably influencing perfusion of renal tubules. As illustrated in Fig. 38-3, frequent transfusions of whole blood or albumin to a hypoproteinemic patient can greatly increase the response to a diuretic agent.

Effect of bed rest and low sodium diet on loss of weight (edema) and sodium in a cirrhotic patient.   **FIG. 38-2**

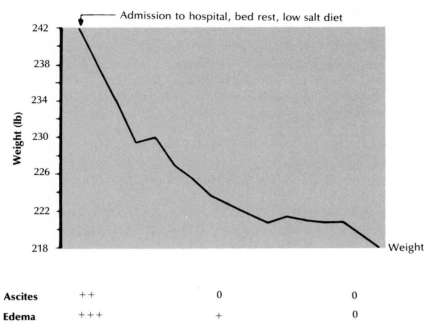

Ascites	++		0	0
Edema	+++		+	0

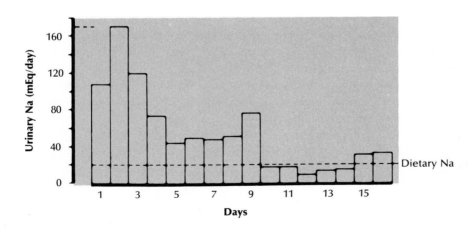

FIG. 38-3 *Effect of intermittent transfusions of whole blood or albumin, or both, on diuretic response to daily oral administration of ethacrynic acid. In the top panel, output (△) and intake (■) of water are depicted relative to each other.*

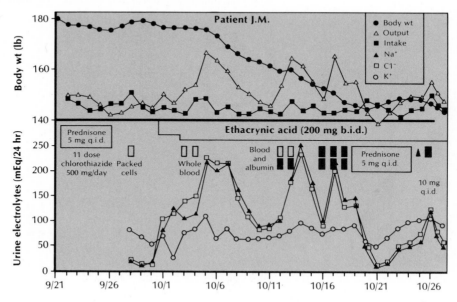

INTRARENAL
ASPECTS

The rate of glomerular ultrafiltration can be increased by plasma volume expansion or increased systemic blood pressure, or both. It can be reduced by decreased systemic arterial pressure or renal afferent arteriolar constriction. Diuretic agents do not affect glomerular filtration directly, though they can have indirect effects. Diuretic-induced volume depletion can increase release of the endogenous vasoconstrictors angiotensin and catecholamines, which in turn decrease glomerular filtration rate and limit the diuresis.

The proximal portion of the renal tubules is responsible for reabsorption of 70% or more of filtered monovalent electrolytes and water.[12,14,21] At the initial portions of the proximal tubule, filtered organic solutes including amino acids and glucose are actively reabsorbed with salt and water following passively.[22] The only diuretics (osmotic) that block this pathway do so indirectly. The proximal tubules actively reabsorb sodium ions in exchange for hydrogen ions (Fig. 38-4). The H^+ is made available by dissociation of $H_2CO_3 \rightleftharpoons H^+ + HCO_3^-$ under the influence of an enzyme, carbonic anhydrase, located on the luminal side of the cell membrane. The H^+ that enters the lumen combines with filtered HCO_3^-:

$$H^+ + HCO_3^- \rightarrow H^+ + OH^- + CO_2$$

The CO_2 then diffuses into the cell where the reverse reaction can occur. The net result is reabsorption of $NaHCO_3$. This exchange can be blocked by suitable carbonic

Diagram of a nephron to illustrate electrolyte and water transport across the cells and the   FIG. 38-4
site or sites of action of some diuretic agents.

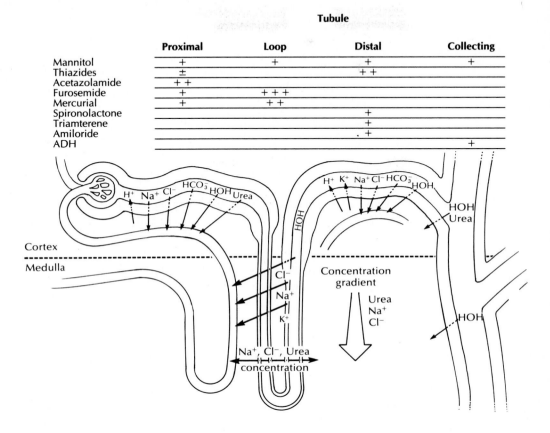

anhydrase inhibitors with a characteristic NH_2SO_2—R structure. Removal of $NaHCO_3$ leaves a favorable concentration gradient for passive Cl^- reabsorption with accompanying Na^+ and water movement to maintain charge and osmotic neutrality.[12] Finally, there also appears to be additional, poorly characterized active Na^+ reabsorption in the proximal tubule. Osmotic diuretics can indirectly inhibit all these pathways. Na^+ and K^+ balance within the cells is sustained by the action of Na^+,K^+-dependent ATPase located at the peritubular border of the cell. Water is not actively reabsorbed but undergoes passive diffusion with the electrolytes so as to maintain an isosmotic relationship. Urea is also substantially reabsorbed proximally, but its transport is even less well understood.

The permeability and physical characteristics of the loop of Henle combine with those of the vasa recta to sustain an increasing concentration gradient of Na^+, Cl^-, and urea from the cortex to the papilla of the medulla[7] (Fig. 38-4). The contributions to this phenomenon of proximity of descending and ascending limbs of the loop and vasa recta are variously explained in terms of the countercurrent multiplier and countercurrent exchange theories of function respectively. Most critical to this concentration gradient of Na^+ and Cl^- is their reabsorption by the thick segment of the ascending limb of the loop, which is impermeable to water. Reabsorption of electrolyte by the thick segment occurs as two Cl^- coupled to one Na^+ and one K^+.[7] It is Cl^- reabsorption that is the determinant. Because this segment is impermeable to water, selective removal of solute occurs, resulting in hypotonic luminal contents; hence this segment is also called the diluting segment. The loop is permeable to diffusion of urea into the interstitium in such a manner that the countercurrent mechanism can sustain the increasing gradient from cortex to inner medulla.

In the distal cortical portion of the tubule, Na^+ undergoes active reabsorption by exchange with H^+ made available by the action of carbonic anhydrase. The H^+ contributes to urine acidification so that little or no HCO_3^- escapes reabsorption, and Cl^- remains as the principal anion excreted. In addition, active reabsorption of Na^+ is facilitated by the action of aldosterone, the hormone of the adrenal cortex that also causes K^+ secretion. Ordinarily, the reabsorption of Na^+ is almost complete at this site.

In the collecting tubules antidiuretic hormone (ADH) facilitates reabsorption of urea and water to the extent of some 99% of the amount filtered. This diffusion of water is driven by the high osmotic gradient of Na^+ and Cl^- in the medulla, to which urea also contributes. If secretion of ADH by the hypothalamus is depressed by alcohol or by a high consumption of water, water reabsorption is prevented and urine flow increases.

OSMOTIC DIURETICS

Mannitol is the prototype osmotic diuretic.[21] Its chemical structure resembles that of glucose. Like glucose it is completely filtered at the glomeruli and is tolerated in large amounts by intravenous injection, but there the resemblance ends. Mannitol is not absorbed to any useful extent when given orally; its distribution in the body is limited to extracellular fluid; and, when filtered, it is not reabsorbed by the renal tubules. Consequently an osmotic equivalent of water passes along the renal tubules with mannitol to increase the volume of urine excreted.

$$\begin{array}{c}
\text{CH}_2\text{OH} \\
|\\
\text{H}-\text{C}-\text{OH} \\
|\\
\text{H}-\text{C}-\text{OH} \\
|\\
\text{HO}-\text{C}-\text{H} \\
|\\
\text{HO}-\text{C}-\text{H} \\
|\\
\text{CH}_2\text{OH}
\end{array}$$

Mannitol

The main use of mannitol, rather than as a diuretic, is to decrease intracranial pressure. Because mannitol increases extracellular osmolality, water is drawn from the intracellular space, and this is useful for treating cerebral edema.[21] On the other hand, the same effect can also be hazardous by expanding intravascular volume and causing hyponatremia (by drawing water into the vascular space). For example, mannitol is not ordinarily employed for reduction of edema associated with heart failure because expansion of the intravascular space in this setting can be disastrous. In such cases a diuretic that acts directly on the tubules to increase salt and water excretion is more desirable.

Mannitol (Osmitrol) is administered intravenously in hypertonic concentrations, greater than 5% and up to 25%, in from 50 to 1000 ml of distilled water. Its duration of action is short (2 or 3 hours) if glomerular filtration rate is normal and depends on mannitol concentration, the volume administered, and the duration of infusion.

Urea and ammonium chloride have also been employed as osmotic diuretics in the past. However, urea is not so effective, mole for mole, since its distribution is not confined to the vascular space. Ammonium chloride causes gastric irritation and induces hyperchloremic acidosis if employed to excess.

In 1920 Saxl and Heilig[15] reported that when syphilitic patients were injected with the antisyphilitic (organomercurial) drug merbaphen, they tended to excrete more urine. Until the 1950s, the organomercurials were the only diuretics that could be relied upon. Today these agents are no longer used. Nevertheless, a general discussion ensues to provide a perspective for modern diuretic therapy.

ORGANO-MERCURIAL DIURETICS

Mercaptomerin sodium

In general, organomercurials were administered intramuscularly. The onset of action was delayed, requiring about 2 hours for maximum effect, and the duration was prolonged (a day or two, depending on dose, edema state, and renal function). Ordinarily, they were administered intermittently, every few days or more frequently if needed.

Typically, organomercurials increased excretion (inhibited reabsorption) of Na^+ and Cl^-. Their effect on K^+ was variable. Water excretion was in excess of electrolyte, an increased *free water clearance*. The mercurials existed in the body and urine as cysteine adducts and were secreted by the proximal tubules by the same active transport system as for *p*-aminohippuric acid and certain other organic acids.

The preponderant action of mercurials was on the thick segment of the loop of Henle, in the manner of loop diuretics (see discussion on loop diuretics, p. 488).

Their effectiveness was enhanced by acidifying agents such as ammonium chloride and was depressed by alkalinization of the urine.

The propensity of these compounds to cause renal tubular damage to the point of necrosis, if administered in too high dosage too frequently, limited their utility. Fortunately, there are safer potent diuretics today that are more convenient to use.

CARBONIC ANHYDRASE INHIBITORS

Shortly after sulfanilamide introduced the modern era of antibiotic chemotherapy (see Chapter 51), it was noted to cause alkaline urine and a metabolic acidosis.[18] Mann and Keilin[10] showed that sulfanilamide inhibited carbonic anhydrase, which is present in the cortex but not the medulla of the kidney. Schwartz[16] in 1949 reported the clinical use of sulfanilamide for relief of edema in decompensated cardiac patients, though increased excretion of HCO_3^- limited its utility. The stage for modern diuretic therapy was set by this report and by Kreb's publication[9] on chemical structure-activity relationships to the effect that (1) irreversible substitution of the sulfamoyl-nitrogen of sulfanilamide destroyed activity, (2) heterocyclic sulfonamides were more active, and (3) acetylation of the *p*-amino group enhanced activity of sulfanilamide.

$$H_2N \!-\!\!\! \bigcirc \!\!\! -\!\! \overset{\overset{\displaystyle O}{\|}}{\underset{\underset{\displaystyle O}{\|}}{S}}\!-\! NH_2$$

Sulfanilamide

The development of diuretics based on carbonic anhydrase inhibition then took two directions: (1) the search for more potent carbonic anhydrase inhibitors as such and (2) the search for carbonic anhydrase inhibitors that would increase Cl^- excretion as the predominant anion with Na^+, a saluretic compound.

Predominantly proximal carbonic anhydrase diuretics

The search for more potent carbonic anhydrase inhibitors culminated in **acetazolamide**,[11] a heterocyclic acetylaminosulfonamide, the clinical utility of which was reported in 1953. Its in vitro activity is about 1000 times greater than that of sulfanilamide; their pharmacodynamic profiles are otherwise similar.

$$H_3C\!-\!\underset{\underset{\displaystyle O}{\|}}{C}\!-\!\underset{\underset{\displaystyle N-N}{}}{NH}\!-\!\!\!\bigcirc\!\!\!-\!\overset{\overset{\displaystyle O}{\|}}{\underset{\underset{\displaystyle O}{\|}}{S}}\!-\!NH_2$$

Acetazolamide

Acetazolamide was the first potent diuretic to be well absorbed and well tolerated when administered orally. It is filtered at the glomeruli and also actively secreted by the proximal renal tubules. It is also reabsorbed; reabsorption is least at alkaline urinary pH.

Typically, acetazolamide increases urinary pH and excretion of Na^+, K^+, HCO_3^-, and water. Little or no Cl^- appears in the urine. Its site of action is primarily the proximal tubules. The increase in K^+ excretion is a compensatory effort by the nephron to conserve (reabsorb) Na^+ more distally in the nephron where Na^+ reabsorption occurs in exchange for K^+.

Acetazolamide (Diamox, Ak-Zol) is available as tablets of 125 and 250 mg and as a 500 mg sustained-release formulation. It is also available for parenteral use in vials containing 500 mg of the cryodesiccated sodium powder.

When acetazolamide is administered as a diuretic, it should be given intermittently to permit recovery of plasma HCO_3^- concentration between doses. Otherwise, continuous therapy soon induces a metabolic (hyperchloremic) acidosis, in which condition acetazolamide becomes ineffective.

In present practice, reduction of intraocular tension in glaucoma is the main indication for carbonic anhydrase inhibitors (see Table 11-1) because more useful diuretics have been developed.

Because of the ubiquitous distribution of carbonic anhydrase in the nervous system, side effects of drugs of this type may include paresthesias, which are reversible on withdrawal of the agent.

Thiazides and related diuretics

Early it was found among sulfanilamide analogs that its *p*-carboxy congener was weakly chloruretic. A long-term search ensued with the description in 1957 of **chlorothiazide,** which predominantly increases excretion of Na^+, Cl^-, and water.[3]

Chlorothiazide and related compounds act from the tubular lumen. They reach this site by secretion at the proximal tubules, and to the extent that they are not bound to plasma albumin they are also filtered at the glomeruli. These agents retain a mild activity to decrease solute reabsorption in the proximal nephron, presumably by inhibiting carbonic anhydrase. However, their predominant effect is a reduction of solute reabsorption in the cortical segment of the thick ascending limb of the loop of Henle by unknown mechanisms, perhaps by inhibition of a Na^+, K^+, two-Cl^- transport pump.[22]

In general, thiazides induce the same maximum natriuretic response regardless of dosage (Fig. 38-5), and their activity is not sensitive to urine pH.

Hypokalemia secondary to increased K^+ excretion can occur. This may manifest as complaints of weakness or fatigue. Patients receiving digitalis are likely to manifest greater sensitivity to digitalis toxicity. Ordinarily, patients with good renal function on a normal diet should not become potassium depleted. In some settings, such as the secondary hyperaldosteronism of heart failure or cirrhosis, sufficient K^+ loss can occur to require treatment.

Hyperuricemia and increased BUN may occur as a manifestation of the phar-

TABLE 38-1   Thiazide diuretics

Name	Structure	Formulation (mg)	Adult daily dose (mg)	Duration of action (hours)
Chlorothiazide (Diuril, others)		T: 250, 500; S: 250/5 ml	250-1000	6-12
Chlorothiazide sodium (Sodium Diuril)		I: 500		
Hydrochlorothiazide (HydroDIURIL, others)		T: 25-100; S: 50, 100/5 ml	25-100	6-12
Bendroflumethiazide (Naturetin)		T: 2.5-10	2 5-15	18-24
Benzthiazide (Aquatag, Exna)		T: 25, 50	50-200	12-18
Cyclothiazide (Anhydron)		T: 2	1-2	18-24
Hydroflumethiazide (Diucardin, others)		T: 50	25-200	18-24
Methyclothiazide (Aquatensen, others)		T: 2.5, 5	2.5-10	24-48

I, Injection (powder for reconstitution); *S*, suspension or solution (oral); *T*, tablets.
*Structurally not thiazides but with virtually identical pharmacology.

TABLE 38-1   Thiazide diuretics—cont'd

Name	Structure	Formulation (mg)	Adult daily dose (mg)	Duration of action (hours)
Polythiazide (Renese)		T: 1-4	1-4	24-48
Trichlormethiazide (Metahydrin, others)		T: 2, 4	2-4	24
Chlorthalidone* (Hygroton, others)		T: 25-100	25-100	24-72
Quinethezone* (Hydromox)		T: 50	2.5-20	12-24
Metolazone* (Diulo, Zaroxolyn)		T: 2.5-10	2.5-20	12-24
Indapamide* (Lozol)		T: 2.5	2.5-5	to 36

FIG. 38-5 *Single-dose response curve for trichlormethiazide, hydrochlorothiazide, and chlorothiazide.*

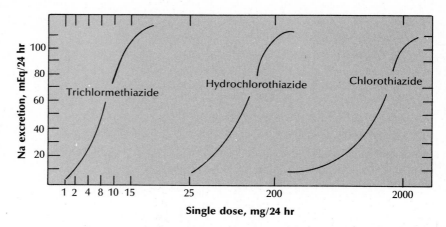

macodynamic effects of these drugs (volume depletion). Impaired glucose tolerance may not be indicative of diabetes in the presence of thiazide therapy.

Since the development of chlorothiazide, numerous analogs that differ only in dose administered and duration of action have been marketed. **Chlorthalidone** and some other agents, though structurally distinct, are pharmacologically indistinguishable from the thiazides. The thiazides are well tolerated and effective when administered orally or parenterally to edematous patients with normal or moderate impairment of renal function. They are also useful alone or as adjuncts to other antihypertensive therapy.

See Table 38-1 for the different thiazide preparations, their doses, formulations, and durations of effect.

LOOP DIURETICS   Current loop diuretics derive from two structural types (other than the organomercurials mentioned previously): (1) sulfonamides, in the instance of **furosemide**[19] and **bumetanide**[20] and (2) a sulfhydryl-reactive agent, **ethacrynic acid**.[5] Both types

Ethacrynic acid

Furosemide

Bumetanide

have severalfold greater efficacy than the thiazides at optimum dosage. All three loop diuretics are well absorbed and active when administered by mouth or intravenously. The loop diuretics are equieffective at optimum dosage.

Their spectrum of electrolyte excretion is essentially the same as for thiazides, but urine volume is likely to be greater and specific gravity less after administration of the loop diuretics. These drugs extend therapy to edematous patients that may not be adequately controlled by thiazides.[6]

These compounds are secreted by the proximal segment of the renal tubules.[13] Since more than 95% of drug in the plasma is bound to albumin, their glomerular filtration is negligible. Their principal site of action is the thick segment of the loop of Henle (both medullary and cortical segments), hence their designation as *loop diuretics*. They act from the luminal side of the tubule; thus secretion by the proximal nephron is essential for their effectiveness.[13] Reduced renal function prolongs the action of these drugs by slowing their entry into the lumen of the tubule.

Loop diuretics reduce or abolish the osmotic gradient of the medulla by inhibiting reabsorption of two Cl^- coupled with one Na^+ and one K^+ at the thick segment of the ascending limb.[2,4,7,8] Whereas the thiazides act predominantly in the cortical segment of the thick limb and do not affect the medullary concentration gradient, all loop diuretics decrease Na^+, Cl^-, and urea gradients in the medulla as well. In so doing, these drugs decrease the osmotic force responsible for water reabsorption from the collecting duct to an extent that cannot be overcome by the facilitatory effect of ADH. Consequently these compounds decrease the ability to concentrate urine. Since the thiazides do not affect the medullary concentration gradient, they do not depress water reabsorption as the loop diuretics do.

Because of their impressive activity, these drugs can be lifesaving, as in acute pulmonary edema, or threatening if misused. Like thiazides, they cause hyperuricemia. Furosemide can alter glucose tolerance, but this seems less well established for ethacrynic acid. When employed at high dosage, as in an attempt to prevent acute renal failure, loop diuretics may induce temporary or permanent vestibular dysfunction or loss of hearing.

Except for an equivalent dosage of bumetanide being only one fortieth that of furosemide, and the bioavailability of bumetanide being about 80% compared to 40% for furosemide, the two drugs seem essentially the same with respect to effects on electrolyte and water excretion, oral efficacy, duration of action, and side effects.

Furosemide (Lasix) is supplied as 20 to 80 mg tablets and as oral and intravenous solutions in various sizes with 10 mg/ml. Ethacrynic acid (Edecrin) is available as 25 and 50 mg tablets. Intravenous ethacrynate sodium is a dry white powder supplied in vials equivalent to 50 mg of ethacrynic acid. Bumetanide (Bumex) is supplied as 0.5 and 1.0 mg tablets. It is also available in sterile solution for intravenous or intramuscular administration as a 2 ml ampule containing 0.25 mg/ml.

ANTIKALIURETIC (POTASSIUM-SPARING) AGENTS

The saluretic diuretic agents discussed to this point cause a concomitant increase in K^+ excretion. Efforts to discover diuretics that would increase Na^+ excretion by inhibiting its exchange with K^+ in the distal convoluted tubule have resulted in two classes of antikaliuretic agents: (1) aldosterone antagonists and (2) agents that act directly to inhibit Na^+ reabsorption and secondary K^+ secretion.

Aldosterone antagonists

Spironolactone is the only available antagonist of aldosterone. It may be administered orally. A parenteral dosage form is not marketed in the United States.

Aldosterone   **Spironolactone**

As an aldosterone antagonist, spironolactone is most effective in settings where enhancement of Na^+ reabsorption and increased K^+ excretion induced by aldosterone are greatest, namely, cirrhosis of the liver, aldosterone-secreting tumors, and high-renin hypertension. It is not active in adrenalectomized animals.[17] The effect of the drug is sustained but slow to develop and is not so great as for other categories of saluretic agents. The spectrum of saluretic effect is one of increased Na^+ and Cl^- and reduced K^+ excretion. Water excretion is isotonic.

Side effects relate to both mode of action and to the chemistry of progestational hormones from which spironolactone was developed. Perhaps the most common undesirable effect is hyperkalemia from excessive K^+ retention. Spironolactone is related to progesterone, which had been observed to have aldosterone antagonist activity. Although spironolactone is at most very weakly progestational, it can cause gynecomastia, which may or may not be reversible. Spironolactone has been reported to be tumorigenic in chronic toxicity studies in rats.

Spironolactone (Aldactone) is supplied as 25 to 100 mg tablets.

Directly acting antikaliuretic agents

Presently, two directly acting antikaliuretic agents are available: **triamterene** and **amiloride**.[1] They are administered orally.

Triamterene   **Amiloride**

Unlike spironolactone, these basic compounds promptly inhibit Na^+ reabsorption and K^+ secretion in the distal cortical segment of the nephron. They are effective regardless of aldosterone status. This tends to make them more reliable than spironolactone.

These agents are filtered at the glomeruli and are secreted by the organic base transport system of the proximal convoluted tubules. This is essential to their activity, for they are effective only when presented to their distal site of action from the luminal side of the tubule.

Amiloride is the more potent of these compounds.[1] Both are inherently less active than thiazides because of the lesser magnitude of sodium reabsorption in the distal nephron.

These compounds are well tolerated except that their propensity to retain K^+ can result in hyperkalemia. Their saluretic, antikaliuretic characteristics make them natural adjuncts to thiazide therapy. The different modes of action of the two types of compounds (these and the thiazides) make their combined saluretic effects additive or even synergistic, whereas their qualitatively opposite actions on K^+ excretion summate to offset the risk of changes in K^+ concentration. This has resulted in the availability of several thiazide plus amiloride or triamterene combined formulations. Although the basic rationale for combining a loop diuretic with one of these agents is the same as for thiazides, the greater difference in potency and duration of action between the loop and antikaliuretic drugs has precluded such a formulation (from a practical standpoint).

Triamterene (Dyrenium) is supplied as 50 and 100 mg capsules. Amiloride (Midamor) is available as the hydrochloride in 5 mg tablets.

REFERENCES

1. Baer, J.E., Jones, C.B., Spitzer, S.A., and Russo, H.F.: The potassium-sparing and natriuretic activity of N-amidino-3,5-diamino-6-chloropyrazinecarboxamide hydrochloride dihydrate (amiloride hydrochloride), J. Pharmacol. Exp. Ther. **157**:472, 1967.

2. Beermann, B., and Groschinsky-Grind, M.: Clinical pharmacokinetics of diuretics, Clin. Pharmacokinet. **5**:221, 1980.

3. Beyer, K.H., Jr., and Baer, J.E.: The site and mode of action of some sulfonamide-derived diuretics, Med. Clin. North Am. **59**:735, 1975.

4. Burg, M.B.: Tubular chloride transport and the mode of action of some diuretics, Kidney Int. **9**:189, 1976.

5. Burg, M., and Green, N.: Effect of ethacrynic acid on the thick ascending limb of Henle's loop, Kidney Int. **4**:301, 1973.

6. Frazier, H.S., and Yager, H.: The clinical use of diuretics, N. Engl. J. Med. **288**:246 and 455, 1973.

7. Hebert, S.C., and Andreoli, T.E.: Control of NaCl transport in the thick ascending limb, Am. J. Physiol. **246**:F745, 1984.

8. Jacobson, H.R., and Kokko, J.P.: Diuretics: sites and mechanisms of action, Annu. Rev. Pharmacol. Toxicol. **16**:201, 1976.

9. Krebs, H.A.: Inhibition of carbonic anhydrase by sulphonamides, Biochem. J. **43**:525, 1948.

10. Mann, T., and Keilin, D.: Sulphanilamide as a specific inhibitor of carbonic anhydrase, Nature [Lond.] **146**:164, 1940.

11. Maren, T.H.: Carbonic anhydrase: chemistry, physiology, and inhibition, Physiol. Rev. **47**:595, 1967.

12. Neumann, K.H., and Rector, F.C., Jr.: Mechanism of NaCl and water reabsorption in the proximal convoluted tubule of rat kidney: role of chloride concentration gradients, J. Clin. Invest. **58**:1110, 1976.

13. Odlind, B.: Relation between renal tubular secretion and effects of five loop diuretics, J. Pharmacol. Exp. Ther. **211**:238, 1979.

14. Rector, F.C., Jr.: Sodium, bicarbonate, and chloride absorption by the proximal tubule, Am. J. Physiol. **244**:F461, 1983.

15. Saxl, P., and Heilig, R.: Ueber die diuretische Wirkung von Novasurol- und anderen Quecksilberinjektionen, Wien. Klin. Wochenschr. **33**:943, 1920.

16. Schwartz, W.B.: The effect of sulfanilamide on salt and water excretion in congestive heart failure, N. Engl. J. Med. **240**:173, 1949.

17. Seller, R.H., Swartz, C.D., Ramirez-Muxo, O., et al.: Aldosterone antagonists in diuretic therapy: their effect on the refractory phase, Arch. Intern. Med. **113**:350, 1964.

18. Southworth, H.: Acidosis associated with the administration of para-amino-benzene-sulfonamide (Prontylin), Proc. Soc. Exp. Biol. Med. **36**:58, 1937.

19. Suki, W., Rector, F.C., Jr., and Seldin, D.W.: The site of action of furosemide and other sulfonamide diuretics in the dog, J. Clin. Invest. **44**:1458, 1965.

20. Tuzel, I.H., editor: Perspectives on bumetanide (symposium), J. Clin. Pharmacol. **21**(11 and 12, Part 2), 1981.

21. Warren, S.E., and Blantz, R.C.: Mannitol, Arch. Intern. Med. **141**:493, 1981.

22. Windhager, E.E., and Giebisch, G.: Proximal sodium and fluid transport, Kidney Int. **9**:121, 1976.

Chapter 39

Pharmacologic approaches to atherosclerosis

Both clinical and experimental research indicate a probable causal relationship between hyperlipidemia and arterial disease. The incorporation of lipids from blood (triglyceride, phospholipids, and cholesterol) into the arterial wall to form the lesions of *atherosclerosis* can lead to coronary artery disease, myocardial infarction, and occlusion of cerebral and peripheral arteries. Although it is recognized that other factors, such as vessel wall injury, also contribute to the pathologic process, the rationale for reducing concentrations of circulating blood lipids is that high concentrations of cholesterol-rich lipoproteins can accelerate atherosclerosis.

There are several drugs that lower abnormally elevated serum lipoproteins by reducing their production or enhancing their removal. *Clofibrate* and *gemfibrozil* inhibit release of lipoproteins from the liver and also inhibit cholesterol biosynthesis. *Cholestyramine* and *colestipol* are resins that bind bile acids and prevent their absorption. *Nicotinic acid* decreases secretion of very-low-density lipoprotein (VLDL) and consequently synthesis of low-density lipoprotein (LDL) cholesterol. *Probucol* reduces LDL and high-density lipoprotein (HDL) cholesterol and apolipoprotein A-I. None of these drugs is completely satisfactory, but when used in combination with dietary control of lipid intake and treatment of concomitant disease (hypertension, diabetes, hypothyroidism) or elimination of other significant risk factors (smoking, high alcohol intake), they may reduce development of atherosclerotic lesions.

Pathogenesis of atherosclerosis

Many factors are believed to contribute to development of atherosclerosis. A recent concept is that atherosclerotic lesions develop subsequent to an inflammatory insult. It has also been proposed that factors from adherent platelets stimulate the growth of smooth muscle cells. The exact mechanisms are still not clear, but formation of atherosclerotic plaques probably involves both inflammatory cells and growth factors.[13] The rationale for lowering plasma lipids is that some of the cellular events appear to be influenced by high concentrations of plasma cholesterol.

Lipoproteins and lipid transport

The two major indices used to assess hyperlipoproteinemias are blood cholesterol and triglyceride concentrations.[7] These lipids are transported in the blood in *lipoproteins*. The lipoproteins consist of macromolecular assemblies of lipids and specialized *apolipoproteins* that function as recognition sites for interactions of lipopro-

FIG. 39-1   *All plasma lipoproteins are spherical particles consisting of a disorganized core of tri-glycerides and cholesterol esters surrounded by a thin lipid monolayer of cholesterol and phospholipid. Apolipoproteins are embedded in the surface lipid shell, with their hydro-phobic domains oriented toward the core and their hydrophilic domains oriented outwards. This configuration is highly stable and facilitates the solubilization of these microdroplets of nonpolar lipids.*

From Weinberg, R.B.: Lipoprotein metabolism: hormonal regulation, Hosp. Pract. 22(6):223, 1987; this illustration was drawn by Alan Iselin, New York, N.Y.

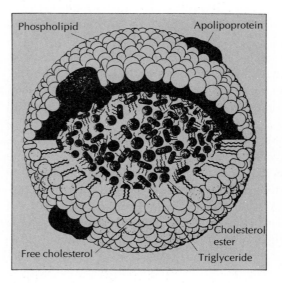

teins with tissues.[16] There are several kinds of lipoproteins, which vary in size and density, but all are spherical particles with a lipid core. The apoproteins and phospholipids that surround the core control the interactions and eventual fate of the particle (Fig. 39-1).

When dietary fat is absorbed from the intestine, it is incorporated into the largest of the lipoprotein particles, the *chylomicrons*, which are formed in the intestinal mucosal cells. These particles are composed primarily of triglycerides and apoproteins A, B, C, and E. Once in the circulation, the chylomicrons are catabolized by the action of *lipoprotein lipase* associated with vessel walls. The free fatty acids released from the triglycerides enter the metabolic pool or are stored as fat.[12] The chylomicron *remnants* are then taken up by cells in the liver, broken down further, and used for synthesis of triglycerides.

Classes of lipoproteins can be separated by analytic methods on the basis of size and density. They range in diameter from 5 nm to more than 500 nm. The larger the particle, the greater is its lipid content and the lower its density.[11] Fig. 39-2 indicates the relative size and density of the lipoproteins. The continuous re-

Relative densities of the lipoproteins as they would appear on ultracentrifugation, along with their physical dimensions. The largest are the least dense because they have the highest lipid content, which weighs less than protein.

From Kreisberg, R.A.: Consultant 23:197, Oct. 1983.

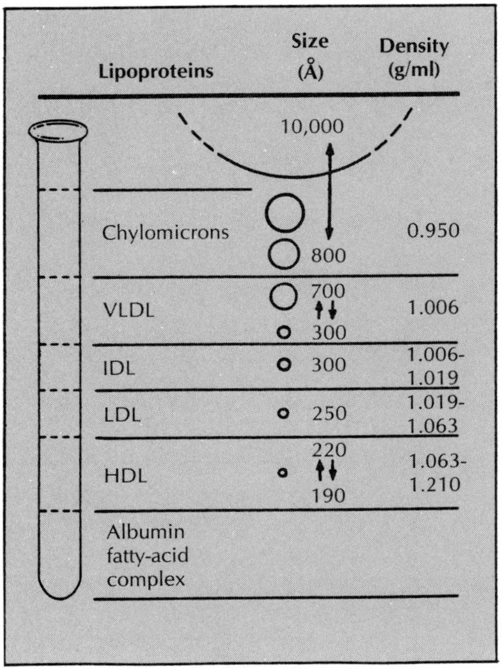

FIG. 39-2

Lipoproteins	Size (Å)	Density (g/ml)
	10,000	
Chylomicrons	800	0.950
VLDL	700 / 300	1.006
IDL	300	1.006–1.019
LDL	250	1.019–1.063
HDL	220 / 190	1.063–1.210
Albumin fatty-acid complex		

moval of free fatty acids from the triglyceride core results in an increasingly dense particle.

The very-low-density lipoproteins (VLDL) are triglyceride-rich particles formed in the liver. These particles, which are smaller than chylomicrons, function as the major form of transport for endogenously synthesized triglycerides. They contain some cholesterol as well. As the VLDL circulate they are degraded by lipoprotein lipase, and triglycerides are removed. The remaining apoproteins, phospholipids, and cholesterol form a particle of intermediate density, the IDL. With further removal of triglycerides, the smaller, cholesterol-rich low-density lipoprotein (LDL) is formed. These particles are destined for peripheral tissues and the liver. High-density lipoproteins (HDL) are small lipoproteins, formed in the intestine, liver, and vascular tissue, that transport cholesterol from peripheral tissues to the liver where it is either excreted or processed into bile salts. Fig. 39-3 shows the schema for removal and transport of fats in lipoproteins. Table 39-1 summarizes the classes and functions of the plasma lipoproteins.

LDL contains the major portion of plasma cholesterol and is believed to be the

FIG. 39-3   *Schema for origin and removal of lipids and lipoproteins.*

From Kuske, T.T., and Feldman, E.B.: Arch. Intern. Med. **147**:*357, copyright 1987, American Medical Association.*

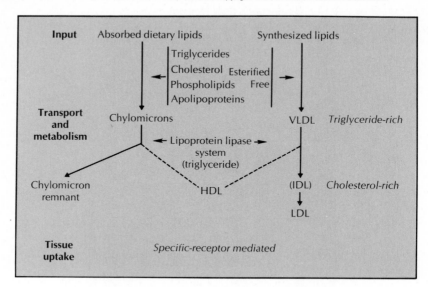

TABLE 39-1   Classes of plasma lipoproteins

	Origin	Major apolipoproteins	Core lipids	Function	Destination
Chylomicrons	Intestine	Apo B, apo C, apo E	Triglycerides	Transport of dietary triglyceride	Triglyceride storage cells, triglyceride metabolizing cells, liver
Very-low-density lipoproteins (VLDL)	Liver (intestine)	Apo B, apo C, apo E	Triglycerides (cholesterol esters)	Transport of endogenously synthesized triglyceride (and some cholesterol)	Triglyceride storage cells, triglyceride metabolizing cells
Low-density lipoproteins (LDL)	Intravascular metabolism of VLDL	Apo B	Cholesterol esters	Transport of cholesterol esters of hepatic and intravascular origin	Peripheral cells (liver)
High-density lipoproteins (HDL)	Intestine, liver, intravascular metabolic reactions	Apo A-I, apo A-II	Cholesterol esters	"Reverse" transport of cholesterol of peripheral origin	Liver, steroidogenic tissues

Modified from Weinberg, R.B.: Lipoprotein metabolism: hormonal regulation, Hosp. Pract. **22**(6):223, 1987.

Route of the low-density-lipoprotein (LDL) receptor in mammalian cells. The receptor be- **FIG. 39-4**
gins life in the endoplasmic reticulum from which it travels to the Golgi complex, cell
surface, coated pit, and endosome and back to the surface. Vertical arrows, *Direction of*
regulatory effects.

From Brown, M.S., and Goldstein, J.L.: Curr. Top. Cell Regul. 26:3, 1985.

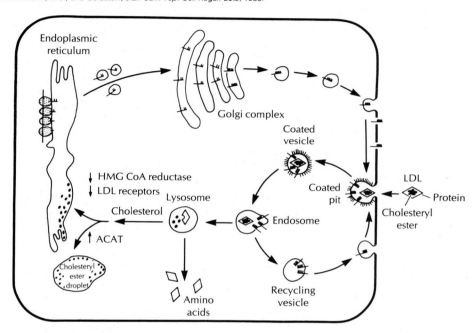

most harmful lipoprotein because risk of coronary disease correlates directly with high concentrations of LDL.[11]

The apolipoproteins associated with circulating lipoproteins are particularly important. Many of the 13 identified apolipoproteins affect lipoprotein metabolism by acting as enzyme cofactors, inhibitors, or receptors.[6] For example, apo C-II is an activator of lipoprotein lipase.[12] Apolipoproteins also function as ligands for cell receptors, directing uptake of lipoprotein particles by the liver and other tissues. Genetic deficiencies of apolipoproteins have been described and related to disorders of lipid metabolism.

The regulation of cholesterol in blood depends largely on the disposition of LDL; elevation of plasma cholesterol is usually attributable to increased LDL.[1] LDL receptors in tissues intercept circulating LDL and carry it into cells by receptor-mediated endocytosis (Fig. 39-4). Cholesterol, in the form of cholesteryl esters, is used by the cell for synthesis of plasma membranes, bile acids, or steroid hormones. The liver contains the highest number of LDL receptors, but they are found on many different types of cells.

Regulation of
cholesterol through
LDL receptors

The number of LDL receptors expressed at the cell surface is a key control mechanism for plasma cholesterol. When LDL receptors are saturated, the removal of LDL is proportional to the number of receptors. LDL receptors are continuously recycled. Once the complex is within the cell, a decrease in intracellular pH dissociates LDL from its receptor, and the receptor returns to the cell surface. A reduced number of receptors results in elevated plasma LDL. A second important function of LDL receptors is suppression of cholesterol synthesis in the liver. After LDL is internalized, the core cholesteryl esters are hydrolyzed by an acid lipase. The free cholesterol inhibits activity of 3-hydroxy-3-methylglutaryl (HMG) CoA reductase, the rate-limiting enzyme in cholesterol synthesis, and suppresses the expression of LDL receptors at the cell surface. Thus the LDL receptor controls not only uptake of cholesterol in the form of LDL but also its synthesis. LDL receptors can also bind IDL, the precursor of LDL, thus effectively limiting generation of circulating LDL.[1]

One genetic factor in man linked to enhanced risk for atherosclerosis is a defect of LDL receptors. A deficiency of LDL receptors is the basis of familial hypercholesterolemia, a genetic disease in which there are very high concentrations of circulating cholesterol and an increased incidence of myocardial infarction. There are four subgroups of this genetic defect, and 10 different mutations have been defined. All result in defective binding of LDL to cells.[1]

High-density lipoproteins	HDL plays an important role in both metabolism of lipoproteins and their transport. HDL is a heterogeneous group of particles that consist of a core of apolar cholesterol ester and triglyceride enveloped by a shell of specific apoproteins and phospholipids. One important function of these particles is to bind free cholesterol.[2] It is generally accepted that the extracellular concentrations of LDL and HDL regulate the concentration of cellular cholesterol. LDL transports cholesterol from the liver and gastrointestinal tract to peripheral tissues, and HDL removes cholesterol from cells and transports it back to the liver, which is the only organ that can efficiently catabolize and excrete cholesterol.[14] Apoprotein C-II is a minor component of HDL, but it has an important function, the activation of lipoprotein lipase, which catabolizes VLDL and chylomicrons. The catabolic fragments can pick up free cholesterol from tissues and convert it to cholesteryl ester. Apoprotein A-I activates lecithin cholesterol acetyl transferase (LCAT), which is required for esterification of cholesterol and transport by HDL.
THERAPY OF HYPERLIPIDEMIA *Therapeutic implications for receptor regulation*	The regulation of LDL is of obvious concern in therapy of hyperlipidemias. There are no selective means of controlling LDL formation, but factors such as heredity, sex hormones, diet, and exercise are believed to be important. One way to lower plasma cholesterol would be to increase the number of LDL receptors in the liver, the major site of LDL receptor expression. A diet high in fat reduces the number of LDL receptors.[1] A decrease in fat intake would thus aid in maintaining LDL receptor number.

An alternative strategy is to inhibit intestinal absorption of bile acids. Since the liver must continually synthesize bile acids from cholesterol, the demand for cholesterol uptake and thus the need for LDL receptors increase. However, this approach has limited efficacy because the liver then increases its HMG-CoA reductase activity in an attempt to enhance cholesterol synthesis.

A more effective strategy is to inhibit hepatic cholesterol synthesis directly by blockade of HMG-CoA reductase. This results in a complex regulatory adjustment that lowers plasma LDL-cholesterol through synthesis of new LDL receptors. **Lovastatin** (Mevacor; formerly called mevinolin), a competitive inhibitor of HMG-CoA reductase, is used in patients who are heterozygous for familial hypercholesterolemia. When administered with inhibitors of bile acid reabsorption, it can cause an even greater lowering of plasma cholesterol. Most patients are helped by this combined therapy. Neither of these therapeutic interventions works, however, with homozygotes because they lack LDL receptors and the attendant regulatory mechanisms controlled by LDL receptors.

Clofibrate is hydrolyzed during gastrointestinal absorption to the active compound chlorophenoxyisobutyric acid (CPIB). The resulting anion is transported in plasma bound largely to albumin. It is particularly effective in lowering serum triglycerides and less so cholesterol, presumably by enhancing activity of lipoprotein lipase, which increases clearance of VLDL.[5] Gemfibrozil, a newer, structurally related agent, also inhibits secretion of VLDL from the liver.[10] These agents are effective in treatment of familial dysbetalipoproteinemia (hyperlipidemia, type III) and may reduce LDL concentration in mild hypercholesterolemia. Moderate increases in HDL cholesterol are reported in some patients with hypertriglyceridemia, but this does not occur in most persons with normal concentrations of triglycerides.

Clofibrate and gemfibrozil

Clofibrate

Gemfibrozil

Despite reduction of body cholesterol pools, the effect of clofibrate on coronary events is still debatable. Primary prevention trials produced equivocal results and indicate that there may be increased risk of gastrointestinal malignancy, cholelithiasis, and pancreatitis.[8] Clofibrate decreases clearance of coumarin anticoagulants so that its use requires downward adjustment of anticoagulant dosage. Other side effects of clofibrate include myopathy, gastrointestinal disturbances, and decreased libido. Because of the potential for myopathy and because it is eliminated by the kidney, clofibrate is not used in patients with impaired renal function.

Clofibrate (Atromid-S) and gemfibrozil (Lopid) are available as 500 and 300 mg capsules respectively.

Bile acid–binding resins

Cholestyramine (Questran) and colestipol (Colestid) are anion-exchange resins that bind bile acids in the intestinal lumen, in exchange for chloride. Since the resin is not absorbed, it promotes the fecal excretion of bile acids. The liver then increases bile acid synthesis to replace the lost acids. Since cholesterol is the precursor for bile acids, the net result is increased utilization of cholesterol and, usually, a lowering of the plasma concentration. The effectiveness of bile acid–binding resins in lowering plasma LDL cholesterol concentration appears to depend on the ability of the liver to increase the population of LDL receptors that supply cholesterol.[9] Cholestyramine, which acts by the same mechanism, may be used for relief of pruritus associated with biliary tract obstruction.

Cholestyramine and colestipol are powder and granular preparations respectively that should be mixed with juice or other liquid, allowed to hydrate for a few minutes, and then taken with meals. They are available in bulk or in individual packets containing 4 g of cholestyramine or 5 g of colestipol. One packet of the former is taken up to six times a day; the daily dose of 15 to 30 g of the latter is divided over two to four doses. The major side effects of these preparations are constipation and bloating. They also interfere with absorption of fat-soluble vitamins and numerous drugs (see Table 63-1).

Nicotinic acid

Nicotinic acid (niacin) acts primarily by inhibiting secretion of VLDL without accumulation of triglycerides in the liver.[4] This in turn decreases production of LDL. The drug also inhibits lipolysis in adipose tissue, but this effect may not be sustained with chronic administration.[8] Another pharmacologic effect of nicotinic acid is a decrease in the fractional catabolic rate of HDL, which results in higher concentrations of HDL and apolipoprotein A-I. In one large-scale clinical trial, nicotinic acid was the only agent of those studied that significantly reduced the incidence of coronary events.[9]

The usefulness of nicotinic acid is, however, limited by troublesome side effects. Flushing occurs in practically all patients initially and may persist in some. This side effect appears to be prostaglandin mediated and can be blocked by pretreatment with aspirin. Activation of peptic ulcer and hepatic dysfunction are toxic effects that can occur with large doses. Although nicotinic acid is available in tablets of 20 to 500 mg and in timed-release capsules of 125 to 500 mg, only the larger sizes are useful for treating hyperlipidemia; the usual dosage is 1 to 2 g three times daily. To minimize side effects, patients begin taking small doses and gradually increase the amount. Occasionally nicotinic acid is used in combination with bile acid–binding resins.[5]

Probucol

Probucol (Lorelco) is a cholesterol-lowering agent that is unrelated chemically to other lipid-lowering drugs. It is believed to increase uptake of LDL by receptor-*independent* pathways.[15] It reduces serum cholesterol concentration in laboratory animals by inhibiting cholesterol synthesis.[3] It has also been shown to increase fecal excretion of bile acids in some human studies. Patients treated with probucol dem-

TABLE 39-2 Nondietary treatment of primary hyperlipidemias	
Disorder	Drugs
Monogenic or oligogenic	
Familial hypercholesterolemia	
Heterozygous	Resin + nicotinic acid*
	Resin + neomycin
Homozygous	Resin + nicotinic acid
Familial multiple hyperlipoproteinemia	
Elevated LDL	Resin, nicotinic acid, or combination
Elevated VLDL	Nicotinic acid or clofibrate
Elevated VLDL + LDL	Resin, nicotinic acid, or combination
Familial hypertriglyceridemia	
Mild	Clofibrate or nicotinic acid
Severe (with chylomicronemia)	Nicotinic acid*
Familial dysbetalipoproteinemia	Clofibrate (small doses)*
	Nicotinic acid
Familial lipoprotein lipase or apolipoprotein C-II deficiency	None
Other	
Polygenic or unclassified hypercholesterolemia	Resin*
	Nicotinic acid or clofibrate
Sporadic or unclassified hypertriglyceridemia	Clofibrate or nicotinic acid

Modified from Havel, R.J., and Kane, J.P.: Annu. Rev. Med. **33**:417, copyright 1982, reproduced with permission from Annual Reviews, Inc.
*Drug of choice.

onstrate reductions in both LDL and HDL cholesterol. Since HDL is believed to exert a protective effect in terms of atherosclerotic disease, a reduced concentration could theoretically be detrimental. Serious cardiotoxicity has been demonstrated in animal studies.[8] Consequently, the use of probucol in treatment of hypercholesterolemia appears to be limited. The drug is taken as 250 mg tablets.

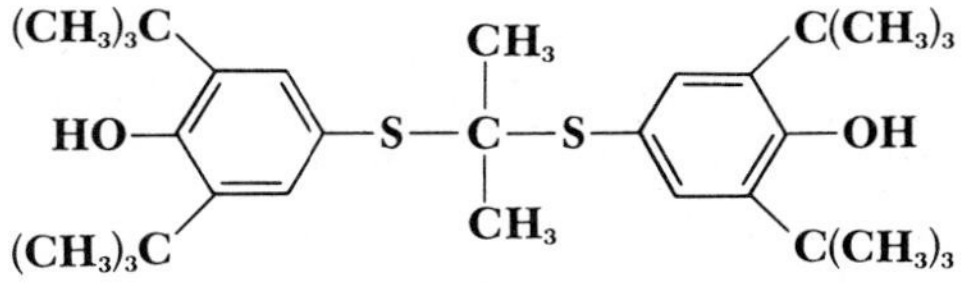

Probucol

Combined drug regimens

    Certain combinations of drugs are more effective than the individual agents, indicative of complementary mechanisms. For example, nicotinic acid administered with cholestyramine or colestipol is more effective than either agent alone. The combination of a bile acid–binding resin with an HMG-CoA reductase inhibitor lowers LDL concentration into the normal range in patients with heterozygous familial hypercholesterolemia or familial multiple hyperlipidemia.[8] Table 39-2 lists some of the combinations used to treat hyperlipidemias.

DIETARY MODIFICATION AND EXERCISE

It is now recognized that a diet rich in fats is associated with development of atherosclerosis. Sustained elevation of triglycerides and cholesterol in the blood indicates a need for dietary modification and possibly for drug therapy. Alteration of a traditionally atherogenic diet is, however, a first step in therapy of hyperlipidemia. Other measures include the correction of ongoing metabolic defects; for example, hyperlipidemia is a common accompaniment of diabetes.

Saturated animal fats contain large amounts of cholesterol. A diet rich in these fats will increase blood cholesterol, whereas substitution by polyunsaturated fats tends to lower cholesterol and triglyceride concentrations. Removal of refined sugars from the diet and substitution of complex carbohydrates is also beneficial. Some studies indicate that increased fiber content in the diet aids in lipid reduction. The mechanism is believed to involve trapping and elimination of cholesterol (in the form of bile acids) within the intestinal contents.[12]

The first goal of any dietary regimen, however, is maintenance of ideal body weight. Obesity is an additional risk factor for cardiovascular disease. To this end, exercise combined with caloric restriction tends to shift the ratio of LDL to HDL to a more favorable setting (reduced LDL and increased HDL). Even when combined with drug therapy, dietary counseling and supervision will play an important role in management of hyperlipidemia.

REFERENCES

1. Brown, M.S., and Goldstein, J.L.: A receptor-mediated pathway for cholesterol homeostasis, Science 232:34, 1986.
2. Glomset, J.A.: High-density lipoproteins in human health and disease, Adv. Intern. Med. 25:91, 1980.
3. Glueck, C.J.: Colestipol and probucol: treatment of primary and familial hypercholesterolemia and amelioration of atherosclerosis, Ann. Intern. Med. 96:475, 1982.
4. Grundy, S.M., Mok, H.Y.I., Zech, L., and Berman, M.: Influence of nicotinic acid on metabolism of cholesterol and triglycerides in man, J. Lipid Res. 22:24, 1981.
5. Havel, R.J., and Kane, J.P.: Therapy of hyperlipidemic states, Annu. Rev. Med. 33:417, 1982.
6. Hoeg, J.M., Gregg, R.E., and Brewer, H.B., Jr.: An approach to the management of hyperlipoproteinemia, J.A.M.A. 255:512, 1986.
7. Illingworth, D.R.: Lipid-lowering drugs: an overview of indications and optimum therapeutic use, Drugs 33:259, 1987.
8. Kane, J.P., and Havel, R.J.: Treatment of hypercholesterolemia, Annu. Rev. Med. 37:427, 1986.
9. Kane, J.P., and Malloy, M.J.: Treatment of hypercholesterolemia, Med. Clin. North Am. 66:537, 1982.
10. Kesäniemi, Y.A., and Grundy, S.M.: Influence of gemfibrozil and clofibrate on metabolism of cholesterol and plasma triglycerides in man, J.A.M.A. 251:2241, 1984.
11. Kreisberg, R.A.: High-density lipoproteins: a 'delicate balance' helps the HDL help us to prevent CHD, Consultant 23:197, Oct. 1983.
12. Kuske, T.T., and Feldman, E.B.: Hyperlipoproteinemia, atherosclerosis risk, and dietary management, Arch. Intern. Med. 147:357, 1987.
13 Majno, G., Zand, T., Nunnari, J.J., and Joris, I.: The diet/atherosclerosis connection: new insights, J. Cardiovasc. Med. 9:21, 1984.
14. Miller, G.J.: High density lipoproteins and atherosclerosis, Annu. Rev. Med. 31:97, 1980.
15. Naruszewicz, M., Carew, T.E., Pittman, R.C., et al.: A novel mechanism by which probucol lowers low density lipoprotein levels demonstrated in the LDL receptor-deficient rabbit, J. Lipid Res. 25:1206, 1984.
16. Weinberg, R.B.: Lipoprotein metabolism: hormonal regulation, Hosp. Pract. 22(6):223, 1987.

section seven

Drug effects on the respiratory and gastrointestinal tracts

40   *Drug effects on the respiratory tract, 506*

41   *Drug effects on the gastrointestinal tract, 518*

Chapter 40

Drug effects on the respiratory tract

<table>
<tr>
<td>GENERAL
CONCEPT</td>
<td>The respiratory system includes the upper airway passages, the nasal cavities, pharynx, and trachea, as well as the bronchi and bronchioles. Diseases of the respiratory tract range from the common cold to potentially lethal disturbances of respiratory function. Pulmonary disorders may result from an acute insult, such as infection or hypersensitivity reactions, a genetic abnormality, as in cystic fibrosis, or a chronic condition, such as smoking or occupational exposure to chemicals or dusts.</td>
</tr>
</table>

Drug therapy of pulmonary disorders is generally directed toward altering a specific physiologic function. For example, *bronchodilators* relax constricted bronchiolar smooth muscle and open blocked airways; *mucolytic agents* alter the characteristics of respiratory tract fluids; *antibiotics* combat infections; *corticosteroids* reduce inflammation within the respiratory tract. These various agents may be used in combination, particularly with persistent infection or chronic airway disease. In addition, *nasal decongestants,* which constrict dilated vessels of the nasal mucosa, and *antitussive agents,* which reduce coughing, are commonly used by the public in over-the-counter preparations.

DRUGS THAT AFFECT UPPER AIRWAYS
Nasal decongestants

Air entering the nasal passages is warmed and humidified before reaching the lungs. The resistance to airflow within the upper respiratory tract is regulated by autonomic control of vascular smooth muscle within mucosal blood vessels. Nasal congestion, which results from dilatation of mucosal vessels, is a common feature in allergic, viral, and inflammatory conditions. Vasoconstrictors reduce congestion without influencing the underlying cause. The many readily available nasal decongestants act by the same mechanism but vary in duration of action. Direct application to engorged membranes of the nasal passages relieves stuffiness by causing vasoconstriction through α-adrenergic mechanisms. Examples of commonly used drugs are phenylephrine, ephedrine, pseudoephedrine, propylhexadrine, and oxymetazoline. The pharmacology of this class of drugs is discussed in detail in Chapter 15.

USE

Nasal decongestants provide temporary relief of nasal stuffiness associated with acute rhinitis of viral or allergic origin. The addition of other chemicals, including preservatives, antihistamines, antibiotics, or anticholinergic drugs, is a common but questionable practice. Antihistamines of the H_1 class are useful in relieving symptoms of an allergic rhinitis but not those of the common cold. Anticholinergic agents are included to diminish nasal secretion, but there is danger of excessive drying and the potential for systemic absorption. There is no justification for inclusion of antibiotics in a decongestant mixture.

Nasal decongestants may be applied topically or taken in an oral preparation. Although the topical form, usually administered as drops or sprays, is convenient and has a rapid onset of action, frequent use can result in rebound vasodilatation. This condition is characterized by chronic swelling of the nasal mucosa and a need to increase the frequency of application of the decongestant. Oral administration can offer a more prolonged action through timed-release preparations but may cause unwanted cardiovascular or central nervous system effects.

Cough remedies

Coughing is a protective mechanism through which foreign materials, irritants, and secretions are cleared from the respiratory tract. Thus complete suppression of coughing is undesirable; however, when coughing is severe and prolonged, it can be painful and exhausting. Cough suppressants depress the cough reflex, which arises from irritated pharyngeal tissues. Mechanical or chemical stimulation of receptors within these tissues initiates impulses that are carried by vagal and glossopharyngeal afferent pathways to a region within the medulla. Efferent pathways from this central cough center are through peripheral nerves to the abdomen, thoracic muscles, and the diaphragm.

MECHANISMS OF ANTITUSSIVE ACTION

Coughing may be inhibited by reduction of the amount of respiratory secretions, elimination of the source of irritation, or decreasing the sensitivity of irritant receptors within the respiratory tract. Some drugs act at one or more of these sites; others act at the medullary cough center to inhibit activation of the efferent limb of the response.

The volume of respiratory secretions can be reduced by anticholinergic agents, such as atropine or scopolamine. These drugs are sometimes used before surgery or intubation, but they are not generally used in treatment of irritated airways because retention of viscous or impacted secretions can worsen asthma or infectious bronchitis. However, ipratropium, a new anticholinergic agent, is beneficial in asthma (see p. 515).

Some antitussive agents have a local anesthetic action. **Benzonatate** (Tessalon) is chemically related to tetracaine. It is believed to act by two mechanisms: the selective anesthesia of stretch receptors within the lungs and central suppression of cough without decreasing respiration.

Other antitussives act primarily through central mechanisms. The opioid compounds codeine and hydrocodone and the synthetic nonopiate derivative dextromethorphan act on the medullary cough center to suppress the efferent limb of the response. The pharmacology of the opioid compounds is discussed in Chapter 29.

Interventions that decrease bronchoconstriction and drying of respiratory secretions will help to reduce the frequency and severity of coughing. For example, mists and vapors that moisturize the airways blunt the reactivity to irritant stimuli. Bronchodilators aid in mobilizing dried or impacted secretions and ultimately relieve a dry, unproductive cough. *Expectorants* and *mucolytic agents* help to remove irritant material from the lower respiratory tract toward the pharynx by increasing the volume and reducing the viscosity of respiratory secretions. Their mode of action is not clearly understood, but some expectorants stimulate secretion reflexly by vagal pathways. **Guaifenesin** (glycerol guaiacolate) and **potassium iodide** or **sodium iodide** solutions are examples of expectorant drugs.

$$O-CH_2-\overset{\overset{\displaystyle OH}{|}}{CH}-CH_2-OH$$

Guaifenesin

Mucolytic agents aid in reducing the viscosity of sputum by depolymerizing mucopolysaccharides into smaller, more soluble molecules. **Acetylcysteine** (Mucomyst) is used as adjunctive therapy of asthma and other diseases in which viscous secretions compromise air exchange. It is usually administered several times daily by nebulization as a 10% solution. Because it releases hydrogen sulfide, acetylcysteine has an unpleasant odor and reacts with rubber and certain metals. It may also irritate the airways to cause rhinorrhea and, possibly, bronchospasm in susceptible persons.

USE   Antitussive agents are used to suppress coughing when the cough is disturbing or debilitating rather than productive. They are frequently used in the common cold or in other acute upper respiratory infections to afford relief from chronic irritation of the airways. They should not be used in patients with acute bronchial asthma because inspissation of mucus may worsen the disease. Often a combination of mucolytic, vapor, and expectorant therapy will suppress coughing. For continuing unproductive and potentially exhausting coughing, however, agents such as codeine or dextromethorphan are indicated. Codeine is sometimes administered in an elixir of terpin hydrate. This vehicle is a volatile oil believed to act on bronchial secretory cells, but the alcohol in the preparation is also an expectorant.

DRUGS THAT AFFECT LOWER AIRWAYS   Bronchoconstriction is an important feature of diseases that affect the lower airways. These include bronchial asthma, acute and chronic bronchitis, viral infections, and, occasionally, bacterial respiratory infections. Bronchoreactivity in these conditions is intimately linked to autonomic innervation and secretory activity of cells along the tracheobronchial tree.[6] The primary therapeutic modalities are administration of bronchodilator drugs and anti-inflammatory steroids, though the mucolytic and expectorant agents may facilitate removal of secretions. When release of mediators from lung mast cells is likely, cromolyn sodium is sometimes effective in *prevention* of bronchospasm, but it does not affect contraction of bronchial smooth muscle.

TABLE 40-1	Drugs that act on bronchial smooth muscle
Cause contraction	Cause relaxation or block contraction
Muscarinic agonists	Muscarinic antagonists
Histamine	H_1 antagonists
β-Adrenergic receptor antagonists	β-Adrenergic receptor agonists
α-Adrenergic receptor agonists	Methylxanthines (theophylline)
Leukotrienes (SRS-A)	Prostaglandin E_2
Prostaglandins D_2 and $F_{2\alpha}$	Prostacyclin (prostaglandin I_2)
Thromboxane A_2	
Kinins	

Pharmacology of bronchial smooth muscle

The entire tracheobronchial tree is invested with smooth muscle to a greater or lessor degree. Bronchial smooth muscle is innervated exclusively by parasympathetic fibers.[9] Parasympathetic stimulation results in bronchoconstriction, whereas adrenergic agonists generally exert a relaxing action through β-adrenergic receptors. There are α-adrenergic receptors, however, that mediate contraction of bronchial smooth muscle. At the molecular level, activation of either cholinergic or α-adrenergic receptors increases the concentration of guanosine 3′,5′-monophosphate (cyclic GMP) via a calcium-dependent cyclase system. These events are associated with muscle contraction through a series of phosphorylation and dephosphorylation steps. By a similar mechanism, enhanced formation of adenosine 3′,5′-monophosphate (cyclic AMP) within bronchial smooth muscle after β-adrenergic receptor stimulation promotes relaxation.[11]

Various drugs and vasoactive mediators can cause contraction or relaxation of bronchial smooth muscle. The more important ones are listed in Table 40-1.

Agents that cause bronchoconstriction are of no therapeutic value but are important as mediators of allergic, inflammatory, or infectious processes. It is believed that the generation of *slow-reacting substance* (SRS-A, leukotrienes C_4 and D_4) by lung mast cells causes bronchospasm in acute asthmatic episodes. Because asthmatics are unusually sensitive to histamine and kinins, release of these mediators may also contribute to the process. Some drugs, such as the α-adrenergic receptor agonists or β-adrenergic receptor antagonists, cause bronchoconstriction. Although these agents may be useful for other purposes, as a general rule they should be avoided in persons with asthma and other airway diseases.

Bronchodilators

The major drugs used to treat bronchospasm are the β-adrenergic receptor agonists and the methylxanthines. Drugs of either class relax bronchial smooth muscle cells. The mechanism of the relaxation caused by β-adrenergic receptor agonists is believed to involve changes in cyclic nucleotides. These agonists activate adenylate cyclase within the cell membrane, and in the presence of Mg^{++} this enzyme catalyzes formation of cyclic AMP from cytoplasmic ATP. The catabolism of cyclic AMP depends on phosphodiesterase, an enzyme that is inhibited in vitro by high concentrations of methylxanthines. However, the methylxanthines are now believed to cause bronchodilatation by another as yet unknown mechanism.[7]

| β-ADRENERGIC RECEPTOR AGONISTS | The effectiveness of epinephrine and other sympathomimetic drugs in treatment of bronchial asthma is well recognized. Ephedrine is the oldest member of this class, and its use in respiratory disease dates back many centuries. As described in Chapter 15, sympathomimetic drugs exhibit profiles of activity that can be related to activation of α, β₁, and β₂ classes of receptors. |

The effectiveness of epinephrine and other sympathomimetic drugs in treatment of bronchial asthma is well recognized. Ephedrine is the oldest member of this class, and its use in respiratory disease dates back many centuries. As described in Chapter 15, sympathomimetic drugs exhibit profiles of activity that can be related to activation of α, β_1, and β_2 classes of receptors. The relaxant action on bronchial smooth muscle is attributable to stimulation of β_2-receptors, and β_2-agonists are safer and thus more useful in therapy of acute obstructive airway disease than drugs that stimulate both β_1- and β_2-receptors. Bronchodilatation is the major effect of β_2-agonists in the lung, though some studies indicate that these agonists also promote ciliary movement and diminish release of mediators from mast cells.[11]

Possible unwanted effects of these agents are predictable from their adrenergic pharmacology. Agonists with both β_1 and β_2 activity can cause tachycardia. The most limiting effect of β_2-agonists is tremor. Those drugs with α-adrenergic actions cause vasoconstriction and perhaps central nervous system stimulation.

The chemical structure affects the selectivity of β-adrenergic receptor agonists for bronchial smooth muscle. The basic structure is that of a catecholamine (epinephrine, isoproterenol) or phenethylamine (ephedrine). Other compounds have been developed with substitutions along the ethanolamine side chain or on the aromatic ring to convey selectivity for β_2-receptors (terbutaline, albuterol). The drugs and their relative selectivity for receptors are listed in Table 40-2.

Side effects and complications of therapy with these agents stem primarily from actions on β_1-receptors. These include central nervous system activation (nervousness, wakefulness, anxiety), cardiac stimulation, and alteration of blood pressure. α-Adrenergic receptor stimulation (epinephrine, ephedrine) may increase blood pressure slightly. Tolerance and refractoriness to further administration can occur with frequent use of epinephrine and isoproterenol. This is less pronounced with the β_2-selective agents. Muscle tremor may occur with extended use of metaproterenol or terbutaline, but these are infrequent with albuterol. Excessive use of inhalers containing any of the β-adrenergic drugs may cause drying of mucous membranes and possibly irritation of the airways.

Specific agents. **Epinephrine** is a highly effective bronchodilator, and it is widely used in emergencies to relieve acute bronchoconstriction. Epinephrine is not selective for β-receptors however, and it is not effective by mouth. The α-adrenergic component can cause a beneficial vasoconstriction that may reduce edema within the airways and thus improve airflow. Epinephrine has a short duration of action (approximately 20 minutes) when injected or administered by inhalation. The major mechanisms terminating its action are discussed in Chapter 10. Why tachyphylaxis develops with continued use is not clear.

TABLE 40-2 β_2-Adrenergic receptor agonist selectivity and dosage forms

Drug	β_2-Receptor selectivity	Dosage forms
Epinephrine	0	See Chapter 15
Ephedrine	0	See Chapter 15
Isoproterenol hydrochloride (Isuprel)	0	See Chapter 15
Isoetharine hydrochloride (Bronkosol)	+ +	A: 340 µg as mesylate; SN: 0.062-1%
Metaproterenol sulfate (Alupent, Metaprel)	+ +	A: 225 mg as powder; S: 10; SN: 0.6, 5%; T: 10, 20
Terbutaline sulfate (Brethine, Bricanyl)	+ + +	A: 200 µg; I: 1; T: 2.5, 5
Albuterol (Proventil, Ventolin)	+ + +	A: 90 µg; S: 2 as sulfate; T: 2, 4 as sulfate
Bitolterol mesylate (Tornalate)	+ + +	A: 370 µg

A, Aerosol, dose per actuation except for metaproterenol; *I*, injection, mg/ml; *S*, syrup, mg/5 ml; *SN*, solution for nebulization; *T*, tablets, mg.

Ephedrine is the oldest of the adrenergic agents used to treat asthma. It is less commonly used today, since the amounts available in over-the-counter preparations are usually insufficient and larger doses commonly cause side effects. Ephedrine is active by either oral or parenteral routes. Although its onset of action is slower than that of epinephrine, the effect persists for several hours. Ephedrine is not so effective as epinephrine for acute attacks of asthma. In addition, tachyphylaxis to ephedrine can develop with continued use.

Isoproterenol was introduced in the 1940s as a pure β-agonist, and it was widely used as a bronchodilator. Administration by inhalation contributed to its popularity. Isoproterenol has some disadvantages, however. It stimulates the heart by its action on β_1-receptors, and its bronchodilatory action is short lived.

Isoetharine was the first of the β_2-selective drugs. Like isoproterenol, it is a catecholamine with a short duration of action. Isoetharine is used in aerosol form, but its brief action makes it less popular than other selective agents.

Metaproterenol is an analog of isoproterenol with a moderately long duration of action. The placement of hydroxyl groups in the *meta* position on the benzene ring provides resistance to degradation by catechol-*O*-methyltransferase and conveys enhanced β_2-receptor selectivity. The drug can be administered orally or by inhalation. Its therapeutic action lasts up to 4 hours.

Terbutaline has a slightly greater selectivity for β_2-receptors. It is slower in onset of action than metaproterenol, but with oral administration the bronchodilator action persists for as long as 8 hours. Terbutaline appears to have little or no action on β_1-receptors. Some degree of tolerance to the β_2 activity may develop, but less than with isoproterenol or ephedrine.[10]

Albuterol is also a relatively selective β_2-adrenergic agent. Modification of the catecholamine structure makes it resistant to degradation and prolongs its action. In equieffective bronchodilator doses albuterol causes fewer cardiac effects than isoproterenol, and the bronchodilator action persists for 4 to 8 hours.

Use. β-Adrenergic receptor agonists are used primarily for relief of bronchospasm. The development of agents with greater β_2-receptor selectivity and prolonged duration of action has advanced therapy of asthma beyond the relief of acute spasm that can be achieved with isoproterenol. Inhalation is usually the preferred route because the onset of action is rapid and the dosage can be regulated by the patient. Oral administration of β_2-agonists is indicated only in chronic asthma and is frequently limited by side effects, such as tremor.

METHYLXANTHINES   The methylxanthine group includes caffeine (see Chapter 27), theophylline, and theobromine. Their general pharmacologic effects include relaxation of smooth muscle, cardiac stimulation, central nervous system stimulation, and diuresis. Of these compounds, only **theophylline** and its salts, **aminophylline** and **oxtriphylline,** are used as bronchodilators.

Mechanism of action. For many years the major mechanism of bronchodilatation by theophylline and related drugs was believed to be inhibition of phosphodiesterase to permit accumulation of cyclic AMP within bronchial smooth muscle cells. However, several derivatives of theophylline with a potent phosphodiesterase inhibitory action have little efficacy as bronchodilators. Although it has been suggested that theophylline is an antagonist at adenosine receptors,[12] **enprophylline,** also a potent bronchodilator, is not. Hence it appears that neither phosphodiesterase inhibition nor adenosine antagonism is a satisfactory explanation for the bronchodilator action of methylxanthines. Other proposed mechanisms involve interactions with prostaglandins, calcium, or cyclic AMP–mediated protein kinase activation.[7] Some studies indicate that theophylline may increase diaphragmatic contractility, which may be especially important in chronic obstructive pulmonary disease (COPD) and in some apneic syndromes.[3]

Use. Theophylline is used to treat moderate to severe reversible bronchospasm that occurs in asthma or COPD. Theophylline is especially useful in prophylaxis of bronchospasm, but therapeutic effectiveness depends on the careful control of plasma concentration. A novel use for the drug is to combat diaphragmatic muscle fatigue in patients with COPD or after upper abdominal surgery.[1] Theophylline, as well as caffeine, is also used to alleviate apneic episodes in neonates.

Administration and dosage. Theophylline is effective after either oral or parenteral administration, as is its congener **dyphylline** (Dilor, Lufyllin). Salt forms, aminophylline and oxtriphylline (Choledyl), are slightly more soluble but have no major therapeutic advantage. These salts, in which theophylline is combined with ethylenediamine or choline respectively, contain about 85% theophylline. Aminophylline is available for intravenous injection, but cautious dosing must be employed to avoid acute toxicity with the rapid elevation of blood concentration that can occur.

Theophylline is well absorbed on oral administration, with an onset of activity from 45 to 60 minutes. Since it is rapidly inactivated, its duration of action is on the order of 5 to 6 hours. Because both efficacy and toxicity depend on the plasma concentration of theophylline, determination of this concentration is an integral part of therapy. Bronchodilatation is generally achieved between 10 and 20 μg/ml, and toxic effects begin to occur above 20 μg/ml. The dosage required to achieve a therapeutic concentration varies greatly among persons and must be carefully determined for each individual patient. Once a maintenance regimen is established, however, sustained-release oral preparations (Theo-Dur, Slo-Phyllin, others) are effective and well tolerated, and they generally improve patient compliance.[13] Theophylline is available in a wide variety of forms for oral administration: capsules, 100 to 250 mg; tablets, 100 to 300 mg; elixirs, solutions, and syrups, 80 to 160 mg in 15 ml; timed-release capsules, 50 to 300 mg; and timed-release tablets, 100 to 500 mg.

The duration of action also shows considerable variation among persons. Theophylline is predominantly metabolized by hepatic microsomal enzymes. Thus other drugs, diseases, or environmental factors that affect metabolism will alter the duration of action of this drug. For example, clearance of theophylline and related compounds is increased by smoking and by phenytoin, both of which induce hepatic microsomal enzymes. The action of theophylline is prolonged in patients with congestive heart failure, liver disease, or alcoholism. Similarly, concomitant therapy with drugs that inhibit its biotransformation, such as erythromycin and cimetidine, can increase plasma concentration and prolong the action of theophylline.

Toxicity and adverse effects. As indicated above, therapeutic and toxic doses of theophylline vary widely among persons. Even at therapeutic concentrations, the drug may cause some gastrointestinal distress, which is believed to be central in origin. Many persons experience central nervous system stimulation, which is sometimes accompanied by headache. Other side effects include tachycardia, hypotension, and diuresis.

Serious toxicities involve the central nervous and cardiovascular systems.[5] These can occur at a plasma concentration only twice the usual therapeutic concentration. Central nervous system excitation is reflected by increasing irritability and hyperexcitability that can extend to generalized convulsions. Cardiac toxicity includes arrhythmias and, in extreme cases, circulatory collapse. A pronounced increase in body temperature may also develop.

Many pulmonary diseases are treated with corticosteroids (glucocorticoids) as a means of reducing the inflammatory process. The basic pharmacology of these agents is discussed in Chapter 43. The benefit of steroid therapy for many pulmonary disorders is controversial. Steroid therapy remains, however, an integral part of the management of asthma. Administration of systemic glucocorticoids is highly effective in reducing the frequency and severity of attacks in chronic asthma, but, because of the potential for serious side effects with extended use, these agents are generally used after other measures have proved ineffective. Unfortunately, not all forms of asthma and not all persons respond adequately to glucocorticoid therapy.

There are several agents available, but all have the same actions and the same basic potential for adverse effects. *Prednisone* or *methylprednisolone* are used for oral administration; *beclomethasone* and *flunisolide* can be given by inhalation. The

Anti-inflammatory steroids

latter route is particularly attractive because it enhances delivery of the drug to the affected organ while decreasing the potential for systemic absorption and side effects.

Mechanism of action. As described in Chapter 43, the glucocorticoid agents have similar actions that depend on chemical substitutions onto the four-ring steroid structure. All clinically useful anti-inflammatory steroids have a 17α-hydroxy substitution in ring D. Glucocorticoids have several biologic actions that affect the inflammatory process, but the basic mechanism through which they reduce bronchoreactivity is still not established. Two possibilities have been suggested. First, there is some evidence that glucocorticoids can enhance the action of adrenergic agonists on β_2-receptors within bronchial smooth muscle, either through modification of receptors or by influencing the molecular events that occur between receptor stimulation and muscle contraction. A second possible mechanism is through modulation of eicosanoid production. One action of glucocorticoids is to suppress release of arachidonate, thereby reducing production of prostaglandins and leukotrienes. As leukotrienes C_4 and D_4 are potent bronchoconstrictors, suppression of leukotriene production would clearly be beneficial in asthma. Additional mechanisms may involve inhibition of release of mediators from mast cells or leukocytes and alteration of the immune response.[15]

Specific agents. **Prednisone** (Deltasone, others) is the drug generally used for oral administration. It is converted in the liver to prednisolone, an active congener, and has a relatively slow onset of action. As with any steroid therapy, continued use may result in several undesirable side effects, some of which are not reversible with cessation of therapy. These include development of osteoporosis, cataract formation, and stunting of growth in children.

Methylprednisolone (Medrol, others) is used for intravenous administration, as in emergency treatment of status asthmaticus, a life-threatening exacerbation of asthma, which consists in persistent, unrelieved bronchospasm. Methylprednisolone is also available in oral form, and its effects may last as long as 24 hours. Adverse effects are the same as for prednisone.

Beclomethasone (Beclovent, Vanceril) is a topically active glucocorticoid that can be administered as an aerosol. This helps to limit its action to the site of application. Beclomethasone aerosol appears to be effective in control of asthma without producing systemic effects. Moreover, therapy with this agent usually enables patients to discontinue or minimize doses of oral steroids.

Flunisolide (AeroBid) can also be used by inhalation. It has a longer duration of action than beclomethasone, but greater systemic absorption occurs with this agent.

See Table 43-2 for preparations of these agents.

Use. The major use of glucocorticosteroids in respiratory disease is in management of serious, chronic asthma. They are sometimes used to treat bronchitis, particularly when there is an associated asthmatic component. Hypersensitivity alveolitis and allergic rhinitis may also be helped by a short course of glucocorticoid treatment, but steroid therapy for pulmonary infections should be avoided.

Adverse effects and toxicity. The short-term use of glucocorticoids in asthma does not usually produce serious systemic side effects. Extended use or use of high doses, however, can produce a spectrum of unpleasant and serious effects. Details of steroid toxicity are given in Chapter 43. The most common side effects in adults include weight gain, capillary fragility (easy bruising), osteoporosis, and development of cataracts. In addition, users of inhalers experience dryness of the mouth and throat with an increased risk of oral candidiasis (thrush). Inhalant forms have been reported to trigger asthmatic attacks in some persons, probably as a result of direct irritation of airways.

Alternative therapy of asthma

Although bronchodilators and steroids remain the basic therapeutic modalities for management of asthma, there are subsets of asthmatic persons in whom a prophylactic approach is beneficial; for example, in exercise-induced asthma. Blockade of mediator release is believed to be the mechanism through which cromolyn and related drugs reduce the incidence and severity of asthmatic attacks in some persons. Cromolyn does not relax bronchial smooth muscle, nor does it block histamine receptors. It inhibits release of histamine and SRS-A (leukotrienes) from mast cells within the mucosa and along bronchial vessels. It appears effective in both immediate and late asthmatic reactions to inhaled or absorbed antigens.

Cromolyn sodium (disodium cromoglycate, Intal) may be inhaled in the form of a dry powder. The particles are deposited on the respiratory mucosa and absorbed. The drug is also used as an inhalation aerosol and in aqueous form in a nebulized spray. The latter is recommended for children under 5 years of age, who may not be able to use the inhaler. An ophthalmic solution (Opticrom) and a nasal solution (Nasalcrom) are also available. Cromolyn must be used several times a day, and poor patient compliance may limit its effectiveness. In addition, there is no means of predicting which patients will respond to the drug without a trial of several weeks. Other agents with mediator release–blocking actions are currently under investigation.[2]

Cromolyn sodium

Ipratropium (Atrovent) is an anticholinergic agent. It has been used in Europe to treat asthma but is still not widely used in the United States. The drug appears to act predominately on central airways rather than on smaller peripheral airways and thus is not as effective as β-adrenergic receptor agonists against stimulus-induced bronchospasm.[8] Ipratropium does, however, have less of a depressant effect than atropine on mucociliary function.[14] Thus it may prove to be of use in situations in which β-agonists and theophylline are undesirable. Ipratropium has been used successfully in combination with β-agonists.

Ipratropium bromide

Other approaches to the prevention or reversal of asthmatic bronchoconstriction are experimental. The rationale for use of *α-adrenergic receptor antagonists* is that α-receptors have been implicated in bronchial hyperreactivity. It is not yet known if α-antagonists will be effective in clinical asthma. Similarly, since bronchoconstriction is a calcium-mediated process, *calcium channel–blocking agents* may have some application. These agents are used to treat various cardiac disorders (see Chapters 35 and 36), but as yet none appear helpful in management of bronchoconstriction. Finally, *nonsteroidal anti-inflammatory drugs,* such as aspirin and ibuprofen, may prove to be useful, particularly when tissue inflammation is a contributing factor.

ELABORATION AND METABOLISM OF MEDIATORS WITHIN THE LUNGS

Although the primary function of the lung is gas exchange, it is now well known that this organ is metabolically active and can process many different vasoactive substances from blood or tissues.[4] The pulmonary vascular bed is a vast surface across which blood is filtered. Serotonin and epinephrine are rapidly removed from pulmonary circulation by active uptake. Prostaglandins E_2 and $F_{2\alpha}$ and bradykinin are completely removed during a single passage through the pulmonary vascular bed. The angiotensin I converting enzyme that is localized on the luminal surface of the pulmonary endothelium both activates angiotensin I to angiotensin II and inactivates circulating kinins by cleaving a dipeptide from the carboxyl terminus of either peptide substrate.

The lung is also a source of various autacoids, including histamine, prostaglandins, thromboxane, and leukotrienes. Histamine from the mast cells of the lung is released during acute allergic reactions and may contribute to the bronchospasm of acute asthma. Histamine released from mast cells of the nasal mucosa is clearly involved in the symptoms of allergic rhinitis and possibly in additional inflammatory reactions involving the upper airways. Prostaglandin release during lung inflation is believed to play a regulatory role in respiration, and the release of SRS-A, now recognized as a mixture of leukotrienes (see p. 235), is likely a key factor in both allergic and intrinsic asthma.

1. Dureuil, B., Desmonts, J.M., Mankikian, B., and Prokocimer, P.: Effects of aminophylline on diaphragmatic dysfunction after upper abdominal surgery, Anesthesiology **62**:242, 1985.

2. Falliers, C.J., and Tinkelman, D.G.: Alternative drug therapy for asthma, Clin. Chest Med. **7**:383, 1986.

3. Galko, B.M., and Rebuck, A.S.: Therapeutic use of respiratory stimulants: an overview of newer developments, Drugs **30**:475, 1985.

4. Gillis, C.N., and Roth, J.A.: Pulmonary disposition of circulating vasoactive hormones, Biochem. Pharmacol. **25**:2547, 1976.

5. Jacobs, M.H., Senior, R.M., and Kessler, G.: Clinical experience with theophylline: relationships between dosage, serum concentration, and toxicity, J.A.M.A. **235**:1983, 1976.

6. Marin, M.G.: Pharmacology of airway secretion, Pharmacol. Rev. **38**:273, 1986.

7. Miech, R.P., and Stein, M.: Methylxanthines, Clin. Chest Med. **7**:331, 1986.

8. Morris, H.G.: Review of ipratropium bromide in induced bronchospasm in patients with asthma, Am. J. Med. **81**(suppl. 5A):36, 1986.

9. Nadel, J.A., and Barnes, P.J.: Autonomic regulation of the airways, Annu. Rev. Med. **35**:451, 1984.

10. Plummer, A.L.: The development of drug tolerance to beta$_2$ adrenergic agents, Chest **73**:949, 1978.

11. Popa, V.: Beta-adrenergic drugs, Clin. Chest Med. **7**:313, 1986.

12. Satchell, D., and Smith, R.: Adenosine causes contractions in spiral strips and relaxations in transverse strips of guinea-pig trachea: studies on mechanism of action, Eur. J. Pharmacol. **101**:243, 1984.

13. Spector, S.L.: Advantages and disadvantages of 24-hour theophylline, J. Allergy Clin. Immunol. **76**:302, 1985.

14. Wanner, A.: Effect of ipratropium bromide on airway mucociliary functions, Am. J. Med. **81**(suppl. 5A):23, 1986.

15. Ziment, I.: Steroids, Clin. Chest Med. **7**:341, 1986.

REFERENCES

Chapter 41

Drug effects on the gastrointestinal tract

GENERAL CONCEPT   Disorders of the gastrointestinal tract are among the most common of medical problems. Approximately 4 to 5 million persons suffer from peptic ulcer disease, and many more, who may or may not seek therapy, suffer from minor gastrointestinal disturbances. Drugs for management of gastrointestinal disorders are best grouped by their therapeutic indications. Therapy of disorders of the upper gastrointestinal tract is directed primarily at correction of esophageal dysfunction and treatment of peptic ulcer. The drugs used include *antispasmodics* and *antisecretory agents* as well as *antacids*. In addition, *metoclopramide* promotes gastric emptying, and *sucralfate* is used to foster ulcer healing. Important adjunctive measures include avoidance of agents, such as alcohol and caffeine, that increase gastric acid secretion and drugs such as aspirin and glucocorticoids, which can alter the normal protective properties of the gastric mucosa.

Drugs for treatment of disorders of the lower gastrointestinal tract include *laxatives*, *antidiarrheal agents*, and *antispasmodics*. Since the underlying causes of diarrhea or spasm vary, appropriate therapy may include drugs directed at eradication of infectious agents, correction of malabsorption, or reversal of inflammatory disorders, such as ulcerative colitis or Crohn's disease (regional enteritis).

DRUGS USED IN DISORDERS OF THE UPPER GASTRO-INTESTINAL TRACT   The general management of acid-peptic disorders involves (1) agents that inhibit secretion of gastric acid and pepsin, (2) those that neutralize secreted acid, and (3) those that enhance mucosal resistance to erosion.[5] Because they are much more effective and have fewer side effects, the histamine (H_2) antagonists have essentially replaced anticholinergic agents for reducing the volume and acidity of gastric secretion. Antacids remain an effective means of neutralizing secreted acid, and sucralfate enhances mucosal resistance by complexing with proteins at the ulcer site to prevent acid diffusion.

Agents that inhibit gastric secretion of acid and pepsin
HISTAMINE ANTAGONISTS   Antagonists of H_2-receptors (see also Chapter 20) are among the most widely used drugs in the United States. Cimetidine (Tagamet), ranitidine (Zantac), and famotidine (Pepcid) reduce the volume and acidity of gastric secretions in both the resting state and after stimulation by food, histamine, or pentagastrin. They neither neutralize gastric acid nor affect secretion of gastrin. Their basic mechanism of action is competitive antagonism of histamine at H_2-receptors within the parietal cells of the gastric mucosa to reduce histamine-stimulated secretion of acid and intrinsic factor. The concomitant reduction of gastric secretory volume decreases secretion of

pepsin from chief cells. Because these agents are highly effective, they are widely used to treat peptic ulcer and reflux esophagitis. They can be administered orally, and serious side effects are uncommon. Cimetidine has been used extensively, and much is known about its pharmacology. Ranitidine, a newer, structurally similar agent, is more potent and can be given less frequently. Famotidine was only recently approved by the FDA. This agent is more potent and longer acting than either cimetidine or ranitidine.[6] Neither ranitidine nor famotidine inhibits hepatic metabolism of other drugs to the extent that cimetidine does (see Chapter 63).

Before development of the H_2-receptor antagonists, drugs that antagonize acetylcholine at muscarinic receptors in the gastric mucosa were used to suppress gastric secretion and motility. Although their antisecretory effectiveness is less than that of H_2-receptor antagonists, when given in sufficient doses muscarinic antagonists such as atropine or propantheline decrease by 30% to 50% both nocturnal (unstimulated) acid secretion and secretion stimulated by histamine, pentagastrin, or a meal. The use of these drugs is limited by dryness of the mouth, loss of visual accommodation, and reduction of smooth muscle motility, which occur at doses required to inhibit gastric secretion. Contraindications to anticholinergic drugs include glaucoma, prostatic hypertrophy, and gastric retention. **ANTICHOLINERGIC AGENTS**

Many experimental and clinical observations indicate that antacids are among the most useful drugs for relief of hyperacidity. Adequate dosage accelerates the healing of ulcers.[7] The goal is to increase the pH of gastric contents to a range of 3.5 to 4.5, at which pepsin activity is greatly diminished. This, however, necessitates that large enough doses be taken frequently enough to maintain the increase in pH, a regimen that is often difficult to maintain. The buffering action of various preparations depends on their composition. Antacid effectiveness may be predicted by the measured neutralizing capacity; as shown in Table 41-1, this varies considerably as does the sodium content among preparations. *Antacids*

Effective doses of antacids contain at least 75 to 150 mEq of buffer; patients with hypersecretion of acid, as in duodenal ulcer, may need larger quantities than those with gastric ulcer or with esophageal reflux. In addition to excessive production of acid, patients with duodenal ulcers are reported to have rapid gastric emptying, which results in loss of buffering by food.[3]

Antacid preparations are weakly basic and consist of metal salts, most commonly aluminum hydroxide, magnesium hydroxide, calcium carbonate, or sodium bicarbonate. These salts dissociate to neutralize gastric acid and form neutral salts within the stomach. Calcium carbonate has the greatest neutralizing capacity and aluminum hydroxide the least.

Antacid preparations have been defined as *absorbable* or *nonabsorbable*, depending on the degree of systemic absorption. Sodium bicarbonate is readily absorbed, whereas aluminum hydroxide and magnesium trisilicate are not. The long-term use of any antacids, however, may result in some systemic effects. For example,

TABLE 41-1   Characteristics of various antacids

Antacid	Composition	Buffering capacity* (mEq of hydrochloric acid per ml)	Sodium content (mg/5 ml)
Aludrox	Magnesium and aluminum hydroxides, simethicone	2.81	4.5
Amphojel	Aluminum hydroxide gel	1.93	8.1
Gelusil	Aluminum hydroxide gel, magnesium trisilicate	1.33	6.5
Gelusil M	Aluminum hydroxide gel, magnesium hydroxide, magnesium trisilicate	2.23	5.7
Maalox	Aluminum hydroxide gel, magnesium hydroxide	2.58	2.5
Magaldrate (Riopan)	Magnesium and aluminum hydroxides	2.21	0.7
Mylanta	Magnesium and aluminum hydroxides, simethicone	2.38	3.9
WinGel	Aluminum hydroxide gel, magnesium hydroxide, stabilized with hexitol	2.25	1.25

*From Fordtran, J.S., Morawski, S.G., and Richardson, C.T.: N. Engl. J. Med. **288:**923, 1973.

patients treated with calcium carbonate can absorb sufficient calcium to cause renal impairment. This has been called the milk-alkali syndrome. Similarly, the chronic use of aluminum-containing antacids by patients with renal insufficiency can result in accumulation of the metal and central nervous system toxicity. Antacids may also cause electrolyte imbalances, and with sodium-containing compounds the absorption of sodium contributes to volume expansion.

INDIVIDUAL PREPARATIONS   **Sodium bicarbonate** (baking soda) is a popular agent used (and misused) for self-medication by the lay public. Although it is an effective and rapidly acting antacid, its absorption can cause metabolic alkalosis; it should not be taken repeatedly. This antacid is found in some over-the-counter medications, such as Alka Seltzer. Because of its systemic effects, it is not prescribed for medical management of acid-peptic disease.

Aluminum salts, such as aluminum hydroxide or aluminum hydroxide gel, are found in many preparations. Aluminum hydroxide gel forms aluminum chloride after interaction with gastric acid, but the chloride is reabsorbed within the more alkaline intestine. As a consequence, there is no alteration in systemic acid-base balance. The gel will increase the pH of the stomach contents only to about 4. Aluminum hydroxide is slightly more effective. Aluminum salts are relatively insoluble and can cause constipation. They may deplete phosphate with excessive use; in fact, they are administered to patients with renal insufficiency to prevent phosphate absorption. In addition, aluminum salts can impair absorption of various drugs.

Magnesium salts, such as magnesium hydroxide or trisilicate, can cause diarrhea. They form compounds that retain water and thus exert an osmotic action within the gut. They are effective antacids, and bowel disturbances are minimized when they are combined with potentially constipating aluminum salts. Magnesium trisilicate is changed in the stomach to magnesium chloride and silicon dioxide. The chloride is absorbed in the intestine, and magnesium carbonate is formed. Magnesium salts can elevate the pH of the stomach contents to 7 or higher. An 8% aqueous suspension of magnesium hydroxide (milk of magnesia) is one of the most effective antacids available.[8]

Absorption of magnesium may be of concern in patients with renal disease. In normal persons the small amounts of magnesium that are absorbed are rapidly cleared by the kidney. However, in patients with poor renal function, retention of magnesium may cause neurologic, cardiovascular, and neuromuscular toxicity.

MIXTURES

Combinations of aluminum and magnesium hydroxides, though more acceptable for normal bowel function, have less neutralizing power than the magnesium salt alone.[7] Such mixtures are frequently used, however, because they minimize the disadvantages of the individual agents, increase the duration of buffering, and improve palatability. *Simethicone* is a defoaming agent that is sometimes combined with antacids. It is said to relieve painful distention caused by formation of gas in the gastrointestinal tract, but there is little clinical evidence for this.

Sucralfate

Sucralfate (Carafate) is a complex of sulfated sucrose and aluminum hydroxide. This disaccharide becomes hydrated when it contacts the gastric contents and forms complexes with albumin, fibrinogen, and globulin on the ulcer surface to create a protective barrier to acid and pepsin. In addition, sucralfate binds pepsin directly. The drug is not absorbed, and its action is limited to the ulcer surface. It may be used with antacids, and it is highly effective in promoting healing. The rate of ulcer healing with sucralfate is similar to that with H_2-receptor antagonists.[10] Sucralfate has very few side effects, though mild constipation may occur with continued use. One drawback is the requirement for administration four times daily, in contrast to the newer H_2-receptor antagonists, which are taken once or twice daily.

$$R = SO_3[Al_2(OH)_5]$$

Sucralfate

Prostaglandins

Prostaglandin E_2 (PGE_2) is believed to play an important role in protection of the gastric and duodenal mucosa from acid and pepsin. This metabolite of arachidonic acid inhibits gastric secretion, and it helps maintain the cellular integrity of the mucosa, probably by promoting secretion of the mucus barrier between mucosal cells and the gastric contents.[4] Although PGE_2 has been used only experimentally, several analogs appear promising as therapy for peptic ulcers.[2] These agents should be available for clinical use in the near future.

Metoclopramide	Metoclopramide is a dopamine antagonist that enhances motility of the upper gastrointestinal tract. Its effect is antagonized by anticholinergic drugs. The drug is used in therapy of reflux esophagitis, in disorders of intestinal motility, such as diabetic gastroparesis, and as an antiemetic. Metoclopramide elevates lower esophageal sphincter pressure, increases resting esophageal tone, and hastens gastric emptying. It facilitates procedures such as endoscopy and intubation and is useful in radiologic examination of gastrointestinal motility. This drug has been particularly useful as an antiemetic in patients receiving chemotherapy for cancer. In this setting very large doses may be required. Adverse reactions to metoclopramide include drowsiness, fatigue, insomnia, dizziness, and bowel disturbances. The drug is contraindicated in patients with pheochromocytoma in whom it may cause hypertension. Metoclopramide hydrochloride (Reglan) is available in tablets containing 10 mg of the base, as a syrup (5 mg/5 ml), and in vials for injection (5 mg/ml).

$$CONHCH_2CH_2N(C_2H_5)_2$$

$$OCH_3$$

Cl

$$NH_2$$

Metoclopramide

DRUGS USED IN DISORDERS OF THE LOWER GASTRO-INTESTINAL TRACT	Most disorders of the lower gastrointestinal tract involve abnormalities of fluid and electrolyte transport or smooth muscle responsiveness. Diarrhea may have many causes, including infection with bacteria or parasites, toxins, inflammation, and malabsorption. Constipation is sometimes caused by organic disease, such as tumors of the bowel, and sometimes by drugs, such as aluminum hydroxide, opioid analgesics, and tricyclic antidepressants or other anticholinergic agents. When not attributable to organic causes, however, constipation is generally caused by poor dietary habits, lack of bulk-producing foods, and inattention to the stimulus for defecation. A sedentary life style with lack of regular exercise will also promote constipation. Correction of such factors will often relieve chronic constipation without the need for laxative treatment.[1]
Antidiarrheal agents	Acute severe diarrhea causes water and electrolyte depletion, which may progress to dehydration and electrolyte imbalance. Even mild chronic diarrhea can cause hypokalemia. The basic management of diarrhea is directed toward elimination of the cause, if possible, and replacement of fluid and electrolytes.[9] In addition, drugs may be given that act nonspecifically to decrease loss of water and electrolytes through

fecal excretion. Small doses of opioids can decrease gastrointestinal motility. Opioid analgesics and anticholinergic drugs are also used to reduce pain and diarrhea associated with inflammatory bowel disease.

Adsorbants coat the lining of the gastrointestinal tract to adsorb bacteria and toxic products, which are then eliminated in the feces. *Bismuth subsalicylate* (Pepto-Bismol) binds toxins produced by *Vibrio cholerae* and *Escherichia coli* and reduces intestinal inflammation and hypermotility. Other agents, such as kaolin, activated charcoal, and pectin, are also used for their adsorbant activity. Unfortunately adsorbants can also bind other drugs, and they may produce constipation after a course of treatment for diarrhea. SPECIFIC AGENTS

Cholestyramine (Questran) and *colestipol hydrochloride* (Colestid) are affinity resins that bind acidic materials. They are used to bind cholesterol in some types of hyperlipidemias (see Chapter 39), but development of constipation is a major side effect. Although these agents also bind toxins from bacterial organisms, their main use is as an aid in control of diarrhea caused by malabsorption of bile acids, such as that after ileal resection. They can adsorb vitamins and other nutrients as well.

Opioids are the most effective and rapidly acting agents for relief of diarrhea. They increase the tone and segmenting activity of both the large and small intestine; this provides resistance to transit of material. In addition, they reduce propulsive motility of the bowel, increase sphincter tone, and decrease secretory activity along the gastrointestinal tract. Decreased motility enhances fluid reabsorption and decreases the volume of intestinal material. Paregoric (camphorated tincture of opium) is a schedule III drug because it has potential for misuse and addiction. Codeine is an effective antidiarrheal agent, but it also carries risk of abuse. The opiate-like drug *diphenoxylate* in combination with atropine (Lomotil, others) is recommended for treatment of chronic diarrhea; in this case the more addictive opiate compounds are undesirable. Diphenoxylate has a low potential for producing physical dependence, but it may enhance the effects of other central nervous system depressants.

Loperamide hydrochloride (Imodium) is an antiperistaltic, antidiarrheal agent. It has a structure similar to that of haloperidol, and it can affect opiate receptors. Loperamide is very effective in reducing diarrhea, but, as with any of the opioid compounds, it should not be used in infectious diarrhea, in which retention of organisms may result in bacterial invasion of the intestinal wall.

Loperamide

Psyllium hydrophilic mucilloid (Metamucil, others) is a powder that swells in water to form a bland, nonirritating bulk. It is used in treatment of irritable bowel syndrome, which is one of the most common causes of diarrhea. Paradoxically, this substance is also used as a bulk laxative to relieve constipation (Table 41-2).

Cathartics and laxatives

Laxatives, agents that produce a soft, but formed, stool, and cathartics, those that produce a fluid or semifluid stool, increase accumulation of water and electrolytes in the lumen of the small bowel. There are several mechanisms by which they achieve these effects. Drugs in both groups promote defecation. The terminology reflects a difference in the intensity and latency of the effect.

Laxatives promote and ease defecation by influencing the consistency of the stool. Soft stools and lack of straining during defecation are especially desirable in some clinical settings, as in postsurgical patients or those with diseases of coronary or cerebral vessels. Cathartics are used to speed elimination of toxic materials or parasites after treatment with anthelmintics and to prepare the bowel for radiologic or surgical procedures. A technique involving ingestion of a large volume (4 liters) of a solution containing nonabsorbable polyethylene glycol with sodium sulfate and other salts (CoLyte, GoLYTELY) promises to be a superior means of cleansing the bowel.

MECHANISMS

The various laxative-cathartics act by several mechanisms (Table 41-2). There is some overlap among the various groups in that more than one mechanism may contribute. In general, hydrophilic (bulk-forming) and osmotic agents increase the bulk of the intestinal contents and the rate of transit. Agents that stimulate motility also expand intestinal contents, in this case by decreasing absorption of electrolytes and fluids. Contact laxative-cathartics have a direct action on intestinal mucosa. They inhibit cyclic AMP—mediated absorption of fluid and electrolytes. Other drugs act as emollients or stool softeners. There is generally no indication for laxative-cathartic combination preparations, since the individual agents are just as effective.

SPECIFIC AGENTS

Bulk laxatives are not absorbed from the intestine. Some dietary components, such as bran fiber, contribute to normal bowel function by adding bulk to the stool. *Carboxymethylcellulose*, when mixed with water, forms a hydrophilic colloid that retains a considerable quantity of water; as a consequence, it softens the stool, distends the colon, and stimulates evacuation. The action of some bulk laxatives may depend, in part, on osmotically active metabolites. Bulk laxatives are generally safe but can occasionally cause obstruction of a narrowed intestinal lumen.

TABLE 41-2	Common laxative-cathartics

Agent	Mechanism
Hydrophilic agents	
Dietary fiber (bran)	Absorb water to form softened but formed stools by increasing
Carboxymethylcellulose	bulk of intestinal contents; decrease intestinal transit time
Psyllium colloid	
Osmotic laxatives	
Magnesium salts	Hypertonic solutions draw fluid into intestinal lumen by osmosis
Lactulose	Low molecular weight metabolites have an osmotic action within the intestinal lumen
Contact laxatives	
Bisacodyl	Decrease fluid and electrolyte absorption in small intestine
Phenolphthalein	
Cascara sagrada	Stimulates peristalsis
Castor oil	Lipolysis in intestine liberates ricinoleic acid
Lubricant-emollients	
Mineral oil	Coat fecal mass, soften stool, and facilitate passage
Glycerin	
Wetting agents	
Docusate salts	Allow entry of water and lipids to soften stool

Osmotic laxatives include such diverse substances as magnesium salts, hypertonic saline, and lactulose. By increasing the water content in the intestinal lumen, the osmotic laxatives also increase bulk. Magnesium sulfate is widely used, as is magnesium in the form of milk of magnesia.

Lactulose (Chronulac) is a semisynthetic disaccharide that is not hydrolyzed in the small intestine but is metabolized, by bacteria in the large bowel, to lactate and other compounds that are not well absorbed. Because it acts within the large bowel, its onset of action is slow. Lactulose is administered in the form of a syrup. Excessive dosage can produce diarrhea and electrolyte loss. In addition to its laxative effect, lactulose is used in portal systemic encephalopathy, in which it reduces blood ammonia.

Glycerin suppositories, which are useful in children or elderly or debilitated persons, promote defecation within a short period of time. Glycerin stimulates evacuation reflexly by a hyperosmotic action on the rectal mucosa. In addition, it is a lubricant for hardened fecal material.

Contact agents should not be used as laxatives because their irritant effects stimulate vigorous intestinal motility. They promote formation of watery stools and can cause cramping and pain. An exception is *bisacodyl* (Dulcolax, others), which produces a soft stool associated with little colic. This agent stimulates the large intestine, and it is useful for preparation of patients for proctoscopic or colonoscopic procedures. Preparations of bisacodyl include enteric-coated tablets and suppositories. The suppository form should not be used in patients with a fissure or ulcerations because systemic absorption may occur.

Another contact agent, *phenolphthalein*, is found in various nonproprietary preparations. This substance acts primarily in the large intestine, and it will color alkaline feces. It is partially absorbed and can cause undesirable skin eruptions and prolonged discoloration. The phenomenon of fixed eruption by this agent probably has an allergic mechanism because even small doses cause the dermal response in sensitive persons.

Surface-active agents include *docusate* (dioctyl sulfosuccinate) salts (Colace, others). They are mild laxatives because of a surface effect on the intestinal contents. They act as dispersing or wetting agents that permit water and lipids to enter the mass and soften it. Wetting agents are otherwise inert. They are slow in onset of action, and the full effect may require as long as 2 days to develop. Diarrhea is an occasional adverse reaction.

1. Binder, H.J.: Pharmacology of laxatives, Annu. Rev. Pharmacol. Toxicol. **17**:355, 1977.

2. Deakin, M., Ramage, J., Paul, A., et al.: Effect of enprostil, a synthetic prostaglandin E_2 on 24 hour intragastric acidity, nocturnal acid and pepsin secretion, Gut **27**:1054, 1986.

3. Fordtran, J.S., and Walsh, J.H.: Gastric acid secretion rate and buffer content of the stomach after eating: results in normal subjects and in patients with duodenal ulcer, J. Clin. Invest. **52**:645, 1973.

4. Grossman, M.I.: Peptic ulcer: new therapies, new diseases, Ann. Intern. Med. **95**:609, 1981.

5. Holt, K.M., and Isenberg, J.I.: Peptic ulcer disease: physiology and pathophysiology, Hosp. Pract. **20**(1):89, 1985.

6. Howard, J.M., Chremos, A.N., Collen, M.J., et al.: Famotidine, a new, potent, long-acting histamine H_2-receptor antagonist: comparison with cimetidine and ranitidine in the treatment of Zollinger-Ellison syndrome, Gastroenterology **88**:1026, 1985.

7. McCarthy, D.M.: Peptic ulcer: antacids or cimetidine? Hosp. Pract. **14**(12):52, 1979.

8. Morrissey, J.F., and Barreras, R.F.: Antacid therapy, N. Engl. J. Med. **290**:550, 1974.

9. Netchvolodoff, C.V., and Hargrove, M.D., Jr.: Recent advances in the treatment of diarrhea, Arch. Intern. Med. **139**:813, 1979.

10. Richardson, C.T.: Sucralfate, Ann. Intern. Med. **97**:269, 1982.

section eight

Drugs that influence metabolic and endocrine functions

42 Insulin, glucagon, and oral hypoglycemic agents, 530

43 Adrenal steroids, 543

44 Thyroid hormones and antithyroid drugs, 557

45 Parathyroid extract and vitamin D, 567

46 Posterior pituitary hormones—vasopressin and oxytocin, 573

47 Anterior pituitary gonadotropins and sex hormones, 580

48 Pharmacologic approaches to gout, 599

49 Antianemic drugs, 605

50 Vitamins, 614

Insulin, glucagon, and oral hypoglycemic agents

GENERAL
CONCEPT

Insulin, the hormone elaborated by the β cells of the pancreas, is a key regulator of metabolic processes. Its major role is to promote storage of fuel for energy. Insulin stimulates glucose transport and metabolism, enhances glycogen synthesis, and stimulates lipogenesis. It also has important growth-promoting actions in a variety of tissues. Although its action on carbohydrate metabolism has received the most attention, an absolute or relative deficiency of insulin results in other serious metabolic changes. *Glucagon*, the hormone produced by the α cells of pancreatic islets, opposes the anabolic effects of insulin by stimulating glycogenolysis and producing hyperglycemia. The ratio of these two hormones may determine the overall metabolic effect. Glucagon also has a positive inotropic action on the heart, probably caused by stimulation of cyclic AMP formation. The orally active *sulfonylurea* drugs promote release of insulin from β cells and improve peripheral utilization of glucose. They are useful therefore only in patients with functional β cells.

INSULIN
Current concepts

Insulin is the most widely studied peptide hormone. Since its initial isolation and characterization, much has been learned about its actions and importance in normal physiology. *Diabetes mellitus* and other disorders of carbohydrate metabolism characterized by abnormal insulin secretion or activity are among the most common metabolic diseases.

In 1889 surgical removal of the pancreas from dogs was shown to cause diabetes, and approximately 30 years later insulin was isolated from the canine pancreas. It was not until the 1960s, however, that its amino acid sequence was established, and insulin was synthesized. The introduction of insulin as a replacement hormone in diabetes mellitus revolutionized treatment of this disease, and insulin therapy greatly prolonged the lives of juvenile diabetic patients. Long-lasting forms of the hormone extended its duration of action. The most recent advances include the cloning and production of human insulin through genetic engineering and the development of continuous-delivery systems for synthetic insulin.

Biosynthesis and
release of insulin

Insulin is formed in the β cells of the pancreatic islets as part of a larger protein, *proinsulin* (Fig. 42-1). This precursor, approximately 1.5 times the molecular weight of insulin, is one of a family of peptides that includes the somatomedins or insulin-like growth factors. Within acidified secretory vesicles of the islet cells, proinsulin

Structure of bovine proinsulin showing A and B chains and C-peptide. Human proinsulin differs in three amino acids in the chains and several amino acids in the C-peptide.   **FIG. 42-1**

From Steiner, D.F.: TRIANGLE, the Sandoz Journal of Medical Science 2(2):52, 1972.

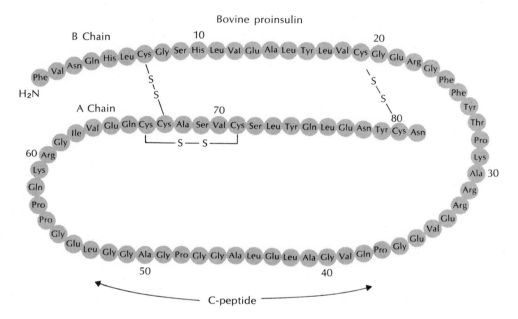

is proteolytically processed to insulin and a C-peptide (connecting peptide).[9] Insulin consists of two polypeptide chains joined by disulfide linkages. It circulates as free hormone with a half-life of approximately 9 minutes and is degraded in the liver and kidneys.

Proinsulin is also released to some extent into the circulation; normally about 6% to 8% of plasma insulin is in this precursor form. In some islet adenomas the percentage is higher. The C-peptide released from proinsulin has no biologic activity, but it can be used to assess insulin secretion. This is important in persons who may have decreased insulin activity attributable to circulating antibodies.

Regulation of blood glucose is a complex process that integrates hormonal and neural mechanisms in the central nervous system, the pancreas, and the autonomic nervous system.[3] It was recognized in early experimental studies that insulin deficiency caused the metabolic derangements in diabetes and that replacement of insulin alleviated the symptoms and changes associated with the disease. Recent research has indicated, however, that neural influences and counterregulatory hormone secretions are important factors in determining insulin secretion as well as target cell response.

Two regions in the hypothalamus regulate glucose production in the liver. Stimulation of the *ventromedial* hypothalamus rapidly increases glycogenolysis, whereas

Regulation of blood glucose

stimulation of the *ventrolateral* region leads to hepatic glycogenesis; it is believed that the former pathways involve β-adrenergic receptor mechanisms and that the latter pathways are primarily cholinergic. This neural regulation is independent of pancreatic or adrenal hormones.

Neural regulation of insulin secretion from the pancreas is mediated by both sympathetic and parasympathetic pathways. The islet β cells contain both α- and β-adrenergic as well as muscarinic cholinergic receptors. Vagal stimulation and stimulation of β-receptors increase insulin secretion, whereas sympathetic nerve activity and circulating catecholamines can inhibit secretion through α-adrenergic receptors.

The primary physiologic stimulus for insulin secretion is glucose, but certain amino acids, gastrointestinal hormones, ketone bodies, and α-adrenergic receptor antagonists also enhance insulin release. Inhibitors of insulin release include muscarinic antagonists, α-adrenergic receptor agonists, β-receptor antagonists, and diazoxide.

Somatostatin, a polypeptide found in the central nervous system, the gastrointestinal tract, and the pancreas, also plays a role in glucoregulation. It affects glucose absorption from the gut and production by the liver, but its primary effects are inhibition of glucagon and insulin secretion by a paracrine mechanism that involves inhibition of a cyclic AMP–mediated process. Somatostatin is synthesized in the D cells of the pancreas, which constitute about 10% of the islet cells. Excessive production of somatostatin from pancreatic tumors is associated with mild carbohydrate intolerance and relative hypoinsulinemia.[3]

Growth hormone from the anterior pituitary gland (Chapter 47) has complex effects on carbohydrate and lipid metabolism. It has a diabetogenic effect in man and in experimental animals. By promoting lipolysis and utilization of fats rather than carbohydrates as a source of fuel, an excess of growth hormone worsens hyperglycemia and ketosis in diabetic patients.

Insulin receptors

The receptor for insulin, like those for other peptide hormones, has two fundamental functions: recognition and binding of the hormone and transmission of a signal to alter intracellular metabolic pathways. Insulin binds to a glycoprotein receptor on target tissues, where one portion, the α subunit, serves the binding function and the other, the β subunit, signals the intracellular changes. The rates of internalization, biosynthesis, and turnover of insulin receptors are also important determinants of the hormone action. A current model of the insulin receptor is shown in Fig. 42-2. The insulin receptor, unlike many other hormone receptors, is not restricted to target tissues for insulin but is found on most mammalian cells.

How the insulin-receptor complex mediates the biologic effects of the hormone is still unknown. The observation that the β subunit of the receptor is a tyrosine-specific protein kinase indicates that kinase activation may be important for the metabolic action of insulin. Tyrosine kinase is also associated with proteins that participate in cell growth. Based on its protein sequence, the insulin receptor appears similar to certain other growth factors and viral oncogenes.[7]

Insulin receptor.

From Kahn, C.R.: Annu. Rev. Med. **36:**429, copyright 1985; reproduced with permission from Annual Reviews, Inc.

FIG. 42-2

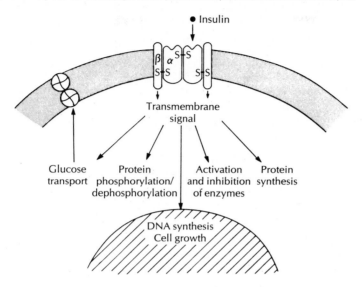

Another possibility is that insulin binding to its receptor generates a "second messenger," which then exerts biologic activity. However, in contrast to glucagon, insulin does not appear to act through formation of cyclic AMP. In fact, insulin may inhibit cyclic AMP–dependent protein kinase.[11]

The link between genetic obesity and a deficiency of insulin receptors in experimental animals indicated that alterations of the hormone receptor could be involved in disease. It is now recognized that the most common disorders of glucose metabolism involve the target cell rather than the pancreas. Even when secretory defects occur, as in insulin-dependent diabetes, changes in target cell receptors can modify the clinical state. Antibodies to insulin receptor proteins can decrease the response to the hormone. Moderate insulin resistance attributable to a deficiency of insulin receptors can occur in obesity, non–insulin dependent diabetes, and acromegaly. On the other hand, supersensitivity caused by an enhanced number of insulin receptors has been reported in anorexia nervosa.[10]

Actions of insulin

The action of secreted or injected insulin ultimately affects carbohydrate, lipid, and protein metabolism. Basically, insulin has metabolic and growth-promoting properties. Metabolic effects, such as increased glucose transport, phospholipid turnover, and activation of intracellular enzymes, occur within minutes of hormone-receptor interaction in the target tissues. These reactions are stimulated by relatively low concentrations of the hormone. Growth-promoting effects, including enhanced protein, lipid, and nucleotide synthesis, are expressed over hours or days and require higher insulin concentrations. These anabolic effects appear to be particularly important during fetal growth and organogenesis, as well as in tissue repair and regeneration.[7]

When insulin is injected into a normal or diabetic person, it causes several changes in blood chemistry: (1) a reduction in blood glucose, (2) increased pyruvate and lactate, (3) decreased inorganic phosphate, and (4) decreased potassium. In diabetics insulin also lowers free amino acid concentrations in circulation by promoting uptake and incorporation into protein. The effect on blood glucose may be explained by enhanced uptake of glucose by tissues such as muscle and fat. Insulin also inhibits glycogenolysis in the liver. The changes in pyruvate and lactate concentration are generally attributed to greater glucose utilization. As more glucose 6-phosphate is produced, more metabolic products accumulate. The fall in phosphate concentration is believed to reflect increased glucose phosphorylation. A decrease in plasma potassium concentration accompanies glycogen deposition in the liver though the mechanism is not well understood.

Insulin deficiency	When the formation of insulin is inadequate, as in insulin-dependent diabetes, and glucose uptake is severely decreased, additional hormones act to provide alternative sources of fuel. Epinephrine, glucagon, growth hormone, and hydrocortisone mobilize free fatty acids, which are converted into ketone bodies by the liver. These agents also accelerate gluconeogenesis in the liver. Major problems arise when these counterregulatory mechanisms are inadequate when they produce large amounts of harmful metabolites. When glucose is not available, enhanced conversion of protein to glucose increases urea and ammonia. Increased lipolysis leads to elevation of fatty acids, formation of ketones, and the eventual development of metabolic acidosis.
GLUCAGON	The hyperglycemic effect of pancreatic extracts was noted by Banting and Best at the time of their signal studies on insulin. Later, a hyperglycemic factor was separated from pancreatic extracts and named "glucagon," the mobilizer of glucose. It was only many years later that its contribution to the physiology of the pancreas was recognized.
Synthesis and secretion	Glucagon is synthesized as a prohormone in pancreatic α cells and converted proteolytically to a polypeptide of 29 amino acids. In contrast to insulin, glucagon is a single chain that does not contain disulfide linkages. It is degraded by liver and kidney and has a plasma half-life of approximately 5 minutes. Glucagon is believed to be one of a family of peptide hormones that includes secretin, VIP (vasoactive intestinal polypeptide), and gastrointestinal inhibitory peptide (GIP).
Actions and relation to diabetes	The actions of glucagon generally oppose those of insulin, but the coordinated secretion of both hormones prevents significant fluctuations in blood glucose concentration. The mechanism through which this occurs is complex and involves paracrine regulation of insulin secretion by both glucagon from the α cells and somatostatin from D cells.

Glucagon promotes hepatic glycolysis and lipolysis, with the subsequent development of hyperglycemia and ketosis, to produce a diabetic state in which there is a relative or absolute decrease in the amount of circulating insulin. The metabolic actions of glucagon involve interaction with specific cellular receptors that activate adenylate cyclase. As a result, cyclic AMP concentration increases and cyclic AMP–dependent protein kinases are activated.[2] These effects culminate in the mobilization of fuels to meet energy requirements of the brain and other tissues in the absence of circulating glucose.

Normally, glucagon secretion is suppressed by insulin, and insulin secretion is stimulated by a small increase in glucagon concentration. Because of the insulin deficiency in insulin-dependent diabetes mellitus the normal suppression of glucagon is lost. Thus the development of the disease depends on a defect in both hormones. Somatostatin, which suppresses both insulin and glucagon secretion, has been used experimentally to decrease glucagon concentrations in insulin-dependent diabetes. Unfortunately, both the hyperglycemia and the ketonemia characteristic of glucagon excess reappear on cessation of somatostatin infusion.[11]

DRUG THERAPY OF DIABETES

It is currently accepted that diabetes mellitus is a heterogeneous group of hyperglycemic disorders. Hyperglycemia can result from a relative or absolute insulin deficiency in the presence of a relative excess of glucagon. Prolonged elevation of blood glucose in an uncontrolled manner leads to complications that involve the retina, kidney, nerves, and blood vessels.

Classification of diabetes

Diabetes is divided into two major categories based on whether endogenous insulin secretion is sufficient to prevent ketoacidosis. The type 1 diabetic, the patient with insulin-dependent diabetes mellitus (IDDM), lacks β cell function and requires insulin therapy to prevent diabetic ketoacidosis. The common form of IDDM is believed to have a genetic basis, and over 90% of affected persons express particular major histocompatibility antigens. The development of the disease, however, appears to require both the genetic background of susceptibility and certain environmental factors, such as viral infection. The onset of the disease is generally sudden. An autoimmune mechanism has been proposed, and studies with animal models indicate that T-cells are involved in both destruction of islet cells and rejection of islet implants.[5] It is still unclear whether the circulating anti-islet antibodies found in experimental or clinical diabetes are a cause or a result of the disease process.[11]

Type 2 diabetes, in which there are functional β cells, is generally referred to as non–insulin dependent diabetes mellitus (NIDDM). This, the more common of the hyperglycemic disorders, occurs in 70% to 80% of patients with diabetes.[8] These persons do not usually require exogenous insulin to prevent ketosis, and their symptoms ordinarily appear gradually during adult life. They are, however, at high risk for the same complications that affect patients with IDDM. Although a genetic basis for NIDDM appears likely, the mode of inheritance in most cases remains unknown. An insulin receptor defect appears likely in some patients, particularly in obese persons.

The therapeutic objectives in NIDDM do not differ from those in IDDM, but there are several subcategories of NIDDM, and there is a broad spectrum of islet cell function. Although insulin may not be required to prevent life-threatening ketoacidosis in these patients, it is part of the therapeutic regimen for some. Others may be maintained by dietary restrictions and weight loss. Only patients with functional β cells can be treated with the oral antihyperglycemic agents, the sulfonylureas (see pp. 538 to 540).

Rationale for metabolic control	Therapy in either IDDM or NIDDM is based on the assumption that the degenerative processes of long-term diabetes are caused, either directly or indirectly, by hyperglycemia. Although it is hoped that correction of the metabolic and hormonal abnormalities of diabetes will prevent development of complications, this is not clearly established. Benefits of glycemic control, however, include a return to normal of blood glucose, amino acid, free fatty acid, triglyceride, cholesterol, lactate, and pyruvate concentrations. Plasma glucagon concentration is normalized, and most patients experience an improved sense of well-being. Healing of foot ulcers is accelerated, and gastroparesis may improve. Meticulous control during pregnancy is clearly indicated to protect the fetus from metabolic abnormalities associated with diabetes, as well as to minimize maternal complications.
Insulin therapy	Several factors make therapy of diabetes more than simply replacement of a deficient hormone. First, the half-life of insulin is short, since insulin is readily metabolized and removed from circulation. Second, the intricate control of insulin secretion by neural, endocrine, and paracrine influences makes the normal pattern of insulin secretion difficult to duplicate with exogenously administered hormone. Third, administration of insulin by injection differs from the normal secretion from the pancreas into the portal circulation. Finally, institution of insulin therapy requires a commitment to implement the therapeutic regimen because control of hyperglycemia involves at least some inconvenience to the patient.[1]
PREPARATIONS AND CLINICAL USE	Insulin preparations differ mainly in their rate of absorption after subcutaneous injection. The rapidly absorbed and short acting *regular insulin* is the only preparation that can be given intravenously. It has been modified by two methods to form less readily absorbed suspensions. First, protamine, a basic compound, has been added to raise the isoelectric point of the acidic insulin peptide. This combination produces protamine insulin. A second approach is to use high concentrations of zinc and acetate buffer to prepare insulin with various particle sizes. Aside from regular insulin, the most widely used insulins are isophane insulin suspension (NPH insulin) and insulin zinc suspension (lente insulin), which are intermediate in onset and duration. The properties of various insulin preparations are listed in Table 42-1.

| Action | Preparation | Hours after subcutaneous injection | | Units/ml |
		Peak action	Duration of action	
Rapid	Insulin injection (regular, crystalline zinc)	2.5-5	6-8	40, 100, 500
	Prompt insulin zinc suspension (semilente)	5-10	12-16	40, 100
Intermediate	Isophane insulin suspension (NPH)	4-12	24	40, 100
	Insulin zinc suspension (lente)	7-15	24	40, 100
Long	Protamine zinc insulin suspension	14-24	36	40, 100
	Extended insulin zinc suspension (ultralente)	10-30	36	40, 100

TABLE 42-1   Insulin preparations

In addition to USP insulins, which may contain up to 6% proinsulin, single-component insulins are available that are more than 99% pure with activities of 26 to 30 units of activity per milligram. The latter insulins are less likely to cause antibody formation; thus they reduce the chance of insulin resistance.

Precise glucoregulation can be achieved by insulin delivery through continuous infusion devices. These can be programmed to provide insulin at a constant basal rate with boluses administered just before meals.[11] Because of the constant monitoring necessary and the potential for hypoglycemia during nighttime fasting, these devices should be used only by highly motivated and adequately trained persons.

MONITORING

Although the degree of glycemic control needed to prevent complications is still not established, most clinicians expect that maintenance of blood glucose within a normal range will at least retard progression of neuropathic and vascular sequelae. To this end, close monitoring of blood glucose (for example, up to four times a day) is required. This can be done at home with kits that use capillary blood and a glucose oxidase–coated paper strip. The color of the exposed paper indicates the glucose concentration. Other means of control that can be used in an office or hospital setting include biochemical assays of blood glucose.[8] In addition, the degree of glycosylation of hemoglobin provides a measure of overall blood glucose regulation and, in effect, serves as an integrated function of control of blood glucose.

ADVERSE EFFECTS OF INSULIN

Adverse effects of insulin include hypoglycemia, local or systemic allergic reactions, lipoatrophy, and visual disturbances. The most serious of these is hypoglycemia, which can cause brain damage. Patients with IDDM are vulnerable to insulin-induced hypoglycemia during exercise or fasting. Normal persons are protected from hypoglycemia by a decrease in insulin and a rise in glucagon or catecholamine concentration, which modulate further islet hormone secretion. Diabetics cannot marshal

FIG. 42-3 *1, Control; 2, glucagon and epinephrine deficiency; 3, glucagon deficiency with α- and β-adrenergic receptor blockade. Hypoglycemia counterregulation is governed by glucagon and epinephrine. Plasma glucose in controls with normal glucagon and epinephrine concentrations rebounds quickly after moderate drop. Glucose concentrations in glucagon- and epinephrine-deficient subjects plunge dangerously low; adrenergic blockade in glucagon-deficient subjects causes significant fall with early partial recovery.*

Data of P.E. Cryer and J.E. Gerick; modified from Levin, P.A., McLaughlin, J., and Kowarski, A.A.: Hosp. Pract. **19**(10):137, 1984.

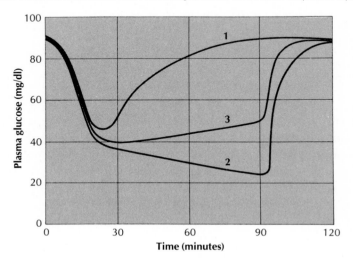

these defenses, and, furthermore, during sleep they may be unaware of symptoms of hypoglycemia, such as tachycardia and sweating. Thus continuous insulin infusion should be used with great caution in patients who are unable to generate a counterregulatory response to hypoglycemia.[8] Fig. 42-3 shows changes in blood glucose in subjects who lack this response. Research is currently focusing on implantable glucose sensors that can monitor extracellular glucose. These could be inserted within an infusion system to alter insulin delivery by a closed-loop system. Additional complications of infusion therapy include cutaneous abscesses from the indwelling needle and severe diabetic decompensation attributable to undetected interruption of insulin delivery.[11]

Oral hypoglycemic agents

The introduction of hypoglycemic sulfonylurea compounds was a notable development in management of diabetes. Loubatières observed in 1942 that some sulfonamides, administered to patients suffering from typhoid fever, produced symptoms and signs of hypoglycemia. It was then established through extensive investigation by numerous laboratories that certain sulfonylureas produce hypoglycemia in normal animals but not in animals made diabetic by administration of alloxan. Later, it was noted that biguanide compounds, such as phenformin, cause similar effects. Because of a high incidence of lactic acidosis in patients receiving phenformin, the biguanides are no longer used in the United States. Since most diabetics have NIDDM and no loss of β cells, the search for additional hypoglycemic agents has been extensive. At present, however, the only such drugs available are the sulfonylureas.

To the sulfonylureas that were widely used initially to control hyperglycemia in patients with NIDDM have been added second-generation compounds. The latter are more potent than the first-generation drugs, but there are no substantive improvements in efficacy or differences in mechanism of action. The major advantage appears to be that they offer a wider range of options, and some may cause fewer side effects. In addition, some studies indicate that patients who do not respond to first-generation sulfonylureas may respond to the newer agents. The structures of the available agents are given below.

First generation

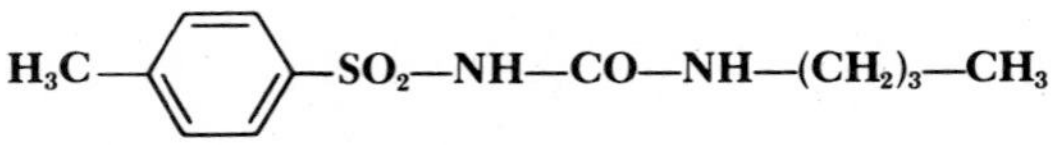

H_3C—⟨benzene⟩—SO_2—NH—CO—NH—$(CH_2)_3$—CH_3

Tolbutamide

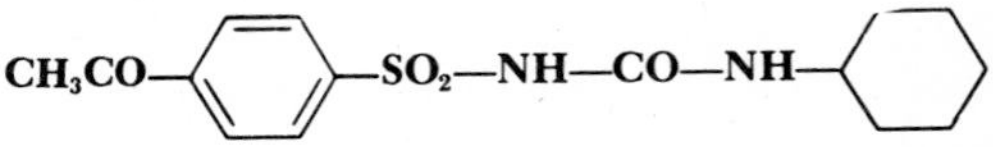

CH_3CO—⟨benzene⟩—SO_2—NH—CO—NH—⟨cyclohexyl⟩

Acetohexamide

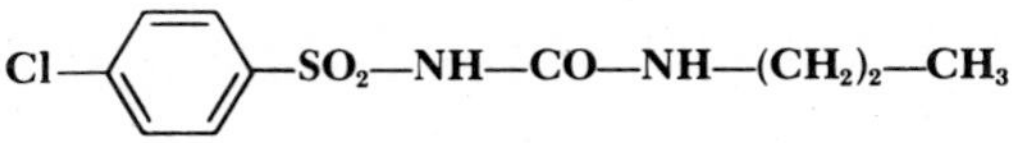

Cl—⟨benzene⟩—SO_2—NH—CO—NH—$(CH_2)_2$—CH_3

Chlorpropamide

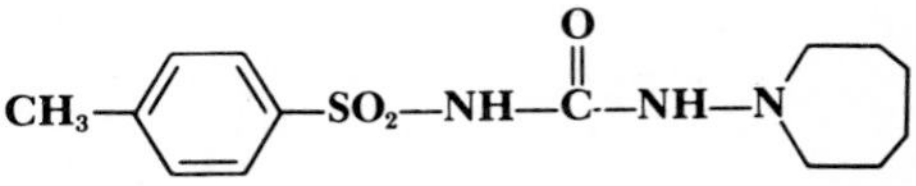

CH_3—⟨benzene⟩—SO_2—NH—$\overset{O}{\overset{\|}{C}}$—NH—N⟨ring⟩

Tolazamide

Second generation

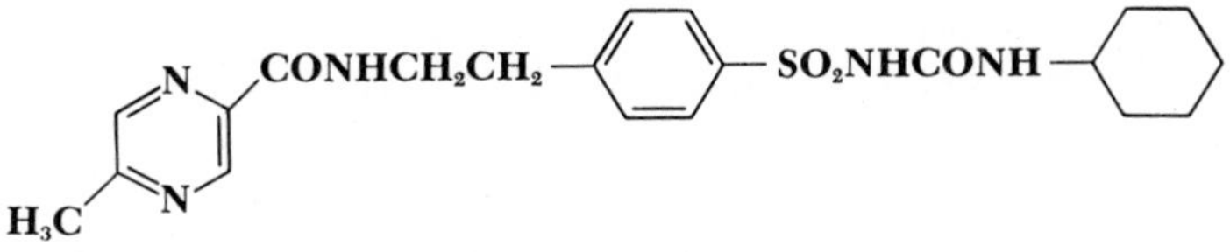

⟨pyrazine with H_3C⟩—$CONHCH_2CH_2$—⟨benzene⟩—$SO_2NHCONH$—⟨cyclohexyl⟩

Glipizide

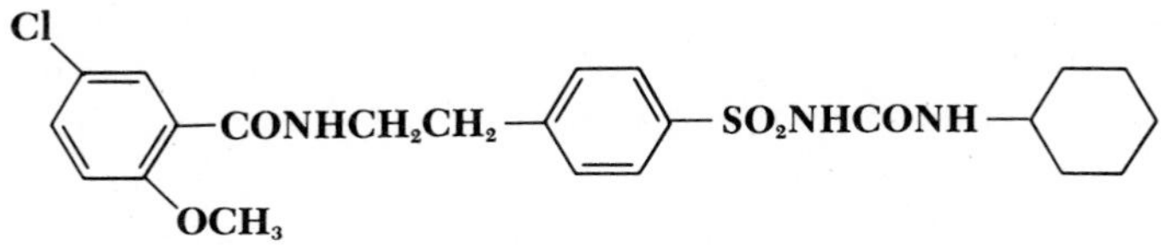

⟨benzene with Cl and OCH_3⟩—$CONHCH_2CH_2$—⟨benzene⟩—$SO_2NHCONH$—⟨cyclohexyl⟩

Glyburide

Despite earlier arguments to the contrary, intact pancreatic β cells are essential for the hypoglycemic action of sulfonylureas. Acute administration of these drugs stimulates insulin release, which has been shown to correlate with degranulation in the β cells. It has been suggested that sulfonylurea drugs lower the glycemic threshold for the β-cell secretory response. However, additional mechanisms that may con-

MECHANISM OF ACTION

TABLE 42-2	Characteristics of oral sulfonylurea drugs		
Name	Half-life (hours)	Duration of action (hours)	Tablet size (mg)
First generation			
Tolbutamide (Orinase, Oramide)	4-6	6-12	250, 500
Acetohexamide (Dymelor)	6-8*	12-24	250, 500
Chlorpropamide (Diabenese, Glucamide)	24-42	24-60	100, 250
Tolazamide (Ronase, Tolinase)	7	10-14	100-500
Second generation			
Glipizide (Glucotrol)	3-7	24	5, 10
Glyburide (DiaBeta, Micronase)	10	24	1.25-5

*Active metabolite.

tribute to lowering of blood glucose include release of somatostatin to suppress glucagon secretion and enhanced binding of insulin to target cell receptors. In addition, sulfonylurea compounds appear to act synergistically with insulin, and it has been proposed that they promote insulin sensitivity at a postreceptor level.[6]

In general, patients with a fasting glucose concentration above 330 mg/100 ml do not respond to sulfonylurea drugs. Those with a lower glucose concentration have at least a partial response though as many as 25% of these eventually become unresponsive. Loss of responsiveness may be caused by infections or stress. Failure of dietary control and weight gain may also play a part.[11]

PREPARATIONS AND CLINICAL USE

The characteristics of oral hypoglycemic drugs are listed in Table 42-2. The major differences in half-life and duration of action are determined by their fate in the body. Tolbutamide and tolazamide are rapidly metabolized. Acetohexamide is also rapidly metabolized, but its metabolite is more potent than the original drug. Chlorpropamide is long-acting because it is less completely metabolized.

ADVERSE EFFECTS

With sulfonylureas, hypoglycemia is generally not so great a danger as with insulin, but in some cases it may be serious and of long duration. The longer-acting drugs have a propensity to cause this adverse effect. Intolerance to alcohol similar to the disulfiram reaction may occur, and gastrointestinal and allergic skin reactions have been reported.

Drug interactions complicate therapy with sulfonylureas. The metabolism of tolbutamide can be inhibited by several drugs (see Chapter 63). Although some sulfonylureas are highly protein bound and may therefore be susceptible to displacement interactions, such interactions are transient and usually of little or no clinical significance. Thiazide diuretics reduce the activity of sulfonylureas.

Pathway of sorbitol in the lens.   *FIG. 42-4*

From Kinoshita, J.H.: Ann. Intern. Med. 101:83, copyright 1984; reproduced with permission from American Medical Association.

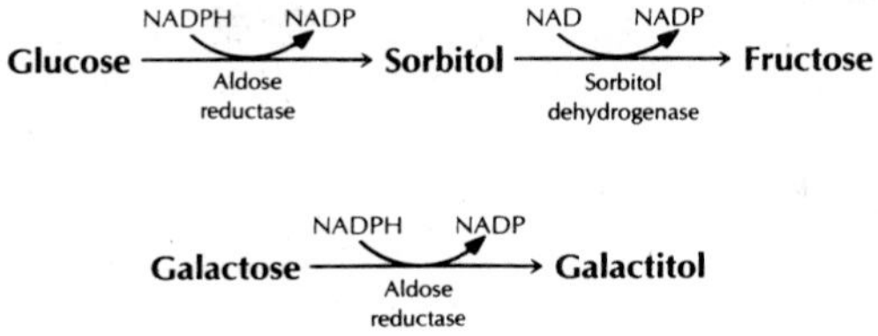

Other aspects of diabetes management, such as diet, have been reevaluated in recent years. Some patients with NIDDM can be controlled by dietary measures alone, particularly if obesity is corrected. Although for many years a low-carbohydrate diet was considered mandatory for diabetic control, a diet containing up to 60% total calories in carbohydrates is acceptable, provided that simple sugars are avoided. Fat intake should be limited, and foods with a high fiber content are recommended.

Potential means of control include inhibitors of gluconeogenesis and inhibitors of counterregulatory hormones. These approaches are still experimental, but some analogs of somatostatin and glucagon appear promising as inhibitors of glucagon secretion.[6]

One particularly promising approach is the use of *aldose reductase inhibitors* to combat development of diabetic complications. The underlying mechanism of diabetic retinopathy and neuropathy is believed to be related to accumulation of sorbitol formed from glucose by the action of aldose reductase.[4] The tissues that bear the brunt of diabetic complications, the lens, retina, nerves, kidney, and blood vessels, do not require insulin for uptake as muscle and adipose tissues do. The former tissues are therefore continually exposed to high concentrations of glucose in the hyperglycemic state. Continued conversion of glucose to sorbitol and subsequently to fructose leads to accumulation of these products within the tissues (Fig. 42-4). Galactose is an even better substrate for aldose reductase, and the product galactitol is not further metabolized. Because sorbitol and other polyols do not readily pass through cell membranes, they cause osmotic swelling and eventual cell disruption.

Evidence obtained from studies of experimental diabetes in animals and clinical disease in humans implicates aldose reductase in cataract formation, retinopathy, and diabetic neuropathy. The first clinical trial of an aldose reductase inhibitor, in 1982, indicated that both motor and sensory nerve conduction were improved in patients treated with *sorbinil*. Aldose reductase inhibitors therefore may prove to be important agents in long-term management of diabetes and its complications.

Alternative therapies and new approaches

REFERENCES

1. Dupré, J.: Insulin therapy: progress and prospects, Hosp. Pract. **18**(11):171, 1983.
2. Farah, A.E.: Glucagon and the circulation, Pharmacol. Rev. **35**:181, 1983.
3. Frohman, L.A.: CNS peptides and glucoregulation, Annu. Rev. Physiol. **45**:95, 1983.
4. Gabbay, K.H.: The sorbitol pathway and the complications of diabetes, N. Engl. J. Med. **288**:831, 1973.
5. Janeway, C.: The immune destruction of pancreatic β cells, Immunol. Today **6**:229, 1985.
6. Johnson, D.G., and Bressler, R.: New pharmacologic approaches to the treatment of diabetes, Spec. Top. Endocrinol. Metab. **6**:163, 1984.
7. Kahn, C.R.: The molecular mechanism of insulin action, Annu. Rev. Med. **36**:429, 1985.
8. Levin, P.A., McLaughlin, J., and Kowarski, A.A.: Diabetes mellitus: customizing management, Hosp. Pract. **19**(10):137, 1984.
9. Orci, L., Ravazzola, M., Storch, M.-J., et al.: Proteolytic maturation of insulin is a post-golgi event which occurs in acidifying clathrin-coated secretory vesicles, Cell **49**:865, 1987.
10. Roth, J., and Taylor, S.I.: Receptors for peptide hormones: alterations in diseases of humans, Annu. Rev. Physiol. **44**:639, 1982.
11. Unger, R.H., and Foster, D.W.: Diabetes mellitus. In Wilson, J.D., and Foster, D.W., editors: Williams textbook of endocrinology, ed. 7, Philadelphia, 1985, W.B. Saunders Co., p. 1018.

Chapter 43

Adrenal steroids

Since the observation by Hench in 1949 of a dramatic response to *cortisone* in patients with rheumatoid arthritis, adrenal steroids and synthetic *corticosteroids* have become widely used and sometimes overused in medicine. Cortisone and related corticosteroids owe their popularity to their anti-inflammatory and immunosuppressive effects. More rarely, these drugs are used for substitution therapy in adrenal insufficiency, which is often iatrogenic.

Aldosterone, the main *mineralocorticoid* of the adrenal gland, stimulates sodium reabsorption and potassium and hydrogen secretion by the distal renal tubule and collecting ducts. It is not used therapeutically though a synthetic derivative is occasionally used in patients with autonomic insufficiency and orthostatic hypotension. On the other hand, aldosterone antagonists have important therapeutic applications.

During the 1940s there was an intense search for the active principles responsible for the life-sustaining role of the adrenal glands. In 1937 Reichstein and von Euw synthetically prepared desoxycorticosterone. They later demonstrated its presence in the adrenal glands.[10] Although this steroid has powerful effects on salt and water reabsorption by the kidney and became useful in management of Addison's disease, it was obvious that extracts of adrenal cortex also contained compounds that, in addition to affecting salt transport, could influence the metabolism of carbohydrates and proteins.

Hench observed that patients with rheumatoid arthritis tended to improve when jaundiced or when pregnant. He attributed this improvement to an "antirheumatic" factor from the adrenal gland. Subsequently, Kendall at the Mayo Clinic isolated *hydrocortisone* (cortisol). A milestone in the history of adrenal steroids was the report of Hench and co-workers[8] on the effectiveness of cortisone in rheumatoid arthritis.

Results of clinical trials in rheumatoid arthritis were dramatic, and soon cortisone was found to cause symptomatic improvement in an amazing number of disease conditions. It was recognized at the same time that cortisone was not a cure for these many diseases. It seemed "to provide the susceptible tissues with a shieldlike buffer against the irritant."[7]

Although hydrocortisone was largely responsible for the glucocorticoid activity of adrenal extracts, it was suspected that the extracts still contained some material whose mineralocorticoid activity was much greater than that of desoxycorticosterone.

The compound responsible for this activity was isolated in 1953 and was named "aldosterone."

Subsequent research on glucocorticoids led to development of a variety of new steroids that have significantly greater anti-inflammatory potency than cortisone. Their influence on carbohydrate metabolism generally parallels their anti-inflammatory activity. A significant advantage of the newer steroids such as prednisone, methylprednisolone, triamcinolone and dexamethasone is that they exert little effect on renal sodium reabsorption while possessing potent anti-inflammatory activity.

PITUITARY-ADRENAL RELATIONSHIPS

ACTH

ACTH (adrenocorticotropic hormone, corticotropin) is released from the anterior pituitary gland and stimulates adrenal steroid synthesis. The release of ACTH is promoted by a polypeptide isolated from the hypothalamus, called corticotropin-releasing factor (CRF) (Fig. 43-1).

Regulation of ACTH release is determined largely by the influence of blood hydrocortisone concentration on CRF production through negative feedback. Stressful stimuli, including drugs such as epinephrine, can override the feedback inhibition, release CRF and ACTH, and elevate the hydrocortisone concentration. In addition to these important regulatory influences, there is a diurnal variation in ACTH release.

The polypeptide ACTH was isolated from the anterior pituitary and eventually synthesized. Human ACTH consists of 39 amino acids, but not all of these are essential for biologic activity. The first 19 amino acids (counting from the N-terminus) are sufficient for stimulating hydrocortisone production. The first 13 amino acids in ACTH are the same as those in melanocyte-stimulating hormone (α-MSH), and so it is not surprising that ACTH exerts an effect on melanocytes. CRF has also been isolated and consists of 41 amino acids.

ACTH promotes synthesis of hydrocortisone from cholesterol by stimulating conversion of cholesterol to pregnenolone. This effect of ACTH is mediated by cyclic AMP (adenosine 3',5'-monophosphate). Cyclic AMP has been shown to act similarly to ACTH both in vitro and on the perfused dog adrenal gland. Other compounds, such as forskolin and cholera toxin, that increase intracellular cyclic AMP also promote synthesis of hydrocortisone.

Oral administration of ACTH is ineffective since the polypeptide is broken down in the gastrointestinal tract. When injected intravenously, ACTH is destroyed in minutes. For this reason, the hormone is administered either by intravenous infusion or as a repository injection (Cortrophin Gel, others) by intramuscular or subcutaneous routes. Corticotropin zinc hydroxide suspension is also given intramuscularly.

ACTH is used to diagnose disturbed adrenocortical function. An intravenous infusion of the hormone will increase the excretion of hydrocortisone metabolites if the adrenal glands are normal or hyperplastic.

Diagrammatic summary of the principal factors regulating ACTH secretion.   *FIG. 43-1*

From Ganong, W.F., Alpert, L.C., and Lee, T.C.: Review of medical physiology, ed. 6, Los Altos, Calif., 1973, Mange Medical Publications.

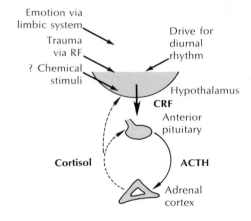

BIOSYNTHESIS OF ADRENAL STEROIDS

   Adrenal steroids are not stored in the adrenal cortex but are synthesized as needed. In the zona fasciculata and zona reticularis, cholesterol is changed to pregnenolone, which is metabolized to progesterone, to desoxyhydrocortisone and then to hydrocortisone. Another product of pregnenolone is androstenedione, the precursor of testosterone. In the zona glomerulosa, the sequence of events is cholesterol → pregnenolone → progesterone → desoxycorticosterone → aldosterone.

Inhibitors of steroid synthesis

   Certain toxic compounds such as amphenone B and the insecticide tetrachlorodiphenylethane (DDD) may damage the adrenal cortex. Amphenone B blocks several hydroxylation steps, whereas DDD is believed to inhibit cholesterol esterase. Aminoglutethimide (Cytadren) also blocks steroidogenesis by interfering with cholesterol side-chain cleavage and the conversion of cholesterol to pregnenolone. Trilostane and cyanoketone are experimental drugs that block synthesis of hydrocortisone and aldosterone by inhibiting the conversion of pregnenolone to progesterone.

   Metyrapone (Metopirone) is used as a diagnostic tool in patients with disorders of adrenal function. It inhibits 11β hydroxylation and blocks biosynthesis of hydrocortisone, corticosterone and aldosterone. The 11-desoxycorticosteroids that accumulate after blockade by metyrapone do not inhibit ACTH release. Thus the decrease in hydrocortisone and corticosterone enhances ACTH release from the anterior pituitary gland in normal persons. In this circumstance, ACTH stimulates production of 11-desoxyhydrocortisone and 11-desoxycorticosterone. The metabolites of these steroids, 17-hydroxycorticosteroids and 17-ketosteroids, can be measured in the urine (Fig. 43-2). If anterior pituitary function is deficient, metyrapone administration will not increase excretion of these metabolites. Hence metyrapone can be used to identify

FIG. 43-2 *Pituitary-adrenal feedback system and its inhibition by metyrapone.*

Modified from Coppage, W.S., Jr., Island, D., Smith, M., and Liddle, G.W.,: J. Clin. Invest. 38:2101, 1959.

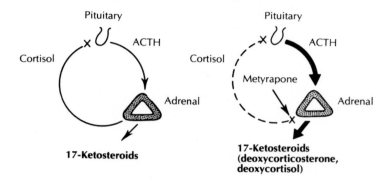

adrenal insufficiency that arises from pituitary, as opposed to adrenal, dysfunction. As would be predicted, however, the metyrapone test is useless if adrenocortical function is defective. This is ascertained beforehand by determining the influence of an ACTH infusion on urinary steroid output.

Metyrapone

In adults, metyrapone is administered orally in doses of 750 mg every 4 hours for six doses. Urinary steroids are determined in the subsequent 24 hours.

GLUCOCOR-TICOIDS

Hydrocortisone and corticosterone

Hydrocortisone and corticosterone are the principle glucocorticoids of the adrenal cortex. Hydrocortisone predominates in the human adrenal cortex, whereas in some species, such as the rat and rabbit, hydrocortisone is not synthesized and so corticosterone is the major glucocorticoid. Human adrenal glands contain 2.3 to 5.5 μg of hydrocortisone per gram of wet tissue. In the plasma of normal persons its concentration is about 80 ng/ml. The rate of secretion follows a characteristic rhythm or diurnal variation. Secretion increases in the early hours of the morning, before

Hydrocortisone

Corticosterone

Steps in glucocorticoid action. St, Steroid; R, specific glucocorticoid receptor; the dissimilar **FIG. 43-3**
shapes of R are intended to represent different conformations of this protein.

From Baxter, J.D., and Forsham, P.H.: Am. J. Med. **53**:573, 1972.

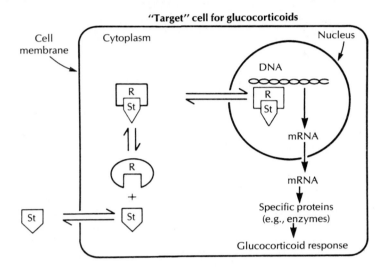

the person awakens, and gradually declines toward late evening. The reasons for this
anticipatory secretion before daily activities begin are not known. Normal daily output
of hydrocortisone in human beings is about 25 mg.

Corticosteroids act by controlling the rate of protein synthesis (Fig. 43-3).[1] The **PHARMACOLOGIC EFFECTS**
steroid diffuses into the cell and binds to a cytosolic receptor. The steroid-receptor
complex undergoes a conformational change and is translocated to the nucleus. In
the nucleus, the complex binds to chromatin and stimulates transcription of certain
messenger RNAs that code for synthesis of specific proteins or enzymes. These
proteins mediate the biologic effects of the steroids.

The three major effects of adrenal steroids are on (1) carbohydrate, protein and
fat metabolism, (2) mineral metabolism, and (3) inflammation.

Effects on carbohydrate and protein metabolism. The primary effects of hydrocortisone on carbohydrate and protein metabolism follow and are shown in Fig. 43-4:[1]

1. Carbohydrate metabolism
   a. An increase in gluconeogenesis (synthesis of glucose from protein)
   b. An increase in liver glycogen
   c. An increase in plasma glucose concentration
   d. A decrease in peripheral glucose utilization
2. Protein metabolism
   a. Mobilization of amino acids from tissues, mainly skeletal muscle
   b. An increase in nitrogen excretion in the urine because of protein metabolism

FIG. 43-4 *Glucocorticoid action on carbohydrate, lipid, and protein metabolism. Arrows, General flow of substrate in response to the catabolic and anabolic actions of glucocorticoids when unopposed by secondary secretions of other hormones. Not shown is increased gluconeogenesis by kidney. + or −, Stimulation or inhibition respectively.*

From Baxter, J.D., and Forsham, P.H.: Am. J. Med. **53:**573, 1972.

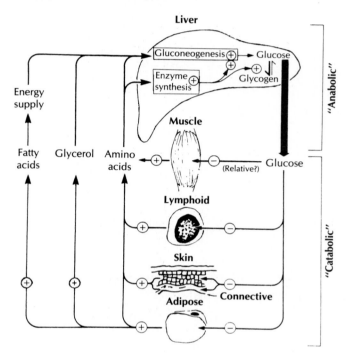

Little is known about the basic action of hydrocortisone on fat metabolism. Unusual accumulations of fat occur in the patient treated with glucocorticoids. Fat is redistributed from the periphery to the face giving a "moon face," to the back of the neck giving a "buffalo hump," and in the supraclavicular region. The glucocorticoids promote fat mobilization[8] and exert complex effects on ketone metabolism. For example, hydrocortisone has a *permissive* effect on free fatty acid release from adipose tissue by catecholamines.

Effects on electrolyte and water metabolism. Glucocorticoids exert much less effect on renal handling of electrolytes than desoxycorticosterone and aldosterone do; nevertheless, administration of hydrocortisone or cortisone increases sodium retention and potassium excretion and causes hypokalemic alkalosis in patients receiving prolonged treatment. On the other hand, patients with Addison's disease cannot be maintained in electrolyte balance with glucocorticoids alone. Adrenalectomized animals cannot excrete a large water load. Cortisone will restore this particular function.

TABLE 43-1	Effects of bilateral adrenalectomy
Circulatory	Decreased blood pressure Decreased blood volume Hyponatremia, hypochloremia, hypoglycemia, and hyperkalemia Increased nonprotein nitrogen
Renal	Increased excretion of sodium and chloride Decreased excretion of potassium
Digestive	Loss of appetite, nausea, and vomiting
Muscular	Weakness Decreased sodium and increased potassium and water in muscle
Miscellaneous	Decreased resistance to all forms of stress Hypertrophy of lymphoid tissue and thymus Death unless treatment is instituted

The cardiovascular actions of corticosteroids and mineralocorticoids can be accounted for by their effects on salt and water balance. For example, patients with Cushing's syndrome or primary aldosteronism retain sodium and have hypokalemia and hypertension. In contrast, patients with Addison's disease excrete an excess of sodium and have hyperkalemia, and cardiovascular collapse may develop because of volume depletion (Table 43-1).

Calcium metabolism is also affected by hydrocortisone. It promotes the renal excretion of calcium, and it may reduce calcium absorption from the intestine.

Anti-inflammatory action. Most clinical use of glucocorticoids and ACTH may be attributed to the remarkable ability of the steroids to inhibit the inflammatory process and act as immunosuppressants.

The mechanisms of the anti-inflammatory and immunosuppressant actions of the corticosteroids remain mysterious though there is no lack of theories on this subject.[2,4] The effects of corticosteroids that contribute to the therapeutic benefit include the following:

Lymphocytopenia, eosinophilia, and monocytopenia. Corticosteroids promote sequestration of lymphocytes and monocytes in the spleen, lymph nodes, and bone marrow. This reduces the number of these cells that reach the site of inflammation and thereby inhibits cell-mediated immunity and inflammation (Fig. 43-5).

A decrease in migration of polymorphonuclear leukocytes. Corticosteroids inhibit adherence of neutrophils to vascular endothelium and thereby reduce their movement from the vasculature into the site of inflammation.

Inhibition of macrophage processing of antigens. Antigens must be modified or processed before they can stimulate T- or B-lymphocytes. Corticosteroids inhibit the ability of macrophages to perform this function.

Inhibition of the actions of lymphokines. Lymphocytes release *lymphokines*, proteins that are chemotactic and cytotoxic (see Chapter 61). Corticosteroids do not modify synthesis of the lymphokines but instead inhibit their actions.

FIG. 43-5 *Effect of hydrocortisone administration on circulating lymphocytes and monocytes. Hydrocortisone, 400 mg, was administered intravenously in a single dose to a normal volunteer.*

From Fauci, A.S., Dale, D.C., and Balow, J.E.: Ann. Intern. Med. **84**:304-315, copyright 1976; reproduced with permission from American Medical Association.

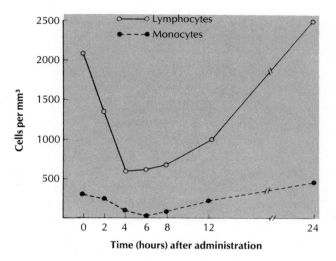

Inhibition of antibody-dependent cell-mediated cytotoxicity. Antibodies directed against a target cell will bind to the cell surface and coat the cell. Macrophages have receptors to the Fc portion of the antibody. This allows the macrophage to attach to the target cell by an antibody bridge that facilitates phagocytosis. Corticosteroids prevent this process by inhibiting binding of the antibodies to the Fc receptor of the macrophage.

Inhibition of arachidonic acid metabolism. Prostaglandins are vasodilators and promote pain, whereas leukotrienes promote chemotaxis and increase capillary permeability (see Chapter 22). Thus these arachidonic acid metabolites are believed to be mediators of inflammation. Corticosteroids promote synthesis of lipomodulin, a protein that inhibits phospholipase A_2. Calpactins are another group of proteins that were believed to be identical to lipomodulin. However, corticosteroids do not promote their synthesis. Calpactins bind to phospholipids so that they are no longer substrates for phospholipases.[3,5] These actions on phospholipase or phospholipids, in turn, prevent release of arachidonic acid and synthesis of prostaglandins, leukotrienes, and related compounds.

Miscellaneous effects. There is little doubt that cortisone exerts actions on the central nervous system. There may occur euphoria and other behavioral abnormalities that cannot be explained by clinical improvement of the primary disease. Psychoses may also develop. In addition, there is evidence that glucocorticoid treatment may lower convulsive thresholds.

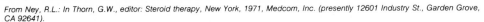

Pattern of plasma ACTH and hydrocortisone values in patients recovering from prior long-term daily glucocorticoid suppression of the pituitary-adrenal axis.   **FIG. 43-6**

From Ney, R.L.: In Thorn, G.W., editor: Steroid therapy, New York, 1971, Medcom, Inc. (presently 12601 Industry St., Garden Grove, CA 92641).

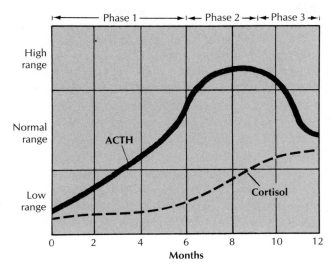

The glucocorticoids improve muscle strength in adrenalectomized animals. On the other hand, they can cause muscle weakness with prolonged treatment, perhaps because of potassium loss or mobilization of muscle protein.

Adverse effects. The effect of corticosteroid treatment to increase the risk of infection is poorly understood. Varicella and herpes can disseminate, herpes of the eye may be more severe, tuberculosis may be reactivated, and fungal diseases may develop after prolonged steroid therapy. Infection must be viewed as an added factor to consider, rather than as an absolute contraindication, when risks of using corticosteroids are appraised.

Excessive doses of glucocorticoids over a prolonged period of time produce the various manifestations of Cushing's disease. The most serious systemic complications that result from clinical use of high doses of steroids are the diabetogenic effects; dissolution of supporting tissues such as bone, muscle, and skin; hypertension; and impairment of defense mechanisms against serious infections.

Prolonged therapy with corticosteroids may produce a long-term suppression of the adrenal-pituitary axis (Fig. 43-6).[6] Suppression may occur when high doses are given for periods as short as 2 weeks. Lower doses require a longer period of therapy for this effect to occur, and use of alternate-day administration can often avoid this effect entirely. After discontinuation of therapy, adrenal and pituitary function may not return to normal for 9 to 12 months; patients may not respond normally to stress for up to 2 years. Thus after long-term therapy abrupt withdrawal of the corticosteroid may result in adrenal insufficiency because of the inability of the adrenal or pituitary to respond normally.

METABOLISM   Cortisone and other synthetic corticosteroids are absorbed rapidly and completely from the gastrointestinal tract. After oral administration, maximum plasma concentrations are reached in 1 to 2 hours. Hepatic degradation of corticosteroids leads to a fairly rapid fall in plasma concentrations, and so after 8 hours only 25% of the peak value can be demonstrated, and the active drug disappears completely in about 12 hours.

Drugs that promote the activity of microsomal enzymes in the liver tend to accelerate metabolism of corticosteroids. These drugs, which include phenobarbital and phenytoin, may necessitate an increase in corticosteroid dosage.

PREPARATIONS AND   **Hydrocortisone** is available in tablets containing 5 to 20 mg. It is also available
CLINICAL USAGE   for injection by various routes, including intravenous, and in lotions and ointments for topical application.

Cortisone is used almost entirely in tablet form or in suspension for intramuscular injection.

Certain principles may be derived concerning therapeutic use of adrenal steroids, as follows:

1. These drugs do not cure any disease. They are used predominantly for their anti-inflammatory properties and provide only symptomatic relief. They do not represent replacement therapy, as insulin does in diabetes, except in the rare conditions of Addison's disease or hypoadrenocorticism.

2. Adrenal steroid therapy is particularly useful in disease processes that occur in episodes and therefore do not require extended treatment. They are also very useful in conditions in which topical application is sufficient.

3. Every effort should be made to use other drugs or procedures before prolonged steroid treatment is undertaken. With continued use, hyperadrenocorticism resembling Cushing's syndrome may be inevitable. Cessation of treatment with these steroids may acutely exacerbate various diseases. Suppression of the pituitary-adrenal axis can present a serious danger if the patient encounters stressful situations.

4. Despite their many disadvantages, adrenal glucocorticoids are of great therapeutic importance in self-limiting diseases and in chronic disabling processes that fail to respond to any other treatment. The systemic use of these drugs is a calculated risk that is often worth taking in the presence of incapacitating and otherwise incurable disease.

Comparison of   Several glucocorticoids have been introduced into therapeutics on the basis of
various   having anti-inflammatory potency greater than hydrocortisone without also having a
glucocorticoids   corresponding increase in their tendency to retain sodium.

The chemical relationships among these newer glucocorticoids may be summarized in comparison with the structural formula of cortisone:

Cortisone

Hydrocortisone has the same structural formula as cortisone except that OH is in position 11.

Prednisone is the same as cortisone except that there is a double bond between positions 1 and 2. It is therefore 1,2-dehydrocortisone.

Prednisolone is the same as hydrocortisone except that there is a double bond between positions 1 and 2. It is therefore 1,2-dehydro-hydrocortisone.

Methylprednisolone is the same as prednisolone except that an α-CH_3 is in position 6.

Triamcinolone is the same as prednisolone except that an α-F is in position 9 and there is an additional α-OH in position 16. It is therefore 9α-fluoro-16α-hydroxyprednisolone.

Dexamethasone is the same as prednisolone except that there is an α-F in position 9 and an α-CH_3 in position 16. It is therefore 9α-fluoro-16α-methylprednisolone.

Betamethasone is the same as dexamethasone except that the CH_3 in position 16 is a β substitution instead of α. It is therefore 9α-fluoro-16β-methylprednisolone.

Fludrocortisone is the same as hydrocortisone except that an α-F is in position 9. It is 9α-fluorohydrocortisone.

Paramethasone is the same as dexamethasone except that the α-F is in position 6 rather than position 9. It is 6α-fluoro-16α-methylprednisolone.

Halcinonide (Halog) differs from triamcinolone by substitution of a chlorine for the hydroxyl group in position 21 and reduction of the double bond at positions 1 and 2.

The introduction of prednisone and prednisolone into therapeutics was of great practical importance, since their high anti-inflammatory activity is not coupled with a correspondingly high sodium-retaining potency. This separation of effects allows the physician to use these compounds without special salt-free diets and potassium supplementation.

The synthetic analogs of hydrocortisone are usually administered orally in the form of tablets (Table 43-2). Suspensions of some of the drugs are available for intramuscular and intra-articular administration. Although they are of low solubility,

TABLE 43-2   Comparison and dosage forms of various steroids

Steroid	Anti-inflammatory potency	Sodium retention	Daily dose (mg)	Dosage forms (mg)
Cortisone (Cortone)	0.8	0.8	50-100	T: 5-25; I: 25, 50
Hydrocortisone (Cortef, Hydrocortone)	1	1	50-100	T: 5-20; I: 25, 50*
Prednisone (Orasone, others)	2.5	0.8	10-20	T: 1-50; S: 5
Prednisolone (Cortalone, others)	3	0.8	10-20	T: 5; S: 15; I: *
Methylprednisolone (Medrol)	4	0	10-20	T: 2-32; I: *
Triamcinolone (Aristocort, Kenacort)	5	0	5-20	T: 1-8; S: 2, 4; I: *
Dexamethasone (Decadron)	20	0	0.75-3	T: 0.25-6; S: 0.5; I: *
Paramethasone (Haldrone)	6	0	4-6	T: 1, 2
Betamethasone (Celestone)	20	0	0.6-3	T: 0.6; S: 0.6; I: *
Desoxycorticosterone (DOCA, Percorten)	0	10-25	1-3	I: 5; P: 125; RI: 25
Fludrocortisone (Florinef)	12	100	0.1	T: 0.1
Aldosterone	0.2	250		
For oral inhalation				
Beclomethasone (Beclovent, Vanceril)				A: 0.042
Dexamethasone (Decadron)				A: 0.084
Flunisolide (AeroBid)				A: 0.250
Triamcinolone (Azmacort)				A: 0.100
For nasal inhalation				
Beclomethasone (Beconase, Vancenase)				A: 0.042
Dexamethasone (Decadron)				A: 0.084
Flunisolide (Nasalide)				A: 0.025

A, Aerosol or spray (approximate dose per actuation); *I*, injection (per milliliter); *P*, pellets for subcutaneous implantation; *RI*, repository injection (per milliliter); *S*, syrup, elixir, or oral solution (per 5 ml); *T*, tablet.
Various salts are available for injection by various routes.

water-soluble preparations of some of the steroids, such as succinates or 21-phosphates, are available for intravenous use. In addition, some preparations can be inhaled into the sinus cavities or into the lungs to relieve rhinitis or asthma respectively.

Dermatologic and other topical applications

The topical treatment of dermatologic, ophthalmologic, and otologic diseases has been revolutionized by the introduction of the anti-inflammatory corticosteroids. The percutaneous absorption, particle size, and vehicle composition of these preparations are important determinants of their topical activity.[9] Excessive use of these preparations over a large surface area may cause systemic effects.

Aldosterone is the main mineralocorticoid of the adrenal cortex. *Primary aldosteronism,* characterized by hypertension and potassium depletion, results from its excessive secretion. Aldosterone itself is not used therapeutically. Instead, desoxycorticosterone is used clinically to correct electrolyte abnormalities in adrenal insufficiency, and fludrocortisone is occasionally used to treat patients with autonomic insufficiency accompanied by severe orthostatic hypotension.

Aldosterone   **Desoxycorticosterone**

Although aldosterone can affect carbohydrate metabolism, its salt-retaining potency is so great and its concentration in blood is so small in relation to hydrocortisone that it has no effect on carbohydrate metabolism in physiologic concentrations. The release of aldosterone is regulated mainly by these three factors: ACTH, the renin-angiotensin system, and the plasma concentration of potassium, all of which stimulate the zona glomerulosa cells to synthesize aldosterone. A reduction in blood pressure or extracellular fluid volume is sensed by the kidney and promotes release of renin (see Chapter 18). This causes synthesis of angiotensin and, in turn, aldosterone release. By enhancing retention of sodium and water, aldosterone may then indirectly feed back to suppress renin release.

Aldosterone production is increased in either "primary" or "secondary" hyperaldosteronism. The former may be caused by adenoma or hyperplasia of the adrenal glands. Secondary hyperaldosteronism occurs with renal artery constriction, malignant hypertension, pregnancy and toxemia of pregnancy, cirrhosis of the liver, nephrotic edema, and in some patients congestive heart failure.

Spironolactone (Aldactone) antagonizes aldosterone at the level of the renal tubules (see Chapter 38). Spironolactone is a synthetic steroid that competes with aldosterone for its receptor in the distal tubule and collecting duct. Blocking the action of aldosterone increases sodium excretion and diminishes potassium secretion.

Desoxycortico-sterone and fludrocortisone

Desoxycorticosterone and fludrocortisone are mineralocorticoids with little or no glucocorticoid activity. Their main action is exerted on the renal tubules. Like aldosterone, they increase reabsorption of sodium and loss of potassium. Prolonged, intensive treatment with desoxycorticosterone in experimental animals can produce hypertension and necrotic changes in the heart and skeletal muscle. It is believed that these actions result from potassium loss and sodium retention. Fludrocortisone acetate has largely replaced desoxycorticosterone acetate in therapeutic usage.

ANDROGENS

In addition to glucocorticoids and aldosterone, the adrenal cortex produces androgenic steroids such as dehydroepiandrosterone. The production of androgenic steroids is greatly increased in the *adrenogenital syndrome* in which an enzymatic defect channels much of the steroid production toward androgens. Exogenous glucocorticoid administration tends to depress the androgen output of the adrenal gland through inhibition at the level of the pituitary gland.

REFERENCES

1. Baxter, J.D., and Forsham, P.H.: Tissue effects of glucocorticoids, Am. J. Med. **53**:573, 1972.
2. Claman, H.N.: Corticosteroids and lymphoid cells, N. Engl. J. Med. **287**:388, 1972.
3. Davidson, F.F., Dennis, E.A., Powell, M., and Glenney, J.R., Jr.: Inhibition of phospholipase A_2 by "lipocortins" and calpactins: an effect of binding to substrate phospholipids, J. Biol. Chem. **262**:1698, 1987.
4. Fauci, A.S., Dale, D.C., and Balow, J.E.: Glucocorticosteroid therapy: mechanisms of action and clinical considerations, Ann. Intern. Med. **84**:304, 1976.
5. Flower, R.J., and Blackwell, G.J.: Anti-inflammatory steroids induce biosynthesis of a phospholipase A_2 inhibitor which prevents prostaglandin generation, Nature **278**:456, 1979.
6. Graber, A.L., Ney, R.L., Nicholson, W.E., et al.: Natural history of pituitary-adrenal recovery following long-term suppression with corticosteroids, J. Clin. Endocrinol. **25**:11, 1965.
7. Hench, P.S.: Introduction: cortisone and ACTH in clinical medicine, Proc. Staff Meet. Mayo Clin. **25**:474, 1950.
8. Hench, P.S., Slocumb, C.H., Barnes, A.R., et al.: The effects of the adrenal cortical hormone 17-hydroxy-11-dehydrocorticosterone (compound E) on the acute phase of rheumatic fever: preliminary report, Proc. Staff Meet. Mayo Clin. **24**:277, 1949.
9. Leibsohn, E., and Bagatell, F.K.: Halcinonide in the treatment of corticosteroid responsive dermatoses, Br. J. Dermatol. **90**:435, 1974.
10. Reichstein, T., and von Euw, J.: Constituents of the adrenal cortex: isolation of substance Q (desoxy-corticosterone) and R with other materials, Helv. Chim. Acta **21**:1197, 1938.

Chapter 44

Thyroid hormones and antithyroid drugs

The structural formulas of the various organic iodine compounds in the thyroid are shown below:

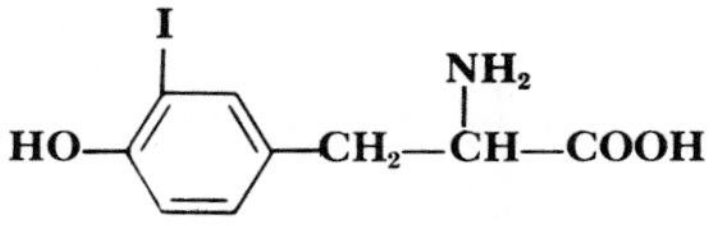

$$HO\!-\!\langle\rangle\!-\!CH_2\!-\!\overset{NH_2}{\underset{\ \ }{CH}}\!-\!COOH$$

Monoiodotyrosine

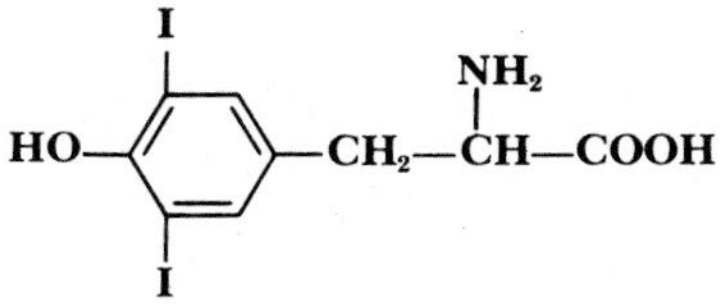

$$HO\!-\!\langle\rangle\!-\!CH_2\!-\!\overset{NH_2}{\underset{\ \ }{CH}}\!-\!COOH$$

Diiodotyrosine

$$HO\!-\!\langle\rangle\!-\!O\!-\!\langle\rangle\!-\!CH_2\!-\!\overset{NH_2}{\underset{\ \ }{CH}}\!-\!COOH$$

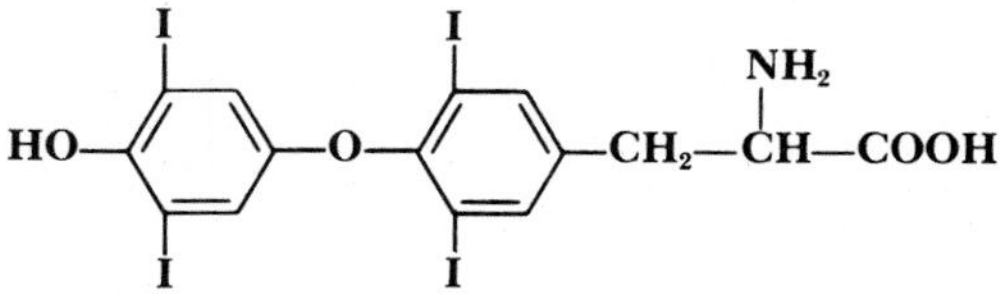

Thyroxine (T_4): 3,5,3',5'-tetraiodothyronine

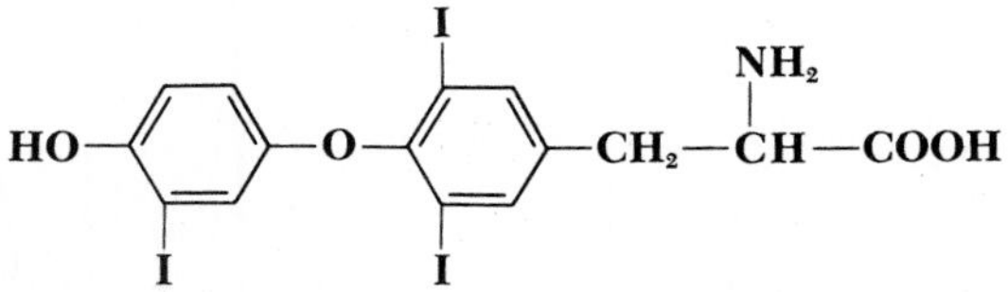

$$HO\!-\!\langle\rangle\!-\!O\!-\!\langle\rangle\!-\!CH_2\!-\!\overset{NH_2}{\underset{\ \ }{CH}}\!-\!COOH$$

3,5,3'-Triiodothyronine (T_3)

These compounds are present in the gland primarily as peptide-linked amino acids within thyroglobulin, a large (660,000-dalton) protein unique to the thyroid gland. T_4 and T_3 are the active hormones secreted by the gland. DIT (diiodotyrosine) and MIT (monoiodotyrosine) are hormonally inactive precursors for T_4 and T_3.

Iodine enters the thyroid follicular cells as inorganic I^- and is transformed through a series of metabolic steps into the thyroid hormones, as illustrated in Fig. 44-1. The steps in this sequence are (1) active transport of I^-, resulting in an intracellular concentration of I^- in the gland 20 to 40 times greater than that in plasma, (2) iodination of tyrosyl residues of thyroglobulin catalyzed by thyroid peroxidase, a membrane-bound hemoprotein that, in the presence of H_2O_2, oxidizes I^- to an active iodinating form, presumably I^+, and (3) conversion of DIT and MIT to T_4 and T_3

FIG. 44-1   *Schema depicting some of the more important steps in thyroid hormone biosynthesis, secretion, and metabolism. ALB, Albumin; DIT, diiodotyrosine; I, iodine; MIT, monoiodotyrosine; PA, prealbumin; PBI, protein-bound iodine; rT_3, 3,3',5'-triiodothyronine, or reverse T_3; T_3, 3,5,3'-triiodothyronine; T_4, thyroxine; TBG, thyroxine-binding globulin; Tg, thyroglobulin; TPO, thyroid peroxidase.*

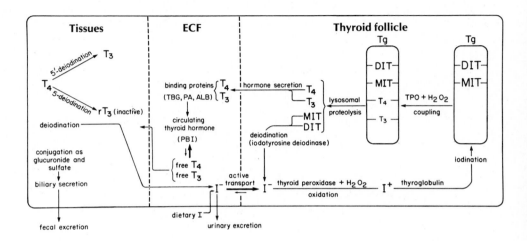

within the matrix of thyroglobulin. Coupling of two molecules of DIT forms T_4, whereas T_3 is formed by coupling one molecule of DIT with a molecule of MIT. Thyroid peroxidase catalyzes coupling as well as iodination. In the normal human thyroid the ratio of T_4 to T_3 in thyroglobulin is about 10:1.

Thyroglobulin contains the bulk of the iodine in the normal thyroid. In a typical human thyroid, about 60% of thyroglobulin iodine is present as DIT and MIT and less than 40% as T_4 and T_3. Only two to four residues of T_4 are normally present per molecule of thyroglobulin. Inorganic I^- generally represents less than 1% of total glandular iodine.

Secretion of thyroid hormones

Thyroglobulin must be hydrolyzed to release T_4 and T_3 for secretion into the circulation. As illustrated in Fig. 44-1, this is accomplished by lysosomal proteases. Digestion of thyroglobulin presumably releases all the iodoamino acids in the free form. The iodotyrosines DIT and MIT are deiodinated by an iodotyrosine deiodinase, which removes the bound iodine as I^- and preserves it for reutilization within the gland. T_4 and T_3 are not substrates for the deiodinase and are free to diffuse into the blood. Thyroglobulin itself normally enters the circulation only in small amounts, but increased concentrations of thyroglobulin are found in the sera of persons with various thyroid disorders.

In normal subjects, activity of the thyroid is largely controlled by thyrotropin (thyroid-stimulating hormone, TSH), a glycoprotein secreted by the anterior pituitary. In hypophysectomized rats all steps in thyroid hormone biosynthesis and secretion are greatly reduced. TSH acts at the level of the thyroid cell membrane by activating the adenylate cyclase system. Many of the effects of TSH on the thyroid can be duplicated by dibutyryl cyclic AMP or by forskolin, a potent activator of adenylate cyclase.

Hypothalamic-pituitary-thyroid interrelationships

TSH secretion is controlled by two major factors: (1) thyrotropin-releasing hormone (TRH), a tripeptide produced in the hypothalamus, which stimulates TSH secretion, and (2) feedback inhibition on the pituitary by circulating T_4 and T_3. Excessive thyroid hormone concentrations in the circulation inhibit secretion of TSH, whereas deficient concentrations increase TSH secretion.

In the hyperthyroidism of Graves' disease, the thyroid gland secretes excessive amounts of T_4 and T_3. In this condition circulating TSH concentration becomes very low, and pituitary secretion of TSH becomes unresponsive to TRH. Graves' disease is an autoimmune disease in which the thyroid gland is stimulated by a circulating abnormal immunoglobulin instead of by TSH, bypassing the normal feedback control by circulating T_4 and T_3.

T_4 is the major circulating thyroid hormone with a mean concentration in normal human serum of 80 to 90 ng/ml. Even though the mean concentration of T_3 is only 1 to 1.5 ng/ml, most of the hormone action at the receptor level is mediated by T_3. Both T_4 and T_3 are transported in plasma largely bound to protein (>99%). Three proteins are involved: thyroxine-binding globulin (TBG), prealbumin, and albumin. Approximately two thirds of plasma T_4 is carried by TBG, even though it is the least abundant of the three proteins. This can be attributed to its extremely high affinity for T_4 (association constant $= 1 \times 10^{10} M^{-1}$). TBG is also the major carrier for T_3, though the association constant is about one twentieth that for T_4. Association constants are intermediate for prealbumin and lowest for albumin. However, because of the high concentration of albumin in plasma, an appreciable fraction of T_4 and T_3 is bound to this protein.

Thyroid hormones in the circulation

There is good reason to believe that it is the free hormone fraction in plasma that is available to tissues; the bound form is primarily an inert reservoir. Measurement of free T_4 and T_3 concentrations is best performed by equilibrium dialysis, though this is not a readily available clinical procedure. Results of such measurements, combined with measurements of total T_4 and T_3 concentrations by routine radioimmunoassay procedures, indicate that free T_4 is only about 0.03% of the total T_4 in serum. For T_3 the corresponding value, though significantly higher, is still only about 0.3%.

These low values for free T_4 and free T_3 largely account for the long half-lives of these hormones in plasma. The half-life for plasma T_4 in humans is about 6 days, whereas that for T_3 is about 1 day. These half-lives are much longer than those for other hormones.

Indirect procedures have been developed for estimating free T_4 and T_3 concentrations. One such method makes use of a T_3 resin–uptake test that measures the distribution of ^{125}I-T_3 between serum proteins and a specially prepared resin. From this procedure one can derive a free thyroxine index that, in many cases, correlates fairly well with free T_4 concentrations measured by equilibrium dialysis.

Peripheral metabolism of thyroid hormones

T_4 is produced exclusively in the thyroid gland. T_3 is also secreted but only to the extent of about 0.1 mole per mole of T_4. In peripheral tissues a major pathway for T_4 metabolism is deiodination, in both the 5' and 5 positions (Fig. 44-1). 5'-Deiodination forms T_3, which displays 5 to 10 times the potency of T_4 in most tests of thyroid hormone activity. Much more T_3 is produced by deiodination of T_4 than is secreted by the thyroid gland. About 80% of the total T_3 in the human body arises from peripheral deiodination of T_4. Since T_3 is responsible for most of the hormonal activity, it is obvious that factors controlling T_4 to T_3 conversion are of major interest in studies of thyroid function. Deiodination of T_4 in the 5 position yields the isomer of T_3, 3,3',5'-triiodothyronine, known as reverse T_3 (rT_3). Reverse T_3 displays little or no hormonal activity and is thus a pathway of T_4 inactivation. Measurement of rT_3 concentration has proved useful in the study of factors controlling T_4 conversion to T_3.

Estimates of mean serum concentrations, metabolic clearances, and production rates for a 70 kg human are listed below.* The production rate of approximately 100 µg of T_4 per day is important in determining the replacement dose for treatment of hypothyroidism.

COMPOUND	SERUM CONCENTRATION (ng/ml)	METABOLIC CLEARANCE (liters/day)	PRODUCTION RATE (µg/day)
T_4	86	1.2	103
T_3	1.35	23.6	32
rT_3	0.38	111	42

Deiodination of T_4 also releases I^-, which is then available for reentry into the thyroid. Similarly, further deiodination of T_3 and rT_3 makes additional I^- available for recycling. Such metabolism conserves iodine, which is a trace element available in short supply in many areas of the world. The optimum iodine requirement for adults is 150 to 300 µg/day.

T_4 and T_3 also undergo conjugation with glucuronic acid and sulfate, primarily in the liver. The conjugates are secreted into the bile. Conjugation of T_3 with sulfate greatly facilitates deiodination.

---

*Data modified from Chopra, I.J., in Ingbar, S.H., and Braverman, L.E., editors: Werner's the thyroid: a fundamental and clinical text, ed. 5, Philadelphia, 1986, J.B. Lippincott Co.

The thyroid hormones do not have discrete target organs. Their effects are manifest throughout the body. Following is a list of some of the physiologic functions on which thyroid hormones exert significant actions:

Physiologic effects of thyroid hormones

1. Growth and differentiation
2. Calorigenesis and thermoregulation
3. Cardiovascular system
4. Neuromuscular system
5. Endocrine and reproductive systems
6. Carbohydrate, protein, and lipid metabolism
7. Enzyme synthesis
8. Vitamin metabolism

Deficiency or excess of thyroid hormones may affect any or all of these.

Much effort has been expended in recent years to determine the molecular basis for thyroid hormone activity. The area that has received the most attention is the cell nucleus. There is good evidence that binding of T_3 to specific receptors in the nucleus initiates hormone action through control of gene expression. In support of this view is the good correlation that exists between the biologic potency of various thyroid hormone analogs and their binding affinity for nuclear receptors. It has also been proposed that specific receptors for T_3 exist in mitochondria and in the plasma membrane and that these are additional sites for initiation of hormone action.

The most commonly used thyroid function test is measurement of serum T_4 concentration by radioimmunoassay. It is important to recognize that the results of this test may be affected by some commonly used drugs. In patients receiving these drugs alterations in serum T_4 and T_3 concentrations may not reflect thyroid dysfunction. The most widespread drugs of this type are those that alter plasma protein binding of T_4 and T_3. This may occur by two mechanisms: (1) by changing the plasma concentration of TBG and (2) by competing with T_4 and T_3 for binding sites on TBG.

PHARMACOLOGY Drugs that affect thyroid hormone concentrations

Increased concentrations of TBG are seen most often in pregnancy and in women receiving exogenous estrogens, including birth control pills. In this situation serum T_4 and T_3 concentrations may be above the normal range. However, the proportion of free T_4 and T_3 is reduced, and the net effect is that the free hormone concentrations remain essentially unchanged. Since it is the free hormone concentration available to tissues that determines the distribution and fractional turnover rate of the hormones, the subject remains euthyroid despite elevated concentrations of total serum T_4 and T_3.

Decreased TBG may occur in subjects receiving androgens or glucocorticoids in pharmacologic doses. The consequences are the converse of those associated with increased TBG. Serum concentrations of T_4 and T_3 are reduced, accompanied by an increase in the proportion of free hormone. The concentration of free hormone is essentially unchanged, and the subject is euthyroid.

Several drugs inhibit binding of T_4 and T_3 to TBG. This occurs in patients taking large doses of salicylates, for example, in rheumatoid arthritis. The effect is an increase in the proportion of free hormone and a decrease in total serum hormone concentration. Free hormone concentrations remain essentially unchanged, and the patients are euthyroid. Phenytoin also inhibits binding of T_4 to TBG and lowers total serum T_4. However, in this case the serum free T_4 fraction remains unchanged so that the free T_4 concentration is also reduced. Serum T_3 concentration, in contrast, is in the normal range. Patients with a low serum T_4 concentration while receiving phenytoin are not hypothyroid, as indicated by normal basal and TRH-stimulated serum TSH concentrations. Phenytoin probably alters thyroid hormone economy in vivo by multiple mechanisms. The predominant effect may be an acceleration of some of the pathways of intracellular T_4 metabolism, possibly leading to an increase in T_4 conversion to T_3. These effects of phenytoin probably involve induction of enzymes in the smooth endoplasmic reticulum.

As indicated for phenytoin, an important site of drug action, in addition to effects on serum binding proteins, is on peripheral conversion of T_4 to T_3. Drugs that have been reported to reduce peripheral T_4 to T_3 conversion include iopanoic acid and ipodate (oral cholecystographic agents), amiodarone, propranolol and propylthiouracil. In general, drugs of this type lead initially to a decreased concentration of serum T_3 and to increased concentrations of T_4 and rT_3. The metabolic consequences may be quite complex, especially in the case of amiodarone.

Changes in circulating thyroid hormone concentrations are also observed in severe nonthyroid illness, in surgical stress, and in caloric deprivation. Under these conditions both total and free T_3 concentrations are reduced, whereas total and free T_4 concentrations may be increased, unchanged, or decreased. Total and free rT_3 concentrations are increased. This condition is referred to as the "low T_3 syndrome," or the "euthyroid sick syndrome." The decrease in T_3 and the increase in rT_3 occur primarily because of slower peripheral 5'-deiodination of T_4. There is generally a diminished or absent TSH response to decreased thyroid hormone concentrations and to TRH. In the presence of severe nonthyroidal illness therefore, the task of diagnosing intrinsic disease of the pituitary-thyroid axis is particularly challenging and requires a clear understanding of the limitations of thyroid function tests and of the assumptions underlying their use.

Clinical preparations and diagnostic tests

REPLACEMENT THERAPY

Several preparations are available when treatment with thyroid hormone is indicated for hypothyroidism:

Thyroid tablets, derived from porcine thyroid glands, contain both T_4 and T_3, in a molar ratio of approximately 4:1. Most adult patients require 60 to 120 mg once daily.

Thyroglobulin tablets (Proloid), obtained from a purified extract of hog thyroid, contain both T_4 and T_3 in a molar ratio similar to that in thyroid tablets. The usual dose should be about half that for thyroid tablets.

Levothyroxine sodium (Synthroid, Levothroid), a synthetic salt of l-T_4, is chemically identical to the major form of circulating thyroid hormone. The usual adult dosage is 100 to 200 μg once daily.

Liothyronine sodium (Cytomel), a synthetic salt of l-T_3, is more rapidly acting than l-T_4 and may be injected intravenously in myxedema coma, for which it is the drug of choice.

Even though liothyronine is several times more potent than levothyroxine, most thyroidologists recommend levothyroxine for replacement therapy in hypothyroidism. Levothyroxine is also preferred over the crude preparations, which contain both T_4 and T_3 and may vary in composition and potency.

This hypothalamic tripeptide (pyroglutamyl-histidyl-prolinamide) stimulates release of TSH and prolactin from the anterior pituitary. Intravenous administration of TRH to normal subjects promptly increases serum TSH concentration. This response is exaggerated in hypothyroidism and greatly blunted in hyperthyroidism. The TRH stimulation test has proved useful in diagnosis of mild cases of decreased or increased thyroid function and also in differential diagnosis of primary, hypothalamic, and pituitary hypothyroidism.

THYROTROPIN-RELEASING HORMONE (TRH)

Inhibition of TSH secretion by exogenous thyroid hormone is a characteristic feature of normal pituitary-thyroid regulation. The thyroid suppression test is usually performed by measurement of thyroid $^{131}I^-$ or $^{123}I^-$ uptake before and at the end of a 7-day course of treatment with T_3, 75 to 100 μg daily, or 7 days after a single dose of 3 mg of T_4. A normal response is a 50% or greater decrease in thyroid radioiodide uptake. However, in patients with hyperthyroidism resulting from Graves' disease or from autonomous thyroid function there is little or no suppression of radioiodide uptake. This test is most useful in patients in whom the diagnosis is not readily established by simpler tests.

THYROID SUPPRESSION TEST

There are several classes of drugs that act directly on the thyroid gland to depress function.

General aspects of antithyroid agents

The most important drugs in this class are the thioureylenes (propylthiouracil, methimazole, and carbimazole) that are used clinically to treat Graves' disease and are discussed in detail on the next page. Miscellaneous agents that inhibit organic iodine formation when administered in vivo include resorcinol, p-aminosalicylic acid, aminotriazole, and derivatives of sulfanilamide.

INHIBITORS OF ORGANIC IODINE FORMATION

Perchlorate and thiocyanate inhibit I^- concentration by the thyroid as well as by other tissues that actively concentrate I^- (salivary and mammary glands, gastric mucosa).

INHIBITORS OF IODIDE TRANSPORT

IODIDE

In large doses, I^- inhibits hormone release from the thyroid, especially in patients with Graves' disease. This effect is believed to involve inhibition of thyroglobulin endocytosis, possibly through an effect on the adenylate cyclase system. Pharmacologic doses of I^- may also greatly decrease the rate of thyroid hormone synthesis, possibly through inhibition of peroxidase-catalyzed iodination. The antithyroid effects of I^- are somewhat paradoxical in view of the fact that a smaller intake of I^- is essential for thyroid hormone biosynthesis. In patients with Graves' disease undergoing treatment with large doses of I^-, the combined effects of iodide-mediated inhibition of hormone synthesis and secretion usually lead to an abrupt and striking improvement in symptoms. Within a few weeks, however, there is a loss of these beneficial effects, and so I^- alone is not generally used for long-term therapy. It is very useful, however, in preparation of patients for surgical removal of the thyroid.

RADIOLABELED IODINE

Because I^- is so greatly concentrated in the thyroid, administration of large doses of $^{131}I^-$ can provide sufficient internal radiation to destroy thyroid tissue. This procedure is widely used to treat Graves' disease. Smaller doses of $^{131}I^-$, or preferably of the more short-lived $^{123}I^-$, can be used diagnostically for thyroid uptake tests or for thyroid scintiscans.

Thioureylene drugs

STRUCTURE

The development of the thioureylene drugs in the 1940s was based on earlier studies of naturally occurring antithyroid substances in plants. The first drug to receive clinical trials for treatment of Graves' disease was thiourea. More extensive tests were soon performed with thiouracil, but its use led to a significant incidence of agranulocytosis. The continued search for antithyroid compounds with high clinical effectiveness but minimal side effects led to development of **propylthiouracil** and soon thereafter to **methimazole** (1-methyl-2-mercaptoimidazole) and its carbethoxy derivative, **carbimazole**.

Propylthiouracil **Methimazole** **Carbimazole**

Propylthiouracil and methimazole are available in the United States, whereas carbimazole is widely used in the United Kingdom and elsewhere. Carbimazole is rapidly metabolized to methimazole and for therapeutic purposes is essentially identical to it.

MECHANISM OF ACTION

Propylthiouracil and methimazole are concentrated severalfold by the thyroid. After entry into the thyroid cell they inhibit thyroid peroxidase-catalyzed iodination of thyroglobulin. They compete with tyrosyl residues of thyroglobulin for the active iodinating agent I^+ (Fig. 44-1), which also acts as a potent drug oxidant. Additional inhibitory mechanisms may involve inactivation of thyroid peroxidase and direct inhibition of the coupling reaction. The thioureylene drugs, unlike perchlorate and thiocyanate, do not inhibit active I^- transport.

When given in sufficient doses, thioureylene drugs may completely prevent hormone formation in the thyroid. These drugs therefore are commonly used in the research laboratory to produce "chemical thyroidectomy" in rats. Under these circumstances, serum T_4 and T_3 are reduced to very low concentrations, thus greatly increasing TSH secretion by the pituitary. This causes considerable enlargement of the thyroid, but the goitrous gland remains essentially unable to secrete hormones as long as the drug is continued. For therapeutic use in humans, however, the aim is not to eliminate hormone secretion but to reduce it to a normal rate. Overtreatment and undertreatment are to be avoided.

Methimazole is approximately 10 times more potent than propylthiouracil. The usual starting dose for methimazole (Tapazole) is 30 to 60 mg per day, whereas that for propylthiouracil is 300 to 600 mg daily. The average dose required to maintain the euthyroid state is 5 to 20 mg daily for methimazole and 50 to 200 mg per day for propylthiouracil. The choice of drug and the dose to be used depend on several factors. Propylthiouracil, but not methimazole, inhibits T_4 to T_3 conversion in peripheral tissues and for this reason may be selected for patients with more severe hyperthyroidism, in whom more rapid improvement is sought. With both drugs several weeks are usually required to reach a euthyroid state. It has generally been recommended that propylthiouracil and methimazole be given in divided doses (3 or 4 times daily) based on their short half-lives in plasma. However, it is the half-life in the thyroid that determines the biologic effect of these agents, and it is now accepted that a majority of patients can be well controlled with once-a-day therapy, especially with methimazole.

Although thioureylene drugs are definitive therapy for Graves' disease, only 40% to 50% of patients so treated remain in remission when the drug is withdrawn after a 12- to 18-month course of treatment. To explain this observation, it has been proposed that, in addition to the mechanism described above, thioureylene drugs exert an immunosuppressive action localized to thyroid gland lymphocytes and that successful long-range treatment depends on this action. Many tests have been used at the end of the treatment period (suppression tests, TRH stimulation tests, measurement of TSH antibodies in serum, and others) to try to predict which patients will relapse; so far these have met with only limited success. For patients who relapse, subtotal thyroidectomy or treatment with $^{131}I^-$ may be used. Indeed, many thyroidologists prefer primary treatment with $^{131}I^-$ or surgery. Many factors, beyond the scope of this chapter, enter into the choice of antithyroid drugs, $^{131}I^-$, or surgery as the primary mode of therapy for a given patient with Graves' disease.

In addition to their use for definitive therapy, thioureylene drugs are frequently used to prepare hyperthyroid patients for surgical removal of the gland. After the patient is made euthyroid by the drugs, iodine in the form of Lugol's solution is administered daily for 1 to 2 weeks before surgery. The addition of iodine reduces the vascularity and friability of the gland and facilitates the surgical procedure.

Propranolol

It has been recognized for many years that some of the abnormalities of hyperthyroidism bear a resemblance to overstimulation of the sympathetic nervous system; these include tachycardia, palpitations, tremor, sweating, nervousness, and irritability. It is a common belief in medicine that the myocardium in patients with hyperthyroidism is hypersensitive to catecholamines.

When sympatholytic agents were introduced into medicine, they were tested for their effects in hyperthyroid patients. Reserpine was first used and then guanethidine and most recently the more specific β-adrenergic receptor blockers, such as propranolol. Clinically, propranolol and other β-blockers produce prompt and pronounced improvement in symptoms of hyperthyroidism. These drugs are generally used as adjuncts to more definitive forms of therapy, such as thioureylenes, to provide symptomatic relief until the patient reaches a euthyroid state.

Propranolol has no direct action on the thyroid, and its inhibitory effect on T_4 to T_3 conversion requires larger doses than those that are effective in relieving symptoms of hyperthyroidism. The mechanism of its action is still under investigation. There is evidence that excess thyroid hormone increases the number of β-adrenergic receptors in the myocardium. This could account for amelioration of cardiac symptoms by propranolol in hyperthyroid patients. However, in liver and in adipose tissue thyroid hormones act in some other manner to modulate the effects of β-receptor activation.

Perchlorate

Perchlorate is a potent inhibitor of the iodide-concentrating mechanism of the thyroid. It has been tested as a therapeutic agent in treatment of Graves' disease. Although perchlorate is very effective in decreasing excessive hormone production, its therapeutic use has been limited because of rare but serious side effects, including aplastic anemia.

Perchlorate discharges inorganic I^- previously accumulated by the thyroid. This property makes it useful for diagnosis of defects in organic iodine formation in the thyroid. In such conditions, radioiodine accumulated by the thyroid remains largely in the form of inorganic I^-, whereas ordinarily radioiodide is rapidly bound to thyroglobulin (Fig. 44-1). Discharge by perchlorate of an appreciable fraction of the radioiodine previously accumulated in the gland is diagnostic for an iodination defect.

Lithium

Lithium carbonate has been used successfully to treat manic-depressive psychosis. This drug inhibits thyroid-hormone release, probably through inhibition of the adenylate cyclase system, and chronic use may lead to hypothyroidism.

REFERENCES

Hennemann, G., editor: Thyroid hormone metabolism, New York, 1986, Marcel Dekker, Inc.

Ingbar, S.H.: The thyroid gland. In Wilson, J.D., and Foster, D.W., editors: Williams textbook of endocrinology, ed. 7, Philadelphia, 1985, W.B. Saunders Co., p. 682.

Ingbar, S.H., and Braverman, L.E., editors: Werner's the thyroid: a fundamental and clinical text, ed. 5, Philadelphia, 1986, J.B. Lippincott Co.

Oppenheimer, J.H., and Samuels, H.H., editors: Molecular basis of thyroid hormone action, New York, 1983, Academic Press, Inc.

Chapter 45

Parathyroid extract and vitamin D

The concentration of ionized calcium in plasma is maintained by absorption from the intestine, rapid exchange with bone calcium, and excretion by the kidney. Parathyroid hormone and vitamin D have the major roles in calcium homeostasis. A fall in plasma calcium concentration promotes parathyroid secretion, whereas a rise in the concentration inhibits secretion.

Hypercalcemia is treated with furosemide and saline, phosphate, calcitonin, and glucocorticoids. *Hypocalcemia* is treated with calcium salts intravenously or orally and by vitamin D or related agents.

Parathyroid hormone is an 84 amino acid polypeptide that, like insulin, is derived from a prohormone (proparathyroid hormone), which in turn is a product of cleavage of a *prepro*hormone.[8] Secretion by the parathyroid gland is under negative-feedback regulation by the plasma ionized-calcium concentration and possibly by activated vitamin D_3. Only a small reserve of parathyroid hormone is stored, and variation in the rate of cytosolic degradation may be more important than variation in synthesis in determining hormone secretion.[11] Pharmacologically, several agents that stimulate adenylate cyclase, such as isoproterenol, epinephrine, and prostaglandin E_2, can increase parathyroid hormone secretion.[5,11] Although parathyroid extract was once used for diagnosis of pseudohypoparathyroidism, it is no longer commercially available.

Parathyroid hormone stimulates adenylate cyclase and rapidly increases cyclic AMP content of bone and the kidney. Apparently as a consequence, the hormone promotes renal reabsorption of calcium, decreases renal reabsorption of phosphate, and stimulates the conversion of vitamin D_3 to *calcitriol*, the major regulator of intestinal absorption of calcium and phosphate.[1,3] A very important effect of the hormone is an increase in osteoclastic and osteocytic resorption, that is, mobilization of calcium and phosphate from bones. This effect does not require the kidney; it has been demonstrated with parathyroid extract in nephrectomized animals. Furthermore, parathyroid transplants can cause local bone resorption.

A variety of factors contribute to maintenance of extracellular calcium concentration within narrow limits. The daily diet contributes about 1 g of calcium, the absorption of which is enhanced by calcitriol and indirectly, by formation of calcitriol, by parathyroid hormone. Antacids containing aluminum promote calcium absorption indirectly by binding and reducing the absorption of phosphate from the intestine;

hypophosphatemia then enhances formation of calcitriol. In contrast, the phosphate, oxalate and phytate content of the diet will form nonabsorbable salts with calcium.

Extracellular calcium is in equilibrium with the exchangeable calcium of bone. When extracellular calcium concentration falls, the exchangeable portion of bone calcium aids in returning it toward normal. In addition, renal reabsorption of calcium and excretion of phosphate are important in opposing decreases in extracellular calcium concentration.

CALCITONIN

Calcitonin (thyrocalcitonin) is a second polypeptide that affects calcium homeostasis, though a physiologic role in adult mammals has not been demonstrated. Calcitonin is secreted by the parafollicular (C) cells of the thyroid. By directly inhibiting bone resorption calcitonin produces hypocalcemia, an effect more apparent in children and patients with Paget's disease than in normal adults.

Calcitonin is normally present in blood, and its concentration increases when the calcium concentration is excessive (>90 μg/ml), as after eating or when calcium salts are administered. Its release by calcium is greatly enhanced in patients with medullary carcinoma of the thyroid.

Synthetic salmon calcitonin (Calcimar) is used clinically to treat Paget's disease[7] and hypercalcemia, and it has been tried in postmenopausal osteoporosis. Resistance may develop with continued administration, especially in patients who have a high antibody titer to the polypeptide. Adverse reactions include allergic responses, nausea, vomiting, and inflammation at injection sites. This preparation is available for subcutaneous or intramuscular administration, 200 IU/ml. Depending on the indication, injections are given at 6- to 48-hour intervals. Synthetic human calcitonin (Cibacalcin) is now available, in syringes containing 0.5 mg with mannitol, for subcutaneous administration to patients with Paget's disease. Hypersensitivity reactions and loss of effectiveness because of formation of antibodies are not expected to be problems with this preparation.

VITAMIN D
Current nomenclature

It was discovered more than 40 years ago that irradiation of plant sterols could yield antirachitic compounds. What was originally called "vitamin D_1" was a mixture of products. The active sterol produced by irradiation of ergosterol became known as "vitamin D_2," or *ergocalciferol*. The vitamin that is produced in the skin by irradiation of 7-dehydrocholesterol[9] was named "vitamin D_3," or *cholecalciferol*. This

Vitamin D₃

Dihydrotachysterol

vitamin is also present in fish liver oils, eggs, and milk. Vitamin D must be activated by metabolism, and the metabolites constitute most of the circulating vitamin. Vitamin D_2, found in yeast, differs from vitamin D_3 only in having a double bond between C-22 and C-23 and a methyl group at position 24.

Metabolic activation

Vitamin D_3 is hydroxylated in the C-25 position by microsomal and, in higher doses, mitochondrial enzymes in the liver. The former, but not the latter, metabolic pathway is under feedback inhibition by the product, 25-hydroxycholecalciferol, or *calcifediol*, which is bound in the circulation to a specific α-globulin. A further activating step occurs in the kidney where 25-hydroxycholecalciferol is hydroxylated to 1,25-dihydroxycholecalciferol, or *calcitriol;* this is the step stimulated by parathyroid hormone. Calcitriol is the most active form of vitamin D_3, can act on receptors in a wide variety of organs,[6] and has a half-life in plasma of 2 to 4 hours.[4]

Binding of the vitamin to intestinal receptors is believed to cause formation of calcium- and phosphate-binding proteins, which transport these ions across the intestinal mucosal cells.[4] In severe renal disease administration of calcitriol bypasses its lack of production by the failing kidney.

Vitamin D_2 and **dihydrotachysterol,** a vitamin D analog, are also hydroxylated in the liver. The 25-hydroxy derivative of dihydrotachysterol is the active form and does not require further activation in the kidney. This drug, given in high doses, is much more effective than cholecalciferol in promoting bone resorption and is commonly used to treat hypoparathyroidism.

Functions

The main function of vitamin D is to promote absorption of calcium and phosphorus from the intestine. It also appears to have a permissive role that potentiates the action of parathyroid hormone to release calcium from bone[4] and may act in concert with parathyroid hormone to facilitate calcium reabsorption by the kidney. In the presence of sufficient plasma concentrations of calcium and phosphate, mineralization of bone proceeds without a direct influence of vitamin D.[4]

Deficiency of the vitamin brings forth the various manifestations of rickets in growing children and animals. There is a disturbance in calcification of bones and teeth. The bones may become soft. Swollen epiphyses and lack of normal calcification are demonstrable by radiologic examination.[2] Osteomalacia can occur in adults with vitamin D deficiency.[10]

The daily requirement of vitamin D depends on the calcium needs of the person. The international unit is 0.025 μg of vitamin D_3. Normal adults require 400 units of vitamin D in 24 hours. Infants, children, and also pregnant or lactating women may require as much as twice this amount because their daily calcium absorption must be increased. In the treatment of hypoparathyroidism or refractory rickets, vitamin D_2 may be administered in very large doses (50,000 to 500,000 IU) initially, and maintenance doses may vary from 100,000 to 200,000 IU/day. Dihydrotachysterol may be administered initially in doses of 3 to 8 mg (compared with 10 mg or more of vitamin D_2), and for maintenance a dose of about 1 mg/day is usually sufficient.

TABLE 45-1   Vitamin D preparations

Vitamin or product	Alternative name	Oral dosage forms (μg)
D₂ (Calciferol, Drisdol)	Ergocalciferol	C: 625, 1250 (25,000, 50,000 IU) O: 200/ml (8000 IU/ml) T: 1250 (50,000 IU)
D₃	Cholecalciferol	T: 10, 25 (400, 1000 IU)
Calcifediol (Calderol)	25-Hydroxycholecalciferol (25-hydroxy-vitamin D₃)	C: 20, 50
Calcitriol (Rocaltrol)	1,25-Dihydroxycholecalciferol (1,25-dihydroxy-vitamin D₃)	C: 0.25, 0.5
Dihydrotachysterol (DHT, Hytakerol)		C: 125; O: 250/ml T: 125-400

C, Capsules; *IU*, international units; *O*, oral solution or suspension; *T*, tablets.

The vitamin may be administered in the form of fish liver oils or as the preparations listed in Table 45-1. Vitamin D₂ is also available in oil for intramuscular injection in a concentration of 500,000 IU/ml.

Drug interactions

Phenobarbital and phenytoin are known to increase microsomal hydroxylase activity in the liver. Development of rickets or osteomalacia in patients taking anticonvulsants may be a consequence of increased enzymatic transformation of vitamin D₂ or D₃ to inactive metabolites or, alternatively, of direct inhibition of calcium absorption or decreased tissue sensitivity to the vitamin.[8]

TOXIC EFFECTS OF PARATHYROID EXTRACT AND VITAMIN D

Toxic effects of parathyroid injection and of vitamin D are manifested as (1) hypercalcemia with numerous clinical consequences, (2) demineralization of bones, and (3) renal calculi and metastatic calcifications of soft tissues.

Hypercalcemia is associated with several clinical manifestations such as anorexia, vomiting, diarrhea, fatigue, and lack of muscle tone. The electrocardiographic changes that may occur at various concentrations of serum calcium are shown in Fig. 45-1. Serious toxic manifestations may be seen at a concentration of 150 μg/ml. Signs of hypocalcemia are tetany, cataracts, and mental lethargy.

OTHER DRUGS THAT INFLUENCE PLASMA CALCIUM CONCENTRATION

Phosphates, sodium sulfate, sodium citrate, and **edetate disodium** (Endrate, others), when given by intravenous infusion, lower blood calcium concentration. Their administration should not be undertaken without consideration of their adverse effects.

Glucocorticoids antagonize the effects of vitamin D on calcium absorption from the intestine. They are useful in hypercalcemia caused by sarcoidosis, certain neoplastic diseases such as lymphomas and myelomas, or hypervitaminosis D.

Effect of varying calcium concentration on electrocardiogram.   *FIG. 45-1*

From Burch, G.E., and Winsor, T.: A primer of electrocardiography, Philadelphia, 1960, Lea & Febiger.

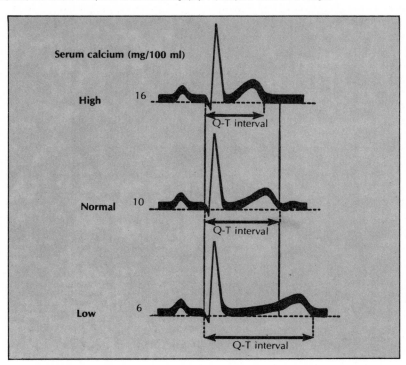

Etidronate is a diphosphonate used in treatment of Paget's disease and more recently in control of hypercalcemia secondary to malignancy.[12] It seems to slow both osteoclastic and osteoblastic activity. The drug can cause hyperphosphatemia and diarrhea and may increase arthralgia. Etidronate disodium (EHDP, Didronel) is available in tablets of 200 and 400 mg.

The loop diuretics, such as **furosemide,** tend to promote calcium excretion, whereas the **thiazides** have the opposite effect and may cause hypercalcemia.

Plicamycin (Mithracin), an antibiotic used to treat testicular neoplasms, lowers calcium concentration, perhaps by a toxic effect on osteoclasts. It has been used successfully to treat Paget's disease.

For the initial treatment of *hypocalcemia,* an intravenous infusion of a 10% solution of **calcium gluconate** (Kalcinate) is highly effective. **Calcium gluceptate** may also be given, intramuscularly as well as intravenously. Salts used orally include calcium gluconate, glubionate, lactate, carbonate, and dibasic and tribasic calcium phosphate.

REFERENCES

1. Agus, Z.S., Wasserstein, A., and Gold-farb, S.: PTH, calcitonin, cyclic nucleo-tides and the kidney, Annu. Rev. Physiol. **43:**583, 1981.
2. Anast, C.S., Carpenter, T.O., and Key, L.L.: Rickets. In Krieger, D.T., and Bardin, C.W., editors: Current therapy in endocrinology and metabolism, 1985-1986, St. Louis, 1985, The C.V. Mosby Co., p. 310.
3. Cohn, D.V., Kumarasamy, R., and Ramp, W.K.: Intracellular processing and secretion of parathyroid gland pro-teins, Vitam. Horm. **43:**283, 1986.
4. DeLuca, H.F.: The metabolism, physi-ology, and function of vitamin D. In Kumar, R., editor: Vitamin D: basic and clinical aspects, Boston, 1984, Martinus Nijhoff Publishing, p. 1.
5. Habener, J.F.: Regulation of parathyroid hormone secretion and synthesis, Annu. Rev. Physiol. **43:**211, 1981.
6. Haussler, M.R.: Vitamin D receptors: nature and function, Annu. Rev. Nutr. **6:**527, 1985.
7. Horwith, M.: Paget's disease of bone. In Krieger, D.T., and Bardin, C.W., edi-tors: Current therapy in endocrinology and metabolism, 1985-1986, St. Louis, 1985, The C.V. Mosby Co., p. 350.
8. Kronenberg, H.M., Igarashi, T., Free-man, M.W., et al.: Structure and expres-sion of the human parathyroid hormone gene, Recent Prog. Horm. Res. **42:**641, 1986.
9. Lawson, D.E.M., and Davie, M.: As-pects of the metabolism and function of vitamin D, Vitam. Horm. **37:**1, 1979.
10. Marks, J.: The vitamins: their role in medical practice, Lancaster, 1985, MTP Press Ltd.
11. Porat, A., and Sherwood, L.M.: Disor-ders of mineral homeostasis and bone. In Kohler, P.O., editor: Clinical endocri-nology, New York, 1986, John Wiley & Sons, p. 377.
12. Symposium: Etidronate disodium: a new therapy for hypercalcemia of malignancy, Am. J. Med. **82**(2A), 1987.

Chapter 46

Posterior pituitary hormones—vasopressin and oxytocin

The posterior lobe of the pituitary gland, the neurohypophysis, contains hormones that have vasoactive, antidiuretic, and oxytocic properties. The original material was separated into two fractions as early as 1928. One contained most of the vasoactive and antidiuretic activities, whereas the other was predominantly oxytocic. Both active components, vasopressin (antidiuretic hormone, ADH) and oxytocin, have now been synthesized.

Vasopressin and oxytocin are peptides of nine amino acid residues with a disulfide link between two cysteines. Human vasopressin and that from several other species contains the sequence shown below. In vasopressin from hog pituitary, arginine is replaced by lysine.

Cys-Tyr-Phe-Gln-Asn-Cys-Pro-Arg-GlyNH$_2$

Vasopressin (human)

Cys-Tyr-Ile-Gln-Asn-Cys-Pro-Leu-GlyNH$_2$

Oxytocin

VASOPRESSIN
Antidiuretic effect

The only clearly established physiologic function of vasopressin is its antidiuretic action on the kidney. The antidiuresis is generally attributed to an increase in the size or number of channels for flow of water along osmotic gradients in the distal tubules and collecting ducts. Support for this hypothesis has been derived from studies on isolated systems such as toad urinary bladder.[7] Vasopressin, by stimulating a receptor designated as "V$_2$," activates adenylate cyclase in the serosal membrane of epithelial cells. A proposed sequence of events is depicted in Fig. 46-1. In physiologic doses the hormone does not influence electrolyte absorption.

Vasopressin is synthesized in hypothalamic structures such as the supraoptic and paraventricular nuclei and is then transported to the neurohypophysis where it is stored.[16] It is generally accepted that certain hypothalamic regions are sensitive to changes in the osmolarity of extracellular fluid and act as osmoreceptors.[2] Thus ingestion of water and dilution of the extracellular fluid lead to inhibition of vaso-

FIG. 46-1 *View of a collecting duct cell or an amphibian bladder granular cell. ADH (vasopressin) activates adenylate cyclase, AD Cyc, at the basolateral membrane. The cyclic AMP generated stimulates a protein kinase. Ultimately, cytoplasmic tubules fuse with the luminal membrane and deliver particles to the membrane (A, B, and C). These particles are believed to conduct water. Elements of the terminal web and tight junction are included, as well as a large subluminal granule, Gr.*

From Hays, R.M., Sasaki, J., Tilles, S.M., et al.: In Schrier, R.W., editor: Vasopressin, New York, 1985, Raven Press.

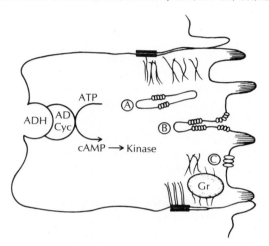

pressin secretion, whereas hypertonic solutions promote secretion. Since exercise, pain, and emotional excitement also inhibit water diuresis, it is likely that some central control mechanism of antidiuretic hormone release is very susceptible to neural and neurohumoral influences. Similarly, the release of vasopressin that occurs in diseases such as congestive heart failure, cirrhosis, and nephrotic syndrome appears to be mediated by the autonomic nervous system.[12,13] This "nonosmotic" release of vasopressin contributes to the hyponatremia in these conditions.

Diabetes insipidus, occurring spontaneously or produced experimentally by pituitary stalk section, is attributable to the lack of vasopressin and is characterized by failure of distal tubular water reabsorption. As a consequence, persons with this condition excrete large amounts of dilute urine (polyuria) and drink large quantities of water (polydipsia).

Clofibrate and chlorpropamide are used for their therapeutic antidiuretic activity in diabetes insipidus.[11] They enhance the release or potency of vasopressin and therefore are more likely to be useful in moderate forms of the disease. Thiazide diuretics, in contrast, can be effective treatment in *nephrogenic* diabetes insipidus, a disorder in which the kidney is unresponsive to circulating vasopressin. The thiazides act, in part, by reducing the dilution of tubular fluid that normally occurs in the cortical portion of the thick ascending loop of Henle (see p. 485). A less hypotonic urine is excreted. The mild degree of volume depletion that occurs causes a greater proportion of water to be reabsorbed with salt at more proximal sites. Thus overall urinary volume decreases. Sodium intake must be concurrently restricted.

Certain hyponatremic syndromes are associated with "inappropriate" secretion of the antidiuretic hormone. They are characterized by primary water retention unassociated with sodium retention or edema. Underlying causes include a variety of cancers, neurologic disorders, and drugs.[8]

The existence of a cholinergic mechanism for vasopressin release was indicated by experiments in which injection of acetylcholine or isoflurophate (DFP) into supraoptic nuclei released the antidiuretic hormone. Nicotine has been shown to inhibit water diuresis in humans, probably through the release of vasopressin. There is increasing interest in the regulatory role of endogenous opioid peptides and a variety of other possible mediators in vasopressin secretion.[4] Antidiuresis after general anesthesia or injection of histamine, morphine, or barbiturates (but not thiopental) has also been attributed to release of the hormone.

Alcohol inhibits release of the antidiuretic hormone in response to dehydration and produces inappropriate water diuresis in a dehydrated person. Alcohol does not block the action of nicotine on vasopressin release. Phenytoin can also block release of vasopressin[12] and has been used for this purpose in cases of inappropriate secretion of the hormone.[14]

The effect of vasopressin can also be blocked at its effector sites,[12] namely, the distal tubule and collecting duct. Lithium carbonate,[15] in particular, and demeclocycline[6] have been used to treat patients with hyponatremia and inappropriate release of vasopressin. Similarly, lithium-ion therapy is frequently associated with nephrogenic diabetes insipidus.[1]

MISCELLANEOUS FACTORS THAT AFFECT VASOPRESSIN ACTIVITY

Although the antidiuretic action of vasopressin is of primary therapeutic interest, the hormone can also stimulate another type of receptor (V_1), on smooth muscle of blood vessels, for instance. This action does not elicit formation of cyclic AMP but rather appears linked to increases in phosphatidylinositol turnover and intracellular calcium concentration, perhaps similar to the response to norepinephrine stimulation of α_1-adrenergic receptors (see Fig. 15-3). When posterior pituitary preparations are used to treat diabetes insipidus, smooth muscle stimulation is undesirable and usually indicates overdosage. Constriction of coronary arteries is dangerous in persons with coronary disease. Although intravenous injection of posterior pituitary extract or vasopressin into animals causes considerable peripheral vasoconstriction, blood pressure often increases only moderately. This is attributed to a baroreceptor-mediated decrease in cardiac output. Previously, the vasoconstricting action of vasopressin was utilized in attempts to decrease gastrointestinal bleeding. Infusions of the hormone into the mesenteric vasculature or intravenously have for the most part been abandoned because of lack of efficacy.

As with a wide variety of other peptides, there has been increasing interest in possible roles of vasopressin and oxytocin in other functions, including neurotrans-

Extrarenal effects

mission.[3] The Brattleboro rat, a strain that cannot synthesize vasopressin, has been a useful experimental tool in many such studies.

Vasopressin also increases coagulation factor VIII activity to a clinically useful extent in patients with hemophilia A or with von Willebrand's disease,[10] provided that the concentration of this factor is at least 5% of normal before treatment.

Antidiuretic
preparations

The treatment of choice for diabetes insipidus is now **desmopressin acetate** (1-desamino-8-D-arginine vasopressin, DDAVP), a vasopressin analog that has a prolonged action. Furthermore, its antidiuretic effect in relation to its vasopressor effect is much greater than is the case for other vasopressin preparations. The drug is usually taken intranasally with a calibrated catheter, as a solution containing 100 μg/ml. Its antidiuretic effect lasts 8 to 20 hours. The drug is also available for subcutaneous or intravenous injection (DDAVP, Stimate; 4 μg/ml). The parenteral form of desmopressin can be given prophylactically, for example, before tooth extraction, to minimize bleeding in patients with von Willebrand's disease or hemophilia A.

Lypressin (8-lysine-vasopressin, Diapid) is a synthetic lysine vasopressin. It is administered by intranasal spray up to six times daily and can cause adverse vasoconstriction.

Posterior Pituitary, intranasal (Posterior Pituitary) is available as a powder in capsules (40 mg = 45 units of antidiuretic activity plus <70 units of oxytocin) for intranasal inhalation three or four times a day. It may cause mucosal irritation. Posterior pituitary may cause abortion and should be used with caution in patients with coronary artery disease.

Vasopressin injection (8-arginine-vasopressin, Pitressin), a synthetic preparation, produces an antidiuretic effect lasting 2 to 8 hours when administered by subcutaneous or intramuscular injection. The solution may also be applied intranasally. Vasopressin may cause fluid retention, hypertension, myocardial ischemia, gastrointestinal and uterine contraction, and allergic reactions. The available solution for injection contains 20 pressor units/ml.

Vasopressin tannate (Pitressin Tannate in Oil) is a suspension of the insoluble tannate of the hormone, suitable for intramuscular administration. Its action lasts 1 to 4 days. The preparation in peanut oil contains 5 pressor units/ml.

DRUGS THAT ACT
ON THE UTERUS

The uterus receives sympathetic and parasympathetic innervation. α_1-Adrenergic receptors mediate stimulation; β_2-adrenergic receptors mediate inhibition. In addition, muscarinic receptors are stimulatory. The uterus is also susceptible to endocrine influences. Estrogens enhance responsiveness, whereas progesterone may decrease responsiveness.

The drugs most commonly used to enhance contractions of the uterus are *oxytocin*, *prostaglandins*, and certain ergot preparations, particularly *ergonovine*.

Comparison of the uterine sensitivity of oxytocin throughout pregnancy in different species.   **FIG. 46-2**

From Dawood, M.Y.: In Amico, J.A., and Robinson, A.G., editors: Oxytocin: clinical and laboratory studies, Amsterdam, 1985, Excerpta Medica (Elsevier Science Publishers BV), p. 391.

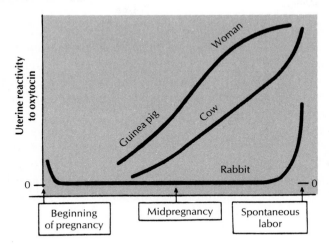

Although some physiologic activities of oxytocin are related to reproduction in the female, its presence in the male indicates that it must also have other functions.

Oxytocin differs from vasopressin in the following respects:

1. It contains isoleucine and leucine in place of phenylalanine and arginine respectively.
2. It has much weaker antidiuretic activity, but it can cause water intoxication, usually when given parenterally in a large volume of fluid.[5]
3. It is a potent stimulant of the gravid uterus at term and post partum (Fig. 46-2).
4. It usually does not produce vasoconstriction and may even lower blood pressure. However, hypertension has occurred in association with oxytocin administration.
5. It contracts the myoepithelial cells of lacteal glands to produce milk letdown during the postpartum period.[9]
6. It has little effect on intestinal smooth muscle and coronary arteries.

Oxytocin

Oxytocin injection (Pitocin, Syntocinon; 10 units/ml) is a synthetic preparation infused intravenously to induce or enhance uterine contractions in labor. It is also used to control postpartum uterine atony, but for this purpose ergonovine is often preferred. To control postpartum bleeding, oxytocin may be administered intra-

PREPARATIONS

muscularly, 10 units, or infused. For intravenous drip, oxytocin, 10 to 40 units, is added to a liter of normal saline. To facilitate milk ejection a nasal spray (Syntocinon; 40 units/ml) can be administered into one or both nostrils 2 to 3 minutes before nursing.

Other uterine stimulants	**Ergonovine** (Ergotrate) **maleate** and **methylergonovine maleate** (Methergine) are used to decrease uterine bleeding by causing contraction of uterine muscle after delivery of the placenta. Both are available for intramuscular or, occasionally, intravenous injection (0.2 mg/ml); tablets (0.2 mg) can be swallowed or taken sublingually to control delayed postpartum bleeding. Prostaglandin preparations are used to produce abortion by the induction of uterine contractions. Carboprost tromethamine (Prostin/15 M; 250 µg/ml) is the 15-methyl derivative of prostaglandin $F_{2\alpha}$. It is injected intramuscularly and is effective from the thirteenth to the twentieth week of pregnancy. Dinoprost tromethamine (Prostin F2-alpha; 5 mg/ml) is administered intra-amniotically. Dinoprostone (Prostin E2) is available in the form of 20 mg vaginal suppositories. Frequent adverse reactions to these agents include nausea, vomiting, diarrhea, and fever.

Uterine relaxants	β-Adrenergic receptor agonists, intravenous ethanol, and prostaglandin synthesis inhibitors, such as indomethacin, may be useful for prevention of premature delivery. **Ritodrine hydrochloride** (Yutopar), which preferentially stimulates β_2-adrenergic receptors, is currently a preferred uterine relaxant in premature labor. Contraindications include maternal eclampsia, cardiovascular problems, hyperthyroidism, and uncontrolled diabetes mellitus. Ritodrine is available in tablets, 10 mg, and for injection, 10 mg/ml.

REFERENCES

1. Baylis, P.H., and Heath, D.A.: Water disturbances in patients treated with oral lithium carbonate, Ann. Intern. Med. **88:**607, 1978.
2. Baylis, P.H., and Robertson, G.L.: Physiological control of vasopressin secretion. In Baylis, P.H., and Padfield, P.L., editors: The posterior pituitary: hormone secretion in health and disease, New York, 1985, Marcel Dekker, Inc., p. 119.
3. Buijs, R.M.: Vasopressin and oxytocin: their role in neurotransmission, Pharmacol. Ther. **22:**127, 1983.
4. Carter, D.A., and Lightman, S.L.: Neuroendocrine control of vasopressin secretion. In Baylis, P.H., and Padfield, P.L., editors: The posterior pituitary: hormone secretion in health and disease, New York, 1985, Marcel Dekker, Inc., p. 53.
5. Dawood, M.Y.: Oxytocin, vol. 2, Montreal, 1984, Eden Press.
6. Forrest, J.N., Jr., Cox, M., Hong, C., et al.: Superiority of demeclocycline over lithium in the treatment of chronic syndrome of inappropriate secretion of antidiuretic hormone, N. Engl. J. Med. **298:**173, 1978.
7. Goodman, D.B.P., and Davis, W.: The mode of action of antidiuretic hormone: membrane reorganization, recycling, and intracellular transport. In Reichlin, S., editor: The neurohypophysis: physiological and clinical aspects, New York, 1984, Plenum Medical Book Co., p. 51.
8. Hou, S.: Syndrome of inappropriate antidiuretic hormone secretion. In Reichlin, S., editor: The neurohypophysis: physiological and clinical aspects, New

York, 1984, Plenum Medical Book Co., p. 165.

9. Leake, R.D., and Fisher, D.A.: Oxytocin secretion and milk ejection in the human. In Amico, J.A., and Robinson, A.G., editors: Oxytocin: clinical and laboratory studies, Amsterdam, 1985, Excerpta Medica (Elsevier Science Publishers BV.), p. 200.

10. Lusher, J.M., and Warrier, A.I.: dDAVP in von Willebrand's disease and in moderately severe hemophilia A. In Reichlin, S., editor: The neurohypophysis: physiological and clinical aspects, New York, 1984, Plenum Medical Book Co., p. 201.

11. Moses, A.M.: Drug-induced states of impaired water excretion. In Baylis, P.H., and Padfield, P.L., editors: The posterior pituitary: hormone secretion in health and disease, New York, 1985, Marcel Dekker, Inc., p. 227.

12. Schrier, R.W., and Berl, T.: Nonosmolar factors affecting renal water excretion, N. Engl. J. Med. **292:**81 and 141, 1975.

13. Schrier, R.W., Berl, T., and Anderson, R.J.: Osmotic and nonosmotic control of vasopressin release, Am. J. Physiol. **236:**F321, 1979.

14. Tanay, A., Yust, I., Peresecenschi, G., et al.: Long-term treatment of the syndrome of inappropriate antidiuretic hormone secretion with phenytoin, Ann. Intern. Med. **90:**50, 1979.

15. White, M.G., and Fetner, C.D.: Treatment of the syndrome of inappropriate secretion of antidiuretic hormone with lithium carbonate, N. Engl. J. Med. **292:**390, 1975.

16. Zimmerman, E.A., Hou-Yu, A., Nilaver, G., and Silverman, A.-J.: Anatomy of pituitary and extrapituitary vasopressin secretory systems. In Reichlin, S., editor: The neurohypophysis: physiological and clinical aspects, New York, 1984, Plenum Medical Book Co., p. 5.

Chapter 47

Anterior pituitary gonadotropins and sex hormones

The cells of the anterior pituitary produce hormones that regulate the activity of other endocrine glands. The anterior pituitary hormones include peptides such as somatotropin (growth hormone), prolactin, ACTH (corticotropin; see Chapter 43), melanocyte-stimulating hormones, and lipotropins, as well as glycoproteins such as TSH (thyrotropin), LH (luteinizing hormone), and FSH (follicle-stimulating hormone). The secretion of these hormones is regulated, in turn, by a multimessenger neuroendocrine system that includes hormones from various target organs and neurotransmitters from the hypothalamus and the median eminence.[21]

Secretion of hormones from the anterior pituitary is stimulated by polypeptide-releasing factors that originate in the hypothalamus. These factors have both neurotransmitter and neuroendocrine roles. Releasing factors include thyrotropin-releasing hormone, corticotropin-releasing factor, gonadotropin-releasing hormone, prolactin-inhibiting factor, and growth hormone–releasing factor. In addition, a growth hormone release–inhibiting factor (somatostatin) also regulates growth hormone secretion.[2]

The releasing factors are secreted by neural cells in the ventral hypothalamus in response to neural or humoral signals. They are transported via a capillary plexus to the venous portal system of the pituitary stalk where they reach cells in which thyrotropin, gonadotropin, ACTH, and somatotropin are stored. These hormones are secreted from five different types of pituitary cells. Additional regulation occurs at the level of adrenergic, dopaminergic, and tryptaminergic transmitters in the hypothalamus. Drugs that affect the concentrations of these amines within the hypothalamus can be expected to influence hormone secretion as well.

The isolation, characterization, and synthesis of releasing factors has firmly established their role in the physiology of endocrine secretion. In addition, these hormones influence behavior, and they affect neuronal excitability within the hypothalamus.[12] The synthesis of some of these releasing factors has provided important research tools as well as the possibility of therapeutic intervention in various endocrine disorders.[20]

TRH (thyrotropin-releasing hormone). TRH was the first hypothalamic releasing hormone to be isolated, fully characterized, and synthesized, through the independdent efforts of Drs. R. Guillemin and A.V. Schally, who shared a Nobel prize in medicine for their work on the hypothalamic regulation of the pituitary gland.[18] The structure of TRH was determined by amino acid sequencing, and this facilitated the preparation of synthetic TRH as well as various structural analogs. **Protirelin** (Relefact TRH, Thypinone) is a synthetic tripeptide, 5-oxo-L-prolyl-L-histidyl-L-proline amide, which is identical to naturally occurring TRH. It is available in solutions containing 0.5 mg/ml. Protirelin is used in diagnosis of thyroid and pituitary disorders, and it was found to stimulate prolactin secretion in experimental studies. TRH is currently being investigated as treatment for amyotrophic lateral sclerosis[20] and for spinal cord injury.[10]

CRF (corticotropin-releasing factor). CRF is a polypeptide of 41 residues. It is a potent stimulant of pituitary secretion of ACTH and other pro-opiomelanocortin products.[15,23] CRF has been used to test for abnormalities of the hypothalamic-pituitary-adrenal axis, and it may function as a neurotransmitter in stress responses. CRF has been used to evaluate ACTH release in depressed persons and in patients with anorexia nervosa. In such patients there is a blunted ACTH response to CRF injection, presumably because of an elevated concentration of hydrocortisone.[6] Dextroamphetamine releases CRF, and this response is blocked by α-adrenergic receptor antagonists. Reserpine transiently increases basal secretion. Phenothiazines reduce secretion of CRF in response to hypoglycemia, metyrapone, and pyrogens, perhaps through blockade of adrenergic, dopaminergic, or serotonergic receptors. The recent development of CRF receptor antagonists should help define the multiple roles of CRF.[16]

Gn-RH (gonadotropin-releasing hormone), also called luteinizing hormone–releasing hormone, LH-RH, is a decapeptide that stimulates release of the pituitary gonadotropins FSH and LH. In addition to its potential for regulation of conception and steroidogenesis,[7] Gn-RH is used for treatment of hypothalamic amenorrhea, isolated gonadotropin deficiency, and carcinoma of the prostate.[8] Intermittent administration of the hormone, which mimics the pulsatile nature of endogenous release, causes sustained secretion of both FSH and LH. Continuous intravenous administration, however, inhibits secretion of both gonadotropins. Analogs of Gn-RH that are more potent and longer lasting than the parent molecule are being used to desensitize the pituitary and thus reduce gonadotropin and sex steroid concentrations in men with prostatic carcinoma. This technique avoids the use of estrogens and may obviate the need for orchiectomy. **Leuprolide acetate** (Lupron) is available for subcutaneous injection, 5 mg/ml. The usual dose is 1 mg daily.

Neuronal regulation of Gn-RH secretion is important in controlling onset of puberty, as well as in determining reproductive potential in the adult. Neural signals from the arcuate nucleus in the hypothalamus stimulate the oscillatory release of Gn-RH from peptidergic neurons in the median eminence. Adrenergic, dopaminergic, tryptaminergic, and opioid neurotransmitters, as well as circulating concentrations of sex steroids, modulate Gn-RH release. Experimental evidence indicates that dopamine stimulates release of Gn-RH whereas serotonin inhibits secretion, as reflected by changes in plasma gonadotropins. Levodopa increases plasma FSH concentration and causes a variable rise in plasma LH. Dopaminergic agonists, such as bromocriptine, can also release Gn-RH.

Prolactin-inhibiting factor (PIF). There is good evidence for a hypothalamic mediator that controls prolactin secretion. More recent research indicates that dopaminergic neurons from the tuberoinfundibular region may complete a negative feedback loop to the anterior pituitary to provide a stable, low basal concentration of circulating prolactin. Alterations of dopamine release probably account for the effects of various drugs on prolactin secretion. For instance, neuroleptic agents can cause pseudo-pregnancy and lactation in experimental animals and menstrual disorders in clinical use. Dopamine inhibits prolactin synthesis and release from pituitary cells in vitro, and there is some indication that neuroleptics cause a delayed increase in dopamine turnover in hypothalamic neurons.[21]

Hyperprolactinemia is associated with a syndrome of gonadal dysfunction, galactorrhea, hirsutism, and obesity. Galactorrhea is a common side effect of psychotropic drugs such as phenothiazines, haloperidol, reserpine, methyldopa, and imipramine. The semisynthetic ergot alkaloid bromocriptine, which stimulates dopamine receptors, has been used to control galactorrhea as well as to influence puerperal lactation, hyperprolactinemia, hypogonadism, acromegaly, and parkinsonism.[22] Bromocriptine mesylate (Parlodel) is available in 2.5 mg tablets and 5 mg capsules.

GRF (growth hormone–releasing factor, GH-RF). Secretion of growth hormone (GH) from the anterior pituitary is under dual control by the stimulatory GRF and the inhibitory factor somatostatin (see next page). GRF has only recently been isolated, characterized, and synthesized. It is composed of 44 amino acids, of which the first 29 contain full biologic activity. Although several other hypothalamic peptides, such as TRH, Gn-RH, neurotensin, substance P, and opioid peptides, can stimulate release of GH under certain conditions, it is currently believed that GRF is the primary physiologic stimulus for secretion.

Release of GRF is regulated by a complex interaction with somatostatin. The secretion of somatostatin is inversely correlated with GRF release. Dopaminergic stimulation enhances basal GH secretion in man and in experimental animals, probably by an action at the level of the pituitary somatotroph, but drugs that affect dopaminergic receptors also influence GRF. Additional evidence indicates possible adrenergic control of GRF secretion. For example, dextroamphetamine stimulates GRF secretion; this effect is enhanced by propranolol. In general, GRF secretion is stimulated by α-adrenergic and inhibited by β-adrenergic mechanisms.

GROWTH HORMONE AND SOMATOSTATIN

Growth hormone (GH), *somatotropin*, is the most abundant hormone of the anterior pituitary. It constitutes approximately 10% of the weight of the gland in the human. It has several different functions. Some actions of GH are probably mediated by *somatomedin C* (insulin-like growth factor), which is derived from the liver and stimulates bone and peripheral tissue growth.[20] One of the physiologic roles of GH is to promote protein synthesis at the expense of carbohydrate and fat. GH decreases glucose utilization and antagonizes insulin. It increases amino acid transport and protein synthesis. GH release is stimulated by hypoglycemia and by exercise. Release also increases during REM sleep and is enhanced by dopaminergic stimulation.[21] Glucocorticoids oppose the anabolic actions of GH. In humans GH and gonadal steroid secretion occur in unison throughout the life cycle. During childhood GH secretion is much lower than during puberty, when both GH and gonadal hormone concentrations increase dramatically.

Human GH, extracted from pituitaries or prepared by recombinant DNA technology, provides a means of treating GH deficiency. Because several persons who received the pituitary extract developed a fatal neurologic disease (Creutzfeldt-Jakob disease),[3] that preparation was withdrawn. However, the recombinant form of GH (somatrem, Protropin) is now available. Except for the few cases in which human pituitary material was contaminated with Creutzfeldt-Jakob virus, GH administration has been remarkably free of side effects. Neutralizing antibodies decreased the effect in some persons, but the major limitation was epiphyseal fusion. A recent review on GH deficiency emphasized that treatment of the deficiency at an early age was the most successful in achieving accelerated growth.[11] No significant growth occurred in persons who had achieved mature bone age (15 to 16 years in males and 14 to 15 years in females).

The hypothalamus has a tonic stimulatory effect on GH production, since hypothalamic lesions decrease GH production and retard growth. Early research on control of GH secretion by GRF led to the discovery of a substance that inhibited GH release.[12] Later studies resulted in isolation and purification of somatostatin, a tetradecapeptide found not only in the hypothalamus but also in the pancreas and in the gastrointestinal tract.[2,13] Somatostatin is a powerful suppresser of GH release both in vitro and in vivo. It blocks the GH response to exercise, insulin-induced hypoglycemia, and levodopa injection. Neurotransmitters and neuropeptides that modify somatostatin release also affect GH concentration. Although it was originally believed to be primarily a regulator of GH secretion, somatostatin is found in many cells that have nothing to do with GH, and it inhibits secretion of several other hormones, including TSH, ACTH, glucagon, and insulin. Somatostatin has an extensive distribution within the nervous system and in many peripheral tissues, including the gastrointestinal tract, and endocrine and exocrine glands. It is believed to be involved in virtually all sensory systems, including those subserving nociception, light, touch, temperature, vision, hearing, and possibly visceral afferents.[13]

GONADOTROPINS AND SEX HORMONES

The sex hormones are produced by specific target cells in the ovaries, testes, and adrenal cortex in response to stimulation by gonadotropins from the anterior pituitary. The secretion of gonadotropins is in turn regulated by hypothalamic centers that communicate with the anterior pituitary via Gn-RH and by the concentrations of sex steroids in circulation. FSH (follicle-stimulating hormone) and LH (luteinizing hormone), which is also the interstitial cell–stimulating hormone (ICSH) of the testes, are found in the placenta and urine as well as in the pituitary.

Gonadotropins   In the female, FSH and LH act in concert to regulate hormone production during the ovarian cycle and during pregnancy. FSH promotes growth of the ovarian follicle and stimulates secretion of estrogen. LH promotes ovulation and stimulates secretion of progesterone from the corpus luteum after ovulation. In the male, the two major testicular functions, testosterone secretion and spermatogenesis, are under control of pituitary gonadotropins. FSH secretion in the male is controlled by two mechanisms: negative feedback by sex steroids and inhibition by a nonsteroidal factor (inhibin) produced by Sertoli cells in the testes. Both FSH and testosterone act directly on the seminiferous tubular epithelium to promote spermatogenesis. FSH also regulates the number of LH receptors expressed by the Leydig (interstitial) cells and thus indirectly influences androgen synthesis. LH interacts with these Leydig cell receptors to stimulate synthesis of androgens from cholesterol. Although androgen synthesis involves several enzymatic steps, expression of LH receptors is a crucial control mechanism. The number of LH receptors is influenced by the gonadotropin concentration, and the secretion of LH is controlled by the testosterone concentration. This negative feedback maintains a relatively constant secretion of testosterone.

Gonadotropins have been used therapeutically to induce ovulation in women with ovarian failure. Extracts (menotropins) prepared from urine of menopausal women are highly effective in promoting ovulation. These extracts contain large amounts of both FSH and LH, and continued therapy results in ovarian enlargement, often with multiple follicles. Multiple births may occur in as many as 20% of patients treated with menotropins.

Human chorionic gonadotropin (HCG) is a glycoprotein extracted from the urine of pregnant women. Its action is nearly identical to that of LH, but there is slight FSH activity as well. It stimulates androgen production in testes and progesterone production by ovaries. HCG is used to replace LH in prepubertal cryptorchism, hypogonadotropic hypogonadism, and failure of ovulation.

Ovulatory cycle   The normal reproductive function in the female involves complex interactions between the brain, the pituitary, and the ovaries. The unique cyclic formation and secretion of estrogen and progesterone in a precisely timed manner depends on both neural signals from the hypothalamus and feedback signaling of ovarian steroids to the hypothalamic-pituitary axis.

Gonadotropin secretion is both tonic and cyclic. The tonic or basal secretion is regulated by inhibitory mechanisms, such as changes in circulating sex steroids. Cyclic secretion involves stimulatory feedback mechanisms. For example, elevation of circulating estrogens to a critical concentration initiates a synchronous, pulsatile burst of LH and FSH secretion during the ovarian cycle.[14]

Before puberty the low, basal secretion of Gn-RH results in low concentrations of FSH and LH. As puberty approaches in both sexes gonadotropin concentrations rise. The specific mechanisms that result in timing of puberty and subsequent sexual maturation are still not completely understood, but they may depend on nutritional

Hormonal control of menstruation.

FIG. 47-1

From Riley, G.M.: Gynecologic endocrinology, New York, 1959, Harper & Row, Publishers, Inc.

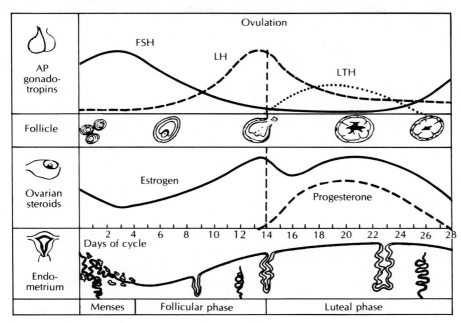

factors or on the rate of steroid synthesis. Many investigators have noted that a minimal amount of body fat is required for menarche and the pubertal growth spurt, and states of chronic illness or malnutrition delay sexual maturation. One interesting hypothesis is that the activation of the adrenal androgen-secreting system that precedes gonadal maturation primes the hypothalamic-pituitary-gonadal axis for sexual maturation at puberty.[14]

The ovarian cycle in the mature female reflects changes in gonadotropins, in steroid synthesis, and in the histology of the ovaries and endometrium. The traditional schema for these changes is shown in Fig. 47-1, whereas the actual measurements of serum hormone concentrations are depicted in Fig. 47-2.

Follicular phase. The release of FSH and LH in the early (follicular) phase of the cycle is believed to be responsible for the growth and development of ovarian follicles. Maturation of the oocyte influences hormone synthesis within the ovary. FSH initially induces proliferation of the granulosa cells and induces an aromatizing enzyme that converts androgens to estradiol. Estradiol acts synergistically with FSH to stimulate proliferation of granulosa cells and to induce LH receptors. LH then acts on the thecal cells to produce the androgen precursor of estradiol, thus providing a continual source of estrogen.

Ovulation. Episodic or pulsatile release of LH is characteristic of the adult pattern of gonadotropin secretion. The simultaneous increase ("midcycle surge") in the go-

FIG. 47-2 *Serum concentrations of progesterone plotted against mean concentrations of FSH and LH determined in normal women. Centered according to day of LH peak (day 0).*

From Yen, S.S.C., Vela, P., Rankin, J., and Littell, A.S.: J.A.M.A. **211**:1513, 1970.

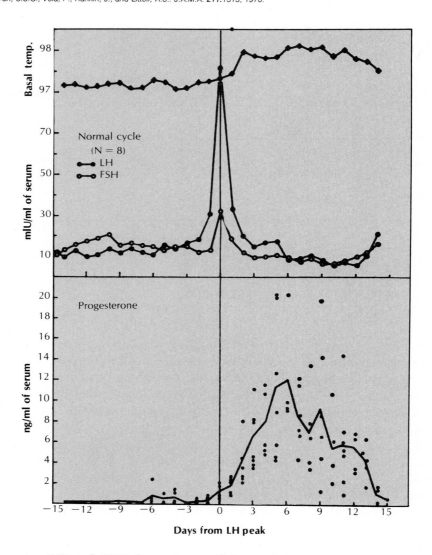

Days from LH peak

nadotropins LH and FSH that is required for ovulation depends on the positive feedback of increased estrogen for a sufficient length of time during the latter part of the follicular phase. The positive feedback affects gonadotropin-secreting cells, which are also exposed to Gn-RH.

Luteal phase. After ovulation there are significant changes in the histologic appearance of the ovarian follicle, and progesterone synthesized from the corpus luteum dominates in the latter part of the cycle. Although progesterone secretion begins before ovulation, the rising concentration of LH at ovulation greatly enhances progesterone synthesis. Despite the limited life-span of the corpus luteum, if pregnancy occurs, the implanted trophoblast secretes HCG (see p. 584). This hormone maintains a high rate of progesterone synthesis by the ovary until placentation occurs.

Menses. The decline of estrogen and progesterone concentrations at the end of the luteal phase results in degenerative changes in the arteries that supply the endometrium. They undergo spasm, which may be attributable to prostaglandin formation, and the subsequent necrosis and desquamation cause menstruation. The decrease in circulating estrogen permits secretion of FSH, and the follicular phase begins anew.

Biosynthesis of steroids

One action of gonadotropins is to promote synthesis of enzymes that catalyze various steps in synthesis of steroid hormones. Androstenedione, the common precursor of androgens and estrogens, is formed by the same mechanism in testis, ovary, and adrenal cortex. The synthetic schema is shown below:

Acetate → Cholesterol → Δ^5-Pregnenolone

Δ^5-Pregnenolone → Progesterone → 17α-OH-progesterone

Δ^5-Pregnenolone → 17α-OH-pregnenolone → Dehydroepiandrosterone

17α-OH-progesterone → Androstenedione ← Dehydroepiandrosterone

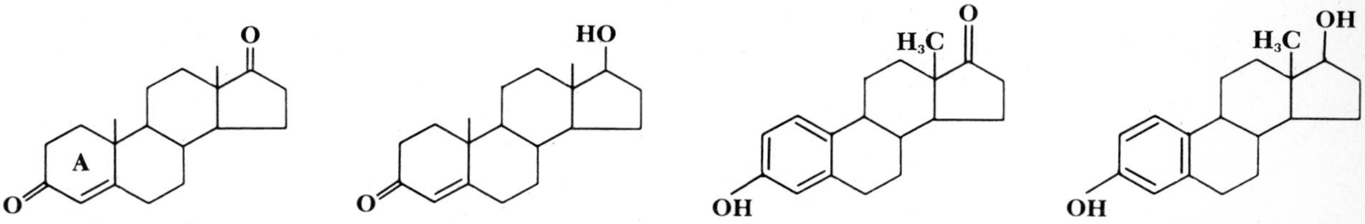

Androstenedione **Testosterone** **Estrone** **Estradiol**

ESTROGENS

Chemistry

Estrogens are formed from androgenic precursors, androstenedione and testosterone. Androstenedione is converted by the ovary to testosterone, which is then aromatized and demethylated to estrogens. Aromatization of the A ring of the steroid is required for estrogenic activity. If this reaction is defective, the circulating androgenic precursors can cause virilization.

The major product of the ovary and the most potent estrogen is estradiol-17β. This compound is also synthesized by the placenta during pregnancy. A less potent estrogenic compound, estrone, may be formed directly from androstenedione in adipose tissue and other extragonadal sites or from oxidation of estradiol by the liver. Estriol, a metabolite of estrone, also has limited estrogenic activity. All three of these estrogens are excreted in urine as glucuronides and sulfates.

Actions   Estrogens are the growth hormones of reproductive tissues in the female. In addition, they share some actions of androgens on the skeleton and other tissues. The increase in estrogen synthesis at puberty occurs in response to stimulation of the ovary by FSH. Estrogen is the dominant hormone both in the earliest part of reproductive life and as menopause approaches.

Circulating estrogens act in concert with androgens and progesterone to establish the changes of puberty: the molding of body contours caused by redistribution of fat, growth of breast tissue, growth and shaping of the skeleton, and maturation of the sexual organs. Cyclic secretion of estrogen and progesterone induces the onset of menstruation, and the continued sequential action of both hormones is required for normal menstrual cycles.

In the early part of the ovarian cycle (follicular or proliferative phase) estrogen stimulates protein synthesis in uterine tissues to increase the myometrial mass and vascularity. There is a simultaneous increase in contractile activity of both the uterus and the fallopian tubes. This proliferative phase is dedicated to rebuilding the endometrium that was sloughed during the previous menstrual period.

In the breast, estrogens stimulate proliferation of ductal epithelium and fibrous stroma. They promote elasticity of the skin by an effect on connective tissues, and they enhance deposition of calcium in bone. Like androgens, they are anabolic agents, and they stimulate rapid skeletal growth at puberty. Similarly, estrogens can promote closure of the epiphyses, but they are less potent than androgens.

All the actions of estrogens on target tissues are mediated through specific tissue receptors. High concentrations of estrogen-binding protein are found in the uterus, vagina, and mammary glands, but receptors are also found in many other tissues.[5] The ultimate mechanism of steroid hormone action, much as in the case of the glucocorticoids (see p. 547), involves transport of the steroid-receptor complex to the nucleus where it directs protein synthesis.

Estrogen receptors are measured in certain forms of metastatic carcinoma to assess the potential response to hormone therapy. Without estrogen receptors, metastases will not respond to treatment with antagonistic estrogens.

Metabolism   The naturally occurring estrogens, estradiol and estrone, are rapidly inactivated by the liver, and neither is effective orally. Semisynthetic and totally synthetic estrogens are less readily metabolized and can be taken by mouth. The attachment of an ethinyl group at the 17α position of estradiol (ethinyl estradiol) slows hepatic metabolism and produces a derivative highly effective for oral administration.

Therapeutic uses   All estrogenic compounds elicit the same responses, even though not all are steroids. The choice of an estrogenic agent depends on its convenience and on its cost.

The most prevalent use of estrogens is in combination with progestins in oral contraceptive preparations. The rationale is that steroid-induced inhibition of Gn-RH through a negative feedback loop should prevent the changes in the ovary required for ovulation. The constant concentrations of circulating hormones suppresses basal secretion of FSH and LH and also the midcycle surge of LH just before ovulation. As a consequence, follicle maturation is retarded and the stimulus for ovulation is suppressed.[9] Estrogens are also used in combination with progestins to treat menstrual disorders. Endometriosis often responds favorably to combined steroid therapy, and there is regression of tissues that are stimulated by naturally cycling hormones.

Estrogens are used as replacement therapy in ovarian failure or at menopause to relieve symptoms of estrogen deficiency.[4] With decreased estrogen secretion at menopause, estrogen-responsive target tissues atrophy. The menopausal symptoms may include vasomotor instability ("hot flashes"), drying and atrophy of the vaginal mucosa, insomnia, irritability, and other mood changes. As ovarian function declines with age, androstenedione from the adrenal cortex becomes the primary source of estrogen, and estrone is the dominant circulating estrogen. Because the naturally occurring concentration of androstenedione and the efficiency of its conversion may vary considerably among persons, estrogen replacement therapy is frequently provided to ease the transition into menopause.

There is considerable controversy about the use of estrogens to prevent or treat osteoporosis, a disorder characterized by reduction of bone mass with resultant fragility and risk of fracture. In a double-blind study of oophorectomized women, estrogen was shown to prevent bone loss during a year of continuous therapy.[17] Estrogen is also effective in retarding bone loss in menopausal women. However, all the studies up to now indicate that estrogen is effective only with continued administration; cessation of therapy results in accelerated bone loss. Estrogen is believed to retard bone resorption by influencing the action of parathyroid hormone, possibly through calcitonin (see Chapter 45). There is little evidence that estrogen can reverse bone loss once osteoporosis is established.[17]

Estrogens are used as androgen antagonists in certain types of androgen-sensitive cancers. The doses required are much higher than those needed for hormone replacement, and adverse effects are limiting.

All compounds with estrogenic activity have virtually the same side effects and risks. Preparations differ in their duration of action and route of administration. Side effects of estrogen therapy are usually minimal but can decrease patient acceptance. Nausea is the most prominent and may be associated with loss of appetite, diarrhea, and vomiting. Other undesirable effects include fluid retention and breast tenderness. The severity of the symptoms, which usually subside with continued use, is related to the potency of the compound used.

Adverse effects of estrogen therapy

There have been reports of increased endometrial neoplasia in patients on long-term estrogen therapy, but a direct association between estrogen and death from carcinoma has never been proved. Several studies indicate that addition of progestins to the therapeutic regimen eliminates the risk of estrogen-induced neoplasia.[17] Other serious risks of estrogen therapy include an increased tendency toward thromboem-

TABLE 47-1 Estrogen preparations	
Preparation	Dosage forms (mg)
Estradiol (Estrace)	T: 1, 2; V: 0.1/g of cream
Polyestradiol phosphate (Estradurin)	I: 40 as powder
Estradiol cypionate (Depestro, others)	I: 1, 5/ml
Estradiol valerate (Delestrogen, others)	I: 10-40/ml
Conjugated estrogens (Premarin, others)	T: 0.3-2.5; V: 0.625/g of cream
Esterified estrogens (Menest, others)	T: 0.3-2.5
Ethinyl estradiol (Estinyl, Feminone)	T: 0.02-0.5
Diethylstilbestrol	T: 1, 5
Diethylstilbestrol diphosphate (Stilphostrol)	I: 250/5 ml; T: 50
Chlorotrianisene (Tace)	C: 12-72
Dienestrol (Estraguard, others)	V: 0.01%
Estrone (Bestrone, others)	I: 2, 5/ml
Estropipate (Ogen)	T: 0.75-6; V: 1.5/g of cream
Quinestrol (Estrovis)	T: 0.1

C, Capsules; *I*, injection; *T*, tablets; *V*, vaginal cream.

bolic disease and a link to hypertension in a small number of persons. Interestingly, women who undergo an early menopause or loss of ovulatory function have an increased incidence of cardiovascular disease. Clearly, more studies are needed to determine the role of estrogens in these conditions.

Contraindications to estrogen therapy include estrogen-dependent neoplasia, prior or active thromboembolic disease, coronary or cerebral arterial disease, active liver disease, or severe liver damage. Relative contraindications include hypertension, fibrocystic breast disease, cholecystitis, uterine leiomyoma, and familial hyperlipoproteinemia. Diethylstilbestrol is absolutely contraindicated in pregnancy because there appears to be a clear association between maternal therapy with this compound and the later development of adenocarcinoma in the offspring.

Specific agents   **Estradiol-17β** can be administered in a variety of forms (Table 47-1), including a polyester form (Estradurin) that can be injected intramuscularly for therapy of prostatic carcinoma.

Conjugated estrogens are a mixture of estrone sulfate and equine estrogens (equilin sulfate) derived from the urine of pregnant mares. These compounds are water soluble and can be taken orally. **Esterified estrogens** are similar to conjugated estrogens.

Ethinyl estradiol, a semisynthetic compound, is the most potent estrogen available. Ethinyl estradiol and its 3-methyl ether derivative, **mestranol,** are commonly used in oral contraceptive combinations. Mestranol is metabolized to ethinyl estradiol.

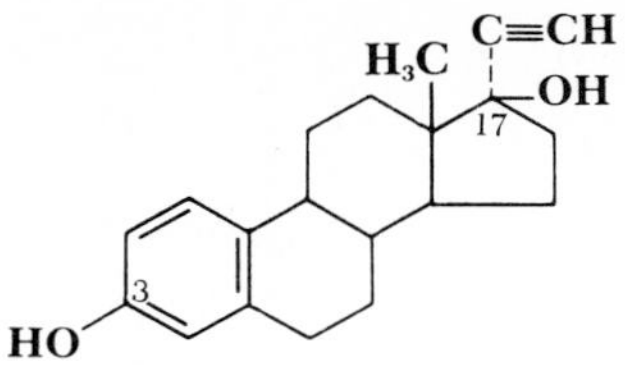

Ethinyl estradiol

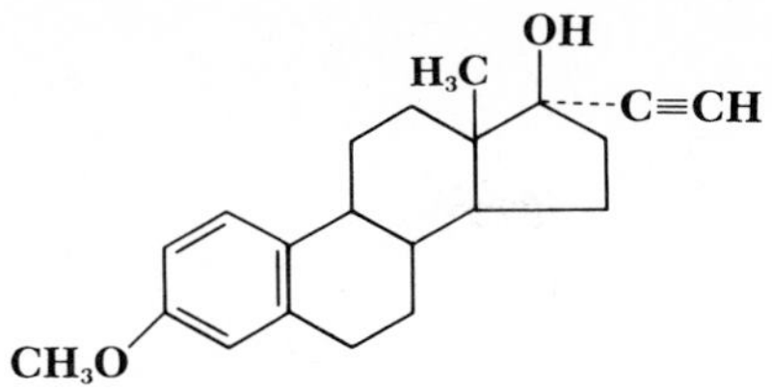

Mestranol

Diethylstilbestrol is a potent nonsteroidal compound with estrogenic actions. It is active on oral administration and is also available for intravenous injection.

Chlorotrianisene has a very long duration of action, probably because it is stored in fat. It is an inactive compound that is metabolized to an active estrogen.

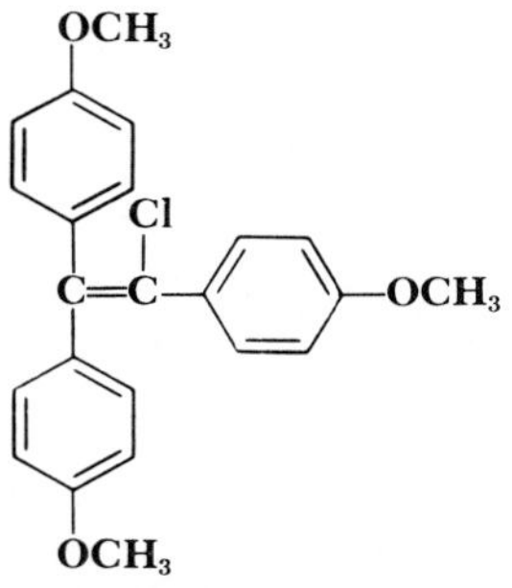

Chlorotrianisene

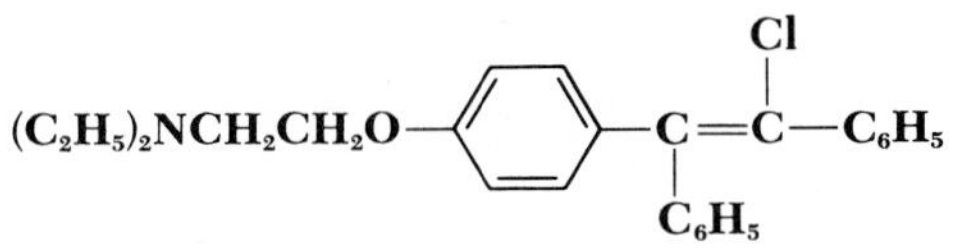

Clomiphene

Clomiphene citrate (Clomid, Serophene) is structurally related to chlorotrianisene but has an antiestrogenic action. It blocks the negative feedback action of estrogen at the level of the hypothalamus and thus promotes pituitary gonadotropin secretion. It has been used to induce ovulation in women who are infertile because they fail to ovulate. An abnormally high incidence of multiple births accompanies the use of clomiphene. It can also cause adverse effects related to estrogen blockade, including hot flashes, enlargement of the ovaries, and atrophy of vaginal mucosal cells. The recommended initial course is one 50 mg tablet each day for 5 days.

PROGESTINS

Progesterone is formed from steroid precursors in the ovary, testis, placenta, and adrenal cortex. It is the hormone produced in the corpus luteum that stimulates development of a secretory endometrium in the latter part of the ovarian cycle. In pregnancy progesterone is secreted in large amounts by the placenta. Semisynthetic derivatives, *progestins*, are used in oral contraceptives and as replacement for the naturally occurring hormone in conditions of ovarian failure or dysfunction.

FIG. 47-3   *Chemical structures of important progestins related to testosterone and 19-nortestosterone that are used as progestational agents. Arrows, Points where the basic norethindrone structure has been modified to produce new compounds.*

From Batzer, F.R.: J. Reprod. Med. **29**(suppl.):503, 1984; adapted with permission from Edgren, R.A., Progestagens. In Given, J.R., editor: Clinical use of sex steroids, Chicago, copyright 1980, Year Book Medical Publishers, Inc.

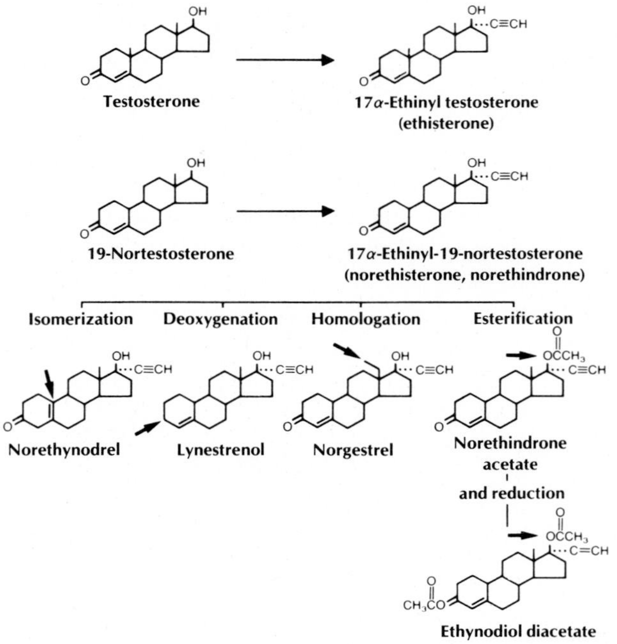

Chemistry

The synthetic oral progestins are derivatives of testosterone. Removal of the 19-methyl group of testosterone greatly reduces its androgenic properties and unmasks progestational activity. Acetylation at the 17α position also conveys progestational activity and produces compounds that are less rapidly metabolized by the liver. Acetylation at the 17β position further enhances progestational activity. These orally active progestins are 19-norsteroids; they are primarily used in oral contraceptive preparations.[9] Some chemical modifications are shown in Fig. 47-3.

Actions

Progesterone and progestins act on specific receptors in estrogen-primed target tissues. The effects of progestins are generally opposite to those of estrogens. They decrease myometrial contractions, increase glandular development of the breast and endometrium, and promote secretion of a viscous mucus from cervical glands. Priming with estrogen is essential for development of an adequate secretory endometrium.

Progestins, like estrogens, inhibit LH secretion through a negative feedback on the hypothalamic–anterior pituitary axis. This is one of the mechanisms by which these synthetic hormones prevent conception. In addition, other activities of progestins may be equally important for contraception. First, alteration of cervical mucus from a watery, nonviscous secretion to a viscous, cellular secretion provides a physical barrier to sperm penetration. Furthermore, progestational stimulation early in the ovarian cycle causes premature development of endometrial glands and involution. The estrogen component of the preparation stimulates stromal development, and the resulting endometrium is unsuitable for implantation.

Use

Progestins are primarily used in oral contraceptive formulations. They are usually combined with a semisynthetic estrogen, but some compounds are used alone. Progestins are used to treat menstrual dysfunction, such as irregular cycles, protracted uterine bleeding, dysmenorrhea, amenorrhea, and endometriosis. It is believed that poorly cycling estrogens may promote hypertrophy of the endometrium. The addition of a progestin can help to repair the necrotic endometrium and promote natural shedding once the hormone is withdrawn. Progestins alone will not promote menstrual bleeding, but in patients who either have endogenous estrogen or are treated first with estrogen, the cyclic treatment with progestin will help restore normal cycling.

Adverse effects

Many of the minor side effects associated with use of oral contraceptives or progestational agents are similar to the symptoms associated with pregnancy. The effects generally attributed to the progestational component include weight gain, depression, fatigue, acne, and hirsutism. These are probably related to the androgenic action of the progestational compound, and, in contrast to the nausea caused by estrogens, the symptoms do not usually subside with continued use. One of the more annoying side effects attributable to progestins is development of candidiasis.

Although reports of increased risk of neoplasia in long-term progestin users continue to appear, there is no convincing evidence linking these hormones to cancer. In fact, there is considerable evidence that oral contraceptives prevent some forms of cancer. A recent review of this issue[19] indicated that blockade of ovulation by pregnancy, lactation, or hormonal suppression may protect against endometrial and ovarian cancer. The case for cervical cancer is, however, less clear.

The oral contraceptive preparations, as well as individual hormones, can affect measurements of plasma lipids, but there is, as yet, no clear link between these drugs and arterial disease.

Specific agents

There are many compounds with progestational activity. The semisynthetic derivatives of progesterone include **medroxyprogesterone** (Depo-Provera; 100 mg/ml) and **hydroxyprogesterone caproate** (Delalutin; 125 and 250 mg/ml). These have little estrogenic or androgenic activity and can be injected intramuscularly in depot form. Medroxyprogesterone acetate (Provera, others) is also available in tablets, 2.5 to 10 mg.

The 19-norsteroids have slight estrogenic potency, probably because of metabolism to estrogenic compounds. Some have androgenic actions as well. The most commonly used agents are those included in oral contraceptives: **ethynodiol diace-**

TABLE 47-2 Formulations of combined oral contraceptives containing less than 50 μg of estrogen, by brand

	Estrogen (μg)	Progesterone (mg)
Ortho-Novum 1/35		Norethindrone, 1.0
Norinyl 1/35		Norethindrone, 1.0
Demulen 1/35		Ethynodiol diacetate, 1.0
Brevicon		Norethindrone, 0.5
Modicon	Ethinyl estradiol, 35	Norethindrone, 0.5
Ovcon-35		Norethindrone, 0.4
Ortho-Novum 10/11		Norethindrone, 0.5/1.0
Ortho-Novum 7/7/7		Norethindrone, 0.5/0.75/1.0
Tri-Norinyl		Norethindrone, 0.5/1.0/0.5
Nordette		Levonorgestrel, 0.15
Loestrin 1.5/30	Ethinyl estradiol, 30	Norethindrone acetate, 1.5
Lo-Ovral		Norgestrel, 0.3 (0.15 D-norgestrel)
Loestrin 1/20	Ethinyl estradiol, 20	Norethindrone, 1.0

Modified from Batzer, F.R.: J. Reprod. Med. **29**(suppl.):503, 1984.

tate, **norethindrone, norethynodrel, norgestrel,** and **levonorgestrel.** Table 47-2 gives the composition of some oral contraceptives.[1]

ANDROGENS
The principle androgen of the testes, testosterone, is formed in the Leydig (interstitial) cells. It is not stored but is continually synthesized and released into the circulation, where it is complexed with a specific β-globulin. Testosterone is also synthesized in the ovaries and adrenal cortex, but plasma testosterone concentrations in males are approximately 10 times higher than those in females.

Chemistry
Testosterone is the precursor of both estradiol and the 5α reduced androgen, dihydrotestosterone. The latter compound is a more potent androgen, and it mediates most of the androgenic effects attributed to testosterone. Orally effective derivatives of testosterone include methyltestosterone, fluoxymesterone, and methandrostenolone.

Testosterone is metabolized in the liver, and the metabolites, androsterone and etiocholanolone, are excreted in the urine. The 17-methyl–substituted compounds, such as methyltestosterone and fluoxymesterone, are not readily inactivated by the liver and are effective orally. Esters of testosterone, such as the propionate, must be administered parenterally and are slowly absorbed.

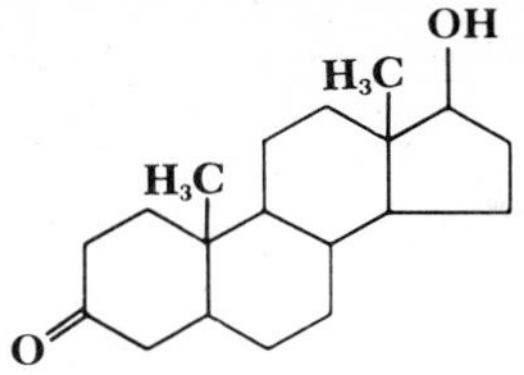

Dihydrotestosterone

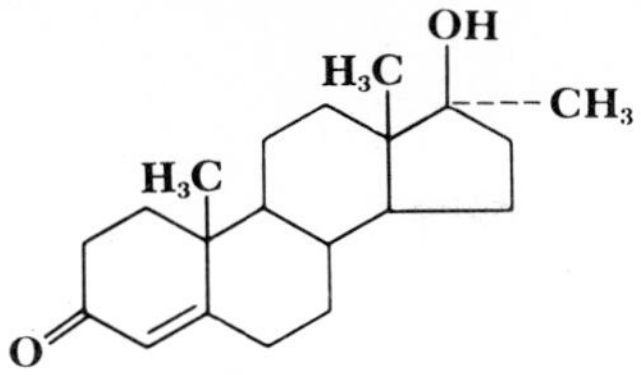

Methyltestosterone

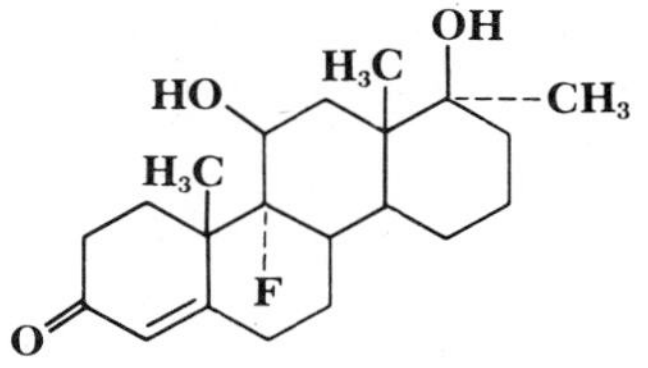

Fluoxymesterone

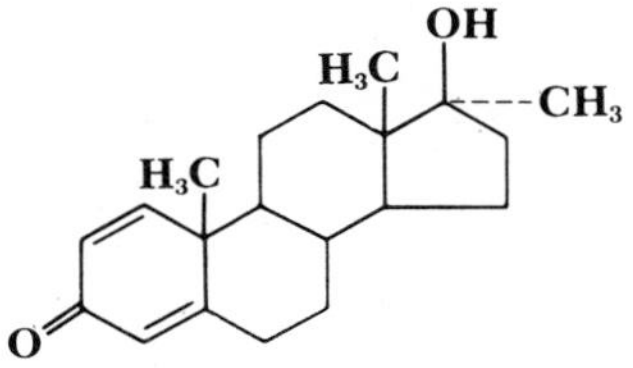

Methandrostenolone

Actions

Androgenic steroids can affect all tissues of the body. There are basically two general actions: androgenic and anabolic. All natural and synthetic androgens have both types of action to some degree. The androgenic actions are responsible for the changes associated with sexual maturation and for stimulation of spermatogenesis. Early in embryonic life androgens promote development of the male phenotype. They are also responsible for the growth spurt at puberty and for the increase in muscle mass that accompanies maturation of the male. In addition, androgens stimulate growth and secretion of sebaceous glands.

The mechanism of androgenic action is similar to that of the other sex hormones. The hormone is bound to a cytoplasmic receptor and transported to the nucleus where it directs synthesis of selected proteins. Feminization can occur in males who lack androgenic receptors, despite high concentrations of circulating testosterone.

The anabolic steroids, compounds that cause nitrogen retention and enhance protein synthesis, are of particular interest. It has not been possible to dissociate completely the anabolic and androgenic actions, but some steroids, such as nandrolone, have a greater action on nitrogen retention than would be predicted by androgenic assays.

Use

The major indication for androgen therapy is deficiency because of testicular or pituitary failure. Androgens have been used in hypogonadism in the male and in certain types of infertility with some degree of success. Testosterone propionate is also used as an estrogen antagonist in estrogen-sensitive tumors, such as metastatic carcinoma of the breast. Its virilizing action, however, makes this hormone less acceptable than other types of therapy.

TABLE 47-3 Androgen preparations	
Preparation	Dosage forms (mg)
Testosterone (Histerone)	I: 25-100/ml; P: 75
Testosterone cypionate (Duratest, others)	I: 50-200/ml
Testosterone enanthate (Everone, others)	I: 100, 200/ml
Testosterone propionate (Androlan, Testex) (Oreton)	I: 25-100/ml BT: 10; T: 10, 25
Methyltestosterone (Oreton-Methyl, others)	BT: 10, 15; C: 10; T: 10, 25
Fluoxymesterone (Halotestin, others)	T: 2-10
Nandrolone phenpropionate (Durabolin, others)	I: 25, 50/ml
Ethylestrenol (Maxibolin)	E: 2/5 ml; T: 2
Methandrostenolone (Methandroid)	T: 2.5, 5
Oxandrolone (Anavar)	T: 2.5
Oxymetholine (Anadrol-50)	T: 50
Stanozolol (Winstrol)	T: 2

BT, Buccal tablet; *E*, elixir; *I*, injection; *P*, pellet for subcutaneous implantation; *T*, tablet.

Anabolic steroids are used in conditions in which there is a negative nitrogen balance: wasting diseases, malnutrition, severe anemia, or severe trauma. There is no indication that they are of any value in persons with adequate nutrition and a normal nitrogen balance. Despite this lack of effect, anabolic steroids are widely misused by athletes in attempts to improve strength and performance.

Adverse effects   Androgen use in the female can cause virilization, acne, and symptoms of estrogen deficiency. Androgen administration in the immature male can cause precocious puberty and all the structural changes to the mature male phenotype. Premature closure of long-bone epiphyses may occur in children who receive androgens. Retention of water and sodium can worsen hypertension in athletes who misuse anabolic steroids, and cholestatic jaundice has occurred in patients treated with compounds containing a 17α-alkyl substitution. In addition, the androgenic actions may worsen hormone-sensitive neoplasms, such as carcinoma of the prostate.

Specific agents   **Testosterone** (Table 47-3) is used for correction of male hypogonadism and for palliative treatment of breast carcinoma. It is administered by intramuscular injection or as regular or buccal tablets. **Methyltestosterone** is quite similar.

Fluoxymesterone is a synthetic halogenated derivative of methyltestosterone. It is more potent than the parent compound with respect to both androgenic and anabolic actions. It is used for androgen replacement and for its nitrogen-retaining effect.

Nandrolone has greater anabolic than androgenic activity and is used when nitrogen retention is desirable.

Nandrolone phenpropionate

REFERENCES

1. Batzer, F.R.: Formulation and noncontraceptive uses of the new, low-dose oral contraceptive, J. Reprod. Med. **29** (suppl.):503, 1984.

2. Brazeau, P., and Guillemin, R.: Somatostatin: newcomer from the hypothalamus, N. Engl. J. Med. **290**:963, 1974.

3. Brown, P., Gajdusek, D.C., Gibbs, C.J., Jr., and Asher, D.M.: Potential epidemic of Creutzfeldt-Jakob disease from human growth hormone therapy, N. Engl. J. Med. 313:728, 1985.

4. Carr, B.R., and MacDonald, P.C.: Estrogen treatment of postmenopausal women, Adv. Intern. Med. **28**:491, 1983.

5. Chan, L., and O'Malley, B.W.: Mechanism of action of the sex steroid hormones, N. Engl. J. Med. **294**:1322, 1976.

6. Chrousos, G.P., Schuermeyer, T.H., Doppman, J., et al.: Clinical applications of corticotropin-releasing factor, Ann. Intern. Med. **102**:344, 1985.

7. Conn, P.M., Staley, D., Harris, C., et al.: Mechanism of action of gonadotropin releasing hormone, Annu. Rev. Physiol. **48**:495, 1986.

8. Cutler, G.B., Jr., Hoffman, A.R., Swerdloff, R.S., et al.: Therapeutic applications of luteinizing-hormone–releasing hormone and its analogs, Ann. Intern. Med. **102**:643, 1985.

9. Durand, J.L., and Bressler, R.: Clinical pharmacology of the steroidal oral contraceptives, Adv. Intern. Med. **24**:97, 1979.

10. Faden, A.I.: Pharmacotherapy in spinal cord injury: a critical review of recent developments, Clin. Neuropharmacol. **10**: 193, 1987.

11. Frasier, S.D.: Human pituitary growth hormone (hGH) therapy in growth hormone deficiency, Endocrine Rev. **4**:155, 1983.

12. Krulich, L., Dhariwal, A.P.S., and McCann, S.M.: Stimulatory and inhibitory effects of purified hypothalamic extracts on growth hormone release from rat pituitary *in vitro*, Endocrinology **83**:783, 1968.

13. Reichlin, S.: Somatostatin, N. Engl. J. Med. **309**:1495 and 1564, 1983.

14. Reiter, E.O., and Grumbach, M.M.: Neuroendocrine control mechanisms and the onset of puberty, Annu. Rev. Physiol. **44**:595, 1982.

15. Rivier, C., and Vale, W.: Effects of corticotropin-releasing factor, neurohypophyseal peptides, and catecholamines on pituitary function, Fed. Proc. **44**:189, 1985.

16. Rivier, J., Rivier, C., and Vale, W.: Synthetic competitive antagonists of corticotropin-releasing factor: effect on ACTH secretion in the rat, Science **224**:889, 1984.

17. Ryan, K.J.: Postmenopausal estrogen

use, Annu. Rev. Med. **33**:171, 1982.

18. Schally, A.V.: Aspects of hypothalamic regulation of the pituitary gland: its implications for the control of reproductive processes, Science **202**:18, 1978.

19. Stubblefield, P.G.: Oral contraceptives and neoplasia, J. Reprod. Med. **29** (suppl.):524, 1984.

20. Thorner, M.O.: Hypothalamic releasing hormones: clinical possibilities, Hosp. Pract. **21**(12):63, 1986.

21. Tuomisto, J., and Männistö, P.: Neurotransmitter regulation of anterior pituitary hormones, Pharmacol. Rev. **37**:249, 1985.

22. Vaisrub, S.: The many faces of bromocriptine (editorial), J.A.M.A. **235**:2854, 1976.

23. Vale, W., and Greer, M.: Corticotropin-releasing factor, Fed. Proc. **44**:145, 1985.

Chapter 48

Pharmacologic approaches to gout

Gout is characterized by hyperuricemia and arthritis. The disease may be *primary*—caused by overproduction or defective renal excretion of uric acid. The *secondary* form develops during some other disease, such as leukemia, or is caused by drugs such as the thiazide diuretics.

In general, patients with gout may be divided into those who overproduce uric acid and those who underexcrete it.[1,5] Overproducers excrete about 1 g of uric acid daily and have a large increase in their body pool of uric acid. Daily excretion of more than 750 mg indicates overproduction.[5] Underexcretors have only a moderately increased pool of uric acid.

The pharmacologic approach to an acute attack is different from management of the chronic disease. The acute attack is a form of arthritis that traditionally has been treated with *colchicine*. More recently, it has become apparent that virtually any of the nonsteroidal anti-inflammatory drugs (NSAIDs) can be used effectively.[1,3,6]

The aim of management of the chronic form of the disease is to reduce the uric acid content of the body. This can be accomplished with uricosuric drugs such as *probenecid* and *sulfinpyrazone* or by use of *allopurinol*, a xanthine oxidase inhibitor.[1] The latter may have advantages over the uricosuric drugs in some cases.

GENERAL CONCEPTS

Colchicine is an alkaloid obtained from *Colchicum autumnale*, the meadow saffron, a plant belonging to the lily family. *Colchicum* has been used for centuries for arthralgia that is presumably of gouty origin.

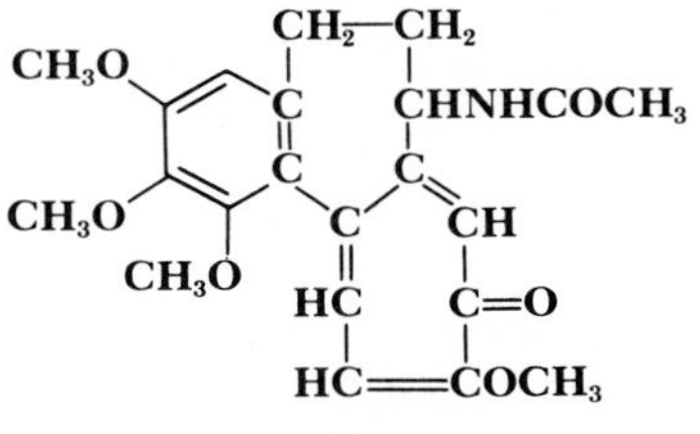

COLCHICINE

Colchicine

Colchicine is well absorbed from the gastrointestinal tract and has a short half-life in plasma. However, it may be retained in cells such as leukocytes. Also, since the kidney is an important route of elimination of this drug, patients with renal disease eliminate colchicine more slowly than normal persons do.

When colchicine is given in doses of 0.5 to 1 mg every hour to a patient having an attack of acute gouty arthritis, relief occurs in 2 to 3 hours. In severe attacks a somewhat longer period may be required. It is quite common for gastrointestinal disturbances such as anorexia, nausea, vomiting, diarrhea, and abdominal pain to appear with about the same dosage as that required for relief. As a consequence, colchicine is administered every hour until relief is obtained or until significant gastrointestinal symptoms develop. In addition to gastrointestinal side effects, colchicine may also cause, though rarely, fever, alopecia, liver damage, and neural and hematopoietic complications.

Colchicine interferes with the microtubular system of cells.[2] In gout, it is believed that this action is exerted on leukocytes, which accumulate in affected joints and ingest the sharp urate crystals. It is quite possible, however, that the action of colchicine is also exerted on synovial cells.

In chronic gout the administration of colchicine has prophylactic value to reduce the incidence of acute exacerbations.[7] Colchicine is available as tablets, 0.5 to 0.65 mg, and for injection, 1 mg/2 ml.

NONSTEROIDAL ANTI-INFLAM-MATORY DRUGS	NSAIDs (see Chapter 31) are replacing colchicine in management of acute gouty arthritis.[1,3,5,6] Phenylbutazone was first shown to be beneficial; four doses of 150 mg every 6 hours are usually sufficient. This drug currently is used infrequently, however, because it has been associated with bone marrow depression. It is important to note that this adverse effect would probably be unlikely to occur with short-duration therapy of gout. Indomethacin can also be used as an initial dose of 75 to 100 mg followed by 50 mg every 6 to 8 hours. After resolution of symptoms, the dose is tapered over 3 to 4 days. These doses of indomethacin can cause headache, light-headedness, and, less frequently, confusion and fluid retention.

Efficacy has also been demonstrated with other NSAIDs, and it is likely that all can be used. In this regard, however, it is important to realize that NSAIDs with a short half-life will have a quicker onset and offset of action and may be preferable to longer-acting agents.

PROBENECID	Even if colchicine is taken chronically for prophylaxis of acute gouty arthritis, it is generally accepted that promotion of uric acid excretion through the use of uricosuric drugs or reduction in synthesis with allopurinol is beneficial in the gouty patient. The most effective uricosuric agents are probenecid and sulfinpyrazone.

Probenecid (Benemid, others) was used originally to inhibit tubular secretion of penicillin G. Currently, probenecid is seldom needed for this purpose because penicillin is readily available; a higher blood concentration can be achieved simply by an increase in the dosage of the antibiotic.

$$CH_3CH_2CH_2 \diagdown$$
$$NSO_2 \diagup\!\!\!\diagdown\!\!\!\!\longrightarrow\!\!\!COOH$$
$$CH_3CH_2CH_2 \diagup$$

Probenecid

Schema of the effects of drugs on uric acid excretion. 1, Below normal; 2, normal; 3, above normal. By decreasing secretion of uric acid, thiazide diuretics, relatively low doses of salicylates, other nonsteroidal anti-inflammatory drugs (NSAIDs), and probenecid can exacerbate preexisting hyperuricemia or may actually be the initiating cause of hyperuricemia. Filtration of uric acid will return to normal as hyperuricemia is resolved by "high" doses of probenecid (or another uricosuric agent).   FIG. 48-1

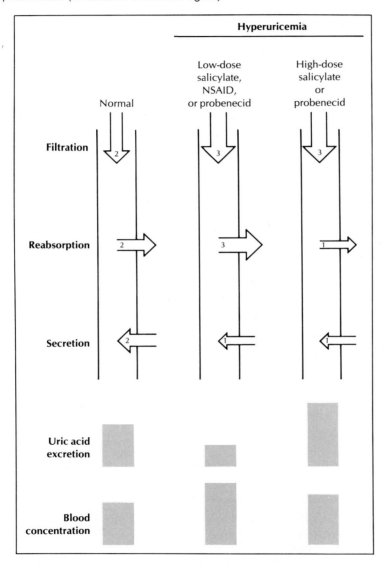

Probenecid greatly increases excretion of uric acid in gouty patients. Doses of 0.5 g three or four times daily lower serum uric acid over extended treatment periods. The increased urinary concentrations of uric acid that result incur a risk of formation of urate stones (urolithiasis). This risk is lessened if patients drink large volumes of fluid to maintain low urinary urate concentrations or if they alkalinize the urine, preferably by ingestion of potassium citrate. With the latter, the high urine pH increases the solubility of urate, and the citrate itself inhibits stone formation.[4]

Renal handling of uric acid involves glomerular filtration, tubular reabsorption, and tubular secretion (Fig. 48-1). Low doses of organic anions such as probenecid itself, salicylates, or other NSAIDs cause retention of uric acid. It is likely that in small doses these anions compete with uric acid for secretion, thereby decreasing excretion and increasing serum concentration; in contrast, with high doses of salicylates or probenecid, blockade of reabsorption predominates to increase uric acid excretion and decrease serum concentration.

Thiazide diuretic- and pyrazinamide-induced uric acid retention may also be attributable to interference with uric acid secretion. In addition, the thiazide diuretics decrease filtration of uric acid secondary to a decline in glomerular filtration rate consequent to volume depletion.

The effect of probenecid on transport of uric acid reflects its general action on organic acid transport. Many other drugs used clinically are organic acids, and their renal excretion can be affected by probenecid. In contrast to uric acid, however, transport of organic acid drugs is predominantly in the secretory direction. Hence probenecid inhibits secretion and decreases excretion of these drugs, and a reduction of their dosage may be necessary. Examples include the penicillins, many cephalosporins, methotrexate, and many NSAIDs.

Probenecid is rapidly absorbed from the stomach and reaches peak plasma concentration in 4 hours. Urinary excretion of the drug is greater in alkaline urine. Treatment should begin with small doses, 250 mg twice a day, to decrease the potential for renal stone formation. Dosage must be gradually increased to a 1 or 1.5 g maintenance level; the ultimate dosage is determined with the use of serum uric acid determinations. The drug is available in tablets, 500 mg. Colchicine is often administered concurrently with probenecid to decrease the likelihood of acute gouty attacks.

Probenecid may cause adverse effects in a small percentage of patients. The figure generally given is less than 2%, but in some series adverse reactions have developed in 8% of patients. Nausea and vomiting, skin rash, and drug fever may occur. Urate stones may cause renal colic.

SULFINPYRAZONE
Sulfinpyrazone (Anturane), which is structurally related to phenylbutazone, also prevents tubular reabsorption of uric acid. Its action is antagonized by salicylates but not by probenecid. As with probenecid the sharp increase in urate excretion may predispose to urolithiasis. An acute gouty attack may occur at the beginning of treatment, and epigastric distress has been reported. The dosage is initially 50 mg

four times daily, which may be increased gradually to as much as 400 mg daily. Sulfinpyrazone can be taken in tablets, 100 mg, or in capsules, 200 mg.

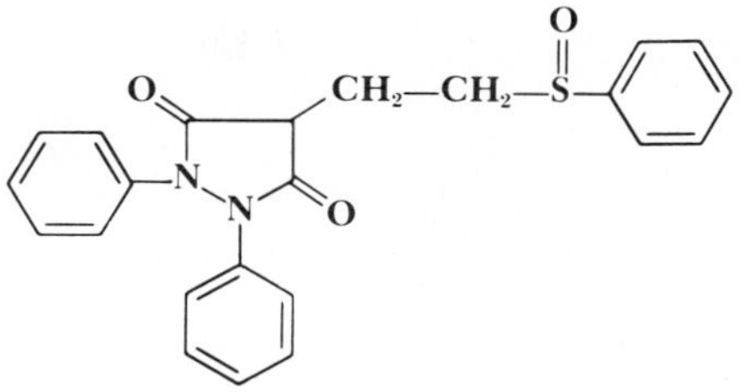

Sulfinpyrazone

ALLOPURINOL

Another approach to treatment of gout is to use an inhibitor of *xanthine oxidase*, an enzyme that converts hypoxanthine to uric acid. Allopurinol (Zyloprim, Lopurin) was originally developed to protect 6-mercaptopurine from rapid inactivation in the body by this enzyme. Allopurinol causes a sharp decrease in both serum uric acid concentration and in urinary uric acid excretion. As a result, the metabolic precursors xanthine and hypoxanthine replace uric acid in the urine.

Allopurinol is rapidly oxidized in the body to oxypurinol, which is then excreted by the kidney. Patients with renal insufficiency retain this metabolite, which can be toxic.

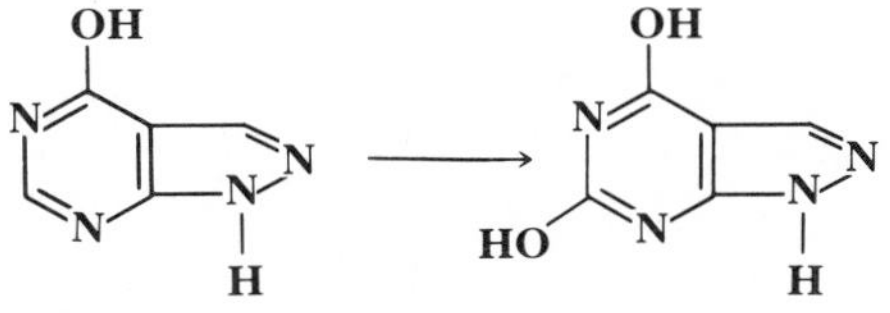

Allopurinol   **Oxypurinol**

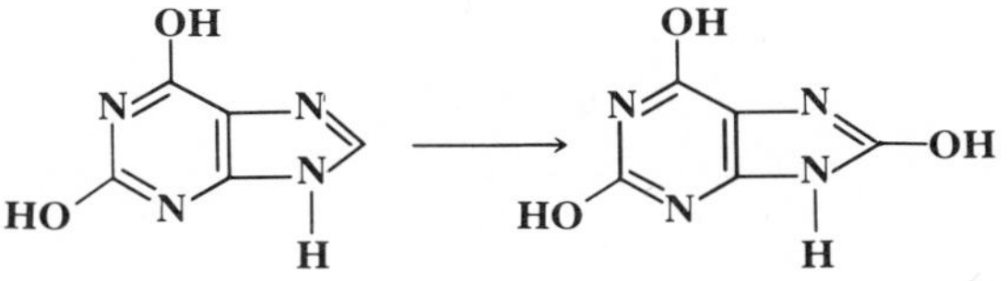

Xanthine   **Uric acid**

In gouty patients intolerant or unresponsive to uricosuric agents, normal serum urate concentrations are achieved with 200 to 600 mg/day of allopurinol. Tablets contain 100 or 300 mg of the drug.

Although uricosuric agents are effective in controlling hyperuricemia in most gouty patients, allopurinol may be more useful for a number of reasons. Gouty nephropathy and formation of urate stones are theoretically less likely with allopurinol therapy because the drug *reduces* the amount of uric acid excreted. In patients with impaired renal function or with urate stones, allopurinol is the agent of choice.

Reactions to allopurinol have been mild or moderate though about 3% of patients taking the drug may develop skin eruptions, fever, hepatomegaly, leukopenia, gastrointestinal distress, diarrhea, pruritus, rash, headache, or alterations of liver function.

REFERENCES

1. Boss, G.R., and Seegmiller, J.E.: Hyperuricemia and gout: classification, complications and management, N. Engl. J. Med. **300**:1459, 1979.
2. Bryan, J.: Biochemical properties of microtubules, Fed. Proc. **33**:152, 1974.
3. Emmerson, B.T.: Drug control of gout and hyperuricaemia, Drugs **16**:158, 1978.
4. Pak, C.Y.C., and Fuller, C.: Idiopathic hypocitraturic calcium-oxalate nephrolithiasis successfully treated with potassium citrate, Ann. Intern. Med. **104**:33, 1986.
5. Rastegar, A., and Thier, S.O.: The treatment of hyperuricemia in gout, Ration. Drug Ther. **8**(3), 1974.
6. Simkin, P.A.: Management of gout, Ann. Intern. Med. **90**:812, 1979.
7. Yü, T.-F.: The efficacy of colchicine prophylaxis in articular gout: a reappraisal after 20 years, Semin. Arthritis Rheum. **12**:256, 1982.

Chapter 49

Antianemic drugs

The normal oxygen-carrying capacity of blood depends on maintenance of an adequate number of erythrocytes and continual synthesis of hemoglobin and stromal (structural) proteins, the synthesis of which normally adjusts to accommodate physiologic loss of blood elements. Anemia results when there is excessive loss or diminished replacement of erythrocytes or when the circulating cells have inadequate hemoglobin. Anemia can result from chronic blood loss, abnormal shape or size of erythrocytes, nutritional deficiencies, chronic disease, or malignancies. Differential diagnosis to determine the underlying cause of the anemia is essential. For example, although a common cause is nutritional deficiency of iron, deficiency of either vitamin B_{12} or folic acid can also cause anemia. Correction of the specific deficiency successfully ameliorates the anemia, provided that an early and accurate diagnosis is made.

Erythrocytes

The mature erythrocyte is a biconcave disk with a diameter of approximately 8 μm. Its large surface-to-volume ratio facilitates gas exchange, and its flexibility enables it to pass easily through capillaries. The normal life-span is about 120 days; aging cells are replaced by maturation of reticulocytes from the bone marrow. Erythropoietin, which is produced in the kidney in response to decreased oxygenation of blood, circulates to the bone marrow to stimulate erythropoiesis, the process of differentiation of stem cells into mature erythrocytes.

Erythrocyte maturation requires multiple nutritional factors, including vitamins B_{12} and folic acid. These two substances are important for synthesis of nuclear DNA by the immature erythrocyte. They are therefore necessary for adequate cell replication and the eventual synthesis of heme, the porphyrin that combines with globulin to form hemoglobin. Hemoglobin synthesis is regulated by the nucleus as well.

Most anemias are attributable to nutritional deficiency of iron, folate, or vitamin B_{12}. Diagnosis and therapy may be confounded by the interdependence of these factors for erythrocyte maturation and replication. The nutritional anemias are, however, generally treatable with replacement of the deficient factor or factors. Often, inadequate intake of these factors is coupled with increased demand to produce a relative deficit. Pregnancy, for example, may increase the need for iron severalfold.

FIG. 49-1   *Metabolism of iron.*

Courtesy Lederle Laboratories, American Cyanamid Co., Pearl River, N.Y.

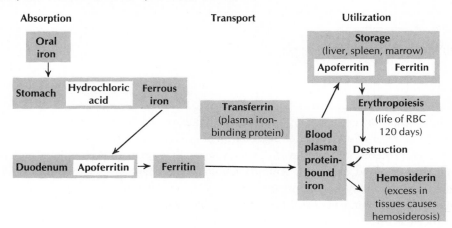

IRON
Distribution

Iron is an integral part of hemoglobin, which in turn constitutes the bulk of the erythrocyte mass. Normal blood contains about 130 to 150 mg of this protein per milliliter, and each gram of hemoglobin contains 3.4 mg of iron. Although the major portion of iron in the body is in the form of hemoglobin, iron is also stored in tissues as *hemosiderin* and *ferritin*, and in blood it is bound to *transferrin*, a carrier protein. Minute quantities of iron are found in myoglobin and in cytochrome enzymes. Total body iron amounts to about 35 mg/kg of body weight. Approximately 70% of body iron is functional (hemoglobin, myoglobin, or enzymes); the remainder is in less readily available storage forms. Iron from tissue stores, however, can replace as much as half of the circulating hemoglobin.[4]

Absorption,
metabolism,
and excretion

Iron is absorbed in the intestine by a carefully regulated transport process (Fig. 49-1). The mucosal cells of the duodenum and proximal jejunum take up iron but transfer only a small amount of it to the blood. The remainder is stored as ferritin and excreted when mucosal cells are sloughed. Thus the intestine is the primary site for both absorption and excretion of iron. Iron is absorbed in the ferrous (Fe^{++}) form; the rate of absorption is influenced by gastric acidity, the presence of reducing substances, such as ascorbic acid, and food intake. Substances such as antacids and phosphates decrease absorption. Excessive iron intake or decreased marrow activity will lower absorption. On the other hand, mucosal absorption is stimulated in conditions of iron deficiency and when erythropoiesis is increased.

Iron is rigidly conserved in the body. Most of the iron released from breakdown of hemoglobin in the liver is reused, and the daily iron requirement of a normal adult is only about 1 mg. Since the diet usually contains about 20 mg of iron, of which approximately 10% is absorbed, this is sufficient to offset small daily losses.

From Herbert, V.: Hosp. Pract. **15**(3):75, 1980. *Illustration by Irwin Kuperberg; data from Hillman, Bothwell, and Finch, 1962 and 1974.* **FIG. 49-2**

Biochemical and hematologic sequence of events in iron deficiency				
	Normal	*Iron depletion*	*Iron-deficient erythropoiesis*	*Iron-deficiency anemia*
RE marrow iron	2-3 +	0-1 +	0	0
Transferrin iron-binding capacity (μg/100 ml)	330 ± 30	360	390	410
Plasma ferritin (ng/ml)	100 ± 60	20	10	< 10
Iron absorption (%)	5-10	10-15	10-20	10-20
Plasma iron (μg/100 ml)	115 ± 50	115	< 60	< 40
Transferrin saturation (%)	35 ± 15	30	< 15	< 10
Sideroblasts (%)	40-60	40-60	< 10	< 10
RBC protoporphyrin (μg/100 ml of RBC)	30	30	100	200
Erythrocyte morphology	Normal	Normal	Normal	Microcytic/ hypochromic

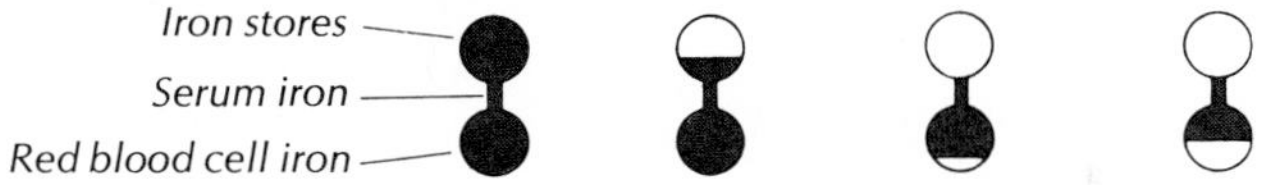

☐ Abnormal

The increased demands of growth, menstruation, or pregnancy, however, coupled with an inadequate intake can eventually lead to a deficiency state. Once iron deficiency has developed, with depletion of iron stores, a normal dietary intake is no longer sufficient to correct the anemia and to replace the stores.

Transferrin transports iron to sites of hemoglobin synthesis. This protein is normally less than saturated with iron. As the amount of iron bound to transferrin decreases, iron from tissue stores is mobilized and absorption increases. When tissue iron stores decrease, changes in erythrocyte morphology slowly develop to produce the characteristic microcytic, hypochromic anemia of iron deficiency. Fig. 49-2 shows the progression of biochemical and hematologic events in iron-deficiency anemia.

Iron-deficiency anemia

Iron deficiency is by far the most common of the nutritional anemias, occurring in 25% of infants, 6% of children, 15% of menstruating women, and 30% of pregnant women in the United States.[4] Women athletes appear to be particularly susceptible because they must offset not only menstrual blood loss but also increased destruction of erythrocytes. In males or postmenopausal females the most common cause of iron-deficiency anemia is chronic blood loss, usually from the gastrointestinal tract. This may be compounded by an inadequate or restricted diet. Ingestion of drugs that cause intestinal blood loss or that cause vitamin loss with subsequent suppression of erythrocyte formation can contribute, as alcoholism can. The hallmark of iron-defi-

TABLE 49-1	Oral iron preparations
Preparation	Dosage
Ferrous sulfate (Feosol, others)	300 mg three times a day
Ferrous gluconate (Fergon, others)	600 mg three times a day
Ferrous fumarate (Ircon, others)	500 mg three times a day

ciency anemia is the microcytic, hypochromic erythrocyte. These cells contain less hemoglobin than normal and are smaller than normal as well. Physical signs include pallor of the skin and mucous membranes, and patients complain of fatigue and loss of appetite. A decreased concentration of serum ferritin also indicates iron-deficiency anemia.[6]

TREATMENT

The goal of iron supplementation in iron-deficiency anemia is to provide immediately available iron for synthesis of hemoglobin and to replenish tissue stores. Iron therapy for as long as 6 months is usually required to replace depleted stores, but many of the laboratory tests may become normal within a few weeks.[4] On the average, the hemoglobin concentration will increase approximately 10 mg/ml per week.

Although many different preparations of iron are available, there is little indication that any are better than orally administered ferrous salts. The oral preparations differ mainly in their rate of absorption from the gastrointestinal tract. Most are administered in excessive doses to assure an adequate amount, but no more than 15% of an oral dose of iron is absorbed, even in deficiency. Recommended adult doses are tailored to provide daily absorption of 15 to 25 mg. The most popular preparations are listed in Table 49-1. All have the same mode of action and produce similar side effects.

Injectible forms of iron are also available but are seldom used. Iron-dextran injection (Imferon) is a complex of ferric hydroxide with dextrans. It is used for patients who are unable to take oral medications or in formulas for parenteral nutrition. The iron is released only after the complex is taken up by cells in the reticuloendothelial system. Parenteral administration of iron can readily restore tissue depots because absorption is not a limiting step. However, it carries the danger of more serious toxicity, including iron overload and anaphylactic shock.

Side effects and toxicity

Both the therapeutic and the adverse effects of iron therapy depend on the amount of elemental iron released. Oral iron preparations frequently irritate the gastrointestinal tract and may be poorly tolerated by debilitated patients. The most common complaints are abdominal cramping and diarrhea. Nausea, gastric pain, and headache are not uncommon. Gastrointestinal irritation can be reduced by administration of iron salts after meals.

Serious reactions to parenteral iron can occur, particularly if oral iron is administered concurrently. Saturation of transferrin elevates the blood concentration of unbound metal, and there is no adequate means of excretion. Excess iron is deposited in tissues where it can cause hemochromatosis. Acute overdose can cause cardiovascular collapse. Such toxicity is rare with oral preparations in adults, whereas children who ingest excessive amounts are at risk.

The potent and specific iron-chelating agent deferoxamine (Desferal) is used to treat acute toxic reactions to iron and to remove iron from patients with overload. It is a water-soluble compound that contains three molecules of trihydroxamic acid. One molecule of deferoxamine binds one molecule of ferric iron. This removes iron from ferritin and blocks further absorption of iron from the gastrointestinal tract. The figure shows the iron-binding site of deferoxamine.

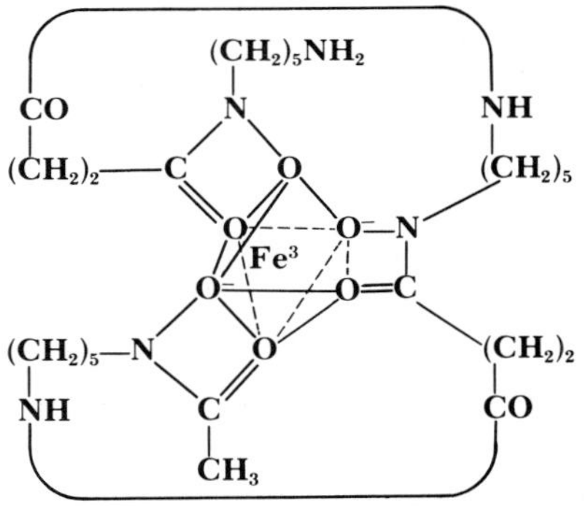

Deferoxamine

Deferoxamine (in combination with iron)

Deferoxamine can be administered by gastric tube to patients with acute poisoning, or it may be injected intramuscularly or intravenously. Repeated doses may be required in pediatric patients.

Nutritional anemias caused by deficiency of either vitamin B_{12} or folate are much less common than iron-deficiency anemia.[4] A deficiency of either factor causes anemia that is characterized by distinctive cytologic appearance and functional abnormalities because of impaired DNA synthesis and subsequent inadequate erythropoiesis. Because of the interrelationship of replicative and synthetic processes, deficiency of folate may cause vitamin B_{12} deficiency and vice versa. Furthermore, anemia from a deficiency of either factor responds to treatment with the other. To compound the problem further, cells with slowed DNA synthesis are inefficient in the use of iron for hemoglobin synthesis.[4] Thus a compound anemia may present with iron overload. Because an untreated deficiency of vitamin B_{12} can cause progressive neurologic damage, it is essential to establish the cause of the megaloblastic anemia before treatment.

MEGALOBLASTIC ANEMIAS

Vitamin B$_{12}$ Vitamin B$_{12}$ is the collective name for cyanocobalamins, cobalt-containing compounds that are synthesized by microorganisms and ingested through animal products in the food chain.[2] Unlike many other vitamins, vitamin B$_{12}$ is not found in plants.

Vitamin B$_{12}$

To become biologically active, cyanocobalamin must be converted to either of two biologically active forms, methylcobalamin or adenosylcobalamin. Methylcobalamin is an essential cofactor in conversion of homocysteine to methionine. Adenosylcobalamin is involved in conversion of methylmalonyl coenzyme A to succinyl coenzyme A. Both active forms of the vitamin are required for erythropoiesis, and a defect in production of succinyl coenzyme A is believed to contribute to the neurologic complications of vitamin B$_{12}$ deficiency.[2] The primary defect found only in vitamin B$_{12}$ deficiency and not in folate deficiency is the inability to synthesize myelin. The lack of vitamin B$_{12}$ results in a demyelinating neuropathy that eventually causes deterioration of the nerve. The process is partially reversible, if replacement therapy begins before deterioration occurs.

The isolation of vitamin B$_{12}$ from liver and its identification as the missing extrinsic factor in pernicious anemia were major discoveries. Pernicious anemia is characterized by megaloblastic anemia, a sharp reduction in gastric secretions, and neurologic damage. This condition was once incurable and inevitably fatal. It was recognized by Castle that the gastric mucosa is the source of an *intrinsic factor* needed for absorption of the extrinsic factor supplied by animal meats and that liver is a rich source of this extrinsic factor. It was subsequently found that both intrinsic factor from gastric secretions and extrinsic factor are needed for erythropoiesis.[3] When folic acid was isolated in 1943, it was believed that a deficiency might cause pernicious anemia. However, it was soon realized that whereas folic acid could correct the hematologic manifestations of the disease it had no effect upon or aggravated the neurologic symptoms. Since liver extract was effective against both hematologic and neurologic defects in pernicious anemia, it was clear that folic acid deficiency was not involved.

The picture was clarified when vitamin B_{12} was isolated, synthesized, and found to correct both hematologic and neurologic deficiencies, as long as intrinsic factor is available. Later it was established that intrinsic factor, which is a thermolabile glycoprotein, is required for adequate absorption of vitamin B_{12}.

ABSORPTION AND FATE

There is no lack of vitamin B_{12} in a normal diet. It is a water-soluble compound that is conserved in the body by enterohepatic recycling; only about 1 μg is lost each day. Since the total body store is normally about a milligram, a long time is required for anemia to develop, even after gastrectomy. Absorption of vitamin B_{12} from dietary sources or from orally administered nutritional supplements requires intrinsic factor from the gastric mucosa. This glycoprotein remains bound to the vitamin until it reaches the lower ileum where the vitamin is absorbed. Gastric resection or gastric malignancy can limit absorption because of loss of gastric mucosal cells that secrete intrinsic factor. Histamine H_2-receptor antagonists, such as cimetidine, also decrease secretion of intrinsic factor.[1] Subnormal intestinal absorption of the vitamin can occur from malabsorption syndromes, such as tropical sprue, celiac disease, or regional enteritis. Finally, coadministration of other drugs or vitamins can affect absorption and utilization of vitamin B_{12}. Megadoses of vitamin C, for example, may destroy vitamin B_{12} during transit through the gastrointestinal tract.[5]

MECHANISM OF ACTION

The characteristic delayed nuclear maturation in megaloblastosis results from inadequate DNA synthesis, which can be corrected by vitamin B_{12} and folic acid. The pathway affected by these vitamins involves synthesis of thymidine from deoxyuridylate (dUMP):

$$\text{Deoxyuridine} \rightarrow \text{Deoxyuridylate} \rightarrow \text{Thymidylate} \rightarrow \text{DNA thymidine}$$

The methylation of deoxyuridylate to thymidylate requires 5,10-methylenetetrahydrofolic acid (Fig. 49-3). This explains the folate requirement in DNA synthesis. Vitamin B_{12} also serves as a cofactor in the regeneration of tetrahydrofolate from the 5-methylated form. This reaction is responsible for conversion of homocysteine to methionine. Additional transfers of one-carbon fragments include conversion of serine to glycine, a reaction that utilizes pyridoxal phosphate as a cofactor.

THERAPEUTIC USE

Vitamin B_{12} is indicated for treatment of megaloblastic anemia caused by nutritional deficiency, which seldom results from inadequate intake; it usually results from defective absorption. Pernicious anemia is the most prevalent cause of vitamin B_{12}

FIG. 49-3   *Pathways for DNA thymine synthesis.*

From Waxman, S., Corcino, J., and Herbert, V.: J.A.M.A. 214:101, copyright 1970; reproduced with permission from American Medical Association.

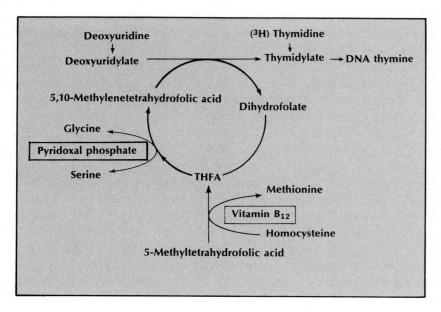

deficiency. Other causes include gastrectomy or extensive damage to the gastric mucosa, malabsorption, as in tropical sprue, and competition by parasites. In the latter condition, for example, the fish tapeworm *(Diphyllobothrium latum)* concentrates much of the vitamin supplied through the diet.

Persons who require vitamin B_{12} therapy for pernicious anemia must be treated parenterally because absorption is negligible without added intrinsic factor. The vitamin is injected intramuscularly (or subcutaneously) in a dosage of 100 μg, repeated daily for a week, then every other day for 2 weeks, then twice weekly for an additional 2 or 3 weeks, and finally monthly for life to prevent progression of neurologic damage. Those who suffer from malnutrition or from a correctable disorder may be treated with oral forms of the vitamin.

Folic acid
CHEMISTRY

Folic acid is pteroylglutamic acid, a combination of pteridine, *p*-aminobenzoic acid, and glutamic acid.

Folic acid

The reactions in which folic acid participates are important for the synthesis of DNA (Fig. 49-3). Folic acid is essential in tissues in which DNA synthesis and turnover is rapid, as in hematopoietic tissues, the mucosa of the gastrointestinal tract, and the developing embryo. For this reason, an increased demand (as in pregnancy) coupled with inadequate intake can lead to deficiency.

Pteroylglutamic acid is the pharmaceutical form of folic acid, but folates in foods are conjugated to six additional glutamic acid residues and are stored as polyglutamates. These naturally occurring folates are destroyed by prolonged cooking. Folates are cleaved to a monoglutamate form during absorption and are converted to several coenzymes that differ structurally in substitution on the pteridine moiety and in the number of glutamate residues. Each of these forms has a specific action in metabolic processes. For example, the interrelationship with vitamin B_{12} involves 5-methyltetrahydrofolic acid as a methyl donor in conversion of homocysteine to methionine.

FUNCTIONS

Folic acid is well absorbed from the proximal intestine. Injectable forms are seldom used except in parenteral alimentation. Like vitamin B_{12}, folic acid is conserved by enterohepatic recycling, and conditions that produce malabsorption in the intestine diminish its absorption. Enterohepatic recycling is compromised in conditions, such as alcoholism, in which there is liver damage.

ABSORPTION, METABOLISM, AND EXCRETION

Folic acid is used as a dietary supplement when there is clearly a nutritional deficiency. Conditions such as chronic alcoholism, pregnancy, lactation, sprue, and ileal disease are indications for supplementation. Conditions in which there is a need for increased erythropoiesis, such as hemolytic anemia or malnutrition, may also be treated with folic acid. Long-term use of certain drugs may lead to folate deficiency. These include anticonvulsants, antimalarial compounds, and steroids. Folic acid should not be used in multiple vitamin preparations because it may obscure diagnosis of pernicious anemia. The danger is that the folic acid can improve the megaloblastic anemia without affecting the demyelinating defect. Thus folate therapy may permit undetected progression of the neurologic damage to an irreversible stage. Even if folic acid is administered with vitamin B_{12} to a person with pernicious anemia, the defect will not be corrected because vitamin B_{12} cannot be adequately absorbed.

THERAPEUTIC USE

REFERENCES

1. Binder, H.J., and Donaldson, R.M., Jr.: Effect of cimetidine on intrinsic factor and pepsin secretion in man, Gastroenterology **74**:371, 1978.
2. Bunn, H.F., Lee, G.R., and Wintrobe, M.M.: Pernicious anemia and other megaloblastic anemias. In Thorn, G.W., Adams, R.D., Braunwald, E., et al., editors: Harrison's principles of internal medicine, ed. 8, New York, 1977, McGraw-Hill Book Co., p. 1656.
3. Castle, W.B.: Current concepts of pernicious anemia, Am. J. Med. **48**:541, 1970.
4. Herbert, V.: The nutritional anemias, Hosp. Pract. **15**(3):65, 1980.
5. Herbert, V., and Jacob, E.: Destruction of vitamin B_{12} by ascorbic acid, J.A.M.A. **230**:241, 1974.
6. Lipschitz, D.A., Cook, J.D., and Finch, C.A.: A clinical evaluation of serum ferritin as an index of iron stores, N. Engl. J. Med. **290**:1213, 1974.

Chapter 50

Vitamins

GENERAL CONCEPT   The early discoveries of vitamins followed observations on naturally occurring diseases such as scurvy and beriberi. The improvement observed in these diseases when modifications were made in the diet indicated that some deficiency may have been the cause of the pathologic process. Feeding experiments were subsequently performed on experimental animals, and soon the essential nature of many vitamins was recognized. Vitamin D (see Chapter 45), folic acid, and vitamin B_{12} (see Chapter 49) are discussed elsewhere.

WATER-SOLUBLE VITAMINS   Many of the water-soluble vitamins are coenzymes or components of coenzymes that have an essential function in the enzymatic machinery of cells.[5]

Thiamine   Thiamine (vitamin B_1) in the form of thiamine pyrophosphate plays important roles in decarboxylation of α-keto acids and in transketolation reactions.

Thiamine hydrochloride

DEFICIENCY   Severe deficiency results in the disease beriberi, which may be characterized by peripheral neuritis, high-output heart failure, or cerebral involvement with Wernicke's encephalopathy. Symptoms include paresthesia, muscle weakness, depression, confusion, and memory deficits. Alcoholism is a major cause of deficiency.

OCCURRENCE   Thiamine is present in sufficient quantities in yeast, wheat germ, and pork.

Niacin   Niacin (nicotinic acid) is an integral part of at least two important coenzymes, nicotinamide-adenine dinucleotide (NAD), and nicotinamide-adenine dinucleotide phosphate (NADP).[2]

Niacin   **Niacinamide**

NAD and NADP exist in an oxidized or a reduced state and can thus act as hydrogen acceptors or donors in many enzymatic reactions of intermediary metabolism. Microsomal enzymes requiring NADP play an important role also in the metabolism of many drugs.

DEFICIENCY

Pellagra is the disease caused by niacin deficiency. It is characterized by pigmentation and lesions of exposed skin, by gastrointestinal mucosal changes with glossitis, stomatitis, anorexia, and diarrhea, and by mental symptoms similar to those with thiamine deficiency.

OCCURRENCE

Niacin is found in significant amounts in yeast, cereals, nuts, liver, and other meats. Mammals can synthesize niacin from tryptophan. Pellagra can occur in patients having carcinoid tumor as a consequence of use of tryptophan for serotonin (5-hydroxytryptamine) synthesis.

PHARMACOLOGY

Niacin, but not nicotinamide, produces noticeable dilatation of small vessels (facial flushing), a transient effect that may be severe with parenteral administration. On a purely empiric basis, niacin is used to lower plasma cholesterol and triglyceride concentrations (see Chapter 39).

Riboflavin

Riboflavin (vitamin B_2) is present in flavin-adenine dinucleotide (FAD), a coenzyme of flavoprotein enzymes important for hydrogen transfer. There is also a flavin mononucleotide (FMN).

DEFICIENCY

A deficiency of riboflavin can cause cheilosis, stomatitis, dermatitis, photophobia, and anemia.

OCCURRENCE

Riboflavin is present in significant quantities in green vegetables, liver, eggs, and milk.

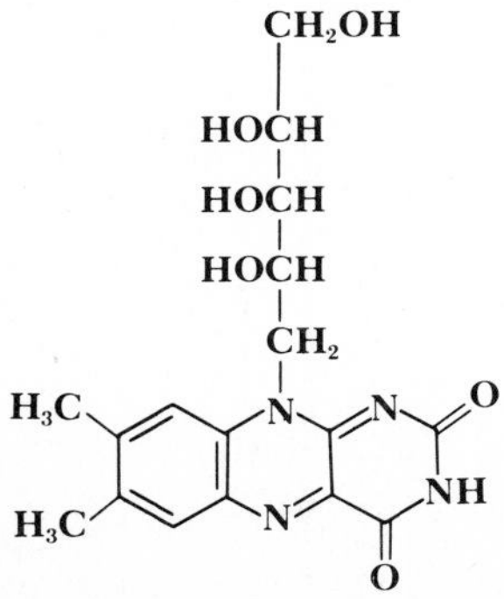

Riboflavin 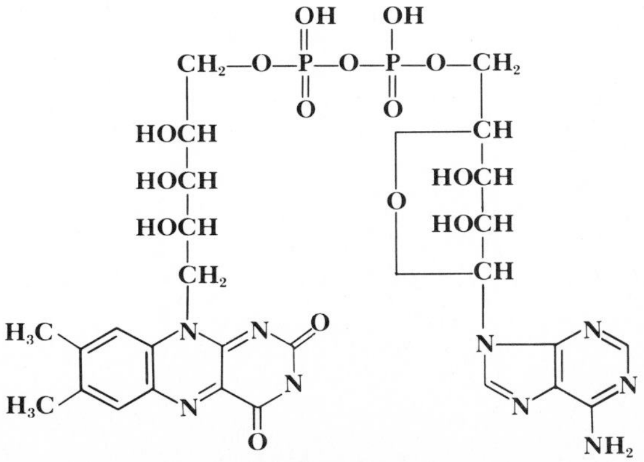   **Flavin-adenine dinucleotide**

Pyridoxine   Pyridoxine, pyridoxal, and pyridoxamine are various forms of vitamin B_6.[3] Pyridoxal 5'-phosphate functions as a coenzyme in many reactions, including transamination between amino acids and keto acids and decarboxylation of amino acids, which is necessary for their conversion to such agents as catecholamines, histamine, and serotonin.

Pyridoxine   **Pyridoxal**   **Pyridoxamine**

DEFICIENCY   A deficiency of pyridoxine in infants can result in convulsions. Deficient patients taking isoniazid may exhibit peripheral neuritis.

OCCURRENCE   Pyridoxine is present in significant amounts in yeast, liver, rice, bran, and wheat germ.

Pantothenic acid   Pantothenic acid is a constituent of the very important coenzyme A. Acetyl coenzyme A is essential for a variety of reactions such as the acetylation of choline to acetylcholine and acetylation of *p*-amino compounds. The coenzyme plays an important role in the Krebs cycle, since citric acid is formed from oxaloacetic acid, acetyl coenzyme A, and water; the reaction regenerates coenzyme A. The coenzyme also plays an important role in fatty acid metabolism.

DEFICIENCY   Pantothenic acid deficiency is not well recognized in humans except for a burning sensation from the feet. In animals it may cause dermatitis, adrenal degeneration, and central nervous system symptoms.

Coenzyme A

Pantothenic acid is found particularly in yeast, bran, egg yolk, and liver. *OCCURRENCE*

Vitamin C (ascorbic acid) is a reducing agent whose exact biologic function is not *Vitamin C*
understood. It may be a free-radical scavenger as well as a cofactor for transformation
of folic to folinic acid, for dopamine β-hydroxylase, for glucocorticoid formation, and
for maintenance of normal connective tissue.[4,5] The benefit of vitamin C in prevention
of the common cold has not been established; large-scale, controlled clinical trials
are not available for proving or disproving its efficacy. In contrast, its purported
efficacy for preventing or treating cancer has been disproved.

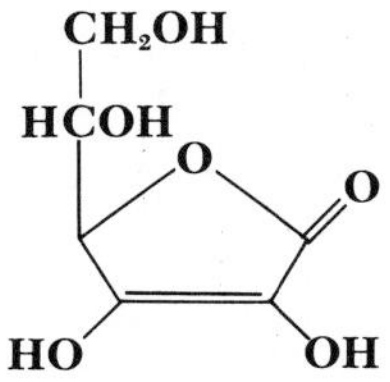

$$CH_2OH$$
$$HCOH$$

Vitamin C

The classical disease scurvy is characterized by abnormalities in the connective *DEFICIENCY*
tissue. Capillary involvement leads to hemorrhage by the gums, skin, and other
tissues. Teeth may become loose, and anemia can develop.

Ascorbic acid is present in high concentrations in citrus fruits, green peppers, *OCCURRENCE*
tomatoes, and fruits and vegetables in general.

There are also other water-soluble factors, such as biotin, essential for experi- *Other water-soluble*
mental animals and presumably for humans. *vitamins*

Vitamin A (retinol) performs an important function in connection with dark ad- *FAT-SOLUBLE*
aptation, being part of the visual purple of the retina. It also maintains the integrity *VITAMINS*
of various epithelial structures. *Vitamin A*
Deficiency of vitamin A produces night blindness, dryness and thickening of the
conjunctiva (xerosis), and ulcerations of the cornea (keratomalacia).[8] The skin may
become rough because of hyperkeratosis.

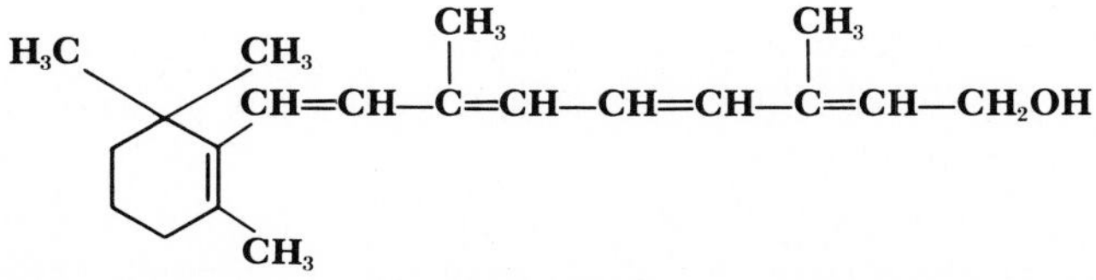

$$H_3C \quad CH_3 \quad CH_3 \quad CH_3$$
$$CH=CH—C=CH—CH=CH—C=CH—CH_2OH$$

Vitamin A

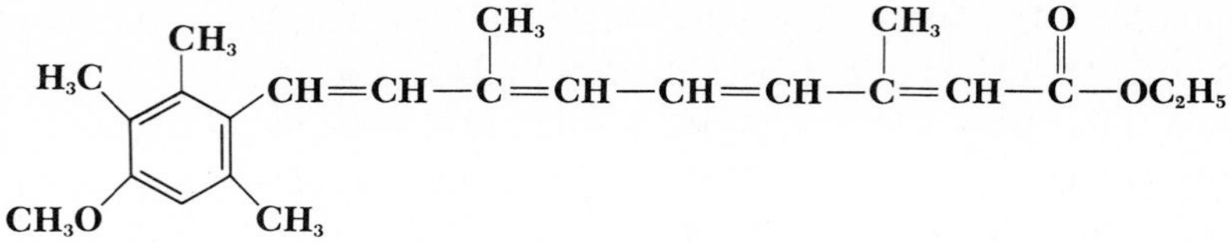

Etretinate

OCCURRENCE

Vitamin A occurs particularly in eggs, milk, and fish liver oils and is also formed in the intestine from vegetable carotenoids (β-carotene).

PHARMACOLOGY AND TOXICITY

Vitamin A is stored in the liver. In toxic quantities it may cause anorexia, irritability, loss of hair, bone disease, and, rarely, hepatomegaly or seizures. **Isotretinoin** (Accutane) and **etretinate** (Tegison), compounds related to the retinol derivative retinoic acid, are now available for chronic treatment of severe acne, psoriasis, and disorders of keratinization. The potential of these agents for adverse effects, such as dry mucus membranes, peeling of the skin, phototoxicity, and arthralgia, is considerable. The danger of teratogenicity is such that pregnancy must be avoided while one is taking these drugs and, because of their long half-lives, for years after therapy is stopped.[1] Etretinate may persist in plasma for over 2 years after a course of treatment and in tissues even longer.

Vitamin E

Vitamin E is present in wheat-germ oil and in many foods. Its role in animal reproduction has been well established, and the term *toco*pherol implies its importance in childbearing. There are several tocopherols, but α-tocopherol has the highest activity.

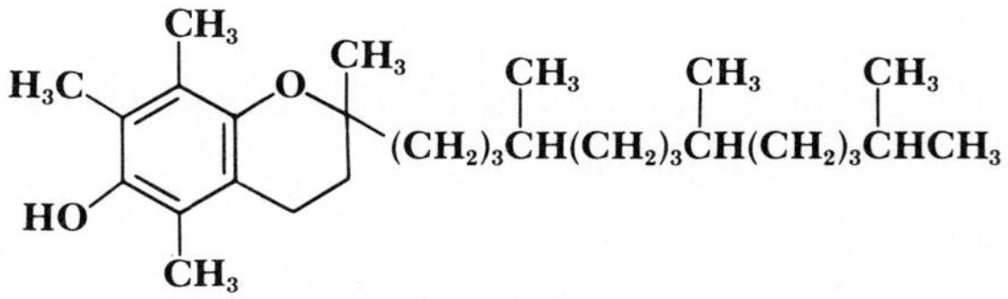

α-**Tocopherol**

Deficiency of vitamin E produces abortion in females and degeneration of the germinal epithelium in males. Muscular dystrophy also develops in animals on a vitamin E–deficient diet. Many other functions have been claimed for α-tocopherol, and the vitamin may be of benefit for minimizing the risk of retrolental fibroplasia in premature infants receiving oxygen.[5]

The feeding of large amounts of unsaturated fats may increase the tocopherol requirement. It has been suggested that tocopherol is a biologic antioxidant whose function becomes particularly important when tissues contain high concentrations of polyunsaturated lipids.

Vitamin K is essential for production of prothrombin and other coagulation factors by the liver,[6] and in its absence hemorrhagic manifestations occur. Various 1,4-naphthoquinones have vitamin K activity. Vitamin K_1 (phytonadione, phylloquinone) is 2-methyl-3-phytyl-1,4-naphthoquinone.

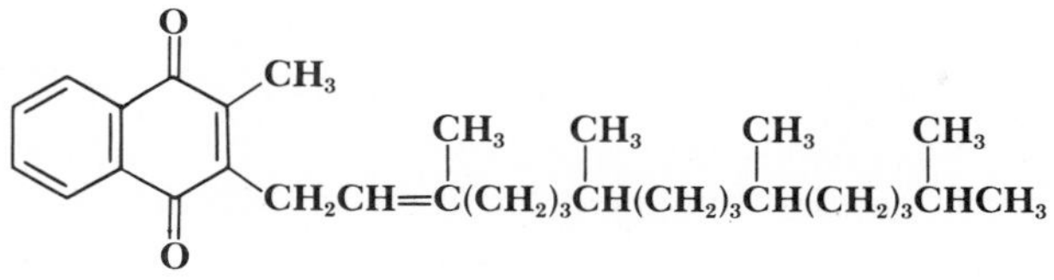

Vitamin K

Vitamin K₁

These naphthoquinone compounds are very insoluble in water and are suitable primarily for oral administration. Emulsions of vitamin K_1, however, can be injected intravenously in hemorrhagic emergencies caused by hypoprothrombinemia.

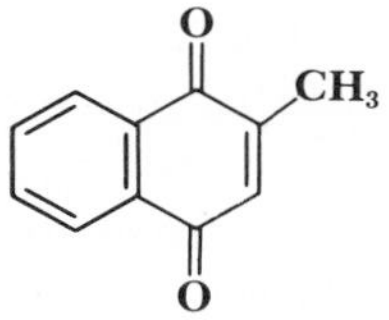

Menadione

Water-soluble derivatives of naphthoquinones have also been prepared. The structural formulas of two such compounds, menadiol sodium diphosphate and menadione sodium bisulfite, are shown below.

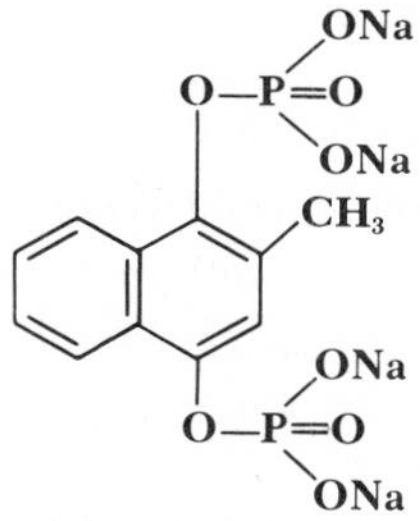

Menadiol sodium diphosphate 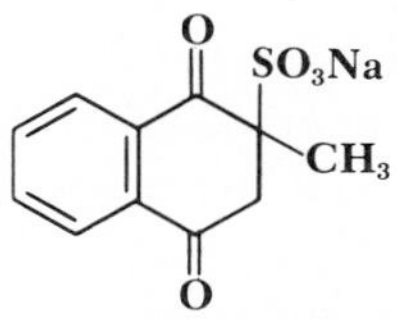   **Menadione sodium bisulfite**

The daily requirement for vitamin K is not certain because considerable quantities are synthesized by the bacterial flora of the intestine. The dosage may vary greatly, depending on the nature and severity of prothrombin deficiency.[6] On the other hand, very large doses may have to be administered in emergency situations when prothrombin concentration has been depressed by anticoagulant drugs. As much as 50 mg or more of vitamin K_1 emulsion has been used in this situation by the intravenous route.

Vitamin K preparations are useful in bleeding caused by hypoprothrombinemia. Causes of hypoprothrombinemia include severe liver disease, biliary obstruction, malabsorption syndromes, coumarin and indanedione drugs, salicylates in large doses, reduction of intestinal flora by chemotherapeutic agents, as well as poor uptake of vitamin K through the placenta and the absence of intestinal flora in premature or newborn infants.[6]

Commonly used preparations are vitamin K_1 (AquaMEPHYTON, Konakion, Mephyton), vitamin K_3 (menadione), or menadiol sodium diphosphate (Synkayvite). The latter two are ineffective treatment for hypoprothrombinemia induced by oral anticoagulants; they are also more likely than vitamin K_1 to cause adverse reactions, such as hyperbilirubinemia and hemolytic anemia, in neonates and should not be given to infants or women near delivery.

TOXICITY   Persons who are subject to primaquine-sensitive anemia may react with hemolysis to large doses of menadione. Such doses can also aggravate liver disease and produce jaundice, particularly in infants.

MEDICAL USES   Vitamins should be used in medicine in (1) those with poor dietary history, (2) deficiency diseases, (3) special disease states, or (4) hereditary vitamin-dependency states. Table 50-1 indicates vitamin requirements for males over 10 years of age and for pregnant or lactating women.[5] Recommended intakes for younger children and nonpregnant females are similar or lower than those for men. Low oral therapeutic dose ranges are also listed.

Persons with a deficient dietary history include vegetarians who do not consume dairy products, persons who do not consume fruits and green vegetables, and also infants and pregnant or lactating women. Ascorbic acid should be given to persons who do not eat fruits and green vegetables. Lactating women should probably take at least 80 mg of ascorbic acid daily, and their increased thiamine requirements should be met by proper food intake. Pyridoxine, folate, and riboflavin should be given to pregnant women. Infants fed cow's milk should receive about 35 mg of ascorbic acid daily. The newborn of mothers taking phenytoin or phenobarbital may be deficient in vitamin K–dependent clotting factors and should receive prophylactic vitamin K_1;[6] so should low birth weight newborns who may also need supplementation with vitamins C, D, E, folic acid, and pyridoxine.[5]

Deficiency diseases include not only those attributable to poor dietary habits but also those attributable to alcoholism, pernicious anemia, total or partial gastrectomy, chronic pancreatitis, celiac disease (nontropical sprue), tropical sprue, and short bowel syndrome.[7]

	Adult requirement		Daily oral therapeutic dose (mg)
Vitamin	Males (mg)	Pregnant or lactating females (mg)	
Water soluble			
Folic acid	0.4	0.5-0.8	5-10
Niacin	16-19	15-19	10-100
Pantothenic acid	4-7	4-7	100-200
Pyridoxine	1.8-2.2	2.5-2.6	20-50
Riboflavin	1.4-1.7	1.5-1.8	5-10
Thiamine	1.2-1.4	1.4-1.6	10-100
Vitamin B_{12}	0.003	0.004	0.1-0.25*
Vitamin C	50-60	80-100	100-200
Fat soluble			
Vitamin A	1.0	1.0-1.2	3-18
Vitamin D	0.005-0.01	0.01-0.0125	0.125
Vitamin E	8-10	10-11	10-100
Vitamin K	0.07-0.14	0.07-0.14	5-10

TABLE 50-1 Recommended daily dietary allowances and therapeutic doses of vitamins

*Weekly by intramuscular injection.

Additional special disease states include infection with *Diphyllobothrium latum,* hypoparathyroidism, and the carcinoid syndrome. The corresponding supplementations are vitamin B_{12}, vitamin D_2, and niacin.

Hereditary vitamin-dependency states have been recognized in which the apoenzyme fails to react normally with the coenzyme; this condition is partially overcome by large doses of the corresponding vitamin. For example, an inborn error in the apoenzyme pyruvate carboxylase can produce lactic acidosis and is treated with 20 mg of thiamine daily. There are several rare diseases of this type, which provide some justification for the search for conditions that might be benefited by the megavitamin concept.[7] It should be remembered that the effectiveness of levodopa in parkinsonism would not have been discovered without someone trying unusually large doses of the drug. This, however, should not be considered an endorsement of megavitamin therapy, which is potentially toxic and in most cases is unnecessary and not based on sound theory or controlled clinical trials.

ADVERSE EFFECTS   Although small excesses of vitamin intake are more wasteful than dangerous, large doses of several of the vitamins can produce adverse effects.

The water-soluble vitamins are generally harmless except in special circumstances. Thiamine injected intravenously has produced a shocklike state, and an anaphylactic type of sensitization to it has been suspected. Nicotinic acid is a potent vasodilator, and for that reason nicotinamide, which does not affect blood vessels, is preferred. Ascorbic acid is remarkably nontoxic. When given in large quantities, the vitamin is rapidly cleared by the kidney. Pyridoxine promotes the peripheral decarboxylation of levodopa and decreases its effectiveness in the treatment of parkinsonism.

The fat-soluble vitamins are more likely to produce distinct pathologic changes when given in excessive quantities.

Hypervitaminosis A has been described as occurring in children when doses of about 100,000 units or more are administered for many days. Changes in skeletal development, hepatomegaly, anemia, loss of hair, and other symptoms have been described in these patients.

Hemolytic anemia and jaundice have been reported after parenteral use of large doses of the various vitamin K preparations.

The occurrence of these adverse reactions is an additional reason for maintaining a rational attitude toward the use of vitamins in cases in which their indications are not clear.

1. Etretinate for psoriasis, Med. Lett. Drugs Ther. **29**:9, 1987.
2. Henderson, L.M.: Niacin, Annu. Rev. Nutr. **3**:289, 1983.
3. Ink, S.L., and Henderson, L.M.: Vitamin B₆ metabolism, Annu. Rev. Nutr. **4**:455, 1984.
4. Levine, M., and Morita, K.: Ascorbic acid in endocrine systems, Vitam. Horm. **42**:1, 1985.
5. Marks, J.: The vitamins: their role in medical practice, Lancaster, 1985, MTP Press Ltd.
6. Olson, R.E.: The function and metabolism of vitamin K, Annu. Rev. Nutr. **4**:281, 1984.
7. Taylor, K.B.: Uses and abuse of vitamin therapy, Ration. Drug Ther. **9**(10):1, 1975.
8. Wittpenn, J., and Sommer, A.: Clinical aspects of vitamin A deficiency. In Bauernfeind, J.C., editor: Vitamin A deficiency and its control, Orlando, Florida, 1986, Academic Press, Inc., p. 177.

REFERENCES

Chemotherapy

51   Introduction to chemotherapy; mechanisms of antibiotic action, 626

52   Sulfonamides, 632

53   Antibiotic drugs, 642

54   Antiviral agents, 667

55   Drugs used to treat mycobacterial and fungal infections, 672

56   Antiseptics and disinfectants, 683

57   Drugs used to treat amebiasis and other intestinal protozoal infections, 687

58   Drugs used to treat malaria and other extraintestinal protozoal infections, 690

59   Anthelmintic drugs, 697

60   Drugs used in chemotherapy of neoplastic disease, 702

Introduction to chemotherapy; mechanisms of antibiotic action

Before 1935 systemic bacterial infections could not be effectively treated with drugs. There were many antiseptics and disinfectants that could eradicate infections when applied topically, but their systemic use was precluded by an unfavorable margin of safety. Certain parasitic infections, such as malaria, amebiasis, and spirochetal infections, could be treated effectively. This was an indication that the concept of "chemotherapy" as envisioned by Ehrlich was not unreasonable. Still, systemic bacterial infections, whether in patients or produced experimentally in animals, were beyond the reach of existing agents.

In 1935 a paper appeared in the German medical literature claiming that the red azo dye **Prontosil** protected mice against systemic streptococcal infection and was curative in patients suffering from such infections.[5] This was a milestone in chemotherapy though in vitro Prontosil was ineffective against bacteria.

It was soon demonstrated that Prontosil is cleaved in the body to release *p*-aminobenzenesulfonamide, known later as **sulfanilamide.** It was also shown that the chemotherapeutic activity of Prontosil is attributable entirely to this metabolite.

These observations initiated a new era in medicine. Numerous derivatives of sulfanilamide were synthesized, and soon a considerable number of systemic infections could be controlled by these compounds. Not only was treatment of many infectious diseases revolutionized, but also the study of these agents greatly advanced knowledge of bacterial metabolism. Furthermore, the discoveries of carbonic anhydrase inhibitors, thiazide diuretics, and oral hypoglycemic drugs were dependent on basic studies on sulfonamides.

Prontosil   **Sulfanilamide**

The successes with the new sulfonamides revived interest in *antibiotics*, which are compounds produced by microorganisms that inhibit the growth of other microorganisms. Fleming discovered that a mold of the genus *Penicillium* prevented multiplication of staphylococci and that culture filtrates of this mold had similar properties.[2] A concentrate of this antibacterial factor was eventually prepared, and its remarkable activity and lack of toxicity were demonstrated by a team at Oxford led by Florey. These properties of penicillin turned the attention of many investigators to antibiotics as potentially useful chemotherapeutic compounds. Soon hundreds of antibiotics were discovered. Although most were too toxic for clinical use, some of them had a satisfactory margin of safety. In the 1940s and 1950s streptomycin, the tetracyclines, chloramphenicol, polymyxin, bacitracin, and neomycin greatly increased the range of effectiveness of antibacterial chemotherapy. However, toxicity presented a significant hazard, and organisms developed resistance to many of these agents. The continued search for effective antimicrobial drugs with less toxicity has led to newer antibiotics of many classes.

GENERAL
CONCEPTS

With the availability of large numbers of effective antimicrobial agents, there have evolved several principles that must guide the physician in selection of the most appropriate drug and dosage for a given patient. The choice of the class of drug may depend principally on the clinical situation, based on probabilities of bacteriologic diagnosis, but the specific compound and dosage relate to such host factors as renal function, age, and disease state. For instance, a patient with a bacterial infection who is receiving antineoplastic chemotherapy for leukemia has requirements different from those of an elderly person with pneumonia. Susceptibility tests do not automatically dictate the kind of agent to be used. This is particularly true because laboratories can now report *minimal inhibitory concentrations* (MIC) rather than just susceptibilities.

Several important concepts have been derived from extensive studies on antibacterial chemotherapy.[5]

Antibacterial spectrum refers to the range of activity of a compound. A broad-spectrum antibacterial drug can inhibit a wide variety of microorganisms, usually including both gram-positive and gram-negative bacteria.

Antimicrobial or *bacteriostatic activity* of a chemotherapeutic agent is usually expressed as the lowest concentration (the MIC) at which the drug inhibits multiplication of the susceptible microorganism.[5]

Bactericidal activity refers to the ability to kill the microorganism, expressed as *minimal bactericidal concentration* (MBC). This requires more complex techniques than the usual plate or tube-dilution methods used to determine MIC. In certain clinical situations, as in treating bacterial endocarditis or the aforementioned leukemic patient, it is essential to use bactericidal agents. Antibacterial substances, such as penicillin or vancomycin, that bind to proteins in the microbial cell wall to disturb the synthesis or function of the cell wall are usually bactericidal. In contrast, drugs, such as tetracyclines, that inhibit protein synthesis by attachment to ribosomal binding sites are *bacteriostatic;* that is, they inhibit growth but do not kill bacteria.

Antibiotic synergism and *antibiotic antagonism* are further concepts. Bacteriostatic combinations are indifferent (no more effective than either drug alone) or additive. However, if two antibiotics, such as penicillin and streptomycin, exert enhanced bactericidal activity in vitro when tested in combination relative to either alone, as in the case of *Streptococcus fecalis*, synergism is said to exist.[6] If, on the other hand, a bacteriostatic antibiotic interferes with the killing action of a bactericidal agent, the phenomenon is known as *antibiotic antagonism*. Clinical situations illustrating this latter phenomenon are difficult to document, but a combination of penicillin with tetracycline is clinically less effective than penicillin alone in treatment of bacterial meningitis.[6] The following three indications for combinations of antibiotics are justified: (1) to prevent emergence of resistant organisms during therapy, (2) to take advantage of a synergistic killing effect, and (3) to broaden the antibacterial spectrum in presumed mixed infections pending bacteriologic diagnosis.

There are also many disadvantages to the combined use of antibiotics.[6] Combinations expose the patient to adverse effects of multiple drugs, and, in rare instances, antibiotic antagonism can occur. Furthermore, enhanced cost is incurred as multiple delivery vials are required and nursing expenses increase. Hence the search continues for agents that can deliver broader antimicrobial activity at lower cost.

RESISTANCE	Bacterial resistance to antibiotics may be present naturally *(nongenetic)* or may develop on a *genetic* basis during therapy.[5] Nongenetic resistance is most frequently attributable to the absence of targets for the drug in the bacteria. If the bacteria have no receptors that bind to the drug or lack a metabolic pathway necessary for drug activity, the bacteria are intrinsically insensitive. Inadequate permeability to a compound may also account for its ineffectiveness against gram-negative bacteria or fungi. Finally, certain microorganisms can escape the consequences of drug action by (1) synthesizing an enzyme that destroys the antibiotic (for example, the β-lactamase that cleaves the β-lactam rings of penicillin and cephalosporin), (2) modifying the antibiotic so that their cell wall is impermeable to it (acetylation of chloramphenicol by acetyltransferase), and (3) altering macromolecules to which the antibiotic binds (methylation of large ribosomal subunits by a plasmid-coded RNA methylase to decrease binding of erythromycin or changing the β-subunit of bacterial RNA polymerase to prevent binding of rifampin).[5]
Genetic drug resistance	Genetic resistance may be of chromosomal origin or may be transmitted by extrachromosomal *plasmids*.[1] Chromosomal resistance can arise from spontaneous mutations. However, an important method of development of resistance was discovered by Japanese investigators in the 1950s. They showed that resistance to several unrelated antibiotics can be transferred to susceptible organisms by cell-to-cell contact or conjugation. The bacteria contain extrachromosomal DNA or resistance (R) plasmids, which act like viruses without coats.[1] These R plasmids are found in a variety of gram-negative bacilli, including *Shigella, Salmonella, Klebsiella, Vibrio, Pasteurella,* and *Escherichia coli*. Emergence of drug-resistant enteric pathogens has been attributed to the feeding of subtherapeutic amounts of antimicrobial compounds to animals.[3] This may be a major factor in transmission of bacterial resistance. In

addition to gram-negative organisms, staphylococci may also contain plasmids, which are transferred from cell to cell by phages, a form of *transduction*.[5]

Most of the commonly used antibacterial agents act by one of the following basic mechanisms: (1) competitive antagonism of some metabolite, (2) inhibition of bacterial cell wall synthesis, (3) an action on cell membranes, (4) inhibition of protein synthesis, or (5) inhibition of nucleic acid synthesis.

ANTIBACTERIAL CHEMOTHERA-PEUTIC AGENTS— MECHANISMS OF ACTION

There are a few examples in which antibacterial compounds act as antimetabolites. Certain bacteria require *p*-aminobenzoic acid (PABA) for synthesis of folic acid precursors. Sulfonamide antimicrobials compete with PABA for binding to the appropriate microbial enzymes, an action that prevents synthesis of folic acid. Since mammalian organisms do not synthesize folic acid but require it as a vitamin, sulfonamides do not interfere with metabolism of mammalian cells.

Competitive antagonism

p-Aminobenzoic acid **Sulfanilamide** **Folic acid**

Another example of competitive antagonism in antibacterial chemotherapy involves the infrequently administered drug *p*-aminosalicylate, which also competes with PABA to produce its effect against mycobacteria.

Several antibiotics inhibit synthesis of the bacterial cell wall.[5] This cell wall, in contrast to mammalian cell membranes, is rigid, so that bacteria can maintain a very high internal osmotic pressure. The structural element of the cell wall is known as *murein;* its synthesis occurs in three steps (see p. 646). Penicillin actively binds to proteins in the cell membrane. After binding, transpeptidation and cell wall synthesis are inhibited and cell wall autolytic enzymes are released into the medium.[8] These enzymes degrade preformed cell wall to cause lysis and death.

Inhibition of bacterial cell wall synthesis

Some antibiotics alter the permeability of cell membranes. This mechanism is sometimes referred to as a detergent-like action.[5] The best examples of this mechanism are provided by polymyxins and antifungal polyene antibiotics (Table 51-1).

Although antibiotics that act on cell membranes have some selective toxicity for microorganisms, they may also be toxic for mammalian cells. The polymyxins, which nowadays are rarely used clinically, are an example.

The interaction of the polyene antibiotics amphotericin B and nystatin with er-

Action on cell membranes

TABLE 51-1	Inhibitors that act on cell membrane
Antibiotic	**Mechanism**
Amphotericin B Nystatin	Preferentially bind to ergosterol, the principal sterol in fungal cell membrane; show much less affinity for cholesterol, the sterol in animal cell membrane; results in cell disruption
Polymyxin B	Cationic detergent; destroys lipoprotein cell membrane

TABLE 51-2	Inhibitors of protein synthesis
Antibiotic	**Mechanism**
Aminoglycosides	Bind to 30 S ribosomal subunit; details of mechanism of action not elucidated
Tetracyclines	Inhibit binding of aminoacyl-tRNA to 30 S ribosomal subunit; also known to have strong affinity for polycations, which might have bearing in their ability to block protein synthesis
Chloramphenicol Lincomycin Clindamycin	Inhibit peptidyl synthetase on 50 S ribosomal subunit and thus prevent formation of initial dipeptide
Erythromycin	Inhibits translocation of peptidyl tRNA from "A" site to "P" site
Cycloheximide	Interacts directly with enzyme translocase involved in the translocation reaction

TABLE 51-3	Inhibitors of nucleic acid synthesis pertaining to bacteria or virus, or both
Antibiotic	**Mechanism**
Idoxuridine (5 IUdR)	Is converted to IDUTP, which in turn is incorporated into viral DNA, rendering this DNA more susceptible to breakage
Cytarabine (ara-C)	Ara-CTP competitive with respect to dCTP in DNA polymerizing reaction; potent inhibitor of virally induced DNA polymerase
Vidarabine (ara-A)	Ara-ATP competitive with respect to dATP in DNA synthesis; also inhibits polyadenylation of RNA in vitro and in vivo
Acyclovir (acycloguanosine)	Phosphorylated by virus-specific thymidine kinase; viral DNA replication specifically blocked by active triphosphate derivative
Nalidixic acid	Inhibits bacterial DNA gyrase, enzyme implicated in DNA replication and transcription
Novobiocin	Inhibits DNA gyrase
Rifampin	Inhibits prokaryotic DNA-dependent RNA polymerase

gosterol results in loss of cations and fungal cell death.[5] These polyenes also bind to mammalian cell sterols and thus are quite toxic, particularly for red blood cell and kidney tubular membranes.

Many of the commonly used antibiotics inhibit protein synthesis (Table 51-2). Generally, these antibiotics can selectively inhibit protein synthesis in microorganisms, usually by binding to ribosomal subunits.[5] However, chloramphenicol is also a potent inhibitor of mitochondrial protein synthesis. In addition, highly toxic experimental drugs such as cycloheximide are potent inhibitors of protein synthesis in both microorganisms and mammals.

Inhibition of protein synthesis

Inhibitors of nucleic acid synthesis that are effective antimicrobial or antiviral agents of recent use can be classified as follows: (1) nucleoside analogs, (2) those that bind to RNA polymerase, (3) those that interact directly with DNA, and (4) those that inhibit DNA gyrase (Table 51-3).[4,7] These drugs are relatively selective inhibitors of nucleic acid synthesis in bacteria or viruses.

Inhibition of nucleic acid synthesis

---

1. Benveniste, R., and Davies, J.: Mechanisms of antibiotic resistance in bacteria, Annu. Rev. Biochem. **42**:471, 1973.
2. Fleming, A.: On antibacterial action of cultures of penicillium, with special reference to their use in isolation of *B. influenzae*, Br. J. Exp. Pathol. **10**:226, 1929.
3. Holmberg, S.D., Osterholm, M.T., Senger, K.A., and Cohen, M.L.: Drug-resistant Salmonella from animals fed antimicrobials, N. Engl. J. Med. **311**:617, 1984.
4. Kaufman, H.E.: Antiviral drugs, Int. J. Dermatol. **16**:464, 1977.
5. Pratt, W.B., and Fekety, R.: The antimicrobial drugs, New York, 1986, Oxford University Press.
6. Rahal, J.J., Jr.: Antibiotic combinations: the clinical relevance of synergy and antagonism, Medicine (Baltimore) **57**:179, 1978.
7. Schinazi, R.F., and Prusoff, W.H.: Antiviral drugs: modes of action and strategies for therapy, Hosp. Pract. **16**(6):113, 1981.
8. Tomasz, A.: Penicillin-binding proteins in bacteria, Ann. Intern. Med. **96**:502, 1982.

REFERENCES

Chapter 52

Sulfonamides

GENERAL
CONCEPT

The discovery of the antibacterial action of sulfanilamide and initial clinical trials in the 1930s are landmarks in the use of pharmacologic agents to treat infections. Sulfonamides are true *antimetabolites;* they block a specific step in the biosynthetic pathway of folic acid. Despite recent development of many effective antibiotics, sulfonamides still have important uses (as for acute urinary tract infections, conjunctivitis, and prevention of infection in burns). Development of the trimethoprim-sulfamethoxazole combination, which provides sequential blockade in the pathway of folic acid synthesis, has extended the usefulness of sulfonamides. This chapter also discusses nonsulfonamide drugs used to treat urinary tract infections.

SULFONAMIDE
DRUGS
Chemistry

The initial sulfonamide studied was Prontosil (Table 52-1). Prontosil is active only in vivo after it is cleaved at the diazo bond to yield sulfanilamide. Thus Prontosil is an early example of a *prodrug*. Nearly all currently used sulfonamides are derivatives of sulfanilamide. Table 52-1 depicts structures of the more important ones. Important structure-activity relationships are (1) no substitution on the benzene nucleus at positions 2, 3, 5, and 6; (2) a free amino group is required in the *para* position—sulfonamides substituted in this amino group become active only if the substituent is removed in vivo; (3) a sulfur molecule must be attached directly to the benzene ring. Substitution on the R_2 amide group can alter absorption, distribution, and solubility.

Antibacterial
spectrum

Sulfonamides are effective against a broad range of microorganisms.[18] Sensitive gram-positive organisms are *Streptococcus pyogenes*, *Streptococcus pneumoniae*, and *Bacillus anthracis*. Susceptible gram-negative organisms include some strains of meningococcus and *Vibrio cholerae*. The sulfonamides are also active against *Actinomyces*, *Nocardia*, *Chlamydia*, and some protozoa. Although efficacious in vitro, they are no longer the drugs of choice to treat a variety of infections because more effective agents are now available.

Short-acting sulfonamides such as sulfisoxazole are among the drugs of choice for treatment of acute urinary tract infections caused by susceptible bacteria such as *Escherichia coli*. They are also useful in treatment of nocardiosis, trachoma, and chancroid. Otitis media (especially in children) and lower respiratory infections may respond to sulfonamides, but other antimicrobials are usually more effective.[11] Derivatives that are poorly absorbed from the gastrointestinal tract have been used for preoperative bowel "sterilization."

TABLE 52-1 Structures of sulfonamides

Prontosil	Sulfanilamide	
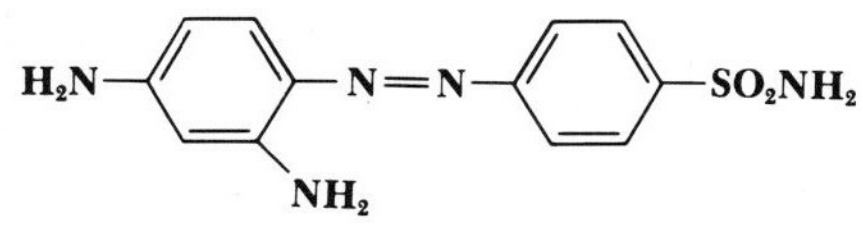H₂N
N=N
SO₂NH₂
NH₂	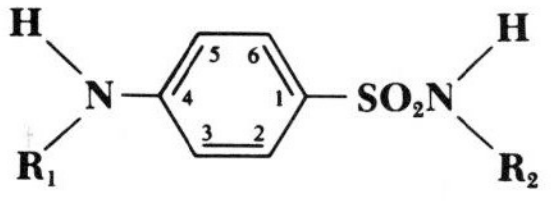H
N
R₁
SO₂N
H
R₂	
	R_1 substitution	**R_2 substitution**
Sulfadiazine (Microsulfon)	—H	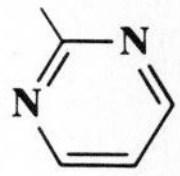
Sulfisoxazole (Gantrisin, others)	—H	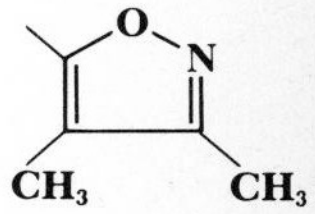
Sulfamethoxazole (used with trimethoprim) (Gantanol, others)	—H	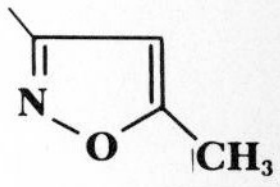
Succinylsulfathiazole	—$COCH_2CH_2COOH$	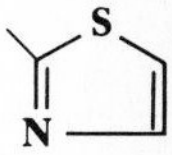
Phthalylsulfathiazole	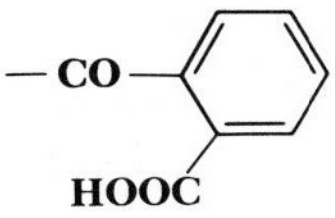—CO
HOOC	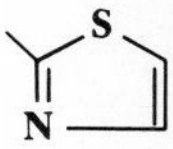
Sulfacetamide (Cetamide, others)	—H	—$COCH_3$
Mafenide (Sulfamylon)	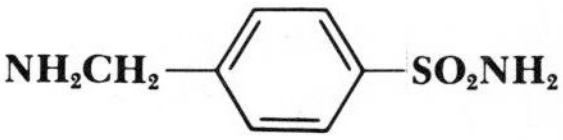NH₂CH₂
SO₂NH₂	
Sulfasalazine (salicylazosulfapyridine) (Azulfidine, Azaline)	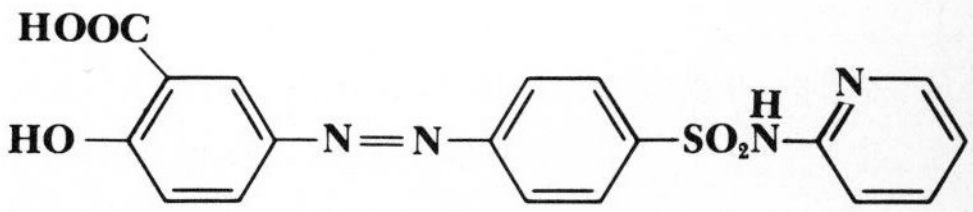HOOC
HO
N=N
SO₂N
H
N	

FIG. 52-1   *Biosynthetic reactions blocked by sulfonamides and trimethoprim.*

(Hydroxymethyl) dihydropteridine + *p*-Aminobenzoic acid (PABA)

Sulfonamides ⟿⟿ Dihydropteroate synthase

Dihydropteroic acid

plus glutamic acid

Dihydrofolic acid

Trimethoprim ⟿⟿ Dihydrofolate reductase

Tetrahydrofolic acid

The potency of sulfonamides is such that growth inhibition may be achieved at concentrations of about 100 μg/ml in simple media and in blood. Potency in vitro is greatly influenced by the nature of the culture medium. Enrichment with yeast extract or *p*-aminobenzoic acid (PABA) greatly decreases the effectiveness of sulfonamides.[18] Even in a simple synthetic medium, their potency is much less than that of widely used antibiotics.

For theoretical reasons, it is unlikely that any sulfonamide that competes with PABA will have greater antibacterial activity than sulfadiazine. Other sulfonamides are more likely to offer advantages in increased solubility, less toxicity to the kidney, or reduced sensitizing properties.

Mode of action   Sulfonamides are competitive inhibitors of the enzyme (dihydropteroate synthase) responsible for synthesis of dihydropteroic acid, a precurser of folic acid.[4] Sulfonamides are structurally similar to PABA, which combines with a dihydropteridine to form dihydropteroic acid (Fig. 52-1). Only organisms that use PABA to form folic acid are sensitive to sulfonamides.[18] Sulfonamides have a higher affinity for the microbial enzyme than PABA does. With decreased folic acid synthesis, there is a reduction in bacterial nucleotides and inhibition of growth. Mammalian cells require preformed folic acid and cannot use PABA.[1]

Resistance   A large proportion of organisms, particularly *Staphylococcus* and those of the family Enterobacteriaceae, are resistant to sulfonamides. The mechanism of resistance may be related to the ability of the bacteria to produce antagonists or to lower the affinity of their enzyme for the drug.[10] In some cases the resistant organism increases PABA production. Resistance can also be mediated by plasmids (R factors).

Pharmacokinetics   Short-acting sulfonamides (**sulfisoxazole** and **sulfadiazine**) are absorbed rapidly from the gastrointestinal tract. They are given in oral doses of 1 to 4 g initially, followed by 1 g every 4 to 6 hours to maintain a serum concentration of approximately 100 μg/ml.[18] The pediatric dosage is 150 mg/kg/day. Serum concentrations of sulfonamides can be determined to monitor serious infections requiring intravenous therapy or for patients with renal failure. The half-life of these drugs varies from 4 to 7 hours, sulfadiazine having a somewhat shorter half-life. **Sulfamethoxazole,** an intermediate-duration drug, has a half-life of up to 12 hours.

The volume of distribution of most sulfonamides approaches that of total body water, and they penetrate cells. Sulfisoxazole is an exception that is distributed only in extracellular water. Hence serum sulfisoxazole concentrations are twice as high as those reached after the same dose of sulfadiazine. Metabolism involves acetylation of the free *p*-amino group. Genetically controlled differences in activity of the acetylase cause large variations in rates of metabolism of these drugs. The acetylated product has no antimicrobial activity and may be less soluble in urine; it retains the capacity to cause toxicity and may accumulate in patients with renal failure.[1]

Sulfisoxazole is readily excreted in human milk.[7] The milk-plasma ratio is 0.06 for the parent compound and 0.22 for the metabolite. Less than 1% of the maternal dose is excreted in milk, but all of this will be absorbed by a nursing infant. An alternative antimicrobial should be used for the lactating mother during an infant's first several weeks of life and also during the last month of pregnancy. Sulfonamides bind to plasma proteins and compete for bilirubin-binding sites; thus in an infant they can displace bilirubin from protein, thereby increasing its free concentration and the risk of kernicterus.[1]

Unbound sulfonamides are filtered through renal glomeruli, and the tubules reabsorb a portion of the filtered drug. The urinary concentration of sulfonamides may be 25 to 50 times higher than that in plasma, a circumstance that contributes to their usefulness as urinary antimicrobials.

Toxicity and hypersensitivity

Virtually every organ system has been involved in toxic reactions to sulfonamides. Gastrointestinal effects (nausea, vomiting, and loss of appetite) are fairly common. Hepatitis and bone-marrow depression occur infrequently as do hemolytic anemia and other blood dyscrasias. However, patients who are deficient in *glucose-6-phosphate dehydrogenase*, such as one third of American blacks, are at risk of hemolysis.

Early in the use of sulfonamides, their precipitation in the urine with subsequent nephropathy was a problem. Sulfonamides behave as weak acids because of dissociation of the sulfamyl group ($-SO_2NH-$). Substitutions on the sulfamyl nitrogen can produce acids considerably stronger than sulfanilamide. Since salts (ions) of sulfonamides are much more soluble than the molecular (acid) form, the solubility of these drugs increases greatly when the pH of the environment exceeds the pK_a of the drug. Hence alkalinization of the urine has been used to decrease precipitation. In addition, when several sulfonamides are dissolved in water or urine, the presence of one does not influence the solubility of the others.[9] The antibacterial effects of such mixtures are additive. Consequently, such a mixture can produce a higher total sulfonamide concentration in urine with less tendency for crystal formation. In the past then, mixtures of poorly soluble compounds (triple sulfas) were used to circumvent precipitation. Currently, however, the high solubility of sulfisoxazole has eliminated the need for combination products. Similarly, if urinary volume is adequate, alkalinization of the urine with bicarbonate is usually no longer necessary.[18]

Hypersensitivity reactions are rare but of great clinical import. These include syndromes that resemble arteritis and lupus erythematosus. Skin eruptions may range from a diffuse morbilliform rash or erythema multiforme to exfoliative dermatitis (Stevens-Johnson syndrome). This latter complication is especially dreaded because of its high mortality. Some longer-acting sulfonamides were removed from the market when the Stevens-Johnson syndrome was associated with their use. Only one long-acting agent, sulfadoxine, is available for use in prophylaxis and treatment of malaria. However, its use has also been associated with Stevens-Johnson syndrome. Other serious hypersensitivity reactions include urticaria, a serum sickness—like syndrome and frank anaphylaxis.

Drug interactions   Sulfonamides and methenamines (see p. 639) should not be administered simultaneously to treat urinary tract infections, since the formaldehyde liberated from methenamine in an acid urine forms a precipitate with some sulfonamides. Binding of sulfonamides by plasma proteins, especially albumin, may displace other drugs. Thus the potencies of tolbutamide, coumarins, thiazides, phenytoin, and uricosuric agents may be transiently enhanced until the increased free drug concentration returns to "normal."

Clinical usage   Sulfonamides are most commonly used to treat acute urinary tract infections. In otherwise healthy persons most of these infections are caused by gram-negative enteric bacteria, especially *E. coli*, usually susceptible to sulfisoxazole. The preferred oral drugs are sulfisoxazole or sulfamethoxazole. A parenteral form (rarely used) is the sodium salt of sulfadiazine. Sulfisoxazole has antibacterial properties similar to those of sulfadiazine, but its solubility at pH 6 is more than 10 times greater. At pH 5.5 its solubility in human urine is only about 1200 μg/ml, but this still exceeds by fourfold the solubility of sulfadiazine. This offers no certain guarantee against crystal formation in renal tubules, since sulfisoxazole reaches high urinary concentrations. Sulfisoxazole in doses of 500 mg twice daily is used for prophylaxis of acute otitis media in children who experience repeated attacks during a short time.[11] **Sulfacetamide** is available in an ophthalmic preparation (10% and 30%) to treat bacterial conjunctivitis. The pH of the solution is 7.4, thereby producing minimal conjunctival irritation.

TRIMETHOPRIM-SULFAMETHOXAZOLE   The trimethoprim-sulfamethoxazole preparation (co-trimoxazole) exerts truly synergistic actions on bacteria. The sulfonamide inhibits PABA utilization in folic acid synthesis, whereas trimethoprim is a competitive inhibitor of dihydrofolate reductase, another enzyme important in folic acid synthesis[14] (Fig. 52-1). Thus the preparation inhibits two steps in bacterial metabolism. For 50% inhibition the mammalian enzyme requires 50,000 times the trimethoprim concentration needed for the bacterial enzyme.[15] This most likely explains the relative lack of toxicity of trimethoprim observed up to now.

Trimethoprim-sulfamethoxazole is effective against a large variety of gram-positive and gram-negative microorganisms.[15] Acute and chronic urinary tract infections are again prime indications. The combination has expanded the clinical spectrum of sulfonamide activity to infections caused by *Shigella* and *Pneumocystis carinii*.[14] The preparation is also effective in treatment of typhoid and paratyphoid fever (for organisms resistant to ampicillin and chloramphenicol), bacterial infections of the lower respiratory tract, otitis media, uncomplicated gonorrhea, and vivax and falciparum malaria. Parenteral drug is now available for severe infections caused by susceptible organisms.[15]

Absorption of trimethoprim-sulfamethoxazole is rapid. Effective concentrations may be present in plasma for 6 to 8 hours.[14] Both drugs are excreted mostly unchanged in the urine, though sulfamethoxazole is also partially acetylated.

Any of the adverse effects of sulfonamides may occur when trimethoprim-sulfamethoxazole is used. Trimethoprim alone can cause skin rashes and bone-marrow toxicity. Crystalluria is rare. The preparation is contraindicated in patients with blood dyscrasias, hepatic damage, and severe renal impairment. It should be used cautiously in patients with low folic acid concentrations caused by malnutrition or chronic administration of phenytoin.

Trimethoprim-sulfamethoxazole is available in single-strength tablets containing trimethoprim, 80 mg, and sulfamethoxazole, 400 mg, as double-strength preparations with twice as much of each and for injection as 16/80 mg/ml. Pediatric suspensions contain 40 mg of trimethoprim and 200 mg sulfamethoxazole per 5 ml. The 1:5 ratio produces a concentration ratio of 1:20 trimethoprim to sulfamethoxazole in serum.[14]

Mafenide was widely used as a topical agent in seriously burned patients to prevent wound contamination, especially by *Pseudomonas* species.[1] Three problems occur with this drug: (1) it is painful on application; (2) resistant organisms emerge during treatment; (3) it is a carbonic anhydrase inhibitor and can cause metabolic acidosis if enough is absorbed through the skin. Mafenide has been replaced by silver sulfadiazine (Silvadene), which is painless and appears to have very low systemic toxicity. Bacterial resistance to silver sulfadiazine has not yet proved to be the problem that it is with mafenide.

TOPICAL SULFONAMIDES

Sulfonamides that are poorly absorbed from the intestine were once used to decrease intestinal bacterial flora. Succinylsulfathiazole and phthalylsulfathiazole are substituted in the *p*-amino portion of the sulfathiazole molecule. As a consequence, they have no antibacterial activity in vitro. Hydrolysis occurs after they reach the large intestine, and free sulfathiazole reaches a high local concentration. Sulfathiazole is not well absorbed from the large intestine. Because of resistance and other problems, these agents are no longer available in the United States.

SULFONAMIDES AS INTESTINAL ANTISEPTICS

Sulfasalazine is used in treating inflammatory bowel disease, such as ulcerative colitis and regional enteritis. It is a *prodrug* for delivery of active 5-aminosalicylate to the lower gastrointestinal tract (the site of the inflammatory process).[2] 5-Aminosalicylate cannot be given as such because it is completely absorbed in the proximal small intestine and is rapidly excreted by the kidney.

Dermatitis herpetiformis is the only indication for sulfapyridine. In this instance sulfapyridine acts by a mechanism unrelated to its antibacterial activity.[8]

In addition to sulfonamides, several antibacterial agents are used almost exclusively to treat urinary tract infections. Their major characteristics are summarized in Table 52-2.

Nitrofurantoin

Nitrofurantoin, one of a series of nitrofurans, is absorbed rapidly, and much of it is excreted unchanged in the urine. Its mechanism of action is unknown, but it may inhibit a variety of enzyme systems in bacteria. It has a wide antibacterial spectrum; both gram-positive and gram-negative bacteria can be inhibited at concentrations attained in urine after daily oral administration of 5 to 10 mg/kg. Its use is limited to short-term treatment or low-dose suppression of urinary tract infection.[6] Nitrofurantoin may cause numerous adverse reactions. Nausea and vomiting are common; the frequency is lessened by concomitant administration with food or milk. Skin sensitization, peripheral neuritis, and cholestatic jaundice also occur. Hemolytic anemia can develop in patients deficient in glucose-6-phosphate dehydrogenase. An acute, dramatic pulmonary reaction occurs rarely.[5] It is particularly likely in the elderly and may represent the most common noncardiac cause of pulmonary edema. Interstitial fibrosis can develop with chronic therapy and is a reason for limiting even low-dose suppression to 6 months of administration. Although bacteriostatic blood concentrations are not produced by oral administration of nitrofurantoin, the drug can accumulate if renal function is impaired and should be avoided in this setting.[5]

Preparations of microcrystalline nitrofurantoin include tablets and capsules, 50 and 100 mg, and a suspension, 25 mg/5 ml. Nitrofurantoin sodium is available for intravenous injections, 180 mg of powder in 20 ml sterile vials. A macrocrystalline preparation (Macrodantin), which may be less nauseating, is available in capsules, 25 to 100 mg.

Nitrofurazone (Furacin, 0.2%) is used topically for infections of the skin, but it may cause sensitization.

TABLE 52-2   Antimicrobial agents used principally for urinary tract infections

Drug	Oral dosage	Activity
Sulfonamides	1 g every 4 to 6 hours	First-time infections in the young; resistance develops in fecal organisms, and so recurrent infections are likely resistant
Trimethoprim-sulfamethoxazole (Bactrim, Septra, others)	160/800 mg	First time, as single dose for lower or for 14 days for upper tract infection (relapse in 1 month in women or any in men may require a 6- to 12-week course); to prevent recurrences in women use 80/400 mg after sexual intercourse or three times weekly for 6 to 12 months; in men alternate every 6 months with nitrofurantoin
Nitrofurantoin (Furadantin, others)	50 to 100 mg every 6 hours	Best as preventive or for recurrent lower tract infection (ineffective for upper tract); use to prevent recurrence in bacteriuric pregnant women or for 6-month periods in nonpregnant women; do not use longer than 6 months because of toxicity; to prevent recurrence, it can be given on a full stomach to women the morning after intercourse
Methenamine mandelate (Mandelamine, others)	1 g every 6 hours	Rarely used since must have very acid urine; toxic in renal insufficiency
Quinolones Nalidixic acid (NegGram, others)	1 g every 6 hours	Rarely used since resistance develops rapidly; difficult to swallow; replaced by other quinolines
Norfloxacin (Noroxin)	400 mg twice daily	Resistant infections; especially recurrent
Cinoxacin (Cinobac)	500 mg twice daily	
Ciprofloxacin (investigational drug)	750 mg twice daily	

Methenamine mandelate is a combination of two old urinary antiseptics, methenamine and mandelic acid.

Methenamine mandelate

In acid urine methenamine liberates formaldehyde. If the pH of the urine is low, mandelic acid is bactericidal. If urinary pH is higher than 6, ascorbic acid or ammonium chloride must be taken in amounts of 0.5 to 1 g three or four times daily to acidify the urine.

Methenamine mandelate is relatively nontoxic, but gastric irritation may occur. This is probably related to production of formaldehyde in the stomach. Because of bladder irritation urinary frequency may develop. A variety of dosage forms containing from 0.25 to 1 g of the compound are available for oral administration. The usual dose is 0.5 to 1 g four times a day. The drug is used primarily as a suppressive agent, though clinical efficacy has been difficult to establish.[17]

In addition to methenamine mandelate, the hippurate salt of methenamine (Hiprex) is also available in tablets, 1 g.

The quinolones are synthetic chemotherapeutic agents that inhibit bacterial DNA gyrases. The gyrases, or topoisomerases, are required to supercoil strands of bacterial DNA into the bacterial cell.[16] Several compounds related to nalidixic acid (Table 52-2) have recently been approved or will likely be available shortly. **Nalidixic acid** is well absorbed from the gastrointestinal tract and is excreted in the urine largely unchanged or as an active metabolite, hydroxynalidixic acid. Nalidixic acid is effective against a variety of gram-negative bacteria, but resistance to the drug develops readily.[3,13] It should not be used for systemic infections. Other quinolones under investigation are very effective for a host of infections.[12] **Norfloxacin** and **cinoxacin** are presently approved for use in urinary tract infections but do not have as broad a range of activity as ciprofloxacin, an investigational compound.

Nausea, vomiting, diarrhea, allergic reactions, and neurologic disturbances may occur after nalidixic acid administration. The drug may cause increased intracranial pressure in children and central nervous system reactions, particularly in those with convulsive disorders or parkinsonism. Toxicity with the new quinolones is quite low.[12]

Preparations of nalidixic acid include tablets of 0.25 to 1 g. A pediatric suspension contains 250 mg/5 ml. Capsules of cinoxacin contain 250 or 500 mg, and norfloxacin is available as tablets of 400 mg.

Nalidixic acid

Cinoxacin

enzyme that breaks the lactam ring (ring A) in the penicillin structure (below), are resistant to penicillins G and V. Substitution of bulky groups at the R site, as in methicillin and oxacillin, protects the lactam ring through steric hindrance. Other substitutions at the R site expand the antimicrobial spectrum to gram-negative organisms. Unfortunately, the "broad-spectrum" penicillins such as ampicillin and car-

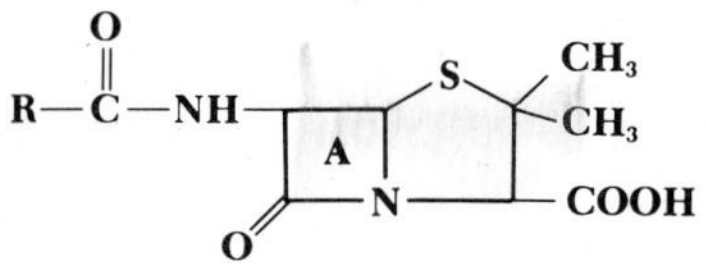

Basic penicillin structure

R side chain

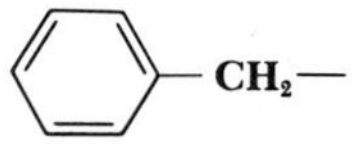

Penicillin G (benzylpenicillin)

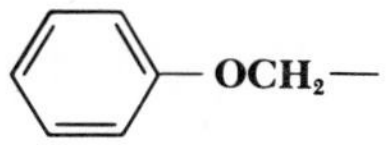

Penicillin V (phenoxymethylpenicillin)

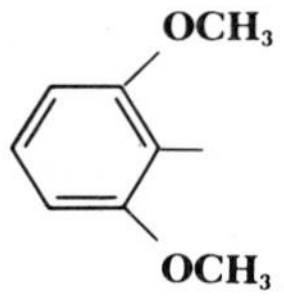

Methicillin (Staphcillin)

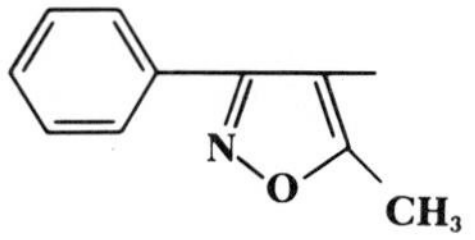

Oxacillin (Bactocill, Prostaphlin)

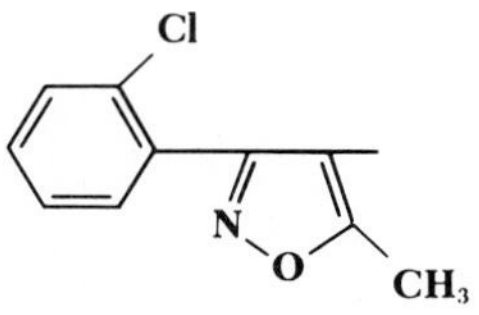

Cloxacillin (Cloxapen, Tegopen)

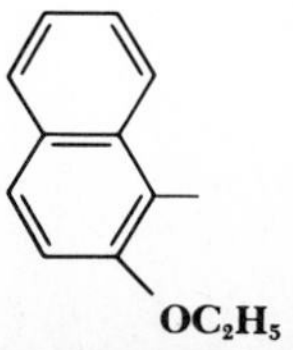

Nafcillin (Nafcil, Unipen)

benicillin are sensitive to destruction by penicillinase. Also, resistance can develop if they are used alone, and so they are frequently combined with another antibiotic, such as an aminoglycoside.[1] Synergism is often noted with combinations of these drugs.

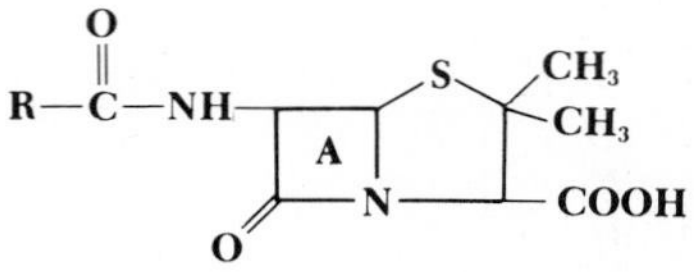

Basic penicillin structure

R side chain

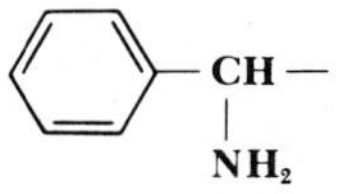

Ampicillin (Polycillin, Omnipen, others)

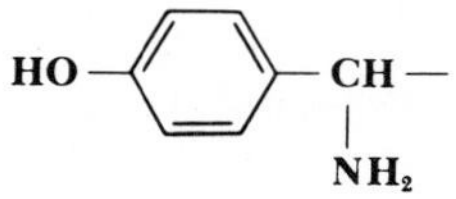

Amoxicillin (Amoxil, Polymox, others)

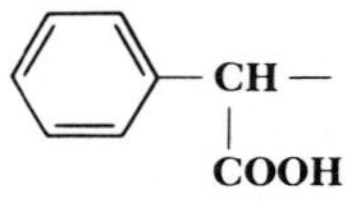

Carbenicillin (Geopen, Geocillin)

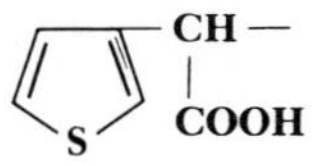

Ticarcillin (Ticar, Timentin)

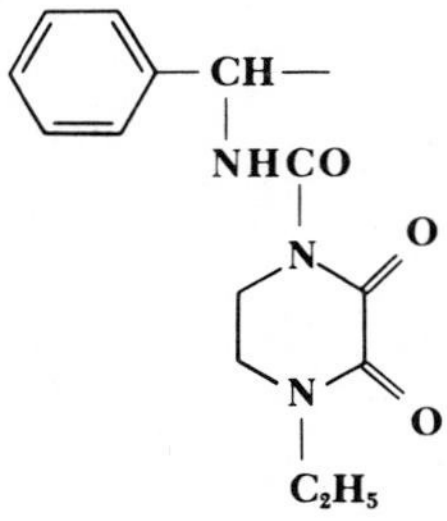

Piperacillin (Pipracil)

Penicillin preparations are standardized on the basis of their capacity to inhibit *Potency*
the growth of test organisms such as *Bacillus subtilis* or sensitive staphylococci.
Activity was initially expressed in units and measured in comparison with a standard
preparation. One milligram of penicillin G equals 1667 units; conversely 1 unit is
equivalent to 0.6 μg of penicillin G. The dose of all penicillins is now usually indicated
in milligrams (or grams). Microorganisms inhibited by less than 1 μg of penicillin
per milliliter may be considered moderately susceptible since in clinical practice
blood concentrations exceeding 1 μg/ml can be readily achieved. Highly susceptible
microorganisms are usually inhibited by less than 0.1 μg/ml.

Penicillins are bactericidal drugs that attach to penicillin-binding proteins (PBPs) *Mode of action*
to interfere with synthesis of the cell wall.[26] The simplified description below illustrates where penicillin and related antibiotics block cell wall synthesis.

The bacterial cell wall consists of strands of a linear peptidoglycan made up of
alternating building blocks of *N*-acetylglucosamine and *N*-acetylmuramic acid. The
latter compound has a "tail" consisting of a pentapeptide ending in alanine-D-alanine.
These peptidoglycans are cross-lined by a pentaglycine bridge.

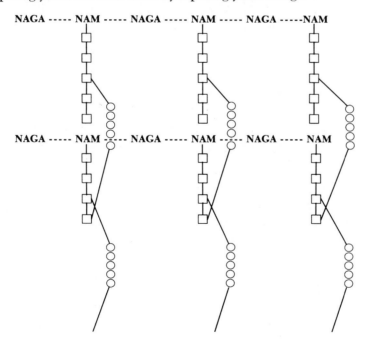

In the early experiments of Park,[29] a nucleotide accumulated in the culture broth of penicillin-treated bacteria. Synthesis of this nucleotide (UDP–*N*-acetylmuramic acid–pentapeptide) is the first step in development of the cell wall. The second step is formation of the linear peptidoglycans. The final step is cross-linking of these linear strands. Compounds (several of which are clinically useful antibiotics) that inhibit enzymatic reactions at each step in cell wall synthesis are known.

Cross-linking is done by a transpeptidase, which also cleaves a terminal D-alanine. The penicillins and cephalosporins bind to this enzyme and act as competitive inhibitors. In addition, changes in the cellular shape of bacteria occurs after binding of penicillins to various PBPs in the cell wall. Finally, cell lysis occurs after release of murein hydrolases, which degrade preformed cell wall.[44] These hydrolases are present in cell walls, but their activity is normally suppressed. Autolysin-deficient mutants that are inhibited, but not killed, by penicillins have been formed. Lysis by antibiotics also depends on pH and on components in the medium, such as Mg^{++}. Hence, β-lactams may produce a variety of changes in bacteria, such as swelling, elongation, and "large-body" formation or, under optimal conditions, lysis and death. These morphologic changes may relate to which PBP the β-lactam binds, since these proteins determine a variety of activities, including elongation, cell division, and size. Derivatives, such as aztreonam, that fail to bind to PBPs lack activity against gram-positive organisms.

Pharmacokinetics   Absorption of penicillin G from the gastrointestinal tract is incomplete and variable (Table 53-1). Also, penicillin G is inactivated by gastric juice so that penicillin V (Veetids, Pen-Vee K, others), which is more resistant to acid, is the preferred oral form.

Serum concentrations after administration of 100,000 units (60 mg) of penicillin G by various routes are illustrated in Fig. 53-1. Concentrations reaching 2 to 4 units/ ml (about 1.25 to 2.5 μg/ml) can be obtained by intravenous or intramuscular injection, but the same dose given orally produces a concentration of only about 0.4 units/ml. Since intramuscular injection of penicillin of any type is quite painful, only one or two injections a day are indicated, as for treatment of streptococcal pharyngitis or syphilis. Seriously ill patients should receive penicillin compounds intravenously because absorption of oral preparations is less reliable.

Elimination of penicillin from the body is primarily by renal mechanisms; little or none is metabolized. The decline in blood concentration results from rapid clearance of the antibiotic. With severe renal failure ($Cl_{Cr} < 10$ ml/min) the half-life increases (Table 53-1) so that the dosage interval must be prolonged. Penicillin is actively secreted by renal tubules, apparently by the same mechanism as *p*-aminohippurate. Probenecid, which blocks this tubular secretory mechanism, is occasionally used with penicillin when an extremely high concentration of the antibiotic is required after intramuscular or oral administration. Since penicillin's half-life is approximately 30 minutes, dosing every 2 to 4 hours is indicated for bacteremia or serious infections.

Relative serum concentrations of penicillin after intravenous, intramuscular, and oral ad-   **FIG. 53-1**
ministration of 100,000 units of crystalline sodium penicillin G.

From Welch, H., et al.: *Principles and practice of antibiotic therapy,* New York, 1954, Medical Encyclopedia, Inc.

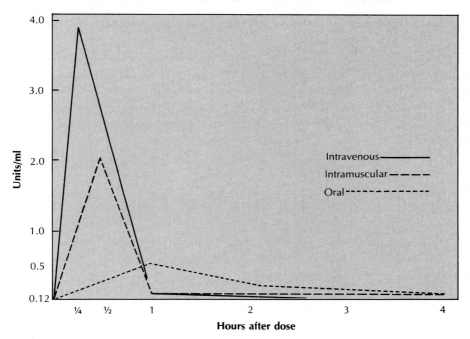

TABLE 53-1   Pharmacologic properties of penicillins

Drug	Oral absorption	Effective serum concentration (µg/ml)	Plasma half-life (hr)		Dosage reduction with renal failure
			Normal	Renal failure	
Oral					
G	Fair	2	0.5	10	Yes
V	Good	4	1	4	Slight
Nafcillin	Fair	1	0.5	1.5	None
Cloxacillin, dicloxacillin	Good	10	0.5	1	None
Ampicillin	Good	3	1	8	Yes
Amoxicillin	Excellent	7	1	8	Yes
Parenteral					
G		5-10	0.5	10	Yes
Methicillin		70	0.5	4	Slight
Nafcillin		20	0.5	4	Yes
Carbenicillin, ticarcillin		100+	1	15	Yes
Piperacillin, mezlocillin		250-300	1	4	Yes

Repository preparations, such as procaine penicillin G (Crysticillin, Duracillin, others) and benzathine penicillin G (Bicillin L-A, Permapen) can be used when sustained blood concentrations, in the range of 0.03 μg/ml or so, are required for 10 days or longer. This concentration is sufficient to treat streptococcal infections and syphilis or to prevent recurrent streptococcal infections in high-risk patients (as with rheumatic fever).

Penicillin is not uniformly distributed to most regions of the body, since it is partially bound to plasma proteins. Penicillin penetrates poorly into cerebrospinal fluid and aqueous humor but adequately reaches pleural and synovial spaces. However, inflammation at the former sites increases permeability so that effective penicillin concentrations can be achieved within 24 hours of administration for treatment of meningitis.

Table 53-1 indicates the extent of absorption after ingestion, the elimination half-life, and the effect of renal failure on elimination of the penicillins.

Toxicity and hypersensitivity

The toxicity of penicillin G is extremely low, but very high doses can cause myoclonic seizures or platelet dysfunction with bleeding (Table 53-2). This is most likely to occur when doses greater than 20 million units are given to persons with impaired renal function. A significant percentage of patients develops hypersensitivity to penicillin. The prevalence varies from 1% to 8% in the general population, but reactions actually occur in fewer than 1% of all treatments.[36] The reactions are diverse, ranging from immediate anaphylactic reactions (<0.1%) to late manifestations of the serum sickness type. These latter reactions are mediated by IgE antibody, which develops to "minor" penicillin determinants that combine with proteins to form haptens. After sensitization to the hapten-protein complex, administration of the parent compound can then induce a reaction.

Penicillin skin tests are done exclusively by research laboratories with a mixture of penicillin, penicilloate, and other "minor" determinants. Hence, clinicians have to rely primarily on a history of previous penicillin reaction. It is best to be prepared for an anaphylactic reaction whenever the antibiotic is injected. Patients allergic to one penicillin must be assumed to be allergic to all since cross-reactions occur frequently between compounds with varied side-chains. If penicillin is required in an allergic patient, desensitization, beginning with small quantities orally, can be performed successfully.[43]

Other adverse effects are much more likely with the newer penicillins. These include leukopenia, hepatitis (oxacillin), interstitial nephritis, diarrhea (oral preparations of ampicillin and amoxicillin), and platelet dysfunction (carbenicillin, ticarcillin, and methicillin). Penicillins are irritating to tissue and even to endothelial surfaces so that care must be taken during intravenous therapy. Certain ones, such as nafcillin, are particularly prone to elicit phlebitis.

TABLE 53-2	Toxicity and hypersensitivity of penicillins	
Type of reaction	Frequency of reaction	Most frequently seen with:
Hypersensitivity		
Anaphylaxis	<0.1%	Penicillin G, all others
Serum sickness	Rare	Penicillin G
Skin rash	Common	All
Idiopathic		
Skin rash	Common	Ampicillin
Fever	Rare	All
Gastrointestinal		
Diarrhea	Common	Ampicillin
Enterocolitis	Infrequent	All
Hematologic		
Neutropenia	Infrequent	Nafcillin, piperacillin
Platelet dysfunction	Infrequent	Carbenicillin (all, high doses)
Hemolytic anemia	Rare	Penicillin G
Electrolyte		
Hypokalemia	Infrequent	Carbenicillin, piperacillin
Liver function		
Elevated enzyme	Infrequent	Cloxacillin
Renal function		
Interstitial nephritis	Infrequent	Methicillin
Neurologic		
Seizures	Rare	Penicillin G (in renal failure)

Ampicillin is more acid resistant and has a broader antimicrobial spectrum than penicillin G. It is effective against many gram-negative microorganisms. **Amoxicillin trihydrate** is a congener of ampicillin that reaches higher serum concentrations on a milligram for milligram basis. Ampicillin is used to treat urinary tract infections caused by susceptible organisms, in treatment of respiratory infections, and intravenously for meningitis caused by *Listeria monocytogenes* and susceptible strains of *Haemophilus influenzae*. Ampicillin may cause skin rash, with a 100% frequency noted in patients with infectious mononucleosis. Most persons who develop rash with ampicillin do not appear to be allergic to the drug.

Ampicillin and amoxacillin are available in 250 and 500 mg capsules and in pediatric suspensions of 125 or 250 mg/5 ml. The sodium salt of ampicillin is available for parenteral administration.

Broad-spectrum penicillins susceptible to penicillinase

Carbenicillin disodium and **ticarcillin disodium** have greater activity than ampicillin against *Pseudomonas aeruginosa, Enterobacter, Serratia,* and *Proteus* organisms. Carbenicillin and ticarcillin are usually used in combination with an aminoglycoside to treat serious gram-negative infections,[1] particularly in leukopenic patients, since resistance develops if the penicillins are used alone. Since carbenicillin has a high sodium content (1 g of carbenicillin contains 6 mEq of sodium), care in administration must be observed because overload could occur. The drug is excreted as a nonreabsorbable anion that enhances potassium excretion, and so hypokalemia can develop.[1] Platelet function may be adversely affected with resultant bleeding if high doses are given to patients with renal failure; consequently, dosages must be altered.

Carbenicillin indanyl sodium is available in tablets of 382 mg for oral administration in treatment of urinary tract infections and prostatitis, but resistance frequently develops during therapy.

Piperacillin is an acylureidopenicillin that has a wider spectrum of activity than carbenicillin for gram-negative bacilli, including *Pseudomonas, Serratia, Enterobacter,* and *Klebsiella* species.[10] Although it can be administered alone, it is better given in combination with an aminoglycoside, since resistance or relapse, or both, can occur when piperacillin is used alone.

Mezlocillin (Mezlin) and **azlocillin** (Azlin) resemble piperacillin in clinical activity and use, but azlocillin is more active than mezlocillin against *Pseudomonas* species.[10] All these drugs cause adverse effects similar to those of carbenicillin.[1]

Penicillins resistant to penicillinase

Penicillinase-resistant penicillins are very useful against organisms resistant to penicillin G, especially staphylococci. Although these drugs are resistant to penicillinase, strains of "methicillin-resistant" (not based on inactivation by penicillinase) *Staphylococcus aureus* have appeared.[42] Most staphylococcal infections are resistant to treatment by penicillin G or V.

Methicillin sodium is administered intramuscularly or intravenously and is unstable in solution. Its only advantage is in treating infections caused by penicillin G–resistant staphylococci. The drug may cause interstitial nephritis, limiting its use.[19]

Nafcillin sodium can be administered orally, intramuscularly, or intravenously. Nafcillin reaches spinal fluid well and is largely excreted in the bile.

Oxacillin sodium is very similar to nafcillin. It is given orally or parenterally. **Cloxacillin sodium** and **dicloxacillin sodium** (Dynapen, Dycill) resemble oxacillin and are preferred for oral therapy of staphylococcal infections.

Uses of penicillins

Penicillins are the standard of therapy in both outpatient and inpatient treatment of infections. For many infectious agents, they remain medications of choice (Table 53-3).[41] For serious infections they must be combined with other antibiotics, since their activity is not universal and resistance can develop on therapy. A perusal of guide-to-therapy booklets (for example, Sanford, J.B.: *Guide to Antimicrobial Therapy,* San Antonio, Texas, 1987, Antimicrobial Therapy, Inc.) will illustrate the usefulness of penicillin for many conditions.

TABLE 53-3   Antimicrobial spectrum and dosage of penicillins

Penicillin	Susceptible organisms	Route: dosage
G	*Streptococcus* (aerobic and anaerobic) *Gonococcus*	IV: 4-10 million U/day IM: 4.8 million U (single dose)
V	*Streptococcus* (aerobic only)	PO: 250-500 mg 4× daily
Ampicillin	*Streptococcus, Haemophilus* species *Listeria,* some *Escherichia coli*	IV: 1-2 g 6× daily PO: 500 mg 4× daily
Amoxicillin	Same as above	PO: 250-500 mg 3-4× daily

Nafcillin,
  cloxacillin,
  dicloxacillin
	Staphylococcus aureus	IV: 1-2 g 4-6× daily,
		PO: 1-2 g daily

Carbenicillin	*Streptococcus,* anaerobic bacilli (facultative
	  and obligate), *E. coli, Enterobacter,*
	  Pseudomonas
		IV: 5 g 6× daily

Ticarcillin	Same as above	IV: 3 g 6× daily
Piperacillin, mezlocillin	Same as above	IV: 3-4 g 4× daily

IM, Intramuscularly; *IV,* intravenously; *PO,* by mouth; *U,* units.

The cephalosporins are β-lactam antibiotics obtained originally from a *Cephalosporium* mold. These antibiotics have the same mechanism of action as the penicillins but differ in antibacterial spectrum, resistance to β-lactamase, and pharmacokinetics.[40] Whereas penicillins are derivatives of 6-aminopenicillanic acid, the cephalosporins are derivatives of 7-aminocephalosporanic acid. The related cephamycins have a 7-methoxy group, which may increase their resistance to β-lactamases. New cephalosporins are being introduced at a rapid rate. Although the newer compounds offer certain advantages in range of activity, pharmacokinetics, and penetration into cerebrospinal fluid, they also retain certain limitations of the group and are extremely costly.[25]

The antibacterial spectrum of the original, so-called first-generation, cephalosporins (Table 53-4) is similar to that of the penicillinase-resistant penicillins with slightly greater gram-negative coverage.[25] Cefaclor and cefuroxime (second generation) are active against *Haemophilus influenzae,* an important pathogen in the pediatric age group. The most recently developed, third-generation cephalosporins are active against a wide spectrum of gram-negative organisms, including *Escherichia coli,* species of *Proteus, Klebsiella, Serratia,* and *Enterobacter.*[40] Certain cephalosporins, such as cefoxitin and moxalactam, are also active against *Bacteroides fragilis.*[25] Some second- and third-generation cephalosporins attain sufficient penetration into cerebrospinal fluid to treat meningitis caused by gram-negative organisms.[21,34] However, cephalosporins are ineffective for penicillin-resistant *Streptococcus pneumoniae,* methicillin-resistant *Staphylococcus aureus, Listeria monocytogenes, Streptococcus fecalis, Legionella pneumophila, Clostridium difficile, Campylobacter jejuni,* and certain *Pseudomonas* species.[25,40] Furthermore, organisms such as *Enterobacter, Serratia,* and *Pseudomonas* species can develop resistance and then display resistance to all β-lactam therapy.[35]

CEPHALOSPORINS

TABLE 53-4	Selected cephalosporins and dosage	
	Proprietary name	Adult dose for serious infection
First generation		
Parenteral		
Cefazolin sodium	Ancef, Kefzol	1-2 g q6-8h
Cephalothin sodium	Keflin, Seffin	2 g q4h
Cephapirin sodium	Cefadyl	2 g q4h
Oral		
Cefadroxil	Duricef, Ultracef	0.5-1 g q12h
Cephalexin monohydrate	Keflex	0.5-1 g q6h
Cephradine	Anspor, Velosef	0.5-1 g q6h
Second generation		
Parenteral		
Cefamandole nafate	Mandol	2 g q4h
Cefonicid sodium	Monicid	2 g q24h
Cefoxitin sodium	Mefoxin	2 g q4h
Cefuroxime sodium	Kefurox, Zinacef	3 g q8h
Cefotetan disodium	Cefotan	2 g q12h
Oral		
Cefaclor	Ceclor	0.5-1 g q8h
Third generation		
Parenteral		
Cefoperazone sodium	Cefobid	3 g q6h
Cefotaxime sodium	Claforan	2 g q4h
Ceftazidime	Fortaz, others	2 g q6h
Ceftizoxime sodium	Cefizox	4 g q8h
Ceftriaxone sodium	Rocephin	1 g q12h
Moxalactam disodium	Moxam	2 g q4h

Most cephalosporins are eliminated by the kidney by glomerular filtration and tubular secretion. Elimination half-lives of the cephalosporins are variably prolonged with renal failure, and so individual drugs require specific alterations in dosage. Some of the newer cephalosporins are excreted in bile, and their dosage may need adjustment with hepatic disease (for example, cefoperazone in patients with elevated globulin with cirrhosis).[40]

Toxicity   The cephalosporins share all the toxicities of the penicillins.[40] Approximately 10% of patients with a history of reaction to penicillin will react to cephalosporins with hives, rash, or anaphylaxis, and so they should be used with caution in such persons.[31] Certain special toxic reactions occur when particular cephalosporins are used; for example, a disulfiram-like reaction and bleeding abnormalities attributable to hypoprothrombinemia can occur with drugs that have the "methylthiotetrazole-leaving" group (moxalactam, cefamandole, cefoperazone).[7,39]

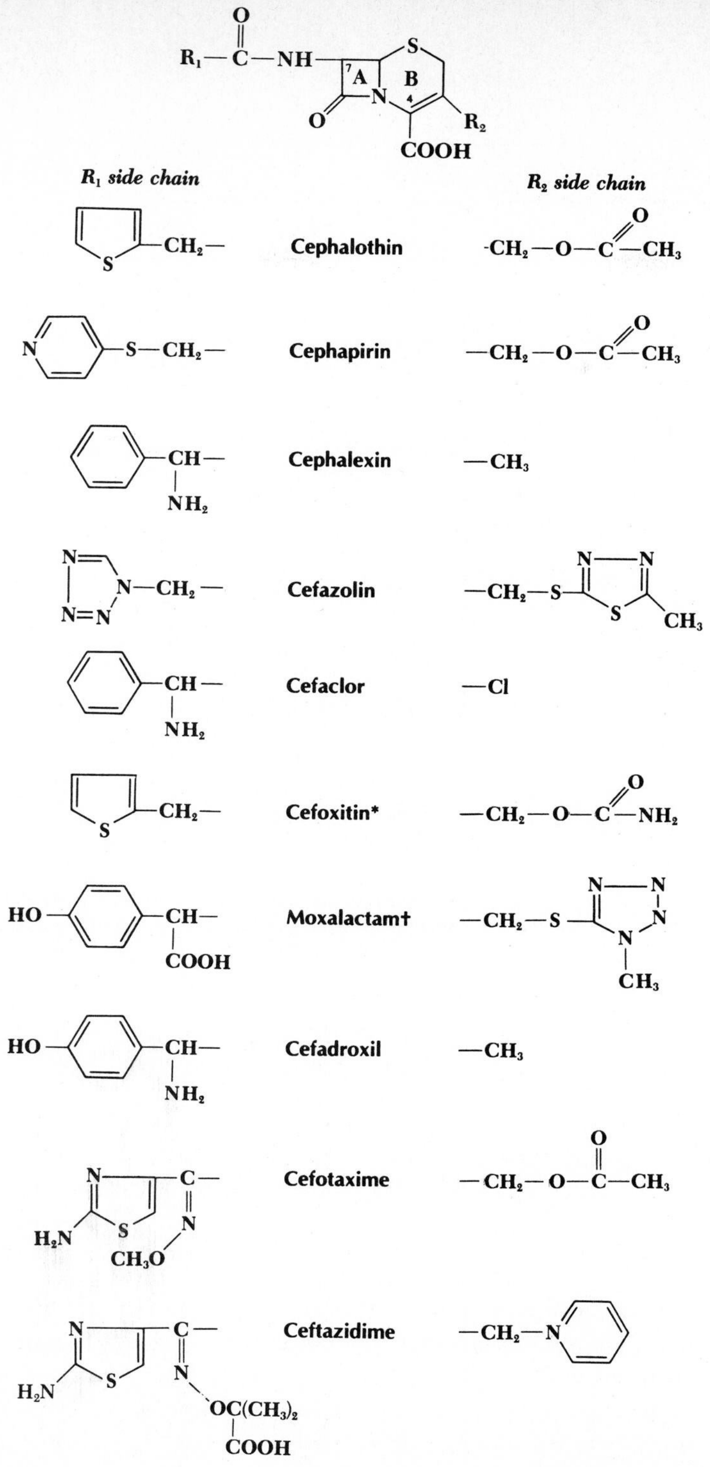

R₁ side chain — R₂ side chain

Cephalothin
Cephapirin
Cephalexin
Cefazolin
Cefaclor
Cefoxitin*
Moxalactam†
Cefadroxil
Cefotaxime
Ceftazidime

---

*Cefoxitin has a methoxy group at position 7 of the β-lactam ring.

†Moxalactam has a methoxy group at position 7 of the β-lactam ring. The sulfur atom in ring B is replaced by an oxygen atom.

TABLE 53-5	Drugs of choice for various infections
Causative agent	Drugs

Gram positive

Streptococcus pyogenes	Penicillin, erythromycin, cephalosporin
Streptococcus viridans*	Penicillin with streptomycin; ampicillin; vancomycin
Enterococcus*	Penicillin with streptomycin; vancomycin with streptomycin or gentamicin
Pneumococcus	Penicillin, erythromycin
Staphylococcus aureus (penicillinase producing)	Oxacillin, nafcillin, cloxacillin, vancomycin
Clostridium	Penicillin, erythromycin
Corynebacterium diphtheriae	Penicillin, erythromycin
Actinomyces	Penicillin or ampicillin; tetracycline

Gram negative

Neisseria meningitidis	Penicillin, chloramphenicol
Neisseria gonorrhoeae	Penicillin, tetracycline, spectinomycin, ceftriaxone
Salmonella	Chloramphenicol, ampicillin
Shigella	Trimethoprim-sulfamethoxazole; ampicillin
Escherichia coli*	Aminoglycoside; ampicillin; trimethoprim-sulfamethoxazole
Enterobacter*	Aminoglycoside; third-generation cephalosporin
Klebsiella*	Cephalosporin, aminoglycoside
Brucella	Tetracycline with rifampin
Haemophilus influenzae	Ampicillin; second-generation cephalosporin
Haemophilus ducreyi	Trimethoprim-sulfamethoxazole; erythromycin
Bordetella pertussis	Erythromycin; trimethoprim-sulfamethoxazole
Pseudomonas*	Aminoglycoside; third-generation cephalosporin
Proteus*	Aminoglycoside; third-generation cephalosporin
Bacteroides	Clindamycin, metronidazole, cefoxitin
Legionella	Erythromycin, rifampin

Miscellaneous

Fusobacterium (Vincent's angina)	Penicillin, erythromycin, tetracycline
Treponema pallidum	Penicillin, tetracycline
Leptospira	Penicillin, tetracycline
Rickettsia	Tetracycline, chloramphenicol
Psittacosis (lymphogranuloma group)	Tetracycline, chloramphenicol)

*Susceptibility tests may be essential.

Uses of cephalosporins   These drugs are becoming commonly used in many clinical situations, since they offer a lower frequency of toxicity than other antibiotics such as the aminoglycosides. Orally administered members of the group (Table 53-4) are indicated when gram-negative coverage is necessary (proved by culture) or for persons allergic to cloxacillin who have skin or bone infections. Cephalosporins are useful in the following clinical settings:

1. As therapy for persons allergic to penicillin they may be acceptable. However, one must proceed with caution in this situation.

2. For treatment of patients with gram-negative infections, such as the elderly with pneumonia or for hospital-acquired bacteremia caused by *Klebsiella* species (cefotaxime or ceftriaxone) or *Pseudomonas* infections (cefoperazone or ceftazidime).

3. For therapy of mixed infections or initial treatment of certain infections of unknown causes (cefoxitin for postoperative abdominal infections).

4. For prophylaxis before surgery, especially for gastrointestinal, pelvic, or orthopedic surgery (the latter involving plastic or metal implants). Here, the least expensive drug, such as cefazolin, given preoperatively is as effective as the more expensive ones.[9]

5. For meningitis potentially caused by either gram-positive or gram-negative organisms (cefotaxime or ceftriaxone).

Use of these antibiotics should be gauged by sensitivity testing of the microorganism isolated from the patient. Presently, testing shows that second- and third-generation cephalosporins are effective for a majority of gram-negative bacilli (Table 53-5). However, resistance can appear rapidly. Only cefoxitin, moxalactam, and cefotetan are satisfactory for obligate anaerobes. Furthermore, the greater the gram-negative spectrum, the less satisfactory the efficacy against staphylococci. Hence use of these agents must be accompanied by microbiologic evaluation, with consideration given to the likelihood of infection with organisms that are not susceptible to them.

Several newly introduced β-lactam drugs differ slightly from penicillin and cephalosporins. **Imipenem** (Primaxin) is a carbapenem with excellent in vitro and in vivo activity for gram-positive and gram-negative (facultative and obligate) bacilli. To prevent destruction by enzymes in the kidney, it is combined with the inhibitor cilastatin. Side effects are similar to those of other β-lactams. Seizures may occur in patients with renal failure even if dosage is adjusted. Clinical efficacy is yet to be determined, though the agent appears to be useful for serious aerobic and anaerobic infections. However, resistance can develop, especially with *Pseudomonas* infections. Monobactams, such as **aztreonam** (Azactam), have activity only for Enterobacteriaceae and *Pseudomonas* species. Aztreonam has also been used to treat serious infections, particularly of the urinary tract, with good success and low toxicity. Finally, certain β-lactamase inhibitors, such as **clavulanic acid,** have been combined with amoxicillin (Augmentin) and ticarcillin (Timentin) with therapeutic benefit.[1] The appropriate role for these agents remains to be established, but treatment of animal bites and recurrent sinusitis are examples.

Imipenem

Aztreonam

Clavulanic acid

OTHER ANTIBIOTICS THAT INHIBIT CELL WALL SYNTHESIS

Vancomycin

Vancomycin (Vancocin) is a complex glycopeptide obtained from an actinomycete. It inhibits the second stage of cell wall formation—polymerization of the peptidoglycan polymer. It is bactericidal against gram-positive bacteria. Vancomycin is poorly absorbed when administered orally but can be used to treat enterocolitis (pseudomembranous colitis) caused by staphylococci and *Clostridium difficile*. The drug is given intravenously for serious systemic infections caused by staphylococci resistant to other drugs and for streptococcal infections in patients allergic to penicillins.[42] Its half-life is about 6 hours. The drug is eliminated through renal mechanisms, and so dosage must be reduced in persons with renal failure.[23] Weekly administration has been used successfully in patients on hemodialysis. Vancomycin is quite irritating to veins and can also cause ototoxicity, nephrotoxicity, and neutropenia.[42] It also must be given slowly intravenously, or it can cause flushing (red-neck syndrome) and hypotension.

Bacitracin

Bacitracin is a mixture of polypeptides that inhibits the second stage of cell wall synthesis. It is used only topically for skin infections caused by gram-positive organisms.

Polymyxin B

Polymyxins are basic peptides that act as cationic detergents to cause lysis of the lipoprotein cell membrane. Polymyxin B (Aerosporin) is particularly active against gram-negative bacteria, but serious nephrotoxicity has limited its internal use. It is used chiefly to treat local infections: external otitis, eye infections, and skin infections with sensitive organisms. Colistin sulfate (Coli-Mycin S) is a very similar compound that can be given parenterally with risks of ototoxicity and nephrotoxicity.[30]

AMINOGLYCOSIDES

The bactericidal aminoglycoside antibiotics (aminocyclitols) are commonly used to treat serious infections caused by many gram-negative bacilli and some gram-positive organisms. Streptococci, pneumococci, clostridia, anaerobes, and fungi are resistant. Aminoglycosides inhibit bacterial protein synthesis by interfering with binding of bacterial aminoacyl transfer ribonucleic acids (tRNAs) to the 30 S ribosomal subunit (see Chapter 51).

General features

The aminoglycosides are important antibiotics for serious, usually systemic, infections caused by gram-negative organisms.[32] The most commonly used agent in this group has been gentamicin.

Aminoglycosides, being polar cations, are poorly absorbed after oral administration and do not reach the central nervous system. Accordingly they are usually injected intramuscularly or intravenously, except for neomycin, which has been given orally to decrease intestinal flora. The aminoglycosides are not highly bound to plasma proteins. They are well distributed in the body, except to the central nervous system, and are excreted by glomerular filtration. Renal elimination is rapid and plasma half-lives are 2 to 3 hours.

The aminoglycosides are ototoxic and nephrotoxic and may cause neuromuscular blockade. Ototoxicity manifests itself in vestibular and auditory disturbances caused by damage to hair cells in the cochlea. Whereas streptomycin and neomycin primarily affect vestibular function, kanamycin, gentamicin, and amikacin have relatively greater auditory toxicity. These drugs may cause dose-related changes in vestibular and auditory function, ranging from disturbances in equilibration and tinnitus to permanent deafness. The risk of ototoxicity is greater in patients with decreased renal function because such patients tend to accumulate aminoglycosides if concentrations are not monitored.[13,17] Ototoxicity is minimized if trough (predose) plasma concentration is maintained below 2 µg/ml.[13]

Manifestations of nephrotoxicity, which is usually reversible, may range from only mild proteinuria to severe azotemia. In patients with preexisting renal dysfunction adjustment of dosage schedules is mandatory, and this can be accomplished by a variety of methods including the use of computer-generated programs.[8]

The neuromuscular blocking action of aminoglycosides may cause apnea, particularly in patients with myasthenia gravis or if large intravenous doses are given rapidly or instilled into the peritoneal cavity.

Resistance develops rapidly to the antibacterial action of streptomycin and more slowly to the other aminoglycosides. Resistance is acquired by (1) a single mutational step (streptomycin), (2) inability to transport the drug to an intracellular site, or (3) the induction of enzymes that metabolize the drug and render it inactive. The latter form of resistance is carried by R factors (plasmids), which may also confer resistance to several other nonaminoglycoside antibiotics. Resistance to one aminoglycoside does not necessarily mean resistance to all. The plasmids induce production of enzymes that acetylate or phosphorylate the aminoglycoside. These enzymes may be specific for some but not all aminoglycosides. For example, organisms such as *Pseudomonas* may be resistant to gentamicin but susceptible to amikacin.

Streptomycin is used in treatment of tuberculosis (see Chapter 55) and with penicillin to treat endocarditis caused by streptococcal species, especially *Streptococcus fecalis*.[37] It is also useful in treatment of tularemia and plague. Resistance may emerge rapidly (induced by R factors), especially when streptomycin is used alone.

Streptomycin

Streptomycin

Gentamicin and tobramycin

Gentamicin sulfate (Garamycin) and tobramycin sulfate (Nebcin) are the most commonly used aminoglycosides. Tobramycin is more effective against *Pseudomonas aeruginosa* and should be used for *Pseudomonas* species known to have lower MIC (minimal inhibitory concentrations). Gentamicin is much less expensive and probably has no greater toxicity, especially if serum concentration is monitored closely.[8] Netilmicin (Netromycin) has similar antimicrobial activity but is reputed to have less nephrotoxicity.[18]

These drugs are used to treat systemic infections caused by susceptible gram-negative bacteria, especially *Pseudomonas*, *Klebsiella*, and *Serratia* species (Table 53-5). Serum concentrations of these aminoglycosides should be monitored every 3 days; trough concentrations predict nephrotoxicity and should not exceed 2 μg/ml.[13] The peak predicts clinical efficacy, and concentrations between 5 and 7 μg/ml should be attained.[24]

Initial dosage of either drug for adults with normal renal function is 1.5 mg/kg every 8 hours. Dosage should then be adjusted according to plasma concentrations in the individual patient. One method of doing so is by a computer-assisted Bayesian feedback program.[8]

Amikacin sulfate (Amikin) is a semisynthetic aminoglycoside with a modification that confers resistance to enzymes that inactivate gentamicin and tobramycin. Amikacin is used to treat infections caused by gram-negative bacteria that are resistant to other aminoglycosides; resistance to amikacin rarely develops or remains at a low level. It is available for intramuscular and intravenous administration in solutions containing 50 and 250 mg/ml. The drug should be administered at 7.5 mg/kg every 12 hours (less in renal failure) to give a peak serum concentration of 25 to 30 μg/ml and a trough below 5 μg/ml (reduce dosage if trough exceeds 10 μg/ml).

Amikacin

Spectinomycin (Trobicin) is an aminocyclitol used as a single 2 g intramuscular injection to treat penicillin-resistant gonorrheal infections or penicillin-allergic patients with gonorrhea. This drug is *not* effective against syphilis. The drug is neither ototoxic nor nephrotoxic and has few side effects.

Spectinomycin

Tetracycline antibiotics are produced by soil organisms. They are broad-spectrum bacteriostatic antibiotics that inhibit protein synthesis in bacteria by blocking the binding of tRNA to the 30 S ribosomal subunit. Tetracyclines tend to suppress an infection and require phagocytes to complete eradication of bacteria. They are highly effective in treatment of *Mycoplasma pneumoniae,* cholera, rickettsial disease, brucellosis, and nongonococcal urethritis caused by chlamydias.[14] They may also be useful in gonorrhea and for first-time urinary tract infections. Tetracycline is used in low doses to treat acne. Combination therapy with other agents has limited application, since tetracyclines occasionally interfere with the killing effect of a bactericidal antibiotic, such as penicillin for pneumococcal meningitis.[33]

TETRACYCLINES

In addition to the three well-known tetracycline antibiotics tetracycline (Acromycin, others), chlortetracycline (Aureomycin), and oxytetracycline (Terramycin, others), other derivatives have been introduced. Of these, demeclocycline (Declomycin) is rarely used, except to treat inappropriate antidiuretic hormone secretion, since it can cause severe photosensitization. Doxycycline (Vibramycin, others) hyclate requires less frequent administration than other tetracyclines because of slower elimination and is safe in renal failure. It may cause phototoxicity. Another slowly excreted member of the tetracycline family is minocycline (Minocin), which has been touted for infrequent dosing. It may cause severe vertigo and nausea, particularly in women.

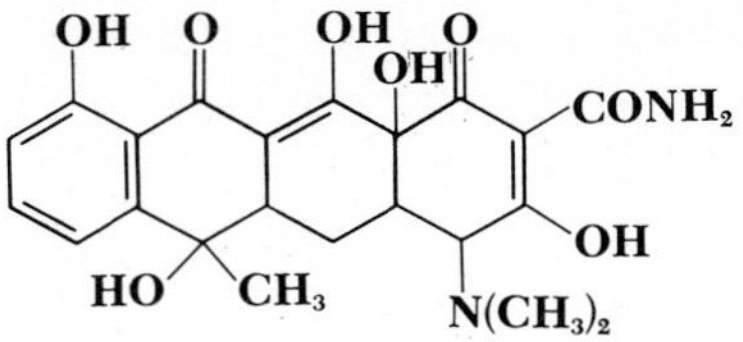

Tetracycline

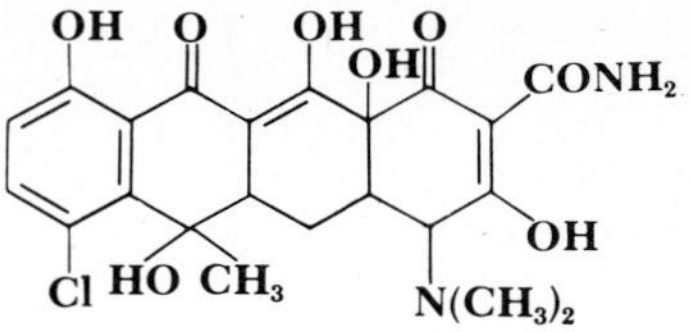

Chlortetracycline

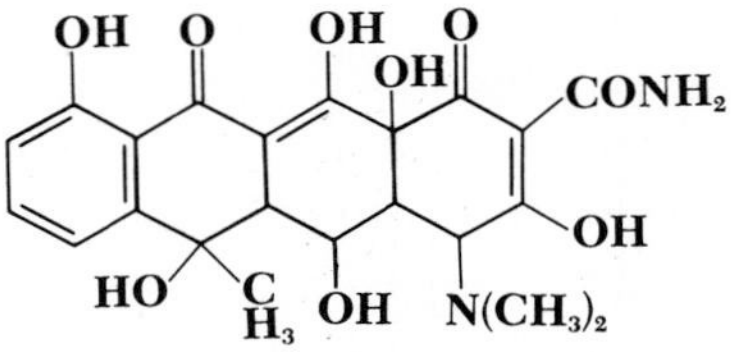

Oxytetracycline

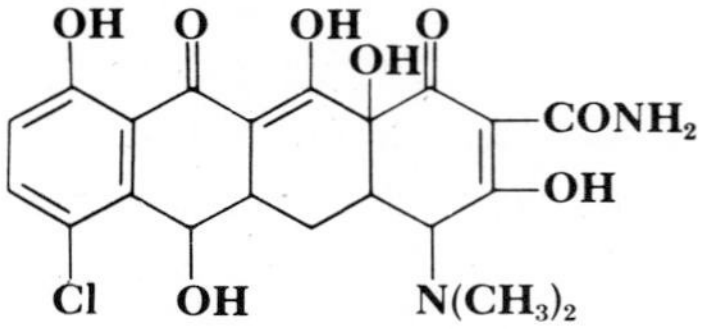

Demeclocycline

Pharmacokinetics   All the aforementioned drugs are absorbed rapidly but incompletely from the gastrointestinal tract.[14,15] Calcium salts and antacids inhibit their absorption, and so the drug should always be taken 30 minutes before meals and antacids should be avoided for at least an hour afterwards.

Tetracycline is widely distributed in most tissues and probably enters cells. However, its concentration is low in cerebrospinal fluid, and so the drug is not indicated for meningitis. As a consequence of its chelating properties, tetracycline tends to localize in bones and teeth, where it may be detected by its fluorescence.[28]

Adverse effects   Adverse effects of tetracyclines include nausea, vomiting, enterocolitis, stomatitis, and superinfections. Deposition in developing teeth can cause permanent discoloration, and so these agents should be avoided by pregnant women and by children up to 8 years of age. Phototoxicity may occur after the administration of demeclocycline and doxycycline. Large intravenous doses of tetracyclines have produced liver damage with fatty infiltration, and so they are no longer used for parenteral therapy of serious infections. Parenteral administration is indicated only for instillation into pleural surfaces to sclerose metastatic foci.

CHLORAM-PHENICOL   Chloramphenicol (Chloromycetin) has a broad antibacterial spectrum similar to that of tetracyclines.[14,22] It has been the drug of choice for treatment of typhoid fever.

Chloramphenicol is a bacteriostatic derivative of nitrobenzene. It binds exclusively to the 50 S ribosomal subunit, thereby interfering with protein synthesis (see Chapter 51). It also interferes with protein synthesis in human bone marrow cells in tissue culture.

Chloramphenicol

An adequate plasma concentration is reached 30 minutes after oral administration, and peak concentration occurs in 2 hours. Chloramphenicol is poorly absorbed after intramuscular administration but can be given intravenously.

Because of its toxicity and the availability of third-generation cephalosporins, the major use of chloramphenicol has been limited to serious rickettsial disease, such as spotted fevers, typhoid fever, other *Salmonella* infections with septicemia, an occasional anaerobic infection, and invasive *Haemophilus influenzae* infections (sepsis, meningitis, pneumonia, epiglottitis, arthritis, and cellulitis).[22]

Chloramphenicol treatment is associated with gastrointestinal disturbances, glossitis, skin rash, and superinfection. Rarely, optic neuritis and encephalopathy may develop with high doses. However, the use of chloramphenicol is severely restricted primarily because of its tendency to produce blood dyscrasias.[5] The frequency of aplastic anemia (1 per 24,000 cases) is low, but it has led physicians to be extremely cautious in using chloramphenicol. The nitrobenzene moiety may be responsible for the anemia, possibly in those with a genetic predisposition. Chloramphenicol is metabolized chiefly (90%) by conjugation to the monoglucuronide. Elevated plasma concentrations of free drug and metabolites can cause toxicity in older patients with significant hepatic disease.[22] The "gray baby" syndrome (cyanosis and vascular collapse) occurs in premature and newborn infants who lack hepatic glucuronyl transferase, which normally detoxifies the antibiotic by changing it to the inactive glucuronide.[45] Concentrations of drug in neonates and young children should be carefully monitored (10 and 25 µg/ml respectively).[22]

Toxicity

Erythromycin (Erythrocin, others), a *macrolide* antibiotic, is a bacteriostatic organic base. It is used mainly to treat pulmonary infections caused by mycoplasma, *Legionella,* and gram-positive organisms in patients allergic to penicillin.[14] In addition, *Chlamydia* and *Haemophilus* species (such as *H. ducreyi,* chancroid) are effectively treated.

Enteric-coated preparations and erythromycin stearate are well absorbed (>50%), and so erythromycin can attain effective blood concentrations of 2 µg/ml or more in an hour or so.[27] Erythromycin diffuses rapidly into tissues and distributes in total body water, though penetration to cerebrospinal fluid is poor. Its excretion is mostly gastrointestinal, with only 5% to 15% eliminated in the urine. Gastrointestinal upset is the most common side effect. Allergic reactions are very rare.

Erythromycin estolate (Ilosone) can be taken with food and can provide longer-lasting therapeutic concentrations than comparable doses of erythromycin base. How-

ANTIBIOTICS FOR GRAM-POSITIVE ORGANISMS
Erythromycin

ever, a higher incidence of cholestatic jaundice has been reported for this drug, particularly in pregnant women and other adults, than for other esters of erythromycin, and so caution is necessary.[6]

Lincomycin	Lincomycin (Lincocin) has an antibacterial spectrum similar to that of erythromycin, but it is also effective against *Bacteroides* species. However, with the usual adult dose of 0.5 g every 6 to 8 hours sufficient gastrointestinal irritation occurs to limit its use.

Clindamycin	Clindamycin (Cleocin) was introduced to replace lincomycin, since its spectrum of activity is similar. Clindamycin can be administered by mouth (150 to 450 mg every 6 hours) or intravenously (250 to 750 mg every 6 hours). The drug is bactericidal for gram-positive organisms and bacteriostatic for anaerobic bacilli.[4] Gastrointestinal irritation is less frequent than with lincomycin but is potentially severe. In addition, neutropenia, eosinophilia, rashes, and elevated hepatic enzymes can occur, especially in those with underlying liver disease.

Clindamycin

Pseudomembranous colitis (caused by toxin from *Clostridium difficile*) is a serious complication that limits the usefulness of clindamycin.[3] Hence any patient on this drug (or any other antibiotic) who develops diarrhea (more than five stools per day) must have the antibiotic discontinued. Pseudomembranous infiltrates can be visualized in the colon, but examination of stools for leukocytes and toxin provide indirect evidence of the condition. If either is present, vancomycin or metronidazole should be administered orally.

METRONIDAZOLE	Metronidazole (Flagyl, others), originally introduced as an oral agent against *Trichomonas* organisms, is also effective in treatment of amebiasis and giardiasis (see Chapter 57). An intravenous form of metronidazole is available for treatment of serious anaerobic bacterial infections (especially *Bacteroides fragilis*).[4] The antimicrobial properties of metronidazole appear to be mediated by a partially reduced interme-

diate.[12] DNA breakage may be its mechanism of action. The drug diffuses well to all tissues, including the central nervous system. Toxicity includes gastrointestinal disturbances, thrombophlebitis, seizures, peripheral neuropathy, and a disulfiram-like reaction to ethanol. It may be a potential mutagen and carcinogen.[12]

Certain generalizations apply to the use of antimicrobial agents for various infections:[9,16] (1) Penicillin derivatives remain the treatment of choice for most respiratory tract infections and are used in combination for other infections. (2) Cephalosporins are effective agents, particularly for patients with hospital-acquired pneumonia and community-acquired gram-negative meningitis. (3) Expense should be considered particularly in outpatient therapy, and expensive albeit broad-spectrum agents should be avoided except in situations in which susceptibility testing shows one to be the only effective agent. There is no evidence that once or twice daily drug administration improves compliance or saves money in the long run. The daily cost to the patient should be considered. (4) Certain drugs fail even when the organism is susceptible to the drug. Some causes of therapeutic failure are listed below:[41]

Incorrect clinical or bacteriologic diagnosis
Improper drug administration or inadequate dose
Poor patient compliance
Alteration in bacterial flora during drug administration and superinfection with a resistant organism
Infection in a location inaccessible to the drug administered
Failure to use indicated surgical drainage
Development of drug resistance by mutant forms of the infecting organism
Deficiency in host defenses
Drug toxicity and hypersensitivity

Poor gastrointestinal absorption of antibiotics such as penicillin G may necessitate administration by another route. If certain agents are given with meals, they may lose much of their effectiveness. Cations in antacids and milk reduce absorption of the tetracyclines. Gastrointestinal complications, such as enterocolitis caused by *Clostridium difficile,* may occur in patients who receive various antibiotics and can cause severe electrolyte disturbances or even death.[3]

Their pharmacokinetics are an important feature in selecting antimicrobial agents, since maintenance of therapeutic blood and tissue concentrations is critical for eradicating infectious agents. For example, the aminoglycosides have therapeutic activity only in relation to their concentration in blood, whereas cephalosporins have a postantibiotic effect. Furthermore, tissue factors affect metabolism, and so some agents (aminoglycosides) are not effective at the pH present in an abscess cavity, whereas others such as metronidazole are just as effective in this environment.

Alterations in microbial flora can occur with antibiotics, as in the development of vaginal candidiasis in patients treated with penicillin or broad-spectrum antibiotics. Usually replacement of normal flora with new organisms (such as pharyngeal flora with gram-negative organisms) is not equivalent to disease. Hence a positive sputum culture is to be considered valid only if accompanied by a new pulmonary infiltrate and fever. Development of resistance in therapy is more likely to occur in immunocompromised patients or with certain infections attributable to gram-negative organisms. In general, to treat a leukopenic patient, a β-lactam agent is combined with an aminoglycoside to achieve bactericidal activity and to prevent emergence of resistance to the β-lactam drug.[33] Certain organisms, including *Enterobacter, Serratia,* and *Pseudomonas* species, have inducible β-lactamases that limit use of a β-lactam antibiotic alone for serious infections of bone or for bacteremia.[35]

Serious toxicity, particularly drug fever, eruptive skin lesions, and liver disease, may limit use of certain antibiotics. Many agents cause a chemical hepatitis, but they only rarely cause severe hepatic dysfunction. Nevertheless, if disorders of liver function are noted, drugs may need to be discontinued.

Effectiveness and safety of antibiotic therapy depend on several host factors. Renal and hepatic elimination need to be considered (see Appendix C), and dosing intervals for many antibiotics may need to be altered when hepatic or renal function is impaired.

Defense mechanisms of the host greatly influence success or failure of any treatment. Debilitating diseases, poor nutrition, or administration of large doses of corticosteroids or other immunosuppressant drugs may affect responses to antibiotic therapy. Nevertheless, many immunocompromised patients can be cured with use of the appropriate agent or agents. Duration of treatment and dosage are important factors, since these patients tend to relapse more easily.

The age of the patient also influences the effectiveness and safety of antibiotic therapy. Infants in the first month of life metabolize or excrete many drugs more slowly, presumably because of less well developed hepatic and renal tubular secretory mechanisms. Serum concentration of an agent should be monitored, and dosage must be adjusted for many antibiotics. Like infants, the elderly or those with hepatic disease may exhibit a reduced capacity to conjugate drugs (such as chloramphenicol) by glucuronidation.

Pregnancy is a contraindication to the use of several antibiotics, including tetracyclines, erythromycin estolate, and various agents that may be teratogenic (metronidazole). Pregnant women are also more sensitive to the hepatotoxicity of tetracyclines.

Liver disease may be aggravated by chloramphenicol, the tetracyclines, and erythromycin. Diminished renal function causes accumulation of aminoglycosides, sulfonamides, some tetracyclines, and most β-lactams. Dosage needs to be altered for these agents, and, for some, blood concentration should be followed. Computer-assisted dosage schemes are available for many drugs, particularly aminoglycosides and vancomycin.

Obstruction or abscess formation can affect the response to antibiotics and make eradication of infection very difficult. Hence surgical drainage needs to be considered if a favorable response to a drug alone does not occur.[2]

Genetic predisposition can affect metabolism or toxicity. Glucose-6-phosphate dehydrogenase deficiency may predispose a person to hemolytic anemia from antimicrobial drugs such as the sulfonamides and nitrofurantoin. Genetic predisposition also may explain rare but fatal reactions to chloramphenicol.

REFERENCES

1. Allan, J.D., and Eliopoulos, G.M.: The newer penicillins: pharmacologic properties and clinical experience, Hosp. Formulary **21**:290, 1986.

2. Antimicrobial prophylaxis for surgery, Med. Lett. Drugs Ther. **27**:105, 1985.

3. Bartlett, J.G.: Antibiotic-associated pseudomembranous colitis, Rev. Infect. Dis. **1**:530, 1979.

4. Bartlett, J.G.: Anti-anaerobic antibacterial agents, Lancet **2**:478, 1982.

5. Best, W.R.: Chloramphenicol-associated blood dyscrasias: a review of cases submitted to the American Medical Association Registry, J.A.M.A. **201**:181, 1967.

6. Braun, P.: Hepatotoxicity of erythromycin, J. Infect. Dis. **119**:300, 1969.

7. Buening, M.K., and Wold, J.S.: Ethanol-moxalactam interactions in vivo, Rev. Infect. Dis. **4**(suppl.):S555, 1982.

8. Burton, M.E., Brater, D.C., Chen, P.S., et al.: A Bayesian feedback method of aminoglycoside dosing, Clin. Pharmacol. Ther. **37**:349, 1985.

9. The choice of antimicrobial drugs, Med. Lett. Drugs Ther. **26**:19, 1984.

10. Drusano, G.L., Schimpff, S.C., and Hewitt, W.L.: The acylampicillins: mezlocillin, piperacillin, and azlocillin, Rev. Infect. Dis. **6**:13, 1984.

11. Fleming, A.: On antibacterial action of cultures of penicillium, with special reference to their use in isolation of *B. influenzae*, Br. J. Exp. Pathol. **10**:226, 1929.

12. Goldman, P.: Metronidazole, N. Engl. J. Med. **303**:1212, 1980.

13. Goodman, E.L., Van Gelder, J., Holmes, R., et al.: Prospective comparative study of variable dosage and variable frequency regimens for administration of gentamicin, Antimicrob. Agents Chemother. **8**:434, 1975.

14. Kucers, A.: Chloramphenicol, erythromycin, vancomycin, tetracyclines, Lancet **2**:425, 1982.

15. Kunin, C.M., and Finland, M.: Clinical pharmacology of the tetracycline antibiotics, Clin. Pharmacol. Ther. **2**:51, 1961.

16. Kunin, C.M., Tupasi, T., and Craig, W.A.: Use of antibiotics: a brief exposition of the problem and some tentative solutions, Ann. Intern. Med. **79**:555, 1973.

17. Lau, W.K., Young, L.S., Black, R.E., et al.: Comparative efficacy and toxicity of amikacin/carbenicillin versus gentamicin/carbenicillin in leukopenic patients: a randomized prospective trial, Am. J. Med. **62**:959, 1977.

18. Lerner, A.M., Reyes, M.P., Cone, L.A., et al.: Randomized, controlled trial of the comparative efficacy, auditory toxicity, and nephrotoxicity of tobramycin and netilmicin, Lancet **1**:1123, 1983.

19. Linton, A.L., Clark, W.F., Driedger, A.A., et al.: Acute interstitial nephritis due to drugs: review of the literature with a report of nine cases, Ann. Intern. Med. **93**:735, 1980.

20. Macfarlane, G.: Howard Florey: the making of a great scientist, Oxford, Eng., 1979, Oxford University Press.

21. McCracken, G.H., Jr., Nelson, J.D., and Grimm, L.: Pharmacokinetics and bacteriological efficacy of cefoperazone, cefuroxime, ceftriaxone, and moxalactam in experimental *Streptococcus pneumoniae* and *Haemophilus influenzae* meningitis, Antimicrob. Agents Chemother. **21**:262, 1982.

22. Meissner, H.C., and Smith, A.L.: The current status of chloramphenicol, Pediatrics **64**:348, 1979.

23. Moellering, R.C., Jr., Krogstad, D.J., and Greenblatt, D.J.: Vancomycin therapy in patients with impaired renal function: a nomogram for dosage, Ann. Intern. Med. **94**:343, 1981.

24. Moore, R.D., Smith, C.R., and Lietman, P.S.: The association of aminoglycoside plasma levels with mortality in patients with gram-negative bacteremia, J. Infect. Dis. **149**:443, 1984.

25. Neu, H.C.: Clinical uses of cephalosporins, Lancet **2**:252, 1982.

26. Neu, H.C.: Relation of structural properties of beta-lactam antibiotics to antibacterial activity, Am. J. Med. **79**(suppl. 2A):2, 1985.

27. Nicholas, P.: Erythromycin: clinical review I. Clinical pharmacology, N.Y. State J. Med. **77**:2088, 1977.

28. Owen, L.N.: Fluorescence of tetracyclines in bone tumours, normal bone and teeth, Nature **190**:500, 1961.

29. Park, J.T.: Uridine-5'-pyrophosphate derivatives, J. Biol. Chem. **194**:877, 885, and 897, 1952.

30. Petersdorf, R.G., and Plorde, J.J.: Colistin: a reappraisal, J.A.M.A. **183**:123, 1963.

31. Petz, L.D.: Immunologic cross-reactivity between penicillins and cephalosporins: a review, J. Infect. Dis. **137**(suppl.):S74, 1978.

32. Phillips, I.: Aminoglycosides, Lancet **2**:311, 1982.

33. Rahal, J.J., Jr.: Antibiotic combinations: the clinical relevance of synergy and antagonism, Medicine **57**:179, 1978.

34. Rahal, J.J., and Simberkoff, M.S.: Host defense and antimicrobial therapy in adult gram-negative bacillary meningitis, Ann. Intern. Med. **96**:468, 1982.

35. Sanders, C.C.: Novel resistance selected by the new expanded-spectrum cephalosporins: a concern, J. Infect. Dis. **147**:585, 1983.

36. Saxon, A.: Immediate hypersensitivity reactions to β-lactam antibiotics, Rev. Infect. Dis. **5**(suppl. 2):S368, 1983.

37. Schatz, A., Bugie, E., and Waksman, S.A.: Streptomycin, a substance exhibiting antibiotic activity against gram-positive and gram-negative bacteria, Proc. Soc. Exp. Biol. Med. **55**:66, 1944.

38. Sheehan, J.C., and Henery-Logan, K.R.: A general synthesis of the penicillins, J. Am. Chem. Soc. **81**:5838, 1959.

39. Shenkenberg, T.D., Mackowiak, P.A., and Smith, J.W.: Coagulopathy and hemorrhage associated with cefoperazone therapy in a patient with renal failure, South. Med. J. **78**:488, 1985.

40. Shibl, A.M., and Sande, M.A.: New cephalosporin antibiotics: selection and uses, Hosp. Formulary **20**:802, 1985.

41. Smith, J.W.: Proper use of antibiotics, Texas Med. **73**:37, Sept. 1977.

42. Sorrell, T.C., Packham, D.R., Shanker, S., et al.: Vancomycin therapy for methicillin-resistant *Staphylococcus aureus*, Ann. Intern. Med. **97**:344, 1982.

43. Sullivan, T.J.: Antigen-specific desensitization of patients allergic to penicillin, J. Allergy Clin. Immunol. **69**:500, 1982.

44. Tomasz, A.: From penicillin-binding proteins to the lysis and death of bacteria: a 1979 view, Rev. Infect. Dis. **1**:434, 1979.

45. Weiss, C.F., Glazko, A.J., and Weston, J.K.: Chloramphenicol in the newborn infant: a physiologic explanation of its toxicity when given in excessive doses, N. Engl. J. Med. **262**:787, 1960.

Chapter 54

Antiviral agents

Several drugs with proved efficacy are available for therapy of viral infections (Table 54-1). Amantadine has been available for two decades for prevention and amelioration of influenza A infections. It appears to inhibit an early stage of viral replication, possibly leading to uncoating of the viral genome.

AMANTADINE

Amantadine (Symmetrel) and rimantadine are synthetic compounds of unusual structure that inhibit influenza A virus replication in host cells.[8] In vitro they are effective against both influenza and rubella viruses. Clinically they have value as chemoprophylactic agents for influenza A2 virus infection and, if used within 2 days, for therapy of the early infection.[7,15] Amantadine reduces the duration of clinical illness and diminishes systemic complaints. It also has some therapeutic effect in parkinsonism (see Chapter 12).

Amantadine can produce central nervous system symptoms, including nervousness, difficulty concentrating, insomnia, and, rarely, grand mal seizures. Neurotoxicity is enhanced by concomitant antihistamine and caffeine ingestion. Rimantadine, an investigational drug, has a lower frequency of side effects.[5] Amantadine dosage must be reduced in renal failure.[6] It is available in 100 mg capsules, to be taken twice daily.

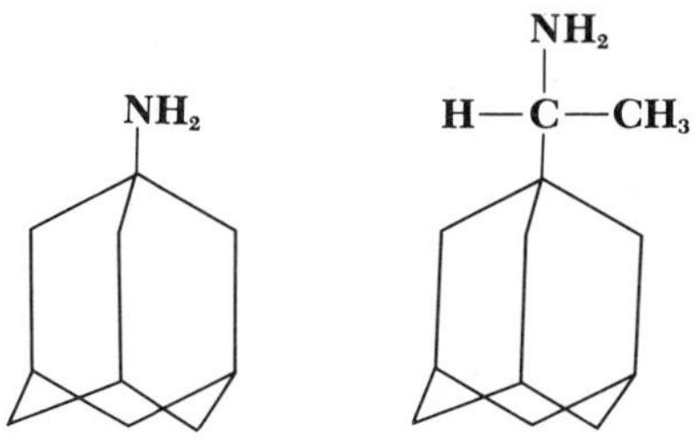

$$NH_2$$

$$H-C-CH_3$$

$$NH_2$$

Amantadine   **Rimantadine**

IDOXURIDINE

The initial antiviral drug for herpes infection was idoxuridine (Stoxil), an inhibitor of nucleic acid synthesis, which produced spectacular results after topical application in herpetic keratitis. However, it is too toxic for systemic use and is available only for herpes simplex virus (HSV) keratitis. Other recently introduced drugs have better safety margins for therapy of herpetic infections.

TABLE 54-1   Treatment of viral infections

Infection	Antiviral drug	Route of administration	Dosage schedule		
			Dose	Interval (hours)	Duration (days)
Influenza A[7,15]	Amantadine	Oral	200 mg	24	5
	Rimantadine†	Oral	200 mg	24	5
Herpes simplex virus (HSV) conjunctivitis[1]	Vidarabine	Topical	3% ointment	5	10-14
	or idoxuridine	Topical	0.5% ointment	5	10-14
	or trifluridine	Topical	1% ointment	2	10-14
HSV encephalitis[13]	Acyclovir	Intravenous	10 mg/kg	8	10
	or vidarabine	Intravenous	15 mg/kg	24	10
HSV mucocutaneous infections*[12]	Acyclovir	Intravenous	250 mg/m²	8	7
		or topical	Thin film	4	7
Genital HSV[9]	Acyclovir	Topical	Thin film	4	7
		or oral	200 mg	5	10
Herpes zoster*[10]	Vidarabine	Intravenous	10 mg/kg	24	7
	or acyclovir†	Intravenous	500 mg/m²	8	5
Human immunodeficiency (HIV, AIDS) virus*[14]	Zidovudine	Oral	200 mg	4	Indefinite

*Immunocompromised.
†Not approved by the FDA for this use.

VIDARABINE   Vidarabine, or adenine arabinoside, inhibits DNA viruses such as HSV and varicella-zoster virus. Its action is poorly understood. Topically, vidarabine is used to treat ocular herpes simplex.[1] When administered intravenously, it is effective treatment for herpes encephalitis and systemic herpes infections in neonates and immunocompromised patients, though recent studies indicate that acyclovir is more effective in these conditions.[10,13] Vidarabine (Vira-A) is infused over 12 to 24 hours at a dosage of 10 to 15 mg/kg/24 hours. It may cause nausea, diarrhea, weight gain because of the large amount of fluid infused, and, rarely, hematologic and metabolic effects.

Vidarabine

Trifluridine (Viroptic) is a trifluoro analog of thymidine. An ointment is instilled into the eye to treat herpes simplex keratitis and keratoconjunctivitis.[1]

TRIFLURIDINE

O

HN   CF$_3$

O   N

HO — CH$_2$ O

OH

Trifluridine

O

HN   N

H$_2$N   N   N

CH$_2$OCH$_2$CH$_2$OH

Acyclovir

Acyclovir (acycloguanosine) is a purine nucleoside analog that is active against herpes viruses. Cells infected with herpes simplex phosphorylate the drug to yield acycloguanosine triphosphate, which preferentially inhibits virus-specified DNA polymerase.[4] Both topically and orally administered acyclovir (200 mg five times daily) have been beneficial in primary genital HSV infections, but they have been less useful for recurrences. Recent trials have shown that low oral doses (400 mg per day), if given chronically, will prevent recurrence.[2] Intravenous acyclovir is now considered the drug of choice for HSV encephalitis.[13] The parenteral drug reduces illness and viral shedding by immunosuppressed patients with HSV disease[12] and has also been found effective for herpes zoster infections in immunocompromised patients, though it is not yet approved for this indication.[9] Acyclovir is excreted principally by glomerular filtration, and dosage must be reduced in patients with renal failure. Adverse responses have included phlebitis at intravenous sites of injection, rash, hematuria, and less frequently central nervous system toxicity (especially in transplant patients) with lethargy and confusion.[11] Reversible renal dysfunction and crystalline nephropathy may also occur.[13] Acyclovir (Zovirax) is available in 200 mg capsules and a 5% ointment. The sodium salt, in 10 ml vials as a powder equivalent to 500 mg of acyclovir, can be dissolved for slow infusion over several hours.

ACYCLOVIR

The advent of acquired immunodeficiency syndrome (AIDS) caused by human immunodeficiency virus (HIV) has spurred research with a wide variety of antiviral compounds for treatment of this lethal infection. Since initial phase I trials with 3'-azido-3'-deoxythymidine (AZT) were encouraging, this drug has been released specifically for adult AIDS victims with *Pneumocystis carinii* pneumonia or HIV-positive patients with an absolute helper/inducer (CD4$^+$, T4$^+$) T-cell count of less than 200/mm^3. AZT has recently been renamed **zidovudine** (Retrovir) and is available as 100 mg capsules. The drug interrupts elongation of DNA chains, making it impossible

ANTI–HUMAN IMMUNO-DEFICIENCY VIRUS AGENTS

for the virus to complete DNA synthesis and reproduce.[14] In doses of at least 200 mg every 4 hours, patients had fewer infectious complications than untreated controls, had a transient rise in circulating T4 lymphocytes, and could manifest delayed hypersensitivity.[14] Serious side effects, such as severe anemia necessitating transfusions, headache, and gastrointestinal intolerance, were observed.

INTERFERON INDUCERS	Inducers of endogenous interferon represent a novel approach to antiviral chemotherapy. Interferons are antiviral proteins that exist in multiple molecular forms in different cells where they arise as a consequence of viral infections. Bacteria and their products are also capable of inducing formation of interferons by host cells. In addition, it has been shown that chemically defined substances, such as a polyanionic pyran copolymer or double-stranded RNA from a synthetic source, can induce demonstrable serum interferon concentrations in humans and animals. Recently, synthetically produced interferon has been demonstrated to prevent the common cold when used in exposed family members.[3]

REFERENCES

1. Coster, D.J., McKinnon, J.R., McGill, J.I., et al.: Clinical evaluation of adenine arabinoside and trifluorothymidine in the treatment of corneal ulcers caused by herpes simplex virus, J. Infect. Dis. **133**(suppl.):A173, 1976.
2. Douglas, J.M., Critchlow, C., Benedetti, J., et al.: A double-blind study of oral acyclovir for suppression of recurrences of genital herpes simplex virus infection, N. Engl. J. Med. **310**:1551, 1984.
3. Douglas, R.M., Moore, B.W., Miles, H.B., et al.: Prophylactic efficacy of intranasal alpha₂-interferon against rhinovirus infections in the family setting, N. Engl. J. Med. **314**:65, 1986.
4. Elion, G.B.: Mechanism of action and selectivity of acyclovir, Am. J. Med. **73**:7, July 20, 1982.
5. Hayden, F.G., Hoffman, H.E., and Spyker, D.A.: Differences in side effects of amantadine hydrochloride and rimantadine hydrochloride relate to differences in pharmacokinetics, Antimicrob. Agents Chemother. **23**:458, 1983.
6. Horadam, V.W., Sharp, J.G., Smilack, J.D., et al.: Pharmacokinetics of amantadine hydrochloride in subjects with normal and impaired renal function, Ann. Intern. Med. **94**:454, 1981.
7. Little, J.W., Hall, W.J., Douglas, R.G., Jr., et al.: Amantadine effect on peripheral airways abnormalities in influenza: a study in 15 students with natural influenza A infection, Ann. Intern. Med. **85**:177, 1976.
8. Oxford, J.S., and Galbraith, A.: Antiviral activity of amantadine: a review of laboratory and clinical data, Pharmacol. Ther. **11**:181, 1980.
9. Powers, R.D., and Hayden, F.G.: Herpesvirus infections: current antiviral therapy, Hosp. Formulary **19**:1040, 1984.
10. Shepp, D.H., Dandliker, P.S., and Meyers, J.D.: Treatment of varicella-zoster virus infection in severely immunocompromised patients: a randomized comparison of acyclovir and vidarabine, N. Engl. J. Med. **314**:208, 1986.
11. Wade, J.C., and Meyers, J.D.: Neurologic symptoms associated with parenteral acyclovir treatment after marrow transplantation, Ann. Intern. Med. **98**:921, 1983.
12. Wade, J.C., Newton, B., McLaren, C., et al.: Intravenous acyclovir to treat mucocutaneous herpes simplex virus infection after marrow transplantation: a double-blind trial, Ann. Intern. Med. **96**:265, 1982.

13. Whitley, R.J., Alford, C.A., Hirsch, M.S., et al. and the NIAID Collaborative Antiviral Study Group: Vidarabine versus acyclovir therapy in herpes simplex encephalitis, N. Engl. J. Med. 314:144, 1986.

14. Yarchoan, R., Klecker, R.W., Weinhold, K.J., et al.: Administration of 3'-azido-3'-deoxythymidine, an inhibitor of HTLV-III/LAV replication, to patients with AIDS or AIDS-related complex, Lancet 1:575, 1986.

15. Younkin, S.W., Betts, R.F., Roth, F.K., and Douglas, R.G., Jr.: Reduction in fever and symptoms in young adults with influenza A/Brazil/78 H1N1 infection after treatment with aspirin or amantadine, Antimicrob. Agents Chemother. 23:577, 1983.

Chapter 55

Drugs used to treat mycobacterial and fungal infections

Tuberculosis remains a frequently encountered disease. After the advent of effective chemotherapy in the late 1940s, a dramatic decrease in the incidence of pulmonary disease occurred, a continuation of the decrease attributable to improved public health measures.[10] Systemic forms, such as miliary and bone tuberculosis, have also decreased but remain as frequent in proportion to cases of pulmonary disease as previously. Now both pulmonary and systemic forms are most commonly seen in alcoholics or the elderly. Tuberculosis must be included in the differential diagnosis of patients with fever of unknown origin, subacute meningitis, or chronic infection at any site.

The slow multiplication of the tubercle bacillus (*Mycobacterium tuberculosis*), its relatively protected intracellular location, and its propensity to become drug resistant, especially on single-drug therapy, make chemotherapy difficult.[10] However, bactericidal activity is accomplished rapidly with combination chemotherapy.[21] The major current problem is failure of compliance,[22] especially among alcoholic patients. In addition, persons from Southeast Asia and Central America are likely to harbor resistant organisms.[4]

The primary agents used in treatment are isoniazid, ethambutol, rifampin, streptomycin, and pyrazinamide.[1,21] Isoniazid and rifampin are highly effective if used in combination.[21] Streptomycin is recommended as a third drug, especially because it can be injected twice weekly to guarantee compliance. However, it is toxic, especially in the elderly, and resistance may develop. Other compounds, particularly pyrazinamide, are becoming frequently included in primary treatment of persons with *M. tuberculosis* infections.[17] Secondary alternatives include *p*-aminosalicylic acid, ethionamide, cycloserine, and capreomycin. These agents are generally more toxic and slightly less effective, but they may be indicated in selected cases (Table 55-1), especially if the patient has organisms resistant to the primary drugs.

Combinations of drugs are necessary to treat tuberculosis but not for prophylaxis. The purpose of combinations is to prevent development of resistant bacilli.

Isoniazid

The effect of isoniazid (INH) on the tubercle bacillus was discovered accidentally during routine screening of chemical intermediates in synthesis of thiosemicarbazones of nicotinamide (a known inhibitor of tubercle bacilli in vitro). Isoniazid kills actively dividing tubercle bacilli and inhibits growth in vitro at concentrations of less than 1

TABLE 55-1   Drugs for treatment of *Mycobacterium* infections

Drug	Effect	Dosage forms (mg)	Daily dosage	Elimination	Infectious treatment
Primary					
Isoniazid (INH) (Izonid, others)	Cidal	T: 50-300; I: 100/ml; S: 50/5 ml	A: 300 mg Ch: 10-20 mg/kg	Hepatic (metabolism)	*M. tuberculosis, M. kansasii;* included for others but less active
Ethambutol hydrochloride (Myambutol)	Static	T: 100, 400	15 mg/kg	Renal (excretion)	*M. tuberculosis, M. kansasii;* less active for others; used if isoniazid resistance possible
Rifampin (Rifadin, Rimactane)	Cidal	C: 150, 300	A: 600 mg Ch: 10-20 mg/kg	Biliary (excretion)	*M. tuberculosis, M. kansasii, M. leprae;* variable for others
Streptomycin sulfate	Cidal	I: 400, 500/ml	1 g (to twice weekly)	Renal	*M. tuberculosis;* daily or twice weekly for 3 months (for compliance); not to exceed 120 g
Pyrazinamide	Cidal	T: 500	20-35 mg/kg	Hepatic	Short course, daily or twice weekly, or for 12 months for drug-resistant varieties of *M. tuberculosis*
Secondary					
Aminosalicylic sodium (Teebacin)	Static	T: 500; P: 4180	10-12 g/day	Renal	Combination therapy in developing countries
Ethionamide (Trecator)	Static	T: 250	500-750 mg	Hepatic	Retreatment of *M. tuberculosis;* in combination for others
Cycloserine (Seromycin)	Cidal	C: 250	500 mg	Renal	Retreatment of *M. tuberculosis, M. avium/intracellulare* complex, *Nocardia*
Capreomycin sulfate (Capastat)	Static	P: 1000	1 g	Renal	Retreatment of resistant strains
Dapsone	Static	T: 25, 100	1-100 mg	Renal	*M. leprae*
Clofazimine (Lamprene)	Cidal	C: 100	100-300 mg	Biliary (slow)	*M. leprae, M. avium/intracellulare* complex

Cidal and *static,* Combining forms for 'bactericidal' and 'bacteriostatic' respectively.
A, Adult; *Ch,* children; *C,* capsule; *I,* injection; *P,* powder for reconstitution; *S,* syrup; *T,* tablet.

μg/ml.[23] The drug acts presumably to inhibit synthesis of mycolic acid. Isoniazid is bactericidal for extracellular populations in body cavities and is also active against intracellular mycobacteria, though it kills them less readily. If used alone for an active infection (usually associated with more than 10^6 bacilli), resistance will develop in a majority of cases within 3 months. Resistance to antitubercular drugs is occurring in many regions of the world and is more likely in those who relapse after previous treatment.[4,22] Initial therapy is usually started with two drugs to which the organism is likely to be sensitive, such as isoniazid and rifampin. If the patient lives in a geographical region known to have resistant organisms or is being treated after relapse, isoniazid is combined with at least two drugs not previously used, such as rifampin and pyrazinamide, pending susceptibility testing.[17,22]

Isoniazid

Isoniazid is rapidly absorbed from the gastrointestinal tract, is widely distributed in the body, and penetrates efficiently into the cerebrospinal fluid.[13,23] It is primarily acetylated initially, and various metabolites are cleared by the kidney. Persons with slow acetylating ability (an autosomal recessive trait) may be more subject to hepatotoxicity, particularly if they receive rifampin concomitantly, because of enhanced conversion of isoniazid to hydrazine.[9]

Isoniazid is given to adults in doses of 3 to 5 mg/kg once a day with a maximal dose of 300 mg. Larger doses have been used in tuberculous meningitis but are not necessary. Parenteral administration can be used if patients cannot take oral drug.

Adverse effects of isoniazid include peripheral neuritis, sensory disturbances, hepatic necrosis, arthritic reactions, and hematologic disturbances.[3,16] Neurotoxicity can be prevented by pyridoxine, which does not affect antimycobacterial activity. However, the most feared complication is hepatitis. Transaminase elevations are common, but the incidence of significant hepatotoxicity with clinical symptoms increases with age to 2% in persons over 50. Patients should be warned to discontinue the drug if abdominal pain or nausea ensue.

Drug interactions may be significant. Rifampin increases the hepatotoxicity of isoniazid, and so they must be discontinued by 3% of patients.[21] Isoniazid interferes with metabolism of phenytoin; reduction of phenytoin dosage is usually necessary.

Ethambutol   Ethambutol, though bacteriostatic, is highly effective in combination with other drugs in treatment of tuberculosis.[21] Its mechanism of action is unknown, but it may affect RNA synthesis. Primary resistance is rare but has been increasing in the past decade.[4] Secondary resistance in previously treated patients is low. Ethambutol is absorbed rapidly from the gastrointestinal tract and is excreted to a large extent unchanged by the kidney.[13] The drug does not normally cross the blood-brain barrier but may do so if the meninges are inflamed.

The major adverse effect of ethambutol is a dose-dependent optic neuritis. This manifests as loss of visual acuity and alterations in color perception. These responses are reversible and are uncommonly experienced if dosage is limited to a single 15 mg/kg dose each day. Patients receiving ethambutol should be warned to return if visual impairment occurs; otherwise prospective ophthalmologic testing is not indicated when 15 mg/kg/day is taken. Visual symptoms commonly precede a measurable decrease in visual acuity.[1] The half-life is prolonged in patients with renal failure and so the drug accumulates; the dosage in this setting should be reduced to 5 to 8 mg/kg.

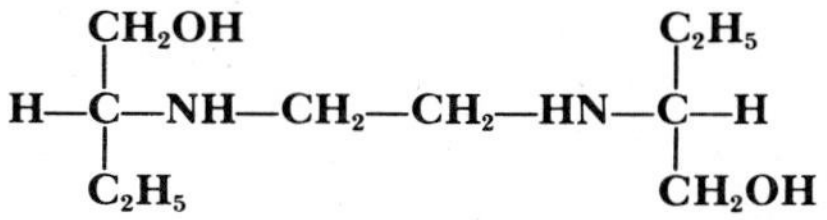

$$H-\underset{\underset{C_2H_5}{|}}{\overset{\overset{CH_2OH}{|}}{C}}-NH-CH_2-CH_2-HN-\underset{\underset{CH_2OH}{|}}{\overset{\overset{C_2H_5}{|}}{C}}-H$$

Ethambutol

Rifampin, a semisynthetic derivative of rifamycin B produced by *Streptomyces mediterranei*, is bactericidal for tubercle bacilli.[10] The drug inhibits DNA-dependent RNA polymerase.[11] Oral administration of 600 mg of rifampin produces an effective serum concentration of 8 μg/ml in less than 2 hours, and antibacterial activity is often still present 10 hours later.[6] Combinations of isoniazid and rifampin are now the standard therapy for short treatments of pulmonary and extrapulmonary tuberculosis.[1,8,21]   *Rifampin*

Resistance to rifampin is increasing, and so it is imperative to use two or more antituberculosis agents concurrently if one is treating relapse.[17,22]

Rifampin is absorbed well from the gastrointestinal tract and distributed throughout body fluids, including the cerebrospinal fluid. It is metabolized in the liver and excreted mostly in the bile.[13] Rifampin and its metabolites may stain body fluids (urine, sweat, tears) orange.[6]

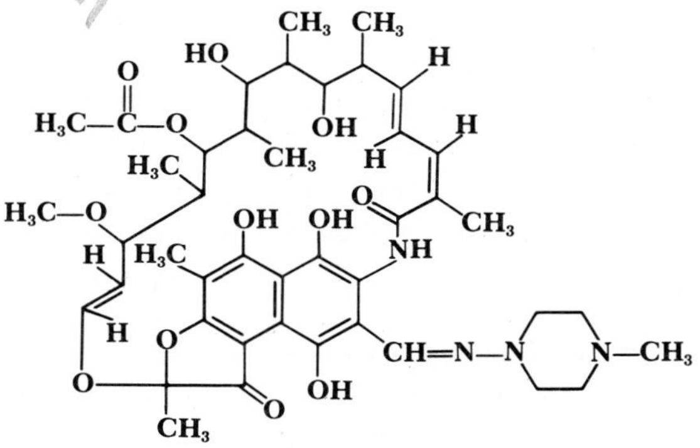

Rifampin

Adverse effects are infrequent (in about 2%) but include hepatotoxicity, abdominal symptoms, leg cramps, and an influenza-like hypersensitivity reaction, especially if the drug is taken intermittently. Drug interactions are numerous. Rifampin increases hepatotoxicity of isoniazid and induces the metabolism of many drugs (see Chapter 63).

Streptomycin

Streptomycin was the first effective drug for treatment of tuberculosis. It must be administered intramuscularly and produces numerous toxic effects, particularly in adults.[19] It is most often used in combination with other drugs to retreat pulmonary infections in the early months of therapy. The dose is 20 mg/kg once daily (20 to 40 mg/kg/day in children, up to 1 g/day) for 4 weeks. The total amount given should not exceed 120 g.[1] Streptomycin can also be injected twice weekly in outpatients to improve compliance.

Pyrazinamide

Pyrazinamide (pyrazinoic acid amine), an analog of nicotinamide, is bactericidal at high concentrations for rapidly dividing tubercle bacilli and for organisms in macrophages.[1] Because of this latter activity, it has achieved status as a first-line drug for the first 2 months of therapy or when 6-month courses are used.[17,21] The drug is well absorbed and distributed throughout the body. It can cause hepatic damage, but this is infrequent at the recommended dosage of 20 to 35 mg/kg/day. Pyrazinamide can also be given twice weekly (at dosages up to 50 mg/kg/day).

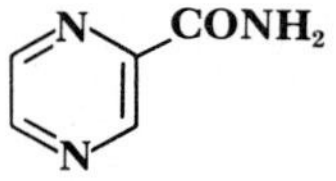

Pyrazinamide

SECOND-LINE ANTITUBERCU-LOSIS DRUGS

Some other compounds are available as alternatives to the aforementioned agents. However, their use should be limited to retreatment of infections proved resistant to the primary agents.

p-Aminosalicylic acid at concentrations as low as 1 µg/ml inhibits growth of tubercle bacilli, but it must be administered in very large doses, up to 15 to 20 g/day.[19] It is well absorbed and distributes throughout total body water. Compliance is often poor, and it is used today only when drug cost is a priority.

Adverse effects of p-aminosalicylic acid include gastrointestinal disturbances (which may warrant termination of therapy), occasional skin rash, and, rarely, hepatic damage and interference with thyroid function.

Ethionamide, like isoniazid, is a pyridine derivative. Its limitation is frequent side effects, especially gastrointestinal upset and peripheral neuropathy, which necessitate its discontinuation.

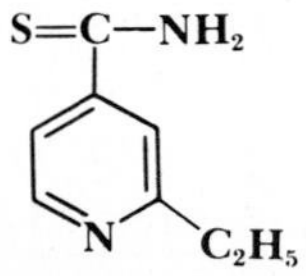

Ethionamide

Cycloserine in combination with other drugs has been effective in treatment of some cases of tuberculosis. Unfortunately, it is neurotoxic.[20] Frequent side effects, such as nausea, vomiting, hypotension, seizures, behavioral changes, and peripheral neuritis, limit its usefulness.

$$H_2C\!-\!CH\!-\!NH_2$$

Cycloserine

The mechanism of action of cycloserine involves competition for D-alanine as a precursor of some bacterial cell wall component.[12] As a consequence, the drug induces protoplast formation. Cycloserine has some usefulness as a second-line drug to treat nontubercular mycobacterial and nocardial infections.

Cycloserine is well absorbed from the gastrointestinal tract, is widely distributed in the body, and penetrates well into the spinal fluid. It is excreted to a considerable extent unchanged in urine.

Capreomycin is a polypeptide antibiotic like viomycin that is particularly effective for retreatment of resistant infection. Renal damage and ototoxicity limit its usefulness, but it is less toxic than kanamycin and amikacin. Capreomycin is given parenterally for 2 to 4 months. Since eighth-nerve damage can be severe, hearing tests should be performed prospectively.

DRUGS USED FOR NONTUBERCULOSIS INFECTIONS

Mycobacteria other than *Mycobacterium tuberculosis* may be sensitive to some of the aforementioned agents. *M. kansasii* infections usually respond to isoniazid and rifampin, but *M. avium/intracellulare* complex forms are more difficult to treat. Combinations of four to five drugs, including rifampin, isoniazid, ethambutol, and pyrazinamide or cycloserine, are employed. Recently some success has been reported with two other substances: anisomycin (a congener of rifampin) and clofazimine. However, they have not been approved by the FDA. *M. fortuitum* and *M. chelonii* (rapid growers) are resistant to the usual antituberculosis drugs but are variably susceptible to amikacin, cefoxitin, or trimethoprim-sulfamethoxazole (susceptibility testing can be performed rather readily to guide the choice of drug).

DRUGS USED IN TREATMENT OF LEPROSY

Chemotherapy of leprosy (Hansen's disease), a disease afflicting 12 to 15 million persons worldwide, has relied on **dapsone** (4,4'-diaminodiphenylsulfone) for over 40 years. This drug has been used in both lepromatous (disseminated) and tuberculoid leprosy (Table 55-1). Unfortunately, single-drug therapy has led to emergence of resistant organisms, and so multidrug therapy with dapsone and rifampin or clofazimine is now standard for lepromatous leprosy.

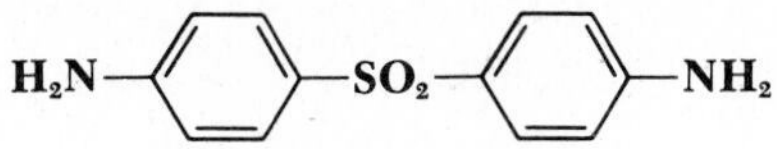

Dapsone

The precise mechanism of action of dapsone is unknown, but it probably acts like sulfonamides to inhibit bacterial metabolism of *p*-aminobenzoic acid. The drug is administered once daily, since it has a half-life of 20 to 40 hours. Initially, however, it is given in low doses (one tablet weekly) to minimize adverse reactions. Erythema nodosum of leprosy may be accelerated by the drug (a reaction prevented by thalidomide). A syndrome of severe skin lesions, hepatomegaly, and psychosis can also develop.[2] Otherwise the toxicity of dapsone is similar to that of sulfonamides, with added risk of methemoglobinemia, leukopenia, and agranulocytosis.[15]

Antitubercular drugs, including rifampin and ethionamide, are bactericidal for the bacilli and rapidly decrease the number of organisms. Since relapse can occur with single-drug therapy, treatment is begun with dapsone and rifampin for 6 months. Clofazimine, an experimental drug in the United States, is effective in patients with borderline-lepromatous and lepromatous leprosy.[2] It is weakly bactericidal and takes some time to decrease bacilli. Its major side effect is skin discoloration, a red-brown pigmentation that clears when the drug is discontinued.

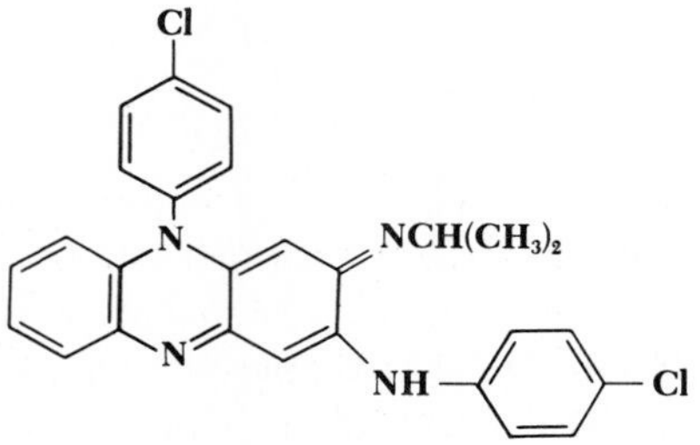

Clofazimine

Treatment of leprosy may lead to reversal reactions and erythema nodosum leprosum. In the reversal reaction, the patient experiences an acute neuritis, which is responsive to corticosteroids. Erythema nodosum leprosum is an inflammatory complication with acute onset of painful skin nodules and iridocyclitis. Thalidomide, corticosteroids, and clofazimine are effective therapy for this condition.[2] Thalidomide must not be used in women of childbearing age because of its teratogenic activity. It must be discontinued gradually or reactions will recur.

	Tablets or capsules (mg)	Vaginal tablets or suppositories (mg)	Topical preparations*
TABLE 55-2 Dosage forms of antifungal agents			
Drug			
A			
Nystatin (Mycostatin, others)	500,000 units	100,000 units	100,000 units
Amphotericin B (Fungizone)			3%
B			
Flucytosine (Ancobon)	250,500		
Miconazole nitrate (Monistat, Micatin)		100, 200	2%
Ketoconazole (Nizoral)	200		
Griseofulvin (Fulvicin, others)	125-500		
C			
Clotrimazole (Lotrimin, Mycelex)		100, 500	1%
Tolnaftate (Tinactin, others)			1%
Haloprogin (Halotex)			1%
Ciclopirox olamine (Loprox)			1%
Clioquinol (Vioform)			3%
Econazole nitrate (Spectazole)			1%
Triacetin (Enzactin)			25%

*Creams, gels, lotions, ointments, solutions.

Nystatin and amphotericin B (Table 55-2, *A*) are *polyene* antibiotics that complex with sterols, principally ergosterol, in fungal membranes.[14] Bacterial membranes are not injured by polyenes. However, mammalian membranes with cholesterol, such as red blood cells, may sustain injury, causing a reutilization type of anemia.

Nystatin used topically is effective against *Candida albicans* and some other fungi. When nystatin is given orally, its absorption is minimal and its action is restricted to the intestine.

Amphotericin B has been an effective antibiotic against deep-seated mycotic infections,[5] such as aspergillosis, mucormycosis, histoplasmosis, cryptococcosis, blastomycosis, coccidioidomycosis, and candidiasis. The drug is given intravenously for a total dose of 1 to 2 g over 4 to 8 weeks. Fever and chills may occur early; so test doses of 1 to 5 mg are injected on the first day.[14] If no untoward reaction occurs, a daily dose of 20 to 50 mg (not to exceed 0.5 mg/kg/day) is given over 2 to 5 hours. Adverse reactions include thrombophlebitis at the site of injection, gastrointestinal upset, and renal toxicity, such as renal tubular acidosis, hypocalcemia, and K^+ loss. Amphotericin B has a long elimination half-life (about 15 days), but serum concentration rarely exceeds 2 μg/ml. It is available as 50 mg vials that contain 41 mg of desoxycholate. The drug is reconstituted in dextrose in water because it aggregates in saline solution. If a long-term infusion (24 hours) is given, the drug must be shielded from light.

ANTIFUNGAL ANTIBIOTICS
Nystatin and amphotericin B

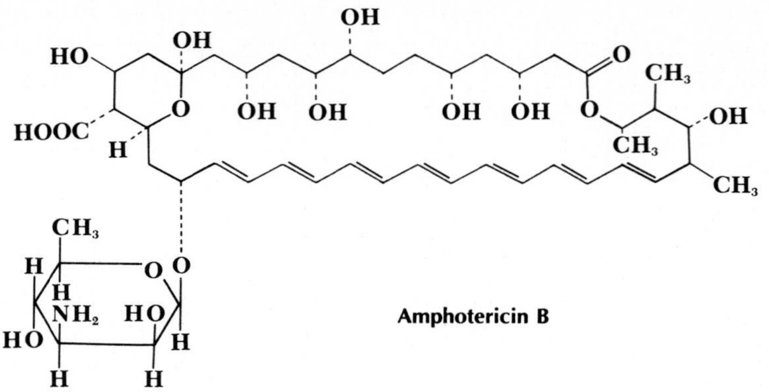

Amphotericin B

---

*Miscellaneous
antifungal agents*

Certain other antifungal agents are useful for systemic infections (Table 55-2, *B*).

Flucytosine is a fluorinated compound administered orally to treat infections caused by *Candida albicans,* especially of the urinary tract or localized infections.[14] For treatment of cryptococcal infections and central nervous system and bone infections caused by *Candida,* the drug is highly effective when combined with amphotericin B. Flucytosine may cause blood dyscrasias, especially leukopenia, hepatic toxicity, and diarrhea.[14] The usual dosage is 100 to 150 mg/kg/day, but serum concentration must be monitored so as not to exceed 100 μg/ml.

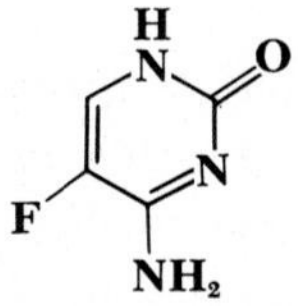

Flucytosine

Miconazole is an imidazole derivative that interferes with formation of the fungal plasma membrane sterol. It is rarely used intravenously, save for *C. albicans* infections in patients allergic to amphotericin B and infections with *Petriellidium boydii.* It is available for topical treatment of dermatophytosis and cutaneous candidal infections or as vaginal suppositories used daily for a week to treat candidiasis. Miconazole may cause intense pruritus.

Ketoconazole, another imidazole, is very effective for chronic mucocutaneous candidiasis, dermatophytosis, and mild systemic fungal infections, such as histoplasmosis and blastomycosis.[18] The drug is given orally, usually 400 mg/day for prolonged periods (6 to 12 months). It is generally well tolerated at this dose or less,[7] but infrequent toxicity includes gastrointestinal and hepatic manifestations, gynecomastia, and decreased libido. Ketoconazole blunts the adrenal response to ACTH but does not produce adrenal insufficiency.[18]

Griseofulvin, produced from a *Penicillium* mold, represents a novel approach to treatment of certain dermatomycoses. When given orally for long periods of time, griseofulvin is incorporated into the skin, hair, and nails where it exerts a fungistatic activity against various species of *Microsporum, Trichophyton,* and *Epidermophyton.* Prolonged administration is necessary because ringworm of the skin may require several weeks for improvement. In fungal infections of the nails, treatment may be needed for several months. The most common side effects are gastric discomfort, diarrhea, and headache. Urticaria and skin rash may also occur.

Griseofulvin

Still other antifungal agents have principal use as topical drugs for cutaneous mycotic infections (Table 55-2, *C*).

Clotrimazole, related structurally to miconazole, is used primarily as a topical fungicide or as vaginal tablets for candidiasis.

Tolnaftate, though effective in epidermophytosis, does not eliminate candidal organisms and is inadequate for fungal infections of the nails, scalp, and soles of the feet.

Undecylenic acid and its zinc salt are topical agents for mild epidermophytosis.

Natamycin (Natacyn), a polyene antibiotic, is used in a 5% ophthalmic suspension for fungal keratitis, blepharitis, and conjunctivitis.

REFERENCES

1. American Thoracic Society Statement: Treatment of tuberculosis and tuberculosis infection in adults and children, Am. Rev. Respir. Dis. **134**:355, 1986.
2. Binford, C.H., Meyers, W.M., and Walsh, G.P.: Leprosy, J.A.M.A. **247**: 2283, 1982.
3. Byrd, R.B., Horn, B.R., Soloman, D.A., and Griggs, G.A.: Toxic effects of isoniazid in tuberculosis chemoprophylaxis: role of biochemical monitoring in 1,000 patients, J.A.M.A. 241:1239, 1979.
4. Carpenter, J.L., Obnibene, A.J., Gorby, E.W., et al.: Antituberculosis drug resistance in South Texas, Am. Rev. Respir. Dis. **128**:1055, 1983.
5. Cohen, J.: Antifungal chemotherapy, Lancet **2**:532, 1982.
6. Deal, W.B., and Sanders, E.: Efficacy of rifampin in treatment of meningococcal carriers, N. Engl. J. Med. **281**:641, 1969.
7. Dismukes, W.E., Stamm, A.M., Graybill, J.R., et al.: Treatment of systemic mycoses with ketoconazole: emphasis on toxicity and clinical response in 52 patients; National Institute of Allergy and Infectious Diseases Collaborative Antifungal Study, Ann. Intern. Med. **98**:13, 1983.
8. Dutt, A.K., Moers, D., and Stead, W.W.: Short-course chemotherapy for extrapulmonary tuberculosis. Nine years' experience, Ann. Intern. Med. **104**:7, 1986.
9. Gangadharam, P.R.J.: Isoniazid, rifampin, and hepatotoxicity, Am. Rev. Respir. Dis. **133**:963, 1986.

10. Glassroth, J., Robins, A.G., and Snider, D.E., Jr.: Tuberculosis in the 1980s, N. Engl. J. Med. **302**:1441, 1980.

11. Hartmann, G., Honikel, K.O., Knüsel, F., and Nüesch, J.: The specific inhibition of the DNA-directed RNA synthesis by rifamycin, Biochim. Biophys. Acta **145**:843, 1967.

12. Hoeprich, P.D.: Alanine: cycloserine antagonism, Arch. Intern. Med. **112**:405, 1963.

13. Holdiness, M.R.: Clinical pharmacokinetics of the antituberculosis drugs, Clin. Pharmacokinet. **9**:511, 1984.

14. Medoff, G., and Kobayashi, G.S.: Strategies in the treatment of systemic fungal infections, N. Engl. J. Med. **302**:145, 1980.

15. Millikan, L.E.: Sulfones: a review of approved and investigational indications, Hosp. Formulary **17**:102, 1982.

16. Mitchell, J.R., Zimmerman, H.J., Ishak, K.G., et al.: Isoniazid liver injury: clinical spectrum, pathology, and probable pathogenesis, Ann. Intern. Med. **84**:181, 1976.

17. Mitchison, D.A., and Nunn, A.J.: Influence of initial drug resistance on the response to short-course chemotherapy of pulmonary tuberculosis, Am. Rev. Respir. Dis. **133**:423, 1986.

18. National Institute of Allergy and Infectious Diseases Mycoses Study Group: Treatment of blastomycosis and histoplasmosis with ketoconazole: results of a prospective randomized clinical trial, Ann. Intern. Med. **103**:861, 1985.

19. Robson, J.M., and Sullivan, F.M.: Antituberculosis drugs, Pharmacol. Rev. **15**:169, 1963.

20. Ruiz, R.C.: D-Cycloserine in the treatment of pulmonary tuberculosis resistant to the standard drugs: a study of 116 cases, Dis. Chest **45**:181, 1964.

21. Stead, W.W., and Dutt, A.K.: Chemotherapy for tuberculosis today, Am. Rev. Respir. Dis. **125**(suppl.):94, 1982.

22. Suwanogool, S., Smith, S.M., Smith, L.G., and Eng, R.: Drug-resistance encountered in the retreatment of *Mycobacterium tuberculosis* infections, J. Chronic Dis. **37**:925, 1984.

23. Youatt, J.: A review of the action of isoniazid, Am. Rev. Respir. Dis. **99**:729, 1969.

Chapter 56

Antiseptics and disinfectants

Antiseptics are drugs that are applied to living tissues to kill or inhibit growth of bacteria. *Disinfectants* are able to kill bacteria when applied to nonliving materials.[4] Related terms are defined as follows:

germicide Anything that destroys bacteria but not necessarily spores.
fungicide Anything that destroys fungi.
sporicide Anything that destroys spores.
sanitizer An agent that reduces the number of bacterial contaminants to a safe level, as may be judged by public health requirements.
preservative An agent or process that, by either chemical or physical means, prevents decomposition.

Disinfectants were used long before the discovery of bacteria. The first germicides were deodorants, since foul odors were associated with disease. Chlorinated soda (NaCl and NaClO) was used on infected wounds in the nineteenth century and was recommended to purify drinking water, since the soda appeared to diminish bacterial growth. Phenol was used as a deodorant and later as an antiseptic for infected wounds, long before the nature of infections was understood. The use of ethanol as an antiseptic was delayed for many years because Koch (1881) had reported that it did not kill anthrax spores. However, the fact that 70% ethanol had superior germicidal properties was established by Beyer (1912). Tincture of iodine was introduced into the *United States Pharmacopeia* in 1830 and was used extensively by the beginning of the Civil War.

Semmelweis, an assistant at the Lying-in Hospital in Vienna, demonstrated the benefits of cleansing the hands with chlorine-containing solutions for prevention of puerperal fever. He noted that the incidence of mortality attributable to puerperal sepsis was lower in women delivered by midwives than in those delivered by medical students (the first case-control study). The students delivered babies after performing autopsies, as noted by Semmelweis because of the odor in the delivery room when the students were present. He suspected that students were carrying "decomposing organic matter" (actually group A streptococci) from the autopsy room to the delivery room. Although he proved his hypothesis when cleansing of the students' hands with a solution of chloride and lime reduced fatalities, he was ostracized by the medical community, was hospitalized with psychiatric illness, and ultimately committed suicide.

The activity of antiseptics has been standardized by use of the *phenol coefficient,* the ratio of dilutions compared to phenol necessary to kill test organisms in vitro. Antiseptics were found to be useless for treating systemic infections, and so they are used only as external agents to prevent growth of bacteria.

ANTISEPTICS AND DISINFECTANTS

The only acceptable disinfectants for initial sterilization of equipment (Table 56-1) are 30-minute exposure to 8% formaldehyde (20% formalin) or 2% alkalinized glutaraldehyde.[4] Organic material, such as blood, exudates, and stool, will totally inactivate other germicides, precluding their use for instrument sterilization.[3] The alkalinized form of glutaraldehyde is as effective as other aqueous forms but less corrosive. These agents, if adequate contact is allowed, will kill all bacteria and all viruses, including hepatitis B and HIV. The causative agent of Creutzfeldt-Jakob disease is relatively resistant to formaldehyde, and so instruments used in surgery on possible cases (dementia) must be autoclaved for 60 minutes at 121° C. Inanimate objects can be treated with 5000 ppm hypochlorite solution.[4]

Alcohol and **iodine preparations** (iodophors) are commonly used for preoperative preparation of the skin. Ethanol is most bactericidal at 70% concentration by weight. Since tincture of iodine leaves stains on the skin and is irritating, povidone-iodine has been introduced for surgical scrubbing. It releases iodine slowly and is somewhat less irritating than tincture of iodine. It must be diluted to be effective. Recently, it has been shown to be the most active disinfectant for methicillin-resistant staphylococci, a common pathogen.[1]

Sodium hypochlorite releases chlorine. It is quite effective for cleaning spills and for killing viruses as well as bacteria.

Halazone, tetraglycine hydroperiodide (Globaline), and **aluminum hexaurea sulfate triiodide** (Hexadine-S) are used to disinfect water by means of halogen release.

The most widely used phenol derivative, **hexachlorophene,** is incorporated into soaps and creams. In a 3% solution, hexachlorophene (pHisoHex) causes a sharp reduction of gram-positive bacterial counts on the skin without being irritating. Hexachlorophene was formerly used for preoperative scrubbing but has been supplanted by iodophors with more generalized activity. Furthermore, the safety of hexachlorophene preparations, particularly for newborn infants, has been questioned because of potential absorption through the skin.

Chlorhexidine gluconate (Hibiclens, others) is a safe antiseptic, comparable to the iodophors, with broad antimicrobial activity against microorganisms. Its major advantage is its prolonged action, particularly against regrowth of resident flora.[2]

TABLE 56-1	Disinfection of medical equipment		
Level of disinfection	Germicidal	Sporicidal	Agents
High	Yes	Yes (long exposure)	8% formaldehyde 2% glutaraldehyde
Intermediate	Yes	No	70% ethanol 1% iodine 5000 ppm hypochlorite or iodophor
Low	Yes (not fungicidal or mycobactericidal)	No	75 ppm iodophor 1% phenolic quaternary ammonium compounds

From Simmons, B.P.: Infect. Control Urological Care 6:14-25, 1981.

Surface-active compounds have been popular but are weakly active agents. Their use as disinfectants is limited to use in soaps for hand washing (if surface action is obvious, people think that more disinfection takes place).

Anionic detergents, such as sodium lauryl sulfate and sodium ethasulfate, are antibacterial against gram-positive organisms but are not important bactericidal agents.

Quaternary ammoniums, such as benzalkonium (Zephiran), kill both gram-positive and gram-negative organisms but have little activity against many hospital strains. They should no longer be used in hospitals.

Surface-active compounds

Derivatives of mercury and silver have been widely used as skin antiseptics. They are largely bacteriostatic.

Silver nitrate in 1% solution has been traditionally used to prevent ophthalmia neonatorum caused by gonococci but is being replaced by application of penicillin or tetracycline to the conjunctival sac of the newborn infant. Silver is combined with a sulfonamide (Silvadene) as a successful antibacterial cream for burn patients.

Zinc sulfate ointment is used in some types of conjunctivitis, and zinc oxide ointment is a traditional remedy in a variety of skin diseases. Calamine lotion USP contains mostly zinc oxide with a small amount of ferric oxide. Phenolated calamine lotion USP also contains 1% phenol.

Metal-containing antiseptics

Acids   Acids, such as benzoic, salicylic, and undecylenic, have been used for many years as fungistatic agents. Whitfield's ointment is a mixture of 6% benzoic acid and 3% salicylic acid used to treat fungal infections of the feet.

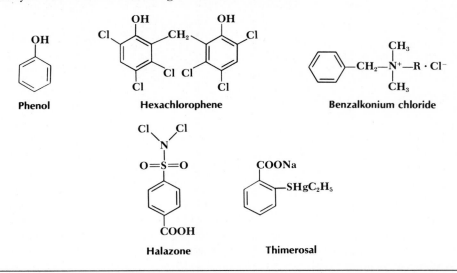

Phenol   **Hexachlorophene**   **Benzalkonium chloride**

Halazone   **Thimerosal**

REFERENCES

1. Haley, C.E., Marling-Cason, M., Smith, J.W., et al.: Bactericidal activity of antiseptics against methicillin-resistant *Staphylococcus aureus*, J. Clin. Microbiol. **21**:991, 1985.
2. Peterson, A.F., Rosenberg, A., and Alatary, S.D.: Comparative evaluation of surgical scrub preparations, Surg. Gynecol. Obstet. **146**:63, 1978.
3. Sanford, J.P.: Disinfectants that don't, Ann. Intern. Med. **72**:282, 1970.
4. Simmons, B.P.: Guidelines for hospital environmental control, Infect. Control Urological Care **6**:14, 1981.

Chapter 57

Drugs used to treat amebiasis and other intestinal protozoal infections

Amebiasis is caused by the protozoon *Entamoeba histolytica*. Its manifestations vary from asymptomatic carriers to dysentery and extraintestinal disease, particularly liver abscess. Antiamebic and other antiprotozoal drugs, which are usually given in courses of several days, are listed in Table 57-1.

METRONIDAZOLE

Drug therapy of moderate to severe amebiasis has been facilitated by use of metronidazole (Flagyl, others), which is safe, inexpensive, and effective for both intestinal and extraintestinal forms of the disease.[3,6] The drug also kills *Trichomonas* and *Giardia* (Table 57-1).[7] Metronidazole acts as an artificial electron acceptor after accumulating within the cell as the reduced compound.[4] This diverts electrons from normal pathways of the protozoon. Metronidazole also impairs the ability of DNA to function as a template. Although it is active against cysts and trophozoites, metronidazole is more effective in symptomatic or invasive amebiasis. It is also active in treatment of amebic liver abscess, but complications can occur. These are usually attributable to the size and position of the abscess and not to lack of activity of the drug.[3,5] Some, however, recommend use of emetine if there is no dramatic clinical improvement within 72 hours of therapy with metronidazole.[8] Side effects of metronidazole include gastrointestinal symptoms, stomatitis, a disulfiram-like reaction with ethanol, a change in urine color, and, rarely, neuropathy.[7] It should not be used during pregnancy. The drug is taken as tablets containing 250 or 500 mg.

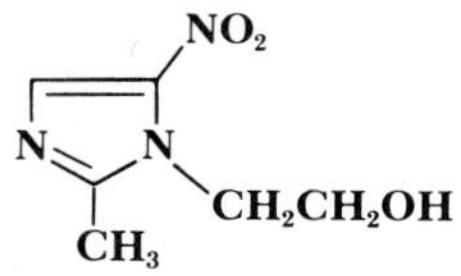

Metronidazole

EMETINE

Although emetine has been used for centuries to treat dysentery, toxicity limits its use for treatment of amebiasis.[3] This alkaloid of ipecac is amebicidal in vitro and on trophozoites localized in tissues. Emetine inhibits protein synthesis in the parasites and in mammalian cells by blocking translocation of peptide chains.[1]

TABLE 57-1	Drugs used to treat amebiasis, other intestinal protozoal infections, and *Trichomonas*			
	Drug	Dosage (mg)	Interval (hours)	Duration (days)
Amebiasis *(Entamoeba histolytica)*				
Asymptomatic (cyst passers)	Iodoquinol	650	8	20
	Paromomycin	25-35/kg/d	8	7
	Diloxanide furoate*	500	8	10
Symptomatic intestinal disease or hepatic abscess	Metronidazole	750	8	10
	If no response: dehy-droemetine*†	1-1.5/kg	24	≤5
	or			
	emetine*†	1/kg	24	≤5
Giardia lamblia	Quinacrine hydrochloride	100	8	5
	Metronidazole‡	250	8	5
	Furazolidone	100	6	7-10
		1.25/kg§	6	7-10
Balantidium coli	Tetracycline‡	500	6	10
Trichomonas vaginalis	Metronidazole	250‖	8	7

Primary source: Drugs for parasitic infections, Med. Lett. Drugs Ther. **28**:9, 1986.
*Available from the Centers for Disease Control, Atlanta, GA 30333 (telephone 404-329-3670, extension 3496, 8:00 AM to 4:30 PM EST, Monday through Friday).
†Intramuscular (others oral).
‡Considered investigational for this condition.
§Pediatric dose.
‖Or single 2 g dose.

Emetine

Emetine and dehydroemetine (Mebadin), a slightly less toxic moiety, are extremely toxic to cardiac and skeletal muscle.[1] Even at 1 mg/kg/day electrocardiographic changes such as T-wave inversion may occur. Emetine also causes gastrointestinal problems in 50% of patients, neurologic effects, and muscular pain and weakness after treatment of symptomatic disease. Patients should remain sedentary and have daily electrocardiograms performed before daily intramuscular administration.

IODOQUINOL   Iodoquinol (diiodohydroxyquin, Yodoxin, others) is recommended as an intestinal amebicide and for asymptomatic carriers. The related drug iodochlorhydroxyquin caused an epidemic of subacute myelo-optic neuropathy in Japan and is not used in the United States. In rare cases iodoquinol also causes this syndrome, but its most common adverse effects are related to the gastrointestinal tract. Tablets of 210 or 650 mg are available.

The mechanism of action of iodoquinol is not known. It is not well absorbed and so is therapeutic only for intestinal infection. Although the drug is recommended for additional therapy after metronidazole,[2] it is not readily available.

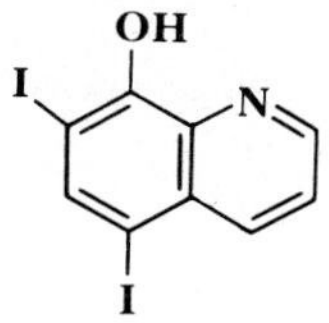

Iodoquinol

CHLOROQUINE

Chloroquine (Aralen) is a well-known antimalarial compound that has been combined with emetine to treat amebic abscess of the liver.[5] Chloroquine does not affect the intestinal form of *Entamoeba histolytica*.

The dosage of chloroquine as an alternative treatment is 1 g daily for 2 days, followed by 500 mg twice daily for 2 weeks.[2]

ANTIBIOTICS

Patients with intestinal amebiasis improve more rapidly when drugs such as tetracyclines are added to the usual antiamebic regimen. However, tetracyclines are not sufficient to effect a cure. Paromomycin (Humatin) and erythromycin are directly amebicidal, whereas tetracyclines modify the bacterial flora to influence amebas indirectly. Paromomycin is an alternative for asymptomatic carriers. Diloxanide furoate is amebicidal with minimal side effects, and so it probably should be the drug of choice for asymptomatic intestinal infections.[3]

REFERENCES

1. Balamuth, W., and Lasslo, A.: Comparative amoebacidal activity of some compounds related to emetine, Proc. Soc. Exp. Biol. Med. **80**:705, 1952.
2. Drugs for parasitic infections, Med. Lett. Drugs Ther. **28**:9, 1986.
3. Krogstad, D.J., Spencer, H.C., Jr., Healy, G.R., et al.: Amebiasis: epidemiologic studies in the United States, 1971-1974, Ann. Intern. Med. **88**:89, 1978.
4. Lindmark, D.G., and Müller, M.: Antitrichomonad action, mutagenicity, and reduction of metronidazole and other nitroimidazoles, Antimicrob. Agents Chemother. **10**:476, 1976.
5. Most, H.: Treatment of common parasitic infections of man encountered in the United States, N. Engl. J. Med. **287**:698, 1972.
6. Powell, S.J.: Therapy of amebiasis, Bull. N.Y. Acad. Med. **47**:469, 1971.
7. Roe, F.J.C.: Metronidazole: review of uses and toxicity, J. Antimicrob. Chemother. **3**:205, 1977.
8. Thompson, J.E., Jr., Forlenza, S., and Verma, R.: Amebic liver abscess: a therapeutic approach, Rev. Infect. Dis. **7**:171, 1985.

Chapter 58

Drugs used to treat malaria and other extraintestinal protozoal infections

MALARIA

For centuries malaria was treated with cinchona bark, from which the alkaloid quinine was extracted and used successfully as an antimalarial drug until World War II. More effective drugs then became available, and new concepts concerning antimalarial therapy evolved.[4] However, adaptation of the parasite to these drugs has created the modern problem of drug-resistant *Plasmodium*.[10]

Classification of antimalarial compounds can be based either on their activity in various stages of the life cycle of *Plasmodium* or on their mechanisms of action. Drugs that cure a clinical attack by eliminating the asexual forms are known as *schizonticides*. They include chloroquine, amodiaquine, quinine, hydroxychloroquine, and pyrimethamine. Tetracycline and combinations of a sulfonamide with pyrimethamine are effective also.

Radical cure implies the elimination from the body of both the asexual forms and the exoerythrocytic forms of the malarial parasite. Since there are no exoerythrocytic forms of falciparum malaria, the usual schizonticides are sufficient to achieve a radical cure. However, primaquine must be added to treatment to obtain a radical cure in *P. vivax* and *P. ovale* infections.

With regard to mechanisms of action, the 4- and 8-aminoquinolines, such as chloroquine and primaquine, appear to act by intercalation (insertion between base pairs) into DNA of the parasite. Another group of antimalarials, including pyrimethamine and sulfonamides, inhibit synthesis of folic acid from *p*-aminobenzoic acid.

Chloroquine

Chloroquine is a 4-aminoquinoline derivative, which was first synthesized in Germany in 1934. Subsequently, extensive studies showed that chloroquine was the most satisfactory of a group of related compounds, and it remains the drug of choice for most forms of malaria.[2]

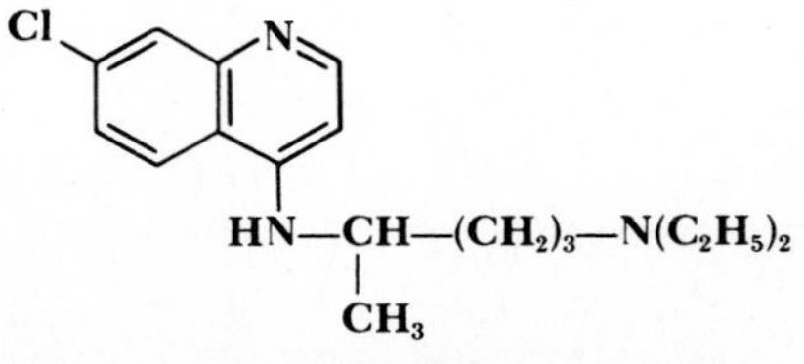

$$HN—CH—(CH_2)_3—N(C_2H_5)_2$$
$$CH_3$$

Chloroquine

TABLE 58-1   Drugs used to treat extraintestinal protozoal infections

	Drug	Dosage (oral unless specified otherwise)
Malaria (except for chloroquine-resistant *Plasmodium falciparum*)		
Chemoprophylaxis	Chloroquine phosphate	500 mg once weekly (from 2 weeks before until 6 weeks after exposure)
If infection very likely	Primaquine phosphate	15 mg daily for 14 days during last 2 weeks of chloroquine
Treatment	Chloroquine phosphate	1 g, then 500 mg in 6 hours and daily for 2 more days
To prevent relapses	Primaquine phosphate	15 mg daily for 14 days; 45 mg weekly for 4 weeks if G-6-PD deficient
Chloroquine-resistant *P. falciparum*		
Chemoprophylaxis	Pyrimethamine +	25 mg weekly and for 6 weeks after exposure
	Sulfadoxine	500 mg weekly and for 6 weeks after exposure
Treatment	Quinine sulfate +	650 mg daily for 3 days
	Pyrimethamine +	25 mg twice daily for 3 days
	Sulfadiazine	500 mg four times daily for 5 days
	or	
	Quinine sulfate +	As above
	Tetracycline	250 mg four times daily for 7 days
	or	
	Quinine sulfate +	As above
	Clindamycin	900 mg three times daily for 3 days
Pneumocystis carinii	Trimethoprim-sulfamethoxazole	5 mg/kg trimethoprim four times daily, orally or intravenously, for 14 days
	or	
	Pentamidine isethionate	4 mg/kg daily for 14 days intramuscularly or intravenously
Toxoplasmosis	Pyrimethamine +	25 mg daily for 4 weeks
	Short-acting sulfonamide	2-6 g daily for 4 weeks
Trypanosomiasis		
Trypanosoma gambiense or *T. rhodesiense*		
Hemolymphatic stage	Suramin*	100-200 mg, then 1 g repeated intravenously on days 1, 3, 7, 14, and 21
	or	
	Pentamidine isethionate	4 mg/kg daily for 10 days
CNS involvement	Melarsoprol*	2 mg/kg daily intravenously for 3 days; after 1 week, 3.6 mg/kg daily for 3 days; repeat in 10 to 21 days
T. cruzi	Nifurtimox*	8-10 mg/kg daily divided into 4 doses, for 120 days
Leishmanial infections	Sodium stibogluconate	20 mg/kg daily intravenously or intramuscularly for 20 days (may be repeated)

Primary source: Drugs for parasitic infections, Med. Lett. Drugs Ther. 28:9, 1986.
*Obtain from the Centers for Disease Control, Atlanta, GA 30333 (telephone 404-329-3670, extension 3496, 8:00 AM to 4:30 PM EST, Monday through Friday).

Chloroquine is highly effective against susceptible strains of *Plasmodium* (Table 58-1). It can produce a radical cure in susceptible falciparum malaria but is suppressive only for *P. vivax and P. ovale,* since it will not eliminate the exoerythrocytic forms. Thus the drug can terminate clinical attacks very efficiently, but relapses occur in vivax malaria.

METABOLISM   Chloroquine is rapidly and almost completely absorbed from the gastrointestinal tract. Its distribution is unusual in that some tissues, such as liver, concentrate the drug; a loading dose must be given.

Chloroquine phosphate (Aralen) is available as 250 and 500 mg tablets (150 and 300 mg base). For treatment a total dose of 2.5 g is given over about 2 days (Table 58-1). Chloroquine (40 mg/ml) as the hydrochloride can be injected by the intramuscular route if necessary for cerebral malaria or severe illness, in a dose of 250 mg. For chronic suppression of sensitive strains in an endemic area, one 500 mg tablet is taken weekly from 2 weeks before exposure until 6 weeks after leaving.

TOXICITY   The toxicity of chloroquine is quite low when a total dose of 2.5 g is given. Rarely, dizziness, blurring of vision, headache, diarrhea, and epigastric distress may occur. The drug should be given cautiously to persons with liver disease but is safe for pregnant women and nonnursing mothers.

RESISTANCE TO CHLOROQUINE   Chloroquine-resistant *Plasmodium falciparum* has been encountered with increasing frequency in South America, Southeast Asia, and Africa. Although chloroquine or quinine therapy reduces parasitemia, patients relapse within 2 weeks. Drug combinations that include quinine with pyramethamine and sulfadiazine or with tetracycline or clindamycin have reasonable success (Table 58-1).

Amodiaquin   Amodiaquin is similar to chloroquine as an antimalarial. It is given by mouth in doses of 0.6 g daily as a suppressive antimalarial or 1.8 g in divided doses the first day, followed by 0.6 g/day for 2 or 3 days for clinical control. Recently its use was associated with several cases of agranulocytosis, with death in some, and so the Centers for Disease Control has recommended against its use for prophylaxis in malaria.[1]

Amodiaquin

Hydroxychloroquine   Hydroxychloroquine sulfate (Plaquenil), another 4-aminoquinoline very similar to chloroquine without significant advantages over the parent drug, is available in tablets, 155 mg.

Certain 8-aminoquinolines act on the exoerythrocytic stage of malarial parasites. *Primaquine* Primaquine is at present considered the most effective representative of this group of drugs.

Primaquine

The development of primaquine was an outgrowth of research on the synthetic antimalarial pamaquine. Related 8-aminoquinolines were synthesized during World War II, of which several were found to be safer than pamaquine.

Primaquine is useful in producing radical cure in *Plasmodium vivax* infections because of its effect on the exoerythrocytic stages.[4] It has some activity against the asexual forms but not enough to make it an efficient suppressive as well as curative drug. For this reason primaquine is nearly always given in combination with a suppressive antimalarial agent. Concomitant administration of chloroquine as a suppressive coupled with primaquine for 14 days will achieve a radical cure of vivax malaria. In a comparable group receiving chloroquine alone, the relapse rate was 39%.[4]

Primaquine is rapidly absorbed from the gastrointestinal tract. In contrast with chloroquine, however, it is also rapidly metabolized and excreted. Primaquine phosphate is available in tablets, 15 mg.

Although primaquine is generally well tolerated at the recommended therapeutic dosages, some patients may complain of anorexia, nausea, abdominal cramps, and other vague symptoms. There may be depression of bone-marrow activity, with leukopenia and anemia. The drug can cause methemoglobinemia that is aggravated by concomitant use of quinacrine.

Hemolytic anemia can follow primaquine therapy in persons with a genetic deficiency of glucose-6-phosphate dehydrogenase (G-6-PD; see p. 55). In persons of Mediterranean origin with the defect, red blood cells of all ages are hemolyzed, whereas in blacks, usually males, only older red blood cells are hemolyzed and the anemia is less severe. Some have recommended weekly doses of 45 mg for 4 to 6 weeks for G-6-PD–deficient patients, especially since they rarely have a fall in hematocrit below 27 or so.[2,3]

Pyrimethamine (Daraprim) inhibits the dihydrofolate reductase of malarial parasites. Resistance to its action develops rapidly when used alone, and for this reason the drug is used, in combination with other drugs, only for prophylaxis and treatment of chloroquine-resistant *P. falciparum* malaria.

Pyrimethamine

Pyrimethamine appears safe in doses of 25 to 50 mg once or twice a week. Megaloblastic anemia of a transient nature has occurred in some persons. This response may be related to metabolic antagonism of folic acid or folinic acid. The drug is taken as tablets of 25 mg.

Pyrimethamine is not recommended for an acute malarial attack because it is slow acting. It is, however, useful in combination with sulfonamides for malaria and toxoplasmosis.[7] A combination of pyrimethamine with sulfadoxine (Fansidar) has been used for prophylaxis against *P. falciparum* in those who stay overnight in rural endemic areas (Asia, South America). However, deaths attributable to severe Stevens-Johnson syndrome have been reported to the Centers for Disease Control; thus caution must be used. It has been recommended that travelers to countries with chloroquine-resistant *P. falciparum* carry three tablets of Fansidar to be taken promptly as a single dose if a febrile illness develops.[8]

| Trimethoprim | Trimethoprim (Trimpex) is a synthetic diaminopyrimidine compound related to pyrimethamine. Both inhibit dihydrofolate reductase. Trimethoprim in combination with sulfamethoxazole has been used for malaria, as treatment for bacterial infections (see p. 636) and most recently as the drug of choice in *Pneumocystis carinii* infections[5] in patients with AIDS. This combination can be given intravenously at a daily dose of 20 mg/kg, as four divided doses, initially and continued orally for 14 days. Skin reactions are increased in patients with AIDS. |

| Other antimalarial drugs | **Quinine,** the traditional antimalarial remedy, is a suppressive drug only. Even as a suppressive, it is not nearly so effective as chloroquine or other newer antimalarial drugs. However, quinine has become very important again, in combination with other agents, in treatment of chloroquine-resistant falciparum malaria. It is rapidly absorbed, and most of it is metabolized, about 20% being excreted unchanged in the urine and the remainder in the form of metabolic products. Metabolism and excretion are both rapid, and no cumulation occurs when it is given daily for long periods of time. Quinine sulfate is available in capsules (130 to 325 mg) and tablets (260 and 325 mg). In a patient who cannot take or tolerate orally administered quinine, the drug may be given as the dihydrochloride by slow intravenous drip. For this purpose 650 mg of quinine is dissolved in 300 ml of saline solution and given over 2 to 4 hours.[2] However, blood concentration must be monitored, particularly in persons with renal failure. Quinidine, an optical isomer of quinine, also can be given intravenously, with a cure achieved in some cases.[9] |

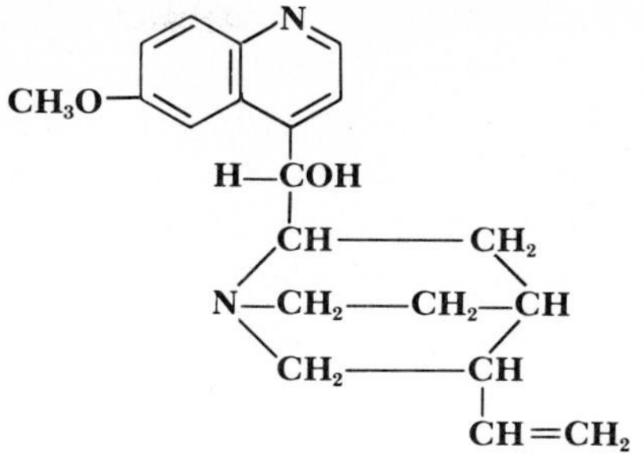

Quinine

Quinine can produce a variety of toxic effects, some of which are known by the collective name *cinchonism*. Headache, nausea, tinnitus, and visual disturbances can occur. Allergic skin rashes and asthmatic attacks have also been reported.

Quinine has other uses in medicine. It is given occasionally to relieve leg cramps, in treatment of myotonia congenita, and as a sclerosing agent.

Quinacrine (Atabrine) is a yellow acridine derivative. It was once an important antimalarial, but chloroquine has so many advantages over quinacrine that the latter is gradually being abandoned. It is used for other purposes, as in treatment of certain tapeworm infestations (see Chapter 59) and *Giardia* infection (see Table 57-1).[2]

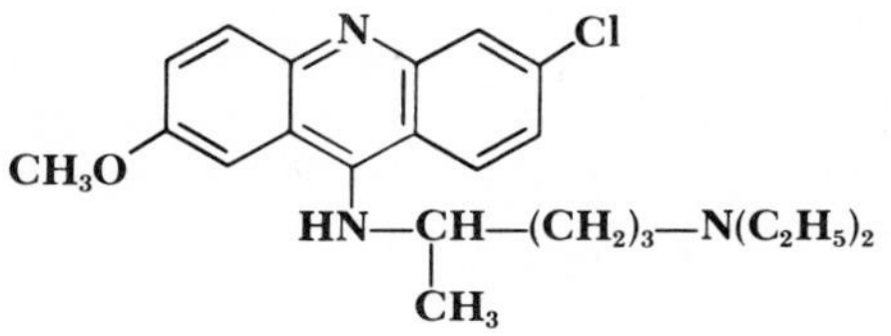

Quinacrine

Tetracycline and doxycycline are effective in treatment of chloroquine-resistant *P. falciparum*.[2] In fact, doxycycline may be effective prophylaxis in persons who are allergic to sulfonamides.[8]

Trypanosomal infections are important diseases in the Southern Hemisphere. Subspecies are responsible for sleeping sickness in tsetse-infested areas of equatorial Africa. Of the three drugs available for routine treatment of human trypanosomiasis, none is well tolerated.[6] **Suramin** (Germanin, others), a nonmetallic dye, is used to treat early cases of both Gambian and Rhodesian forms of the disease. It is given orally first, as a test dose of 0.2 g, to be followed by five 1 g doses intravenously at 3- to 7-day intervals. Renal toxicity is the most severe side effect. **Pentamidine isethionate** (Lomidine, Pentam 300), a diamidine that produces hypoglycemia with an indirect effect on the protozoon, is also useful in early cases of sleeping sickness. It is of more importance now as therapy of *Pneumocystis* pneumonia in patients with

ANTITRYPANO-SOMAL DRUGS

AIDS. Side effects, including hypotension, hypoglycemia, blood dyscrasias, and renal failure, are commonplace. **Melarsoprol** (Arsobal) is an organic compound of arsenic that is effective in treatment of late African trypanosomiasis involvement in the central nervous system. The drug of choice for Chagas disease is **Nifurtimox** (Lampit). It is variably effective for acute cases and is associated with significant side effects that involve the central nervous system and gastrointestinal tract.

Leishmania   Pentavalent antimonials are the drugs of choice for leishmanial infections. Their mechanism of action is unknown. **Sodium stibogluconate** (Pentostam) is given intravenously or intramuscularly (maximum of 800 mg/day).[2] Muscle pain and gastrointestinal side effects occasionally result.

REFERENCES

1. Agranulocytosis associated with the use of amodiaquine for malaria prophylaxis, MMWR **35**:165, 1986.
2. Drugs for parasitic infections, Med. Lett. Drugs Ther. **28**:9, 1986.
3. Health status of Indochinese refugees, MMWR **28**:385, 1979.
4. Howells, R.E.: Advances in chemotherapy, Br. Med. Bull. **38**:193, 1982.
5. Hughes, W.T.: *Pneumocystis carinii* pneumonia, N. Engl. J. Med. **297**:1381, 1977.
6. James, D.M., and Gilles, H.M.: The trypanosomiases. In James, D.M., editor: Human antiparasitic drugs: pharmacology and usage, Chichester, 1985, John Wiley & Sons, p. 72.
7. Krick, J.A., and Remington, J.S.: Toxoplasmosis in the adult: an overview, N. Engl. J. Med. **298**:550, 1978.
8. Outbreak of malaria imported from Kenya, MMWR **35**:567, 1986.
9. White, N.J., Looareesuwan, S., Warrell, D.A., et al.: Quinidine in falciparum malaria, Lancet **2**:1069, 1981.
10. Wyler, D.J.: Malaria: resurgence, resistance, and research, N. Engl. J. Med. **308**:875 and 934, 1983.

Chapter 59

Anthelmintic drugs

GENERAL
CONCEPT

Antiparasitic chemotherapy, especially for intestinal human helmintic infections, has undergone important advances and developments recently. The new anthelmintics are safer and are frequently effective in a single course of therapy (Table 59-1). An effective drug for treatment of schistosomiasis, praziquantel, is now available, and the price has been reduced so that mass application at low cost per unit course of treatment is possible.[1] For all anthelmintics, cost is as important as efficacy in determining which agent is distributed.[9]

INDIVIDUAL
ANTHELMINTICS
Thiabendazole

The first imidazole anthelmintic in general use was thiabendazole. The drug is absorbed rapidly after oral administration, inactivated in the liver by hydroxylation, and excreted as a conjugate in urine and feces. Thiabendazole inhibits fumarate reductase, a key enzyme in ATP production under anaerobic conditions.[3] Vermicidal actions of the drug may be attributable to negative effects on energy metabolism or to microtubular disruption as a consequence of colchicine-like binding to tubulin dimers.

Thiabendazole has a wide spectrum of anthelmintic activity, but side effects (nausea, chills, vertigo, hypotension, hallucinosis, leukopenia, crystalluria) have limited its use. It remains a first-line drug for strongyloidiasis, though after a single use many refuse to take the drug again.[5] The drug is ovicidal and larvicidal.

Thiabendazole (Mintezol) is dispensed as chewable tablets (500 mg) and oral suspensions (500 mg/5 ml). The drug is taken twice daily after meals.

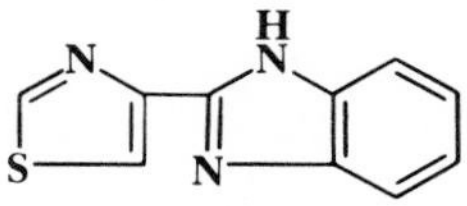

Thiabendazole 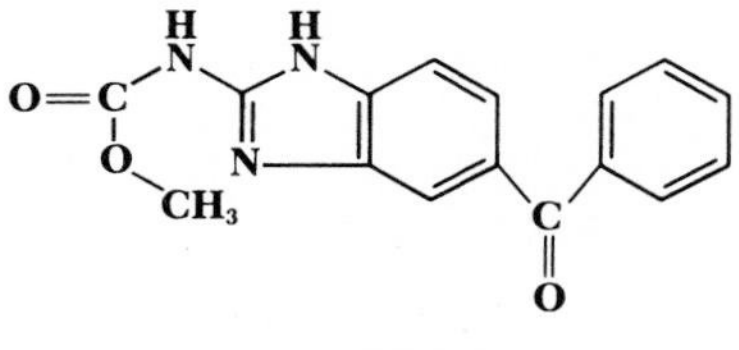   **Mebendazole**

Mebendazole

Mebendazole (Vermox) is one of several thiabendazole congeners that retain the broad spectrum of activity but with fewer untoward reactions. Mebendazole is a first-line drug for *Trichuris, Enterobius, Ascaris,* and hookworm infections.[2] In most of these the cure rate exceeds 90%. Mebendazole, like thiabendazole, depletes hel-

TABLE 59-1   Anthelmintic drug applications

Organism	Drugs of choice	Usual oral* adult dose
Nematodes—intestinal		
Strongyloides stercoralis (threadworm)	Thiabendazole	25 mg/kg twice daily for 2 days
Trichuris trichiura (whipworm)	Mebendazole	100 mg twice daily for 3 days
Enterobius vermicularis (pinworm)	Mebendazole or	100 mg single dose; repeat in 2 weeks
	pyrantel pamoate	11 mg/kg single dose; repeat in 2 weeks
Ascaris lumbricoides (roundworm)	Mebendazole or	100 mg twice daily for 3 days
	pyrantel pamoate	11 mg/kg single dose
Necator americanus and *Ancylostoma duodenale* (hookworms)	Mebendazole or	100 mg twice daily for 3 days
	pyrantel pamoate	11 mg/kg single dose
Trichostrongylus species	Pyrantel pamoate† or	11 mg/kg single dose
	mebendazole†	100 mg twice daily for 3 days
Nematodes—extraintestinal		
Wuchereria bancrofti, W. malayi, Loa loa, Acanthocheilonema perstans (filariasis)	Diethylcarbamazine‡	50 mg first day, 150 mg second day, 300 mg third day, then 6 mg/kg/day for 18 days
Onchocerca volvulus	Diethylcarbamazine‡ followed by	25 mg/day for 3 days, then 50 mg/day for 5 days, then 100 mg/day for 3 days, then 150 mg/day for 12 days
	suramin‡	100-200 mg intravenously, then 1 g/week for 5 weeks
Dracunculus medinensis (guinea worm)	Niridazole‡ or	25 mg/kg/day for 10 days
	metronidazole†	250 mg three times daily for 10 days
Trichinella spiralis (trichinosis)	Thiabendazole (plus corticosteroids)	25 mg/kg twice daily for 5 days
Larva migrans (creeping eruption)	Thiabendazole	25 mg/kg twice daily for 5 days
Trematodes		
Schistosoma haematobium, S. japonicum, S. mekongi	Praziquantel	20 mg/kg three times in 1 day
S. mansoni	Praziquantel or	20 mg/kg three times in 1 day
	oxamniquine	15 mg/kg single dose
Clonorchis sinesis, Fasciola hepatica (flukes)	Praziquantel† or	25 mg/kg three times in 1 day
	bithionol‡	30-50 mg/kg alternate days for 10 to 15 doses
Cestodes		
Diphyllobothrium latum, Taenia saginata, T. solium, Dipylidium caninum (tapeworms)	Niclosamide or	2 g (1 g twice at 1-hour interval)
	praziquantel†	10-20 mg/kg single dose
Hymenolepis nana (dwarf tapeworm)	Praziquantel† or	25 mg/kg single dose
	niclosamide	2 g once daily for 7 days
Cysticercus cellulosae	Praziquantel†	50 mg/kg daily for 15 days

Primary data from Drugs for parasitic infections, Med. Lett. Drugs Ther. **28:**9, 1986.
*Unless otherwise indicated.
†Investigational for this indication.
‡Available from the Centers for Disease Control, Atlanta, GA 30333 (telephone 404-329-3670, extension 3496, 8:00 AM to 4:30 PM EST, Monday through Friday).

minth energy stores and disrupts the capacity for cytoskeletal transport by binding to tubulin.[8] Mebendazole is poorly absorbed, and so colonic concentrations are high. This lack of absorption may account for its fewer side effects. Since it is teratogenic in animals, it should not be given to women who are or may become pregnant.

For most infections, a 100 mg tablet is chewed twice daily for several days. Pinworms can be eradicated with a single dose, but reinfection may necessitate periodic readministration. Filariasis (for which mebendazole is a second-line drug) requires daily therapy for a month.

Pyrantel

Pyrantel is useful against intestinal nematodes by its action to cause neuromuscular blockade in the worms so that they can no longer maintain the tone necessary to attach to host tissues.[6] Pyrantel depolarizes worm muscle. The persistent nicotinic activation by pyrantel paralyzes the worms, and they are expelled by host peristalsis.

Because pyrantel is poorly absorbed, intestinal parasites are exposed to high concentrations after oral administration. The small fraction that is absorbed causes minimal side effects (dizziness, headache, rash, fever). Pyrantel pamoate (Antiminth) is marketed as an oral suspension, 250 mg/5 ml. It can be given as a single dose with over 90% effectivensss for *Ascaris, Enterobius,* or hookworm infection.

Pyrantel   **Diethylcarbamazine**   **Piperazine hexahydrate**

Piperazine

Piperazine citrate is converted in vivo to the hexahydrate. It is now considered alternative therapy for *Ascaris* and *Enterobius* infections. Piperazine can cause gastrointestinal and allergic reactions, since it is readily absorbed from the intestine. Some persons taking piperazine develop an ataxia that has been given the sobriquet "worm wobble." Between 15% and 75% of a dose may be recovered unchanged in the urine. Piperazine paralyzes worms by hyperpolarizing their skeletal muscles.[3] Since pyrantel and piperazine have opposing actions on membrane potentials of muscle fibers, they are never coadministered.

In persons very heavily infested with *Ascaris*, mebendazole has been reported to cause aberrant migration of worms into the bile duct and nasopharyngeal cavities. A suggested preventive measure is to give a single dose of piperazine to paralyze the worms before giving mebendazole to kill them. Piperazine citrate (Antepar) can be taken as tablets, 250 or 500 mg, or as an oral solution of 500 mg/5 ml; tablets containing 500 mg as the tartrate are also available (all in hexahydrate equivalents).

Diethylcarbamazine

The drug of choice for filariasis and *Onchocerca* infections is diethylcarbamazine, a piperazine derivative. Its mode of action is unclear, but it kills microfilariae and may kill adult worms. When microfilariae of *O. volvulus* are killed by the drug, violent allergic manifestations may occur. Reversible allergic reactions to the drug itself are less frequent if the dosage is increased slowly to the desired level (Table 59-1). Diethylcarbamazine citrate (Hetrazan) is dispensed as 50 mg tablets. Antihistamines may be required to reduce allergic reactions. Surgical incision of *Onchocerca* nodules before therapy is recommended by some.

Niclosamide

Tapeworm infections are treated with niclosamide. The drug inhibits oxidative phosphorylation in the mitochondria of cestodes and kills proximal worm segments and the scolex so that these appear in the feces severely damaged.[6] Since mature eggs are still viable, there is a risk that *Taenia solium* ova, the larvae of the pig tapeworm, will become invasive to produce cysticercons. Hence treatment of *T. solium* with niclosamide should be followed in an hour or two by a cathartic purge. The drug should not be used if there is intestinal obstruction. It is not absorbed by the host, and the incidence of side effects (nausea, abdominal pain) is very low.

Niclosamide (Niclocide) is available as 500 mg chewable tablets. Adults and children over 8 take two doses of 1 g each 1 hour apart for treatment of *T. saginata*, *T. solium*, and *Diphyllobothrium latum* (fish tapeworm) infestations.

Niclosamide   **Praziquantel**

Praziquantel

The drug of choice for dwarf tapeworm, *Hymenolepis nana*, and for liver and intestinal flukes is praziquantel. Now available after extensive clinical trials, this compound as a one-time dose has a better cure rate than niclosamide for *H. nana*. Praziquantel is particularly effective against schistosomes that infect humans.[1] Traditionally, schistosomiasis has been one of the more difficult infestations to treat. Praziquantel is readily absorbed from the gut. It is metabolized rapidly by the host but not by the worms, which seem to concentrate the drug. Its action appears to cause changes in integument permeability to monovalent and divalent cations. In the tapeworm, influx of calcium is believed responsible for muscular spasticities that dislocate the worm from the intestinal wall. Side effects thus far have been mild (sedation, headache, nausea, rash), transient (a few minutes to an hour), and infrequent (less than 5% of patients).[1] Praziquantel (Biltricide), in 600 mg tablets, is given three times in 1 day with over 90% effectiveness for all species of schistosomes. It has also been used successfully in investigative trials for treatment of central nervous cysticercosis, 50 mg/kg divided over three doses daily for 15 days.[4]

Pyrvinium pamoate (Povan) is a pink cyanine dye that inhibits tissue respiration and glycolysis in intestinal nematodes. It was formerly used mostly in pinworm infections, but nausea and vomiting led to many discolored sheets.

Suramin (Germanin, others) is used as follow-up therapy to a course of diethylcarbamazine for onchocerciasis. Suramin is given intravenously at weekly intervals to kill circulating microfilariae that persist after diethylcarbamazine administration.

Niridazole (Ambilhar) kills certain extraintestinal worms, specifically *Schistosoma haematobium*, *S. japonicum*, and *Dracunculus medinensis*. The initial effect of the drug is to damage female reproductive tissues and decrease egg production. Presently, it is recommended only for *Dracunculus* infection. It can cause gastrointestinal side effects and headache.

Metronidazole (Flagyl), used primarily for its amebicidal and trichomonacidal activities (see Chapter 57), also has limited utility as an alternative drug for *Dracunculus* infection.

Metrifonate (Bilarcil), an organophosphorus inhibitor of trematode cholinesterase, was once a drug of choice for *Schistosoma haematobium*. Although available from the Centers for Disease Control, it has now been replaced by praziquantel.

Oxamniquine (Vansil) is an alternative for infections with *Schistosoma mansoni*, particularly South American strains. In Brazil more than 7 million people have been treated successfully with the drug.[7] Capsules contain 250 mg of the drug.

Bithionol (Bitin, Lorothidol) was used for lung and liver flukes but seems to be less effective for liver flukes than praziquantel. Side effects include photosensitivity and urticaria.

Paromomycin (Humatin) is a nonabsorbable antibiotic that is cestodicidal. Its main use has been as an alternative for infections with *T. saginata*, *T. solium*, and *H. nana*.

REFERENCES

1. Archer, S.: The chemotherapy of schistosomiasis, Annu. Rev. Pharmacol. Toxicol. **25**:485, 1985.
2. Drugs for parasitic infections, Med. Lett. Drugs Ther. **28**:9, 1986.
3. Mansour, T.E.: Chemotherapy of parasitic worms: new biochemical strategies, Science **205**:462, 1979.
4. Nash, T.E., and Neva, F.A.: Recent advances in the diagnosis and treatment of cerebral cysticercosis, N. Engl. J. Med. **311**:1492, 1984.
5. Pelletier, L.L., Jr.: Chronic strongyloidiasis in World War II Far East ex-prisoners of war, Am. J. Trop. Med. Hyg. **33**:55, 1984.
6. Sheth, U.K.: Mechanisms of anthelmintic action, Prog. Drug Res. **19**:147, 1975.
7. Stürchler, D.: Chemotherapy of human intestinal helminthiases: a review, with particular reference to community treatment, Adv. Pharmacol. Chemother. **19**:129, 1982.
8. Van den Bossche, H., Rochette, F., and Hörig, C.: Mebendazole and related anthelmintics, Adv. Pharmacol. Chemother. **19**:67, 1982.
9. Wang, C.C.: Current problems in antiparasite chemotherapy, Trends Biochem. Sci. **7**:354, 1982.

Chapter 60

Drugs used in chemotherapy of neoplastic disease

The search for pharmacologic approaches to neoplastic disease has made impressive gains during the past 30 years. Drugs can cure patients having choriocarcinoma, Hodgkin's disease, acute lymphatic and myelogenous leukemia, and testicular cancer.[6] In combination with surgery and radiation, drugs have prolonged life in many other forms of cancer, though the quality of life is often impaired.

The current emphasis in cancer chemotherapy is on use of combinations of drugs. Such combinations take into account the phase of the cell cycle affected by each drug and potential synergistic actions in attempts to increase efficacy and decrease emergence of cell resistance.[3] The cell cycle is divided into several phases: G_0, G_1 (gap$_1$), S_1 (synthesis), G_2, M (mitosis). The resting phase is designated as G_0. The G_1 phase ends with a sudden increase in RNA synthesis, which signals the beginning of the S phase. During the S phase there is a pronounced increase in DNA synthesis, which ceases when cells enter the short G_2 phase, which ends with the mitotic process (M phase). Cancer chemotherapeutic agents may be *cell cycle–specific* or *cell cycle–nonspecific*. Resting cells do not respond to cell cycle–specific agents. However, they may respond to alkylating agents or to other agents that combine directly with DNA.

The lack of specificity of cancer chemotherapeutic agents for malignant cells compared to relatively rapidly but normally proliferating cells such as bone marrow, skin, and intestinal mucosa results in a very narrow margin of safety for these agents. Advances in understanding of drug action, of mechanisms of their toxicity, and of tumor biology have continually led to changes in dosing and scheduling of certain drugs. For example, continuous infusion of anthracyclines in attempts to decrease cardiotoxicity, continuous infusion of *Vinca* alkaloids to increase cell kill, and low-, moderate-, or high-dose methotrexate (20 to >20,000 mg/m^2/dose) are all being used or evaluated in current treatment regimens. Therefore, as opposed to prior editions of this text, specific dosage and regimens for different diseases have been omitted. Information as to drug dose and schedule should be obtained by consultation of protocols written to facilitate treatment of the patient.

The antineoplastic activity of nitrogen mustards was discovered during World War II as an outgrowth of earlier observations on the leukopenic effect of mustard gas (bis[2-chloroethyl]sulfide). Subsequently, the less toxic nitrogen mustards (bis[2-chloroethyl]amines) and eventually many other alkylating agents were introduced into chemotherapy of neoplastic diseases.

DEVELOPMENT OF ANTINEOPLASTIC CHEMOTHERAPY

The development of folic acid antagonists and other antimetabolites as potential antitumor agents originated from observations on the role of folic acid in both white cell production and as an "antianemia" factor. It seemed reasonable that compounds structurally related to folic acid could inhibit white cell production, and this was indeed demonstrated. These observations stimulated interest in other metabolic antagonists as possible chemotherapeutic agents, and eventually several purine, pyrimidine, and amino acid antagonists were discovered. Since proliferating cells are the main target for antineoplastic agents, nucleic acid biosynthesis and DNA have been the chief targets of the chemotherapeutic approach to cancer.

The drugs currently used in management of malignant diseases fall into several categories (Table 60-1).

CLASSIFICATION

The sites and mechanisms of action of various cancer chemotherapeutic agents are indicated in Fig. 60-1.

The alkylating agents are highly reactive compounds that transfer alkyl groups to important cell constituents by combining with amino, sulfhydryl, carboxyl, and phosphate groups.[1] They are *cell cycle–nonspecific;* they can combine with cells in any phase of their cycle. It is believed that these drugs alkylate DNA, and more specifically guanine, as a primary mechanism of cell kill. This basic action may explain their preferential toxicity for rapidly multiplying cells.

ALKYLATING AGENTS

Mechlorethamine (nitrogen mustard) must be injected intravenously because it is highly reactive. More recently, attempts have been made to inject the drug intra-arterially, close to the tumor. Because it disappears very rapidly from the blood, the activity of mechlorethamine lasts only a few minutes.

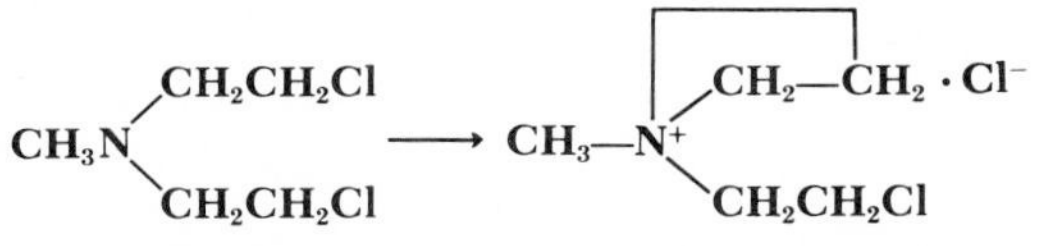

Nitrogen mustard   Ethyleneimmonium intermediate 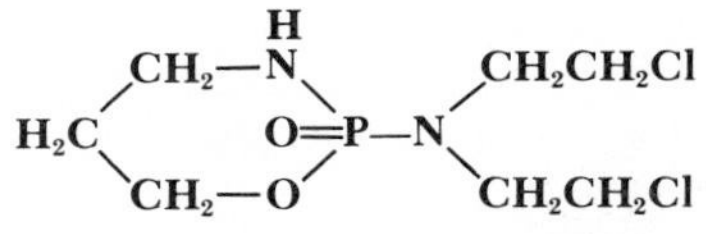   Cyclophosphamide

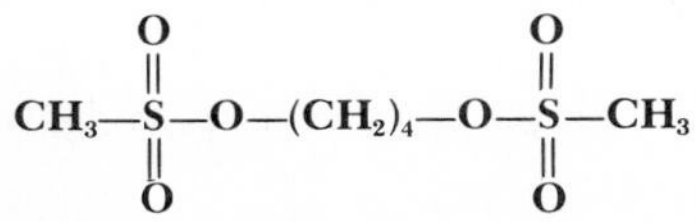

Busulfan 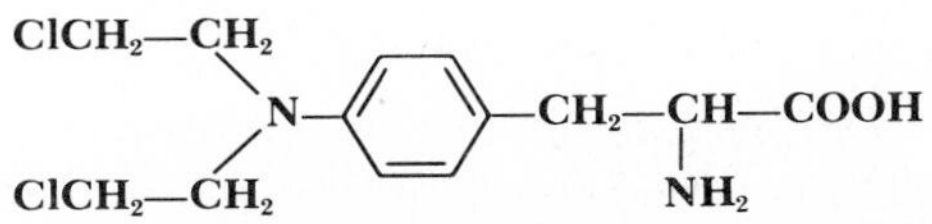   Melphalan

---

TABLE 60-1   Classification of antineoplastic agents

Compound	Abbreviations	Routes of delivery*	Oral dosage forms† (mg)
Alkylating agents			
Mechlorethamine hydrochloride (Mustargen)		IV	
Chlorambucil (Leukeran)		PO	T: 2
Cyclophosphamide (Cytoxan, Neosar)		IV, PO	T: 25, 50
Melphalan (Alkeran)		IV, PO	T: 2
Thiotepa	TSPA, TESPA	IV, IT, IM, SC	
Busulfan (Myleran)		PO	T: 2
Carmustine (BiCNU)	BCNU	IV	
Lomustine (CeeNU)	CCNU	PO	C: 10-100
Antimetabolites			
Methotrexate (Folex, Mexate)	MTX	IV, IM, PO, SC, IT	T: 2.5
Mercaptopurine (Purinethol)	6-MP	PO, IV	T: 50
Thioguanine	6-TG	PO, IV	T: 40
Fluorouracil (Adrucil)	5-FU	IV	
Cytarabine (Cytosar-U)	ara-C	IV, SC, IT	
Hormones			
Adrenal corticosteroids (prednisone)		PO, IV, IT	
Estrogens (Estinyl)		PO	T: 0.02-0.5
Antiestrogens (Nolvadex)		PO	T: 10
Androgens (Halotestin)		PO, IM	T: 2-10
Antibiotics			
Bleomycin sulfate (Blenoxane)	BLM	IV, SC, IM	
Dactinomycin (Cosmegen)	ACT	IV	
Doxorubicin hydrochloride (Adriamycin)	ADR	IV	
Daunorubicin hydrochloride (Cerubidine)	DNR	IV	
Mitoxanthrone (Novantrone)	DHAD	IV	
Plicamycin (Mithracin)		IV	
Mitomycin (Mutamycin)	MTC	IV	
Miscellaneous			
Vinblastine sulfate (Velban)	VLB	IV	
Vincristine sulfate (Oncovin)	VCR, LCR	IV	
Asparaginase (Elspar)		IV, IM	
Procarbazine hydrochloride (Matulane)	MIH	PO, IV, IM	C: 50
Hydroxyurea (Hydrea)		PO, (IV)	C: 500
Cisplatin (Platinol)	*cis*-DDP, DDP	IV	
Dacarbazine (DTIC-Dome)	DTIC, DIC	IV	
Mitotane (Lysodren)	*o,p'*-DDD	PO	T: 500
Teniposide	VM-26	IV	
Etoposide (VePesid)	VP-16	IV	

**IM*, Intramuscular; *IT*, intrathecal; *IV*, intravenous; *PO*, oral; *SC*, subcutaneous.
†*C*, Capsule; *T*, tablet.

Mechlorethamine can induce venous thrombosis, severe vomiting, and delayed depression of the bone marrow. In toxic doses it may cause involution of lymphatic tissues and the thymus, ulcerations of gastrointestinal mucosa, convulsions, and death.

The main indication for mechlorethamine is in treatment of Hodgkin's disease and lymphomas, but it may also be useful in other malignancies. Other alkylating agents have an advantage over mechlorethamine in that they can be administered orally.

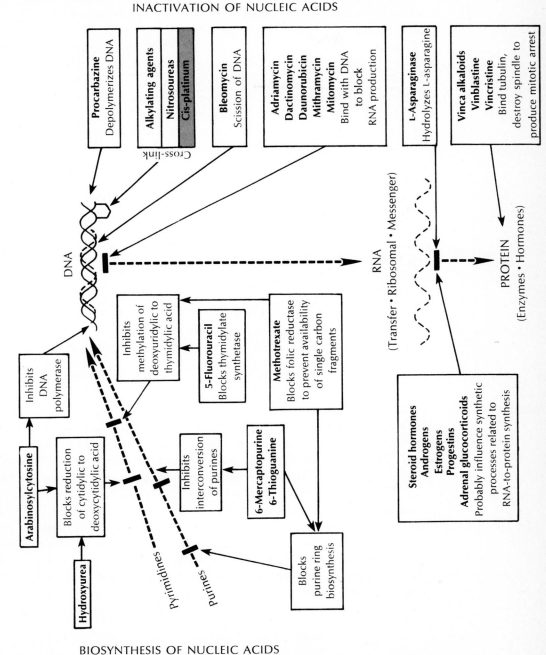

FIG. 60-1   Mechanism of action of antineoplastic drugs.

From Goldberg, R.S., and Krakoff, I.: Hosp. Formulary, I.: Hosp. Formulary, Oct. 1979, p. 891. Reprint from Hospital Formulary, New York, copyright 1980, Harcourt Brace Jovanovich, Inc.

Chlorambucil is used principally in chronic lymphocytic leukemia, Hodgkin's disease, multiple myeloma, and macroglobulinemia. **Cyclophosphamide** is a widely used cytotoxic drug, which is metabolically activated in the liver. This drug is generally useful in therapy of lymphomas, acute lymphocytic leukemia in children, multiple myeloma, and many solid tumors. Hemorrhagic cystitis is a characteristic toxic effect of the cyclophosphamide metabolite acrolein. **Melphalan** (L-sarcolysin) is L-phenylalanine mustard, a derivative of nitrogen mustard. It is used to treat multiple myeloma and some solid tumors, such as those of the ovary, testis, and breast. Occasionally the drug is infused intra-arterially for regional chemotherapy of specific tumors. **Thiotepa** (triethylenethiophosphoramide) is used parenterally in treatment of carcinoma of the ovary and breast. It can also be given intrathecally for therapy of carcinomatosis. **Busulfan** is used mainly to treat chronic myelocytic leukemia, since it has a somewhat selective effect on granulocytes.

Carmustine and **lomustine** are nitrosoureas that alkylate DNA and RNA. Lomustine may have additional effects on DNA synthesis. An important characteristic of the nitrosoureas is their high lipid solubility, which allows them to cross the blood-brain barrier.

Carmustine

Lomustine

ANTIMETABOLITES
Folic acid antagonists

The folic acid antagonists inhibit nucleic acid synthesis by blocking the enzyme dihydrofolate reductase. **Methotrexate,** formerly known as amethopterin, is effective in treatment of acute leukemias in children and of lymphomas.[8] It is curative in women with choriocarcinoma. In combination with other agents, methotrexate is useful in treatment of many solid tumors such as carcinoma of the breast, ovary, or colon. It is also used in high doses (>10 g/m^2) with *leucovorin rescue* to treat osteogenic sarcoma. Leucovorin (5-formyltetrahydrofolate) is a reduced folate that bypasses the metabolic block imposed by methotrexate. Methotrexate produces many toxic effects, such as nausea, vomiting, diarrhea, alopecia, aphthous stomatitis, skin rash, and bone-marrow depression. A long-term sequela may be leukoencephalopathy, especially in children also treated with cranial radiation or intrathecal methotrexate, or both.

Folic acid (pteroylglutamic acid)

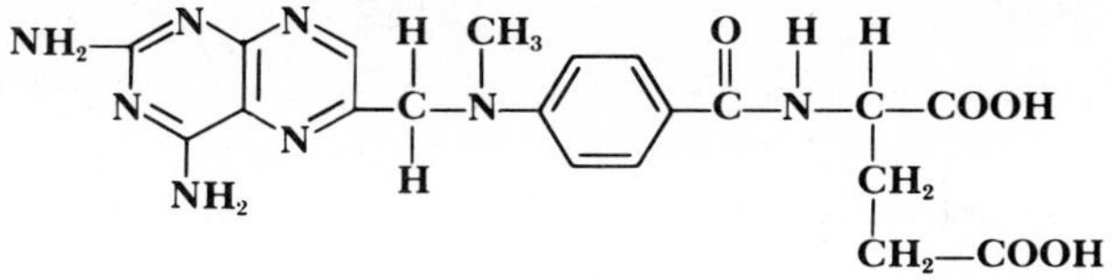

Methotrexate

Mercaptopurine, one of the most important purine antagonists, acts by several *Purine antagonists* mechanisms. After it is converted to its ribonucleotide, it competes with enzymes that convert hypoxanthine ribonucleotide (inosinic acid) to adenine and xanthine ribonucleotides. In addition, mercaptopurine is converted to 6-methyl mercaptopurine and its ribonucleotide. This metabolite inhibits the enzyme that synthesizes phosphoribosylamine, which is required for RNA and DNA synthesis.[11]

Mercaptopurine is effective in therapy of acute lymphocytic[8] and chronic myelocytic leukemias. Its toxic manifestations include bone-marrow depression, gastrointestinal disturbances, and hepatic dysfunction, initially seen as jaundice.

For patients taking allopurinol, a drug that inhibits xanthine oxidase, the dose of mercaptopurine should be decreased.

Thioguanine has essentially the same indications and adverse effects as mercaptopurine. Thioguanine is also metabolized to its ribonucleotide, which enters the pathway of nucleic acid synthesis by substituting for guanine. Thus "fraudulent" polynucleotides that block nucleic acid synthesis are produced.

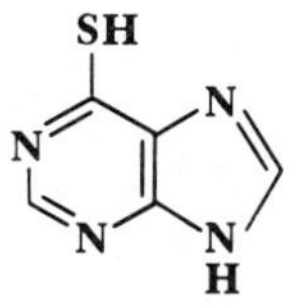

Mercaptopurine

Fluorouracil is a pyrimidine antimetabolite of some usefulness in treatment of *Pyrimidine* carcinoma of the colon, breast, ovary, pancreas, and liver.[9] It is highly toxic and *antagonists* produces hyperpigmentation and photosensitization as well as the same adverse effects as mercaptopurine. Fluorouracil is available as a solution, 50 mg/ml, for intravenous injection. It is also used topically as Efudex solution or cream. The solution contains 2% or 5% fluorouracil, the cream 5%.

Fluorouracil is converted to the ribonucleotide 5-fluorouridine monophosphate (5-FUMP), which may be reduced to 5-fluoro-2′-deoxyuridine-5′-phosphate (5-FdUMP). This enzymatic product inhibits thymidylate synthetase, which is involved in the production of deoxythymidylate from deoxyuridylic acid. Recent data also indicate that disruption of RNA metabolism by 5-FUMP may be an important mechanism of action of fluorouracil.[9]

Cytarabine (cytosine arabinoside) is a pyrimidine antagonist that differs from deoxycytidine (cytosine deoxyriboside) in that it contains arabinose rather than deoxyribose.[14] It is converted to the nucleotide, which then blocks conversion of cytidine nucleotide to deoxycytidine nucleotide. It also prevents formation of DNA by blocking incorporation of deoxycytidine triphosphate.

Cytarabine

Cytarabine is usually injected intravenously, since it is not effective after oral administration. It can also be given subcutaneously as a bolus or continuous infusion. It is used to treat acute lymphocytic and acute myelocytic leukemias. The dose and schedule have ranged from 100 mg/m²/day for 5 days to 3000 mg/m² every 12 hours for 3 days. It was also of interest as a possible antiviral agent; however, its margin of safety is too low for this indication.

HORMONAL AGENTS

Steroid hormones, such as estrogens, androgens, and corticosteroids, are useful in some neoplastic diseases.[10] The estrogens include **diethylstilbestrol diphosphate** (Stilphostrol) and **ethinyl estradiol** (Estinyl, Feminone). Androgens that are widely used, particularly in treatment of carcinoma of the breast, include **testosterone propionate** (Testex, others), **fluoxymesterone** (Halotestin, Android-F), and the recently introduced **calusterone** (Methosarb). The most widely used corticosteroid is **prednisone,** which is effective in various lymphomas and some other malignancies.

The progestins include **medroxyprogesterone** (Provera), **hydroxyprogesterone** (Delalutin), and **megestrol acetate** (Megace). The progestins are sometimes effective treatment for renal and endometrial carcinomas.

Estrogens, along with castration and other measures, are used to treat prostatic carcinoma. Both androgens and estrogens have been employed in management of advanced mammary carcinoma. The choice depends on the age of the patient. Estrogens are used in women well past the menopause, whereas androgens may be helpful in patients who are still menstruating. The main benefit from such therapy is reduction of pain related to metastatic bone lesions. The rationale for use of estrogens and androgens is the belief that prostatic and mammary carcinomas are to some extent "hormone dependent."

Adverse effects of estrogens include gastrointestinal symptoms, hypercalcemia, edema, uterine bleeding, and feminization in males. The adverse effects expected from large doses of androgens in treatment of advanced mammary carcinoma are virilization, edema, and hypercalcemia.

Tamoxifen citrate (Nolvadex), an antiestrogen, apparently competes with estradiol for the estrogen receptor. The drug is not a steroid. Its main usefulness is in carcinomas of the breast in postmenopausal and also premenopausal women.

Bleomycin binds to DNA and has been useful in treatment of squamous cell carcinomas of the head and neck, testicular tumors, and malignant lymphomas.[6] Although bleomycin does not depress the bone marrow, it can cause an unusual toxic manifestation—pulmonary fibrosis.

Dactinomycin (actinomycin D) combines with DNA and blocks RNA production. It is effective treatment for choriocarcinoma of women, Wilms' tumor, and testicular carcinoma.[7] The drug causes bone-marrow depression and gastrointestinal toxicity. It may also have a "radiation recall" effect (that is, an increase in toxicity in irradiated tissue).[5]

Doxorubicin (hydroxydaunorubicin) is an anthracycline antibiotic that combines with DNA and is cell cycle–specific; it inhibits the S phase preferentially. Doxorubicin is used to treat lymphomas, leukemia, sarcomas, and neuroblastoma. Mucositis and bone-marrow depression are common acute toxic effects, and a dose-related cardiomyopathy, often fatal, is a late effect.[15] The incidence of the latter toxicity may be increased with concomitant use of chest irradiation or drugs such as cyclophosphamide. Tissue necrosis is severe in cases of extravasation. Other commonly used anthracyclines include daunorubicin and a newer synthetic compound, mitoxantrone.

Plicamycin (mithramycin) inhibits DNA-dependent RNA synthesis. In addition, the drug affects calcium metabolism, probably by acting on osteoclasts, and it is used to treat the hypercalcemia that occurs with some malignancies. Among numerous toxic effects, thrombocytopenia, bleeding, and gastrointestinal manifestations are most common.

Mitomycin is an alkylating antibiotic that combines with DNA. The drug is used occasionally when other alkylating agents are ineffective. It causes severe bone-marrow depression, gastrointestinal toxicity, and renal toxicity.

ANTIBIOTICS

Vincristine and **vinblastine** are alkaloids from the periwinkle plant *(Vinca)*. Antineoplastic activity is presumably a consequence of mitotic arrest. Nausea, vomiting, leukopenia, unique neurotoxic effects such as loss of deep tendon reflexes, jaw pain, constipation, seizures, and secretion of inappropriate antidiuretic hormone (SIADH) as well as alopecia are side effects of *Vinca* alkaloids.[4] Vinblastine is more marrow suppressive than vincristine. *Vinca* alkaloids are very active agents in combination therapy for lymphomas and solid tumors.

L-Asparaginase is an enzyme used to treat leukemia.[2] Apparently some malignant cells require exogenous asparagine, though normal cells synthesize their own. Thus

MISCELLANEOUS ANTINEOPLASTIC AGENTS

a metabolic difference between normal and neoplastic cells appears to exist for this drug. The discovery of L-asparaginase as an antineoplastic agent resulted from observations on the suppressive effect of guinea pig serum, now known to contain L-asparaginase, on experimental leukemias in vitro. Toxicity includes pancreatitis, hepatitis, bleeding diathesis, and thrombosis. Approximately 10% of patients have a significant allergic reaction to *Escherichia coli* L-asparaginase. A second preparation from *Erwinia* species is available to avoid this problem.

Procarbazine is a synthetic methylhydrazine derivative that finds usefulness in treatment of generalized Hodgkin's disease. It causes numerous adverse effects, including gastrointestinal symptoms, bone-marrow depression, a monoamine oxidase inhibitory action, and disulfiram-like reactions.

Hydroxyurea is one of the few agents that has ribonucleotide reductase, a key enzyme in DNA synthesis, as its target.[16] It may be useful in patients with chronic myelocytic leukemia when there is no response to busulfan. Bone-marrow depression is its most serious adverse effect. The drug is available in capsules, and an intravenous form is available for experimental purposes.

The observation that an electric current delivered through platinum electrodes was cytotoxic led to development of **cisplatin** (*cis*-platinum II) as an antineoplastic drug. Platinum functions as an alkylating agent, forming interstrand and intrastrand DNA cross-links. The dose-limiting toxicity is nephrotoxicity, clinically apparent as decreased glomerular filtration rate and salt wasting. Aggressive prehydration seems to decrease this toxicity. Cisplatin also causes a high-frequency hearing loss and is one of the most emetic compounds used in anticancer therapy. It is used to treat sarcomas, testicular carcinomas, and brain tumors.[12]

Dacarbazine (DTIC, imidazole carboxamide), though structurally similar to purine precursors, also appears to function as an alkylating agent. It causes severe nausea and vomiting as well as bone-marrow suppression. In addition, a "flulike" syndrome and urticarial rashes have been reported. Dacarbazine is primarily used to treat Hodgkin's disease. It also has some activity in therapy of sarcoma, especially in combination with an anthracycline such as doxorubicin.

Mitotane is a synthetic compound related to DDT that has specific toxicity for the adrenal gland. It causes a chemical adrenalectomy.

The epipodophyllotoxins **teniposide** and **etoposide** are derivatives of the mayapple (mandrake). Although related to the podophyllotoxins, these compounds are not tubulin binders (that is, mitotic inhibitors) but interrupt the S and G_2 phases of the cell cycle. They inhibit topoisomerase, a DNA repair enzyme.[13] Etoposide is commercially available. It is especially useful in treatment of lymphomas, leukemia, and testicular cancer and may be helpful in therapy of brain tumors. Teniposide is primarily used to treat acute leukemia.

In addition to the use of surgery and radiation, various drugs may be beneficial in treating malignancies. In fact, chemotherapy is considered the primary method of treatment in the following conditions: choriocarcinoma of the female, Wilms' tumor, acute and chronic leukemias, disseminated lymphomas, multiple myeloma, and polycythemia vera.

As a general rule, the drugs or schedule of choice of these agents for various malignancies are continually in flux as new information is accumulated by cancer chemotherapy study groups performing controlled trials. Several multiagent combinations have withstood the test of time and form the basis for chemotherapy of several types of malignancies. Examples are listed in Table 60-2.

CHOICE OF DRUGS IN CANCER CHEMOTHERAPY

TABLE 60-2   Examples of multiagent protocols*

	Components	Dose (mg/m²)	Days of administration
MOPP	*m*echlorethamine	6	1 and 8
	*O*ncovin (vincristine)	1.4	1 and 8
	*p*rocarbazine	100	1-14
	*p*rednisone	40	1-14
ABVD	*A*driamycin (doxorubicin)	25	1 and 14
	*b*leomycin	10 IU/m²	1 and 14
	*v*inblastine	6	1 and 14
	*D*TIC	375	1 and 14
CHOP	*c*yclophosphamide	750	1
	*h*ydroxydaunorubicin (= doxorubicin)	50	1
	*O*ncovin (vincristine)	1.4	1
	*p*rednisone	100	1-5
COMLA	*c*yclophosphamide	1500	1
	*O*ncovin (vincristine)	1.4	1, 8, 15
	*m*ethotrexate	120	22, 29, 36, 43, 57, 64, 71
	*l*eucovorin	25†	
	*a*ra-C (cytarabine)	300	Same as methotrexate
VAC (pulse)	*v*incristine	1.5	1 (repeat
	*a*ctinomycin D (dactinomycin)	1.25	1 every
	*c*yclophosphamide	750	1 2 to 3 weeks)

*Modifications and variations of these time-tested regimens, based upon empiric or pharmacologic data, may be used.
†Every 6 hours for four doses, 24 hours after methotrexate.

1. Brookes, P., and Lawley, P.D.: The reaction of mono- and di-functional alkylating agents with nucleic acids, Biochem. J. **80**:496, 1961.

2. Capizzi, R.L., Bertino, J.R., and Handschumacher, R.E.: L-Asparaginase, Annu. Rev. Med. **21**:433, 1970.

3. Capizzi, R.L., Keiser, L.W., and Sartorelli, A.C.: Combination chemotherapy: theory and practice, Semin. Oncol. **4**:227, 1977.

4. Carbone, P.P., Bono, V., Frei, E., III, and Brindley, C.O.: Clinical studies with vincristine, Blood **21**:640, 1963.

5. D'Angio, G.J.: Clinical and biologic studies of actinomycin D and roentgen irradiation, Am. J. Roentgenol. **87**:106, 1962.

6. DeVita, V.T., Jr., Hellman, S., and Rosenberg, S.A., editors. Cancer: principles & practice of oncology, ed. 2, Philadelphia, 1985, J.B. Lippincott Co.

7. Frei, E., III: The clinical use of actinomycin, Cancer Chemother. Rep. **58**:49, 1974.

8. Frei, E., III: Acute leukemia in children: model for the development of scientific methodology for clinical therapeutic research in cancer, Cancer **53**:2013, 1984.

9. Heidelberger, C.: Fluorinated pyrimidines and their nucleosides. In Sartorelli, A.C., and Johns, D.G., editors: Antineoplastic and immunosuppressive agents, Part II, New York, 1975, Springer-Verlag, p. 193.

10. Lippman, M.E., and Eil, C.: Steroid therapy of cancer. In Chabner, B.A., editor: Pharmacologic principles of cancer treatment, Philadelphia, 1982, W.B. Saunders Co., p. 132.

11. Nelson, J.A., Carpenter, J.W., Rose, L.M., and Adamson, D.J.: Mechanisms of action of 6-thioguanine, 6-mercaptopurine, and 8-azaguanine, Cancer Res. **35**:2872, 1975.

12. Rosenberg, B.: Fundamental studies with cisplatin, Cancer **55**:2303, 1985.

13. Ross, W., Rowe, T., Glisson, B., et al.: Role of topoisomerase II in mediating epipodophyllotoxin-induced DNA cleavage, Cancer Res. **44**:5857, 1984.

14. Valeriote, F.: Cellular aspects of the action of cytosine arabinoside, Med. Pediatr. Oncol. **10**(suppl. 1):5, 1982.

15. Von Hoff, D.D., Layard, M.W., Basa, P., et al.: Risk factors for doxorubicin-induced congestive heart failure, Ann. Intern. Med. **91**:710, 1979.

16. Yarbro, J.W., Kennedy, B.J., and Barnum, C.P.: Hydroxyurea inhibition of DNA synthesis in ascites tumor, Proc. Natl. Acad. Sci. U.S.A. **53**:1033, 1965.

REFERENCES

Principles of immunopharmacology

61   *Principles of immunopharmacology, 716*

Chapter 61

Principles of immunopharmacology

The rapidly expanding discipline of immunology contributes to the diagnosis, therapy, and prevention of human diseases in many ways. First, immunologic competence enables one to fend off repeated infections with pathogenic organisms, and preventive immunizations are commonplace. The role of immunocompetence in prevention of malignancy is currently of great interest in experimental science as well as in clinical medicine. The ability of an individual to mount an immune response, however, is also the basis of allergic reactions and autoimmune diseases. Selective modification of the immune response is a primary goal in organ transplantation and in therapy of a variety of diseases. The development of methods for monitoring behavior of specific cell populations has aided greatly in understanding basic immunologic mechanisms as well as in predicting the course of diseases with an immunologic cause. Interest in the immune response has been stimulated by the alarming increase in a novel epidemic form of immunodeficiency, the acquired immunodeficiency syndrome (AIDS). Finally, the explosion of molecular and immunologic technologies has had a strong impact on therapeutic as well as basic research. For example, immunochemical measurements of drugs in biologic tissues or fluids is a sensitive means of quantitation as well as a means of identification. Hybridoma technology has made it possible to produce a wide variety of antibodies, hormones, and other biologically active molecules for therapeutics and research.

The control of disease by immunologic means has two primary objectives: the production of desired immunity and the elimination of undesired immune reactions. The first of these is achieved by immunization to selected antigens or the administration of specific antibodies or cytokines. The second objective is generally achieved through drugs that alter immunity and inflammation. This chapter is not intended to be a comprehensive review of immunology and its relationship to therapeutics, but it will emphasize some aspects of immunopharmacology including immunomodulation, autoimmune disease, and selected mediators of the immune response. Immediate hypersensitivity and allergic reactions are discussed in Chapters 19 and 20, which cover histamine and antihistamines, respectively.

Vaccine	Method	Example
Subunit vaccines	Isolation of polypeptide subunits from infectious agent	Hepatitis B virus
Recombinant vaccines	Synthesis of antigen by recombinant DNA	*Escherichia coli* LT toxin Hepatitis B virus
Recombinant infectious vectors	Genome of infectious agent is inserted into infectious vector	Human sarcoma virus *Shigella* Hepatitis B virus Rabies virus
Synthetic peptides	Synthesis of antigenic sequence or conformational determinants	Cholera toxin Poliomyelitis virus Foot and mouth disease virus

TABLE 61-1 Development of new vaccines

Modified form Steward, M.W., and Howard, C.R.: Immunol. Today **8**:51, 1987.

PRODUCTION AND ENHANCEMENT OF THE IMMUNE RESPONSE

Immunization

The modern science of immunology began in 1796 with Edward Jenner's discovery that immunization with vaccinia (cowpox) prevented development of the more lethal smallpox. The derivation of the term *vaccination* is from vaccinia.[8] Since that time the development of safe and effective vaccines for prevention of infectious diseases has been responsible, in part, for the substantial decline in morbidity and mortality associated with smallpox, rabies, diphtheria, pertussis, tetanus, yellow fever, poliomyelitis, measles, mumps, and rubella.[9] As the incidence of these diseases declined, routine immunizations became primarily the concern of pediatricians. With the development of pneumococcal, influenza, and hepatitis vaccines, however, immunization of adults has increased.

Some of the early vaccines made from live or attenuated organisms caused serious reactions, and their efficacy was questionable. The recent development of recombinant DNA technology and the success of peptide sequencing and synthesis have helped in development of new and safer vaccines. Although some of these products are still experimental, they show considerable promise for clinical use (Table 61-1).[21]

Synthetic vaccines

Synthetic vaccines use chemically synthesized antigens (usually peptides) as the immunizing agent. The success of these vaccines depends on the ability of an antibody elicited in response to a small, defined peptide to recognize and bind to that peptide sequence within a larger molecule. Advantages of synthetic vaccines are twofold. First, since they do not rely on live or attenuated viruses, they are quite safe. Second, the antigenic peptides can be synthesized on a large scale. If the sequence of only a few amino acid residues of a viral protein is known, this small peptide can be synthesized and used to immunize against the virus. In practical terms, the amino acid sequence of bacterial or viral proteins can be discerned from the nucleotide sequence of the gene. Once this is known, a variety of peptides can be synthesized as potential immunogens. This technique has been used successfully in protecting animals against foot and mouth disease virus,[23] and it is believed that synthetic vaccines will have some application in immunization against tumor antigens.

ANTIBODIES AS THERAPEUTIC AGENTS
Tumor therapy with antibodies

The idea for immunologic treatment of human disease originated with Paul Ehrlich, who suggested the use of toxic antibody molecules as therapeutic agents.[14] Since Ehrlich's time, advances in molecular biology have revolutionized immunology and medicine. Initially, the use of antibodies as therapeutic agents was limited by their impurity and heterogeneity. More recently, monoclonal antibodies of defined specificity have been used successfully to lyse malignant cells in some types of leukemias and lymphomas.[11] The effect depends on recognition of antigens unique to the tumor cells and the successful removal of antibody-coated cells by the reticuloendothelial system or killing by macrophages. One drawback is that the monoclonal antibodies are obtained from mice; hence they can act as antigens in man and can trigger an immune response. Monoclonal antibody therapy seldom results in hypersensitivity reactions, but in the host it frequently stimulates production of blocking antibodies, which neutralize the therapeutic effect of further antibody administration.[11]

Immunotoxins

Immunotoxins are formed by linking antibodies to polypeptides that inactivate protein synthesis. The rationale is that the cell-binding antibody serves to direct the toxin to the target cells and thus spares normal cells from the chemotherapeutic agent. This approach is particularly relevant for tumors of mesenchymal or epithelial origin. Fig. 61-1 shows the general structure of an immunotoxin.

The toxin portion is usually of plant or bacterial origin. One of these that has been studied extensively is ricin, a plant polypeptide that consists of two chains. One (B chain) is a lectin capable of binding to the cell surface. The other (A chain) inhibits protein synthesis. Since immunotherapy requires binding to specific target cells rather than to surfaces of cells in general, only the A chain is used in preparation of the immunotoxin. Because the ricin A chain is not active outside of the cell, it affects only cells that bind it through the antibody portion of the complex. Immunotoxins containing ricin A chain have been used to kill mouse and human tumor cells.[25] Other toxins that can be coupled to antibodies include diphtheria toxin, abrin (a plant-derived toxin), daunorubicin, vinblastine, and methotrexate. Some of these conjugates can kill human tumor cells at very low concentrations.

The inhibition of protein synthesis requires uptake of the toxin into endosomes and processing within the cell, as indicated in Fig. 61-2.

Although this approach is still experimental, there are at least four different clinical applications for immunotoxins: T-cell depletion in bone-marrow transplantation, intracavitary treatment of tumors such as ovarian carcinoma or bladder carcinoma, systemic therapy of leukemias and lymphomas, and systemic treatment of refractory metastatic tumors.[5]

Schematic structure of immunotoxin.

Reproduced, with permission, from Frankel, A.E., Houston, L.L., Issell, B.F., and Fathman, B.F.: Annu. Rev. Med. **37**:125-142, copyright 1986 by Annual Reviews Inc.

FIG. 61-1

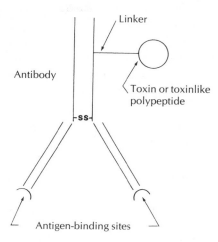

According to its antigen specificity, the immunotoxin binds to its antigen and the complex migrates into coated pits on the cell surface. After invagination, a vesicle is formed that becomes acidified and the endosome eventually is processed by the Golgi complex into lysosomes. At some point in this path, immunotoxin escapes and the toxin (solid circle) (which may or may not be still linked to the antibody) attacks the ribosome (ricin A chain) or elongation factor 2 (diphtheria toxin).

FIG. 61-2

Reproduced, with permission, from Frankel, A.E., Houston, L.L., Issell, B.F., and Fathman, B.F.: Annu. Rev. Med. **37**:125-142, copyright 1986 by Annual Reviews Inc.

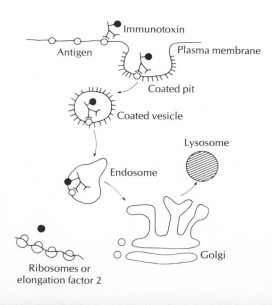

Catalytic antibodies   An approach similar to that for immunotoxins is currently being applied to produce catalytic antibodies, molecules that can share the functions of both antibodies and enzymes.[12] One approach involves chemical modification of the antigen-binding site; a second will apply genetic selection techniques in antibody-producing cells to obtain antibodies with the desired antigen-binding and catalytic specificities. The resultant antibodies, though not directly lytic for tumor or other invading cells, might be used to activate specific cells of the immune system. Antibodies that could both bind to and hydrolyze specific proteins also have potential as fibrinolytic agents. These potential applications are still under investigation.

LYMPHOKINES   Lymphokines and monokines are nonantibody mediators derived from lympho-
AND MONOKINES   cytes or monocytes. They are considered hormones that regulate immune and inflammatory responses. This class of mediators includes interferons, interleukins, and macrophage-activating and inhibition factors. Interferon and interleukins have been used experimentally in immunology of malignancies.

Interleukins   There are two recognized interleukins; these are polypeptides originally described as T-cell mitogens. The term *interleukin* was adopted because these substances are produced by and act on leukocytes. They have several common biologic properties, including enhancement of the thymocyte mitogenic response and stimulation of antigen-dependent, cell-mediated, and humoral immune responses in culture.[4] Later, it became clear that interleukin 2 (IL-2), produced by T-lymphocytes, is the major thymocyte growth factor and that IL-1, which is produced by macrophages, activates specific subsets of lymphocytes and promotes differentiation of antibody-forming cells. IL-1 is not stored preformed in mononuclear phagocytes but is synthesized in response to viruses, bacteria, microbial products, antigens, and inflammatory agents. Most inducers of IL-1 production are pyrogens, and IL-1 appears to be the common mediator of fever caused by infection, immunologic reactions, and inflammation. IL-1 is a key mediator of the host response to microbial invasion, an inflammatory mediator and a modulator of the "acute-phase response." It can also affect several nonleukocytic target cells. Decreased production of IL-1 or an absence of receptors for IL-1 may play a role in susceptibility to some types of tumors.[3]

IL-2 is a growth factor for helper, suppressor, and cytotoxic T-lymphocytes. It is more specific than IL-1 because it acts directly as a growth factor for T-lymphocytes, whereas IL-1 mediates several components of the systemic acute-phase response.[4] The role of IL-2 in immunity is not restricted, however, to that of a growth factor for T-cells. It is necessary for activation of all T-lymphocytes, regardless of class. IL-2 can induce secretion of γ-interferon by T-cells, and it also influences the cytolytic activity of lymphocytes, activates macrophages, and modulates expression of histocompatibility antigens. The human gene for IL-2 has some structural features that indicate homology with the promoter portion of the human γ-interferon gene and viral enhancer elements. These features might be involved in expression of IL-2

The multiple roles of interleukin 2 (IL-2) in various immune responses. Ag, *Antigen;* B-act,   ***FIG. 61-3***
activated B-cell; BCDF, *B-cell differentiation factor;* BCGF, *B-cell growth factor;* γ-IFN,
immune (gamma) interferon; IL-1, *interleukin 1;* LAK, *lymphocyte-activated killer cell;* MHC,
major histocompatibility complex proteins; Mϕ, *macrophage;* NK, *natural killer cell;* T-act,
activated T-cell; T-resp, *IL-2 responsive T-cell.*

From Robb, R.J.: Immunol. Today 5:203, 1984.

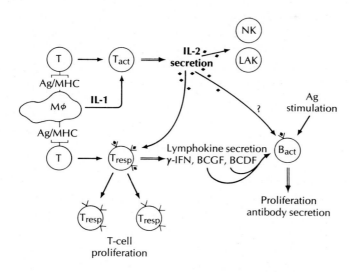

during T-cell activation.[16] Some of the relationships between the interleukins 1 and 2 and immune cells are shown in Fig. 61-3.

One of the important actions of IL-2 is the enhancement of tumoricidal activity of both T-cells and large granular lymphocytes, a subpopulation of lymphocytes that can kill tumor cells without prior sensitization of the donor against tumor antigen and without the expected histocompatibility restriction. These natural killer (NK) cells recognize and lyse a wide variety of target cells, including tumor cells, micro-organisms, and cells infected with viruses.[7] They are believed to play an important role in host resistance at the tissue level against viral infection and metastasis of neoplasms.[1] A promising development in the potential of IL-2 as an antineoplastic agent is its use to activate lymphocytes ex vivo. Additional studies indicate that IL-2 can enhance several parameters of immune function in patients with AIDS, but the efficacy of this agent in AIDS or other immunodeficiency syndromes remains to be demonstrated.

A third proposed interleukin (IL-3) is a multipotential colony-stimulating factor that functions in growth and differentiation of hematopoietic cells from experimental animals. This factor activates naturally occurring cytotoxic cells distinct from NK cells, probably by stimulating production of interferon. Activation of these cytotoxic cells together with NK cells provides a nonspecific application of the immune response.[4]

Interferons

Interferons were first discovered by virologists who were interested in suppression of viral replication. It was recognized that interferons could induce cells to make new RNA and protein as well as to prevent viral replication. They are currently regarded as important immunoregulatory molecules. There are several different proteins classified as interferons (IFN). These differ in molecular weight and also in their source. α-IFN and β-IFN are produced in leukocytes and fibroblasts, respectively, in response to viral or bacterial infections. Immune interferon, or γ-IFN, is produced by lymphocytes after stimulation by antigens, mitogens, or other lymphokines.[6] The activities of the interferons are similar; they inhibit replication of viruses, cell division, and various immunologic reactions, and they enhance phagocytosis and cytotoxicity of lymphocyte subpopulations.

Reports that interferon had antitumor effects in man stimulated considerable interest, and intensive efforts went into preparation of immune interferon for clinical use. Recombinant interferons have been used in clinical studies of acute and chronic viral infections, tumors, and various other disorders. Although interferons have lessened the severity of viral infections in several studies, they have not lived up to expectations as anticancer agents in humans.[22] A recent trial of γ-IFN in treatment of AIDS was disappointing. There may be a potential for combination of IFN with other therapeutic modalities, however, particularly for certain types of malignancies.

Despite initial disappointment when γ-IFN was assessed in therapeutic trials, it is still of great interest because of its role in immunity.[6] IL-2–stimulated production of γ-IFN by NK cells correlates with an increase in cytotoxicity. γ-IFN induces the appearance of new surface markers and receptors associated with differentiation of immune cells. It also enhances the expression of human lymphocyte (MHC or major histocompatibility) antigens (HLA), which are recognition sites for directed cytotoxicity or for replicative signals in various types of cells. Finally, γ-IFN is a maturation factor for B-lymphocytes and thus promotes immunoglobulin synthesis and secretion.[24]

A fully responsive immune system is necessary for survival. However, the expression of an immune response is potentially harmful to the host if directed against host tissues. Because a normal immune response is responsible for rejection of tissue grafts or organ transplants, selective suppression helps to control this unwanted reaction.

IMMUNOSUP-PRESSION

The general concept of autoimmune diseases is that immune reactions to infectious or other agents are extended to include host tissues. Control of such unwanted reactions involves reduction of the number of lymphoid cells. Treatment with cytotoxic drugs or irradiation effectively reduces the total number of lymphoid cells but results in general immunosuppression. An alternative approach is to use antibodies or immunotoxins directed against specific T-cell subpopulations.[18]

Autoimmune disease

Immunosuppressive therapy of immunologic disease or for the purpose of organ transplantation is relatively nonspecific. It is not directed at the cause of the disease, and it can inhibit normal immune and inflammatory responses as well. Agents such as mercaptopurine, azathioprine, cyclophosphamide, and methotrexate are cytotoxins. They interfere with cell replication and metabolism in various ways, but the result is disruption of normal cell function. Interference with replication of rapidly dividing cells results in several undesirable side effects. A further drawback to extended use of cytotoxic drugs for treatment of autoimmune disease or for transplantation is that the risks of developing neoplasms or altering chromosomes are not known. Fig. 61-4 compares mechanisms of several immunosuppressive agents.

Immunosuppressive drugs

Glucocorticoids, such as prednisone, have anti-inflammatory as well as immunosuppressive actions. This might be explained simply by the fact that immune injury causes an inflammatory response and activates cells that produce inflammatory me-

FIG. 61-4 *Diagrams show comparison of sites of action of various immunosuppressive agents. Aza-thioprine inhibits proliferation of effector lymphocytes; prednisone is cytolytic. Since neither is specific for the T-lymphocytes most prominently involved in graft rejection, their untoward effects can include bone marrow suppression and susceptibility to infection. Antilympho-cyte globulin adds immunologic attack but will be directed against B- as well as T-cells, with consequent infection risks. Only cyclosporin is appropriately specific. By inhibiting production or activity of interleukin 2, it aborts the signal for effector T-cell proliferation.*

From Najarian, J.S.: Hosp. Pract. 17(10):61, 1982; this illustration drawn by Nancy Lou Makris, Wilton, Conn.

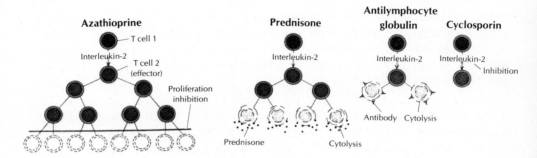

diators.[10] Alternatively, glucocorticoids could inhibit production of mediators, such as arachidonate metabolites, that both augment inflammation and activate immune cells. There is substantial evidence that oxidative products of arachidonic acid are involved in both mechanisms. Both prostaglandins and leukotrienes can alter vascular permeability and activate various leukocyte responses. Leukotriene B_4 is a potent chemoattractant for neutrophils. Other products of arachidonic acid lipoxygenation, the mono-HETES and HPETES, are chemotactic for phagocytes. Experiments with lymphocytes in vitro clearly indicate that lipoxygenase products affect proliferative and cytotoxic responses, probably through production of lymphokines such as IL-2 or γ-IFN.[17]

Azathioprine (Imuran), which has been used successfully in organ transplantation, interferes with nucleic acid synthesis in all replicating cells. It first affects the most actively dividing cells, the lymphocytes, to temporarily prevent rejection of the graft. It also inhibits replication of cells in bone marrow and the gastrointestinal tract. Azathioprine in combination with prednisone, which promotes lysis of lymphocytes, provides even greater immune suppression but does not prevent side effects or the increased incidence of secondary infection.[13]

Cyclosporine (cyclosporin A, Sandimmune) is a fungal metabolite that has proved superior to azathioprine in clinical trials of organ transplantation.[2,15] It is more selective than azathioprine because it primarily affects lymphoid cells and does not cause bone-marrow suppression. It is not directly cytotoxic, but it inhibits the activation of lymphocytes before DNA synthesis begins by preventing production of IL-1 and IL-2. This prevents the formation of cytotoxic lymphocytes. There is also evidence that cyclosporine inhibits antigen activation of B-cells.[20] A major drawback to use of cyclosporine is its nephrotoxicity. Blood concentration must be regulated closely in an attempt to minimize this adverse effect.

Antilymphocytic globulin (ALG), an antibody directed against lymphocytes, was also used to combat rejection episodes after organ transplantation. The binding of antibody to lymphocytes mediates complement-mediated lysis. The early preparations were nonselective for lymphocyte subpopulations and caused many serious side effects. The application of monoclonal antibody technology promises more specific and safer variants of this product. This treatment is usually reserved, however, for patients who are unresponsive to immunosuppressive drugs.[15]

IL-2 antibodies are currently being evaluated as therapy for disease states in which T-cells are involved. One application is in patients with aplastic anemia, in which IL-2 receptors are believed to suppress hematopoiesis. This technique is still experimental, but it shows great promise for autoimmune diseases as well as for organ transplantation.[26]

Histocompatibility antigens and disease

Much has been learned about genetically controlled immune responsiveness and about the relationship between tissue antigens and the development of autoimmunity. The major histocompatibility complex (MHC or HLA) antigens of the host are involved in recognition of foreign antigens. A common application of HLA typing is in transplant-donor matching. It is also used to identify susceptibilities to various autoimmune diseases but not for clinical diagnosis of disease. The observation that certain autoimmune connective tissue diseases were associated with particular MHC antigens indicated that these recognition sites may be involved in pathogenesis of the disease. The associations are particularly strong for rheumatic diseases, such as ankylosing spondylitis and juvenile onset rheumatoid arthritis, and for a group of diseases that are characterized by chronic inflammatory and aberrant immune reactions. This latter group includes myasthenia gravis, insulin-dependent diabetes mellitus, Grave's disease, and Addison's disease. Other diseases with HLA association include pemphigus, multiple sclerosis, pernicious anemia, and psoriasis.[19]

The mechanism by which HLAs contribute to development of these diseases is still not entirely clear. It is known that helper T-cells can recognize only antigen in association with the HLAs on the surface of an antigen-presenting cell. Several hypotheses have been advanced to explain the association between HLAs and susceptibility to disease. One hypothesis is that the molecular similarity between histocompatibility antigens and those of viruses or bacteria enables antibodies to the invading microorganism to cross-react with tissues. Another hypothesis is that cell-surface antigens are modified as a result of exposure to microorganisms or toxins or through neoplastic changes. These alterations would then render the host tissue sufficiently antigenic to stimulate an immune response. In addition, there is evidence that Ir (immune response) genes are involved. Thus the pathogenesis could occur at the level of gene expression for control of antibody production.[19]

Immunopharmacology has clearly expanded as a result of new technologies that aid in development of more selective vaccines for the prevention of disease and newer therapeutic agents for precise and selective control of unwanted or inappropriate immune responses. It may soon be possible to design highly potent drugs or antibodies to interfere with single steps in the immune response.

1. Burns, G.F., Begley, C.G., Mackay, I.R., et al.: 'Supernatural' killer cells, Immunol. Today **6**:370, 1985.

2. Canadian Multicentre Transplant Study Group: A randomized clinical trial of cyclosporine in cadaveric renal transplantation, N. Engl. J. Med. **309**:809, 1983.

3. Dinarello, C.A.: Interleukin-1, Rev. Infect. Dis. **6**:51, 1984.

4. Dinarello, C.A., and Mier, J.W.: Interleukins, Annu. Rev. Med. **37**:173, 1986.

5. Frankel, A.E., Houston, L.L., Issell, B.F., and Fathman, G.: Prospects for immunotoxin therapy in cancer, Annu. Rev. Med. **37**:125, 1986.

6. Friedman, R.M., and Vogel, S.N.: Interferons with special emphasis on the immune system, Adv. Immunol. **34**:97, 1983.

7. Heberman, R.B.: Natural killer cells, Annu. Rev. Med. **37**:347, 1986.

8. Krause, R.M.: The restless tide: the persistent challenge of the microbial world, Washington, D.C., 1981, The National Foundation for Infectious Diseases.

9. Krugman, S., and Katz, S.L.: Childhood immunization procedures, J.A.M.A. **237**:2228, 1977.

10. Larsen, G.L., and Henson, P.M.: Mediators of inflammation, Annu. Rev. Immunol. **1**:335, 1983.

11. Levy, R., and Miller, R.A.: Biological and clinical implications of lymphocyte hybridomas: tumor therapy with monoclonal antibodies, Annu. Rev. Med. **34**:107, 1983.

12. Marx, J.L.: Making antibodies work like enzymes, Science **234**:1497, 1986.

13. Najarian, J.S.: Immunologic aspects of organ transplantation, Hosp. Pract. **17**(10):61, 1982.

14. Parker, C.W.: Drugs and the immune response, Fed. Proc. **33**:1881, 1974.

15. Reemtsma, K., Hardy, M.A., Drusin, R.E., et al.: Cardiac transplantation: changing patterns in evaluation and treatment, Ann. Surg. **202**:418, 1985.

16. Robb, R.J.: Interleukin-2: the molecule and its function, Immunol. Today **5**:203, 1984.

17. Rola-Pleszczynski, M.: Immunoregulation by leukotrienes and other lipoxygenase metabolites, Immunol. Today **6**:302, 1985.

18. Rowley, D.A., Fitch, F.W., Stuart, F.P., et al.: Specific suppression of immune responses, Science **181**:1133, 1973.

19. Schaller, J.G., and Hansen, J.A.: HLA relationships to disease, Hosp. Pract. **16**(5):41, 1981.

20. Shevich, E.M.: Cyclosporine, Annu. Rev. Immunol. **3**:397, 1985.

21. Steward, M.W., and Howard, C.R.: Synthetic peptides: a next generation of vaccines? Immunol. Today **8**:51, 1987.

22. Sun, M.: Interferon: no magic bullet against cancer, Science **212**:141, 1981.

23. Sutcliffe, J.G., Shinnick, T.M., Green, N., and Lerner, R.A.: Antibodies that react with predetermined sites on proteins, Science **219**:660, 1983.

24. Trinchieri, G., and Perussia, B.: Immune interferon: a pleiotropic lymphokine with multiple effects, Immunol. Today **6**:131, 1985.

25. Vitetta, E.S., Krolick, K.A., Miyama-Inaba, M., et al.: Immunotoxins: a new approach to cancer therapy, Science **219**:644, 1983.

26. Waldmann, T.A., and Tsudo, M.: Interleukin-2 receptors: biology and therapeutic potentials, Hosp. Pract. **22**(1):77, 1987.

section eleven

Poisons and antidotes

62   Poisons and antidotes, 730

Chapter 62

Poisons and antidotes

A poison may be defined as any substance causing death, disease, or injury. Poisons arise from various sources, including bacteria (toxins), industrial pollution, burning of fossil fuels (carbon monoxide), and radionuclides. Drugs also fit the definition of a poison and are commonly classified as such. In fact, the word pharmacology derives from the Greek *phármakon*, which means 'drug' or 'poison.' Poisoning by drugs is usually a matter of degree; a relatively small quantity produces a desired (therapeutic) effect, whereas a large amount is likely to induce untoward or toxic effects.

Toxicology is defined as the science of poisons and poisonings. It encompasses diagnosis, treatment, mechanism of action, and identification of poisons. Persons skilled in this area of endeavor are classified as clinical, forensic, or industrial toxicologists. Chemical analysis is central to diagnosis of drug intoxication, and recent advances in analytic chemistry have proved valuable in managing patient treatment.

Currently, in the United States 10% of all ambulance calls are poison related. Of pediatric admissions 2% to 5% and of adult admissions to medical services 10% to 20% are for toxin ingestions.[7]

Today, and even more in the future, every human will experience some loss of quality of life from environmental poisons: (1) air pollutants, such as auto exhausts, excessive ozone, and smog, (2) food and water contaminated with pesticides, bacteria, viruses, and plasticizers, and (3) buildings with mold in air vents and often gases from synthetic building materials.

DIAGNOSIS OF POISONING

The diagnosis of poisoning can be difficult, particularly since the victim is often unconscious. Recognition of the cause and severity of intoxication depends largely on physical examination, history, and chemical identification and quantitation of the compound responsible. The conscious patient may not admit to self-poisoning, and this possibility may not enter the physician's differential diagnosis. A suspicious mind is essential to detect these cases. Intoxication should be suspected when an ill person does not respond to treatment within a reasonable time. Cases of poisoning often mimic the initial signs and symptoms of a disease. On the other hand, symptoms and pathologic changes can be quite characteristic for certain types of poisoning. As an aid to considering the possibility of poisoning, the victim's family should be encouraged to produce bottles of medication, particularly empty or partially empty ones, to which the patient had access.

Since there are more poisons than diseases and almost all medical training is focused on disease, physicians may consider themselves less equipped to handle poisoning than other problems. Physicians in this predicament should consult experts in clinical toxicology at regional poison control centers.

Poisoning demographics can aid in diagnosis. Excluding alcohol, fewer than 20 of the 20,000 different pharmaceutical products currently marketed account for 90% of the *nonaccidental* toxin ingestions.[7] Among the most common intoxicants are antidepressants, benzodiazepines, cocaine, opioids, nonopioid analgesics (aspirin, acetaminophen), barbiturates and other sedative-hypnotics, amphetamines, and the phenothiazines. Designer drugs and special blends of drugs appear in periodic cycles, and the local office of the Drug Enforcement Administration can be very helpful in providing the expected composition of these preparations at any given time.

PRINCIPLES OF TREATMENT

The judicious use of drugs and other therapeutic measures in treating poisonings is of utmost importance. However, overtreatment of the intoxicated patient with large doses of antidote, sedatives, or stimulants can cause more damage than the poison itself.[2]

General principles of poison treatment include (1) stabilization of the patient, (2) removal of the poison from the stomach, except where contraindicated, (3) evaluation as soon as possible of samples of blood, urine, vomitus, and so on for identification of the responsible chemical, (4) symptomatic and supportive therapy, (5) administration of an antidote if there is one, and (6) measures to hasten removal of absorbed intoxicant from the body.

The importance of emptying the stomach cannot be overemphasized; this mainstay of treatment can be lifesaving in most intoxications. Exceptions are if the patient is having a seizure, if the airway cannot be protected to prevent aspiration, if the ingested product is corrosive or a petroleum distillate, or if too much time has elapsed since ingestion of the poison. If vomiting has not occurred, the conscious patient should be made to vomit, since vomiting is more effective than the most intensive gastric lavage.[1] Many poisons are themselves emetics, but if emesis does not happen spontaneously, it can usually be induced by stimulation of the pharynx with a finger, often after having the victim drink a glass of milk or water, or by emetic drugs. If vomiting cannot be induced, gastric lavage should be performed at once.

Emetics

Two drugs used to induce vomiting are syrup of ipecac (not the fluid extracts) and apomorphine. For best results fluids should be given before administration of emetics, since emesis does not readily occur if the stomach is empty.

Ipecac syrup is by far the most widely used emetic.[17] It can be kept at home and is inexpensive and safe. With a dosage of 15 to 20 ml the average time before vomiting is 15 minutes. If one dose does not induce emesis in 20 minutes, another 15 ml dose may be administered. If this fails to cause vomiting, gastric lavage becomes imperative, since ipecac is an irritant and, when absorbed, a cardiotoxin. Syrup of ipecac should never be given simultaneously with charcoal because charcoal absorbs the ipecac, thereby preventing its emetic effect. Charcoal should be given after vomiting has stopped.

Subcutaneous injection of **apomorphine hydrochloride** (6 mg/kg for an adult, 0.066 mg/kg for a child) produces emesis within 5 minutes with expulsion of all gastric contents and promotes reflux of the contents of the upper intestinal tract into the stomach. However, prolonged vomiting and, especially in children, the narcotic effects of apomorphine can be serious disadvantages, even though naloxone can be given (0.01 to 0.1 mg/kg intravenously, intramuscularly, or subcutaneously) as an antidote. Most toxicologists consider apomorphine to be of historic interest, and its use should be discontinued.

ANTIDOTES
Nonsystemic antidotes

One gram of activated charcoal has a surface area that exceeds 3000 m². It is a potent adsorbent for many organic and inorganic poisons, excluding cyanide, strong acids or bases, and some lithium compounds. The adsorbed material is retained on the carbon throughout its passage through the gastrointestinal tract. About 15 g (5 to 6 teaspoons) in a glass of milk or water should be given after emesis.[13] Recently, activated charcoal has also been shown to hasten elimination of some intoxicants after absorption. Drugs such as theophylline, phenobarbital, and tricyclic antidepressants undergo enterohepatic circulation. Charcoal can trap these agents in the intestine after they are secreted with bile, thereby preventing reabsorption. For this use activated charcoal is given every 4 to 6 hours for 24 hours and is usually accompanied by sorbitol, which acts as an osmotic cathartic to purge the intestinal tract.

Tannic acid forms insoluble salts with many alkaloids and heavy metals. Approximately 30 to 50 g/L of water is an effective concentration. Larger amounts than those recommended should be avoided because of hepatotoxicity.

Magnesium oxide is used as a neutralizing agent for acids and has the added advantage of not forming gas. In this regard it differs from sodium bicarbonate. The recommended concentration is approximately 25 g/L.

A universal antidote consisting of these three substances in combination has been recommended in the past. The modern trend is to avoid this practice, since the three together can render each other ineffective.[12] Furthermore, this antidote produces a gastric pH of 9 to 9.5, which will favor the absorption of some drugs. Other locally acting antidotes against unabsorbed poisons include vinegar, potassium permanganate, milk, egg white, sodium sulfate, sodium bicarbonate (aerosol), soap, some calcium compounds, ammonia water, starch, vegetable oil, and normal saline (lavage). For practical purposes, most toxicologists today recommend use of activated charcoal.

Systemic antidotes

In addition to use of supportive measures and nonsystemic antidotes, several antidotes that act systemically as physiologic, or occasionally pharmacologic, antagonists to specific intoxicants are available. The most important ones are listed in Table 62-1,[3,4] and certain of these that have not been considered elsewhere are discussed after the table.

TABLE 62-1 Specific antidotes and their dosages

Drug or toxin	Antidote	Dosage*
Acetaminophen	N-Acetylcysteine	*Loading:* 140 mg/kg orally; *oral maintenance:* 70 mg/kg every 4 hours for 17 doses
Anticholinergics	Physostigmine	*Adult:* 1-2 mg; *child:* 0.5 mg; given slowly
Bromide	Sodium chloride	
Carbon monoxide	Oxygen	
Cyanide	Amyl nitrite perles†	
	Sodium nitrite	*Adult:* 300 mg; *child:* 10 mg/kg
	Sodium thiosulfate	*Adult:* 12.5 g; *child:* 0.3-0.5 g/kg
Ethylene glycol	Ethanol	*Loading:* 1 ml/kg of 95%; *maintenance:* 0.1 ml/kg/hour
Heavy metals	Dimercaprol (BAL), calcium disodium edetate, penicillamine	See text
Isoniazid	Pyridoxine	2 to 5 g slowly
Iron	Deferoxamine	10 to 15 mg/kg/hour for 8 hours
Methanol	Ethanol	Same as for ethylene glycol (above)
Narcotics	Naloxone	*Adult:* 0.4-2 mg; *child:* 0.01-0.1 mg/kg
Nitrites	Methylene blue	1 to 2 ml/kg of 1% solution
Organophosphates	Atropine, pralidoxime	2 mg as needed, 1 g

*Given intravenously unless indicated otherwise
†Gelatinous pills containing a medicine (French 'pearls').

Some antidotes are effective after they have been absorbed. Dimercaprol (2,3-dimercaptopropanol, or BAL) is routinely used to treat mercury, gold, and arsenic poisoning. It was developed during World War II as an antidote to vesicant arsenicals. Arsenicals had been known to combine with sulfhydryl groups. After several sulfhydryl compounds were synthesized, it was found that dimercaprol was a particularly effective antidote because of a pair of adjacent sulfhydryl groups that enable it to form a stable ring structure with the metal.

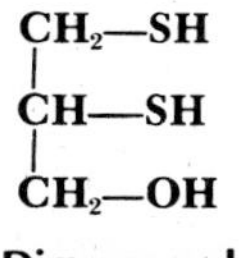

DIMERCAPROL

$$\text{CH}_2\text{—SH}$$
$$|$$
$$\text{CH—SH}$$
$$|$$
$$\text{CH}_2\text{—OH}$$

Dimercaprol

Therapeutic objectives. There are two major objectives in the use of dimercaprol. The first is inactivation of the poison by formation of a complex or a *chelate* (a ringed complex) with it, thus preventing its combination with sulfhydryl groups of essential enzyme systems. The second objective is to promote elimination of the poison from the body; the complex is water soluble at pH 7.5 and is readily excreted.

Toxicity and adverse effects. Dimercaprol is potentially dangerous; side effects include flushing, myalgia, nausea and vomiting, nephrotoxicity, hypotension, pulmonary edema, salivation, lacrimation, and fever. Despite these, dimercaprol has been in use for over 30 years because it remains the most effective antidote.

Metabolism. Dimercaprol is metabolized through S-methylation by a microsomal enzyme. Its use is contraindicated in the presence of liver disease, severe renal disease, or iron poisoning.

Preparations. Dimercaprol (BAL) USP is available as a 10% solution (100 mg/ml) in peanut oil. Dosage varies from 2.5 to 3 mg/kg intramuscularly repeated from one to four times a day, depending on the severity of the intoxication.

CALCIUM DISODIUM EDETATE AND DISODIUM EDETATE

Ethylenediaminetetraacetic acid (EDTA) and its salt, disodium edetate, are powerful chelating agents that form a highly stable complex with calcium. Despite the stability of the chelate, calcium is displaced from it by lead, zinc, chromium, copper, cadmium, manganese, and nickel. Calcium disodium edetate, also called calcium disodium versenate, is used in combination with dimercaprol in treatment of lead poisoning associated with encephalopathy.

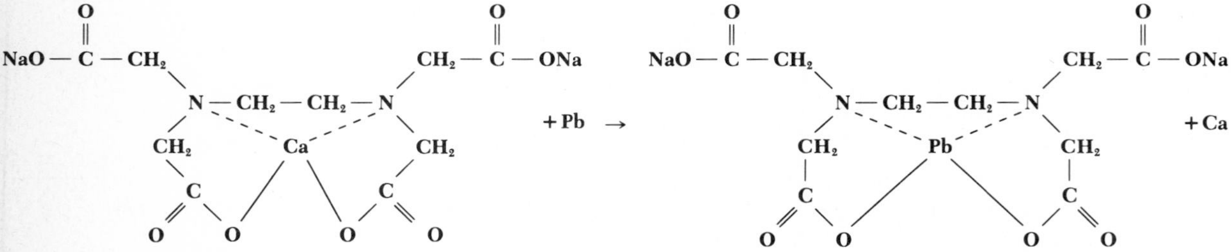

Edetate calcium disodium   Disodium lead edetate

The calcium derivative should be used, since the disodium salt will chelate calcium to produce hypocalcemia. Although the older literature states that the intravenous route of administration is preferred for edetate administration, recent drug schedules for these agents use deep intramuscular injections of dimercaprol and edetate. Severe reactions, such as fever, headache, vomiting, decreased blood pressure, and histamine-like reactions, have been observed with intravenous administration. Oral administration of edetate is unsatisfactory and may be harmful because absorbable edetate-lead complexes can form in the gastrointestinal tract. The rate of urinary lead excretion is enhanced by combined dimercaprol-edetate treatment.

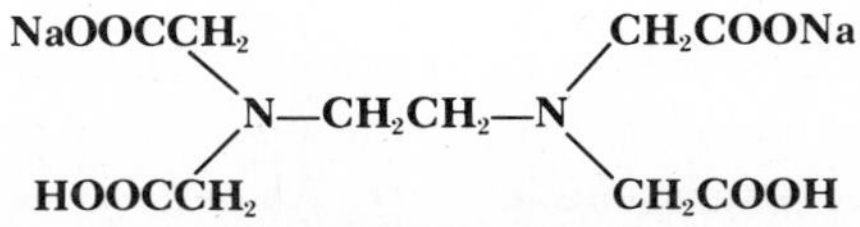

Disodium edetate

Toxicity and adverse effects. The toxicity of edetate is probably caused by binding of essential metal ions. Large doses are nephrotoxic in humans. Edetate is not metabolized; it is excreted by the kidney and is contraindicated in the presence of renal disease.

Preparations. Edetate calcium disodium USP for parenteral use is a 20% solution. To avoid toxic symptoms the total daily dose should not exceed 50 mg/kg of body weight. It is also marketed as 500 mg tablets though it is not usually given orally.

Edetate disodium is marketed in 20 ml ampules that contain 150 mg/ml or 15 ml ampules containing 200 mg/ml. It is used to treat hypercalcemia.

PENICILLAMINE

Therapeutic objectives. Penicillamine (Cuprimine) and its acetyl derivative, N-acetylpenicillamine, can chelate copper and other metals, such as mercury, lead, and iron. Since other drugs are more effective for the latter metals, penicillamine is recommended only for removal of copper in hepatolenticular degeneration (Wilson's disease). The drug is also of value in treatment of nephrolithiasis associated with cystinuria and in treatment of rheumatoid arthritis.

Toxicity and adverse effects. Adverse effects of penicillamine include acute allergic reactions, leukopenia, eosinophilia, thrombocytopenia, and nephrotoxicity. D-Penicillamine is less toxic and is the preferred form, in contrast to former use of the L or D,L forms.

D-Penicillamine USP is marketed as 125 or 250 mg capsules and is administered orally, 1 to 4 g/day divided over four doses.

$$CH_3-\underset{\underset{SH}{|}}{\overset{\overset{CH_3}{|}}{C}}-\underset{\underset{NH_2}{|}}{CH}-COOH$$

Penicillamine

$$CH_3-\underset{\underset{SH}{|}}{\overset{\overset{CH_3}{|}}{C}}-\underset{\underset{\underset{COCH_3}{\diagdown}}{\overset{H}{\diagup}}N}{CH}----COOH$$

N-Acetylpenicillamine

DEFEROXAMINE MESYLATE

Deferoxamine is isolated from *Streptomyces pilosus* and has high affinity for ferric iron and low affinity for calcium. This chelating agent is used to treat iron poisoning and hemochromatosis. It is metabolized by plasma enzymes and is also excreted unchanged in the urine. The drug is toxic and should be used only if the severity of the poisoning justifies it. Reactions include diarrhea, hypotension, and cataract formation. Deferoxamine mesylate USP (Desferal) is available in ampules containing 500 mg. The recommended dose in iron poisoning is 1 g intramuscularly or intravenously, repeated if necessary every 4 to 12 hours. The total dose should not exceed 6 g in 24 hours.

LIFE-SUSTAINING MEASURES

Certain patients with severe drug intoxication or underlying systemic disease in whom the complications of drug overdose are more hazardous may require special interventions to enhance drug removal from the body. These currently include forced diuresis, peritoneal dialysis, hemodialysis, lipid dialysis, hemoperfusion, and exchange transfusion. It is important to stress that such measures are helpful in the minority of cases in contrast, for example, to activated charcoal. When deciding whether to institute such approaches, one must consider if there will be a substantial increase in clearance of the poison. In general, if the intervention does not contribute 30% or more to the total clearance of a drug, it is unlikely to be useful. Lastly, one must also compare the risks of the intervention itself to those of the poisoning. For example, in centers where respiratory and nursing care are expert, the risks of hemoperfusion to remove sedative-hypnotics may be greater than nonintervention.

Forced diuresis	Forced diuresis depends on the kidney's ability to excrete the drug and its metabolites. Many substances with low renal clearance rates are reabsorbed by diffusion across tubular cells. There are two types of diffusion. One is pH independent: in this case excretion can be enhanced when the volume of fluid passing through the renal tubules is increased. Doing so minimizes the time for reabsorption of the drug. Forced diuresis can be accomplished by diuretics (usually osmotic or loop diuretics) or by administration of large volumes of isotonic fluids. The other type of diffusion is pH dependent; by changing urinary pH the excretory rate of the drug is increased (see pp. 25 and 753). Since the urine is normally acidic, if an intervention is needed, it is to alkalinize the urine. This can be accomplished by intravenous administration of isotonic solutions of sodium bicarbonate or by giving of diuretics that inhibit carbonic anhydrase to cause a bicarbonate diuresis.
Peritoneal dialysis	For peritoneal dialysis to be effective the drug or poison should be freely permeable through the peritoneal membrane. Larger molecular weight compounds are not diffusible. Neither are those with a high degree of protein or lipid binding. In general, peritoneal removal of drugs is of insufficient magnitude to be helpful.
Hemodialysis	Hemodialysis can enhance removal of some drugs from the body. For example, 6 hours of hemodialysis can remove as much barbiturate as a 24-hour diuresis. Long-acting barbiturates can be removed with greater efficiency than short-acting ones. This is in part because the short-acting drugs are eliminated quickly enough that dialysis cannot add a substantial increment to clearance. The latter drugs are better removed by lipid dialysis in which soybean oil is circulated on the dialysate side of the membrane, though this intervention is seldom necessary. The use of hemodialysis to treat drug intoxication has waned in recent years because of poor clearance of many drugs by standard procedures.[4]
Hemoperfusion	Hemoperfusion, in which blood is passed through a column containing charcoal or a resin, is now being promoted for removal of numerous poisons. This procedure achieves high clearance rates for most common intoxicants, and its application has been, on occasion, lifesaving. Clearance values obtained by this procedure are substantially higher than those by hemodialysis. The risks of hemoperfusion are decreases

in platelets and other blood cells as they bind to or are damaged in passing through the column. Hence one should not institute this intervention without reconsidering its risks.

The toxic dose is about 30 g or a serum bromide concentration that exceeds 19 mEq/L. Many over-the-counter preparations formerly contained bromide because small doses cause sedation and drowsiness. Excessive chronic intake can lead to mental and respiratory depression, hypotension, and skin rashes. Bromide replaces chloride in the extracellular fluid and is slowly removed from the body when ingestion stops. Treatment of bromide poisoning includes gastric lavage and osmotic diuresis with added chloride. Severe cases may require peritoneal dialysis or hemodialysis.

Ethylene glycol is contained in antifreeze preparations. The lethal dose is about 100 mg. Ethylene glycol is metabolized by alcohol dehydrogenase to oxalate, which can cause severe renal injury and failure. Striking oxalate formation is present throughout the renal tubules. Crystals may even appear in the brain. A metabolic acidosis is caused by formic acid production. Ethylene glycol–induced central nervous system depression can progress to narcosis, coma, and death.

Gastric lavage should be performed to remove the poison. Specific treatment is aimed at correcting the acidosis with sodium bicarbonate. As in methanol intoxication (see p. 298) ethanol greatly slows metabolism and protects against the acute toxicity of ethylene glycol. This represents the mainstay of therapy with administration of sufficient doses of ethanol to maintain serum concentrations of 0.1% to 0.2%. Hemodialysis is effective in reducing the body load of ethylene glycol and should be used.[7] When instituted, however, the dose of ethanol must be increased, since it too is removed by the dialysis. Calcium gluconate should be administered intravenously if hypocalcemia and muscle spasms result from calcium chelation by the oxalate formed.

Diethylene glycol has many industrial uses; however, its ingestion can cause hepatic and renal failure. In the 1930s its use as a solvent in an elixir of sulfanilamide caused 107 fatalities in 15 states among 353 people taking the preparation. From this catastrophe it was estimated that the oral lethal dose is approximately 1 ml/kg.

Carbon monoxide is a highly poisonous, odorless, colorless, flammable gas. Since carbon monoxide does not irritate air passages, its effects are insidious, and a dangerous state of intoxication can arise before the victim becomes aware of it. Carbon monoxide competes with and displaces oxygen from ferrous sites on hemoglobin. Tissue hypoxia and acidosis follow.

Symptoms of carbon monoxide poisoning include headache, dizziness, weakness, nausea, vomiting, loss of muscular control, collapse, unconsciousness, and death. Carbon monoxide affects the cardiac and respiratory systems as a consequence of hypoxia. Cardiac arrhythmias are common, and myocardial infarction often occurs.[11] Coma and death can result when about 60% of the hemoglobin is in the form of carboxyhemoglobin; in cardiac patients lower levels may be fatal. The skin becomes cherry red in color when as little as 25% of the hemoglobin is saturated with carbon monoxide. Retinal hemorrhages have been observed with subacute poisoning.

Oxygen containing 5% to 7% carbon dioxide is used for treatment of carbon monoxide poisoning. Carbon dioxide both increases ventilatory exchange and hastens dissociation of carbon monoxide from hemoglobin. The use of two atmospheres of oxygen results in faster conversion of carboxyhemoglobin to oxyhemoglobin than will breathing 100% oxygen at sea level. Hyperbaric oxygen reduces the carboxyhemoglobin level by one half in 40 minutes. The same effect will not occur for over 4 hours if room air is breathed. Treatment with two atmospheres for 1 hour is usually sufficient.

Cyanide poisoning   Cyanide inhibits cellular respiration by reacting with cytochrome oxidase. Cytotoxic hypoxia results. The minimal lethal dose of cyanide is about 0.5 mg/kg; autopsy data indicate that death predictably results at about 1.4 mg/kg of body weight.

Symptoms of poisoning appear very quickly after cyanide ingestion. They consist in giddiness, headache, palpitations, unconsciousness, convulsions, and death. Diagnosis is usually made by the characteristic odor of oil of bitter almond associated with asphyxia. Death is sometimes delayed so that prompt treatment can be lifesaving; effective antidotes are available.[16]

Treatment of cyanide poisoning is specific and must be given rapidly to be effective. The strategy for treatment relies on the fact that cyanide reacts only with iron in the ferric state. Thus it forms a cytochrome oxidase–cyanide complex that binds with methemoglobin to form cyanomethemoglobin.[18] This reaction draws cyanide away from cytochrome oxidase and can be lifesaving. The objective is to produce a high concentration of methemoglobin ($HbFe^{+++}$) by administration of nitrite.

$$HbFe^{++} + NaNO_2 \rightleftarrows HbFe^{+++}$$

Methemoglobin competes with cytochrome oxidase ($Cyto\text{-}Fe^{+++}$) for cyanide ion. The concentration gradient favors formation of cyanomethemoglobin, and cytochrome oxidase activity is restored. Actual detoxification is achieved by administration of thiosulfate, which reacts with cyanide to form thiocyanate (SCN^-). Thiocyanate is then excreted in the urine.

$$Na_2S_2O_3 + CN^- \rightleftarrows SCN^- + Na_2SO_3$$

This reaction is reversible, and symptoms can return after initial treatment. A solution of 0.5 g of $NaNO_2$ (sodium nitrite) in 15 ml of water is injected intravenously over a 3-minute period, followed by 12.5 g of $Na_2S_2O_3$ (sodium thiosulfate) in 50 ml of water as a slow intravenous infusion over a 10-minute period. If symptoms reappear, the aforementioned procedure is repeated with half the doses. Amyl nitrate should be given while one is waiting for the solutions to be prepared. It is inhaled for 30 seconds every 2 minutes. **Hydroxocobalamin** (alphaREDISOL, others) can also prevent toxicity from cyanide by combining with it to form vitamin B_{12}. Hypoxia resulting from methemoglobinemia should be treated by oxygen inhalation.

Environmental contaminants are the result of our modern life styles. For example, albeit an extreme one, in Canada some totally self-contained homes were built in which no one could live because of gases released from synthetic materials. Similarly, several persons have been forced to move to new locations because of hypersensitivity to formaldehyde. Air ducts in buildings can be sources of bacteria or molds that cause toxic reactions. These areas should be explored when traditional poisons cannot be identified.

ENVIRONMENTAL POISONING

Various metals may produce vastly different symptoms, but one common characteristic is their tendency to accumulate to produce chronic as well as acute poisoning.[15]

Heavy metal poisoning

Lead poisoning was a recognized disease even in colonial times, and in 1723 Massachusetts passed a law preventing the distillation of rum and liquors in retorts or pipes containing lead. In 1975 the Centers for Disease Control reported that more than 28,000 young children suffered from excessive lead absorption. Ingestion is unsafe if it exceeds 0.5 mg/day; 3 months of daily ingestion at this rate is required to reach dangerous concentrations. A few small chips of old paint may contain more than 100 mg of lead.

Early symptoms of lead poisoning include anorexia, apathy, irritability, and perhaps sporadic vomiting. After the early symptoms, acute encephalopathy characterized by ataxia, persistent vomiting, lethargy, stupor, convulsions, and coma can occur rapidly. Children are at greater risk than adults of developing encephalopathy. Twenty-five percent of children who survive encephalopathy suffer severe permanent brain damage. Organic lead produces symptoms predominantly of the central nervous system, whereas inorganic lead poisoning is accompanied by disturbances in hemoglobin synthesis.

The primary screening procedure for lead toxicity is the free erythrocyte protoporphyrin (FEP) test. It is used to detect metabolic evidence of toxicity. Measurements of urinary δ-aminolevulinic acid and coproporphyrin III are also useful for assessing lead poisoning. The toxic concentration of lead in whole blood is above 0.5 μg/ml, whereas concentrations of FEP above 1.1 μg/ml are consistent with lead intoxication. Urine lead concentrations above 0.2 μg/ml, urine coproporphyrin concentrations larger than 0.8 μg/ml, and urinary δ-aminolevulinic acid concentrations higher than 19 μg/ml indicate dangerous amounts of lead absorption.

In patients with encephalopathy, chelation therapy is started with dimercaprol and calcium disodium edetate for 5 to 7 days, depending on severity. Seizures should be controlled with diazepam. If the patient is symptomatic but without encephalopathy, dimercaprol may be omitted. Patients should be separated from the source of lead, since calcium disodium edetate increases absorption of lead from the intestine.

The half-life of lead in blood and soft tissue is about 15 days; in bone it is about 15 years. Of blood lead, 80% to 90% is in the erythrocytes. Over 90% of total body lead is in bone. Chelating agents remove lead from blood and soft tissue but will not remove lead tightly bound to bone.

Most lead enters through the gastrointestinal tract and lungs. Adults consume approximately 300 μg of lead each day but absorb only 10%. Children, on the other hand, absorb about 50% of the lead they ingest.[7] Lead concentrations are many times higher in children compared to adults because children breathe closer to the ground where lead-particle densities are higher. This coupled with a more permeable blood-brain barrier makes children much more susceptible to lead poisoning. Analysis of bones demonstrates over a hundredfold increase in the average total-body lead burden of children compared to unexposed ancestors. As new data are obtained, the level of lead believed to have no effect on children is continually being revised downward.

Mercury contaminates the atmosphere as a result of burning fossil fuels and enters the food chain through fish exposed to water contaminated with mercury compounds. Such a cycle was illustrated by the tragic deaths of those eating mercury-contaminated fish from Minamata Bay in Japan. Mercury wastes from insecticide manufacture were poured into the bay from industrial plants on its shores. Another deplorable event was the death of 459 victims in Iraq who ate bread prepared from wheat treated with a methylmercury fungicide.

The approximate lethal dose of $HgCl_2$ is 1 g, and symptoms of mercury poisoning are first observed at a whole blood concentration of 1 μg/ml. The half-life of methyl mercury is 65 days; therefore repeated exposure leads to accumulation. Methyl mercury is a subtle, difficult to detect, long-lasting poison that easily passes into the central nervous system. Symptoms of chronic mercury poisoning most frequently involve the central nervous system and manifest themselves as tremor and psychotic behavior. Other symptoms include gingivitis, stomatitis, excessive salivation, dermatitis, anorexia, anemia, and weight loss.[5] Acute poisoning produces gastroenteritis with severe abdominal pain and bloody diarrhea. Proteinuria may occur. Anuria and uremia are common.

Depending on the molar ratio of antidote to poison, dimercaprol forms either a chelate or a complex with mercury. The complex is water soluble at pH 7.5, binds mercury more tightly than the chelate does, and is rapidly excreted.

$$H_2C - S$$
$$\quad | \qquad \searrow$$
$$\qquad\qquad Hg$$
$$\quad | \qquad \nearrow$$
$$HC - S$$
$$\quad |$$
$$CH_2OH$$

$$CH_2 - S - Hg - S - CH_2$$
$$\quad | \qquad\qquad\qquad |$$
$$HC - SH \qquad HS - CH$$
$$\quad | \qquad\qquad\qquad |$$
$$CH_2OH \qquad\qquad CH_2OH$$

Mercury chelate   **Mercury complex**

Thallium was used to a greater extent than arsenic for poisoning in antiquity. Acute poisoning currently has been caused by rodenticides and depilatory preparations. Cases of chronic industrial poisoning have involved metal alloys, jewelry, optical lenses, thermometers, electronic equipment, and pigment manufacture. Manifestations of poisoning involve mainly the gastrointestinal tract and the central nervous system. They include hematemesis, bloody diarrhea, mental changes, tremors, choreiform movements, ataxia, convulsions, cyanosis, and death. Among the most lethal of metal poisons, thallium produces one of the highest incidences of long-term neurologic sequelae. The average acute lethal dose of thallium sulfate is about 1 g.

Diagnosis is usually late if it depends only on the alopecia that occurs about 3 weeks after exposure. Hair loss is complete, including hair in the axillary and pubic regions. Black pigmentation around hair roots can be seen as early as 3 days after exposure. Lunule stripes develop as a result of transient disturbances in nail growth. Pronounced tachycardia appears 1 to 4 weeks after initial exposure.

To treat acute intoxication, gastric lavage or emesis should be instituted promptly. Activated charcoal is given in a dose of 0.5 g/kg twice daily for 5 days along with 3 to 5 g of potassium chloride daily for 5 to 10 days. Dimercaprol is used in maximum doses.

Gold in the form of soluble salts has been given intramuscularly for treatment of rheumatoid arthritis for half a century. Its use is empirical, and its mode of action is not understood, but it causes remission in some patients. Dermatitis and stomatitis with fever are the most common manifestations of toxicity. Gold also causes nephritis with albuminuria, gastritis, colitis, and hepatitis. Other organ systems affected are the hematopoietic system, where gold may produce agranulocytosis or aplastic anemia, and the respiratory system, where it initiates a rare pneumonitis characterized by diffuse interstitial inflammation, fibrosis, and lymphocyte and plasma cell infiltration.

Dimercaprol is an effective antidote when given early. Penicillamine, as an oral chelating agent, has also been reported to be effective.

Arsenic, a protoplasmic poison, is found in herbicides, fungicides, and pesticides. Fortunately, its emetic effect can be lifesaving.[6] Other toxic effects are erosion of the gastrointestinal tract, intense diarrhea, and anuria. Inhalation of arsine gas leads to rapid hemolysis and jaundice and the released hemoglobin blocks renal tubules. Even though arsenic crosses the blood-brain barrier slowly and brain levels are among the lowest in the body, it does induce encephalopathy.

Dimercaprol is the antidote of choice,[10] since organic and inorganic trivalent arsenicals have a high affinity for adjacent thiol groups with formation of stable five-membered rings:

$$
\begin{array}{ccccc}
& \text{O} & \text{HS}-\text{CH}_2 & & \text{S}-\text{CH}_2 \\
& \diagup & \mid & & \diagup \quad \mid \\
\text{R-As} & & \text{HS}-\text{CH} \rightarrow & \text{R-As} & \quad + \text{H}_2\text{O} \\
& \diagdown & \mid & & \diagdown \quad \mid \\
& \text{O} & \text{HO}-\text{CH}_2 & & \text{S}-\text{CH} \\
& & & & \mid \\
& & & & \text{HO}-\text{CH}_2
\end{array}
$$

Trivalent arsenical   **BAL**   **BAL-arsenic complex**

Iron in the ferrous form has proved fatal to children. Symptoms include vomiting, erosion of the gastrointestinal tract, hemorrhage, cyanosis, coma, respiratory depression, and shock.

Gastric lavage must be instituted immediately. In severe intoxication calcium disodium edetate is administered orally; if an intravenous dose is used shortly thereafter, the size of the dose must be appropriately reduced. Deferoxamine, also effective in the treatment of severe acute poisoning, can be given orally or intravenously but may produce systemic toxicity. Acidosis and shock occur in severe iron poisoning and necessitate prompt treatment.

Aluminum compounds are widely distributed in nature. Despite an oral intake of 10 to 100 mg daily, little aluminum is absorbed. This barrier may be broken, however, in uremic patients maintained on long-term hemodialysis and receiving aluminum-containing antacids to decrease phosphate absorption. A few such patients develop a peculiar neurologic syndrome characterized by speech abnormalities, dyspraxia, asterixis, myoclonus, personality changes, disordered EEGs, dementia, and psychosis, progressing to death. Lung damage caused by inhalation of fumes containing Al_2O_3 results in shortness of breath, cyanosis, substernal pain, and often spontaneous pneumothorax (Shaver's disease). The use of calcium disodium edetate may be unnecessary, since effects of the metal are self-limited. Its source should be found and eliminated.

Although humans developed pesticides for the deliberate killing of insects and other pests, as fate would have it, these agents can also kill humans. All the organochlorine compounds are central nervous system stimulants, promote convulsions, and are absorbed through the skin as well as from the gastrointestinal tract.

The **cyclodiene** insecticides (for example, dieldrin and chlordane) cause seizures similar to epilepsy along with tremor, nausea, vomiting, and ataxia. Endrin is the most toxic compound in this group.

The **chlorinated ethane derivatives** are related to DDT. Since its ban, DDT has been largely replaced by methoxychlor, which is less toxic and less effective as an insecticide. Sudden death from ventricular fibrillation has been reported after ingestion of these substances, caused by sensitization of the myocardium to endogenous catecholamines. In DDT poisoning, death may also result from respiratory failure secondary to medullary paralysis. These compounds tend to accumulate in fat and induce the microsomal enzyme system.[3]

The **chlorocyclohexanes** are represented by benzene hexachloride and its γ isomer, lindane, which is used to treat pediculosis. In addition to producing severe convulsions, they induce pulmonary edema, liver and kidney damage, and agranulocytosis as well. Like DDT, these substances can sensitize the myocardium. If renal and hepatic damage should occur from the organochlorine compounds, management is the same as when these injuries arise from other causes.

Other types of insecticides are thiocyanates, phosphate esters, organophosphate compounds (anticholinesterases), fluorides, and botanicals such as nicotine, pyrethrins, and rotenoids. For symptoms and treatment of organophosphate poisoning refer to Chapter 11.

Insecticides

In contrast to insecticides, the rodenticides are designed to kill animals with essentially the same major biochemical pathways as humans. These include (1) anticoagulants such as coumarins and indandiones, (2) heavy metals such as arsenicals, thallium, copper, and lead salts, (3) botanicals such as squill and strychnine, and (4) miscellaneous substances such as fluoroacetate, phosphorus, and zinc phosphide. The treatment for rodenticide poisoning varies with the poison because the substances are extremely varied in composition and actions.

Rodenticides

Solvents   A significant number of poisonings occur from solvents used at home and in industrial settings. Since these are fat solvents, they cross lipid cellular membranes quite easily; the brain is a major target organ because of its high lipid content. In the brain these solvents exert narcotic or convulsant actions depending on the molecule. In general, solvents that are aliphatic hydrocarbons induce coma. Reflexes are weak or absent. Aromatic solvents tend to cause motor unrest, tremors, jactitations, and hyperactive reflexes. Intentional gasoline sniffing has been shown to be a major form of abuse.[8]

Toluene in many ways exemplifies the typical solvent; it is extensively used in industrial and household products. Essentially replacing benzene because of its reduced toxicity,[9] toluene (the primary intoxicant in glue-sniffing) is a psychotropic and neurotoxic agent. Neurologic symptoms are its most frequently cited effects. Toluene can produce sudden death, addictive-like behavior, renal abnormalities, hepatic and hematologic illness, and an acute brain syndrome with EEG changes, visual hallucinations, confusion, and seizures. Since it accumulates in bone marrow and has a slow rate of elimination from this tissue, toluene exposure can also cause blood dyscrasias.

The distribution of toluene into various tissues is faster after inhalation than after ingestion. Exercise increases blood concentration and total uptake of inhaled toluene, largely by increasing respiration and cardiac output.

Toluene is sometimes contaminated with benzene, a highly toxic substance. Industrial-grade toluene contains as much as 25% benzene. Toluene in combination with other solvents is more toxic than would be predicted on the basis of the additive toxic action of each component by itself.

1. Arena, J.M.: Poisoning, Emerg. Med. 8(4):171, 1976.

2. Arena, J.M.: Poisoning: toxicology, symptoms, treatments, ed. 4, Springfield, Ill., 1979, Charles C Thomas, Publisher.

3. Bayer, M.J., and Rumack, B.H.: Poisoning & overdose. Rockville, Md., 1983, Aspen Systems Corp.

4. Bryson, P.D.: Comprehensive review in toxicology, Rockville, Md., 1986, Aspen Systems Corp.

5. Burston, G.R.: Self-poisoning, London, 1970, Lloyd-Luke (Medical Books) Ltd.

6. Dreisbach, R.H.: Handbook of poisoning, ed. 11, Los Altos, Calif., 1983, Lange Medical Publications.

7. Goldfrank, L.R., Flomenbaum, N.E., Lewin, N.A., et al.: Goldfrank's toxicologic emergencies, ed. 3, Norwalk, Conn., 1986, Appleton-Century-Crofts.

8. Gossell, T.A., and Bricker, J.D.: Principles of clinical toxicology, New York, 1984, Raven Press Books.

9. Klaassen, C.D., Amdur, M.O., and Doull, J.: Casarett and Doull's toxicology: the basic science of poisons, ed. 3, New York, 1986, Macmillan Publishing Co.

10. Loomis, T.A.: Essentials of toxicology, ed. 3, Philadelphia, 1978, Lea & Febiger.

11. Matthew, H., and Lawson, A.A.H.: Treatment of common acute poisonings, ed. 2, Edinburgh, 1970, E. & S. Livingstone.

12. Moeschlin, S.: Poisoning: diagnosis and treatment, New York, 1965, Grune & Stratton, Inc.

13. Neuvonen, P.J.: Clinical pharmacokinetics of oral activated charcoal in acute intoxications, Clin. Pharmacokinet. 7:465, 1982.

14. Okonek, S.: Hemoperfusion in toxicology: basic considerations of its effectiveness, Clin. Toxicol. 18:1185, 1981.

15. Polson, C.J., Green, M.A., and Lee, M.R.: Clinical toxicology, ed. 3, Philadelphia, 1983, J.B. Lippincott Co.

16. Thienes, C.H., and Haley, T.J.: Clinical toxicology, ed. 5, Philadelphia, 1972, Lea & Febiger.

17. Veltri, J.C., and Litovitz, T.L.: 1983 annual report of the American Association of Poison Control Centers National Data Collection System, Am. J. Emerg. Med. 2:420, 1984.

18. Vennesland, B., Castric, P.A., Conn, E.E., et al.: Cyanide metabolism, Fed. Proc. 41:2639, 1982.

REFERENCES

section twelve

Drug interactions

63   Drug interactions, 748

Chapter 63

Drug interactions

When several drugs are administered concurrently, they may influence each other favorably or unfavorably. Drug interactions may be of great clinical importance when the margin of safety of one or more of the drugs is small. The interactions present as either an enhanced or diminished drug effect. Enhanced drug effects may manifest themselves as idiosyncratic responses that can occasionally have dire consequences. The clinically significant drug interactions can be minimized by avoidance of combinations of drugs known to be incompatible, according to current pharmacologic literature and tables such as those presented in this chapter. Ultimately, however, it is the physician's familiarity with the clinical literature and understanding of the mechanisms underlying drug interactions that are most likely to prevent their occurrence.

Adverse reactions based on drug interactions are not always iatrogenic. Self-medication with over-the-counter drugs may also be causal. In addition, **environmental contaminants** such as the chlorinated insecticides (DDT) may stimulate drug metabolism by hepatic microsomal enzymes and could conceivably contribute to unusual reactions to drugs.

MECHANISMS UNDERLYING ADVERSE EFFECTS OF DRUG INTERACTIONS	Adverse drug interactions may be divided into *pharmacokinetic* and *pharmacodynamic* interactions.[1,2] The pharmacokinetic interactions may be at the level of (1) absorption, (2) distribution, (3) metabolism, or (4) excretion. Pharmacodynamic interactions influence the response to a drug once it reaches its site of action and may occur at the receptor site, may alter response by changing the physiologic milieu, and so forth.
Intestinal absorption	Drug interactions involving absorption are presented in Table 63-1. Important examples include calcium-, magnesium- or aluminum-containing antacids that interfere with absorption of tetracycline, which forms a chelate with the metals. Antacids containing aluminum also interfere with phosphate absorption. Carbonates and phytates (cereals) prevent absorption of iron. Cholestyramine and colestipol (bile acid–binding resins) may interfere with absorption of several drugs, particularly warfarin and digitalis glycosides.

Antacids may also influence drug absorption by changing the lipid-soluble, nonionized fraction of weak acids in the gastrointestinal tract. Recall from p. 21 that the nonionized moiety is much better absorbed from the stomach (as opposed to the |

TABLE 63-1 Drug interactions at sites of absorption

Proposed mechanism	Drug affected	Drug causing effect	Results of interaction
Formation of complexes, chelation, adsorption	Bishydroxycoumarin	Antacids	Increased absorption
	Carbamazepine	Activated charcoal	Decreased absorption, increased elimination
	Cephalexin	Cholestyramine	Decreased absorption
	Chlorothiazide	Cholestyramine	Decreased absorption
	Chlorpromazine	Antacids	Decreased absorption
	Diflunisal	Antacids	Decreased absorption
	Digitoxin	Cholestyramine	Decreased absorption, increased elimination
	Digoxin	Activated charcoal, antacids, cholestyramine, kaolin-pectin	Decreased absorption
	Isoniazid	Antacids	Decreased absorption
	Penicillamine	Antacids	Decreased absorption
	Phenobarbital	Activated charcoal	Decreased absorption, increased elimination
	Phenylbutazone	Cholestyramine	Decreased absorption
	Phenytoin	Activated charcoal	Decreased absorption
	Propranolol	Antacids, cholestyramine	Decreased absorption
	Ranitidine	Antacids	Decreased absorption
	Tetracyclines	Antacids	Decreased absorption
	Theophylline	Activated charcoal	Decreased absorption, increased elimination
	Thyroxine	Cholestyramine	Decreased absorption
	Tolbutamide	Activated charcoal	Decreased absorption
	Valproate	Activated charcoal	Decreased absorption
	Warfarin	Cholestyramine	Decreased absorption, increased elimination
Alteration in gastric pH	Cimetidine	Antacids	Decreased absorption
	Ketoconazole	Cimetidine	Decreased absorption
	Tetracyclines	Cimetidine, sodium bicarbonate	Decreased absorption
Alterations in gastric motility			
Increase	Acetaminophen	Metoclopramide	Increased rate of absorption
	Chlorothiazide	Metoclopramide	Increased rate of absorption
	Cimetidine	Metoclopramide	Decreased absorption
	Digoxin	Metoclopramide	Decreased absorption
	Ethanol	Metoclopramide	Increased rate of absorption
	Lithium	Metoclopramide	Increased rate of absorption
Decrease	Acetaminophen	Narcotic analgesics, propantheline	Decreased rate of absorption
	Benzodiazepines	Antacids	Decreased rate of absorption
	Bishydroxycoumarin	Amitriptyline	Increased absorption
	Chlorothiazide	Propantheline	Decreased rate of absorption
	Digoxin	Propantheline	Increased absorption
	Ethanol	Propantheline	Decreased rate of absorption
	Isoniazid	Antacids	Decreased rate of absorption
	Lithium	Propantheline	Decreased rate of absorption
	Phenytoin	Antacids	Decreased rate of absorption
	Propranolol	Antacids	Decreased rate of absorption
Effects on gastrointestinal mucosa	Aminoglycoside antibiotics	Ethanol	Increased absorption caused by mucosal damage
	Digoxin	Neomycin, sulfasalazine	Decreased absorption
	Furosemide	Phenytoin	Decreased absorption
Effects on gastrointestinal flow	Digoxin	Broad-spectrum antibiotics	Increased absorption

TABLE 63-2	Drug interactions caused by displacement from plasma protein–binding sites	
Drug displaced	Causative agents	
Coumarin anticoagulants	Chloral hydrate, clofibrate, diazoxide, ethacrynic acid, mefenamic acid, nalidixic acid, phenylbutazone, phenytoin, salicylates	
Diazepam	Heparin, valproic acid	
Phenytoin	Phenylbutazone, salicylates, tolbutamide, valproic acid	
Tolbutamide	Phenylbutazone, salicylates, dicumarol	

small intestine where pH-dependent lipid solubility appears to play a lesser role). Because of this, antacids would be expected to diminish gastric absorption of weak acids. Absorption from the small intestine would not be affected.

Other gastrointestinal drug interactions may be of clinical significance. Antibiotics that alter the bacterial flora in the intestine can decrease formation of vitamin K and thus increase the anticoagulant action of the coumarins. Similarly, in some patients gut bacteria metabolize digoxin, decreasing its availability. Certain antibiotics can eliminate the responsible flora and thereby increase the bioavailability of digoxin. Some drugs, such as phenytoin and triamterene, inhibit an intestinal conjugase that breaks down the polyglutamate portion of naturally occurring folic acid and, by this mechanism, cause megaloblastic anemia.

Direct chemical interactions occur not only in the gastrointestinal tract but also when drugs are mixed for intravenous infusions. For example, carbenicillin and other ureidopenicillins inactivate aminoglycosides if mixed for intravenous infusion.

Distribution   Many drugs are bound to plasma proteins to varying degrees, and the bound fraction fails to exert pharmacologic actions. For example, two antibiotics having the same potency in a protein-free culture medium will have different clinical effectiveness if their affinities for plasma proteins differ greatly. The most important adverse drug interactions caused by displacement from plasma proteins occur with the coumarin anticoagulants (Table 63-2). Although in general the increase in concentration of free drug is expected to be transient, in many instances the displacer inhibits drug metabolism as well. For example, phenylbutazone displaces warfarin from its binding sites and also inhibits its metabolism and may thereby cause bleeding.

TABLE 63-3	Examples of drugs that inhibit hepatic metabolism of other drugs
Drug causing inhibition	**Drugs inhibited**
Amiodarone	Digoxin, phenytoin, procainamide, quinidine, flecainide
Bishydroxycoumarin	Tolbutamide
Chloramphenicol	Carbamazepine, chlorpropamide, oral anticoagulants, phenobarbital, phenytoin, tolbutamide
Chlorpromazine	Phenytoin, propranolol
Cimetidine	Benzodiazepines, carbamazepine, 5-fluorouracil, imipramine, lidocaine, meperidine, phenytoin, propranolol, theophylline, warfarin
Disulfiram	Benzodiazepines, phenytoin, warfarin
Erythromycin	Carbamazepine, theophylline
Ethanol (acute ingestion)	Diazepam, meprobamate, pentobarbital, phenytoin, tolbutamide, warfarin
Isoniazid	Carbamazepine, phenytoin
Methylphenidate	Phenobarbital, phenytoin, primidone
Oral contraceptives	Diazepam, imipramine, oral anticoagulants, theophylline
Propoxyphene	Carbamazepine, doxepin, phenytoin
Propranolol	Diazepam, lidocaine
Sulfonamides	Carbamazepine, phenytoin, tolbutamide, warfarin

Tolbutamide can be displaced from plasma binding by dicumarol, resulting in severe hypoglycemia. Chloral hydrate transiently increases the anticoagulant action of warfarin because its metabolite, trichloroacetic acid, competes with the anticoagulant for plasma protein binding.

Metabolism or biotransformation

Inhibition of the metabolism of one drug by another is a well-established mechanism of enhanced drug effect (Table 63-3). By their enzyme-inhibiting action, the anticholinesterases enhance the effects of acetylcholine, succinylcholine, and some other choline esters. Allopurinol inhibits xanthine oxidase and thus increases plasma levels of mercaptopurine and azathioprine. Monoamine oxidase inhibitors have caused severe reactions by preventing destruction of catecholamines in the body. Cimetidine halves the clearance of some drugs with narrow therapeutic margins, such as warfarin, lidocaine, and theophylline. In some instances a drug may diminish hepatic blood flow and inhibit drug metabolism by that mechanism. In this way β-adrenergic receptor blocking agents raise lidocaine concentrations.

TABLE 63-4	Examples of drugs that induce hepatic metabolism of other drugs
Inducing agent	**Drug induced**
Carbamazepine	Oral anticoagulants, phenytoin
Cigarette smoking	Theophylline
Ethanol (chronic, before hepatic impairment)	Meprobamate, oral anticoagulants, pentobarbital, phenytoin, tolbutamide
Glutethimide	Oral anticoagulants
Griseofulvin	Oral anticoagulants
Oral contraceptives	Acetaminophen
Phenobarbital	Chloramphenicol, chlorpromazine, cimetidine, digitoxin, griseofulvin, oral anticoagulants, phenylbutazone, phenytoin, theophylline
Phenytoin	Carbamazepine, clonazepam, cyclosporine, diazepam, digitoxin, doxycycline, glucocorticoids, methadone, oral anticoagulants, quinidine, theophylline, valproic acid
Rifampin	Chloramphenicol, digoxin, digitoxin, glucocorticoids, oral anticoagulants, quinidine, theophylline, tolbutamide

Many drugs can accelerate their metabolism and also that of other drugs by induction of hepatic microsomal enzymes (Table 63-4). Phenobarbital accelerates metabolism of hydrocortisone, estrogens, androgens, progesterone, and many other agents. Phenobarbital combined with phenytoin greatly increases the clearance of quinidine, probably as a consequence of enzyme induction. Other agents that induce hepatic metabolism include glutethimide, phenytoin, rifampin, and chlorinated hydrocarbon insecticides, such as DDT.

Enzyme induction decreases the effectiveness of certain other drugs and may have life-threatening consequences if the inducer is discontinued without changing the dosage of the second drug. For example, if phenobarbital is suddenly discontinued without lowering the dosage of a coumarin anticoagulant, severe hemorrhagic episodes may develop (see Fig. 4-2).

TABLE 63-5	Agents actively secreted by the proximal renal tubules
Organic acids	**Organic bases**
p-Aminohippurate	Amantadine
Captopril	Amiloride
Cephalosporins (most)	Cimetidine
Dyphylline	Ethambutol
Heparin	Mecamylamine
"Loop" diuretics	Mepacrine
Methotrexate	*N*-Methylnicotinamide
Nonsteroidal anti-inflammatory agents	Procainamide
Penicillins	Pseudoephedrine
Probenecid	Tetraethylammonium
Salicylates	
Sulfonamides	
Sulfonylureas	
Thiazide diuretics	

Renal excretion

There are several examples of drug interactions resulting from an influence on renal tubular excretion of drugs. The best is the inhibition of penicillin secretion by probenecid. A variety of organic acids and organic bases (Table 63-5) can compete with each other for renal secretion.

Acidification of the urine after oral administration of ammonium chloride or alkalinization with sodium bicarbonate may have a demonstrable effect on renal clearance of several drugs, but the quantitative importance is not great except in phenobarbital or salicylate intoxication. The excretion of amphetamine is greatly decreased in a relatively alkaline urine. However, since the urine is normally acidic, this phenomenon becomes important only in unusual circumstances.

Another important renal drug interaction involves digoxin and quinidine. Quinidine decreases the distal tubular secretion of digoxin, thus increasing digoxin concentration in the plasma. In addition, quinidine decreases the volume of distribution of digoxin, probably by decreasing the binding of digoxin in muscle.

TABLE 63-6 Examples of pharmacodynamic drug interactions

Drug or condition altering response	Drug response altered	Comments
Acidemia	Sympathomimetics	Decreased effect
Aminoglycoside antibiotics	Neuromuscular blockers	Increased effect
β-Adrenergic receptor antagonists	Clonidine	Blood pressure overshoot during withdrawal
Digitalis	β-Adrenergic receptor antagonists	Profound bradycardia
Disopyramide	Practolol	Profound bradycardia
Diuretics	Antihypertensives	Increased effect
Guanidinium antihypertensives	Directly acting α-adrenergic receptor agonists	Increased effect
Hypercalcemia	Cardiac glycosides	Increased toxicity
Inhibitors of prostaglandin synthesis	Captopril	Decreased effect
	"Loop" diuretics	Predominately decreased effect
	Propranolol	Decreased antihypertensive effect
Magnesium depletion	Cardiac glycosides	Increased toxicity
Methyldopa	Haloperidol	Dementia
Phenytoin	Lithium	Increased effect
Potassium depletion	Cardiac glycosides	Increased toxicity
Reserpine	Indirectly acting α-adrenergic receptor agonists	Decreased effect
Tricyclic antidepressants	Directly and indirectly acting α-adrenergic receptor agonists	Increased effect
	Guanidinium antihypertensives	Decreased effect
	Clonidine	Decreased effect

The numerous pharmacodynamic interactions usually take place at the receptor level. Innumerable synergisms and antagonisms discussed throughout the text are examples of pharmacodynamic interactions. Representative examples are also presented in Table 63-6. These interactions may be at the same receptor or at different receptors.

Pharmacodynamic interactions

Some drug interactions among those listed in Tables 63-1 to 63-6 may be life threatening, whereas others are relatively less important and require only a simple adjustment in the dosage. A major determinant of the seriousness of an interaction is the therapeutic margin of the drugs involved. With anticoagulants, oral hypoglycemic drugs, digitalis, and antiarrhythmic drugs, the margin of safety is not great, and relatively small changes in plasma concentration resulting from drug interactions can have catastrophic results. On the other hand, drugs with large margins of safety do not cause serious problems as a consequence of drug interactions. This principle should be kept in mind when one is examining tables of drug interactions.

Significance of adverse drug reactions

1. Hansten, P.D.: Drug interactions, ed. 5, Philadelphia, 1985, Lea & Febiger.
2. Vasko, M.R., and Brater, D.C.: Drug-drug interactions. In Chernow, B., and Lake, C.R., editors: The pharmacologic approach to the critically ill patient, Baltimore, 1983, The Williams & Wilkins Co., p. 22.

REFERENCES

section thirteen

Prescription writing and drug compendia

64   *Prescription writing and drug compendia, 758*

Chapter 64

Prescription writing and drug compendia

A prescription is a written order given by a physician to a pharmacist. In addition to the name of the patient and that of the physician, the prescription should contain the name or names of the drugs ordered and their quantities, instructions to the pharmacist, and directions to the patient.

Prescription writing has changed in modern medicine as a result of several developments. Most preparations today are compounded by pharmaceutical companies, and the pharmacist's current role in most cases is dispensing. Also, the practice of writing long, complicated prescriptions containing many active ingredients, adjuvants, correctives, and various vehicles has been abandoned in favor of pure compounds. Even when combinations of several active ingredients are desirable, pharmaceutical companies often provide several suitable combinations. The custom of prescribing trademarked mixtures has disadvantages. The physician may be so accustomed to prescribing a mixture of drugs by a trade name that he becomes uncertain about the individual components, some of which may be unnecessary or undesirable in a given case. Physicians should be cautious to avoid this pitfall.

A drug may be prescribed by its official name, which is listed in the *United States Pharmacopeia (USP)*, by its nonproprietary (often called "generic") name or *United States Adopted Name (USAN)*, or by a manufacturer's trade name.[1] The designation USAN has recently been coined for generic or nonproprietary names adopted by the American Medical Association–United States Pharmacopeia Nomenclature Committee in cooperation with the respective manufacturers. Adoption of USAN names does not imply endorsement by these organizations.

There is considerable advantage to prescribing drugs by their official or nonproprietary names. This often allows the pharmacist to dispense a more economical product than a trademarked preparation of one company. It also reduces the expense of each pharmacy's maintaining a multiplicity of very similar preparations, a saving that could ultimately benefit the patient.

On the other hand, the physician may have reasons for prescribing one manufacturer's product. This is often the only way to be certain that the preparation given to the patient will be exactly what is intended, not only in its active ingredients but even to the point of its appearance and taste.

Approval of a generic formulation by the Food and Drug Administration (FDA) requires demonstration of "bioequivalence." This has been defined in regulatory terms as the generic drug's absorption differing no more than 20% from the brand-name product (with drugs having a narrow margin of safety, less variation may be required). This means that a product may have from 80% to 120% absorption compared to the standard. If an individual manufacturer's product is consistent in this regard, substitution of a generic formulation for the brand-name product may cause no problems. However, if a patient's pharmacy switches from a product with 80% absorption to one with 120% bioavailability or vice versa, problems could conceivably ensue. Physicians and patients should be alert to this potential.

There is much discussion at present concerning the relative advantages of prescribing by nonproprietary names rather than by trade names. It is clear that savings to patients can occur. It is equally clear that even greater savings would be possible if pharmacists passed more of their savings to the patient. Whether there is a cost in terms of decreased drug efficacy or increased toxicity is unclear. The outcome of this debate should be of great interest in medical economics.

Traditionally a prescription is written in a certain order and consists of four basic parts:

Parts of a prescription

1. *Superscription*. This is simply *Rx*, the abbreviation for *recipe*, meaning "take thou," the imperative of *recipere*.

2. *Inscription*. This indicates the ingredients and their amounts. If a prescription contains several ingredients in a mixture, it is customary to write them in the following order: (1) the basis, or principal ingredient, (2) the adjuvant, which may contribute to the action of the basis, and (3) the corrective, which may eliminate some undesirable property of the active drug or the vehicle, which is the substance used for dilution.

3. *Subscription*. This contains directions for dispensing. Often it consists only of *M*., the abbreviation for *misce*, meaning "mix (thou)."

4. *Signature*. This is often abbreviated as *Sig*. and contains the directions to the patient, such as "Take one teaspoonful three times a day before meals." It is also helpful to include the indication for the medication, for example, "for ulcers." Wherever possible, instructions of a general nature, such as "take as directed," should be avoided, since the patient may misunderstand or forget oral directions given by the physician.

In addition to these basic parts of a prescription, it should have the patient's name and the physician's signature, followed by the prescriber's degree. The current trend is that the physician may sign his or her name in one of two places to designate whether generic substitution is permitted. Some state laws require that if substitution is to be prohibited, the physician must actually write "dispense as written" or a similar phrase.

Modern trends in prescription writing

The parts of the prescription described in the previous paragraphs represent a tradition that is undergoing considerable change. Latin, even in the form of abbreviations, is not necessary. Its main purpose in the past was to conceal from the patient the nature (and often worthlessness) of a drug. At the present time, prescriptions are written in English. Even such abbreviations as *M.* or *Sig.* may be avoided. It is also advisable to avoid the use of the decimal point and to state the number of milligrams in a dose instead of using the decimal fraction of a gram.

There are other interesting trends in prescription writing.[2] Much confusion results when the name of the drug is not included on the label so that patients know only that they are taking pills having certain physical characteristics. The busy physician wastes much time trying to identify medications given to his patients by other physicians. To avoid this problem, physicians should ask the pharmacist to name the drug on the label, indicating their wish by checking an appropriate box on the prescription form. They also indicate in another box the number of allowable refills.

TABLE 64-1	Criteria for scheduling drugs				
	Schedule I	Schedule II	Schedule III	Schedule IV	Schedule V
Potential for abuse	+ + + +	+ + + +	+ + +	+ +	+
Accepted medical use in U.S.A.	None	Yes, with severe restrictions	Yes	Yes	Yes
Potential dependence:					
Psychologic	+ + + +	+ + + +	+ + +	+ +	+
Physical	+ + + +	+ + + +	+ +	+ +	+
Examples	Heroin LSD Marijuana MDA Methaqualone Phencyclidine THC	Amphetamine Cocaine Codeine Methadone Morphine Pentobarbital Phenmetrazine	Codeine combinations Glutethimide Phendimetrazine	Diazepam Flurazepam Phentermine Propoxyphene*	Cold/cough preparations with codeine Diphenoxylate combinations (Lomotil)†

LSD, Lysergic acid diethylamide; *MDA*, 3,4-methylenedioxyamphetamine; *THC*, tetrahydrocannabinol.
*Bulk chemical in schedule II.
†Prescription necessary.

Until recently, prescriptions for narcotic drugs were regulated by the Harrison Anti-Narcotic Act and the drug abuse control amendments of 1965. These regulations have been replaced by the Federal Controlled Substances Act of 1970 and the regulations issued by the director of the Federal Drug Enforcement Administration (DEA). The drugs controlled by the act are placed in five categories, or schedules (Table 64-1).

All prescriptions for controlled drugs (schedules II to V) must contain the full name and address of the patient, full name, address, and DEA (Drug Enforcement Administration) number of the prescribing doctor, signature of the prescribing doctor, and date. Prescriptions for schedule II drugs are not refillable. Schedules III and IV drugs may be refilled up to five times within 6 months of initial issuance if so authorized by the prescribing physician. Prescriptions for schedule V drugs may be refilled as authorized by the prescribing physician.

Prescriptions and the Federal Controlled Substances Act

Typical prescription

John Doe, M.D.
555 Medical Arts Building
City
Telephone: 361-4282

Name ___David Smith___   Date ___May 9, 1988___

Address ___201 Hall St.___   Age ___42___

    Tetracycline, 250 mg capsules
    Dispense twenty
    Label: Take one capsule four times a day for 5 days

Signature:

Refills _____   *Dispense as written* _____

DEA No. _____   *Substitution permitted* _____

DRUG COMPENDIA   Authoritative information on drugs can be found in the *United States Pharmacopeia* as well as in many textbooks of pharmacology. The *United States Pharmacopeia* was first published in 1820 and became official in 1906, when it was so designated by the first Food and Drug Act. The *United States Pharmacopeia* is revised by physicians, pharmacists, and medical scientists who are elected by delegates to the United States Pharmacopeial Convention. The delegates originate from schools of medicine and pharmacy, from medical and pharmaceutical societies, and from some departments of the government. Its current official position is based on the Federal Food, Drug, and Cosmetic Act of 1938, which recognizes it as an "official compendium." The *United States Pharmacopeia* is published every 5 years. For a drug to be included there must be good evidence for its therapeutic merit or its pharmaceutical necessity.

AMA Drug Evaluations is a valuable source of information, published yearly, on most drugs that are available in the United States. It is particularly useful in describing currently accepted therapeutic practices and available preparations.

If physicians could limit their use of drugs to those that are listed in the *United States Pharmacopeia* or those that have been recommended by *AMA Drug Evaluations*, they would be protected against unfounded claims or the power of advertising. When a new drug represents a therapeutic advance, physicians may be unable to wait for such authoritative reviews. They must often rely on written or verbal statements of recognized experts in the field. In any case, they should not depend solely on advertising literature or drug circulars and package inserts (including the *Physicians' Desk Reference*, or *PDR*).

REFERENCES   1. Cutting, W.: A note on names, Clin. Pharmacol. Ther. **4**:569, 1963.
2. Friend, D.G.: Principles and practices of prescription writing, Clin. Pharmacol. Ther. **6**:411, 1965.

appendixes

A Drug concentrations in blood, 766

B Comparison of selected effects of commonly abused drugs, 773

C Pharmacokinetic characteristics of drugs, 776

Drug concentrations in blood

The concentration of drugs in the blood is of interest in clinical medicine and medicolegal situations. The tabular presentation of drug concentrations in the blood on pp. 768 to 771 is intended as a source of information and as a guide to the available literature.[5] It should be recognized that the figures given are often based on a few cases and are subject to change as more information accumulates. Furthermore, the significance of blood concentrations depends on numerous factors, and the tables should be consulted with full recognition of the role of modifying influences.

IMPORTANCE OF DRUG CONCENTRATIONS IN SERUM

The determination of drug concentrations in serum is not important when the pharmacologic effects of the drug can easily be monitored. For example, in the use of coumarin anticoagulants or antihypertensive drugs the effects of the drugs provide a good indication of adequacy of serum concentrations and dosage. On the other hand, there are drugs, such as phenytoin and quinidine, that are used prophylactically and provide therapeutic problems in the absence of knowledge of their serum concentrations. Studies have demonstrated that the correlation of serum concentration of these drugs with response is closer than the correlation of dose to response.[1-3] The determination of concentrations in the serum is also useful for revealing noncompliance with the physician's instructions.

The relationship between serum concentration and a drug's effects is complicated by numerous factors such as (1) tolerance, (2) drug interactions, (3) the underlying disease, (4) protein binding, and (5) active metabolites. The first three factors in modifying the relationship between concentration and effect are easily understood. The importance of the latter two is not always appreciated.

The role of protein binding is illustrated by the following problem.

PROBLEM A. *The therapeutic concentration of phenytoin is 20 mg/L. It is about 95% bound to serum albumin. In the case of uremia, hypoalbuminemia, or the presence of other drugs that displace phenytoin from its binding sites, the bound fraction can decrease to 90%. What will be the effect on the free drug fraction and the potential toxicity of phenytoin? If the total phenytoin concentration in the serum is reported to be 20 mg/L, the free fraction will now be 2 mg/L, which is twice the concentration with normal albumin binding and could be toxic.*[4]

The complicating effect of active metabolites is demonstrated in the case of procainamide. This drug is metabolized to *N*-acetylprocainamide, which also has antiarrhythmic activity. If one knows only the serum concentration of procainamide, it may not be possible to state the antiarrhythmic effect.

---

therapeutic blood concentration The concentration of drug in blood, serum, or plasma after therapeutically effective dosage in humans. The values in Table A1 are generally those reported with oral administration of the drug. Only agents for which monitoring is clinically necessary or at least useful are included.

toxic blood concentration The concentration of drug in blood, serum, or plasma that is associated with serious toxic symptoms in humans (Table A2).

lethal blood concentration The concentration of drug in blood, serum, or plasma that has been reported to cause death or is so far above therapeutic or merely toxic concentrations that it would be expected to cause death in humans (Table A2).

DEFINITION OF BLOOD CONCENTRATIONS

• • •

The following tables give the therapeutic, toxic, and lethal blood concentrations of a large number of drugs.

TABLE A1	Therapeutic drug concentrations (μg/ml)*		
	Peak	Steady-state average	Trough
Antibiotics			
Amikacin	20-25		<5
Chloramphenicol		10-20	
Gentamicin	5-8		<2
Kanamycin	20-25		<5
Netilmicin	5-8		<2
Tobramycin	5-8		<2
Vancomycin	20-25		<5
Antiarrhythmics			
Procainamide		4-10	
N-Acetylprocainamide		10-20	
Quinidine		2-5	
Amiodarone		1-2.5	
Disopyramide		2-5	
Flecainide		0.2-1	
Lidocaine		1.5-5	
Mexiletine		0.8-2	
Tocainide		3-10	
Psychotherapeutic agents			
Lithium		0.8-1.4 mEq/L	
Imipramine		0.15-0.25	
Amitriptyline		0.12-0.25	
Nortriptyline		0.05-0.15	
Desipramine		0.15-0.25	
Protriptyline		0.07-0.17	
Antiepileptic agents			
Carbamazepine		4-10	
Ethosuximide		40-100	
Phenobarbital		15-40	
Phenytoin		10-20	
Primidone		5-12	
Valproate		50-100	
Miscellaneous			
Aspirin (salicylate)			
Antipyretic, analgesic		20-100	
Anti-inflammatory		100-250	
Cyclosporin A (cyclosporine)		0.2-0.4	
Digitoxin		0.01-0.03	
Digoxin		0.0008-0.002	
Theophylline		10-20	

*Ranges may vary among different laboratories because of different assay methods.

TABLE A2   Toxic and lethal blood concentrations*

Compound	Toxic concentrations (mg/L)†	Lethal concentrations (mg/L)
Acetaminophen	30-300	>160
Acetone	200-300	550
Aminophylline	>20	50-250
Amitriptyline	0.5-3.4	2-20
Amobarbital	8-21	13-96
Amoxapine	>0.2	>0.6
Amphetamine	>0.1	0.5-41
Arsenic	1	9-15
Barbital	60-80	>100
Benzene	>0	0.94
Boron (boric acid)	40	50
Bromide	500-1500	2000
Brompheniramine	>0.05	>1
Butabarbital	10-30	30-88
Butalbital	>7	13-26
Caffeine	>40	79-181
Carbocaine	10	50
Carbamazepine	20-60	
Carbon monoxide	15%-35% (saturation of hemoglobin)	50%
Carbon tetrachloride	20-50	100-200
Carbromal	24-83	100
Carisoprodol	30	100
Chloral hydrate	(see trichloroethanol)	
Chlordane	0.0025	1.7-4
Chlordiazepoxide	5-60	>20
Chloroform	70-250	390
Chlorpheniramine	>0.5	>1
Chlorpromazine	>0.5	3-35
Chlorpropamide	300-750	
Chlorprothixene	>0.2	
Chloroquine	>0.6	3-16
Clonazepam	>0.6	
Cocaine	0.9	1-20
Codeine	0.5	1.4-5.6
Copper	5.4	2.5-63
Cyclizine	0.76	15
Desipramine	>0.5	5-20
Diazepam	>5	>30
Dicyclomine	>0.5	
Digitoxin		0.32
Digoxin	0.0021	0.015
Dinitro-*O*-cresol	0.03-0.04	75
Diphenhydramine	>1	>8
Disopyramide	3	>20
Doxepin	>0.14	0.7-29
Ethanol	1000 (legal)	>3500
Ethchlorvynol	20-100	100-400
Ethinamate		100
Ethosuximide	150	250
Ethyl alcohol (see ethanol)		

Sources

Winek, C.L.: Drug & chemical blood-level data, Pittsburgh, Pa., 1985, Fisher Scientific.

Garriott, J.C.: Interpretation of 112 drug concentrations in blood, San Antonio, 1987, Bexar County Medical Examiners Office.

*The values listed are mostly derived from actual blood assays. The upper range of toxic concentrations may be greater than the listed lethal concentrations because of variation in individual sensitivity or intervening therapy, or both.

†The current convention of toxicologists is to express concentrations as mg/L, which is the same as μg/ml and parts per million.

Continued.

TABLE A2   Toxic and lethal blood concentrations*—cont'd

Compound	Toxic concentrations (mg/L)†	Lethal concentrations (mg/L)
Ethyl chloride		400
Ethyl ether		1400-1890
Ethylene glycol	1500	2000-4000
Fenfluramine	0.2-0.9	6-15
Fentanyl	0.02	0.02
Fluoride		2
Flurazepam	0.2	0.5-4
Glutethimide	5-78	10-100
Haloperidol	0.01	
Halothane		200
Hydrocodone		0.6
Hydrogen sulfide		0.92
Hydromorphone	0.02	0.02-1.2
Hydroxyzine		20
Ibuprofen	>100	
Imipramine	0.5-1.5	2
Iron	6	
Isoniazid	20	70
Isopropyl alcohol	0.34	
Lead	1.3	
Lidocaine	8	6-33
Lithium	13.9	13.9-34.7
Lorazepam	0.3	
Loxapine	0.1	1
Lysergide (LSD)	0.001-0.004	
Magnesium	90-130	
Manganese	4.6	
Maprotiline	0.45-0.8	2-13
Meperidine	5	>5
Meprobamate	60-120	100-300
Mercury (inorganic)	0.18-0.62	0.4-22
Mercury (organic)	>0.2	>0.6
Mesoridazine		>2
Methadone	0.1	0.1-1.8
Methamphetamine	0.1	2
Methanol	200	>890
Methapyrilene		4.4-30
Methaqualone	2-12	5-42
Methohexital		100
Methylphenidate	0.8	2.3
Methyprylon	17	50
Metoprolol	>10	
Morphine	0.2	0.2
Nicotine	10	5-52

TABLE A2	Toxic and lethal blood concentrations*—cont'd	
Compound	Toxic concentrations (mg/L)†	Lethal concentrations (mg/L)
Nortriptyline	0.2	1
Orphenadrine	4	4-75
Oxalate		10
Oxazepam	2.0	
Oxycodone		5
Paraldehyde	200-400	>480
Paraquat	8.5	35
Pentazocine	0.5	1-5
Pentobarbital	>5	10-169
Perphenazine	0.1	1
Phenacetin		100
Phencyclidine	0.09-0.22	0.3-25
Phenmetrazine	0.5	0.5-5
Phenobarbital	40-60	65-116
Phentermine	0.2	1
Phenylbutazone	100	400
Phenytoin	20-50	45
Primidone	50-80	100
Procainamide	10	>20
Procaine	>21	
Prochlorperazine	>1	5
Procyclidine		0.4-7.8
Promazine	>1	>5
Propoxyphene	0.3-0.6	1-17
Propranolol	2	4-29
Protriptyline	0.5-2	>1
Quinidine	9-28	30-50
Quinine	6	12
Salicylate	150-300	>500
Secobarbital	5-12	5-52
Strychnine	2	2.8-12
Thallium	>1	0.5-11
Theophylline	20	63-250
Thiopental	>7	11-26
Thioridazine	2.4	4-13
Tolbutamide		600
Toluene		10
Trazodone		28
Trichloroethanol	>50	100-640
Trifluoperazine	1.2-3	3-8
Trimethobenzamide	>10	
Trimipramine		>5
Tripelennamine		10
Valproic acid	200	

REFERENCES

1. Beller, G.A., Smith, T.W., Abelmann, W.H., et al.: Digitalis intoxication: a prospective clinical study with serum level correlations, N. Engl. J. Med. **284**:989, 1971.

2. Koch-Weser, J.: Serum drug concentrations as therapeutic guides, N. Engl. J. Med. **287**:227, 1972.

3. Koch-Weser, J., and Klein, S.W.: Procainamide dosage schedules, plasma concentrations, and clinical effects, J.A.M.A. **215**:1454, 1971.

4. Reidenberg, M.M., Odar-Cederlöf, I., von Bahr, C., et al.: Protein binding of diphenylhydantoin and desmethylimipramine in plasma from patients with poor renal function, N. Engl. J. Med. **285**:264, 1971.

5. Winek, C.L.: Tabulation of therapeutic, toxic, and lethal concentrations of drugs and chemicals in blood, Clin. Chem. **22**:832, 1976.

Comparison of selected effects of commonly abused drugs

Selected effects of commonly abused drugs are summarized in the table on pp. 774 and 775. This table is intended for quick reference only. Greater detail on the subject is available in Chapter 30 dealing with contemporary drug abuse.

Drug category	Physical dependence	Characteristics of intoxication
Opiates	Pronounced	Analgesia with or without depressed sensorium; pinpoint pupils; patient may be alert and appear normal; respiratory depression with overdose
Barbiturates	Pronounced	Patient may appear normal with usual dose, but narrow margin between dose needed to prevent withdrawal symptoms and toxic dose is often exceeded, and patient appears "drunk," with drowsiness, ataxia, slurred speech, and nystagmus on lateral gaze; pupil size and reaction normal; respiratory depression with overdose
Nonbarbiturate sedatives Glutethimide	Pronounced	Pupils dilated and reactive to light; coma and respiratory depression prolonged; sudden apnea and laryngeal spasm common
Antianxiety agents	Pronounced	Progressive depression of sensorium as with barbiturates; pupil size and reaction normal; respiratory depression with overdose
Ethanol	Pronounced	Depressed sensorium, acute or chronic brain syndrome; odor on breath; pupil size and reaction normal
Amphetamines	Mild to absent	Agitation with paranoid thought disturbance in high doses; acute organic brain syndrome after prolonged use; pupils dilated and reactive; tachycardia, elevated blood pressure, with possibility of hypertensive crisis and cerebrovascular accident; possibility of convulsive seizures
Cocaine	Absent	Paranoid thought disturbance in high doses, with dangerous delusions of persecution and omnipotence; tachycardia; respiratory depression with overdose
Marijuana	Absent	Milder preparations: drowsy, euphoric state with frequent inappropriate laughter and disturbance in perception of time or space (occasional acute psychotic reaction reported); stronger preparations such as hashish: frequent hallucinations or psychotic reactions; pupils normal, conjunctivas injected (marijuana preparations frequently adulterated with LSD, tryptamines, or heroin)
Psychotomimetics LSD, STP, tryptamines, mescaline, morning glory seeds	Absent	Unpredictable disturbance in ego function, manifest by extreme lability of affect and chaotic disruption of thought, with danger of uncontrolled behavioral disturbance; pupils dilated and reactive to light
Phencyclidine	Unknown	Disinhibition, agitation, confusion, chaotic thought disturbance, unpredictable behavior, hypertension, miosis, respiratory collapse, cardiovascular collapse, death
Anticholinergic agents	Absent	Decreased salivary secretion, anhidrosis, hyperthermia, urinary retention, tachycardia; central anticholinergic syndrome with agitation, veridical hallucinations (usually visual), confusion, convulsions, coma, and death
Inhalants*	Unknown	Depressed sensorium, hallucinations, acute brain syndrome; odor on breath; patient often with glassy-eyed appearance

Modified from Dimijian, G.G.: Drug Ther. 1:7, 1971.
*The term *inhalant* is used to designate a variety of gases and highly volatile organic liquids, including the aromatic glues, paint thinners, gasoline, some anesthetic agents, and amyl nitrite. The term excludes liquids sprayed into the nasopharynx (droplet transport required) and substances that must be ignited before administration (such as marijuana).

Characteristics of withdrawal	"Flashback" symptoms	Masking of symptoms of illness or injury during intoxication
Rhinorrhea, lacrimation, and dilated, reactive pupils, followed by gastrointestinal disturbances, low back pain, and waves of gooseflesh; convulsions not a feature unless heroin samples were adulterated with barbiturates	Not reported	An important feature of opiate intoxication, because of analgesic action, with or without depressed sensorium
Agitation, tremulousness, insomnia, gastrointestinal disturbances, hyperthermia, blepharoclonus (clonic blink reflex), acute brain syndrome, major convulsive seizures	Not reported	Only in presence of depressed sensorium or after onset of acute brain syndrome
Similar to barbiturate withdrawal syndrome, with agitation, gastrointestinal disturbances, hyperthermia, and major convulsive seizures	Not reported	Same as in barbiturate intoxication
Similar to barbiturate withdrawal syndrome, with danger of major convulsive seizures	Not reported	Same as in barbiturate intoxication
Similar to barbiturate withdrawal syndrome, but with less likelihood of convulsive seizures	Not reported	Same as in barbiturates intoxication
Lethargy, somnolence, dysphoria, and possibility of suicidal depression; brain syndrome may persist for many weeks	Infrequently reported	Drug-induced euphoria or acute brain syndrome may interfere with awareness of symptoms of illness or may remove incentive to report symptoms of illness
Similar to amphetamine withdrawal	Not reported	Same as in amphetamine intoxication
No specific withdrawal symptoms	Infrequently reported	Uncommon with milder preparations; stronger preparations may interfere in same manner as psychotomimetic agents
No specific withdrawal symptoms; symptoms may persist for indefinite period after discontinuation of drug	Commonly reported as late as 1 year after last dose	Affective response or psychotic thought disturbance may remove awareness of, or incentive to report, symptoms of illness
No specific withdrawal symptoms	Occasionally reported	Same as in LSD intoxication
No specific withdrawal symptoms; mydriasis may persist for several days	Not reported	Pain may not be reported as a result of depression of sensorium, acute brain syndrome, or acute psychotic reaction
No specific withdrawal symptoms	Infrequently reported	Same as in anticholinergic intoxication

Pharmacokinetic characteristics of drugs

Values in this table are derived from multiple publications in the literature. They apply to adults and should be applied to children with caution if at all. When discrepant results were reported from different laboratories, a decision was made as to which methodology (assay, study design, and so on) was likely to be the most accurate. The ranges reflect those reported among the multiple sources reviewed. Drugs in development and available in countries other than the United States are included in anticipation of future availability.

Class / Drug	Bioavailability (%)	Elimination (%) Renal	Elimination (%) Hepatic	Protein bound (%)	V_d (L/kg)	Elimination half-life (hours)	Clearance (ml/min/kg)	ESRD V_d	ESRD Cl	Cirrhosis V_d	Cirrhosis Cl	Other
ANALGESICS AND ANTAGONISTS												
Acetaminophen	75-85	0	100	Negligible	0.8-1.4	2-4	5					
Buprenorphine	30	0	100		2.8	2-3	20					
Butorphanol		<5	>95	80	7	2.5-3	43					
Meperidine	56	5-7	93-95	60-80	4.2-5.2	3-7	7.5-12	No Δ	No Δ	No Δ	5	Bioavailability ↑ to 87% in cirrhosis
Methadone	80-90	25	75	60-90	3.6	30	1.4-2.1					
Morphine	38	10	90	35	2-3.5	1.7-4.5	8-15					
Nalbuphine		<7	>93			5						
Naltrexone	20			20	16	10	18					
Pentazocine	18	<5	>95		5-7	3-5	17-20			No Δ	10	Bioavailability ↑ to 70% in cirrhosis
Propoxyphene		0	100	80	16	8-24	14	No Δ	No Δ			Active metabolite eliminated by the kidney
ANESTHETICS (and other agents used primarily in anesthetic practice)												
Alcuronium		80-95	5-20	40	0.28-0.36	3-3.5	1.3-1.4					
Alfentanil		<1	>99	88-95	0.3-1.0	1.5-2	4.4-6.5				1.5	
Aminopyridine	95	90	10		3.2	3.9	9.3					
Atracurium		0	0		0.15-0.18	0.3-0.4	5.5-6.1		0.4			Metabolized by plasma esterases
Etomidate		2	98	75	2-4.5	4-5.5	11.6-25					
Fazadinium		0	100	17	0.18-0.23	1	1.9-2.3					
Fentanyl		6-8	92-94	79-87	2-5	2.5-3.5	5.7-12.7					
Gallamine		85-100	0-15	30-70	0.21-0.24	2.3-2.7	1.2-1.6		0.3			

CHF, Congestive heart failure; *Cl*, clearance; *Cl$_{Cr}$*, creatinine clearance; *COPD*, chronic obstructive pulmonary disease; *ESRD*, end-stage renal disease; *K$_m$*, Michaelis-Menten constant; *V$_d$*, volume of distribution.

Class / Drug	Bioavailability (%)	Renal	Hepatic	Protein bound (%)	V_d (L/kg)	Elimination half-life (hours)	Clearance (ml/min/kg)	ESRD V_d	ESRD Cl	Cirrhosis V_d	Cirrhosis Cl	Other
Ketamine	80	2-3	97-98		1.8-3.1	2.2-3.5	14-19					
Metocurine		45-60	40-55	70	0.42-0.57	3.5-5.8	1.2-1.8		↓			
Minaxolone					1.6-2.2	0.75	17-25					
Pancuronium		30-40	60-70	70-85	0.15-0.38	1.7-2.2	1.1-2.1	No Δ	0.4			
Sufentanil		1-2	98-99	92	2.4	2.5	10-11					
Thiopental		<1	>99	84	1.9	10	3.2	No Δ	No Δ			
Tubocurarine		40-60	40-60	30-50	0.22-0.39	0.5-4	1.8-2.7	No Δ	↓			
Vecuronium					0.19-0.27	0.4	3.2-5.3					
ANTIANXIETY AGENTS, SEDATIVES, AND HYPNOTICS												
Alprazolam	80	20	80	70	1-1.5	10-20	0.6-1.6					
Barbital		80	20			2.4-3.3						
Buspirone	4	<1	>99	95	5.3	2-8	45		23		↓	Bioavailability probably ↑ in cirrhosis
Chloral hydrate				70-80	0.6	4-10	1.0					
Chlordiazepoxide	100	0	100	94-97	0.3-0.6	6-28	0.25-0.5				0.15	
Clobazam		0	100	90	0.9-1.5	17-50	0.35-0.65					
Clomethiazole	10	<3	>97	64	4.4	4.8	16.4				10	Bioavailability ↑ to 100% in cirrhosis
Clorazepate		0	100		0.33	2	1.8					
Clotiazepam		0	100	99	2.5	9-10	3-4			1.6	2.5	
Diazepam	100	0	100	98	1-2	20-70	0.25-0.5					
Ethchlorvynol		0	100		3.5	19-32	1.7-2.0					
Flunitrazepam	85	0	100	80	3.3	15	3.5					
Flurazepam				97	22	50-100*	4.5					
Glutethimide		<2	>98	50	2.7	5-22	2.3					
Hexobarbital	>90	<1	>99	50	1.2	3.5	3.9					
Lorazepam	93	0	100	85	0.7-1.0	10-20	0.7-1.2					
Lormetazepam		0	100			9-15	2.6-4.3					
Meprobamate		10	90	Negligible		6-17						

Drug								
Methaqualone	40	0		70-90	6	20-60	1.7	
Methohexital		<1	>99		2.2	3.9	11	
Midazolam	40	0	100	94-97	0.8-1.5	1.5-3.5	4-9	
Nitrazepam	80	0	100	87	1.9-2.6	20-28	0.86-1.2	
Oxazepam	>90	0	100	97	0.6-2	4-13	0.9-2	
Paraldehyde		0	100			3.5-10		
Phenobarbital	100	20	80	50	0.9	24-140	0.1	
Prazepam		0	100		14	1.3	140	
Temazepam	>80	0	100	96-98		5-11		
Triazolam	55	0	100	80-90	1.1	2-4.5	3-9	
Zopiclone	80	4-5	95-96	45	1.4	5	3.3	

ANTICHOLINERGICS AND CHOLINERGICS

Drug								
Atropine	10-22				2.7	4.1	7.6	
Edrophonium					1.1	1.8	9.6	
Metoclopramide	60-75	78-90		40	2-3	2.5-5	8-11	No Δ
Neostigmine	10-20	67		Negligible	0.9	1.3	8.4	3
Pirenzepine	26	10		12	3.4	11-14	3.6	1.7
Pyridostigmine	10-20	80-90		10-20	1.5	1.9	9	2

ANTICOAGULANTS, ANTIFIBRINOLYTICS, AND ANTIPLATELET AGENTS

Drug								
Dipyridamole	45			99	2.4	12	2.4	No Δ
Epsilon-aminocaproic acid	70-86	14-30			0.39	4.9	2.7	→
Sulfinpyrazone	100	25-50	>95		0.06	2.2-2.7	0.28	1/8 normal
Tranexamic acid	90	10				1.5		
Warfarin	100	0		99	0.14	35-45	0.045	No Δ

ANTIDEPRESSANTS, ANTIPSYCHOTICS, AND ANTIMANIC AGENTS

Drug								
Amitriptyline	48	<2	>98	95	14	16	12.5	No Δ
Amoxapine			100			8		
Bupropion		0	100		40	7.5-19	57	
Chlorpromazine	40	0	100	95	20	30	8.5	
Clomipramine					7-20	20-80		
Desipramine	50		90		20-60	15-60	30	
Doxepin	13-45		100		9-33	8-25	14	
Fluoxetine		0	98	94	20-40	2	10	No Δ
Fluvoxamine		0	100	77		15		No Δ

CHF, Congestive heart failure; *Cl*, clearance; *Cl_{Cr}*, creatinine clearance; *COPD*, chronic obstructive pulmonary disease; *ESRD*, end-stage renal disease; *K_m*, Michaelis-Menten constant; *V_d*, volume of distribution.
* Active metabolites.

Class / Drug	Bioavailability (%)	Elimination (%) Renal	Elimination (%) Hepatic	Protein bound (%)	V_d (L/kg)	Elimination half-life (hours)	Clearance (ml/min/kg)	ESRD V_d	ESRD Cl	Cirrhosis V_d	Cirrhosis Cl	Other
Haloperidol	45-75	0	100	92	14-21	20	12					
Imipramine	30-75	<2	>98	95	20-40	10-20	15					
Lithium	100	0	100	0	0.67	8-41	0.35		→			
Maprotiline	37-67				15-28	20-60						
Mianserin	30-75			90	16	10-40	8.7					
Nortriptyline	50-80			95	20-30	15-56						
Protriptyline	80-90			90-95	20-55	55-200	3.6					
Tranylcypromine					2.7	2.4	14					
Trazodone		<1	>99	90-95		6.3						
Trimipramine	41			95	31	23	16					
ANTIEPILEPTICS												
Carbamazepine	70	2-3	97-98	75	1	4-6	0.9					Undergoes autoinduction
Clonazepam	98	0	100	86	3.2	24	1.6					
Ethosuximide		17-40	60-83	Negligible	0.7	35-55	0.17					
Phenytoin	100	2	98	90	0.6	24						$V_{max} = 8.4$ mg/kg/d; $K_m = 8.5$ mg/L
Primidone	90-95	40	60	19	0.6	5-15	0.85-1.7					
Valproate	100	3-7	93-97	90	0.19	6-15	0.15					
ANTIHISTAMINES												
Astemizole		0	100	97		20 days						Clearance ⅓ normal in elderly
Brompheniramine	34				11.7	25	6					
Chlorpheniramine		20	80		5.9-11.7	14-24	1.4-4.7					
Cimetidine	60	50-70	30-50	20	1.3	1-5	8-10		3	0.6		Bioavailability ↑ to 75% in cirrhosis
Diphenhydramine	40-60	2	98	78	3.3-6.8	3.4-9.3	8.6-18.6					
Famotidine	37-45	65-80	20-35	15-22	1.1-1.4	2.5-4	6.4		2		6	
Flunarizine	85	0	100	99	43-78	17-18 days						
Hydroxyzine					19.5	20	9.8					
Methapyrilene	14	<2	>98		3.9	1.6	28					
Nizatidine					1.2	1.3	11					
Oxatomide		<1	>99	91		20						
Promethazine	25	<1	>99	93	13.5	12	16					

Drug										Comments
Ranitidine	50	80	20	15	1.2-1.8	1.5-2.5	9-10	2.5		Bioavailability ↑ to 70% in cirrhosis
Terfenadine						16-23				
Tripelennamine		10			10	3-4.5	32			
Tripolidine						5				
ANTI-INFLAMMATORY AGENTS										
Alclofenac		10-50	50-90	>99	0.10	1.5-2.5	0.14			
Auranofin		50	50			70-80 days				
Azapropazone			>99	>99		10-15		0.05	0.03	
Diclofenac		<1	>97	>99	0.15	1-2	3.7			
Diflunisal		<3	100	95	0.12	5-20	0.11			
Etodolac		0	96	>98	0.10	7				
Fenbufen		4	70	>99	0.40	10				
Fenclofenac			>99		0.2-0.25	20-38	0.6-1.3			
Fenoprofen		30	>85	>90	0.10	2-3				
Flufenamic acid		<1	99	99		9				
Flurbiprofen		<15	70	99	0.10	3-5	0.3			
Ibuprofen		1	>99	>90	0.15	2-2.5	0.75			
Indomethacin		30	96-98	99	0.12	6	1-2			
Ketoprofen		<1	>94	>99	0.11	1.5	1.2			
Meclofenamic acid		2-4	>99	>94		3				
Mefenamic acid		<6	>99	99		3-4				
Naproxen		<1	>98	>99	0.10	12-15	0.07	↓		
Oxaprozin	100	<1	75-97	99	0.15-0.25	50-60	0.04	No Δ	No Δ	
Oxyphenbutazone		<2	99	>99		27-64				
Penicillamine		3-25	90		1.5-3		10.7			
Phenylbutazone		1	93		0.17	50-100	0.02			
Piroxicam		10	>92		0.12-0.15	45	0.04			
Pirprofen			85		0.11-0.17	6-7	0.28			
Salicylates (low dose)	70	Dependent on urine pH		80-90	0.15	2-3	0.8			Dose-dependent elimination
Salicylates (high dose)				↑	↑	15-30				
Sulindac sulfide		7		95		16	0.2			
Tiaprofenic acid		<8		98	0.4-1.0	1.5-2.5	0.6-1.4			
Tolfenamic acid				>99	0.16	2.2	2.5			
Tolmetin		15		>99	0.10-0.14	1.8	1-1.5			

CHF, Congestive heart failure; *Cl*, clearance; *Cl$_{Cr}$*, creatinine clearance; *COPD*, chronic obstructive pulmonary disease; *ESRD*, end-stage renal disease; *K$_m$*, Michaelis-Menten constant; *V$_d$*, volume of distribution.

Class / Drug	Bioavailability (%)	Elimination (%) Renal	Elimination (%) Hepatic	Protein bound (%)	V_d (L/kg)	Elimination half-life (hours)	Clearance (ml/min/kg)	ESRD V_d	ESRD Cl	Cirrhosis V_d	Cirrhosis Cl	Other
ANTISPASTICITY AGENTS												
Baclofen	100	70-80	20-30	30	0.84	3-4	2.6		→			
Dantrolene	70	0	100			8						
ANTIULCER AGENT												
Omeprazole	65	0	100	95	0.3-0.4	0.5-1.5	8.6		→			
BRONCHODILATORS												
Albuterol						6.5						
Dyphylline		85	15	<3	0.80	1.8-2.3	4.8					
Enprophylline		90	10	47	0.5-0.6	1.6	3-4					
Prenalterol	27	60	40		3.4	2	21					
Terbutaline	15	50	50	25	0.94	3	3.8					
Theophylline	95	0	100	55	0.4-0.7	4-12	1.0			No Δ	0.7	Clearance is about half normal in COPD
CARDIOVASCULAR AGENTS												
Antianginal agents												
Diltiazem	45	<1	>99	80-85	5	3.5-5	14-20		No Δ			
Felodipine		<1	>99	99	9.5	10	12					
Isosorbide dinitrate	30	0	100	30	1.4	1	32		No Δ			
Nicardipine		0	100			12	8					
Nifedipine	40-50	<1	>99	92-98	0.8	3.5-4	6-15				3	Bioavailability doubles in cirrhosis
Nimodipine						6						
Nitrendipine	16	<1	>99	98	2-6	12-24	3.2		No Δ	→	→	Bioavailability may ↑ in cirrhosis
Nitroglycerin	36	<1	>99		3	3 min	300-1000					
Verapamil	34	3-4	96-97	90	5-6	3-5	14-20			3	5	Bioavailability doubles in cirrhosis
Antiarrhythmic agents												
N-Acetylprocainamide	85	85	15	10	1.6	6	3.1	No Δ	0.5			
Amiodarone	22-86	0	100	96	70	25-50 days	2					
Aprindine	75	2	98		4	50	1					

Drug									Comments
Bretylium	25	100		8-10	5.0	6-11	No Δ	2	
Cibenzoline	100	60		55	4.0	12	→	3.5	
Disopyramide	65-85	40-60	40-60	50-70	0.91	4-10	1-5	2.5	Clearance is about ⅓ normal in CHF
Encainide	30-85	0	100	80	5.7	2-5	15	17	All activity resides in metabolites
Flecainide	90-95	40	60	40	5.5-7.3	10-12	5		
Lidocaine	30	5	95	50	1.6	1.8	No Δ	6	Volume of distribution and clearance are ½ normal in CHF
Lorcainide	Dose-dependent	<3	>97	85	6.5	7.8	No Δ	12	Clearance is about ⅓ normal in CHF
Mexiletine	90	30-55	45-70	50	5.9	10	No Δ	2.3	
Pirmenol	87	25	75	85	1.5	6-12	2.9	→	
Procainamide	75-85	50-70	30-50	15	2.4	2.6-3.5	8.6-9.8	→	
Propafenone	<1	>99	>95	3	2-5	12			
Quinidine	70	15-40	60-85	70-95	2-3.5	5-12	2.5-5	No Δ	Both volume of distribution and clearance are ½ normal in CHF
Tocainide	90-100	60		50	2.2	12-14	2-2.5	No Δ	0.5-1.3
Acebutolol	40	30	70		1.2	3-4	8.8	No Δ	Active metabolite is eliminated by the kidney
Antihypertensives									
Amosulalol	100	35	65		0.75	2.8	1.9	No Δ	
Atenolol	45-55	75-85	15-25	<5	1.2	6-9	1.3-2.1	0.16	
Betaxolol	15	85	55		4.9-9.8	14-22	4.7	No Δ	
Captopril	60-70	24-38	62-76	30	2	2	13.3	1.5-2	
Carteolol	85	65	35	15	4	4.7	10	→	
Clonidine	100	40-50	50-60	20-30	4.0	7-18	3-5	→	
Diazoxide	85-95	20	80	>90	0.18	15-30	0.1	No Δ	
Doxazosin	60	5	95	98	3.5	18-20	2.2	No Δ	
Enalapril			50	50	5	11-19	5		
Guanabenz	<1	>99		90	5	4.3	9	→	2
Guanadrel		20		20		10			
Guanfacine	24-37	63-76	64		3.9-6.5	12-23	2.6-5.2	No Δ	

CHF, Congestive heart failure; *Cl*, clearance; *ClCr*, creatinine clearance; *COPD*, chronic obstructive pulmonary disease; *ESRD*, end-stage renal disease; *Km*, Michaelis-Menten constant; *Vd*, volume of distribution.

Class	Drug	Bioavailability (%)	Elimination (%) Renal	Elimination (%) Hepatic	Protein bound (%)	V_d (L/kg)	Elimination half-life (hours)	Clearance (ml/min/kg)	ESRD V_d	ESRD Cl	Cirrhosis V_d	Cirrhosis Cl	Other
	Hydralazine	10-35	<10	>90		6-8	0.7-1.0	75-140		No Δ			
	Indoramin	31	<10	>90	92	7.4	4-5.5	20			9.5	12	
	Ketanserin	50	<4	>96	94	5-6	6-12	6-10					
	Labetalol	30			50	5.6	3-3.5	21	No Δ	No Δ			Bioavailability doubles in cirrhosis
	Medroxalol	30	8	92	50-60	16	11	16					
	Mepindolol	80	<1	>99			3						
	Methyldopa	25-30	50-65	35-50	<15	0.5-0.6	1.3-1.8	3.3-5.7	No Δ	↓			
	Metoprolol	50	5-10	90-95	12	4.9	2.5-5	10-20	No Δ	No Δ	No Δ	9	Bioavailability ↑ to 85% in cirrhosis
	Minoxidil	95	12	88	0	12	3-4	0.15		No Δ			
	Nadolol	30	60-75	25-40	20-30	1.5	14-24	1-3		0.11			
	Nitroprusside		0	100									Thiocyanate metabolite (toxic) is eliminated by the kidney
	Penbutolol	95	4-6	94-96		3.4	22	9.5		No Δ	2.6	4.9	
	Pinacidil	75	4	96		2.1	4	6.9-7.7		No Δ		No Δ	
	Pindolol	75	36-39	61-64	57	0.57	3-4	2.4-3.3					
	Prazosin	50-70	<10	>90	90-95	4-4.5	2.5-4.5						
	Propranolol	36	0	100	99		2.5-5	12	No Δ		↑	8	Bioavailability doubles in cirrhosis
	Sotalol		60-75	25-40	54	0.7	5-8	1.5		0.45			
	Terazosin		15	85			10	1.1					
	Timolol	50-60	15	85	10	1.7	2.7	7.7					
	Trimazosin	63	<10	>90			2.9	0.9					
Blood lipid-lowering agents	Bezafibrate	95				0.35	2.1	1.4		0.19			
	Clofibrate	95	40-70	30-60	92-97	0.14	15-17.5	0.10		0.05		→	
Cardiac inotropes	Amrinone	90	10-40	60-90	35-50	1.4	2-4.4	3.9-8.8					Both V_d and clearance are about ½ normal in CHF
	Digitoxin	95	33	67	90	0.73	6-8 days	0.05		No Δ			
	Digoxin	75	70-80	20-30	25	3.9	42	1.8	↓	0.45			
	Milrinone	90	85	15		0.32	0.8	6.2					

CENTRAL NERVOUS SYSTEM STIMULANTS											
Cocaine		0	100		2	0.8-1.2	35				
Phencyclidine	65-80	9-10	90-91	60-65	6.2	16	5.4				
CHEMOTHERAPEUTIC AGENTS											
Antibacterials											
Aminocyclitols											
Spectino-mycin		75	25	0	0.15-0.24	1.6	1.0		↓		
Aminoglycosides											
All	0	100	0	0	0.25	2-3	1.2	No Δ			Cl = 0.04 + 0.01 Cl_{Cr}
Carbapenems											
Clavulanic acid		27-32	68-73		0.35	1-1.5	2-5				
Imipenem	0	70	30	20	0.23-0.42	1	3.5		↓		
Cephalosporins											
Cefaclor		62	38		0.36	0.7-0.8	5.5		↓		
Cefadroxil		90-95	5-10	16	0.30	1.3	2.5		↓		
Cefamandole		>95	<5	74	0.19	0.5-1.5	2.8		↓		
Cefatrizine		80	20	60-65	0.30	1	3.2				
Cefazolin		80-100	0-20	85	0.14	1.6-2.3	1.0				Cl = 0.06 + 0.0056 Cl_{Cr}
Cefixime		16	84	63	1.1	3-5	2.4				Cl = 0.82 + 0.013 Cl_{Cr}
Cefmen-oxime		80	20	30	0.17	1	2.8				Cl = 0.29 + 0.02 Cl_{Cr}
Cefonicid		82-96	4-18	98	0.10	3-5	0.3				Cl = 0.02 + 0.003 Cl_{Cr}
Cefoper-azone		25	75	90	0.17	1.6-2.4	1.1		No Δ	↓	
Ceforanide		80-82	18-20	80-82	0.14-0.17	2.5-3.0	0.7-1.0				Cl = 0.074 + 0.086 Cl_{Cr}
Cefotaxime		60	40	20-40	0.48	1-1.5	4-5				Cl = 1.2 + 0.025 Cl_{Cr}
Cefotetan		80	20	80-90	0.12	3	0.46		↓		
Cefotiam		53	47			0.9-1.6	4.2-6.4				Dose-dependent elimination
Cefoxitin		80	20	74	0.27	0.7	4.7				Cl = 0.05 Cl_{Cr}
Cefpiramide		22	78		0.10	4.5	0.27				
Cefroxadine		70	30		0.35	1.0	4.1				Cl = 0.034 Cl_{Cr}
Cefsulodin		50	50	15	0.26	1.6	2.0				Cl = 0.362 + 0.010 Cl_{Cr}

CHF, Congestive heart failure; *Cl*, clearance; *Cl_{Cr}*, creatinine clearance; *COPD*, chronic obstructive pulmonary disease; *ESRD*, end-stage renal disease; *K_m*, Michaelis-Menten constant; *V_d*, volume of distribution.

Class	Drug	Bioavailability (%)	Elimination (%) Renal	Elimination (%) Hepatic	Protein bound (%)	V_d (L/kg)	Elimination half-life (hours)	Clearance (ml/min/kg)	ESRD V_d	ESRD Cl	Cirrhosis V_d	Cirrhosis Cl	Other
	Ceftazidime		70-80	20-30	17	0.25	1.5-3	1.7					$Cl = 0.15 + 0.016\ Cl_{Cr}$
	Ceftizoxime		90-100	0-10	30	0.23-0.35	1.4	1.9-2.5			→		$Cl = 0.007 + 0.0157\ Cl_{Cr}$
	Ceftriaxone		40-65	35-60	83-96	0.16	6	0.15-0.30					
	Cefuroxime		95-100	0-5	33-50	0.20	1-2	1.5-2.1				→	$Cl = 0.28 + 0.013\ Cl_{Cr}$
	Cephacetrile		>90	<10	25-35	0.37	1-1.5	3.4		→			
	Cephalexin	95	90-96	4-10	15	0.33	0.9-1.2	3.6		→			
	Cephalothin		50-80	20-50	65-70	0.32	0.4-0.6	8.2		→			
	Cephapirin		50	50	60	0.22	0.6-0.7	4.3		→			
	Cephradine	>90	80-95	5-20	14	0.32	0.7-0.8	5.3		→			
Chloramphenicol and thiamphenicol													
	Chloramphenicol	75-90	5-10	90-95	25-50	0.5-0.8	3-5	2.5-3.2		→	No Δ	0.7-2.1	
	Thiamphenicol		60-90	10-40	<10		2-3						
Macrolide antibiotics													
	Clindamycin	85	10-15	85-90	60-90	0.66	2.5-3.5	2.1-3.5			No Δ	1.7	
	Erythromycin	33	10-15	85-90	85	0.78	1.1-2.0	6-9	↑	No Δ			
	Lincomycin		5-15	85-95	70	0.54	4.7-5.6	1.2		→		→	
Monobactams													
	Aztreonam		65	35	50-60	0.20	1.7	1.0	No Δ	0.35	No Δ	0.8	
	Carumonam		70-90	10-30	18	0.18	1.5	1.5		0.2			
	Moxalactam		60-80	20-40	50-60	0.28	2-4	1.7		0.14			
Nitroimidazole													
	Ornidazole		<4	>96	5-10	0.86	14	0.7		1.2	No Δ	0.5	
Penicillins													
	Amdinocillin (Mecillinam)		50-70	30-50	5-10	0.5	1	3-6		→			
	Amoxicillin	95	50-70	30-50	17	0.66	0.9-2.3	6.5		→			
	Ampicillin	60	90	10	18	0.30	0.8-1.5	2.7		0.45			
	Azlocillin		65	35	30	0.18	0.8	2.6		→			
	Carbenicillin		80	20	50	0.13	1.0	1.5		0.25			
	Cloxacillin	40	75	25	95	0.10	0.5	2.2		No Δ			
	Dicloxacillin	50-85	60	40	96	0.09	0.7	1.6		No Δ			
	Methicillin		85-90	10-15	30-50	0.45	0.5-0.85	6.1		→			

Effect of diseases

APPENDIX C

Pharmacokinetic Characteristics of Drugs

Drug										Dose-dependent elimination
Mezlocillin		60-70	30-40	16-42	0.14	1	4	No Δ	1.3	1.8
Nafcillin	35	25	75	90	0.35	1-2	7.5	No Δ	No Δ	
Oxacillin	35	45	55	92	0.30	0.5	6.1		No Δ	
Penicillin		90-100	0-10	50-65	0.23	0.5	5.3		1.0	
Piperacillin		53-73	27-47	21	0.18-0.22	1.0	2.6	No Δ	0.7	
Temocillin		85	15	85	0.15-0.24	5-6	0.35		0.15	
Ticarcillin		85-90	10-15	45-65	0.21	1.2-1.5	1.9		↓	
Polymyxins										
Colistin		60-75	25-40	50	0.47	3-4.5	1.4		↓	
Polymyxin B		60-90	10-40			3-6			↓	
Quinolones										
Ciprofloxacin	60-75	30-50	50-70	20	5.0	3.5-6.5	10.5	No Δ	↓	
Enoxacin	87-98	60	40		1.6-4.4	6	6.7	No Δ	1.2	
Norfloxacin		30	70	14		3.5-6.5			↓	
Pefloxacin		9	91		1.9	11	2	No Δ	No Δ	0.6
Sulfonamides										
Sulfadiazine	100	66	34	55	0.3	7.5-9.0	0.5			
Sulfamethoxazole	100	20-30	70-80	65	0.25	9-11	0.32		↓	
Sulfasalazine		10-20	80-90	50		6-14	0.6-2.1			
Sulfisoxazole	95	50-55	45-50	90	0.16	5.5-6.0	0.32		↓	
Trimethoprim	100	50	50	70	2.1	8-11	2.2		↓	
Tetracyclines										
Doxycycline	90	40	60	90	0.75	16	0.53		No Δ	
Tetracycline	80	60	40	65	1.5	6	1.7		↓	
Urinary bacteriostatic										
Cinoxacin		60	40	63	0.25	1-1.5	2.3	No Δ		
Vancomycin										
Vancomycin	90-100	90-100	0-10	<10	0.47-0.90	6-11	0.9-1.2		0.11	
Antifungals										
Amphotericin B		3	97	95	4	15 days	0.43		No Δ	
Flucytosine	85	80-90	10-20	3-4	0.7	3.5-5.5	2.0		0.1	
Ketoconazole	<1	<1	>99	99	1.25	4-7.5	3		No Δ	
Miconazole	0	0	100	98	21	24	10	↓	↓	
Antimalarials										
Chlorguanide		50	50			6-12				

CHF, Congestive heart failure; *Cl*, clearance; *Cl_{Cr}*, creatinine clearance; *COPD*, chronic obstructive pulmonary disease; *ESRD*, end-stage renal disease; *K_m*, Michaelis-Menten constant; *V_d*, volume of distribution.

Class	Drug	Bioavailability (%)	Elimination (%) Renal	Elimination (%) Hepatic	Protein bound (%)	V_d (L/kg)	Elimination half-life (hours)	Clearance (ml/min/kg)	Effect of diseases ESRD V_d	ESRD Cl	Cirrhosis V_d	Cirrhosis Cl	Other
	Chloroquine	90	55	45	55	150	6–50 days	10					
	Halofantizine					100–570	1.3–6.6 days	2.5–3.5					
	Mefloquine		0	100	98	13–29	6.5–35 days	0.26–0.6					
	Primaquine	75	4	96		3	7.6	5					
	Pyrimethamine		<1	>99	85	2.9	35–175	0.4					
	Quinine		20	80	90	1.8	8.5–11						
Antineoplastics and antimetabolites													
	Adriamycin						14						
	Azathioprine (mercaptopurine)	60	<2	>98	20	0.55	1	11					
	Bleomycin		60	40		0.3	9	0.38		↓			
	Busulfan		1	99		1	2.5	4.5					
	Carmustine (BCNU)					3.3	1.5	56					
	Chlorambucil					0.86	1	0.55					
	Cisplatin		27–45	55–73	>90	0.5	0.3–0.5	17		No Δ			Clearance of active metabolites is decreased in renal disease
	Cyclophosphamide	75	10–15	85–90	60	0.62	4–7.5	0.8–1.1		↓			
	Cytarabine		6	94		52	0.5–3.3	17		No Δ			
	Doxorubicin		<15	>85	80–85	0.5	36	17					
	Etoposide		36	64		0.25	6–8	0.5					
	Fluorouracil	30	<5	>95	10	0.6	0.2	16					
	Melphalan	70	12	88		0.76	1.4	5.2					
	Methotrexate	65	80–90	10–20	45–50	15.5	8–12	1–5					
	Mitoxantrone		<7	>93	>95		37	4.7		↓		↓	
	Vinblastine				75	24	1–1.5	10.6					
	Vincristine		12	88	75	8.6	1–2.5	1.8					
Antiparasitics and anthelmintics													
	Metronidazole	100	6	94	10	0.8–1.0	8	0.7–1.3	No Δ	No Δ		0.25	
	Ornidazole		<5	>95	<10	0.7	10	0.7		No Δ ↓			
	Pentamidine		100	0		3							

APPENDIX C

Pharmacokinetic Characteristics of Drugs

Tinidazole	100	25	75	12-20	0.6-0.8	12-17	0.6	No Δ	No Δ
Antituberculosis agents									
p-Aminosalicylic acid		40-60	40-60	50-70	0.24	0.7	4		
Capreomycin				50					
Cycloserine		50	50			8-12			
Ethambutol	75-80	80	20	20-30	2.3	3	8.6		↓
Ethionamide		<1	>99	24		2			
Isoniazid		5-25	75-95	0	0.6	0.7-4.0	2.5-7.0		No Δ
Pyrazinamide			>99			9-10			
Rifampin		<1	>90	90	1.0	3.5	3.5		↓
Thiacetazone				30		13			
Viomycin		<10		85					
Antiviral agents									
Acyclovir	15-30	75-80	20-25	9-22	0.7	2-3	4.2		0.4
Amantadine		100	0	0	5.1	12	4.9		↓
DHPG (dehydroxyphenylglycol)		91	19		0.47	2.5	3		0.3
Vidarabine		40-60	40-60			3.5	2		↓
Zidovudine (AZT)	63	19	81		1.4	1.1	22		
DERMATOLOGIC AGENTS									
Etretinate	40			98	3	80-100 days			
Isotretinoin		0	100	>99		10-30	5		
Methoxsalen		0	100	90	0.9-8.9	0.6-2.4	10.2-157		
DIURETICS									
Acetazolamide						13			
Amiloride		52	48			7-11			↓
Bendroflumethiazide						2.5-5.5			↓
Bumetanide		50	50		0.15	1	2-3.5		↓
Chlorothiazide						15-25			↓
Chlorthalidone						24-55			↓

CHF, Congestive heart failure; *Cl*, clearance; Cl_{Cr}, creatinine clearance; *COPD*, chronic obstructive pulmonary disease; *ESRD*, end-stage renal disease; K_m, Michaelis-Menten constant; V_d, volume of distribution.

Class	Drug	Bioavailability (%)	Elimination (%) Renal	Elimination (%) Hepatic	Protein bound (%)	V$_d$ (L/kg)	Elimination half-life (hours)	Clearance (ml/min/kg)	ESRD V$_d$	ESRD Cl	Cirrhosis V$_d$	Cirrhosis Cl	Other
	Furosemide	40-60	50	50		0.15	1-1.5	1.5-3		↓			
	Hydrochlorothiazide	65-75					3-10			↓			
	Hydroflumethiazide	75					6-10			↓			
	Indapamide						6-15						
	Mannitol		80	20	0	0.5	1.2	7		0.03			
	Polythiazide						25			↓			
	Triamterene	55	7	93	60	3.0	2-5	14		↓			Metabolite accounts for most of activity
	Trichlormethiazide						1-4			↓			
HYPOGLYCEMIC AGENTS													
	Acetohexamide		Minor				1-1.3			↓			Active metabolite is eliminated by the kidney
	Chlorpropamide	>90	47	53	88-96	0.15	24-42	0.03		↓			
	Gliclazide		<20	>80	85-95	0.24	8-11	0.19					
	Glipizide	80	<5	>95	97	0.13	3-7	0.4-0.6					
	Tolbutamide	95	0	100	95-97	0.12	4-6	0.28		No Δ		0.14	
HYPOURICEMIC AGENTS AND COLCHICINE													
	Allopurinol	67	30	70	<5	2.2	2-8			↓			Active metabolite is eliminated by kidney
	Colchicine		5-17	83-95	31	0.15	19	1.3					
	Probenecid	100	<2	>98	85-95	0.15	5-8	0.25-0.4					
MISCELLANEOUS AGENTS													
	Acetylcysteine	6-10	30	70		0.34	2.3	3.5					
	Aminoglutethimide		35-50	50-65	20-25	1.1	9-16	0.8-1.0		↓			
	Clodronate	1-2	70-90	10-30		0.25	1.8	1.7					
	Cyclosporine (cyclosporin)	<5-80	<1	>99	96	3-5	16	6	No Δ	No Δ			
	Dapsone	70-80	5-15	85-95	70-90	1.5	10-30	0.6		↓			
	Dextran 40						10			↓			

Drug									
Dihydroergotamine mesylate	9		89		15	14	25		
Disulfiram						7			
Domperidone	15	11	99	92	5.7	7.5	10	No Δ	
Edetate (EDTA)		1			0.05–0.23	2–3	0.8	No Δ	0.17
Misoprostol				85		1–5			
Nabilone	96								
Pentoxifylline	20	0			2.4	2	0.7		
Tolrestat			99			1.6	19		
Vigabatrin		50	50			7.5	10		
STEROIDS									
Betamethasone	70	5	95	65	1.4	5.5	3		
Budesonide	11	0	100	88	4.3	2	20		
Dexamethasone	80	<3	>97	70	0.8	3	3.5		
Methylprednisolone	80	10	90	40–60	1.2	3.6	4.8		
Prednisone	98	34			2.2	2.5–3.5	10		
Triamcinolone			66		1.4–2.1	1.4	11–16		4.4
SYMPATHOMIMETICS									
Dobutamine					0.2	2.5 min	60		
Ritodrine				38		17			
THYROID AND ANTITHYROID DRUGS									
Methimazole	95	7	93	0	3–6	1.4		No Δ	
Propylthiouracil	75	<10	>90	80	0.3–0.4	1–2	3.9		
Thyroxine						6 days			
Triiodothyronine						1 day			

CHF, Congestive heart failure; *Cl*, clearance; *Cl$_{Cr}$*, creatinine clearance; *COPD*, chronic obstructive pulmonary disease; *ESRD*, end-stage renal disease; *K$_m$*, Michaelis-Menten constant; *V$_d$*, volume of distribution.

Index

A

A fibers
  local anesthetics and, 409
  nonsteroid anti-inflammatory drugs and, 366
Aδ fibers, 366
AAG; *see* α₁-Acid glycoprotein
Abbokinase; *see* Urokinase
Abscess, 664
Absence seizures, 308, 314-315
Absorption, 21-23
  age and, 57-58
  of atropine, 117
  diet and, 64
  disease and, 72-73
  of ganglionic blocking agents, 130
  of salicylates, 370
  of scopolamine, 117
Abstinence syndrome
  alcohol and, 343
  barbiturates and, 351
  heroin and, 340
  morphine and, 340
Abuse; *see* Drug abuse
ABVD; *see* Doxorubicin, bleomycin, vinblastine, and DTIC
Acanthocheilonema perstans, 698
Acatalasia, 52
Accutane; *see* Isotretinoin
Acebutolol, 167, 170
  action of, 169
    sites of, 178
  hypertension and, 192-193
  pharmacokinetics of, 783
Acebutolol hydrochloride, 167
Acetaldehyde dehydrogenase, 296
Acetaminophen, 30, 365, 373-375
  antidote for, 733
  as antipyretic, 366
  caffeine and, 305
  codeine and, 326
  dosage, dosage forms, and indications for, 375
  hepatic or renal dysfunction and, 71
  lethal concentration of, 769
  metabolism of, 374
  metoclopramide and, 749
  narcotic analgesics and, 749
  nonaccidental toxin ingestion of, 731
  oral contraceptives and, 752
  pharmacokinetics of, 777
  propantheline and, 749
  structure of, 373

Acetanilide, 30
Acetate buffer, insulin and, 536
Acetazolamide, 484
  in epilepsy, 310
  infantile spasms and, 316
  pharmacokinetics of, 790
  structure of, 484
Acetohexamide, 539-540, 790
Acetone, 358, 769
Acetophenetidin; *see* Phenacetin
Acetylation, 33
Acetylcholine
  anticholinesterases and, 103, 751
    inhibitors of, 90
  atropine and, 10-11, 46, 116
    scopolamine and, 114
  autonomic nervous system and, 82
  binding sites for, 85, 86
  blood pressure and, 104
  as cholinergic agonist, 102
  denervation sensitivity and, 90
  digitalis and, 422
  discovery of, 83
  epinephrine and, 84
  neurotransmission and, 86, 91
  receptor concept and, 84, 86
  sites of action of, 83, 83
  synthesis, storage, and release of, 87
  tension development and, 115
  upper gastrointestinal tract and, 519
  vasopressin and, 575
Acetylcholine chloride, 102
Acetylcholine receptor, 84, 86
Acetylcholinesterase, 91
  acetylcholine and, 103, 751
  inhibitors of, 90
Acetylcysteine
  coughing and, 508
  pharmacokinetics of, 791
N-Acetylcysteine
  acetaminophen intoxication and, 375
  as antidote, 733
l-α-Acetylmethadol hydrochloride, 330, 341
N-Acetylpenicillamine, 735
N-Acetylprocainamide, 441, 782
  classification of, 434
  procainamide and, 767
  therapeutic concentrations of, 768
Acetylsalicylic acid, 364, 365, 437
Acetylstrophanthidin, 419, 425
ACh; *see* Acetylcholine

Acid
  absorption and, 14, 21
  as disinfectant, 686
  secretion of, 518-519
  as street name for lysergic acid diethylamide, 353
  sympathomimetics and, 754
α₁-Acid glycoprotein
  drug binding to, 73
  lidocaine and, 442
Acidemia, 754
Acquired immunodeficiency syndrome
  antiviral drugs for, 669
  pentamidine isethionate in, 695-696
  trimethoprim for, 694
ACTH; *see* Adrenocorticotropic hormone
Actidil; *see* Triprolidine
Actinomyces, 632, 654
Actinomycin D, 709; *see also* Dactinomycin
Action potential, cardiac, 434
  antiarrhythmics and, 433, 434, 436
Activated charcoal; *see* Charcoal
Active transport, 15
Acute intermittent porphyria, 289
Acycloguanosine, 669; *see also* Acyclovir
  nucleic acid synthesis and, 630
Acyclovir, 669
  nucleic acid synthesis and, 630
  pharmacokinetics of, 789
  viral infections susceptible to, 668
Adalat; *see* Nifedipine
Adapin; *see* Doxepin
Additive effect, 45
Adenine arabinoside, 668; *see also* Vidarabine
Adenosine, 82, 83
Adenosine diphosphate, platelets and, 470
Adenosine triphosphate, release of, 93
Adenosylcobalamin, 610
Adenylate cyclase, 202
ADH; *see* Vasopressin
Adrenal glucocorticoids, mechanism of action of, 705
Adrenal medulla, chemical mediators to, 84
Adrenal steroid(s), 543-556
  adrenocorticotropic hormone in, 544-545
  androgens in, 556
  biosynthesis of, 545-546
  glucocorticoids in, 546-554
  mineralocorticoids in, 555-556
  neoplasms and, 704
  pituitary-adrenal relationship in, 544-545
Adrenalectomy, 549

Adrenal-pituitary axis, 551
Adrenergic agonist(s); *see also* Adrenergic
    drug(s)
  antidepressants and, 753
  bronchial smooth muscle and, 158, 509
  glucocorticoids and, 514
  guanidinium and, 753
  hypertension and, 188-189
  insulin and, 532
  ipratropium and, 516
  lower airway in, 510-512
  reserpine and, 753
  uterus and, 578
α-Adrenergic antagonist(s); *see also* Adrenergic
    drug(s)
  asthma and, 516
  corticotropin-releasing factor and, 581
  hypertension and, 187
  insulin and, 532
β-Adrenergic antagonist(s), 434, 445; *see also*
    Adrenergic drug(s)
  antihypertensives and, 178
  bronchial smooth muscle and, 509
  clonidine and, 753
  digitalis and, 753
  in glaucoma, 105
  hypersusceptibility to, 42
  insulin and, 532
Adrenergic blocking agent(s), 163-171; *see also*
    α-Adrenergic blocking agent(s);
    β-Adrenergic blocking agent(s);
    Adrenergic drug(s)
α-Adrenergic blocking agent(s), 85, 98, 163-
    166, 445
  antidepressants and, 246
  hypertension and, 187
  norepinephrine and, 86
β-Adrenergic blocking agent(s), 85, 98, 166-
    170
  absorption of, 58
  angina and, 450, 454
  antiarrhythmics and, 433, 436
  antidepressants and, 246
  calcium blockers and, 455
  glucocorticoids and, 514
  hypertension and, 190-193
  hyperthyroidism and, 566
  insomnia and, 291
  introduction of, 177
  lidocaine and, 751
  lower airway and, 510-511
  myocardial oxygen requirements and, 451
  nitrates and, 454
  norepinephrine and, 86
  properties, uses, and dosage forms of, 167
Adrenergic drug(s), 98, 142-162; *see also*
    Adrenergic agonist(s)
  as bronchodilators, 158
  catecholamines as, 142-154; *see also*
    Catecholamine(s)
  as central nervous system stimulants and
    anorexiants, 159-161

Adrenergic drug(s)—cont'd
  classification of, 154
  ephedrine as, 154-156
  related to epinephrine or ephedrine, 157-
    158
  structure-activity relationships in, 161
  tachyphylaxis and, 47
  as vasodilators, 159
Adrenergic neuron, 83, 89, 172-176
  bretylium and, 174
  catecholamine release and, 172-173, 175
  guanethidine and, 174
  methyldopa and, 175
  monoamine oxidase inhibitors and, 176
  reserpine and, 174
Adrenergic neuron false transmitters, 175
α₂-Adrenergic receptor agonists, 188-189
Adrenergic receptors, 82
  catecholamines and, 144-146
  corticotropin-releasing factor and, 581
  gonadotropin-releasing hormone and, 581
  growth hormone–releasing factor and, 582
  receptor regulation and, 9
  subclasses of, 144-146
  upper airway and, 506
  uterus and, 576
α₁-Adrenergic receptors, 576
β₂-Adrenergic receptors, 576
Adrenocorticotropic hormone, 544-545
Adrenogenital syndrome, 556
Adriamycin; *see* Doxorubicin
Adrucil; *see* Fluorouracil
Adsorbants as antidiarrheal agents, 523
Adverse effects; *see* specific agent
Advil; *see* Ibuprofen
AeroBid; *see* Flunisolide
Aerosporin; *see* Polymyxin B
Affective disorders, 268
Affinity, 8
Age, 57-62
  antibiotics and, 664
  drug absorption and, 57-58
  drug disposition and, 60
  drug distribution and, 58-60
  drug excretion and, 61
  drug metabolism and, 61
  drug safety and effectiveness and, 44
  investigation problems and, 57
Agonist, 6, 10
  partial, 11
Agonist-antagonists, mixed, 332-333
β-Agonists; *see* Adrenergic agonist(s)
AIDS; *see also* Acquired immunodeficiency
    syndrome
Airway
  lower, 508-516
  upper, 506-507
Akineton; *see* Biperiden hydrochloride
Ak-Pentolate; *see* Cyclopentolate hydrochloride
ALB; *see* Albumin
Albumin, 559
  age and, 58, 59

Albumin—cont'd
  binding of drugs to, 73
  binding of proteins and, 24
  drug disposition and, 70
  ethacrynic acid and, 380
  thyroid hormones and, 558
Albuterol, 510-511, 782
Alclofenac, 781
Alcohol, 292-298
  antihistamines and, 209
  barbiturates and, 289
  blood level of, 294, 295
  in body fluids, 294
  chronic alcoholism and; *see* Alcoholism
  gastrointestinal tract and, 518
  hepatic transformation of, 296
  insomnia and, 291, 292
  intoxication from, 296-297
  kinetics of, 294-296
  methanol as, 298-299
  nerve block and, 294
  nonsteroidal anti-inflammatory drugs and,
    368
  pharmacologic effects of, 293-294
  skin disinfection and, 684
  tolerance of, 296-297
  vasopressin and, 575
  zero-order elimination and, 18
Alcohol dehydrogenation, 32. 296
Alcohol intoxication, 297
Alcohol withdrawal, 290
Alcoholism, 292-298; *see also* Alcohol
  characteristics of, 342-343
  chronic, 297-298
  genetic factors and, 343
Alcuronium, 777
Aldactone; *see* Spironolactone
Aldomet; *see* Methyldopa
Aldose reductase, 541
Aldose reductase inhibitors, 541
Aldosterone, 490, 543-544, 555-556
  adrenal steroid synthesis and, 545
  dosage of, 554
  hypertension and, 180-181
  structure of, 490
Aldosterone antagonists, 490, 543, 555
Aldosteronism, 555
Alfenta; *see* Alfentanil
Alfentanil, 327, 777
ALG; *see* Antilymphocyte globulin
Aliphatic hydroxylation, 30
Alka Seltzer; *see* Sodium bicarbonate
Alkalinized glutaraldehyde, 684, 685
Alkeran; *see* Melphalan
Alkylamines, action of, 208
Alkylating agents, 703-706
Allergy
  drug safety and effectiveness and, 42-43
  histamine release in, 201-203
Allopurinol
  azathioprine and, 751
  gout and, 599, 600, 603-604

Allopurinol—cont'd
  mercaptopurine and, 751
  pharmacokinetics of, 790
  xanthine oxidase and, 751
All-or-nothing response, 42
Alpha receptors; *see* Adrenergic receptors
Alpha$_2$-adrenergic agonists, hypertension and, 188-189
Alpha-adrenergic blocking agents, 85, 98, 163-166
  hypertension and, 187
Alphaprodine, 327, 329
Alphaprodine hydrochloride, 327
AlphaREDISOL; *see* Hydroxocobalamin
Alprazolam, 273
  depression with schizophrenia and, 268
  dosage and forms of, 263
  pharmacokinetics of, 778
  seizures and, 262
  structure of, 261
Alprostadil, 233
Aludrox; *see* Antacid(s)
Aluminum
  poisoning and, 742-743
  tetracyclines and, 748
  upper gastrointestinal tract and, 520
Aluminum hexaurea sulfate triiodide, 684
Aluminum hydroxide
  constipation and, 522
  upper gastrointestinal tract and, 519-520
Aluminum hydroxide gel, 520
Aluminum salts, 520
Alupent; *see* Metaproterenol
Alurate; *see* Aprobarbital
AMA Drug Evaluations, 762
Amantadine, 667
  parkinsonism and, 122, 125
  pharmacokinetics of, 789
  renal excretion of, 753
  viral infections susceptible to, 668
Amantadine hydrochloride, 125
Ambenonium, 106, 108
Ambenonium chloride, 106
Ambilhar; *see* Niridazole
Amdinocillin, 786
Amebiasis, 687-689
American Medical Association Drug Evaluations, 762
Amethopterin; *see* Methotrexate
Amidate; *see* Etomidate
Amides as local anesthetics, 407, 408
Amikacin, 657, 658, 659
  therapeutic concentrations of, 768
Amikin; *see* Amikacin
Amiloride, 490-491
  hepatic or renal dysfunction and, 71
  pharmacokinetics of, 790
  as potassium-sparing diuretics, 194
  renal excretion of, 753
  structure of, 490
Amines, action of, 82
Amino acid antagonists, 703

L-Amino acid decarboxylase, 198
Amino acids
  action of, 82
  intestinal absorption and, 22
p-Aminobenzoic acid
  antibacterial chemotherapy and, 629
  folic acid and, 612
  microsomal oxidations and, 33
  procaine and, 410
  sulfonamides and, 634
γ-Aminobutyric acid, 99, 293, 303, 310
  action of, 82
  barbiturates and, 287
  depressant or stimulant action of, 247-248
  regulation of chloride channels by, 282
  sites of action of, 83
γ-Aminobutyric acid system, 293
γ-Aminobutyric acid–receptor agonists, 310
γ-Aminobutyric acid–receptor mechanisms, 303
7-Aminocephalosporanic acid, 651
Aminocyclitol, 656; *see also* Aminoglycosides
  pharmacokinetics of, 785
ε-Aminocaproic acid, 779
Aminoglutethimide
  adrenal cortex and, 545
  pharmacokinetics of, 791
Aminoglycosides, 656-659
  carbenicillin and, 750
  ethanol and, 749
  neuromuscular blockers and, 753
  organisms susceptible to, 654
  pharmacokinetics of, 785
  protein synthesis and, 630
  ureidopenicillin and, 750
p-Aminohippurate, renal excretion of, 753
γ-Aminolevulinic acid synthetase, 289
6-Aminopenicillanic acid, 642
p-Aminophenol derivatives, 365
Aminophylline
  lethal concentration of, 769
  lower airway and, 512
  visceral smooth muscle relaxation and, 306
Aminopyridine, 777
Aminopyrine
  as adulterant of heroin, 339
  age and, 60
  hepatic or renal dysfunction and, 71
  liver disease and, 74, 75, 76
[14]Aminopyrine, 75
5-Aminosalicylate, 638
p-Aminosalicylate, 629
p-Aminosalicylic acid
  acetylation of, 53
  gastrectomy and, 72
  iodine formation and, 563
  pharmacokinetics of, 789
  tuberculosis and, 672, 676
Aminosalicylic sodium, 673
Aminotriazole, 563
Amiodarone
  classification of, 434

Amiodarone—cont'd
  drugs inhibited by, 751
  pharmacokinetics of, 440, 782
  structure of, 446
  therapeutic concentrations of, 768
  thyroid hormones and, 562
  ventricular arrhythmias and, 448
Amitriptyline, 272
  age and disposition of, 60
  bishydroxycoumarin and, 749
  genetic conditions and, 49
  lethal concentration of, 769
  metabolic reactions of, 54
  pharmacokinetics of, 779
  structure of, 271
  therapeutic concentrations of, 768
  tranylcypromine and, 270
Amitriptyline hydrochloride, 272
Ammonia water as antidote, 732
Ammonium chloride
  disadvantages of, 483
  renal excretion and, 753
Amobarbital
  deficient *N*-glucosidation of, 54
  elimination half-life and clinical data for, 287
  genetic conditions and, 49
  lethal concentration of, 769
Amodiaquine, malaria and, 690, 692
Amosulalol, 783
Amotivational syndrome, 345
Amoxapine, 273-274
  clinical responses and doses of, 272
  extrapyramidal effects and, 271
  lethal concentration of, 769
  pharmacokinetics of, 779
  structure of, 271
Amoxicillin, 644, 649
  adverse effects of, 648
  organisms susceptible to, 651
  pharmacokinetics of, 647, 786
Amoxicillin trihydrate, 649
Amoxil; *see* Amoxicillin
Amphenone B, 545
Amphetamine(s)
  abuse of, 338, 348-349, 774-775
  action of, 172, 173, 246
  catecholamine release and, 94, 98
  as central nervous system stimulants and anorexiants, 159-160, 274
  chlorpromazine antagonism of, 244
  as cocaine adulterant, 350
  disadvantages of, 275
  lethal concentration of, 769
  microsomal oxidations and, 31
  nonaccidental toxin ingestion and, 731
  renal excretion of, 753
  scheduling of, 760
  schizophrenic symptoms and, 242-243, 348
  tachyphylaxis and, 47
d-Amphetamine, 244
Amphetamine psychosis, 242-243, 348

Amphojel, 520
Amphotericin B
  cell membranes and, 629-630
  drug interaction with digoxin, 430
  fungal infections and, 679-680
  pharmacokinetics of, 788
Ampicillin, 643, 644
  adverse effects of, 648-649
  hepatic or renal dysfunction and, 71
  organisms susceptible to, 651, 654
  pharmacokinetics of, 647, 786
Amrinone
  congestive heart failure and, 431
  pharmacokinetics of, 784
  structure of, 431
  toxicity of, 431
Amrinone lactate, 431
Amyl acetate, abuse of, 358
Amyl nitrite, 452
  abuse of, 357
  angina and, 450
  as antidote, 733
  cyanide poisoning and, 738-739
  structure of, 451
Amytal; *see* Amobarbital
Anabolic agent, estrogen as, 588
Anadrol-50; *see* Oxymetholine
Analeptic agents, 302
Analgesics, 319
  nonsteroidal anti-inflammatory agents and;
    see Nonsteroidal anti-inflammatory
    agent(s)
  pharmacokinetics of, 777
  therapeutic concentrations of, 768
Anaphylatoxins, 201, 202
Anaphylaxis, 44, 201-203
Anaprox; *see* Naproxen
Anavar; *see* Oxandrolone
Ancef; *see* Cefazolin
Ancobon; *see* Flucytosine
Ancylostoma duodenale, 698
Androgen(s), 556, 594-597
  mechanism of action of, 705
  neoplasms and, 704, 708-709
  phenobarbital and, 752
Androgen antagonist, estrogen as, 589
Androlan; *see* Testosterone propionate
Androstenedione, 587
  adrenal steroid synthesis and, 545
  menopause and, 589
Androsterone, testosterone and, 594
Anemia
  iron-deficiency, 607-609
  megaloblastic, 609-613
Anemia, 605-613; *see also* Antianemic drug(s)
Anesthesia; *see also* Anesthetic(s)
  balanced, 329, 385, 404
  dissociative, 405
  general, 384-406
    clinical pharmacology of individual, 399-
      403
    efficacy of, 385

Anesthesia—cont'd
  general—cont'd
    intravenous, 385, 403-405
    pharmacologic effects of, 395-399
    potency of, 385
    preanesthetic medication and, 395
    solubility of, 385-388
    stages and signs of, 392-394
    theories of, 394-395
    uptake of, 388-391
  local; *see* Anesthetic(s), local
Anesthetic(s); *see also* Anesthesia
  alcohol and, 293
  biotransformation of, 389
  inhalation, 384, 399-404; *see also* Anesthesia,
    general
  intravenous, 385, 403-405
  local, 407-415
    absorption rate of, 409-410
    administration of, 410
    choice of, 415
    classification of, 407
    clinical characteristics of, 412-415
    dosages of, 412
    excretion of, 409-410
    hydrolysis rates of, 410
    mode of action of, 408-409
    onset and duration of action of, 410
    systemic action of, 411
    toxicity of, 411-412
    uses of, 408
  pharmacokinetics of, 777
  selection of, 384
Angel dust, 352
Angina, 450-458
  propranolol and, 168
Angioneurotic edema, 44
Angiotensin, 99
  diuretics and, 480
  hypertension and, 180-181
  metabolism of, 180
Angiotensin I, 180
Angiotensin I converting enzyme, 220
Angiotensin II, 180, 181
Angiotensin-converting enzyme inhibitors, 177
Anhydron; *see* Cyclothiazide
Animal studies, 39-40
Anionic detergent, 685
Anisindione, 468
Anspor; *see* Cephradine
Antabuse; *see* Disulfiram
Antacid(s)
  benzodiazepines and, 749
  calcium and, 567
  chlorpromazine and, 749
  cimetidine and, 749
  diflunisal and, 749
  digoxin and, 425, 749
  dishydroxycoumarin and, 749
  gastrointestinal tract and, 518
  iron absorption and, 606
  isoniazid and, 749

Antacid(s)—cont'd
  penicillamine and, 749
  phenytoin and, 749
  propranolol and, 749
  ranitidine and, 749
  tetracyclines and, 749
  upper gastrointestinal tract and, 519-521
Antagonism, 6, 10, 45-46
  noncompetitive, 11
Antepar; *see* Piperazine(s)
Anterior pituitary gonadotropins, 580-598
  androgens and, 594-597
  estrogens and, 587-591
  growth hormone and, 582-583
  hypothalamic releasing factors in, 580-582
  progestins and, 591-594
  sex hormones and, 583-587
  somatostatin and, 582-583
Anthelmintics, 697-701, 789
Anthracyclines, 702
Antianemic drug(s), 605-613
  deferoxamine as, 609
  erythrocytes and, 605
  iron in, 606-609
  megaloblastic anemias and, 609-613
    folic acid in, 612-613
    vitamin B_{12} in, 610-612
Antianginal(s), 450-458
  beta-adrenergic receptor blockers as, 454
  nitrates as, 450-454
  nitrites as, 450-454
  pharmacokinetics of, 782
  slow calcium-channel antagonists and, 455-
    457
Antianxiety agent(s), 247-248, 250, 260-265
  abuse of, 338, 774-775
  benzodiazepine drugs as, 262-264
  buspirone as, 264
  meprobamate as, 264-265
  pharmacokinetics of, 778
  as physically addicting drugs, 337
Antiarrhythmic(s), 433-449
  amiodarone as, 446
  aprindine as, 444
  beta-adrenergic receptor agonists as, 445
  bretylium tosylate as, 445
  cardiac electrophysiology and, 433-434
  disopyramide as, 441
  electrophysiology and, 434-436
  encainide as, 444
  flecainide as, 443
  lidocaine as, 441-442
  lorcainide as, 444
  mexiletine as, 442, 443
  pharmacokinetics of, 782
  phenytoin as, 444
  procainamide as, 439-441
  propranolol as, 168
  quinidine as, 436-439
  safety and, 755
  selection as, 447-448
  therapeutic concentrations of, 768

Antiarrhythmic(s)—cont'd
  tocainide as, 443
  verapamil as, 446
Antibacterial chemotherapy, 629-631
Antibacterial spectrum, 627
Antibacterials, 627, 785; *see also* Antibiotic(s)
Antibiotic(s), 642-666, 709
  amebiasis and, 689
  aminoglycosides as, 656-659
  antibacterial chemotherapeutic, 629-631
  bacitracin as, 656
  cephalosporins as, 651-655
  chloramphenicol as, 660-661
  coumarin and, 750
  definition of, 626
  digoxin and, 425-426, 750
  gram-positive organisms and, 661-663
  history of use of, 626-627
  macrolide, pharmacokinetics of, 786
  mechanisms of, 626-631
  nasal decongestants and, 506-507
  penicillin as, 642-651
  polymyxin B as, 656
  polypeptide, histamine and, 201
  resistance to, 628-629
  respiratory tract and, 506
  tetracyclines as, 659-660
  therapeutic concentrations of, 768
  vancomycin as, 656
  vitamin K and, 750
Antibiotic antagonism, 627-628
Antibiotic synergism, 627-628
Antibody(ies)
  corticosteroids and, 550
  as therapeutic agents, 718-720
Anticholinergic(s)
  abuse of, 357, 774-775
  action of, 84
  antidote for, 733
  asthma and, 515-516
  constipation and, 522
  coughing and, 507-508
  disopyramide and, 441
  gastrointestinal disease and, 118
  induction and, 395
  levodopa and, 123
  metoclopramide and, 522
  nasal decongestants and, 506-507
  Parkinson's disease and, 122, 124, 125
  pharmacokinetics of, 779
  smooth muscle relaxant, 119-120
  tricyclic antidepressants and, 273
  upper gastrointestinal tract and, 519
Anticholinesterase(s), 106-112
  acetylcholine and, 86, 751
  choline esters and, 751
  in glaucoma, 105
  as insecticide, 743
  preparations of, 106
  succinylcholine and, 751
Anticoagulant(s), 462-470
  blood concentration of, 766

Anticoagulant(s)—cont'd
  carbamazepine and, 752
  chloramphenicol and, 751
  coumarin, barbiturates and, 289
  ethanol and, 752
  glutethimide and, 752
  griseofulvin and, 752
  oral, as platelet inhibiting agent, 471-472
  oral contraceptives and, 751
  pharmacokinetics of, 779
  phenobarbital and, 752
  phenytoin and, 752
  rifampin and, 752
  as rodenticides, 743
  safety and, 755
Anticonvulsants; *see also* Antiepileptic(s)
  benzodiazepines and, 263-264
  folic acid and, 613
Antidepressant(s), 245-247, 268-276
  α-adrenergic receptor agonists and, 753
  charcoal and, 732
  constipation and, 522
  insomnia and, 291
  monoamine oxidase inhibitors as, 269-270
  nonaccidental toxin ingestion of, 731
  pharmacokinetics of, 779
  psychotomimetic drugs and, 274-276
  second-generation, 273-274
  synaptic effects of, 246
  tricyclic, 98, 270-273
    catecholamines and, 90, 94
    clinical response and doses of, 272
    clonidine and, 189
    constipation and, 522
    discovery of, 269
    serotonin and, 216
    structure of, 271
    tyramine and, 173
Antidiarrheal(s), 522-524
  gastrointestinal tract and, 518
  opioid, 329
Antidiuretic hormone; *see also* Vasopressin
  alcohol and, 293
  morphine and, 324
  renal tubules and, 482
Antidiuretics, vasopressin as, 573-576
Antidote(s), 730-745; *see also* Poison(s)
  atropine, 118-119
  scopolamine, 118-119
Antiepileptic(s), 308-317
  adverse effects of, 310
  benzodiazepines as, 263-264
  classes of, 310-316
  clinical activity of, 311
  clinical pharmacology of, 316-319
  dosage of, 311
  drug interactions of, 310
  folic acid and, 613
  modes of action of, 309-310
  pharmacokinetics of, 311, 780
  therapeutic concentrations of, 768
Antiestrogen, 704

Antifibrinolytics, 779
Antifungals, 679-681, 788
Antihistamine(s), 203-204, 206-212
  antagonism and, 46
  histamine H_1-receptor antagonists as, 206-210
  histamine H_2-receptor antagonists as, 210-211
  nasal decongestants and, 506-507
  nonprescription sleep medication and, 291
  parkinsonism and, 122, 125
  pharmacokinetics of, 780
Antihypertensive(s), 177-196
  α-adrenergic mechanism interference and, 185-189
  β-adrenergic receptor blocking agents as, 190-193
  angiotensin and aldosterone and, 180-181
  benzodiazepines and, 263-264
  blood concentration of, 766
  classification of, 181
  converting enzyme inhibitors as, 184
  direct vasodilators as, 181-184
  diuretics as, 193-194, 753
  ganglionic blocking agents as, 194
  monoamine oxidase inhibitors as, 194
  pharmacokinetics of, 783
  propranolol as, 168
  reflex inhibitors of central sympathetic function as, 195
  site of action of, 178
  slow calcium-channel blockers as, 190
  tricyclic antidepressants and, 273
Anti-inflammatory agent(s)
  nonsteroidal; *see* Nonsteroidal anti-inflammatory agent(s)
  pharmacokinetics of, 781
  steroid, 549
    lower airway and, 508, 513-515
  therapeutic concentrations of, 768
Antikaliuretic agents, 490-491
Antilirium; *see* Physostigmine
Antilymphocyte globulin, 724, 725
Antimalarial(s)
  cellular binding of, 24
  folic acid and, 613
  pharmacokinetics of, 788
Antimanic agents, 779
Antimetabolite(s)
  neoplasms and, 706-708
  pharmacokinetics of, 788
  sulfonamides as, 632
Antimicrobial activity, 627; *see also* Antibiotic(s)
Antiminth; *see* Pyrantel
Antineoplastics, 703, 788; *see also* Chemotherapy
Antiparasitics, 789
Antiparkinsonian drugs, 121-126
Antiplatelet drugs, 470-473, 779
Antipsychotic drugs, 250-259

Antipsychotic drugs—cont'd
abuse of, 352
butyrophenones as, 258-259
choosing, 259
concentrations of, 243
development of, 250-252
pharmacokinetics of, 779
phenothiazine derivatives as, 252-257
thioxanthene derivatives as, 257-258
Antipyretic analgesics
nonsteroidal anti-inflammatory; *see*
Nonsteroidal anti-inflammatory agent(s)
therapeutic concentrations of, 768
Antipyrine
age and, 60
alteration in disposition of, 50, 60, 70
charcoal-broiled beef and, 65
dietary carbohydrate and, 65
hepatic or renal dysfunction and, 71, 74
plasma half-life of, 50
Antischizophrenic drugs, 242-243; *see also*
Antipsychotic drugs
Antisecretory agents, 518
Antiseptic(s), 683-686
definition of, 683
intestinal, sulfonamides as, 637
Antispasmodics, 518, 782
Antithrombin III
heparin and, 463
kallikrein and, 219, 220
Antithyroid drugs, 563-566
Antitrypanosomal drugs, 695-696
Antituberculosis agents, 672-677, 789
Antitussives, 507-508
clinical pharmacology of, 334-335
respiratory tract and, 506
Antiulcer agent, pharmacokinetics of, 782
Antivert; *see* Meclizine
Antiviral agent(s), 667-671
acyclovir as, 669
amantadine as, 667
anti–human immunodeficiency virus agents
as, 669-670
idoxuridine as, 667
interferon inducers as, 670
pharmacokinetics of, 789
trifluridine as, 669
vidarabine as, 668
Anturane; *see* Sulfinpyrazone
Anxiety, rebound, 282
Anxiety disorder, generalized, 261
APC tablets; *see* Aspirin, phenacetin, and
caffeine
Apolipoproteins, 493, 497
Apomorphine, 323, 731, 732
Apomorphine hydrochloride, 731, 732
Apresoline; *see* Hydralazine
Aprindine, 444
classification of, 434
pharmacokinetics of, 782
structure of, 444
Aprobarbital, 287

Aquachloral; *see* Chloral hydrate
AquaMEPHYTON; *see* Phytonadione;
Vitamins, K_1
Aquatag; *see* Benzthiazide
Aquatensen; *see* Methyclothiazide
Arabinosylcytosine, 705
Arachidonic acid, 205
biosynthesis of derivatives of, 228, 230, 231
corticosteroids and, 550
glucocorticoids and, 514
immunosuppression and, 724
leukotrienes and, 237
nonsteroidal anti-inflammatory drugs and,
364
platelet inhibitory drugs and, 459
prostaglandins and, 227
Arachidonic acid lipoxygenases, 235, 236
Aralen; *see* Chloroquine
Arfonad; *see* Trimethaphan
Aristocort; *see* Triamcinolone
Aromatic L-amino acid decarboxylase, 92
Aromatic rings, hydroxylation of, 30
Aromatic solvents, poisoning from, 744
Arrhythmia(s)
anesthesia and, 397-398
digitalis and, 427
supraventricular, 447-448
ventricular, 448
Arsenic, 742
dimercaprol and, 45, 733
lethal concentration of, 769
as rodenticide, 743
Arsobal; *see* Melarsoprol
Artane; *see* Trihexyphenidyl hydrochloride
Arthrolate; *see* Sodium thiosalicylate
Arthropan; *see* Choline salicylate
Arylamine, reductions and, 32
Asbestos exposure, 69
Ascaris lumbricoides, 698
Ascorbic acid, 617; *see also* Vitamin(s), C
Asendin; *see* Amoxapine
L-Asparaginase, 704, 705, 709-710
Aspartic acid, 82, 83, 97
Aspercreme; *see* Trolamine salicylate
Aspirin, 364, 365
absorption of, 23, 370
as anti-inflammatory agent, 367
asthma and, 516
codeine and, 326
dipyridamole with, 473
distribution of, 371
dosage, dosage forms, and indications for,
372, 375
gastrointestinal tract and, 368-369, 518
lethal dose of, 372
mechanisms and sites of action of, 366
metabolism of, 371
migraine and, 368
nonaccidental toxin ingestion and, 731
as platelet inhibiting agent, 471-472
platelet inhibitory drugs and, 459

Aspirin—cont'd
renal toxicity of, 369-370
structure of, 365
therapeutic concentrations of, 768
use of, 473
warfarin and, 469
zero-order elimination and, 18
Aspirin, phenacetin, and caffeine, 369-370
Astemizole, 780
Asthma, 44
β-adrenergic receptor agonists for, 510-512
alternative therapy for, 515
anti-inflammatory steroids for, 513-515
methylxanthines for, 512-513
theophylline in, 306
Atabrine; *see* Quinacrine
Atarax; *see* Hydroxyzine
Atenolol, 170
action of, 169
sites of, 178
hypertension and, 192
myocardial infarction and, 169
pharmacokinetics of, 783
properties and uses of, 167
Atherosclerosis, 493-503
cholesterol regulation and, 497-498
dietary modification and, 502
exercise and, 502
high-density lipoproteins and, 498
hyperlipidemia therapy and, 498-501
lipoproteins and, 493-497
pathogenesis of, 493
Athrombin-K; *see* Warfarin
Ativan; *see* Lorazepam
Atonic seizures, 308
Atracurium, 777
Atrial fibrillation
antiarrhythmic drugs and, 447-448
digitalis and, 427
Atrial flutter
antiarrhythmic drugs and, 447
digitalis and, 427
Atrial muscle, digitalis and, 422
Atrial tachycardia, paroxysmal
antiarrhythmic drugs and, 447
digitalis and, 428
Atropa belladonna, 114
Atropine, 98, 114-119
abuse of, 357
acetylcholine and, 10-11, 46, 86, 104
action of, 84
as antidote, 733
bradycardia and, 118
propranolol-induced, 169
cardiovascular system and, 115
coughing and, 507-508
diphenoxylate and, 329
dosage of, 445
histamine and, 201
hypersensitivity to, 36
Lomotil and, 118
lower gastrointestinal tract and, 118, 523

Atropine—cont'd
 morphine and, 324
 pharmacokinetics of, 779
 as preanesthetic medication, 395
 upper gastrointestinal tract and, 519
Atropine methylbromide, 120
Atropine sulfate, 120
Atropisal; *see* Atropine
Atrovent; *see* Ipratropium
Attention deficit disorder, 269
Attenuated virus vaccine, 717
Atypical plasma cholinesterase, 52
Augmentin; *see* Amoxicillin
Auranofin, 781
Aureomycin; *see* Chlortetracycline
Aurothioglucose, 379
Autacoids of brain and gastrointestinal tract,
 222-225
Autoimmune disease, 723
Autoinduction, 36
Autonomic drugs, 98; *see also* specific agent
Autonomic nervous system, 88, 98
 general anesthesia and, 396
Autoreceptors, 82
Aventyl; *see* Nortriptyline
Azactam; *see* Aztreonam
Azaline; *see* Sulfasalazine
Azapropazone, 781
Azatadine, 209
Azathioprine
 allopurinol and, 751
 immunosuppression and, 723, 724, 725
 pharmacokinetics of, 788
3'-Azido-3'-deoxythymidine, 669, 789
Azlin; *see* Azlocillin
Azlocillin, 650, 786
Azmacort; *see* Triamcinolone
Azoreduction, 32
AZT; *see* 3'-Azido-3'-deoxythymidine
Aztreonam, 655
 pharmacokinetics of, 786
Azulfidine; *see* Sulfasalazine

B

B fibers, 409
Bacillus anthracis, 632
Bacitracin, 626, 656
Baclofen, 139, 782
Bacteria, gastrointestinal, 73
Bactericidal activity, 627
Bacteriostatic activity, 627
Bacteroides, 651, 654
Bactocill; *see* Oxacillin
Bactrim; *see* Trimethoprim-sulfamethoxazole
Baking soda; *see* Sodium bicarbonate
BAL; *see* Dimercaprol
Balanced anesthesia, 329, 385, 404
Balantidium coli, 688
Barbital
 elimination half-life and clinical data for, 287
 lethal concentration of, 769
 pharmacokinetics of, 778

Barbiturate(s), 286-287
 absorption of, 21, 23
 abuse of, 337, 338, 350-351, 774-775
 as adulterant of heroin, 339
 anesthetics and, 385
 antihistamines and, 209
 benzodiazepines and, 263-264
 digitalis intoxication and, 429
 epilepsy and, 313-314
 formulas for, 311
 history of use of, 280
 intermediate acting, 287
 long acting, 287
 nonaccidental toxin ingestion of, 731
 overdose of, 350
 as physically addicting drugs, 337
 poisoning from, 288, 731
  picrotoxin and, 303
 strychnine poisoning and, 304
 ultrashort-acting, 286, 287, 288
  anesthesia and, 403-404
  elimination half-life and clinical data for,
   287
 vasopressin and, 575
 warfarin and, 469
 withdrawal from, 351
Barbiturate abstinence syndrome, 351
Barbiturate poisoning, 288, 731
 picrotoxin and, 303
Barbituric acid, 286
Base
 plasma protein binding of, 73
 as street name for cocaine, 349
BCNU; *see* Carmustine
Beclomethasone
 dosage of, 554
 lower airway and, 513, 514
Beclovent; *see* Beclomethasone
Beconase; *see* Beclomethasone
Beer, 295
Belladonna alkaloids, 122, 124; *see also*
  Atropine; Scopolamine
Benadryl; *see* Diphenhydramine
Bendroflumethiazide, 486, 790
Benemid; *see* Probenecid
Benzalkonium, 685, 686
Benzathine penicillin G, 648
Benzene
 exposure to, 69
 lethal concentration of, 769
 poisoning from, 743
 toluene and, 744
Benzene hexachloride, 743
Benzocaine, 413; *see* Ethyl aminobenzoate
Benzodiazepine(s), 315
 abuse of, 351-352
 action of, 247-248
 adverse effects of, 263-264
 age and, 57, 61
 γ-aminobutyric acid and, 247, 282
 antacids and, 749

Benzodiazepine(s)—cont'd
 antihistamines and, 209
 in anxiety, 261, 262-264
 cimetidine and, 212, 751
 disulfiram and, 751
 as hypnotics, 280-286
 for induction, 385, 395
 insomnia and, 292
 nonaccidental toxin ingestion and, 731
 perioperative, 282
Benzoic acid, 686
Benzonatate, 507-508
Benzthiazide, 486
Benztropine, 124, 125
Benztropine mesylate, 125
Benzyl alcohol, 299
Benzylisoquinolines, 322
Benzylpenicillin, 642; *see also* Penicillin G
Beriberi, 614
Bestrone; *see* Estrone
Beta receptors, 85; *see also* Adrenergic
  receptors
 subclasses of, 144-146
Beta-adrenergic blocking agents; *see* β-
  Adrenergic blocking agent(s)
Beta-adrenergic agonists; *see* Adrenergic
  agonist(s)
Betagan; *see* Levobunolol
Betamethasone
 dosage of, 554
 pharmacokinetics of, 791
 structure of, 553
Betaxolol, 170
 pharmacokinetics of, 783
 properties and uses of, 167
 structures of, 167
Bethanechol chloride, 102, 103
Betoptic; *see* Betaxolol
Bezafibrate, 784
Bhang, 344
Bicillin L-A; *see* Benzathine penicillin G
BiCNU; *see* Carmustine
Bicuculline
 action of, 302
 depressant or stimulant action of, 247
 GABA and, 85
Bilarcil; *see* Metrifonate
Bile acid-binding resins, 500
Bilirubin
 phenobarbital and, 36
 protein binding capacity and, 24
Biltricide; *see* Praziquantel
Bioavailability, 15
Bioequivalence, 759
Biologic variation, 42
Biosynthesis
 catecholamines and, 92-93
 of serotonin, 215-216
Biotin, 617
Biotransformation
 of anesthetics, 389
 drug interactions and, 751-752

Biotransformation—cont'd
general anesthesia and, 398-399
Biperiden hydrochloride, 124
Biperiden lactate, 124
Bipolar disorder, 268
Bisacodyl, 525, 526
Bishydroxycoumarin
amitriptyline and, 749
drugs inhibited by, 751
plasma half-life of, 50
variations in disposition of, 50
Bismuth subnitrate, 454
Bismuth subsalicylate, 523
Bithionol, 698, 701
Bitin; *see* Bithionol
Bitolterol mesylate, 511
Blenoxane; *see* Bleomycin
Bleomycin
mechanism of action of, 705
neoplasms and, 709
pharmacokinetics of, 788
Bleomycin sulfate, 704
Blocadren; *see* Timolol
Blood, drug concentrations in, 766-772
Blood coagulation factors, 460-462
Blood lipid-lowering agents, 784
Blood pressure, 177; *see also*
Antihypertensive(s)
acetylcholine and, 104
anesthesia and, 397
diuretics and, 380
mechanisms regulating, 179
Blood vessels, prostaglandins and, 233
Blood-brain barrier, 24
Blue heavens, 350
Blush area, 452
Bolt, 357
Bonine; *see* Meclizine
Bordetella pertussis, 654
Boric acid, 769
Boron, 769
Botanicals, 743
Botulinum toxin, 98
acetylcholine and, 86, 91
Bradycardia, atropine and, 118
Bradykinin, 99
and kallidin, 219
lungs and, 516
Bran, 525
Breast-fed infant, 25
Breasts, estrogen and, 588
Brethine; *see* Terbutaline
Bretylium, 98, 173, 186, 445
action of, 172
adrenergic neuron and, 174
classification of, 434
norepinephrine and, 86
pharmacokinetics of, 440, 783
structure of, 445
Bretylium tosylate, 174, 445
pharmacokinetics and, 440
structure of, 445

Bretylium-like action, 186
Bretylol; *see* Bretylium
Brevital; *see* Methohexital
Bricanyl; *see* Terbutaline
British antilewisite; *see* Dimercaprol
Broad-spectrum penicillins, 649-650
Bromide(s), 120
abuse of, 352
antidote for, 733
history of use of, 311
intoxication from, 737
lethal concentration of, 769
seizures and, 316
Bromocriptine, 219
galactorrhea and, 582
gonadotropin-releasing hormone and, 582
parkinsonism and, 122, 125, 219
Bromocriptine mesylate, 125, 219
Brompheniramine
doses and sedative property of, 209
lethal concentration of, 769
pharmacokinetics of, 780
Bronchial smooth muscle, 509
Bronchoconstriction, 508-516
Bronchodilatation
coughing and, 507-508
epinephrine and, 148-149
lower airway and, 508, 509-516
norepinephrine and, 148-149
pharmacokinetics of, 782
respiratory tract and, 506
Bronkosol; *see* Isoetharine
Brucella, 654
Brussels sprouts, 66-67
Budesonide, 791
Bulk laxatives, 524, 525
Bumetanide, 488-489
digoxin interaction with, 430
pharmacokinetics of, 790
structure of, 488
Bumex; *see* Bumetanide
Bupivacaine, 407, 408, 414-415
dosage of, 412
history of use of, 407
onset and duration of action of, 410
as preferred local anesthetic, 415
safe dosage of, 412
structure of, 415
uses of, 408
vasoconstriction and, 411
Buprenex; *see* Buprenorphine
Buprenorphine, 333
dosage of, 327
pharmacokinetics of, 777
Bupropion, 779
Burimamide, 210
BuSpar; *see* Buspirone
Buspirone, 264, 778
Buspirone hydrochloride, 264
Busulfan, 703, 704, 706
pharmacokinetics of, 788

Butabarbital, 287, 769
Butacaine, 408
Butazolidin; *see* Phenylbutazone
Butisol; *see* Butabarbital
Butorphanol, 327, 333, 777
Butorphanol tartrate, 327
Butyn; *see* Butacaine
Butyrophenones
dopaminergic receptors and, 85
psychoses and, 258-259
Butyrylcholinesterase, 91

C

C fibers
local anesthetics and, 409
nonsteroidal anti-inflammatory drugs and,
366
Cabbage, 66-67
Cadmium poisoning, 734
Cafergot; *see* Ergotamine
Caffeine, 304-306
abuse of, 360
action of, 302
chemical structure of, 305
as cocaine adulterant, 350
gastrointestinal tract and, 518
insomnia and, 291, 292
lethal concentration of, 769
lower airway and, 512
relative activities of, 305
Caffeine with sodium benzoate, 305
Calamine lotion, 685
Calan; *see* Verapamil
Calcifediol, 569, 570
Calciferol, 570
Calcimar; *see* Salmon calcitonin
Calcitonin, 567, 568
Calcitriol, 569, 570
parathyroid extract and, 567
Calcium
as antidote, 732, 733
blood coagulation and, 462
digitalis and, 422
intoxication from, 429
diuretics and, 477
glucocorticoids and, 549
homeostasis and, 567-568, 570-571
hypocalcemia and, 567
local anesthetics and, 408
parathyroid extract and, 567-568
tetracycline and, 748
vitamin D and, 569
Calcium antagonists, 169
Calcium carbonate
hypocalcemia and, 571
upper gastrointestinal tract and, 519-520
Calcium channel, slow, 433, 436; *see* Calcium-
channel blockers
Calcium cyanamide, 297
Calcium disodium edetate, 733, 734-735
in iron poisoning, 742

Calcium disodium edetate—cont'd
  in lead poisoning, 739
Calcium disodium versenate, 734
Calcium glubionate, 571
Calcium gluceptate, 571
Calcium gluconate
  ethylene glycol intoxication and, 737
  hypocalcemia and, 571
Calcium homeostasis, 570-571
  parathyroid extract and, 567-568
Calcium influx, 433
Calcium lactate, 571
Calcium phosphate, 571
Calcium salts, 567
Calcium-channel blockade, 434
Calcium-channel blocker(s)
  angina and, 450
  antiarrhythmics and, 434
  asthma and, 516
  epilepsy and, 310
  hypertension and, 190
  myocardial oxygen requirements and supply
    and, 451
  nitrates and, 454
Calderol; *see* Calcifediol
Calpactin, 550
Calusterone, 708
Camphorated tincture of opium, 523
Cancer chemotherapy, 711-712
Candida albicans, 679, 680
Cannabinoids, 344-347
Cannabis sativa, 344
Cantharidin, abuse of, 360
Capastat; *see* Capreomycin
Capoten; *see* Captopril
Capreomycin
  Mycobacterium infections susceptible to, 673
  pharmacokinetics of, 789
  tuberculosis and, 672, 677
Captopril
  pharmacokinetics of, 783
  prostaglandin and, 753
  renal excretion of, 753
  sites of action of, 178
  structure of, 184
Carafate; *see* Sucralfate
Carbacel; *see* Carbachol
Carbachol, 98, 102, 103
  acetylcholine and, 86
  histamine and, 204
Carbachol chloride, 102
Carbamazepine, 36, 311-312
  action of, 309
  charcoal and, 749
  chloramphenicol and, 751
  cimetidine and, 751
  clinical activity of, 311
  dosage of, 311
  drugs induced by, 752
  in epilepsy, 310, 316
  erythromycin and, 751
  isoniazid and, 751

Carbamazepine—cont'd
  lethal concentration of, 769
  pharmacokinetics of, 311, 780
  phenytoin and, 752
  propoxyphene and, 751
  structure of, 312
  sulfonamides and, 751
  therapeutic concentrations of, 768
  warfarin and, 469
Carbapenems, 785
Carbenicillin, 643-644, 650
  adverse effects of, 648-649
  aminoglycosides and, 750
  hepatic or renal dysfunction and, 71
  organisms susceptible to, 651
  pharmacokinetics of, 647, 786
Carbenicillin disodium, 650
Carbenicillin indanyl sodium, 650
Carbidopa, 123
Carbimazole, 563, 564-565
Carbocaine; *see* Mepivacaine
Carbohydrate metabolism
  alcohol and, 293
  glucocorticoids and, 547-548
β-Carboline derivatives, 247, 248
Carbon monoxide poisoning, 737-738
  antidote for, 733
  lethal concentration in, 769
Carbon tetrachloride
  abuse of, 358
  lethal concentration of, 769
  liver damage and, 35
Carbonates, 748
Carbonic anhydrase inhibitors, 105, 484-488
Carboprost tromethamine, 578
Carboxymethylcellulose, 524, 525
Carboxypeptidase N, 220
Carbromal, 769
Carcinoid
  kinins and, 221
  serotonin and, 215, 217
Cardiac electrophysiology, 433-434
Cardiac inotropes, 784
Cardiac glycosides, 753, 784
Cardiac output
  β-blockers and, 191
  general anesthesia and, 391
Cardioquin; *see* Quinidine
Cardioselectivity, 169
Cardiovascular agents, pharmacokinetics of,
    782; *see also* specific agent
Cardiovascular system, catecholamines and,
    146-148
Cardizem; *see* Diltiazem
Carisoprodol, 769
Carmustine, 704, 706, 788
Carteolol, 783
Carumonam, 786
Cascara sagrada, 525
Castor oil, 525
CAT; *see* Choline acetyltransferase
Catalytic antibodies, 720

Catapres; *see* Clonidine
Catecholamine(s), 142-154
  adrenergic neuron false transmitters and,
    175
  adrenergic receptors for, 144
  antipsychotic drugs and, 242-243
  cocaine and, 412
  digitalis intoxication and, 429
  discovery of, 83
  diuretics and, 380
  dopamine as, 153-154
  dopaminergic receptors for, 144-146
  drug-receptor interaction and, 6
  epinephrine as, 146-153
  histamine and, 203
  6-hydroxydopamine and, 97
  isoflurane and, 403
  lower airway and, 510-511
  neurotransmission and, 91-97
  norepinephrine and; *see* Norepinephrine
  occurrence of, 143-144
  pathway of synthesis of, 93
  physiologic functions of, 143-144
  release mechanisms of, 172-173
  reuptake of, 94
  storage and release of, 93
Catechol-*O*-methyltransferase, 95, 244
Catechols, 91
Cathartics, 524-526
Catnip, 360
Ceclor; *see* Cefaclor
Cedilanid; *see* Lanatoside C
Cedilanid-D; *see* Deslanoside
CeeNU; *see* Lomustine
Cefaclor, 651, 652, 653
  pharmacokinetics of, 785
Cefadroxil, 652, 653
  pharmacokinetics of, 785
Cefadyl; *see* Cephapirin sodium
Cefamandole, 652, 785
Cefamandole nafate, 652
Cefatrizine, 785
Cefazolin, 652, 653
  hepatic or renal dysfunction and, 71
  pharmacokinetics of, 785
Cefazolin sodium, 652, 653
Cefixime, 785
Cefizox; *see* Ceftizoxime
Cefmenoxime, 785
Cefobid; *see* Cefoperazone sodium
Cefonicid, 652, 785
Cefonicid sodium, 652
Cefoperazone, 652, 785
  alcohol intolerance and, 297
Cefoperazone sodium, 652
Ceforanide, 785
Cefotan; *see* Cefotetan disodium
Cefotaxime, 652, 653
  pharmacokinetics of, 785
Cefotaxime sodium, 652, 653
Cefotetan, 652, 785

Cefotetan disodium, 652
Cefotiam, 785
Cefoxitin, 652, 653
  organisms susceptible to, 654
  pharmacokinetics of, 786
Cefoxitin sodium, 652, 653
Cefpiramide, 786
Cefroxadine, 786
Cefsulodin, 786
Ceftazidime, 652, 653
  pharmacokinetics of, 786
Ceftizoxime, 652, 786
Ceftizoxime sodium, 652
Ceftriaxone, 652, 786
  organisms susceptible to, 654
Ceftriaxone sodium, 652
Cefuroxime, 651, 652
  pharmacokinetics of, 786
Cefuroxime sodium, 652
Celestone; *see* Betamethasone
Cell cycle, chemotherapy and, 702
Cell membranes, antibiotics and, 629-631
Cell wall synthesis, inhibition of, 629
Cellular binding of drugs, 24
Celontin; *see* Methsuximide
Central nervous system
  β-adrenergic blockers and, 190-191
  atropine and, 117
  epinephrine and, 150
  general anesthesia and, 395-396
  norepinephrine and, 150
  reserpine and, 185
  scopolamine and, 117
Central nervous system depressants,
    antidepressants and, 273
Central nervous system stimulants, 274, 302-
    306
  caffeine as, 304-306
  doxapram as, 303
  nikethamide as, 303
  pentoxifylline as, 306
  pentylenetetrazol as, 302
  pharmacokinetics of, 785
  picrotoxin as, 303
  strychnine as, 304
Centrax; *see* Prazepam
Cephacetrile, 71, 786
Cephalexin, 652, 653
  cholestyramine and, 749
  hepatic or renal dysfunction and, 71
  pharmacokinetics of, 786
Cephalexin monohydrate, 652, 653
Cephaloridine, 71
Cephalosporin(s), 651-655
  alcohol intolerance and, 297
  organisms susceptible to, 654
  pharmacokinetics of, 785
  renal excretion of, 753
  uric acid and, 602
Cephalothin, 652, 653
  hepatic or renal dysfunction and, 71

Cephalothin—cont'd
  pharmacokinetics of, 786
Cephalothin sodium, 652, 653
Cephapirin, 652, 653
  pharmacokinetics of, 786
Cephapirin sodium, 652, 653
Cephradine, 652
  pharmacokinetics of, 786
Cerubidine; *see* Daunorubicin
Cestodes, 698
Cetamide; *see* Sulfacetamide
Charas, 344
Charcoal
  as antidote, 732
  carbamazepine and, 749
  digoxin and, 749
  ipecac syrup and, 731-732
  lower gastrointestinal tract and, 523
  phenobarbital and, 749
  phenytoin and, 749
  salicylate intoxication and, 373
  strychnine poisoning and, 304
  theophylline and, 749
  tolbutamide and, 749
  tricyclic antidepressant intoxication and, 273
  valproate and, 749
Charcoal broiling, 65-66
Chemical mediators
  effector response to, 89-90
  sites of action of, 83-84
Chemical neurotransmission, 82-83
Chemical sympathectomy, 95
Chemoreceptor trigger zone, 323
Chemotherapy, 1
  antibiotic, 626-631
    history of, 626-627
    pharmacokinetics of, 785
    resistance to, 628-629
Child, drug dose for, 44
Chlamydia, sulfonamides for, 632
Chloral hydrate, 290
  abuse of, 351-352
  alcohol dehydrogenation of, 32
  coumarin and, 750
  lethal concentration of, 769
  pharmacokinetics of, 778
  structure of, 290
  trichloroacetic acid and, 751
  warfarin and, 751
Chlorambucil, 704, 706
  pharmacokinetics of, 788
Chloramphenicol, 660-661
  alcohol intolerance and, 297
  antibacterial chemotherapy and, 626
  drugs inhibited by, 751
  hepatic or renal dysfunction and, 71
  nitroreduction and, 32
  organisms susceptible to, 654
  pediatric use of, 44
  pharmacokinetics of, 786
  phenobarbital and, 752
  protein synthesis and, 630, 631

Chloramphenicol—cont'd
  rifampin and, 752
  therapeutic concentrations of, 768
Chlordane, 743, 769
Chlordiazepoxide
  age and, 57, 60
  dosage and forms of, 263
  kinetics of, 262
  lethal concentration of, 769
  pharmacokinetics of, 778
  structure of, 261
Chlorguanide, 788
Chlorhexidine gluconate, 684
Chloride
  diuretics and, 477, 485
  intestinal absorption and, 22
  renal tubules and, 482
Chlorinated ethane derivates, 743
Chlorinated soda, 683
Chlorine, 683
Chlormezanone, 262
Chlorocyclohexane, 743
Chloroform
  abuse of, 358
  lethal concentration of, 769
  toxicity and biotransformation of, 398-399
Chloromycetin; *see* Chloramphenicol
p-Chlorophenylalanine, 216, 356
Chloroprocaine, 408, 413
  hydrolysis rates of, 410
  procaine and, 413
  uses of, 408
Chloroquine
  amebiasis and, 689
  extraintestinal protozoa susceptible to, 691
  lethal concentration of, 769
  malaria and, 690-692
  pharmacokinetics of, 788
8-Chlorotheophylline, 208
Chlorothiazide, 485
  cholestyramine and, 749
  diuretics and, 485
  metoclopramide and, 749
  pharmacokinetics of, 790
  potency and efficacy of, 9
  propantheline and, 749
  single dose curve and, 488
  structure of, 486
Chlorothiazide sodium, 486
Chlorotrianisene, 590, 591
Chlorpheniramine
  action of, 208
  doses and sedative property of, 209
  lethal concentration of, 769
  pharmacokinetics of, 780
  structure of, 207
Chlorpromazine
  action of, 242
  d-amphetamine and, 244
  antacids and, 749
  cocaine poisoning and, 412
  drugs inhibited by, 751

Chlorpromazine—cont'd
  lethal concentration of, 769
  microsomal oxidations and, 31
  parkinsonism and, 122
  pharmacokinetics of, 779
  phenobarbital and, 752
  psychomotor stimulants and, 275
  psychoses and, 252-257
Chlorpropamide
  chloramphenicol and, 751
  diabetes insipidus and, 574
  diabetes mellitus and, 539-540
  hepatic or renal dysfunction and, 71
  lethal concentration of, 769
  pharmacokinetics of, 790
Chlorprothixene, 769
Chlortetracycline, 659-660
Chlorthalidone, 193, 488
  pharmacokinetics of, 790
  structure of, 487
Chlor-Trimeton; *see* Chlorpheniramine
Cholecalciferol, 568-569, 570
Cholecystographic agents, thyroid hormones
    and, 562
Cholecystokinin, 222
Choledyl; *see* Oxtriphylline
Cholera
  adrenocorticotropic hormone and, 544
  vaccine for, 717
Cholesterol
  adrenal steroid synthesis and, 544-545
  elevation of, 502
  low-density lipoprotein receptor regulation
    of, 497-498
  prostaglandins and, 230
  thiazide diuretics and, 193
Cholesterol esters, 230
Cholestyramine, 493, 500
  cephalexin and, 749
  chlorothiazide and, 749
  and combined drug regimens, 501
  drug interaction and, 429, 748
    digitoxin in, 749
    digoxin in, 425, 430, 749
  lower gastrointestinal tract and, 523
  phenylbutazone and, 749
  propranolol and, 749
  thyroxine and, 749
  warfarin and, 749
Choline, 91, 102-104, 751
  theophylline and, 512
Choline acetyltransferase, 91
Choline esters, 102-104
  anticholinesterases and, 751
Choline magnesium trisalicylate, 365
Choline salicylate, 365
  absorption of, 370
Cholinergic agonists, directly acting, 102-106
Cholinergic blocking agents, 114-126
  atropine as, 114-119
  atropine substitutes in, 119-126
  scopolamine as, 114-119

Cholinergic crisis, 109
Cholinergic neurotransmission, 83, 89
Cholinergic receptor antagonists, 98
Cholinergics, 98, 102-113
  anticholinesterases as, 106-112
  bronchial smooth muscle and, 509
  cholinergic agonists as, 102-106
  as mediators, 84
  myasthenia gravis and, 112-113
  pharmacokinetics of, 779
Cholinesterases, 91
  atypical plasma, drug metabolism and, 52
CHOP; *see* Cyclophosphamide, doxorubicin,
    oncovin, and prednisone
Christmas trees, 350
Chromium poisoning, 734
Chromogranin, 93
Chromosomal resistance to antibiotics, 628-629
Chronulac; *see* Lactulose
Chylomicron, 494, 496
Chylomicron remnants, 494
Cibacalcin; *see* Calcitonin
Cibalith-S; *see* Lithium citrate
Cibenzoline, 783
Ciclopirox olamine, 679
Cimetidine, 35, 85, 211
  antacids and, 749
  benzodiazepines and, 262
  clinical pharmacology, indications, and
    toxicity of, 211-212
  development of, 210
  dosage of, 211
  drug interactions and, 469-470
  drugs inhibited by, 751
  glomerular filtration and, 26
  ketoconazole and, 749
  metabolism of, 50
  metoclopramide and, 749
  peptic ulcer disease and, 211
  pharmacokinetics of, 780
  phenobarbital and, 752
  renal excretion of, 753
  structure of, 210
  tetracyclines and, 749
  theophylline and, 513
  upper gastrointestinal tract and, 518-519
  vitamin B_{12} and, 611
  warfarin and, 469
Cinchonism, 372
  quinine and, 695
Cinobac; *see* Cinoxacin
Cinoxacin
  pharmacokinetics of, 787
  urinary tract infection and, 639, 640
Cin-Quin; *see* Quinidine
Ciprofloxacin
  pharmacokinetics of, 786
  urinary tract infection and, 639, 640
Circulation
  general anesthesia and, 397-398
  histamine and, 203

Circulation—cont'd
  thyroid hormones in, 559-560
Cisplatin, 704, 710
  mechanism of action of, 705
  pharmacokinetics of, 788
Citanest; *see* Prilocaine
Citrate, blood coagulation and, 462
Citrated caffeine, 305
Claforan; *see* Cefotaxime
Claudication, intermittent, 306
Clavulanic acid
  amoxicillin and, 655
  pharmacokinetics of, 785
  ticarcillin and, 655
Clearance, 16
Clemastine, 209
Cleocin; *see* Clindamycin
Clindamycin, 662
  hepatic or renal dysfunction and, 71
  organisms susceptible to, 654
    extraintestinal protozoal, 691
  pharmacokinetics of, 786
  protein synthesis and, 630
Clinical pharmacology, 41-42
Clinoril; *see* Sulindac
Clioquinol, 679
Clobazam, 778
Clodronate, 791
Clofazimine
  dapsone and, 677
  leprosy and, 678
  Mycobacterium infections susceptible to, 673
Clofibrate, 493, 499
  atherosclerosis and, 499
  coumarin and, 750
  diabetes insipidus and, 574
  pharmacokinetics of, 784
  primary hyperlipidemias and, 501
  structure of, 499
  warfarin and, 469
Clomethiazole, 778
Clomid; *see* Clomiphene citrate
Clomiphene citrate, 591
Clomipramine, 779
Clonazepam
  as anticonvulsant, 262
  clinical activity of, 311
  dosage of, 311
  in epilepsy, 310, 315
  lethal concentration of, 769
  pharmacokinetics of, 311, 780
  phenytoin and, 752
  structure of, 261
Clonidine
  β-adrenergic antagonists and, 753
  antidepressants and, 753
  hypertension and, 189
  introduction of, 177
  nicotine and, 359
  opiate withdrawal and, 340-341
  pharmacokinetics of, 783
  sites of action of, 178

Clonidine—cont'd
structure of, 189
transdermal administration and, 23
Clonorchis sinesis, 698
Clorazepate, 262, 310, 315
dosage and forms of, 263
pharmacokinetics of, 778
structure of, 261
Clorazepate dipotassium, 315
Closed anesthesia system, 393
Clostridium, 654
Clotiazepam, 778
Clotrimazole, 679, 681
Clotting, drug action and, 460-462
Cloxacillin, 643, 650
adverse effects of, 649
hepatic or renal dysfunction and, 71
organisms susceptible to, 651, 654
pharmacokinetics of, 647, 786
Cloxacillin sodium, 650
Cloxapen; *see* Cloxacillin
Coca, 349
Cocaine, 98
abuse of, 338, 349-350, 774-775
cardiovascular effects of, 411
catecholamines and, 86, 90, 94
clinical characteristics of, 412
dosage of, 412
history of use of, 407
lethal concentration of, 769
nonaccidental toxin ingestion of, 731
overdose of, 349
pharmacokinetics of, 785
scheduling of, 760
as stimulant, 274
structure of, 413
tricyclic antidepressants and, 86
tyramine and, 173
uses of, 408
Cocaine-like action, 186
Codeine, 325-326, 327
as antitussive, 334-335
chemistry of, 322
coughing and, 507-508
lethal concentration of, 769
lower gastrointestinal tract and, 523
scheduling of, 760
Codeine phosphate, 327
Codeine sulfate, 327
Coenzyme A, 616
Coffea arabica, 360
Cogentin; *see* Benztropine mesylate
Coke, 349
Colace; *see* Docusate salts
Colchicine
gout and, 599-600
hepatic or renal dysfunction and, 71
pharmacokinetics of, 790
Colchicum autumnale, 599
Cold turkey, 340
Colestid; *see* Colestipol
Colestipol, 493, 500

Colestipol—cont'd
and combined drug regimens, 501
drug interaction and, 429, 748
digoxin and, 430
lower gastrointestinal tract and, 523
Colestipol hydrochloride, 523
Coli-Mycin S; *see* Colistin
Colistimethate, 71
Colistin, 786
CoLyte; *see* Cathartics
COMLA; *see* Cyclophosphamide, oncovin,
methotrexate, leucovorin, and
cytarabine
Competitive versus noncompetitive antagonist,
10
Compound 48/80, 201
COMT; *see* Catechol-*O*-methyltransferase
Concentration effect in general anesthesia,
389-390
Conducting tissue, 421
Congestive heart failure, 427
Conjugated estrogens, 590
Conjugation, 33-34
Contact dermatitis, 43, 44
Contact laxatives, 525, 526
Continuous variation, 37, 38
Contraceptive(s)
drugs induced by, 752
drugs inhibited by, 751
estrogens in, 588-590
progestins in, 591-594
Contragonists, 248
Converting enzyme inhibitors, 184
Convulsions, 262, 308; *see also* Antiepileptic(s)
neuronal connections and, 309
Copper
lethal concentration of, 769
poisoning with, 743
calcium disodium edetate for, 734
penicillamine for, 735
as rodenticide, 743
Cor pulmonale, 428
Coramine; *see* Nikethamide
Corgard; *see* Nadolol
Coronary vessels, prostaglandins and
thromboxane and, 233
Cortalone; *see* Prednisolone
Cortef; *see* Hydrocortisone
Corticosteroid(s), 543-544; *see also* Steroid(s)
erythema nodosum leprosum and, 678
lower airway and, 513-515
neoplasms and, 704, 708
respiratory tract and, 506
Corticosterone, 546-554
Corticotropin, 544-545
in zinc hydroxide suspension, 544
Corticotropin-releasing factor, 544, 581
Cortisol, 543
Cortisone, 543-544
dosage of, 554
preparations of, 552
Cortone; *see* Cortisone

Cortrophin Gel; *see* Adrenocorticotropic
hormone
Corynebacterium diphtheriae, 654
Cosmegen; *see* Dactinomycin
Co-trimoxazole; *see* Trimethoprim-
sulfamethoxazole
Coughing, drugs for, 334-335, 507
Coumadin; *see* Warfarin
Coumarin anticoagulants
antibiotics and, 750
barbiturates and, 289
blood concentration of, 766
hemorrhage and, 466
phenobarbital and, 752
plasma protein displacement and, 750
as rodenticide, 743
sulfonamides and, 636
C-peptide, 531
CPZ; *see* Chlorpromazine
Crack, 349
Crank, 348
Creatinine clearance, endogenous, 77
Creeping eruption, 698
Creutzfeldt-Jakob disease, 583, 684
CRF; *see* Corticotropin-releasing factor
Crigler-Najjar syndrome, 36
Cromolyn sodium, 508, 515
Crystal, 348
Crysticillin; *see* Procaine penicillin G
Crystodigin; *see* Digitoxin
CTZ; *see* Chemoreceptor trigger zone
Cumulation, 46
Cuprimine; *see* Penicillamine
Curare, 201
Cyanide, 733, 738-739
Cyanocobalamin, 610
Cyanoketone, 545
Cyclaine; *see* Hexylcaine
Cyclic adenosine monophosphate
histamine and, 202
phosphodiesterase and, 306
Cyclizine, 210
action of, 208
lethal concentration of, 769
structure of, 207
Cyclodiene, 743
Cyclogyl; *see* Cyclopentolate hydrochloride
Cycloheximide, 630, 631
Cyclomethycaine, 408
Cyclooxygenase
aspirin and, 366
nonsteroidal anti-inflammatory drugs and,
364
patent ductus arteriosus and, 378
platelet function and, 471, 472
prostaglandin synthesis and, 228
sulfinpyrazone and, 472
Cyclooxygenase inhibitors, 378
Cyclopentolate hydrochloride, 119
Cyclophosphamide
immunosuppression and, 723

Cyclophosphamide—cont'd
neoplasms and, 703, 704, 706
pharmacokinetics of, 788
Cyclophosphamide, doxorubicin, oncovin, and
prednisone, 712
Cyclophosphamide, oncovin, methotrexate,
leucovorin, and cytarabine, 712
Cycloplegia, belladonna alkaloids and, 116
Cyclopropane, 400
abuse of, 358
autonomic nervous system and, 396
circulation and, 397
clinical characteristics of, 400
halothane and, 401-402
medical history of, 385
postoperative nausea and, 399
preanesthetic medication and, 395
Cycloserine
Mycobacterium infections susceptible to, 673
pharmacokinetics of, 789
tuberculosis and, 672, 677
Cyclosporin A, 768; *see also* Cyclosporine
Cyclosporine; *see also* Cyclosporin A
immunosuppression and, 724, 725
pharmacokinetics of, 791
phenytoin and, 752
Cyclothiazide, 486
Cylert; *see* Pemoline
Cyproheptadine, 210, 218
doses and sedative property of, 209
Cyproheptadine hydrochloride, 218
Cysticercus cellulosae, 698
Cytadren; *see* Aminoglutethimide
Cytarabine, 704, 708
nucleic acid synthesis and, 630
pharmacokinetics of, 788
Cytochrome P-450, 73, 74
acetaminophen and, 373
age and, 61
microsomal enzymes and, 28
Cytochrome P-450 reductase, 28
Cytomel; *see* Liothyronine sodium
Cytosar-U; *see* Cytarabine
Cytosine arabinoside, 708; *see also* Cytarabine
Cytotoxin, 723
Cytoxan; *see* Cyclophosphamide

D

Dacarbazine, 704
Dactinomycin, 704, 709
mechanism of action of, 705
Dalmane; *see* Flurazepam
Dantrolene, 399, 782
Dapsone
genetic conditions altering response to, 49
leprosy and, 677-678
Mycobacterium infections susceptible to, 673
pharmacokinetics of, 791
Daraprim; *see* Pyrimethamine
Darvon; *see* Propoxyphene
Darvon-N; *see* Propoxyphene
Datura stramonium, 114

Daunorubicin, 704, 705, 709
Daunorubicin hydrochloride, 704
Dazoxiben, 235
DDAVP; *see* Desmopressin acetate
DDD; *see* Tetrachlorodiphenylethane
DDT, 743
DEA; *see* Drug Enforcement Adminstration
N-Dealkylation, 30
O-Dealkylation, 31
S-Dealkylation, 31
Deamination, 31
Debrisoquin, 54, 173
genetic conditions altering response to, 49
polymorphic hydroxylation of, 54
Decadron; *see* Dexamethasone
Decarbazine, 710-711
Decarboxylase, aromatic L-amino acid, 92
Decentralization, 89
Declomycin; *see* Demeclocycline
Defense mechanisms, antibiotics and, 664
Deferoxamine, 735
anemia and, 609
as antidote, 733
iron poisoning and, 742
Deferoxamine mesylate, 735
Dehydroemetine, 688
Dehydroepiandrosterone, 556
Dehydroxyphenylglycol, 789
Delalutin; *see* Hydroxyprogesterone
Delestrogen; *see* Estradiol
Delirium tremens, 343
Deltasone; *see* Prednisone
Delysid; *see* Lysergic acid diethylamide
Demecarium, 110-111
glaucoma in, 106
Demecarium bromide, 106
Demeclocycline, 659-660
vasopressin and, 575
Demerol; *see* Meperidine
N-Demethylate aminopyrine, 76
Denatured alcohol, 298
Denervation supersensitivity, 89-90
Deoxyribonucleic acid, 611, 612, 613
Deoxyuridine, 611
Deoxyuridylate, 611
Depakene; *see* Valproic acid
Depakote; *see* Divalproex sodium
Depestro; *see* Estradiol
Depo-Provera; *see* Medroxyprogesterone
Deprenyl, 122, 124
Depressants; *see also* specific agent
central nervous system, 273
sites of action of, 247
Depression, mental, 268; *see also*
Antidepressant(s)
Dermatitis, contact, 43, 44
Dermatologic agents, 789
Dermatology, corticosteroids and, 554
Desensitization or tachyphylaxis, 9
Desferal; *see* Deferoxamine
Designer drugs, 329

Desipramine, 94, 272
clonidine and, 189
discovery of, 269
lethal concentration of, 769
pharmacokinetics of, 779
structure of, 271
therapeutic concentrations of, 768
Desipramine hydrochloride, 272
Deslanoside, 426
chemistry of, 423
properties of, 424
N-Desmethyldiazepam, 262
Desmopressin acetate, 576
Desoxycorticosterone, 543, 555, 556
adrenal steroid synthesis and, 545
dosage of, 554
Desoxyhydrocortisone, 545
Desulfuration, 32
Desyrel; *see* Trazodone hydrochloride
DET; *see* Diethyltryptamine
Detoxification, 34-35
Dexamethasone, 544
dosage of, 554
pharmacokinetics of, 791
structure of, 553
Dexchlorpheniramine, 209
Dextran, 791
capillary transfer of, 23
as platelet inhibiting agent, 471-472
Dextran 40, 791
Dextroamphetamine
corticotropin-releasing factor and, 581
disadvantages of, 275
growth hormone–releasing factor and, 582
Dextromethorphan, 335, 507-508
Dextromethorphan hydrobromide, 335
Dey-Dose; *see* Atropine
Dey-Lute; *see* Atropine
DFP; *see* Isoflurophate
DHPG; *see* Dehydroxyphenylglycol
DHT; *see* Dihydrotachysterol
Diabenese; *see* Chlorpropamide
DiaBeta; *see* Glyburide
Diabetes insipidus, 574
Diabetes mellitus, 535-541
classification of, 535-536
insulin and, 530, 536-538
oral hypoglycemic agents and, 538-541
Dialysis, peritoneal, 736
Diamox; *see* Acetazolamide
Diapid; *see* Lypressin
Diazepam, 261
age and, 57, 60
as antianxiety drug, 247, 248
depressant or stimulant action of, 247
dosage and forms of, 263
ethanol and, 751
hepatic or renal dysfunction and, 71
as hypnotic, 282
kinetics of, 262, 281
lead poisoning and, 739

Diazepam—cont'd
  lethal concentration of, 769
  oral contraceptives and, 751
  pharmacokinetics of, 778
  phenytoin and, 752
  plasma proteins and, 750
  as preanesthetic medication, 395
  propranolol and, 751
  scheduling of, 760
  seizures and, 262, 310, 315, 412
  structure of, 261
  strychnine poisoning and, 304
  toxicity and, 411-412
Diazepam-binding inhibitor, 248
Diazinon, 111
Diazoxide, 99
  coumarin and, 750
  as direct vasodilator, 181
  hepatic or renal dysfunction and, 71
  hypertension and, 183
  insulin and, 532
  pharmacokinetics of, 783
  sites of action of, 178
  structure of, 183
  warfarin and, 469
Dibasic calcium phosphate, 571
Dibenzyline; *see* Phenoxybenzamine
Dibucaine, 408, 415
  hydrolysis rates of, 410
  structure of, 415
  uses of, 408
Dibucaine number, 52
Dichloroisoproterenol, 166
Dicloxacillin, 650
  hepatic or renal dysfunction and, 71
  organisms susceptible to, 651
  pharmacokinetics of, 647, 786
Dicloxacillin sodium, 650
Dicodid; *see* Hydrocodone
Dicumarol
  absorption of, 23
  daily doses of, 468
  structure of, 466
  tolbutamide and, 750, 751
Dicyclomine, 769
Didronel; *see* Etidronate
Dieldrin, 743
Dienestrol, 590
Diet, 63-68
  atherosclerosis and, 502
  brussels sprouts in, 66-67
  cabbage in, 66-67
  charcoal broiling and, 65-66
  drug absorption and, 64
  drug binding and, 64-65
  drug excretion and, 65
  drug metabolism and, 65
  fiber in, 525
  starvation, 63-64
  theobromine in, 68
Diethyl ether
  abuse of, 358

Diethyl ether—cont'd
  and autonomic nervous system, 396
  circulation and, 397
  clinical characteristics of, 400
  equilibrium curve and, 390
  history of use of, 385
  minimal alveolar concentration of, 388
  postoperative nausea and, 399
  preanesthetic medication and, 395
  respirations and, 397
  signs of anesthesia and, 392
  stages of anesthesia and, 392
  volatile liquid anesthetics and, 401
Diethylaminoethanol, 33, 410
Diethylcarbamazine, 698, 700
Diethylene glycol, intoxication from, 737
Diethylstilbestrol, 590, 591
  neoplasms and, 708
Diethylstilbestrol diphosphate, 708
Diethyltryptamine, 356
Diffusion, 13
  anesthesia and, 389
Diflunisal, 364, 365
  antacids and, 749
  dosage, dosage forms, and indications for,
    375
  pharmacokinetics of, 781
Digitalis, 418-432
  absorption of, 23
  atrial fibrillation and, 447-448
  atrial flutter and, 447
  β-blockers and, 445, 753
  cellular effects of, 422
  chemistry of, 423-424
  in congestive heart failure, 427
  in cor pulmonale, 428
  deslanoside and, 426
  digitalization and, 430-431
  digitoxin and, 426
  digoxin and, 425-426
  diuretics and, 485, 478
  dosages of, 424
    factors modifying, 427
  effects of, 419, 420-421
  extracardiac effects of, 422-423
  heart and, 419-422
  heart rate and, 422
  history of use of, 418-419
  loading dose of, 424, 430
  maintenance doses of, 424
  newer inotropic agents and, 431
  ouabain and, 426
  and paroxysmal atrial tachycardia, 428
  pharmocokinetics of, 424
  poisoning by, 428-430
  preparations of, 425
  propranolol and, 169
  safety and, 755
  sources of, 423-424
  therapeutic indications for, 426-428
  toxicity of, 418, 428-430, 445
  ventricular and atrial muscle and, 422

Digitalis glycosides; *see* Digitalis
Digitalis leaf, 423
Digitalization, 424, 430-431
  congestive heart failure and, 431
Digitoxin, 426
  absorption of, 23
  chemistry of, 423
  cholestyramine and, 749
  digitalis poisoning and, 430
  hepatic or renal dysfunction and, 71
  lethal concentration of, 769
  pharmacokinetics and, 424, 785
  phenobarbital and, 752
  phenytoin and, 752
  properties of, 424
  rifampin and, 752
  structure of, 423
  therapeutic concentrations of, 768
Digoxin, 425-426
  age and, 60
  alteration in drug disposition and, 70
  amiodarone and, 751
  antacids and, 749
  antibiotics and, 750
  charcoal and, 749
  chemistry of, 423
  cholestyramine and, 749
  digitalis poisoning and, 430
  erythromycin and, 749
  excretion of, 61
  gastrointestinal flora and, 73
  hepatic or renal dysfunction and, 71
  kaolin-pectin and, 749
  lethal concentration of, 769
  metoclopramide and, 749
  neomycin and, 749
  pharmacokinetics and, 19, 424-426, 785
  preparations of, 425
  propantheline and, 749
  properties of, 424
  renal excretion and, 45, 753
  rifampin and, 752
  sulfasalazine and, 749
  therapeutic concentrations of, 768
  volume of distribution or clearance and, 17
Dihydroergotamine mesylate, 791
Dihydrostreptomycin, 60
Dihydrotachysterol, 569-570
Dihydrotestosterone, 594-595
1,25-Dihydroxycholecalciferol, 569, 570
1,25-Dihydroxy-vitamin D_3; *see* 1,25-
    Dihydroxycholecalciferol
Diiodohydroxyquin; *see* Iodoquinol
Diiodotyrosin, 557-558
Diisopropyl fluorophosphate; *see* Isoflurophate
Dilantin; *see* Phenytoin
Dilaudid; *see* Hydromorphone
Dilor; *see* Dyphylline
Diloxanide furoate, 688, 689
Diltiazem, 457
  in angina, 450

Diltiazem—cont'd
  dosages of, 456
  pharmacokinetics of, 455, 782
  side effects of, 456
  sites of action of, 178
  slow calcium-channel blockers and, 190
  structure of, 457
Diltiazem hydrochloride, 456
Dimenhydrinate, 208
Dimercaprol, 45, 733-734
  arsenic poisoning and, 742
  gold poisoning and, 742
  lead poisoning and, 739
  mercury poisoning and, 740
  thallium poisoning and, 741
2,3-Dimercaprol, 733-734
Dimetane; *see* Brompheniramine
2,5-Dimethoxy-4-methylamphetamine, 356, 774-775
Dimethyltryptamine, 356
N-Dimethyltryptamine; *see* Psilocybin
Dinitro-*O*-cresol, 769
Dinoprost tromethamine, 234, 578
Dinoprostone, 234, 578
Dioctyl sulfosuccinate, 526
1,3-Diols, 228
Diphenhydramine, 85, 206
  absorption and metabolism of, 209
  action of, 208
  doses and sedative property of, 209
  lethal concentration of, 769
  nonprescription sleep medication and, 291
  Parkinson's disease and, 125
  pharmacokinetics of, 780
  structure of, 207
Diphenoxylate, 329
  dosage of, 327
  lower gastrointestinal tract and, 523
  scheduling of, 760
  structure of, 329
Diphenoxylate hydrochloride, 327
Diphenylan; *see* Phenytoin
Diphenylheptanes, 327
Diphenylpyraline, 209
Diphyllobothrium latum, 698
Dipropylacetic acid, 315
Dipropyltryptamine, 356
Dipylidium caninum, 698
Dipyridamole, 472
  aspirin with, 473
  in hemostasis, 459
  pharmacokinetics of, 779
  as platelet inhibiting agent, 471-472
  uses of, 473
Disalcid; *see* Salsalate
Discontinuous variation, 37, 38
Disease, 69-79
  drug absorption and, 72-73
  drug distribution and, 73
  hepatic metabolism and, 73-76
  histamine and, 204-205
  Parkinson's, 121-126

Disease—cont'd
  renal excretion and, 77
  von Gierke's, 37
Dishydroxycoumarin, 749
Disinfectants, 683-686
Disodium cromoglycate, 203, 515
Disodium edetate, 734-735
Disopyramide, 441
  antiarrhythmic action of, 434-436
  atrial fibrillation and, 447-448
  classification of, 434
  lethal concentration of, 769
  pharmacokinetics of, 440, 783
  practolol and, 753
  structure of, 441
  therapeutic concentrations of, 768
  ventricular arrhythmias and, 448
Disopyramide phosphate, 440
Dissociative anesthesia, 405
Distribution, drug
  age and, 58-60
  disease and, 73
  salicylates and, 371
Disulfiram, 298
  alcohol intolerance and, 297
  alcoholism and, 343
    chronic, 297-298
  drugs inhibited by, 751
  paraldehyde and, 290
  pharmacokinetics of, 791
  structure of, 298
  warfarin and, 469
DIT; *see* Diiodotyrosin
Diulo; *see* Metolazone
Diuresis, forced, 736
Diuretics, 477-492
  action of, 178
  antihypertensives and, 753
  antikaliuretic, 490-491
  carbonic anhydrase inhibitor, 484-488
  extrarenal aspects of, 477-480
  forced diuresis and, 736
  hypertension and, 193-194
  intrarenal aspects of, 480-482
  loop, 488-489
    hypertension and, 194
  organomercurial, 483-484
  osmotic, 482-483
  pharmacokinetics of, 790
  potassium-sparing, 194
  potency and efficacy of, 9
  prostaglandin and, 753
  renal excretion of, 753
  thiazide
    direct vasodilator, 181, 182
    sites of action of, 178
    sulfonylureas and, 540
Diuril; *see* Chlorothiazide
Divalproex sodium, 310, 315
DMT; *see* Dimethyltryptamine
DNA thymidine, 611, 612
DOA, 352

Dobutamine, 431, 791
Dobutamine hydrochloride, 431
Dobutrex; *see* Dobutamine
DOCA; *see* Desoxycorticosterone
Docusate salts, 525, 526
Dolobid; *see* Diflunisal
Dolophine; *see* Methadone hydrochloride
DOM; *see* 2,5-Dimethoxy-4-methylamphetamine
Domperidone, 791
Done nomogram, 372
Dopa; *see also* Dopamine; Levodopa
  methyldopa and, 175
  structure of, 93
Dopamine, 85, 153-154
  action of, 82
  antipsychotic drugs and, 243-245
  brain, 92
    metabolism and, 244
  gonadotropin-releasing hormone and, 581
  localization and, 91
  prolactin-inhibiting factor and, 582
  propranolol and, 169
  psychomotor stimulants and, 274-275
  reserpine and, 174
  schizophrenic symptoms and, 242-243
  sites of action of, 83
  structure of, 93
Dopamine antagonist, 522
Dopamine-β-hydroxylase, 92, 93
Dopaminergic receptors, 85
  catecholamines and, 144-146
  corticotropin-releasing factor and, 581
  gonadotropin-releasing hormone and, 581
  growth hormone and, 583
  growth hormone–releasing factor and, 582
Dopar; *see* Levodopa
Dope, 344
Dopram; *see* Doxapram
Doriden; *see* Glutethimide
Dosage schedules, 26-27
Dose-dumping, diet and, 64
Dose-response curve, log, 9
  competitive antagonism and, 10
Double-sal; *see* Sodium salicylate
Downregulation, 9, 90
Down's syndrome, 36
Doxapram, 302, 303
Doxazosin, 783
Doxepin, 272
  lethal concentration of, 769
  pharmacokinetics of, 779
  propoxyphene and, 751
  structure of, 271
Doxepin hydrochloride, 272
Doxorubicin, 704, 709, 712
  hepatic or renal dysfunction and, 71
  mechanism of action of, 705
  pharmacokinetics of, 788
Doxorubicin, bleomycin, vinblastine, and DTIC, 712

Doxorubicin hydrochloride, 704
Doxycycline, 659
  age and, 60
  chloroquine-resistant *Plasmodium falciparum*
    and, 695
  pharmacokinetics of, 787
  phenytoin and, 752
DPT; *see* Dipropyltryptamine
Dracunculus medinensis, 698
Drisdol; *see* Vitamin(s), D$_2$
Droperidol, fentanyl and, 329, 385, 404
Drug absorption
  age and, 57-58
  diet and, 64
  disease and, 72-73
Drug abuse, 337-361
  alcohol and, 342-343
  amphetamines and, 348-349
  barbiturates and, 289, 350-351
  caffeine and, 360
  cantharidine and, 360
  catnip and, 360
  characteristics of, 354-357
  clinical evaluation and, 360-361
  cocaine and, 349-350
  drug mixing and, 360
  drugs commonly used in, 338
  epidemiology in research of, 338
  inhalants and, 357-359
  marijuana and, 344-347
  nicotine and, 359-360
  nonbarbiturate sedatives and, 351-352
  opiates and, 338-342
  physical dependence and tolerance and, 353
  propoxyphene and, 359-360
  psychomimetic drugs and, 352-353
  side effects of, 337-338, 339
Drug allergy, 42-44
Drug antagonism, 45-46
Drug binding, diet and, 64-65
Drug compendia, 762
Drug concentration in blood, 766-772
  logarithm of, 20
Drug disappearance curves, 19
Drug distribution
  age and, 58-60
  disease and, 73
Drug efficacy, 9-10
Drug elimination, 48, 51
Drug Enforcement Administration, 761
Drug excretion
  age and, 61
  diet and, 65
  renal, disease and, 77
Drug fever, 44
Drug interactions, 748-755
  adrenergic central nervous system stimulants
    and anorexiants and, 161
  anticoagulants and, 469-470
  antiepileptics and, 310
  barbiturates and, 289

Drug interactions—cont'd
  digitalis and, 429
  monoamine oxidase inhibitors and, 270
  propranolol and, 169
  tricyclic antidepressants and, 273
Drug intolerance, 42
Drug intoxication, 730
Drug metabolism, 28-38
  age and, 61
  chemical reactions in, 28-34
  delay of, 35
  detoxification and, 34-35
  dietary manipulation and, 65
  disorders of, 37
  enzyme induction in, 35-36
    occupational factors and, 69
  hepatic, disease and, 73-76
  occupational chemicals and, 69
  pharmacogenetics and, 36-38, 52-55
Drug mixing, abuse and, 360
Drug movement in body, 13
Drug potency, 9-10
Drug response, variability in, 48-51
Drug tolerance, 46
Drug-receptor interactions, 6-11
  affinity in, 8
  agonist in, 10-11
  antagonist in, 10-11
  drug potency and efficacy in, 9-10
  intrinsic activity in, 8
  noncompetitive antagonism in, 11
  partial agonist in, 10-11
  receptor regulation in, 9
  receptor theory in, 6-7
  receptor-related diseases in, 9
DTIC; *see* Dacarbazine
DTIC-Dome; *see* Dacarbazine
Ducardin; *see* Hydroflumethiazide
Ductus arteriosus, 478
Dulcolax; *see* Bisacodyl
Dumpling cactus, 356
Durabolin; *see* Nandrolone
Duracillin; *see* Procaine penicillin G
Duranest; *see* Etidocaine
Duraquin; *see* Quinidine
Duratest; *see* Testosterone cypionate
Duricef; *see* Cefadroxil
Dwarf tapeworm, 698
Dycill; *see* Dicloxacillin
Dymelor; *see* Acetohexamide
Dynapen; *see* Dicloxacillin
Dyphylline
  lower airway and, 512
  pharmacokinetics of, 782
  renal excretion of, 753
Dyrenium; *see* Triamterene

E

Echothiophate, 106, 110-111
Echothiophate iodide, 106
Econazole nitrate, 679
Ecstasy, 355

ED$_{50}$; *see* Median effective dose
Edecrin; *see* Ethacrynic acid
Edema, relief of, 477-482
Edetate, 462, 570; *see also*
    Ethylenediaminetetraacetic acid
  pharmacokinetics of, 791
Edetate disodium, 570
Edrophonium, 109
  curare and, 109
  myasthenia gravis and, 106, 112
  paroxysmal atrial tachycardia and, 447
  pharmacokinetics of, 779
  tubocurarine and, 109
Edrophonium chloride, 106
Edrophonium test, 109
EDTA; *see* Edetate;
    Ethylenediaminetetraacetic acid
Effectiveness; *see* Safety and effectiveness
Effector cell, 173
  chemical mediators and, 89-90
Efficacy, 9-10
  potency versus, 7
Egg white as antidote, 732
EHDP; *see* Etidronate
Eicosanoid compounds, 227
  glucocorticoids and, 514
Eicosapentaenoic acid, 228, 230, 231, 238
5,8,11,14,17-Eicosapentaenoic acid, 228, 230,
    231
Eicosatetraenoic acid, 228, 230, 231
5,8,11,14-Eicosatetraenoic acid, 228, 230, 231;
    see also Arachidonic acid
8,11,14-Eicosatetraenoic acid, 228, 230, 231
Eicosatetraynoic acid, 236
Elavil; *see* Amitriptyline
Electrocardiography, 422
Elimination of drugs, 29
  ganglionic blocking agents and, 130
  variations in, 48, 51
Elimination rate constant, 77
Elspar; *see* L-Asparaginase
Emesis, morphine and, 323
Emetics, 731-732
Emetine, 687-688
Emollients, 524, 525
Enalapril
  hypertension and, 184
  pharmacokinetics of, 783
  sites of action of, 178
  structure of, 184
Encainide, 440, 444
  classification of, 434
  genetic conditions altering response to, 49
  metabolic reactions of, 54
  pharmacokinetics of, 783
Encainide hydrochloride, 440
Encephalopathy, 739
Endogenous depression, 268
Endogenous opioid peptides, 320-321
Endoplasmic reticulum, 29
β-Endorphin(s), 223-224

β-Endorphin(s)—cont'd
action of, 82
pain and, 319-320
End-plate receptor, 85
Endrate; *see* Edetate
Endrin, 743
End-tidal concentration of anesthetic, 386
Enflurane, 402
clinical characteristics of, 400
history of use of, 384
isoflurane and, 403
minimal alveolar concentration of, 388
second gas effect and, 390
Enkaid; *see* Encainide
Enkephalins, 222, 223-224, 320
action of, 82
neurotransmitter studies and, 89
Enoxacin, 786
Enprophylline, 512, 782
Entamoeba histolytica, 687
Enteric-coated tablets
absorption of, 23
aspirin and, 370
Enterobacter, 654
cephalosporins for, 651
penicillin for, 650, 651
sulfonamides and, 634
Enterobius vermicularis, 698
Enterochromaffin cells, 215, 217
Enterococcus, 654
Environmental factors
drug response variations and, 51
poisoning and, 739-744
Enzactin; *see* Triacetin
Enzyme induction, 35-36
Enzyme inhibitors, converting, 184
Enzymes, drug-metabolizing, 28-30, 35-36
occupational factors and, 69
Eosinophil chemotactic factor, 201
Eosinophilia, 549
EPA; *see* 5,8,11,14,17-Eicosapentaenoic acid
Ephedrine, 98, 154-156
abuse of, 349
as cocaine adulterant, 350
gastrointestinal absorption of, 21
lower airway and, 510-511
upper airway and, 506
Epidemiology in drug abuse research, 338
Epidermophyton, 681
Epilepsy, 262, 308; *see also* Antiepileptic(s)
Epinephrine, 34, 98, 146-153
acetylcholine and, 84
action of, 82
adrenocorticotropic hormone and, 544
circulation and, 397-398
in glaucoma, 105
glucagon and, 538
halothane and, 401-402
hypersusceptibility to, 42
insulin and, 534
local anesthetics and, 409, 411
localization and, 91

Epinephrine—cont'd
lower airway and, 510-511
lungs and, 516
metabolism of, 96
parathyroid extract and, 567
reversal of, 163, 164
structure of, 93
Epinephrine reversal, 163, 164
Epipodophyllotoxins, 711
Epsilon-aminocaproic acid, 779
Equanil; *see* Meprobamate
Equipment, sterilization of, 684, 685
Ergocalciferol, 568-569, 570
Ergonovine
isolation of, 218
structure of, 218
uterus and, 576, 577, 578
vascular smooth muscle and, 455
Ergonovine maleate, 455, 578
Ergosterol, 629-631
Ergot alkaloids, 166, 218-219
Ergotamine, 166, 219
caffeine and, 305
isolation of, 218
Ergotrate; *see* Ergonovine
Erythema nodosum leprosum, 678
Erythrityl tetranitrate, 451
Erythrocin; *see* Erythromycin
Erythrocytes, anemia and, 605
Erythromycin, 661-662
amebiasis and, 689
digoxin and, 749
drugs inhibited by, 751
hepatic or renal dysfunction and, 71
organisms susceptible to, 654
pharmacokinetics of, 786
protein synthesis and, 630
theophylline and, 513
Erythromycin estolate, 661-662
Erythroxylon coca, 349
Escherichia coli
cephalosporins for, 651
drugs for, 654
penicillins for, 651
sulfonamides for, 632
vaccine for, 717
Eserine; *see* Physostigmine
Eskalith; *see* Lithium carbonate
Esterified estrogen, 590
Esters as local anesthetics, 407, 408
Estinyl; *see* Estrogen(s); Ethinyl estradiol
Estrace; *see* Estradiol
Estradiol, 587-588, 590
ovulation and, 585
Estradiol cypionate, 590
Estradiol valerate, 590
Estradurin; *see* Polyestradiol phosphate
Estraguard; *see* Dienestrol
Estrogen(s), 587-591
mechanism of action of, 705
neoplasms and, 704, 708-709
ovulation and, 585

Estrogen(s)—cont'd
phenobarbital and, 752
uterus and, 576
Estrone, 587-588, 590
menopause and, 589
Estropipate, 590
Estrovis; *see* Quinestrol
Ethacrynic acid, 488-489
coumarin and, 750
structure of, 488
transfusions and, 480
Ethambutol
gastrectomy and, 72
hepatic or renal dysfunction and, 71
mycobacterial infections susceptible to, 673
pharmacokinetics of, 789
renal excretion of, 753
tuberculosis and, 672, 674-675
Ethanol, 292-298; *see also* Alcohol
abuse of, 338, 358, 774-775
aminoglycoside antibiotics and, 749
as antidote, 733
benzodiazepines and, 263-264
as disinfectant, 683
drugs induced by, 752
drugs inhibited by, 751
equipment sterilization and, 685
ethylene glycol intoxication and, 737
lethal concentration of, 769
methanol intoxication and, 299
metoclopramide and, 749
as physically addicting drug, 337
propantheline and, 749
skin disinfection and, 684
uterus and, 578
warfarin and, 469
Ethanolamines, 208
Ethchlorvynol, 289
lethal concentration of, 769
pharmacokinetics of, 778
Ethinamate, 289, 769
Ethinyl estradiol, 588, 590-591
neoplasms and, 708
Ethionamide
gastrectomy and, 72
mycobacterial infections susceptible to, 673
pharmacokinetics of, 789
tuberculosis and, 672, 676
Ethisterone, 592
Ethopropazine hydrochloride, 125
Ethosuximide, 310, 316
absence seizures and, 314
clinical activity of, 311
dosage of, 311
lethal concentration of, 769
pharmacokinetics of, 311, 780
phenobarbital and, 313
therapeutic concentrations of, 768
Ethotoin, 310, 313
Ethrane; *see* Enflurane
Ethyl alcohol; *see* Ethanol
Ethyl aminobenzoate, 408, 413

Ethyl chloride, 770
Ethyl ether, 770
Ethylene glycol, 299
    antidote for, 733
    intoxication from, 737
    lethal concentration of, 770
Ethylenediamine, 208, 512
Ethylenediaminetetraacetic acid, 734-735; *see also* Edetate
Ethylestrenol, 596
Ethylphenylhydantoin, 313
Ethynodiol diacetate, 592, 593-594
Etidocaine, 408
Etidronate, 571
Etiocholanolone, 594
Etodolac, 781
Etomidate, 405, 777
Etoposide, 704, 711
    pharmacokinetics of, 788
Etretinate, 618, 789
ETYA; *see* Eicosatetraynoic acid
Euthyroid sick syndrome, 562
Eutonyl; *see* Pargyline
Everone; *see* Testosterone enanthate
Excretion, drug, 25-26
    age and, 61
    atropine, 117
    diet and, 65
    renal, disease and, 77
    salicylate, 372
    scopolamine, 117
Exercise, atherosclerosis and, 502
Exna; *see* Benzthiazide
Expectorants, 508
Extracellular fluid, 477, 478
Extrinsic pathway of thrombin formation, 460, 461-462
Eye, atropine and scopolamine and, 116

F

Facilitated diffusion, 15
Factor VIII, 576
FAD; *see* Flavin-adenine dinucleotide
False transmitters, 94
Famotidine, 212
    as antihistamine, 212
    development of, 210
    dosage of, 211
    pharmacokinetics of, 780
    structure of, 211
    upper gastrointestinal tract and, 518-519
Fansidar; *see* Pyrimethamine
Fasciola hepatica, drugs for, 698
Fast sodium channel blockade, 434
Fat
    metabolism of, 548
    solubility of, 389
Fat-soluble vitamins, 617-620
    cholestyramine and colestipol and, 500
Fatty liver, 293-294
Fatty tissues, concentration of drug in, 24

Fazadinium, 777
FDA; *see* Food and Drug Administration
Federal Controlled Substances Act, 761
Feedback regulation, morphine and, 326
Feldene; *see* Piroxicam
Felodipine, 782
Feminone; *see* Ethinyl estradiol
Fenamates, 365, 379
Fenbufen, 781
Fenclofenac, 781
Fenfluramine, 770
Fenoprofen, 365, 376
    dosage, dosage forms, and indications for, 375
    gastrointestinal disturbances and, 376
    pharmacokinetics of, 781
Fentanyl
    dosage of, 327
    with droperidol, 329, 385, 404
    lethal concentration of, 770
    with nitrous oxide and oxygen, 329
    pharmacokinetics of, 777
    as preanesthetic medication, 395
    structure of, 329
Feosol; *see* Ferrous sulfate
FEP test; *see* Free erythrocyte protoporphyrin test
Fergon; *see* Ferrous gluconate
Ferguson's principle, 8
Ferric hydroxide, 608
Ferritin, 606
Ferrous fumarate, 608
Ferrous gluconate, 608
Ferrous sulfate, 608
Fetal alcohol syndrome, 343
Fever, production of, 367
Fibers, nerve, 321
Fibrillation, atrial, 447-448
Fibrin, 460, 462, 473
Fibrinogen, 460, 462
Fibrinolysin, 473
Fibrinolytic agents, 473-475
Filariasis, drugs for, 698
Filtration, 13
First-dose phenomenon, 187
First-order kinetics, 18
First-pass effect, 23
Flagyl; *see* Metronidazole
Flavin mononucleotide, 615
Flavin-adenine dinucleotide, 615
Flecainide, 443
    amiodarone and, 751
    classification of, 434
    pharmacokinetics and, 440, 783
    structure of, 443
    therapeutic concentrations of, 768
    ventricular arrhythmias and, 448
Florinef; *see* Fludrocortisone
Floropryl; *see* Isoflurophate
Fluctuations, 27
Flucytosine
    fungal infections and, 679, 680

Flucytosine—cont'd
    hepatic or renal dysfunction and, 71
    pharmacokinetics of, 788
Fludrocortisone, 555, 556
    dosage of, 554
    structure of, 553
Flufenamic acid, 781
Flukes, 698
Flunarizine, 780
Flunisolide
    dosage of, 554
    lower airway and, 513, 514
Flunitrazepam, 778
Fluoride(s)
    anesthesia and, 398
    as insecticide, 743
    lethal concentration of, 770
    methoxyflurane and, 402
Fluoroacetate, 743
Fluoroalkane gases, sudden sniffing death and, 358-359
Fluorouracil; *see also* 5-Fluorouracil
    neoplasms and, 704, 707
    pharmacokinetics of, 788
5-Fluorouracil; *see also* Fluorouracil
    cimetidine and, 751
    mechanism of action of, 705
Fluothane; *see* Halothane
Fluoxetine, 779
Fluoxymesterone, 594-595, 596, 704, 708
Flurazepam, 283-284
    age and, 60
    effectiveness of, 283
    as hypnotic, 262, 280, 282
    kinetics of, 281
    lethal concentration of, 770
    scheduling of, 760
    structure of, 281
Flurbiprofen, 781
Fluvoxamine, 779
FMN; *see* Flavin mononucleotide
Focal seizures, 308
Folex; *see* Methotrexate
Folic acid
    anemia and, 609, 612-613
    erythrocytes and, 605
    jejunal disease and, 72
    phenytoin and, 750
    recommended daily allowance of, 621
    sulfonamides and, 632
    triamterene and, 750
Folic acid antagonists, neoplasms and, 703, 706-707
Follicle-stimulating hormone, 583-587
Follicular phase of ovulation, 585
Food and Drug Administration, 42, 759
Forane; *see* Isoflurane
Formaldehyde
    equipment sterilization and, 684, 685
    sulfonamides and, 636
Formalin; *see* Formaldehyde

5-Formyltetrahydrofolate; *see* Leucovorin
Forskolin
　adrenocorticotropic hormone and, 544
　thyrotropin-stimulating hormone and, 559
Fortaz; *see* Ceftazidime
Free base, 349
Free erythrocyte protoporphyrin test, 739
Free water clearance, 483
Fructose, 541
FSH; *see* Follicle-stimulating hormone
Fulvicin; *see* Griseofulvin
Fungal infections, 679-681
Fungicide, definition of, 683
Fungizone; *see* Amphotericin B
Furacin; *see* Nitrofurazone
Furadantin; *see* Nitrofurantoin
Furazolidone
　alcohol intolerance and, 297
　intestinal protozoa susceptible to, 688
Furosemide, 488-489
　calcium and, 571
　digoxin and, 430
　hepatic or renal dysfunction and, 71
　hypercalcemia and, 567
　as loop diuretic, 489
　pharmacokinetics of, 790
　phenytoin and, 749
　structure of, 488
Fusobacterium, 654

G

G-6-PD; *see* Glucose-6-phosphate
　　dehydrogenase
GABA; *see* γ-Aminobutyric acid
Galactitol, 541
Galactorrhea, 582
Galactose, 541
Gallamine, 777
Ganglionic blocking agent(s), 127-131
　absorption of, 130
　chemistry of, 128-129
　clinical pharmacology of, 129-130
　denervation sensitivity and, 90
　development of, 128
　elimination of, 130
　ganglionic stimulants and, 128
　hypertension and, 194
　mecamylamine and, 131
　trimethaphan and, 131
　vasopressors and, 90
Ganglionic stimulants, 128
Gantanol; *see* Sulfamethoxazole
Gantrisin; *see* Sulfisoxazole
Garamycin; *see* Gentamicin
Gastric acid, histamine and, 204
Gastric lavage, strychnine poisoning and, 304
Gastric secretion, 518-519
　H₂-receptor antagonists and, 211
　histamine and, 204
　prostaglandins and, 234
Gastrin, 222

Gastrin—cont'd
　histamine and, 204
Gastrointestinal inhibitory peptide, 534
Gastrointestinal tract, 518-527
　absorption from, 21-22
　atropine and, 116
　bleeding in, 368-369
　flora of, 768-369
　flora of, 73
　irritation of, 368-369
　lower, 522-526
　　antidiarrheal agents in, 522-524
　　laxative4-526
　nonsteroidal anti-inflammatory drugs and,
　　368-369
　scopolamine and, 116
　upper, 518-522
　　antacids in, 519-521
　　anticholinergics in, 519
　　histamine antagonists in, 518-519
　　metoclopramide in, 522
　　prostaglandins in, 521-522
　　sucralfate in, 521
Gating mechanism in spinal cord, 223
Gelusil, 520
Gelusil M, 520
Gemfibrozil, 493, 499
Gemonil; *see* Metharbital
General anesthesia; *see* Anesthesia, general
Genetics
　antibiotics and, 628-629, 665
　drug response variations and, 51
Genital herpes simplex virus, 668
Gentamicin, 656, 657, 658-659
　hepatic or renal dysfunction and, 71
　organisms susceptible to, 654
　therapeutic concentrations of, 768
Geocillin; *see* Carbenicillin
Geopen; *see* Carbenicillin
Germanin; *see* Suramin
Germicide, definition of, 683
GH; *see* Growth hormone
GH-RF; *see* Growth hormone–releasing factor
Giardia lamblia, 688
GIP; *see* Gastrointestinal inhibitory peptide
Glaucoma
　muscarinic blocking drugs and, 116-117
　over-the-counter drug hazards with, 291
　pharmacologic approaches to, 105
Glipizide
　diabetes mellitus and, 539-540
　pharmacokinetics of, 790
Globaline; *see* Tetraglycine hydroperiodide
Glomerular ultrafiltration, 477, 478, 480
Glucagon, 530, 534-535
　propranolol and, 168
Glucamide; *see* Chlorpropamide
Glucocorticoid(s), 546-554
　as anti-inflammatory agent, 367
　calcium and, 570
　gastrointestinal tract and, 518
　growth hormone and, 583

Glucocorticoid(s)—cont'd
　hypercalcemia and, 567
　immunosuppression and, 723-724
　inhibition of arachidonic acid release of, 236
　lower airway and, 513-515
　mechanism of action of, 705
　phenytoin and, 752
　as platelet inhibiting agents, 471-472
　prostanoid synthesis inhibitors and, 235
　rifampin and, 752
Glucose
　insulin and, 531-532
　salicylate intoxication and, 372
Glucose-6-phosphate dehydrogenase, 55
　sulfonamides and, 635
Glucose-6-phosphate dehydrogenase
　　deficiency, 37
　genetic control of, 55
Glucotrol; *see* Glipizide
Glucuronic acid, 560
Glucuronide synthesis, 33
Glue-sniffing, 744
Glutamic acid(s), 97
　action of, 82
　　sites of, 83
　folic acid and, 612
Glutaraldehyde, equipment sterilization and,
　684, 685
Glutathione
　acetaminophen intoxication and, 375
　glucose-6-phosphate dehydrogenase
　　deficiency and, 55
　nitrates and, 452, 453
Glutethimide, 289, 289
　abuse of, 351, 774-775
　drugs induced by, 752
　fatty tissue concentration of, 24
　lethal concentration of, 770
　pharmacokinetics of, 778
　poisoning and, 289
　scheduling of, 760
Glyburide, 539-540
Glycerin, 525
Glycerol guaiacolate, 508
Glyceryl trinitrate; *see* Nitroglycerin
Glycine, 99
　action of, 82, 83
　conjugation of, 33
Glycine antagonized by strychnine, 85
Glycopyrrolate, 120
　as preanesthetic medication, 395
Gn-RH; *see* Gonadotropin-releasing hormone
Gold poisoning, 741-742
　dimercaprol for, 733
Gold salts, 367, 379
Gold sodium thiomalate, 379
GoLYTELY, 524
Gonadal steroids, growth hormone and, 583
Gonadotropin-releasing hormone, 581-582
Gonadotropins, anterior pituitary, 580-598; *see
　also* Anterior pituitary gonadotropins
Gonococcus, 651

Gout, 599-604
  allopurinol for, 603-604
  colchicine for, 599-600
  nonsteroidal anti-inflammatory drugs for, 600
  probenecid for, 600-602
  sulfinpyrazone for, 602sulfinpyrazone for,
     602-603
Gram-negative bacteria, 654
Gram-positive organisms, 654, 661-662
Grand mal seizures, 308
Grass, 344
Gray baby syndrome, 661
Gray man syndrome, 446
GRF; *see* Growth hormone–releasing factor
Griseofulvin
  alcohol intolerance and, 297
  drugs induced by, 752
  fungal infections and, 679, 681
  phenobarbital and, 36, 752
  warfarin and, 469
Growth hormone, 582-583
  insulin and, 532, 534
Growth hormone–releasing factor, 582
Guaifenesin, 508
Guanabenz
  hypertension and, 189
  pharmacokinetics of, 783
  sites of action of, 178
  structure of, 189
Guanadrel
  action of, 180
     sites of, 178
  hypertension and, 186-187
  pharmacokinetics of, 783
  structure of, 186
Guanadrel, 174
Guanethidine, 98, 173
  action of, 172, 178, 180
  adrenergic neuron and, 174
  hypertension and, 186-187
  hyperthyroidism and, 566
  introduction of, 177
  sensitization and, 90
  structure of, 186
  tricyclic antidepressants and, 273
Guanethidine monosulfate, 174
Guanfacine, 783
Guanidinium, 753
Guedel's stages of anesthesia, 392
Guinea worm, 698

H

H₁ antagonists, 509
Haemophilus, 649, 651, 654
Haemophilus ducreyi, 654
Haemophilus influenzae
  ampicillin for, 649
  cephalosporins for, 651
  drugs for, 654
Hageman factor, 461
Halazepam
  dosage and forms of, 263

Halazepam—cont'd
  kinetics of, 262
  structure of, 261
Halazone, 684, 686
Halcinonide, 553
Halcion; *see* Triazolam
Haldrone; *see* Paramethasone
Half-life, 15-16, 19
Hallucinogens, 275-276
  serotonin and, 214
Halofantizine, 788
Haloperidol
  dopaminergic cell and, 244
  galactorrhea and, 582
  lethal concentration of, 770
  methyldopa and, 753
  parkinsonism and, 122
  pharmacokinetics of, 780
  psychomotor stimulant blockade and, 275
  warfarin and, 469
Haloprogin, 679
Halotestin; *see* Fluoxymesterone
Halotex; *see* Haloprogin
Halothane, 401-402
  abuse of, 358
  and autonomic nervous system, 396
  circulation and, 397-398
  clinical characteristics of, 400
  enflurane and, 402
  equilibrium and, 389
  gaseous anesthetics and, 400
  history of use of, 384
  isoflurane and, 403
  lethal concentration of, 770
  malignant hyperthermia and, 399
  methods of administration of, 393
  methoxyflurane and, 402
  minimal alveolar concentration of, 388
  second gas effect and, 390
  toxicity and biotransformation of, 398-399
Hansen's disease, 677-678
Harrison Anti-Narcotic Act, 761
Hashish, 344
HCG; *see* Human chorionic gonadotropin
HDL; *see* High-density lipoprotein
Heart
  digitalis and, 419-422
  procainamide and, 440
  quinidine and, 437
Heart block, antidepressants and, 273
Heart rate
  atropine methylbromide and, 120
  digitalis and, 422
Heart-On, 357
Heavenly blue, 356
Heavy metal poisoning, 739-743
Heavy metals
  antidote for, 733
  as rodenticide, 743
Hemicholinium, 98
  acetylcholine and, 86, 91
Hemodialysis, 736

Hemoglobin
  iron in, 606
  nitrites and, 454
Hemoperfusion, poisoning and, 736-737
Hemosiderin, 606
Hemostasis, 459-476
  anticoagulants and, 462-470
  antiplatelet drugs and, 470-473
  drug action and, 460-462
  fibrinolytic agents and, 473-475
Hemp, 344
Heparin, 462-466
  administration of, 463-464
  antithrombin III and, 463
  complications of therapy and, 465
  configuration of, 463
  contraindications of, 469
  diazepam and, 750
  dosage of, 463-464
  as platelet inhibiting agent, 471-472
  renal excretion of, 753
  short duration of, 466
  toxicity and, 465
  use of, 464-465
Hepatic disease, antibiotics and, 664
Hepatic drug metabolism, 73-76
Hepatic dysfunction, 71
Hepatitis B, vaccine for, 717
Heroin, 328
  abstinence syndromes and, 340
  characteristics of abuse of, 339
  death from overdose of, 339
  scheduling of, 760
Heroin hydrochloride, 327
Herpes simplex virus, 668
Herpes zoster, antiviral drugs for, 668
HETEs; *see* Hydroxyeicosatetraenoic acids
Hetrazan; *see* Diethylcarbamazine
Hexachlorophene, 684, 686
Hexadine-S; *see* Aluminum hexaurea sulfate
     triiodide
Hexamethonium, 98
  acetylcholine and, 84, 86
  hypertension and, 194
Hexitol, 520
Hexobarbital, 778
Hexylcaine, 408
5-HIAA; *see* 5-Hydroxyindoleacetic acid
Hibiclens; *see* Chlorhexidine gluconate
High-density lipoprotein, 493, 496
  atherosclerosis and, 498
Hiprex; *see* Methenamine(s)
Hispril; *see* Diphenylpyraline
Histamine, 85, 97, 99, 197-205; *see also*
     Antihistamine(s)
  action of, 82, 83
  antihistaminic drug and, 46
  binding and release of mast cell, 201-203
  bronchial smooth muscle and, 509
  content of human tissues, 199
  degradation of, 199
  first synthesis of, 197

Histamine—cont'd
  histidine decarboxylases and, 198
  hypersusceptibility to, 42
  lungs and, 516
  metabolic pathways of, 200
  pharmacologic effects of, 203-204
  receptors for, 197-198
  role of, in health and disease, 204-205
  structure of, 198
  tissue distribution and formation and, 198
  tolazoline and, 165
  upper gastrointestinal tract and, 519
  vasopressin and, 575
Histamine antagonists, 518-519; *see also*
    Antihistamine(s)
Histamine H$_1$-receptor antagonists, 206-210
Histamine H$_2$-receptor antagonists, 210-211
  vitamin B$_{12}$ and, 611
Histamine receptors, 197-198
  distribution of, 198
Histaminergic receptors, 85
Histerone; *see* Testosterone
L-Histidine decarboxylase, 198
Histidine decarboxylases, 198
Histocompatibility antigens, 726
HIV; *see* Human immunodeficiency virus
HLA; *see* Human lymphocyte antigens
HMG; *see* 3-Hydroxy-3-methylglutaryl
Hog, 352
Homatropine hydrobromide, 119
Hookworm, drugs for, 698
Hormonal agents, neoplasms and, 708-709
HPETE; *see* Hydroperoxyeicosatetraenoic
    acids
Human calcitonin, 568
Human chorionic gonadotropin, 584
Human growth factor, 583
Human immunodeficiency virus, 668, 669-670
Human lymphocyte antigens, 722, 726
Humantin; *see* Paromomycin
Humorsol; *see* Demecarium
Hurricaine, 408; *see* Ethyl aminobenzoate
Hydantoins, 312-313
  formulas of, 311
  nonsteroidal anti-inflammatory drugs and,
    364
Hydralazine, 53, 99
  action of, 178
  as direct vasodilator, 181
  genetics and, 49, 53
  histamine and, 201
  hypertension and, 182
  introduction of, 177
  pharmacokinetics of, 784
  sites of action of, 178
  structure of, 182
Hydralazine hydrochloride, 182
Hydrea; *see* Hydroxyurea
Hydrochlorothiazide, 9
  pharmacokinetics of, 790
  single dose curve and, 488
  structure of, 486

Hydrocodone, 326
  coughing and, 507-508
  lethal concentration of, 770
Hydrocodone bitartrate, 327, 335
Hydrocortisone, 543, 546-554
  adrenal steroid synthesis and, 545
  adrenocorticotropic hormone and, 544
  corticotropin-releasing factor and, 581
  dosage of, 554
  hepatic or renal dysfunction and, 71
  insulin and, 534
  phenobarbital and, 752
  preparation of, 552
  prostaglandin synthesis and, 228
  structure of, 553
Hydrocortone; *see* Hydrocortisone
HydroDIURIL; *see* Hydrochlorothiazide
Hydroflumethiazide, 486
Hydrogen peroxide, 49
Hydrogen sulfide, 770
Hydrolysis, 33
Hydromorphone, 326, 328, 770
Hydromorphone hydrochloride, 327
Hydromox; *see* Quinethazone
Hydroperoxyeicosatetraenoic acids, 235-238
  biologic activities of, 235-236
  chemistry and formation of, 235
  inhibitors of, 236-238
Hydrophilic agents, 524, 525
Hydroxocobalamin, 739
2-Hydroxybenzoic acid; *see* Salicylic acid
Hydroxychloroquine, 690, 692
25-Hydroxycholecalciferol, 569, 570
Hydroxydaunorubicin, 709; *see also*
    Doxorubicin
4-Hydroxydebrisoquin, 54
6-Hydroxydopamine
  catecholamines and, 97
  chemical sympathectomy and, 97
Hydroxyeicosatetraenoic acids, 235
Hydroxyethylflurazepam, 283
5-Hydroxyindoleacetic acid, 97
  daily excretion of, 216
  serotonin and, 215
  structure of, 215
β-Hydroxyketones, 228
Hydroxylation of debrisoquin, 54
4-Hydroxy-3-methoxphenyl(ethylene) glycol,
    95, 96
4-Hydroxy-3-methoxymandelic acid, 97
3-Hydroxy-3-methylglutaryl, 498
p-Hydroxyphenobarbital, 30
Hydroxyprogesterone, 708
Hydroxyprogesterone caproate, 593
15-Hydroxyprostaglandin dehydrogenase, 232
11-Hydroxy-tetrahydrocannabinol, 347
5-Hydroxytryptamine; *see* Serotonin
5-Hydroxytryptophan, 215
Hydroxyurea, 704, 710
25-Hydroxy-vitamin D$_3$; *see* 25-
    Hydroxycholecalciferol
Hydroxyzine, 262

Hydroxyzine—cont'd
  lethal concentration of, 770
  pharmacokinetics of, 780
Hygroton; *see* Chlorthalidone
Hylorel; *see* Guanadrel
Hymenolepis nana, drugs for, 698
Hyoscyamine, 114
Hyoscyamus niger, 114
Hy-Pam; *see* Hydroxyzine
Hyperaldosteronism, 555
Hypercalcemia, 567
  cardiac glycosides and, 753
Hyperglycemia, 535
Hyperlipidemia, 498-501
Hyperprolactinemia, 582
Hypersensitivity
  penicillin and, 648-649
  sulfonamides and, 635-636
Hyperstat; *see* Diazoxide
Hypersusceptibility, 42
Hypertension
  aldosterone and, 180-181
  angiotensin and, 180-181
  drugs for; *see* Antihypertensive(s)
Hyperthyroidism, propranolol and, 566
Hypertonic saline, 525
Hypertrophic subaortic stenosis, 168
Hyperuricemia, 601
Hypervitaminosis A, 622
Hypnotics, 280-292
  alcohol and, 293
  barbiturates as, 286-289
  benzodiazepines as, 280-286
  insomnia and, 291-292
  nonaccidental toxin ingestion of, 731
  nonbarbiturate, nonbenzodiazepine, 289-291
  pharmacokinetics of, 778
Hypocalcemia, 567
  treatment of, 571
Hypochlorite, 684, 685
Hypoglycemia, insulin and, 537-538
Hypoglycemic agents
  diabetes mellitus and, 538-541
  pharmacokinetics of, 790
  safety and, 755
Hypokalemia, 485
Hypoprothrombinemia, 620
Hypotension, orthostatic, 179-180, 271
Hypothalamic releasing factors, 580-582
Hypothalamic-pituitary-thyroid relationship,
    559
Hypothalamus, 531-532
Hypothyroidism, 562-563
Hypouricemic agents, 790
Hypsarrhythmia, 308
6-Hyroxydopamine, 94
Hytakerol; *see* Dihydrotachysterol

I

I; *see* Iodine
Ibuprofen, 365, 376

Ibuprofen—cont'd
  as anti-inflammatory agent, 367
  as antipyretics, 366
  asthma and, 516
  dosage, dosage forms, and indications for,
    375
  gastointestinal disturbances and, 376
  lethal concentration of, 770
  pharmacokinetics of, 781
  as reversable inhibiting agent, 472
  structure of, 376
ICSH; *see* Interstitial cell–stimulating hormone
IDDM; *see* Insulin-dependent diabetes
    mellitus
Idiosyncrasy, drug safety and effectiveness
    and, 42-43
Idoxuridine
  as antiviral agent, 667
  nucleic acid synthesis and, 630
  viral infections susceptible to, 668
IFN; *see* Interferon(s)
IgE, 201, 204
IL-1; *see* Interleukin 1
IL-2; *see* Interleukin 2
IL-3; *see* Interleukin 3
Ilosone; *see* Erythromycin
Imferon; *see* Iron-dextran injection
Imidazole, 235
Imidazole carboxamide, 710; *see also*
    Dacarbazine
Imidazole-*N*-methyltransferase, 199
Imipenem, 655, 785
Imipramine, 245, 270, 272
  cimetidine and, 751
  discovery of, 269
  galactorrhea and, 582
  lethal concentration of, 770
  oral contraceptives and, 751
  pharmacokinetics of, 780
  structure of, 271, 312
  therapeutic concentrations of, 768
Imipramine hydrochloride, 272
Imipramine pamoate, 270, 272
Immune interferon, 722
Immune response, histamine and, 205
Immunization, 717
Immunocompetence, 716
Immunodeficiency, 716
Immunopharmacology, 716-727
  antibodies as therapeutic agents in, 718-720
  immunization in, 717
  immunosuppression in, 723-726
  lymphokines in, 720-722
  monokines in, 720-722
  synthetic vaccines in, 717-718
Immunosuppression, 549, 723-726
Immunotoxins, 718-719
Imodium; *see* Loperamide
Indandione, 743
Indapamide
  pharmacokinetics of, 790
  structure of, 487

Inderal; *see* Propranolol
Indocin; *see* Indomethacin
Indocyanine green
  age and disposition of, 60
  hepatic or renal dysfunction and, 71
Indole derivatives, 365
Indomethacin, 365, 377-378
  as antipyretic, 366
  dosage, dosage forms, and indications for,
    375
  gout and, 600
  patent ductus arteriosus and, 378
  pharmacokinetics of, 781
  platelet function and, 471-472, 459
  as reversable inhibiting agent, 472
  structure of, 377
  uterus and, 578
Indoramin, 784
Induction of anesthesia, premedication and,
    395
Infantile spasms, 308, 316
Inflammation and pain, 334
Inflammatory response, histamine and, 202,
    205
Influenza A
  amantadine and, 667
  antiviral drugs for, 668
INH; *see* Isoniazid
Inhalants, abuse of, 338, 357-359, 774-775
Inhalation anesthetics, 384, 399-404
Inhibitors
  of leukotrienes, 236-238
  of prostaglandins, 235
  of thromboxane, 235
Innovar; *See* Fentanyl with droperidol
Inocor; *see* Amrinone
Inotropic effect, anesthesia and, 397
Inscription, 759
Insecticide, poisoning from, 743
Insomnia
  rebound, 282
  treatment of, 291-292
Insulin, 530-534
  absorption with parenteral administration of,
    22
  biosynthesis of, 530-531
  deficiency of, 534
  diabetes mellitus and, 536-538
  glucose regulation and, 531-532
  receptors of, 532-533
  release of, 530-531
Insulin receptors, 532-533
Insulin zinc suspension, 536
Insulin-dependent diabetes mellitus, 535-537
Insulin-infusion pumps, 22
Insulin-like growth factor, 582
Intal; *see* Cromolyn sodium
Interferon(s), 722
  inducers of, 670
α-Interferons, 722
β-Interferons, 722

γ-Interferons
  immunosuppression and, 724
  neoplasms and, 722
Interleukin(s), 720-721
Interleukin 1, 720-721
Interleukin 2, 720-721
  immunosuppression and, 724, 725
Interleukin 3, 721
Intermediate acting barbiturates, 287
Intermittent claudication, 306
Interstitial cell–stimulating hormone, 583
Intestinal absorption, drug interaction and,
    748-750
Intestinal antiseptics, 637
Intestinal protozoal infection, 687-689
Intolerance, nonsteroidal anti-inflammatory
    drugs and, 368
Intoxication, 737-739
  acetaminophen, 373-375
  alcohol and, 296-297
  barbiturate, 288-289
  digitalis, 428-430
  marijuana, 344-348
  morphine, 325
  organophosphorus, 112
  salicylate, 371, 372-373
  tricyclic antidepressants and, 273
Intravenous anesthetics, 385, 403-405
Intrinsic pathway of thrombin formation, 460-
    461
Intrinsic sympathomimetic activity, 190
Inverse agonists, 247
Iodide, thyroid and, 564
Iodine
  deiodination of thyroxine and, 560
  as disinfectant, 683
  equipment sterilization and, 685
  inhibitors of formation and transport of, 563
  skin disinfection and, 684
  thyroid hormones and, 558
Iodochlorhydroxyquin, 688
Iodophors
  equipment sterilization and, 685
  skin disinfection and, 684
Iodoquinol
  amebiasis and, 688-689
  intestinal protozoa susceptible to, 688
Ion fluxes, 433
Iopanoic acid, thyroid hormones and, 562
Ipecac syrup, 731-732
Ipodate, thyroid hormones and, 562
Ipratropium
  asthma and, 515-516
  coughing and, 507-508
Ircon; *see* Ferrous fumarate
Iris, autonomic innervation of, 116
Iron, 606-609
  anemia and, 605
  antidote for, 733
  lethal concentration of, 770

Iron poisoning, 742
  deferoxamine mesylate for, 735
  penicillamine for, 735
Iron-deficiency anemia, 607-609
Iron-dextran injection, 608
Irreversibility, 6
Irreversible organophosphorus
      anticholinesterases, 109-110
ISA; *see* Intrinsic sympathomimetic activity
Ismelin; *see* Guanethidine
Isobutyl nitrite, abuse of, 357
Isocarboxazid, 269, 272
Isoetharine, 511
Isoflurane, 403
  clinical characteristics of, 400
  medical history of, 384
  minimal alveolar concentration of, 388
  toxicity and biotransformation of, 398-399
Isoflurophate, 98, 99, 109-111
  glaucoma in, 106
  structure of, 110
  vasopressin and, 575
Isoleucine, oxytocin and, 577
Isoniazid
  age and disposition of, 60
  alcohol intolerance and, 297
  antacids and, 749
  antidote for, 733
  diet and, 63
  drug-metabolizing enzymes and, 35
  drugs inhibited by, 751
  enflurane and, 402
  gastrectomy and, 72
  genetics and, 49, 53
  hepatic or renal dysfunction and, 71
  lethal concentration of, 770
  Mycobacterium infections susceptible to, 673
  pharmacokinetics of, 789
  rifampin and, 675
  structure of, 34
  tuberculosis and, 672-674
Isophane insulin suspension, 536
Isopin; *see* Verapamil
Isopropanol, 299
  abuse of, 358
Isopropyl alcohol, 299
  lethal concentration of, 770
Isoproterenol, 98, 158
  and dobutamine hydrochloride, 431
  dosage of, 445
  lower airway and, 510-512
  parathyroid extract and, 567
  propranolol and, 168
  prostaglandins and, 234
Isoptin; *see* Verapamil
Isopto Atropine; *see* Atropine
Isopto Carbachol; *see* Carbachol
Isopto Carpine; *see* Pilocarpine
Isopto Homatropine; *see* Homatropine
      hydrobromide
  dosage of, 453
  oral, 453

Isopto Homatropine—cont'd
  pharmacokinetics of, 782
  structure of, 451
  sublingual, 453
Isosorbide dinitrate
  chewable, 453
Isotonic fluids, diuresis and, 736
Isotretinoin, 618, 789
Isuprel; *see* Isoproterenol
Izonid; *see* Isoniazid

J

J, as slang for marijuana, 344
Jimson weed, 114
Joint, 344
Junctional transmission
  drug action in, 86

K

Kabikinase; *see* Streptokinase
Kalcinate; *see* Calcium gluconate
Kallikrein, 219
  activation of, 220
  clinical significance of, 221
  Hageman factor and, 461
Kanamycin, 657
  absorption of, 23
  age and disposition of, 60
  therapeutic concentrations of, 768
Kaolin
  digoxin absorption and, 425
  lower gastrointestinal tract and, 523
Kaolin-pectin, digoxin and, 749
Keflex; *see* Cephalexin
Keflin; *see* Cephalothin
Kefurox; *see* Cefuroxime
Kefzol; *see* Cefazolin
Kemadrin; *see* Procyclidine
Kenacort; *see* Triamcinolone
Keratomalacia, 617
Ketamine, 385, 405
  pharmacokinetics of, 778
  structure of, 405
Ketanserin, 218, 784
Ketoconazole
  cimetidine and, 749
  fungal infections and, 679, 680
  pharmacokinetics of, 788
Ketocyclazocine, 332
Ketoprofen, 365, 376
  dosage, dosage forms, and indications for,
      375
  pharmacokinetics of, 781
Kidney
  anesthesia and, 399
  damage to, anti-inflammatory drugs and, 369
  drug clearance and, 25-26
Kinetics, 18
Kininase I, 220
Kininase II, 220
Kinins, 219-221
  bronchial smooth muscle and, 509

Kinins—cont'd
  generation of, 220
Klebsiella
  cephalosporins for, 651
  drugs for, 654
  penicillin for, 650
Klonopin; *see* Clonazepam
Konakion; *see* Vitamins, K_1

L

LAAM; *see* *l*-α-Acetylmethadol hydrochloride
Labetalol, 170, 193
  cimetidine and, 212
  pharmacokinetics of, 784
  sites of action of, 178
  structures of, 167
Labetalol hydrochloride, 167
β-Lactam antibiotics, 651
Lactation, 620-621
Lactose as cocaine adulterant, 350
Lactulose, 525
Lampit; *see* Nifurtimox
Lamprene; *see* Clofazimine
Lanatoside C, 423, 426
  deslanoside and, 426
Lanoxicaps; *see* Digoxin
Lanoxin, 426; *see* Digoxin
Larodopa; *see* Levodopa
Larva migrans, 698
Lasix; *see* Furosemide
Laxatives, 518, 524-526
LD_{50}; *see* Median lethal dose
LDL; *see* Low-density lipoprotein(s)
Lead, 45
  lethal concentration of, 770
  poisoning by, 739-740
    calcium disodium edetate for, 734
    penicillamine for, 735
  as rodenticide, 743
Lectins, histamine and, 201
Legionella, drugs for, 654
Leishmania, 696
  drugs for, 691
Lente insulin, 536
Lepromatous leprosy, 677
Leprosy, 677-678
Leptospira, drugs for, 654
Lethal blood concentration, 767
Leucine, 577
Leucovorin, 706
[Leu]enkephalin, 320
Leukemia, antibodies for, 718
Leukeran; *see* Chlorambucil
Leukotriene receptors, antagonists of, 238
Leukotrienes, 235-238
  biologic activities of, 235-236
  biosynthesis of, from arachidonic acid, 237
  bronchial smooth muscle and, 509
  chemistry of, 235
  formation of, 235
  glucocorticoids and, 514

Leukotrienes—cont'd
  histamine and, 204, 205
  immunosuppression and, 724
  inhibitors of, 236-238
  lungs and, 516
Leuprolide acetate, 581
Levallorphan, 341
Levobunolol, 167, 170
Levodopa; *see also* Dopa; Dopamine
  gonadotropin-releasing hormone and, 581-582
  parkinsonism and, 122, 123-124
  propranolol and, 169
Levo-Dromoran; *see* Levorphanol tartrate
Levonorgestrel, 594
Levoprome; *see* Methotrimeprazine
Levorphanol tartrate, 327
Levothroid; *see* Levothyroxine sodium
Levothyroxine sodium, 563
LH; *see* Luteinizing hormone
LH-RH; *see* Luteinizing hormone–releasing hormone
Librium; *see* Chlordiazepoxide
Lidocaine, 408, 413-414, 441-442
  β-adrenergic receptor blocking agents and, 751
  alteration in drug disposition and, 70
  antiarrhythmic action and, 434-436
  binding of, to plasma proteins, 73
  cardiovascular effects of, 411
  cimetidine and, 751
  classification of, 434
  digitalis poisoning and, 430
  digitalis toxicity and, 445
  dosage of, 412
  excretion of, 410
  heart and, 411
  hepatic or renal dysfunction and, 71
  history of use of, 407
  for infiltration, 407
  lethal concentration of, 770
  liver disease and, 75
  mepivacaine and, 414
  miscellaneous effects of, 411
  onset and duration of action of, 410
  pharmacokinetics of, 19, 442, 783
  as preferred local anesthetic, 415
  propranolol and, 751
  safe dosage of, 412
  structure of, 414
  tetracaine and, 414
  therapeutic concentrations of, 768
  toxicity and, 411-412
  uses of, 408
  vasoconstrictors and, 411
  ventricular arrhythmias and, 448
  volume of distribution or clearance and, 17
Lidocaine hydrochloride, 440, 442
Lincocin; *see* Lincomycin
Lincomycin, 662
  pharmacokinetics of, 786

Lincomycin—cont'd
  protein synthesis and, 630
Lindane, 743
Liothyronine sodium, 563
Lipid metabolism
  alcohol and, 293-294
  glucocorticoids and, 548
Lipid transport, 493-497
Lipomodulin, 550
Lipoproteins
  atherosclerosis and, 493-497
  high-density, 498
Lipoxygenase(s)
  arachidonic acid and, 235
  oxygenation of, 236
Liquamar; *see* Phenprocoumon
Liquifilm; *see* Pilocarpine
Listeria, penicillins for, 651
Listeria monocytogenes, 649
Lithane; *see* Lithium carbonate
Lithium
  age and disposition of, 60
  lethal concentration of, 770
  in manic psychosis, 259-260
  metoclopramide and, 749
  pharmacokinetics of, 780
  phenytoin and, 753
  propantheline and, 749
  therapeutic concentrations of, 768
  thyroid and, 566
  vasopressin and, 575
Lithium carbonate, 259-260, 575
Lithium citrate, 260
Lithonate; *see* Lithium carbonate
Lithotabs; *see* Lithium carbonate
Live virus vaccine, 717
Liver
  anesthesia and, 398
  disease of, 73-76
    antibiotics and, 664
  nonsteroidal anti-inflammatory drugs and, 369
Loa loa, drugs for, 698
Loading dose, 16
Local anesthesia; *see* Anesthetic(s), local
Localization, catecholamines and, 91-92
Locker Room, 357
Log dose-response curve, 9, 10
Lomidine; *see* Pentamidine
Lomotil; *see* Atropine, diphenoxylate and; Diphenoxylate
Lomustine, 704, 706
Long-acting barbiturates, 287
Loniten; *see* Minoxidil
Loop diuretics, 488-489
  hypertension and, 194
Loperamide, 329, 523
  dosage of, 327
Loperamide hydrochloride, 327, 523
Lophophora williamsii, 356
Lopressor; *see* Metoprolol
Loprox; *see* Ciclopirox olamine

Lopurin; *see* Allopurinol
Lorazepam
  age and disposition of, 60
  dosage and forms of, 263
  kinetics of, 262, 281
  lethal concentration of, 770
  pharmacokinetics of, 778
  seizures and, 262
  status epilepticus and, 315
  structure of, 261
Lorcainide, 444
  classification of, 434
  pharmacokinetics of, 783
  structure of, 443
Lorelco; *see* Probucol
Lormetazepam, pharmacokinetics of, 778
Lorothidol; *see* Bithionol
Lotrimin; *see* Clotrimazole
Lotusate; *see* Talbutal
Love pill, 355
Low T$_3$ syndrome, 562
Low-density lipoprotein(s), 493, 496, 498
  cholesterol regulation and, 497-498
  therapeutic implications and, 498-499
Lower airway, 508-516
Lower gastrointestinal tract, 522-526
Low-solubility drugs, 391
Loxapine, 770
Lozol; *see* Indapamide
LSD; *see* Lysergic acid diethylamide
LSD psychosis, 355
Lubricants, gastrointestinal tract and, 525
Ludes, 351
Ludiomil; *see* Maprotiline
Lufyllin; *see* Dyphylline
Luminal; *see* Phenobarbital
Lungs, mediators within, 516
Lupron; *see* Leuprolide acetate
Luteal phase of ovulation, 586-587
Luteinizing hormone, 583-587
Luteinizing hormone–releasing hormone, 581-582; *see also* Gonadotropin-releasing hormone
Lymphocytopenia, 549
Lymphokines, 720-722
  corticosteroids and, 549
Lymphoma, 718
Lynestrenol, 592
Lypressin, 576
Lysergic acid, structure of, 218
Lysergic acid diethylamide, 275-276
  abuse of, 352, 353, 774-775
  lethal concentration of, 770
  scheduling of, 760
  serotonin and, 214
  structure of, 276
D-Lysergic acid diethylamide; *see* Lysergic acid diethylamide
Lysergide; *see* Lysergic acid diethylamide
Lysodren; *see* Mitotane
Lysylbradykinin; *see* Bradykinin and kallidin

M

Maalox, 520
Macrodantin; *see* Nitrofurantoin
α_2-Macroglobulin
    kallikrein and, 219, 220
Macrolide antibiotics, 786
Macrophages, 549
Mafenide, 633, 637
Magaldrate, 520
Magan; *see* Magnesium salicylate
Magnesium
    cardiac glycosides and, 753
    diuretics and, 477
    lethal concentration of, 770
    tetracycline and, 748
Magnesium carbonate, 521
Magnesium chloride, 521
Magnesium hydroxide, 519-520
Magnesium oxide as antidote, 732
Magnesium salicylate, 365, 370
Magnesium salt
    lower gastrointestinal tract and, 525
    upper gastrointestinal tract and, 520-521
Magnesium sulfate, 525
Magnesium trisilicate, 520-521
Maintenance regimen of drug, 16-17
Malaria, 690-696
Malathion, 110, 111
Malonic acid, 286
Mandelamine; *see* Methenamine(s)
Mandelic acid, 639
Mandol; *see* Cefamandole
Manganese
    lethal concentration of, 770
    poisoning by, calcium disodium edetate for, 734
Manic psychosis, 259-260
Mannitol, 483-483
    as cocaine adulterant, 350
    as heroin adulterant, 339
    pharmacokinetics of, 790
    structure of, 482
MAO; *see* Monoamine oxidase
MAO inhibitors; *see* Monoamine oxidase inhibitors
Maprotiline, 273-274
    lethal concentration of, 770
    pharmacokinetics of, 780
    structure of, 274
Maprotiline hydrochloride, 272
Marcaine; *see* Bupivacaine
Marezine; *see* Cyclizine
Marijuana, 344-347
    abuse of, 338, 774-775
    scheduling of, 760
Marijuana-induced temporal disintegration, 345-346
Marplan; *see* Isocarboxazid
Mast cells
    histamine and, 201, 202, 204
        binding and release of, 201-203

Mast cells—cont'd
    serotonin and, 215
Matulane; *see* Procarbazine
Maxibolin; *see* Ethylestrenol
MBC; *see* Minimum bactericidal concentration
MDA; *see* 3-Methoxy-4,5-methylenedioxyamphetamine
MDMA; *see* 3,4-Methylenedioxymethamphetamine
Mebadin; *see* Dehydroemetine
Mebaral; *see* Mephobarbital
Mebendazole as anthelmintic, 697-699
Mecamylamine, 98, 131
    hypertension and, 194
    renal excretion of, 753
Mechlorethamine, 703-704
Mecillinam, 786
Meclizine, 210
Meclofenamate, 365
    dosage, dosage forms, and indications for, 375
    gastrointestinal disturbances and, 376
Meclofenamate sodium, 379
Meclofenamic acid, 781
Meclomen; *see* Meclophenamate
Median effective dose, 40
Median lethal dose, 39
Medrol; *see* Methylprednisolone
Medroxalol, 784
Medroxyprogesterone, 593
    neoplasms and, 708
Mefenamic acid, 365, 379
    coumarin and, 750
    dosage, dosage forms, and indications for, 375
    pharmacokinetics of, 781
Mefloquine, 788
Mefoxin; *see* Cefoxitin
Megace; *see* Megestrol acetate
Megaloblastic anemia, 609-613
Megestrol acetate, 708
Melarsoprol
    extraintestinal protozoa susceptible to, 691
    trypanosomal infections and, 696
Melatonin, 97, 215
Melenamic acid, 469
Melphalan
    neoplasms and, 703, 704, 706
    pharmacokinetics of, 788
Membranes, drug passage across, 12-15
Menadiol sodium diphosphate, 619, 620
Menadione, 619; *see* Vitamins, K_3
Menadione sodium bisulfite, 619, 620
Menest; *see* Esterified estrogen
Meningitis, 655
Meningococcus, 632
Menopause, estrogen and, 589
Menstruation
    estrogen and, 588
    hormonal control of, 585, 587
Mental depression, 268; *see also* Antidepressant(s)

Mepacrine
    prostanoid synthesis inhibitors and, 235
    renal excretion of, 753
Meperidine, 328-329
    age and disposition of, 60
    biliary tract and, 324
    cimetidine and, 751
    hepatic or renal dysfunction and, 71
    lethal concentration of, 770
    pharmacokinetics of, 777
    as preanesthetic medication, 395
    structure of, 328
Meperidine hydrochloride, 327
Mephenesin, 264
Mephentermine, 349
Mephenytoin, 313
    in epilepsy, 310
    genetics and, 49
    metabolic reactions of, 54
Mephobarbital, 314
    in epilepsy, 310
    genetics and, 49
    metabolic reactions of, 54
    microsomal oxidations and, 30
Mephyton; *see* Vitamins, K_1
Mepindolol, 784
Mepivacaine, 407, 408, 414
    history of use of, 407
    lethal concentration of, 769
    onset and duration of action of, 410
    structure of, 414
    uses of, 408
    vasoconstrictors and, 411
Meprobamate, 36, 262
    anxiety and, 264-265
    ethanol and, 751, 752
    lethal concentration of, 770
    pharmacokinetics of, 778
    structure of, 264
Meprospan; *see* Meprobamate
Mercaptomerin sodium, 483
Mercaptopurine, 31, 705
    allopurinol and, 751
    immunosuppression and, 723
    neoplasms and, 704, 707
6-Mercaptopurine, 31, 705
Mercapturic acid synthesis, 34
Mercurials, 483-484
Mercury, 45
    lethal concentration of, 770
    poisoning by, 740-741
        dimercaprol for, 733
        penicillamine for, 735
Mesantoin; *see* Mephenytoin
Mescaline
    abuse of, 356-357, 774-775
    structure of, 276
Mesoridazine, 770
Mestinon; *see* Pyridostigmine
Mestinon Timespan; *see* Pyridostigmine
Mestranol, 590-591

Metabolism
  of acetaminophen, 373-375
  of atropine, 117
  drug
    age and, 61
    dietary manipulation and, 65
    hepatic, disease and, 73-76
    pharmacogenetic conditions that alter, 52-
      55
  of epinephrine, 150-151
  of kinins, 219-220
  nonsteroidal anti-inflammatory drugs and,
    369-370
  of norepinephrine, 150-151
  of prostaglandins, 228-232
  of salicylates, 371
  of scopolamine, 117
  of serotonin, 215-216
  of thromboxane, 228-232
Metahydrin; see Trichlormethiazide
Metal-containing antiseptics, 685
Metamucil; see Psyllium hydrophilic mucilloid
Metanephrine, 95, 96
Metaprel; see Metaproterenol
Metaproterenol, lower airway and, 510-511
Metaraminol, 98
  action of, 172
  as false transmitters, 94
[Met]enkephalin, 320, 321
Meth, 348
Methacholine chloride, 102
Methadone, 330-331
  abstinence syndrome and, 340
  drug rehabilitation programs and, 341
  lethal concentration of, 770
  pharmacokinetics of, 777
  phenytoin and, 752
  scheduling of, 760
  structure of, 330
Methadone hydrochloride, 327
Methadose; see Methadone
Methadyl acetate, 330, 341
Methamphetamine, lethal concentration of,
  770
Methandroid; see Methandrostenolone
Methandrostenolone, 594-595, 596
Methanol, 298-299
  antidote for, 733
  lethal concentration of, 770
Methapyrilene
  as adulterant of heroin, 339
  lethal concentration of, 770
Methapyriline, 780
Methaqualone, 289
  abuse of, 351
  lethal concentration of, 770
  pharmacokinetics of, 779
  scheduling of, 760
Metharbital, 314
  in epilepsy, 310
Methdilazine, 209

Methemoglobin, cyanide poisoning and, 738
Methemoglobinemia, 53-54
Methenamine(s), 639-640
  sulfonamides and, 636
Methenamine mandelate, 639-640
Methergine; see Methylergonovine maleate
Methicillin, 643
  adverse effects of, 648-649
  hepatic or renal dysfunction and, 71
  pharmacokinetics of, 647, 786
Methicillin sodium, 650
Methimazole
  pharmacokinetics of, 791
  thyroid and, 563, 564-565
Methohexital, 403, 404
  barbiturates and, 404
  elimination half-life and clinical data for, 287
  etomidate and, 405
  lethal concentration of, 770
  pharmacokinetics of, 779
Methosarb; see Calusterone
Methotrexate
  cancer chemotherapy and, 702
  immunosuppression and, 723
  mechanism of action of, 705
  neoplasms and, 704, 706
  pharmacokinetics of, 789
  renal excretion of, 753
  uric acid and, 602
Methotrimeprazine, 365, 379
  dosage, dosage forms, and indications for,
    375
Methoxamine, tachycardia and, 447
Methoxsalen, 789
3-Methoxy-4,5-methylenedioxyamphetamine,
  355
Methoxychlor, poisoning from, 743
Methoxyflurane; see Penthrane
  clinical characteristics of, 400
  minimal alveolar concentration of, 388
  toxicity and biotransformation of, 398-399
Methscopolamine, 120
Methsuximide
  absence seizures and, 314
  in epilepsy, 310
Methyclothiazide, 486
Methyl alcohol; see Methanol
Methyl mercury, 740
Methyl salicylate, 364, 365
  lethal dose of, 372
  structure of, 365
Methylation, 34
Methylcobalamin, 610
Methyldiamphetamine, 760
Methyldopa, 98
  action of, 172
  adrenergic neuron and, 175
  adverse reactions to, 188
  allergies and, 44
  galactorrhea and, 582
  haloperidol and, 753

Methyldopa—cont'd
  hypertension and, 188
  introduction of, 177
  parkinsonism and, 122
  pharmacokinetics of, 784
  sites of action of, 178
  structure of, 188
  transport of, 94
Methyldopa hydrochloride, 188
Methylene blue as antidote, 733
3,4-Methylenedioxymethamphetamine, 355
Methylergonovine maleate, 578
N-Methylnicotinamide, 753
N-Methylpyridinium-2-aldoxime; see
  Pralidoxime
Methylphenidate, 275
  abuse of, 349
  dose of, 275
  drugs inhibited by, 751
  lethal concentration of, 770
  in narcolepsy, 269
  as stimulant, 274
  structure of, 275
Methylphenidate hydrochloride, 275
1-Methyl-4-phenyl-1,2,3,6-tetrahydropyridine,
  339; see MPTP
1-Methyl-4-phenylpyridinium, 122
N-Methylpiperidine, 322
Methylprednisolone, 544
  dosage of, 554
  lower airway and, 513, 514
  pharmacokinetics of, 791
  structure of, 553
Methyltestosterone, 594-595, 596
6-Methylthiopurine, 31
Methylthiourea, 49
α-Methyltyrosine, 274
Methylxanthine(s)
  action of, 302, 306
  asthma and, 306
  bronchial smooth muscle and, 509-510
  chemical structures of, 305
  lower airway in, 512-513
  relative activities of, 305
  synthetic, 306
Methylxanthine theobromine, 68
Methyprylon, 289
  lethal concentration of, 770
  withdrawal of, 352
Methysergide, 217-218
  serotonin receptors and, 85
  structure of, 217
Methysergide maleate, 218
Metiamide, 210
Metoclopramide
  acetaminophen and, 749
  chlorothiazide and, 749
  cimetidine and, 749
  digoxin and, 749
  ethanol and, 749
  gastrointestinal tract and, 518

Metoclopramide—cont'd
  lithium and, 749
  pharmacokinetics of, 779
  upper gastrointestinal tract and, 522
Metocurine, 778
Metolazone, 193
  structure of, 487
Metopirone; *see* Metyrapone
Metoprolol, 170
  cimetidine and, 212
  genetics and, 49
  hypertension and, 192
  lethal concentration of, 770
  metabolic reactions of, 54
  myocardial infarction and, 169
  pharmacokinetics of, 784
  sites of action of, 178
  structures of, 167
Metoprolol tartrate, 167
Metrazol, 302
Metrifonate as anthelmintic, 701
Metronidazole, 662-663
  alcohol intolerance and, 297
  amebiasis and, 687
  as anthelmintic, 701
  intestinal protozoa susceptible to, 688
  organisms susceptible to, 654
  parasites susceptible to, 698
  pharmacokinetics of, 789
Metyrapone, 545-546
Metyrosine, 98
  norepinephrine and, 86
Mevacor; *see* Lovastatin
Mexate; *see* Methotrexate
Mexican morning glory, 356
Mexiletine, 442
  classification of, 434
  pharmacokinetics of, 440, 783
  structure of, 443
  therapeutic concentrations of, 768
  ventricular arrhythmias and, 448
Mexitil; *see* Mexiletine
Meyer-Overton correlation, 394
Mezlin; *see* Mezlocillin
Mezlocillin, 650
  organisms susceptible to, 651
  pharmacokinetics of, 647, 786
Mianserin, 245
  pharmacokinetics of, 780
MIC; *see* Minimal inhibitory concentration
Micatin; *see* Miconazole
Miconazole, 679
  fungal infections and, 680
  pharmacokinetics of, 788
Miconazole nitrate, 679
Micronase; *see* Glyburide
Microsomal enzymes, drug metabolism and, 28-30
Microsomal hydroxylase, 30
Microsomal oxidation, 30-32
Microsporum, griseofulvin for, 681
Microsulfon; *see* Sulfadiazine

Midamor; *see* Amiloride
Midazolam, 286
  as hypnotic, 280, 282
  pharmacokinetics of, 779
  as preanesthetic medication, 395
  structure of, 281
Migraine headaches, serotonin and, 217
Milk
  as antidote, 732
  drugs in, 25
Milk of magnesia; *see* Magnesium hydroxide
Milk-alkali syndrome, 520
Milontin; *see* Phensuximide
Milrinone
  congestive heart failure and, 431
  pharmacokinetics of, 785
  side effects of, 431
Miltown; *see* Meprobamate
Minaxolone, 778
Mineral oil, 525
Mineralocorticoids, 543, 555-556
Minimal inhibitory concentration, 626
Minimum alveolar concentration, 388
Minimum bactericidal concentration, 627
Minipress; *see* Prazosin
Minocin; *see* Minocycline
Minocycline, 659
Minoxidil
  as direct vasodilator, 181
  hypertension and, 182-183
  pharmacokinetics of, 784
  sites of action of, 178
  structure of, 183
Mintezol; *see* Thiabendazole
Miradon; *see* Anisindione
Misoprostol, 791
MIT; *see* Monoiodotyrosin
Mithracin; *see* Plicamycin
Mithramycin; *see* Plicamycin
Mitomycin
  mechanism of action of, 705
  neoplasms and, 704, 709
Mitotane, 704, 711
Mitoxantrone
  neoplasms and, 704, 709
  pharmacokinetics of, 789
Mixed agonist-antagonists, 332-333
Monicid; *see* Cefonicid
Monistat; *see* Miconazole nitrate
Monoamine, discovery of, 83
Monoamine oxidase, 94, 95
  dopamine metabolism and, 244
  histamine degradation and, 199
  serotonin and, 215
Monoamine oxidase inhibitors, 269-270
  action of, 172, 173
  adrenergic neuron and, 175
  as antidepressants, 245-246, 269
  catecholamine biosynthesis and, 93
  clinical responses and doses of, 272
  hypertension and, 194

Monoamine oxidase inhibitors—cont'd
  levodopa and, 124
  meperidine and, 328
  serotonin and, 216
  tyramine and, 94
Monobactams, 655
  pharmacokinetics of, 786
Monoclonal antibody therapy, 718
Monocytopenia, corticosteroids and, 549
Monoiodotyrosin, 557-558
Monokines, 720-722
Monooxygenases, 61, 73, 74
Monopioid analgesics, poisoning from, 731
MOPEG; *see* 4-Hydroxy-3-methoxyphenyl(ethylene) glycol
MOPP; *See* Mechlorethamine, oncovin, procarbazine, and prednisone
Morning glory seeds, abuse of, 356, 774-775
Morphine, 322-325
  absorption with parenteral administration of, 22
  abstinence from, 326
  abstinence syndromes and, 340
  analgesic action of, 321
  biliary tract and, 324
  bronchial smooth muscle and, 324
  cardiovascular system of, 324
  chemistry of, 322
  contraindications to, 333
  feedback regulation and, 326
  gastrointestinal tract and, 324
  genitourinary tract and, 324
  histamine and, 201
  intoxication and, 325
  lethal concentration of, 770
  medical history of, 385
  methotrimeprazine and, 379
  opioid receptors and, 332
  pharmacokinetics of, 777
  as preanesthetic medication, 395
  pupils and, 324
  scheduling of, 760
  structure of, 322
  tolerance to, 325, 326
  vasopressin and, 575
Morphine receptor, 320
Morphine sulfate, 327
Motrin; *see* Ibuprofen
Moxalactam, 786
Moxam; *see* Moxalactam
MPTP, 122, 339
Mucolytics, 506, 508
Mucomyst; *see* Acetylcysteine
Muscarine, 82, 104-106
Muscarine choline esters, 86
Muscarinic agonists
  bronchial smooth muscle and, 509
  in glaucoma, 105
Muscarinic antagonists
  bronchial smooth muscle and, 509
  glaucoma and, 116-117
  insulin and, 532

Muscarinic antagonists—cont'd
  upper gastrointestinal tract and, 519
Muscarinic blocking agents; *see* Cholinergic
    blocking agents; Muscarinic antagonists
Muscarinic receptors, 84
  uterus and, 576
Muscimol, 247
Muscle
  bronchial smooth, 509
Muscle relaxant(s), 132-141
  neuromuscular blocking agents and, 132-138
  pentylenetetrazol and, 302
  spasticity and, 139-141
  spinal cord and, 138-139
Mustargen; *see* Mechlorethamine
Mutamycin; *see* Mitomycin
Myambutol; *see* Ethambutol
Myasthenia gravis, 112-113
Myasthenic crisis, 109
Mycelex; *see* Clotrimazole
Mycobacterial infection, 672-682
  antituberculosis drugs in, 672-677
  leprosy in, 677-678
  nontuberculosis infections in, 677
Mycobacterium avium/intracellulare complex,
    673, 677
Mycobacterium chelonii, 677
Mycobacterium fortuitum, 677
Mycobacterium kansasii, 673, 677
Mycobacterium leprae, 673
Mycobacterium tuberculosis, 672, 673
Mycostatin; *see* Nystatin
Mydriacyl; *see* Tropicamide
Mydriafair; *see* Tropicamide
Mydriatics
  atropine-like, 119
  belladonna alkaloids and, 116
Myidone; *see* Primidone
Mylanta, 520
Myleran; *see* Busulfan
Myocardial infarction
  atropine and, 118
  β-receptor blockers and, 169
Myochrysine; *see* Gold sodium thiomalate
Myoclonic seizures, 308
Myristica, 357
Mysoline; *see* Primidone
Mytelase; *see* Ambenonium

N

Nabilone, 791
Nadolol, 170
  action of, 169
    sites of, 178
  hypertension and, 192
  pharmacokinetics of, 784
  properties and uses of, 167
NADP; *see* Nicotinamide-adenine dinucleotide
    phosphate
Nafcil; *see* Nafcillin
Nafcillin, 643, 650
  adverse effects of, 649

Nafcillin—cont'd
  hepatic or renal dysfunction and, 71
  organisms susceptible to, 651, 654
  pharmacokinetics of, 647, 786
Nafcillin sodium, 650
Naladixic acid, 469
Nalbuphine, 327, 333, 777
Nalbuphine hydrochloride, 327
Nalfon; *see* Fenoprofen
Nalidixic acid
  coumarin and, 750
  nucleic acid synthesis and, 630
  urinary tract infection and, 639, 640
Nalorphine, 331, 341
Naloxone, 223, 321, 331, 341
  as antidote, 733
  apomorphine hydrochloride and, 732
  dosage of, 327
  fentanyl and, 329
  opioid receptors and, 332
  pentazocine and, 332-333
  propoxyphene and, 331
  structure of, 331
  thebaine and, 322
Naloxone antagonism, 223
Naloxone hydrochloride, 327
Naltrexone, 332
  dosage of, 327
  as narcotic antagonist, 342
  pharmacokinetics of, 777
Nandrolone, 596, 597
  nitrogen and, 595
NAPA; *see* N-Acetylprocainamide
Naphtha, abuse of, 358
Naphthoquinone, 619
Naprosyn; *see* Naproxen
Naproxen, 365, 376
  dosage, dosage forms, and indications for,
    375
  gastointestinal disturbances and, 376
  pharmacokinetics of, 781
  structure of, 376
Narcan; *see* Naloxone
Narcotic(s), 319-335
  acetaminophen and, 749
  action of, 321-322
  addiction to, social consequences of, 339-340
  anesthetics and, 385
  antagonists to, 321, 331-332, 341-342
  antidote for, 733
  antitussive drugs and, 334-335
  contraindications to, 333
  definitions of, 319, 338
  endogenous opioid peptides and, 320-321
  induction and, 395
  meperidine as, 328-329
  methadone as, 330-331
  mixed agonist-antagonists and, 332-333
  natural and semisynthetic derivatives of,
    322-328
  opioid receptors and, 319-320
  pain relief and, 333-334

Narcotic(s)—cont'd
  prescriptions for, 761
Narcotic antagonists, 321, 331-332, 341-342
Narcotine, 335
Nardil; *see* Phenelzine
Nasal decongestants, 157-158, 506-507
Nasalide; *see* Flunisolide
Natacyn; *see* Natamycin
Natamycin, 681
Natural killer cells, 721
Naturetin; *see* Bendroflumethiazide
Nebein; *see* Tobramycin
Necator americanus, 698
NegGram; *see* Nalidixic acid
Neisseria gonorrhoeae, 654
Neisseria meningitidis, 654
Nematodes, 698
Nembutal; *see* Pentobarbital
Neomycin, 657
  absorption of, 23
  antibacterial chemotherapy and, 626
  digoxin and, 749
  gastrointestinal flora and, 73
  primary hyperlipidemias and, 501
Neoplastic disease, 702-713
  alkylating agents for, 703-706
  antibiotics for, 709
  antimetabolites for, 706-708
  hormonal agents for, 708-709
Neosar; *see* Cyclophosphamide
Neostigmine, 99, 108-112
  edrophonium test and, 109
  myasthenia gravis and, 106, 112
  paroxysmal atrial tachycardia and, 447
  pharmacokinetics of, 779
  as reversible anticholinesterase, 107
  substitutes for, 108
Neostigmine bromide, 106
Neostigmine methylsulfate, 106
Nepeta cataria, 360
Nephrogenic diabetes insipidus, 574
Nerve block, 294
Nerve ending effector cell, 173
Nerve impulse, transmission of, 87
Nervous system
  general anesthesia and, 395-396
  impulse transmission in, 87
  neuroeffector junctions and, 85-89
  neurotransmitter kinetics and, 90-97
Nesacaine; *see* Chloroprocaine
Netilmicin, 658, 768
Netromycin; *see* Netilmicin
Neuroeffector junctions, 85-89
Neurohypophysis, 573
Neuroleptanalgesia, 329
Neuroleptanesthesia, 404
Neuroleptics
  barbiturates and, 289
  Parkinson's disease and, 122
Neuromuscular blocking agent(s), 132-138
  aminoglycoside antibiotics and, 753
  anesthetics and, 385

Neuropharmacology, 82-101
  chemical events at synapses and
    neuroeffector junctions and, 85-89
  chemical mediator sites of action and, 83-84
  chemical neurotransmission concept and, 82-
    83
  cholinergic and adrenergic
    neurotransmission and, 89
  effector response to chemical mediators and,
    89-90
  neuropharmacologic agent classification and,
    100
  neurotransmitter kinetics and nervous
    system and, 90-97
  potential neurotransmitters and, 97-100
  receptor concept in, 84-85
Neurotensin, 222
Neurotransmission; *see also* Neurotransmitters
  adrenergic or cholinergic, 89
  kinetics of, 90-97
Neurotransmitters
  action of, 82
  autoreceptors and, 82
  sensitization to, 90
  sites of action of, 83
New drug development, 39-41
Niacin, 614-615; *see also* Nicotinic acid
  recommended daily allowance of, 621
Niacinamide, 303
  adverse effects of, 622
Nicardipine, 782
Nickel poisoning, 734
Niclocide; *see* Niclosamide
Niclosamide, 698, 700
Nicotiana tabacum, 359
Nicotinamide; *see* Niacinamide
Nicotinamide adenine dinucleotide phosphate,
  28, 614-615
Nicotinamide adenine dinucleotide phosphate
  cytochrome P-450 reductase, 28
Nicotine, 98, 128
  abuse of, 359-360
  acetylcholine and, 86
  as cocaine adulterant, 350
  as insecticide, 743
  insomnia and, 291, 292
  lethal concentration of, 770
  receptor concept and, 84
  vasopressin and, 575
Nicotine choline esters, 86
Nicotinic acid, 493, 496, 500, 614-615; *see also*
  Niacin
  adverse effects of, 622
  atherosclerosis and, 500
  and combined drug regimens, 501
  primary hyperlipidemias and, 501
Nicotinic receptors, 84
NIDDM; *see* Non–insulin dependent diabetes
  mellitus
Nifedipine, 457
  in angina, 450

Nifedipine—cont'd
  diltiazem and, 457
  dosages of, 456
  pharmacokinetics of, 455, 782
  side effects of, 456
  sites of action of, 178
  slow calcium-channel blockers and, 190
  structure of, 457
Nifurtimox, 691, 696
Nikethamide, 302, 303
Nimodipine, 782
Nipride; *see* Nitroprusside
Niridazole, 701
  hepatic or renal dysfunction and, 71
  parasites susceptible to, 698
Nisentil; *see* Alphaprodine
Nitrates
  angina and, 450-454
  side effects of, 456
  tachyphylaxis and, 47
Nitrazepam, 60, 779
Nitrendipine, 782
Nitrites, 99
  angina and, 450-454
  antidote for, 733
  myocardial oxygen requirements and supply
    and, 451
  poisoning from, 454
p-Nitrobenzyl alcohol, 32
Nitrodisc; *see* Nitroglycerin
Nitrofurantoin, 638
Nitrofurazone, 638
Nitrogen mustard, 703-704; *see also*
  Mechlorethamine
Nitroglycerin
  in angina, 450
  effects of, 452
  first-pass effect and, 23
  metabolism of, 453
  in ointment, 453
  oral, 453
  pharmacokinetics of, 782
  preparations of, 453
  structure of, 451
  sublingual, 22
  therapeutic aims of, 454
  transdermal, 23
Nitroimidazole, 786
Nitroprusside, 183-184
  pharmacokinetics of, 784
  sites of action of, 178
Nitroreduction, 32
Nitrosoureas, mechanism of action of, 705
Nitrous oxide, 400
  abuse of, 358
  and autonomic nervous system, 396
  circulation and, 397
  clinical characteristics of, 400
  clinical pharmacology of, 399
  concentration effect and, 390
  equilibrium and, 389, 390
  halothane and, 401-402

Nitrous oxide—cont'd
  history of use of, 384
  innovar and, 404
  minimal alveolar concentration of, 388
  and oxygen, 329
Nizatidine, 780
Nizoral; *see* Ketoconazole
NK cells; *see* Natural killer cells
Nocardia, 632
Noctec; *see* Chloral hydrate
Nolahist; *see* Phenindamine
Noludar; *see* Methyprylon
Nolvadex; *see* Tamoxifen citrate
Nonautonomic drugs, 99
Nonbarbiturate sedatives as physically
  addicting drugs, 337
Noncompetitive antagonism, 11
Nonequilibrium blockade, 164
Nongenetic resistance, 628
Non–insulin dependent diabetes mellitus, 535-
  539
Nonmicrosomal oxidation, 32
Nonnarcotic analgesics, 319
Nonrebreathing, nonvalvular anesthesia
  system, 393
Nonsteroidal anti-inflammatory agent(s), 364-
  381
  acetaminophen as, 373-375
  analgesia and, 366
  asthma and, 516
  classification of, 364
  dosage, dosage forms, and indications for,
    375
  fenamates as, 379
  gout and, 599, 600
  indomethacin as, 377-378
  methotrimeprazine as, 379
  piroxicam as, 377
  platelet function and, 471, 472
  platelet inhibitory drugs and, 459
  propionic acid derivatives as, 375-376
  prostanoid synthesis inhibitors and, 235
  pyrazolone derivatives as, 378-379
  renal excretion of, 753
  rheumatic disease and, 379
  salicylates as, 364-373
  sulindac as, 377-378
  tolmetin as, 377
  uric acid excretion and, 601-602
Noraxin; *see* Norfloxacin
Norepinephrine, 34, 84, 98, 146-153
  action of, 82
  adrenergic receptors and, 84
  anesthesia and, 396
  antidepressants and, 245
  autonomic nervous system and, 82
  in brain, 92
  discovery of, 83
  disposition of, 95
  junctional transmission and, 86
  localization and, 91
  monoamine oxidase inhibitors and, 176

Norepinephrine—cont'd
  pathways of metabolism of, 96
  reserpine and, 174
  sites of action of, 83
  structure of, 34, 93
  tachyphylaxis and, 47
  uptake of, 94
Norethindrone, 592, 594
Norethindrone acetate, 592
Norethisterone, 592
Norethynodrel, 592, 594
Norfloxacin
  pharmacokinetics of, 787
  urinary tract infection and, 639, 640
Norgestrel, 592, 594
Normetanephrine, 95, 96
  structure of, 34
Normodyne; see Labetalol
Norpace; see Disopyramide
Norpramin; see Desipramine
19-Nortestosterone, 592
Nortriptyline, 272
  discovery of, 269
  genetic conditions altering response to, 49
  metabolic reactions of, 54
  pharmacokinetics of, 780
  structure of, 271
  therapeutic concentrations of, 768
  toxic and lethal concentrations of, 771
Nortriptyline hydrochloride, 272
Noscapine, 335
Novantrone; see Mitoxantrone
Novobiocin, 630
Novocain; see Procaine
Noxious stimulus, perception of, 321
NPH insulin, 536
NSAID; see Nonsteroidal anti-inflammatory
    agent(s)
Nubain; see Oxymorphone
Nucleic acid synthesis, 630, 631
Number, 344
Nupercaine; see Dibucaine
Nuprin; see Ibuprofen
Nutmeg, abuse of, 357
Nystatin, 679-680
  cell membranes and, 629-630

O
Occupation, drug disposition and, 69
Octopamine, 94
Ocusert Pilo-20 or -40; see Pilocarpine
Ogen; see Estropipate
Oil of wintergreen, 364
Ololiuqui, 356
Omeprazole, 782
Omnipen; see Ampicillin
Onchocerca volvulus, 698
Oncovin; see Vincristine
One-compartment model, 18
On-off phenomenon, 123
Open model, two-compartment, 20
Ophthaine; see Proparacaine

Ophthalmology, corticosteroids and, 554
Opiate(s)
  abuse of, 338-343, 774-775
  benzodiazepines and, 263-264
  physical addiction to, 337
Opioid(s)
  as antidiarrheal agent, 523
  constipation and, 522
  coughing and, 507-508
  definitions of, 319; see also Narcotic(s)
  dosage of, 327
  gonadotropin-releasing hormone and, 581
  histamine and, 201
  nonaccidental toxin ingestion and, 731
Opioid peptides, endogenous, 320-321
Opioid receptors, 223, 224, 319-320
  classification of, 332
Opium, 46
  paregoric and, 324
Opium alkaloid hydrochlorides, 326, 327
Opticrom; see Cromolyn sodium
Optimine; see Azatadine
Oradrate; see Chloral hydrate
Oral administration, 26
Oral contraceptives
  drugs induced by, 752
  drugs inhibited by, 751
  naproxen and, 376
Oral hypoglycemic agents, 538-541
Oramide; see Tolbutamide
Orasone; see Prednisone
Oreton; see Testosterone propionate
Oreton-Methyl; see Methyltestosterone
Organomercurial diuretics, 483-484
Organophosphate(s)
  antidote for, 733
  as insecticide, 743
  intoxication from, 112
  medical uses of, 110-111
Organophosphorus anticholinesterase,
    irreversible, 109-110
Orinase; see Tolbutamide
Ornidazole, 786, 789
Orphenadrine, 125, 771
Orthostatic hypotension, 179-180
  tricyclic antidepressants and, 271
Orudis; see Ketoprofen
Osmitrol; see Mannitol
Osmotic agents, gastrointestinal tract and, 524,
    525
Osmotic diuretics, 482-483
Osteomalacia, 569
Osteoporosis, 465, 589
Otitis media, 636
Otology, corticosteroids and, 554
Ouabain, 94, 426
  chemistry of, 423
  effects of, 423
  pharmacokinetics and, 424
  properties of, 424
  structure of, 423

Overdose, heroin, 339
Ovulatory cycle, 584-587
  estrogen and, 588
Oxacillin, 643, 650
  adverse effects of, 648
  hepatic or renal dysfunction and, 71
  organisms susceptible to, 654
  pharmacokinetics of, 786
Oxacillin sodium, 650
Oxalate, 462, 771
Oxamniquine, 698, 701
Oxandrolone, 596
Oxaprozin, 781
Oxatomide, 780
Oxazepam
  dosage and forms of, 263
  hepatic or renal dysfunction and, 71
  kinetics of, 262, 281
  liver disease and, 74
  pharmacokinetics of, 779
  structure of, 261
  toxic and lethal concentrations of, 771
Oxazolidinediones, 314-315
  formulas of, 311
Oxidation
  microsomal, 30-32
  nonmicrosomal, 32
N-Oxidation, 31
Oxtriphylline, 512
Oxycodone, 326, 327
  toxic and lethal concentrations of, 771
Oxycodone hydrochloride, 327
Oxygen, 44
  as antidote, 733
Oxymetazoline, 506
Oxymetholine, 596
Oxymorphone, 326, 327
  N-allyl derivative of, 331
Oxymorphone hydrochloride, 327
Oxyphenbutazone, 365, 378
  pharmacokinetics of, 781
Oxypurinol, 603
Oxytetracycline, 659-660
Oxytocin, 573, 576-578

P
P.V. Carpine Liquifilm; see Pilocarpine
PA; see Prealbumin
PABA; see p-Aminobenzoic acid
Pain
  with inflammation, 334
  without organic cause determined, 334
  perception of, 320
2-PAM; see Pralidoxime
Pamelor; see Nortriptyline hydrochloride
Pancuronium, 778
Pantopon; see Opium alkaloid hydrochlorides
Pantothenic acid, 616-617
  recommended daily allowance of, 621
Papaverine, 99
PAPS; see 3'-Phosphoadenosine-5-
    phosphosulfate

Paradione; *see* Paramethadione
Paral; *see* Paraldehyde
Paraldehyde, 290-291
  abuse of, 352
  pharmacokinetics of, 779
  structure of, 290
  toxic and lethal concentrations of, 771
Paramethadione, 310, 314
Paramethasone, 553, 554
Paranoid delusions in cocaine abuse, 350
Paraoxon, 32, 110
Paraquat, 771
Parasympathetic nerves, 88
  anesthesia and, 396
  reserpine and, 185
Parathion
  as insecticide, 111
  microsomal oxidations and, 32
  structure of, 110
Parathyroid extract, 567-572
Paregoric, 324
  lower gastrointestinal tract and, 523
Parenteral administration, 22
Parenteral nutrition, iron in, 608, 609
Pargyline, 270
  as antihypertensive, 176
  indirectly acting sympathomimetics and, 194
  sites of action of, 178
Parkinson's disease, 121-126
Parlodel; *see* Bromocriptine
Parnate; *see* Tranylcypromine
Paromomycin, 701
  amebiasis and, 689
  intestinal protozoa susceptible to, 688
Paroxysmal atrial tachycardia, 428, 447
Parsidol; *see* Ethopropazine hydrochloride
Partial agonists, 8, 10, 11
Partial complex seizures, 316
Partial pressure of anesthetic, 386
Partial seizures, 308
Partition coefficient, tissue:blood, 386-388
Patent ductus arteriosus, 378
Paxipam; *see* Halazepam
PBI; *see* Protein-bound iodine
PBP; *see* Penicillin-binding protein
PBZ; *see* Tripelennamine
PCP, 352
PCPA; *see* p-Chlorophenylalanine
PDR; *see* Physicians' Desk Reference
Peace pill, 352
Pearly gates, 356
Pectin, 425, 523
Pediatric anesthesia system, 393
Pefloxacin, 787
Peganone; *see* Ethotoin
Pelecyphora asselliformis, 357
Pellagra, 615
Pemoline, 275
Penbutolol, 784
Penicillamine, 379, 735
  antacids and, 749

Penicillamine—cont'd
  as antidote, 733
  as anti-inflammatory agent, 367
  pharmacokinetics of, 781
Penicillin(s), 642-651
  absorption of, 22
  action of, 626-627
  age and, 60
  alteration in drug disposition and, 70
  blood-brain barrier and, 25
  cerebrospinal fluid and, 25
  glomerular filtration and, 26
  organisms susceptible to, 654
  pharmacokinetics of, 786
  probenecid and, 753
  renal excretion of, 753
  uric acid and, 602
Penicillin G, 643
  absorption of, 23
  adverse effects of, 648-649
  hepatic or renal dysfunction and, 71
  organisms susceptible to, 651
  pharmacokinetics of, 646, 647
  safety of, 642
Penicillin V, 642-643
  organisms susceptible to, 651
  pharmacokinetics of, 646, 647
Penicillinase, 642-643, 644, 649-650
Penicillinase-resistant penicillin, 650
Penicillin-binding protein, 645
Penicillium chrysogenum, 642
Pentaerythritol tetranitrate, 451, 453
Pentagastrin, 216, 519
Pentam 300; *see* Pentamidine
Pentamidine, 695
  extraintestinal protozoa susceptible to, 691
  pharmacokinetics of, 789
Pentamidine isethionate, 691, 695
Pentazocine, 332
  biliary tract and, 324
  dosage of, 327
  pharmacokinetics of, 777
  as street drug, 340
  structure of, 333
  toxic and lethal concentrations of, 771
  with tripelennamine, 340
Pentazocine hydrochloride, 327, 332
Pentazocine lactate, 332
Penthrane, 402
Pentobarbital
  acetylcholine and, 104
  depressant or stimulant action of, 247
  elimination half-life and clinical data for, 287
  ethanol and, 751, 752
  hepatic or renal dysfunction and, 71
  microsomal oxidations and, 30
  as preanesthetic medication, 395
  scheduling of, 760
  thiopental sodium and, 403-404
  toxic and lethal concentrations of, 771
Pentolair; *see* Cyclopentolate hydrochloride

Pentolinium, 194
Pentostam; *see* Sodium stibogluconate
Pentothal; *see* Thiopental
Pentoxifylline, 306, 791
Pentylenetetrazol, 302
  action of, 247, 302
  intoxication and, 325
  structure of, 302
Pen-Vee K; *see* Penicillin V
Pepcid; *see* Famotidine
Pepsin, 204, 518-519
Peptides, 99
  action of, 82
  sites of, 83
  synthetic vaccines and, 717
Pepto-Bismol; *see* Bismuth subsalicylate
PER; *see* Perphenazine
Perception of noxious stimulus, 321
Perchlorate, 563, 566
Percorten; *see* Desoxycorticosterone
Perhexiline, 49, 54
Periactin; *see* Cyproheptadine
Peripheral vascular resistance
  β-blockers and, 191
  hypertension and, 179
Peritoneal dialysis, 736
Permapen; *see* Benzathine penicillin G
Pernicious anemia, 610-611, 612
Perphenazine, 244, 771
Pertofrane; *see* Desipramine
Pesticides, 743
Pethadol; *see* Meperidine
Petriellidium boydii, 680
Peyote, 352, 356
PGDH; *see* 15-Hydroxyprostaglandin
    dehydrogenase
PGE; *see* Alprostadil
PGE₂; *see* Dinoprostone
PGE₃, 228, 230, 231; *see also* Prostaglandin(s)
PGF₂α; *see* Dinoprost tromethamine
pH, 15
Pharmacodynamics, 1
  drug interactions and, 748, 755
Pharmacogenetics, 36-38, 48-56
  drug elimination rates and, 51
  drug interactions and, 55
  drug metabolism and, 52-55
  genetic and environmental factors and, 51
  variability in drug response and, 48-51
Pharmacokinetic parameters, 15-19
Pharmacokinetics, 12-27
  absorption and, 21-23
  dosage schedules and, 36-27
  drug distribution and, 23-25
  drug excretion and, 25-26
  drug interactions and, 748
  drug passage across membranes and, 12-15
  parameters of, 15-19
  principles of, 18, 19
  two-compartment open model and, 19-21
Pharmacology, 1

Pharmacotherapeutics, 1
Pharmacy, 1
Phenacemide, 310, 316
Phenacetin, 31, 365
  acetaminophen and, 373
  charcoal-broiled beef and, 65
  diet and, 66
  genetic conditions altering response to, 49
  hepatic or renal dysfunction and, 71
  metabolic reactions of, 54
  methemoglobinemia induced by, 53-54
  microsomal oxidations and, 31
  renal toxicity and, 369
  structure of, 373
  toxic and lethal concentrations of, 771
Phenanthrenes, 322
Phencyclidine, 385
  abuse of, 352-353, 774-775
  pharmacokinetics of, 785
  toxic and lethal concentrations of, 771
Phencyclidine hydrochloride, 352
Phendimetrazine, 760
Phenelzine, 49, 53, 269
  clinical responses and doses of, 272
  structure of, 269
Phenergan; *see* Promethazine
Phenethylamine, 510
β-Phenethylamine, 276
Phenformin, 538-539
Phenindamine, 209
Phenmetrazine
  abuse of, 349
  scheduling of, 760
  toxic and lethal concentrations of, 771
Phenobarbital
  age and, 60
  alkaline urine and, 25
  charcoal and, 732, 749
  chloramphenicol and, 751
  clinical activity of, 311
  corticosteroids and, 552
  dosage of, 311
  drug interaction and, 429
  drug metabolism and, 36
  elimination half-life and clinical data for, 287
  epilepsy and, 310, 313-314
    history of use in, 311
  ethosuximide and, 313-314
  hepatic metabolism induced by, 752
  methylphenidate and, 751
  microsomal oxidations and, 30
  pharmacokinetics of, 311, 779
    antagonism in, 46
  plasma levels and prothrombin time and, 36
  renal excretion of, 753
  structure of, 313
  therapeutic concentrations of, 768
  toxic and lethal concentrations of, 771
  urinary pH and, 14
  valproic acid and, 315
  vitamin D and, 570

Phenol
  calamine lotion and, 685
  as disinfectant, 683, 686
  exposure to, 69
Phenol coefficient, 684
Phenolphthalein, 525, 526
Phenomenon(a)
  first dose, 187
  triple response of Lewis, 203
Phenothiazine(s)
  action of, 242
  as antipsychotics, 252-257
  corticotropin-releasing factor and, 581
  dopaminergic receptors and, 85
  galactorrhea and, 582
  nonaccidental toxin ingestion of, 731
  propranolol and, 169
Phenoxybenzamine, 98, 163-164
  drug-receptor interaction and, 7
  norepinephrine and, 86
  pheochromocytoma and, 164
  sites of action of, 178
  structure of, 164
Phenoxybenzamine hydrochloride, 163
Phenoxymethylpenicillin, 643; *see also*
    Penicillin V
Phenprocoumon, 468
Phensuximide, 310, 314
Phentermine, 760, 771
Phentolamine, 98, 165
  acetylcholine and, 104
  epinephrine reversal and, 164
  sites of action of, 178
  structure of, 165
Phentolamine mesylate, 165
Phenurone; *see* Phenacemide
Phenycyclidine, 760
Phenylacetone, 31
Phenylbutazone, 378
  age and, 60
  cholestyramine and, 749
  coumarin and, 750
  diet and, 64
  dosage, dosage forms, and indications for,
    375
  gout and, 600
  hepatic or renal dysfunction and, 71
  pharmacokinetics of, 781
  phenobarbital and, 752
  phenytoin and, 750
  tolbutamide and, 750
  toxic and lethal concentrations of, 771
  variations in disposition of, 50
  warfarin and, 469, 750
Phenylbutazone derivatives, 365
l-Phenylcyclohexylpiperidine; *see*
    Phencyclidine
Phenylephrine, 447, 506
Phenylethanolamine-*N*-methyltransferase, 92
γ-Phenyl-*N*-methylproperidine, 321
Phenylpiperidines, 327

Phenylthiocarbamide, 55
Phenylthiourea, 49
Phenytoin, 36
  action of, 309, 310
    depressant or stimulant, 247
  adverse effects of, 312
  age and, 60
  amiodarone and, 751
  antacids and, 749
  antiarrhythmic action and, 434-436
  barbiturates and, 289
  binding to albumin, 73, 750
  blood concentration of, 766
  carbamazepine and, 752
  charcoal and, 749
  chloral hydrate and, 290
  chloramphenicol and, 751
  chlorpromazine and, 751
  cimetidine and, 212, 751
  clinical activity of, 311
  corticosteroids and, 552
  coumarin and, 750
  digitalis toxicity and, 430, 445
  disulfiram and, 751
  dosage of, 311, 444
  epilepsy and, 310, 312, 316
  ethanol and, 751, 752
  folic acid and, 750
  furosemide and, 749
  hepatic dysfunction and, 71
  hepatic metabolism induced by, 752
  isoniazid and, 674, 751
  lithium and, 753
  methylphenidate and, 751
  pharmacokinetics of, 311, 313, 440, 780
  phenobarbital and, 752
  plasma protein displacement and, 73, 750
  propoxyphene and, 751
  renal dysfunction and, 71
  structure of, 313
  sulfonamides and, 636, 751
  theophylline and, 513
  therapeutic concentrations of, 768
  thyroxine-binding protein and, 562
  toxic and lethal concentrations of, 771
  valproic acid and, 315
  vasopressin and, 575
  ventricular arrhythmias and, 448
  vitamin D and, 570
  warfarin and, 469
  zero-order elimination and, 18
Pheochromocytoma, 152, 168
  phenoxybenzamine and, 164
pHisoHex; *see* Hexachlorophene
Phosphate(s)
  aluminum and, 748
  calcium and, 570
  hypercalcemia and, 567
  as insecticides, 743
  iron absorption and, 606
  as rodenticides, 743

Phosphate(s)—cont'd
  vitamin D and, 569
Phosphate ester, 743
3'-Phosphoadenosine-5-phosphosulfate, 33
Phospholine; *see* Echothiophate
Phospholipids, 230, 238
Phosphorus; *see* Phosphate(s)
O-Phosphoryl-4-hydroxy-N,N-
    dimethyltryptamine; *see* Psilocybin
Phthalylsulfathiazole, 633, 637
Phylloquinone, 619
Physical dependence, 337
  barbiturates and, 350
  cocaine and, 349
  lysergide and, 353
  marijuana and, 344
Physicians' Desk Reference, 762
Physostigmine, 98, 99, 107
  as antidote, 733
  in glaucoma, 106
  as reversible anticholinesterase, 107
  tricylic antidepressant intoxication and, 273
Physostigmine salicylate, 107
Physostigmine sulfate, 106
Phytates, iron and, 748
Phytonadione, 468, 619; *see also* Vitamins, K
Picrotoxin, 303
  action of, 302
    depressant or stimulant, 247
  γ-aminobutyric acid and, 247
  barbiturates and, 287
  intoxication and, 325
  morphine and, 323
Picrotoxinin receptor, 287
Picrotoxinin site, 248
PIF; *see* Prolactin-inhibiting factor
Pilocarpine, 104-106
  acetylcholine and, 86
  rate-controlled drug delivery and, 22
Pilopine H.S. Gel; *see* Pilocarpine
Pinacidil, 784
Pindolol, 170
  hypertension and, 192
  pharmacokinetics of, 784
  properties and uses of, 167
  sites of action of, 178
Pinocytosis, 15
Pinworm, 698
Piperacillin, 644, 650
  adverse effects of, 649
  organisms susceptible to, 651
  pharmacokinetics of, 647, 786
Piperazine(s)
  action of, 208
  as anthelmintic, 699
Piperocaine, 410
Pipracil; *see* Piperacillin
Pirenzepine, 120-121
  pharmacokinetics of, 779
  structure of, 121
Pirmenol, 783
Piroxicam, 365, 377

Piroxicam—cont'd
  as anti-inflammatory agent, 367
  dosage, dosage forms, and indications for,
    375
  pharmacokinetics of, 781
  structure of, 377
Pirprofen, 781
Pitocin; *see* Oxytocin
Pitressin; *see* Vasopressin
Pitressin Tannate in Oil; *see* Vasopressin
Pituitary hormones
  anterior, 580-598; *see also* Anterior pituitary
      gonadotropins
  posterior, 573-579
pK values, 14
Placidyl; *see* Ethchlorvynol
Plaquenil; *see* Hydroxychloroquine
Plasma, 477, 478
  calcium in; *see* Calcium
Plasma cholinesterase, atypical, 52
Plasma half-lives in twins, 50
Plasma protein(s)
  binding of drugs to, 24, 750
  diuretic and, 478
Plasma volume expansion, 480
Plasmin, 219, 473
Plasminogen activator, 473
Plasmodium, 690, 691, 692
  primaquine for, 693
Plateau, 27, 46
Platelet adhesion, 470, 471
Platelet-aggregating activity, 232
Platinol; *see* Cisplatin
Plicamycin
  calcium and, 571
  mechanism of action of, 705
  neoplasms and, 704, 709
Pneumococcus, 654
Pneumocystis carinii
  drugs for, 691
  sulfonamides and, 637
  trimethoprim for, 694
Poisons, 730-745
  antidotes for, 732-735
  barbiturates as, 288
    picrotoxin and, 303
  bromide as, 737
  carbon monoxide as, 737-738
  cyanide as, 738-739
  definition of, 730
  diagnosis of, 730-731
  diethylene glycol as, 737
  digitalis as, 428-430
  environmental, 739-744
  ethylene glycol as, 737
  life-sustaining measures for, 735-737
  nitrites as, 454
  organophosphate, 111
  strychnine, 304
  treatment for, 731-732
Polaramine; *see* Dexchlorpheniramine
Poliomyelitis, vaccine for, 717

Polycillin; *see* Ampicillin
Polyestradiol phosphate, 590
Polyethylene glycol, 524
Polymorphic hydroxylation of debrisoquin, 54
Polymox; *see* Amoxicillin
Polymyxin(s), 626; *see also* Polymyxin B
  histamine and, 201
  pharmacokinetics of, 786
  toxicity of, 629
Polymyxin B, 656; *see also* Polymyxin
  cell membranes and, 630
  pharmacokinetics of, 786
Polypeptide antibiotics, 201
Polysaccharides, 201
Polythiazides, 487, 790
Ponstel; *see* Mefenamic acid
Pontocaine; *see* Tetracaine
Porphyrias, 289
Posterior pituitary hormones, 573-579
Pot, 344
Potassium
  aldosterone antagonists and, 490-491
  cardiac glycosides and, 753
  diuretics and, 477
  renal tubules and, 481-482
  salicylate intoxication and, 372
  thiazide diuretics and, 485
Potassium chloride, 430
Potassium iodide, 508
Potassium permanganate, 732
Potassium-sparing diuretics, 490-491
  hypertension and, 194
Potency, 9-10
  efficacy versus, 7
  general anesthesia and, 385-388
Potentiation, 45
Povan; *see* Pyrvinium pamoate
Povidone-iodine, 684
Practolol
  absorption of, 58
  age and, 60
  disopyramide and, 753
Pralidoxime, 111-112, 733
Prazepam
  dosage and forms of, 263
  kinetics of, 262, 779
  structure of, 261
Praziquantel, 698, 700
Prazosin, 165-166
  hypertension and, 187
  introduction of, 177
  pharmacokinetics of, 784
  sites of action of, 178
  structure of, 166
Prazosin hydrochloride, 165, 166
Prealbumin, 559
  thyroid hormones and, 558
Preanesthetic medication, 395
Prednisolone
  dosage of, 554
  lower airway and, 514

Prednisolone—cont'd
structure of, 553
Prednisone, 544
dosage of, 554
hepatic or renal dysfunction and, 71
immunosuppression and, 723, 724, 725
lower airway and, 513, 514
neoplasms and, 704, 708
pharmacokinetics of, 791
structure of, 553
Pregnancy
antibiotics and, 664
vitamin requirements in, 620-621
Pregnenolone, 544-545
Premarin; *see* Conjugated estrogens
Prenalterol, 782
Preprohormone, 567
Prescription writing, 758-761
Preservative, 683
Prilocaine, 407
history of use of, 407
onset and duration of, 410
uses of, 408
vasoconstriction and, 411
Primaquine, 37
extraintestinal protozoa susceptible to, 691
malaria and, 690, 693
pharmacokinetics of, 788
Primaxin; *see* Imipenem
Primidone, 314
clinical activity of, 311
dosage of, 311
in epilepsy, 310
methylphenidate and, 751
pharmacokinetics of, 311, 780
structure of, 313
therapeutic concentrations of, 768
toxic and lethal concentrations of, 771
Prinzmetal's variant angina, 450
Pritocaine, 408
PRO; *see* Promethazine
Probenecid
alteration in drug disposition and, 70
gout and, 599, 600-602
penicillin and, 646
pharmacokinetics of, 790
renal excretion of, 753
Probucol, 493, 500-501
Procainamide, 53, 439-441
N-acetylprocainamide and, 767
alteration in drug disposition and, 70
amiodarone and, 751
antiarrhythmic action of, 434-436
cardiac effects of, 440
classification of, 434
development of, 439-440
genetics and, 49, 53
glomerular filtration and, 26
hepatic dysfunction and, 71
lethal concentrations of, 771
pharmacokinetics of, 440, 441, 783
renal function and, 71, 753

Procainamide—cont'd
structure of, 439
therapeutic concentrations of, 768
toxicity and, 441, 771
ventricular arrhythmias and, 448
Procaine, 408, 413
as adulterant of heroin, 339
p-aminobenzoic acid and, 410
as cocaine adulterant, 350
development of, 439-440
diet and, 63
dosage of, 412
epinephrine and, 411
excretion of, 410
history of use of, 407
hydrolysis rates of, 410
lethal concentrations of, 771
microsomal oxidations and, 33
onset and duration of action of, 410
structure of, 413, 439
tetracaine and, 414
toxicity of, 411-412, 771
uses of, 408
vasoconstrictors and, 411
Procaine penicillin G, 648
Procan; *see* Procainamide
Procarbazine, 704, 710
mechanism of action of, 705
Procardia; *see* Nifedipine
Prochlorperazine, 771
Procyclidine, 124, 771
Progesterone, 591-594
adrenal steroid synthesis and, 545
ovulation and, 585
phenobarbital and, 752
serum concentration of, 586
uterus and, 576
Progestins, 591-594
mechanism of action of, 705
Progestogen, 708
Progressive myoclonic epilepsy, 315
Proinsulin, 530-531
Prolactin-inhibiting factor, 582
Proloid; *see* Thyroglobulin
Promazine, 122, 771
Promethazine
dopaminergic cell and, 244
doses and sedative property of, 209
pharmacokinetics of, 780
structure of, 207
Promine; *see* Procainamide
Pronestyl; *see* Procainamide
Prontosil, 632, 633
antibiotic action of, 626
azoreduction and, 32
Pro-opiomelanocortin, 223
Propafenone, 783
Propantheline, 120
acetaminophen and, 749
chlorothiazide and, 749
digoxin and, 749
ethanol and, 749

Propantheline—cont'd
lithium and, 749
upper gastrointestinal tract and, 519
Propantheline bromide, 120
Proparacaine, 408
Proparathyroid hormone, 567
Propicillin, 60
Propionic acid derivative, 365, 367
Propoxycaine, 408
Propoxyphene, 330
abuse of, 359
dosage of, 327
drugs inhibited by, 751
pharmacokinetics of, 777
scheduling of, 760
structure of, 330
toxic and lethal concentrations of, 771
Propoxyphene hydrochloride, 327
Propoxyphene napsylate, 327
Propranolol, 98, 166-168, 169, 445
adverse effects of, 191-192
age and, 60
in angina, 450
antacids and, 749
chlorpromazine and, 751
cholestyramine and, 749
cimetidine and, 212, 751
digitalis toxicity and, 445
dosage of, 192
drugs inhibited by, 751
genetics and, 49
growth hormone–releasing factor and, 582
hepatic or renal dysfunction and, 71
hypertension and, 191-192
metabolic reactions of, 54
migraine and, 169
norepinephrine and, 86
paroxysmal atrial tachycardia and, 447
pharmacokinetics of, 168, 191, 784
as platelet inhibiting agent, 471-472
properties and uses of, 167
prostaglandins and, 753
as receptor blocking agent, 436
renin release of, 181
sites of action of, 178
structures of, 167
thyroid hormones and, 562, 566
toxic and lethal concentrations of, 771
withdrawal from, 169
Propranolol hydrochloride, 167
Propylhexadrine, 506
Propylthiouracil
pharmacokinetics of, 791
thyroid and, 562, 563, 564-565
Propylthiourea, 49
Prostacyclin, 228
bronchial smooth muscle and, 509
dipyridamole and, 472
in hemostasis, 459
nonsteroidal anti-inflammatory drugs and, 364
as platelet inhibiting agent, 471-472

Prostaglandin(s), 99, 204, 205, 227-235
  actions of, 232
  arachidonic acid and, 230
  disease and, 233-234
  glucocorticoids and, 514
  history of, 227-228
  immunosuppression and, 724
  inhibitors of, 235
  metabolism of, 228-232
  nonsteroidal anti-inflammatory drugs and, 364
  precursors of, 231
  renal function and, 369
  renin release of, 181
  side effects of, 234
  structure of, 228, 229
  synthesis of, 228-232
  upper gastrointestinal tract and, 521-522
  uterus and, 576, 578
Prostaglandin D$_2$
  bronchial smooth muscle and, 509
  histamine and, 204
Prostaglandin E$_2$
  bronchial smooth muscle and, 509
  lungs and, 516
  parathyroid extract and, 567
  upper gastrointestinal tract and, 521-522
Prostaglandin F$_{2\alpha}$
  bronchial smooth muscle and, 509
  carboprost tromethamine and, 578
  lungs and, 516
Prostaglandin I$_2$, 509
Prostaglandin synthesis inhibitors, 578
Prostanoids
  effects of, 233
  inhibitors of, 235
Prostaphlin; see *Oxacillin*
Prostigmin; see Neostigmine
Prostin E$_2$; see Dinoprostone
Prostin F$_{2\alpha}$; *see* Dinoprost tromethamine
Prostin VR Pediatric; *see* Alprostadil
Prostin/15 M; *see* Carboprost tromethamine
Protamine, insulin and, 536
Protamine sulfate, 465
Protein binding of drugs, 24, 73, 750, 766-767
Protein metabolism, glucocorticoids and, 547-548
Protein synthesis, inhibition of, 630, 631
Protein-bound iodine, 558
Proteus, 654
  cephalosporins for, 651
  penicillin for, 650
Prothrombin, 619
Protirelin, 581
Protopam; *see* Pralidoxime
Protoveratrines A and B, 195
Protozoa
  extraintestinal, 690-696
  intestinal, 687-689
  sulfonamides for, 632
Protriptyline
  clinical responses and doses of, 272

Protriptyline—cont'd
  pharmacokinetics of, 780
  structure of, 271
  therapeutic concentrations of, 768
  toxic and lethal concentrations of, 771
Protriptyline hydrochloride, 272
Protropin; *see* Growth hormone
Proventil; *see* Albuterol
Provera; *see* Medroxyprogesterone
Pseudocholinesterase, 91
Pseudoephedrine, 506, 753
Pseudohallucinations, 275
Pseudomembranous colitis, 662
Pseudomonas, 654
  mafenide and, 637
  penicillins for, 650, 651
  tobramycin and, 658
Pseudomonas aeruginosa, 650, 658
Pseudopiperidine ring, disubstituted, 330
Psilocin, 357
Psilocybin, 276, 357
Psittacosis, 654
Psychologic drug dependence, 337
Psychomotor stimulants, 274-275
Psychopharmacology, 242-248
  antianxiety agents and, 247-248
  monoamine basis of, 242-246
Psychotomimetics, 274-276
  abuse of, 338, 352-353, 774-775
  therapeutic concentrations of, 768
Psyllium colloids, 525
Psyllium hydrophilic mucilloids, 524
PTC; *see* Phenylthiocarbamide
Pteridine, 612
Pteroylglutamic acid, 612-613; *see also* Folic acid
Puberty, 588
Pumps, infusion, 22
Purine(s), depressant or stimulant action of, 247
Purine antagonists, 703, 707
Purinethol; *see* Mercaptopurine
Purkinje fibers, 433, 434, 435
Purodigin; *see* Digitoxin
Purple hearts, 350
Pyrantel, 698, 699
Pyrantel pamoate, 698
Pyrazinamide
  isoniazid and, 674
  mycobacterial infections susceptible to, 673
  pharmacokinetics of, 789
  tuberculosis and, 672, 676
  uric acid and, 602
Pyrazinoic acid amine, 676; *see also* Pyrazinamide
Pyrazolone derivatives, 365, 378-379
Pyrethrins, 743
Pyridostigmine, 106, 108
  pharmacokinetics of, 779
Pyridostigmine bromide, 106, 108
Pyridoxal, 616

Pyridoxamine, 616
Pyridoxine, 616
  adverse effects of, 622
  as antidote, 733
  isoniazid and, 674
  levodopa and, 123
  recommended daily allowance of, 621
Pyrilamine
  action of, 208
  doses and sedative property of, 209
  nonprescription sleep medication and, 291
Pyrimethamine, 690, 693-694
  extraintestinal protozoa susceptible to, 691
  pharmacokinetics of, 788
Pyrimidine(s), depressant or stimulant action of, 247
Pyrimidine antagonists, 703, 707-708
Pyroglutamyl-histidyl-prolinamide, 563
Pyrvinium pamoate, 701

Q

Quaalude; *see* Methaqualone
Quaas, 351
Quaternary amines
  blood-brain barrier and, 24
  gastrointestinal absorption of, 21
Quaternary ammonium compounds, 685
  bretylium and, 445
Questran; *see* Cholestyramine
Quinacrine, 35
  alcohol intolerance and, 297
  cellular binding of, 24
  intestinal protozoa susceptible to, 688
  malaria and, 695
Quinacrine hydrochloride, 688
Quinaglute; *see* Quinidine
Quinestrol, 590
Quinethazone, 193, 487
Quinidex; *see* Quinidine
Quinidine, 436-440
  administration of, 439
  adverse effects of, 438
  age and, 60
  amiodarone and, 751
  antiarrhythmic action and, 434-436
  atrial fibrillation and, 447-448
  atrial flutter and, 447
  blood concentration of, 766
  cardiac effects and, 437-438
  cardiotoxicity and, 439
  classification of, 434
  digoxin toxicity and, 429, 430
  gastrectomy and, 72
  history of use of, 437
  malaria and, 694
  pharmacokinetics of, 426, 439, 440, 783
  phenytoin and, 752
  propranolol and, 169
  renal excretion and, 753
  rifampin and, 752
  structure of, 436

Quinidine—cont'd
    therapeutic concentrations of, 768
    toxic and lethal concentrations of, 771
    ventricular arrhythmias and, 448
Quinidine gluconate, 439, 440
Quinidine polygalacturonate, 440
Quinidine sulfate, 439, 440
Quinine
    adverse effects of, 438
    extraintestinal protozoa susceptible to, 691
    gastrointestinal absorption of, 21
    malaria and, 690, 694-695
    pharmacokinetics of, 788
    toxic and lethal concentrations of, 771
Quinolones
    pharmacokinetics of, 786
    urinary tract infection and, 639, 640
Quinora; *see* Quinidine
Quipazine, 216

R

Rabies, vaccine for, 717
Radical cure, 690
Radiolabeled iodide, 564
Radium, exposure to, 69
Ragweed extract, 202
Rainbows, 350
Ranitidine, 212
    antacids and, 749
    as antihistamine, 212
    development of, 210
    dosage of, 211
    pharmacokinetics of, 781
    structure of, 210
    upper gastrointestinal tract and, 518-519
Ranitidine hydrochloride, 212
Rate-controlled drug delivery, 22-23
Rauwolfia alkaloids, 172
Rauwolfia serpentina, 185, 242
Ravocaine; *see* Propoxycaine
Reaction component of pain, 321
Reactive depression, 268
Rebound anxiety, 282
Rebound insomnia, 282
Receptor concept, 6
    drug-receptor interactions and, 9
Receptor-site abnormalities, 37
Recombinant interferons, 722
Red birds, 350
Red devils, 350
Red-neck syndrome, vancomycin and, 656
Reds, 350
Reductions, drug metabolism and, 32
Reefer, 344
Refractory period, antiarrhythmics and, 433
Refractory seizures, 316
Regitine; *see* Phentolamine
Reglan; *see* Metoclopramide
Regonol; *see* Pyridostigmine
Relaxant(s)
    anticholinergic smooth muscle, 119-120
    uterine, 578

Relefact TRH; *see* Protirelin
Renal drug excretion, 25-26, 71, 77
    anesthesia and, 399
    drug interactions and, 753
    nonsteroidal anti-inflammatory drugs and, 369
Renal tubules, 480-481
Renese; *see* Polythiazides
Renin, 180, 191
    hypertension and, 181
Repetitive dosing, 27
Replacement therapy
    estrogen, 589
    thyroid, 562-563
Reserpine, 98
    action of, 172, 173
        sites of, 178
    adrenergic neuron and, 174
    α-adrenergic receptor agonists and, 753
    as antihypertensive drug, 174
    barbiturates and, 289
    corticotropin-releasing factor and, 581
    denervation sensitivity and, 90
    digitalis intoxication and, 429
    digoxin interaction with, 430
    galactorrhea and, 582
    hypertension and, 185-186
    hyperthyroidism and, 566
    introduction of, 177
    norepinephrine and, 86
    parkinsonism and, 122
    serotonin and, 214
    structure of, 185
Reserpine-like action, 186
Resin(s)
    digoxin absorption and, 425
    primary hyperlipidemias and, 501
Resistance to antibiotics, 628-629
Resorcinol, 563
Respirations
    general anesthesia and, 396-397
    morphine and, 323
Respiratory tract, 506-517
    lower, 508-516
        β-adrenergic receptor agonists in, 510-512
        anti-inflammatory steroids in, 513-515
        bronchial smooth muscle in, 509
        methylxanthines in, 512-513
    mediators in lungs and, 516
    upper, 506-508
        antitussives in, 507-508
        cough suppressants in, 507
        nasal decongestants in, 506-507
Resting cell membrane potential, 433
Restoril; *see* Temazepam
Retinol, 617-618; *see also* Vitamins, A
Retrovir; *see* Zidovudine
Reuptake of catecholamines, 94
Reverse T3; *see* Triiodothyronine
Reversibility, 6
Reversible anticholinesterases, 107

Rexolate; *see* Sodium thiosalicylate
Reye's syndrome, 369
Rheumatic disease, 379
Riboflavin, 615, 621
Ricin A chain, 718
Rickets, 569
Rickettsia, 654
Rifadin; see Rifampin
Rifampin
    dapsone and, 677
    drugs induced by, 752
    hepatic or renal dysfunction and, 71
    isoniazid and, 673-674
    mycobacterial infections susceptible to, 673
    nucleic acid synthesis and, 630
    organisms susceptible to, 654
    pharmacokinetics of, 789
        antagonism and, 46
    tuberculosis and, 672, 675
    warfarin and, 469
Rimactane; *see* Rifampin
Rimantadine, 667, 668
Riopan, 520
Ritalin; *see* Methylphenidate
Ritodrine, 578, 791
Ritodrine hydrochloride, 578
Roach, 344
Robinul; *see* Glycopyrrolate
Rocaltrol; *see* Calcitriol
Rocephin; *see* Ceftriaxone
Rock, 349
Rodenticide, 743
Romilar; *see* Dextromethorphan
Ronase; *see* Tolazamide
Root, 344
Rotenoids, 743
Roundworm, 698
rT3; *see* Triiodothyronine
Rufen; *see* Ibuprofen
Rum fits, 343
Rush, 357

S

Safety and effectiveness, 39-47
    clinical pharmacology and, 41-42
    factors in, 42-47
    new drug development and, 39-41
Salicylamide, 33, 364, 365
Salicylate(s), 364-373, 365
    acid-base balance and, 372-373
    adverse effects of, 438
    as antipyretics, 366
    caffeine and, 305
    contraindications to, 368
    coumarin and, 750
    distribution of, 70, 371
    dosage of, 372
    excretion of, 372
    gastrointestinal absorption of, 21
    intoxication from, 371, 372
    metabolic effects of, 369-370

Salicylate(s)—cont'd
  metabolism of, 371
  pharmacokinetics of, 781
  phenytoin and, 750
  platelet function and, 471
  protein binding capacity of, 24
  renal excretion of, 753
  Reye's syndrome and, 369
  thyroxine-binding protein and, 562
  tolbutamide and, 750
  toxic and lethal concentrations of, 771
  uric acid excretion and, 601-602
Salicylate intoxication, 371, 372
Salicylazosulfapyridine, 633; *see also*
    Sulfasalazine
Salicylic acid, 15, 364, 365
  as disinfectant, 686
  distribution of, 371
  metabolism of, 371
  urinary pH and, 14
Salicylism, 372
Saline
  as antidote, 732
  hypercalcemia and, 567
Salmon calcitonin, 568
Salmonella, 654
Salsalate, 365, 370
Sanitizer, 683
Sansert; *see* Methysergide
Saralasin, 180
L-Sarcolysin; *see* Melphalan
Sarcoma virus, vaccine for, 717
Schistosoma haematobium, 698
Schistosoma japonicum, 698
Schistosoma mansoni, 698
Schistosoma mekongi, 698
Schizonticide, 690
Schizophrenia
  chlorpromazine and, social behavior and
    mental symptoms with, 245
  drugs for, 242-243
Scopolamine, 114-119
  abuse of, 357
  cardiovascular system and, 115
  coughing and, 507-508
  motion sickness and, 118
  as preanesthetic medication, 395
  transdermal administration and, 23
Scopolamine hydrobromide, 117
Scurvy, 617
Secobarbital
  elimination half-life and clinical data for, 287
  as preanesthetic medication, 395
  toxic and lethal concentrations of, 771
Seconal; *see* Secobarbital
Second gas effect, 390
Second-generation antidepressants, 273-274
Secretin, 534
Secretory glands, 233
Sectral; *see* Acebutolol

Sedatives
  antihistamines and, 207
  induction and, 395
  nonaccidental toxin ingestion of, 731
  nonbarbiturate, abuse of, 351-352, 774-775
  pharmacokinetics of, 778
Seffin; *see* Cephalothin
Seldane; *see* Terfenadine
Sensitization to neurotransmitters, 90
Sensorcaine; *see* Bupivacaine
Septra; *see* Trimethoprim-sulfamethoxazole
Serax; *see* Oxazepam
Seromycin; *see* Cycloserine
Serophene; *see* Clomiphene citrate
Serotonergic receptors, 581
Serotonin, 85, 99, 214-217, 455
  action of, 172, 216
    sites of, 83
  antidepressants and, 245
  gonadotropin-releasing hormone and, 581
  5-hydroxytryptamine and, 82, 97
  lungs and, 516
  lysergic acid diethylamide and, 276
  monoamine oxidase inhibitors and, 176
  neurotransmission and, 97
  platelets and, 470
  structure of, 215
  transport of, 94
  two subclasses of, 217
Serotonin antagonists, 216, 217-219
Serotonin receptors, 85
Serratia, 650, 651
Serum
  albumin concentrations in, 58
  drug concentrations in, 766-772
    digitalis and, 429
Serum cholesterol, 193
Serum sickness, 44
Sex hormones, 583-587
Shigella
  drugs for, 654
  sulfonamides and, 637
  vaccine for, 717
Side-chain oxidation, 30
Silicon dioxide, 521
Silvadene; *see* Silver sulfadiazine
Silver nitrate, 685
Silver sulfadiazine, 637
Simethicone, 520, 521
Sinemet; *see* Carbidopa
Sinequan; *see* Doxepin
Skeletal muscle relaxants, spinal cord and,
    138-139; *see also* Muscle relaxant(s)
Sleep disturbances, 291-292
Slo-Phyllin; *see* Theophylline
Slow calcium channel, antiarrhythmics and,
    433, 436
Slow calcium-channel antagonists, 455
  hypertension and, 190
  introduction of, 177
Slow-reacting substance of anaphylaxis, 204,
    509

Smoking, 752
Smooth muscle(s)
  bronchial, 509
  epinephrine and, 149-150
  histamine and, 203-204
  norepinephrine and, 149-150
  prostaglandins and, 233
Smooth muscle relaxants, anticholinergic, 119-
    120
Snow, 349
Soap as antidote, 732
Sodium
  aldosterone antagonists and, 490-491
  antiarrhythmics and, 433
  diet low in, 479
  digitalis and, 422
  diuretics and, 477, 485
  influx of, 433
  intestinal absorption and, 22
  lithium and, 260
  local anesthetics and, 408
  renal tubules and, 481-482
Sodium benzoate, caffeine with, 305
Sodium bicarbonate
  as adulterant of heroin, 339
  as antidote, 732
  forced diuresis and, 736
  methanol intoxication and, 299
  phenobarbital excretion and, 25
  renal excretion of, 753
  tetracyclines and, 749
  upper gastrointestinal tract and, 519-520
Sodium chloride, 733
Sodium citrate, 570
Sodium Diuril; *see* Chlorothiazide
Sodium ethasulfate, 685
Sodium hypochlorite, 684
Sodium influx, 433
Sodium iodide, 508
Sodium lauryl sulfate, 685
Sodium nitrate, 738
Sodium nitrite, 452
  as antidote, 733
  structure of, 451
Sodium nitroprusside, 181, 183-184
Sodium salicylate, 365, 366
Sodium stibogluconate, 691, 696
Sodium sulfate
  as antidote, 732
  calcium and, 570
  cathartics and, 524
Sodium thiosalicylate, 365
Sodium thiosulfate, 733, 738
Solfoton; *see* Phenobarbital
Solganal; *see* Aurothioglucose
Solvents, poisoning from, 744
Soman, 111
Somatomedin C, 582
Somatostatin, 582-583
  glucagon and, 535
  growth hormone–releasing factor and, 582

Somatostatin—cont'd
  insulin and, 532
Somatotropin, 582
Somatrem, 583
Somaz; *see* Temazepam
Sorbinil, 541
Sorbitol
  charcoal and, 732
  diabetes mellitus and, 541
Sotalol, 784
Spanish fly, 360
Spasticity, 139-141
Spectazole; *see* Econazole nitrate
Spectinomycin, 659
  organisms susceptible to, 654
  pharmacokinetics of, 785
Speed, 348
Spermatogenesis, 584
Spinal cord
  gating mechanism in, 223
  skeletal muscle relaxants and, 138-139
Spironolactone, 490, 555-556
  digoxin and, 430
  pharmacokinetics and, 426
  as potassium-sparing diuretic, 194
  structure of, 490
Sporicide, 683
Squill as rodenticide, 743
SRS-A; *see* Slow-reacting substance of
      anaphylaxis
Stadol; *see* Butorphanol
Stanozolol, 596
Staphycillin; *see* Methicillin
Staphylococci, 650, 651, 654
  penicillin G resistant, 650
  sulfonamides and, 634
Staphylococcus aureus, 650, 651, 654
Starch as antidote, 732
Starvation, 63-64
Status epilepticus, 262, 317
  lorazepam and, 315
Steroid(s); *see also* Corticosteroid(s)
  adrenal; *see* Adrenal steroid(s)
  anti-inflammatory, lower airway and, 508,
      513-515
  folic acid and, 613
  insomnia and, 291
  mechanism of action of, 705
  pharmacokinetics of, 791
Stevens-Johnson syndrome, 636, 694
Stilphostrol; *see* Diethylstilbestrol
Stimate; *see* Desmopressin acetate
Stimulant(s)
  synaptic effects of, 246
  uterine, 578
Stimulants
  central nervous system, 274, 302-306; *see*
      also Central nervous system stimulants
    pharmacokinetics of, 785
  ganglionic, 128
  insomnia and, 291
  sites of action of, 247

Stomach emptying in poisoning, 731
Stool softeners, 524, 525
Stoxil; *see* Idoxuridine
STP; *see* 2,5-Dimethoxy-4-methylamphetamine
Streptase; *see* Streptokinase
Streptococcus, 651, 654
  antibiotic synergism and, 628
  cephalosporins for, 651
  penicillins for, 651
  sulfonamides for, 632
Streptococcus fecalis, 628
Streptococcus pneumoniae, 632, 651
Streptococcus pyogenes, 654
Streptococcus pyrogenes, 632
Streptococcus viridans, 654
Streptokinase, 459, 474
Streptomycin, 657
  absorption of, 23
  antibacterial chemotherapy and, 626
  hepatic or renal dysfunction and, 71
  mycobacterial infections susceptible to, 673
  organisms susceptible to, 654
  tuberculosis and, 672, 676
Strongyloides stercoralis, 698
Strychnine, 304
  action of, 302
  glycine and, 85
  meprobamate and, 265
  morphine and, 323
  as rodenticide, 743
  structure of, 304
  toxic and lethal concentrations of, 771
Subacute toxicity, 39-40
Subaortic stenosis, hypertrophic, 168
Sublimaze; *see* Fentanyl
Subscription, 759
Substance P, 222
  action of, 82
  enkephalins and, 224
Succinimides, 311, 314
Succinylcholine, 52, 99
  anticholinesterases and, 751
  genetic conditions altering response to, 49
  local anesthetic and, 412
  as neuromuscular blocking agent, 137-138
  pentylenetetrazol and, 302
Succinylsulfathiazole, 633, 637
Sucralfate, 518, 521
Sudden sniffing death, 358-359
Sufenta; *see* Sufentanil
Sufentanil, 329, 778
Sugars, 22
Sulfacetamide, 633, 636
Sulfadiazine, 633, 634-635
  extraintestinal protozoa susceptible to, 691
  pharmacokinetics of, 787
Sulfadimethoxine, 71
Sulfadoxine, 691, 694
Sulfamethazine, 49, 71
Sulfamethoxazole, 633, 635, 636
  hepatic or renal dysfunction and, 71

Sulfamethoxazole—cont'd
  pharmacokinetics of, 787
  trimethoprim and; *see* Trimethoprim-
      sulfamethoxazole
Sulfamethoxypyridazine, 71
Sulfamylon; *see* Mafenide
Sulfanilamide, 484, 632, 633
  antibiotic action of, 626
  iodine formation and, 563
  reductions and, 32
  structure of, 484
Sulfapyridine, 638
Sulfasalazine, 633, 638
  abdominal bacteria and, 73
  digoxin and, 749
  pharmacokinetics of, 787
Sulfate conjugation, 33
  thyroid hormones and, 560
Sulfentanil, 327
Sulfinpyrazone, 378, 472
  gout and, 599, 600, 602-603
  in hemostasis, 459
  pharmacokinetics of, 779
  as platelet inhibiting agent, 471-472
  uses of, 473
Sulfisoxazole, 632, 633, 634-635, 636
  binding capacity of proteins and, 24
  diet and, 63, 65
  gastrectomy and, 72
  pharmacokinetics of, 787
Sulfonamide(s), 632-641
  absorption of, 23
  drug allergies and, 43
  drugs inhibited by, 751
  nonsteroidal anti-inflammatory drugs and,
      364
  pharmacokinetics of, 787
  renal excretion of, 753
  urinary tract infection and, 639
Sulfonylurea(s)
  alcohol intolerance and, 297
  diabetes mellitus and, 538-540
  insulin and, 530
  nonsteroidal anti-inflammatory drugs and,
      364
  renal excretion of, 753
Sulfoxidation, 31
Sulindac, 365, 367, 377-378
  dosage, dosage forms, and indications for,
      375
  gastrointestinal disturbances and, 376
  pharmacokinetics of, 781
  structure of, 377
Sulindac sulfide, 377, 781
Sulindac sulfone, 377, 378
Summation, 45
Superscription, 759
Supersensitivity, denervation, 89-90
Supraventricular arrhythmia, 447-448
Suprofen, 365, 376
  dosage, dosage forms, and indications for,
      375

Suprol; *see* Suprofen
Suramin, 701
   extraintestinal protozoa susceptible to, 691
   parasites susceptible to, 698
   trypanosomal infection and, 695
Surfacaine; *see* Cyclomethycaine
Surface area, dose and, 44
Surface-active agent(s)
   as disinfectants, 685
   lower gastrointestinal tract and, 525, 526
Surital; *see* Thiamylal
Surmontil; *see* Trimipramine
Susceptibility, drug
   biologic variation in, 43
   disease and, 45
Sustained-release preparations, 370
Sweat glands, chemical mediators to, 84
Symmetrel; *see* Amantadine
Sympathectomy, chemical, 95
Sympathetic nervous system, 88
   anesthesia and, 396
Sympathetic neuronal function, peripheral
   impairment of, 185-186
Sympathin, 83
Sympathomimetic(s), 98; *see also* Adrenergic
   drug(s)
   acidemia and, 753
   digitalis intoxication and, 429
   histamine and, 201
   lower airway and, 510-511
   pharmacokinetics of, 791
Synapse, 87
   chemical events at, 85-89
Syndrome
   Down's, 36
   Reye's, 369
Synechiac; *see* Atropine
Synergism, 45
Synkayvite; *see* Vitamins, K_3
Synthroid; *see* Levothyroxine sodium
Syntocinon; *see* Oxytocin
Syrosingopine, 185, 186
Syrup of ipecac, 731-732

T

T_3; *see* Triiodothyronine
T_4; *see* Thyroxine
T's and blues, 332, 340
Tabun, 110, 111
Tacaryl; *see* Methdilazine
Tace; *see* Chlorotrianisene
Tachycardia, paroxysmal atrial, 428, 447
Tachyphylaxis, 47
Taenia saginata, 698
Taenia solium, 698
Tagamet; *see* Cimetidine
Talbutal, 287
Talwin; *see* Pentazocine
Talwin Nx; *see* Pentazocine hydrochloride
Tambocor; *see* Flecainide
Tamoxifen citrate, 704, 709

Tannic acid, 732
Tapazole; *see* Methimazole
Tapeworm, 698
Tavist; *see* Clemastine
TBG; *see* Thyroxine-binding globulin
Teebacin; *see* Aminosalicylic sodium
Tegison; *see* Etretinate
Tegopen; *see* Cloxacillin
Tegretol; *see* Carbamazepine
Temaril; *see* Trimeprazine
Temazepam, 284
   effectiveness of, 283
   as hypnotic, 262, 280, 282
   pharmacokinetics of, 281, 779
   structure of, 281
Temocillin, 786
Teniposide, 704, 711
Tenormin; *see* Atenolol
Tensilon; *see* Edrophonium
Teratogenicity, 618
Terazosin, 784
Terbutaline, 510-511, 782
Terfenadine
   action of, 208
   doses and sedative property of, 209
   pharmacokinetics of, 781
   structure of, 207
Terpin hydrate, 508
Terramycin; *see* Oxytetracycline
Tessalon; *see* Benzonatate
Testex; *see* Testosterone propionate
Testosterone, 594-597
   adrenal steroid synthesis and, 545
   gonadotropins and, 584
   neoplasms and, 708
   progestins and, 592
   structure of, 587
Testosterone cypionate, 596
Testosterone enanthate, 596
Testosterone propionate, 596, 708
Tetracaine, 407, 408, 414
   coughing and, 507-508
   dosage of, 412
   history of use of, 407
   hydrolysis rates of, 410
   onset and duration of action of, 410
   structure of, 414
   toxicity and, 411-412
   uses of, 408
Tetrachlorodiphenylethane, 545
Tetracycline(s), 659-660
   age and, 60
   amebiasis and, 689
   antacids and, 749
   antibacterial chemotherapy and, 626
   chloroquine-resistant *Plasmodium falciparum*
     and, 695
   cimetidine and, 749
   hepatic or renal dysfunction and, 71
   malaria and, 690
   organisms susceptible to, 654

Tetracycline(s)—cont'd
   protein synthesis and, 630
   protozoa susceptible to
     extraintestinal, 691
     intestinal, 688
   sodium bicarbonate and, 749
Tetraethylammonium, 21, 753
Tetraethylthiuram disulfide, 298
Tetraglycine hydroperiodide, 684
Tetrahydrocannabinol, 344-347, 760
l-Δ^9-*trans*-Tetrahydrocannabinol, 344-347
Tg; *see* Thyroglobulin
Thalidomide, 678
Thallium, 741 743, 771
Δ^9-THC; *see* l-Δ^9-*trans*-Tetrahydrocannabinol
Thea sinensis, 360
Thebaine, 322
Theobroma cacao, 360
Theobromine
   action of, 302
   chemical structure of, 305
   dietary, 68
   lower airway and, 512
   methylxanthine abstention and, 67
   relative activities of, 305
Theo-Dur; *see* Theophylline
Theophylline
   action of, 302
   age and, 60
   asthma and, 306
   bronchial smooth muscle and, 509
   carbohydrate in diet and, 65
   charcoal and, 732, 749
   charcoal-broiled beef and, 65
   chemical structure of, 305
   cimetidine and, 751
   diet and, 64, 65, 66
   erythromycin and, 751
   histamine and, 203
   lower airway and, 512-513
   metabolism of, 50
   oral contraceptives and, 751
   pharmacokinetics of, 782
   phenobarbital and, 752
   phenytoin and, 752
   relative activities of, 305
   rifampin and, 752
   smoking and, 752
   therapeutic concentrations of, 768
   toxic and lethal concentrations of, 771
   visceral smooth muscle relaxation and, 306
Therapeutic blood concentration, 767
Therapeutic index, 40-41
Therapeutics, 1
Thiabendazole, 697, 698
Thiacetazone, 789
Thiamine, 614
   adverse effects of, 622
   recommended daily allowance of, 621
Thiamine hydrochloride, 614
Thiamine pyrophosphate, 614
Thiamphenicol, 786

Thiamylal, 287, 404
Thiazide(s)
  calcium and, 571
  diabetes insipidus and, 574
  digoxin and, 430
  as direct vasodilators, 181, 182
  hypertension and, 193-194
  introduction of, 177
  renal excretion of, 753
  sites of action of, 178
  sulfonamides and, 636
  sulfonylureas and, 540
  uric acid excretion and, 601-602
Thimerosal, 686
Thiobarbiturate(s)
  fatty tissue concentration of, 24
  for induction, 385
Thiocyanate
  cyanide poisoning and, 738
  as insecticide, 743
  iodine transport and, 563
Thioguanine, 704, 705, 707
6-Thioguanine, 705
Thiopental, 35, 403, 404
  elimination half-life and clinical data for, 287
  etomidate and, 405
  history of use of, 385
  pharmacokinetics of, 286-287, 778
  toxic and lethal concentrations of, 771
Thiopental sodium, 403
Thioridazine, 771
Thiosulfate, 738
Thiotepa, 704, 706
Thiouracil, 564
Thiourea, 564
Thioureylenes, 563, 564-565
Thioxanthine derivatives, 257-258
Threadworm, 698
Thrombin formation, 460-462
Thrombocytopenia, 465
Thrombolytic agents, 475
Thromboxane, 227-235, 455; *see also*
    Thromboxane A₂
  action of, 232
  disease and, 233-234
  history of use of, 227-228
  inhibitors of, 235
  lungs and, 516
  metabolism of, 228-232
  structure of, 228
  synthesis of, 228-232
Thromboxane A₂; *see also* Thromboxane
  bronchial smooth muscle and, 509
  nonsteroidal anti-inflammatory drugs and,
    364
  platelets and, 459, 470
Thrombus formation, 462, 470, 471
Thymidylate, 611
Thypinone; *see* Protirelin
Thyrocalcitonin, 568; *see also* Calcitonin

Thyroglobulin, 557-558
  hypothyroidism and, 562
Thyroid drugs
  hypothyroidism and, 562
  pharmacokinetics of, 791
Thyroid function test, 561
Thyroid hormone(s), 557-563
  drug-receptor interaction and, 7
  hypothyroidism and, 562
  receptor regulation and, 9
Thyroid peroxidase, 557
  thyroid hormones and, 558
Thyroid suppression test, 563
Thyroid-stimulating hormone, 559
Thyrotropin-releasing hormone, 559, 563, 580-
    581
Thyroxine, 557-563
  cholestyramine and, 749
  pharmacokinetics of, 791
  protein-binding capacity of, 24; *see also*
    Thyroxine-binding globulin
  thyroid hormones and, 558
Thyroxine-binding globulin, 24, 559
  increase or decrease in, 561-562
  thyroid hormones and, 558
TI; *see* Therapeutic index
Tiaprofenic acid, 781
Ticar; *see* Ticarcillin
Ticarcillin, 644, 650
  adverse effects of, 648
  organisms susceptible to, 651
  pharmacokinetics of, 647, 786
Ticarcillin disodium, 650
Timentin; *see* Ticarcillin
Timolol, 170
  genetic conditions altering response to, 49
  hypertension and, 192
  metabolic reactions of, 54
  pharmacokinetics of, 784
  properties and uses of, 167
  sites of action of, 178
  structure of, 167
Timolol maleate, 167
Timoptic; *see* Timolol
Tinactin; *see* Tolnaftate
Tincture of iodine, 683
Tinidazole, 789
Tinnitus, 372
Tissue plasminogen activator, 460, 475
Tissue thromboplastin, 468
Tissue:blood partition coefficient, 386-388
Tissue-metabolism disorders, 37
T-lymphocytes, 720-721
Tobramycin, 658-659
  hepatic or renal dysfunction and, 71
  therapeutic concentrations of, 768
Tocainide, 440
  classification of, 434
  pharmacokinetics of, 783
  structure of, 443
  therapeutic concentrations of, 768

Tocainide—cont'd
  ventricular arrhythmias and, 448
Tocainide hydrochloride, 440
α-Tocopherol, 618
Tofranil; *see* Imipramine
Tofranil-PM; *see* Imipramine pamoate
Tolazamide, 539-540
Tolazoline, 165
Tolazoline hydrochloride, 165
Tolbutamide
  bishydroxycoumarin and, 751
  charcoal and, 749
  chloral hydrate and, 290
  chloramphenicol and, 751
  diabetes mellitus and, 539-540
  ethanol and, 751, 752
  pharmacokinetics of, 790
  phenytoin and, 750
  plasma protein displacement and, 750, 751
  rifampin and, 752
  sulfonamides and, 636, 751
  toxic and lethal concentrations of, 771
  warfarin and, 469
Tolectin; *see* Tolmetin
Tolerance, 46
  alcohol and, 296-297
  barbiturates and, 350
  cocaine and, 349
  lysergide and, 353
  marijuana and, 344
  morphine and, 325
Tolfenamic acid, 781
Tolinase; *see* Tolazamide
Tolmetin, 365, 367, 377
  dosage, dosage forms, and indications for,
    375
  gastrointestinal disturbances and, 376
  pharmacokinetics of, 781
  structure of, 377
Tolnaftate, 679, 681
Tolrestat, 791
Toluene
  abuse of, 358
  poisoning from, 744
  toxic and lethal concentrations of, 771
Tonic-clonic seizures, 308
Tonocard; *see* Tocainide
Tooies, 350
Toot, 349
Tornalate; *see* Bitolterol mesylate
Toxic blood concentration, 767
Toxicity
  of antihistamines, 209-210
  of atropine, 118-119
  of cimetidine, 211-212
  digitalis, 418, 445
  general anesthesia and, 398-399
  heparin and, 465
  new drug development and, 39-40
  nitrates and, 454
  nitrites and, 454
  of organophosphates, 111

Toxicity—cont'd
  procainamide and, 441
  of scopolamine, 118-119
  variations in, 48
Toxicology, 1, 730
Toxoplasmosis, 691
TPA; *see* Tissue plasminogen activator
TPO; *see* Thyroid peroxidase
Trancopal; *see* Chlormezanone
Trandate; *see* Labetalol
Tranexamic acid, 779
Transderm; *see* Nitroglycerin
Transferrin, 606-607
Tranxene; *see* Clorazepate
Tranylcypromine, 269, 272
  amitriptyline and, 270
  clinical responses and doses of, 272
  pharmacokinetics of, 780
  prostanoid synthesis inhibitors and, 235
  structure of, 270
Tranylcypromine sulfate, 272
Trazodone, 245, 273-274
  clinical responses and doses of, 272
  pharmacokinetics of, 780
  structure of, 274
  toxic and lethal concentrations of, 771
Trazodone hydrochloride, 272
Trecator; *see* Ethionamide
Trematodes, 698
Tremorine, 121
Trental; *see* Pentoxifylline
Treponema pallidum, *654*
Trexan; see Naltrexone
TRH; *see* Thyrotropin-releasing hormone
Triacetin, 679
Triamcinolone, 544
  dosage of, 554
  pharmacokinetics of, 791
  structure of, 553
Triamterene, 490-491
  folic acid and, 750
  pharmacokinetics of, 790
  as potassium-sparing diuretic, 194
  structure of, 490
Triazolam, 284-286
  effectiveness of, 283
  efficacy and withdrawal of, 285
  as hypnotic, 262, 280, 281
  pharmacokinetics of, 281, 779
  side effects of, 285
  structure of, 281
Tribasic calcium phosphate, 571
Trichinella spiralis, 698
Trichinosis, 698
Trichlormethiazide
  pharmacokinetics of, 790
  single dose curve and, 488
  structure of, 487
Trichloroacetic acid, 751
Trichloroethane, 358
Trichloroethanol, 290
  chloral hydrate and, 32, 290

Trichloroethanol—cont'd
  toxic and lethal concentrations of, 771
Trichloroethylene, 358
Trichomonas vaginalis, 688
Trichophyton, 681
Trichostrongylus, 698
Trichuris trichiura, 698
Triclofos, 290
Triclos; *see* Triclofos
Tricyclic antidepressant
  discovery of, 269
Tricyclic antidepressant(s), 98, 270-273; *see also* Antidepressant(s)
  catecholamines and, 90, 94
  clinical responses and doses of, 272
  clonidine and, 189
  constipation and, 522
  serotonin and, 216
  structure of, 271
  tyramine and, 173
Tridione; *see* Trimethadione
Triethylenethiophosphoramide, 704, 706
Trifluoperazine, 771
Trifluridine, 668, 669
Triglycerides, 502, 230
Trihexyphenidyl hydrochloride, 124
Triiodothyronine, 557-563
  pharmacokinetics of, 791
  thyroid hormones and, 558
Trilisate; *see* Choline magnesium trisalicylate
Trilostane, 545
Trimazosin, 784
Trimeprazine, 209
Trimethadione, 310, 311
  absence seizures and, 314
Trimethaphan, 131
  hypertension and, 194
  sites of action of, 178
Trimethobenzamide, 771
Trimethoprim
  hepatic or renal dysfunction and, 71
  malaria and, 694
  pharmacokinetics of, 787
  sulfonamides and, 634
Trimethoprim-sulfamethoxazole, 636-637, 694
  extraintestinal protozoa susceptible to, 691
  organisms susceptible to, 654
  urinary tract infection and, 639
3,4,5-Trimethoxyphenethylamine, 356
Trimethylamine, 31
1,3,7-Trimethylxanthine; *see* Caffeine
Trimipramine, 272
  pharmacokinetics of, 780
  structure of, 271
  toxic and lethal concentrations of, 771
Trimipramine maleate, 272
Trimpex; *see* Trimethoprim
Tripelennamine, 206
  doses and sedative property of, 209
  pentazocine and, 332, 340
  pharmacokinetics of, 781
  toxic and lethal concentrations of, 771

Triple response of Lewis, 203
Triprolidine
  doses and sedative property of, 209
  pharmacokinetics of, 781
Triptone; *see* Scopolamine
Trobicin; *see* Spectinomycin
Trolamine salicylate, 365
Tropicamide, 119
Trypanosoma cruzi, 691
Trypanosoma gambiense, 691
Trypanosoma rhodesiense, 691
Trypanosomal infection, 691, 695-696
Trypsin, 219
Tryptaminergic receptors, 581
Tryptamines, abuse of, 774-775
Tryptophan, 215, 615
TSH; *see* Thyrotropin-stimulating hormone
Tuberculoid leprosy, 677
Tuberculosis, 672-677
Tubocurarine, 99
  acetylcholine and, 86
  nicotinic receptors and, 84
  pharmacokinetics of, 778
Tusscapine; *see* Noscapine
Two-compartment open model, 19-21
Tylenol; *see* Acetaminophen
Tyramine, 94, 98
  action of, 172, 173
  drug interactions and, 270
  monoamine oxidase inhibitors and, 194
  norepinephrine and, 86
  sensitization by drugs, 90
  tyramine-like action, 186
Tyrosine, 92, 93
Tyrosine hydroxylase, 92
Tyrosine kinase, 532

U

Ultracef; *see* Cefadroxil
Ultrashort-acting barbiturate(s), 286, 287, 288
  anesthesia and, 403-404
  elimination half-life and clinical data for, 287
Undecylenic acid, 681, 686
Unipen; *see* Nafcillin
United States Adopted Name, 758
United States Pharmacopeia, 758, 762
United States Pharmacopeial Convention, 762
Unsaturated ketones, 228
Upper airway, 506-507
Upper gastrointestinal tract, 518-522
Upregulation, 7
Uracel; *see* Sodium salicylate
Urea, 286, 483
Urecholine; *see* Bethanechol chloride
Ureidopenicillin, 750
Uric acid
  excretion of, 601
  gout and, 599
  nonsteroidal anti-inflammatory drugs and, 368

Uricosuric drugs
  gout and, 599, 600
  sulfonamides and, 636
Urinary bacteriostatics, 787
Urinary tract
  atropine and, 116
  bacteriostatics and, 787; *see also* Urinary
    tract infection
  excretion in, 29
  scopolamine and, 116
Urinary tract infection, 787
  methenamine mandelate for, 639-640
  nitrofurantoin for, 638
  nitrofurazone for, 638
  sulfonamides for, 632-641
Urokinase, 475
  fibrinolytic system and, 474
  hemostasis and, 460
Urolithiasis, 602
Uromide; *see* Salicylamide
Urticaria, 44
USAN; *see* United States Adopted Name
USP; *see* United States Pharmacopeia
Uterus
  drugs acting on, 576-578
  general anesthesia and, 398

V

VAC; *see* Vincristine, dactinomycin, and
  cyclophosphamide
Vaccines
  development of, 717
  synthetic, 717-718
Valium; *see* Diazepam
Valmid; *see* Ethinamate
Valproate
  charcoal and, 749
  pharmacokinetics of, 780
  therapeutic concentrations of, 768
Valproic acid
  age and, 60
  clinical activity of, 311
  diazepam and, 750
  dosage of, 311
  epilepsy and, 310, 315, 316
  pharmacokinetics of, 311
  phenytoin and, 750, 752
  structure of, 316
  toxic and lethal concentrations of, 771
van der Waals forces, 7
Vancenase; *see* Beclomethasone
Vanceril; *see* Beclomethasone
Vancocin; *see* Vancomycin
Vancomycin, 656
  hepatic or renal dysfunction and, 71
  organisms susceptible to, 654
  pharmacokinetics of, 787
  therapeutic concentrations of, 768
Vansil; *see* Oxamniquine
Variegate prophyrias, 289
Vascular smooth muscle, chemical mediators
  to, 84

Vasoactive intestinal polypeptide, 222, 224-225
  glucagon and, 534
Vasoconstrictors, 455
  ganglionic blocking agents and, 90
  local anesthetics and, 411
  upper airway and, 506
Vasodilatation
  alcohol and, 293
  anesthesia and, 397
  hypertension and, 181-184
  prostaglandins and, 233
Vasodilators, direct, hypertension and, 181-184
Vasopressin, 99, 573-576; *see also* Antidiuretic
  hormone
  tachyphylaxis and, 47
Vasopressin tannate, 576
Vasopressors; *see* Vasoconstrictors
Vasotec; *see* Enalapril
Vecuronium, 778
Veetids; *see* Penicillin V
Vegetable oil as antidote, 732
Velban; *see* Vinblastine
Velosef; *see* Cephradine
Ventilation, anesthesia and, 390-391
Ventolin; *see* Albuterol
Ventricular arrhythmia, 448
Ventrolateral hypothalamus, 532
Ventromedial hypothalamus, 531
VePesid; *see* Etoposide
Verapamil, 446, 455-457
  in angina, 450
  atrial fibrillation and, 447-448
  atrial flutter and, 447
  as blocking agent, 436
  as calcium antagonist, 455
  classification of, 434
  digoxin and, 430
  dosages of, 456
  nifedipine and, 457
  paroxysmal atrial tachycardia and, 447
  pharmacokinetics of, 426, 440, 782
  pharmacologic activities of, 455
  side effects of, 456
  sites of action of, 178
  slow calcium-channel blockers and, 190
  structure of, 457
Verapamil hydrochloride, 456
Veratrum alkaloids, 99, 195
  sites of action of, 178
Vermox; *see* Mebendazole
Veronal; *see* Barbital
Versed; *see* Midazolam
Very-low-density lipoprotein, 493, 496
Vibramycin; *see* Doxycycline
Vibrio cholerae, 632
Vicia fava, 37, 55
Vidarabine, 668
  nucleic acid synthesis and, 630
  pharmacokinetics of, 789
  viral infections susceptible to, 668

Vigabatrin, 791
Vinblastine, 704, 709
  mechanism of action of, 705
  pharmacokinetics of, 789
Vinblastine sulfate, 704
Vinca alkaloids, 702, 705
Vincristine, 704, 709
  mechanism of action of, 705
  pharmacokinetics of, 789
Vincristine sulfate, 704
Vincristine, dactinomycin, and
  cyclophosphamide, 712
Vinegar as antidote, 732
Vinyl chloride, 69
Vioform; *see* Clioquinol
Viomycin, 789
VIP; *see* Vasoactive intestinal polypeptide
Vira-A; *see* Vidarabine
Viroptic; *see* Trifluridine
Visken; *see* Pindolol
Vistaril; *see* Hydroxyzine
Vitamins, 614-623
  A, 617-618
    jejunal disease and, 72
    recommended daily allowance of, 621
  adverse effects of, 622
  B_1, 614; *see also* Thiamine
  B_2, 615; *see also* Riboflavin
  B_6, 616; *see also* Pyridoxine
  B_{12}, 72-73
    anemia and, 609, 610-612
    erythrocytes and, 605
    recommended daily allowance of, 621
  C, 617
    adverse effects of, 622
    recommended daily allowance of, 621
    vitamin B_{12} and, 611
  D, 567-572
    hypocalcemia and, 567
    jejunal disease and, 72
    recommended daily allowance of, 621
  D_2, 568-569, 570
  D_3, 568-569, 570
  E, 618
    jejunal disease and, 72
    recommended daily allowance of, 621
  fat-soluble, 617-620
    cholestyramine and colestipol and, 500
  K, 44, 619-620
    adverse effects of, 622
    antibiotics and, 750
    coagulation factors and, 469
    jejunal disease and, 72
    recommended daily allowance of, 621
    warfarin and, 55
    water-soluble form of, 468
  K_1, 619, 620
  K_3, 620
  medical use of, 620-621
  water-soluble, 614-617
Vivactil; *see* Protriptyline

VLDL; *see* Very-low-density lipoprotein
VMA; *see* 4-Hydroxy-3-methoxymandelic acid
Volume of distribution, 16
von Gierke's disease, 37

W

Warfarin, 459
  action of, 466-467
  chloral hydrate and, 290, 751
  cholestyramine and, 749
  cimetidine and, 212, 751
  contraindications to, 469
  disulfiram and, 751
  doses of, 468
  drug interactions and, 469-470
  ethanol and, 751
  genetic conditions altering response to, 49
  hepatic or renal dysfunction and, 71
  laboratory control and, 468
  liver disease and, 74
  pharmacokinetics of, 779
  phenobarbital and, 36
  phenylbutazone and, 750
  ranitidine and, 212
  resistance to, 55
  structure of, 466
  sulfonamides and, 751
  use of, 467-468
Warfarin potassium, 468

Warfarin resistance, 55
Warfarin sodium, 468
Water metabolism, 548-549
Water-soluble vitamins, 614-617
Weed, 344
Weight, drug safety and effectiveness and, 44
Wetting agents, gastrointestinal tract and, 525
Whipworm, 698
Whiskey, 295
White cross, 348
Whitfield's ointment, 686
Whole blood, ethacrynic acid and, 480
Wine, 295
WinGel, 520
Winstrol; *see* Stanozolol
Withdrawal
  barbiturate, 351
  propranolol, 169
Wood alcohol, 298
Wuchereria bancrofti, *698*
Wuchereria malayi, *698*
Wytensin; see Guanabenz

X

X rays, exposure to, 69
Xanax; *see* Alprazolam
Xanthine, structure of, 305
Xanthine oxidase, 603, 751
Xerosis, 617

Xylene, 358
Xylocaine; *see* Lidocaine

Y

Yeast extract, 634
Yellow jackets, 350
Yodoxin; *see* Iodoquinol
Yutopar; *see* Ritodrine

Z

Zanaz; *see* Alprazolam
Zantac; *see* Ranitidine
Zarontin; *see* Ethosuximide
Zaroxolyn; *see* Metolazone
Zephiran; *see* Benzalkonium
Zero-order kinetics, 18
Zero-order reaction, 296
Zidaridine, 668
Zidovudine, 669, 789
Zinacef; *see* Cefuroxime
Zinc
  insulin and, 536
  poisoning from, 734, 743
Zinc phosphide, 743
Zinc sulfate, 685
Zopiclone, 779
Zovirax; *see also* Acyclovir
Zyloprim; *see* Allopurinol